S0-AMP-809

# Craniospinal Magnetic Resonance Imaging

**Stephen J. Pomeranz, M.D.**

Co-director, Magnetic Resonance Imaging
James N. Gamble Institute of Medical Research
Department of Radiology
The Christ Hospital
Cincinnati, Ohio

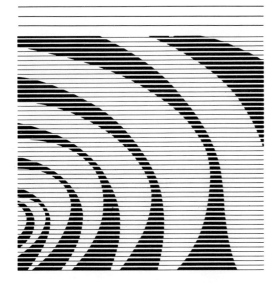

**1989**
**W. B. SAUNDERS COMPANY**

Harcourt Brace Jovanovich, Inc.
Philadelphia London Toronto
Montreal Sydney Tokyo

**W. B. SAUNDERS COMPANY**
Harcourt Brace Jovanovich, Inc.

The Curtis Center
Independence Square West
Philadelphia, PA 19106

**Library of Congress Cataloging-in-Publication Data**

Craniospinal magnetic resonance imaging.

1. Brain—Imaging. 2. Spine—Imaging. 3. Magnetic resonance imaging. 4. Brain—Diseases—Diagnosis. 5. Spine—Diseases—Diagnosis. I. Pomeranz, Stephen J. [DNLM: 1. Brain—pathology. 2. Brain Diseases—diagnosis. 3. Magnetic Resonance Imaging. 4. Spinal Diseases—diagnosis. 5. Spine—pathology. WL 348 C891]

RC386.6.M34C73 1989 616.8′0757 88–6677

ISBN 0–7216–2428–6

*Editor:* Lisette Bralow
*Designer:* Maureen Sweeney
*Production Manager:* Bob Butler
*Manuscript Editor:* Lorraine Zawodny
*Illustration Coordinator:* Lisa Lambert
*Cover Designer:* Sharon Iwanczuk
*Indexer:* Julie Schwager

Craniospinal Magnetic Resonance Imaging ISBN 0–7216–2428–6



Last digit is the print number: 9 8 7 6 5 4 3 2 1

This book is dedicated to my loving wife Penny,
for her patience and support,
and to my four children
Christy, Corbin, Taylor, and Jory.

# CONTRIBUTORS

**WILLIAM S. BALL, Jr., M.D.**
Assistant Professor, Radiology and Pediatrics, University of Cincinnati College of Medicine
Staff Radiologist, Children's Hospital
Attending Radiologist, University Hospital
Cincinnati, Ohio

**BOKYUNG K. HAN, M.D.**
Associate Professor, Radiology and Pediatrics, University of Cincinnati College of Medicine
Staff Radiologist, Children's Hospital
Attending Radiologist, University Hospital
Cincinnati, Ohio

**STEVEN E. HARMS, M.D.**
Director of Magnetic Resonance Division, Baylor University Medical Center
Dallas, Texas

**DOUGLAS A. KAFFENBERGER, M.D.**
Fellow, Neuroradiology, University of South Florida College of Medicine
H. Lee Moffit Cancer Center, Tampa General Hospital
Tampa, Florida

**JAMES G. KEREIAKES, PH.D.**
Professor of Radiology (Chairman, Radiologic Physics),
University of Cincinnati College of Medicine
Cincinnati, Ohio

**JAMES MACFALL, PH.D.**
Senior Physicist, General Electric Medical Systems
Milwaukee, Wisconsin

**JAMES J. MASTERS, M.D.**
Attending Neuroradiologist, The Christ Hospital
Cincinnati, Ohio

**F. REED MURTAGH, M.D.**
Professor, Radiology and Neurology
Directory of Neuroradiology, University of South Florida College of Medicine
H. Lee Moffit Cancer Center, Tampa General Hospital
Tampa, Florida

**STEPHEN F. QUINN, M.D.**
Staff Radiologist, Department of Radiology, Good Samaritan Hospital
Portland, Oregon

**SCOTT D. SCHLESINGER, M.D.**
Clinical Instructor, Department of Radiology
New York University Medical Center
Neuroradiology Fellow, New York University Medical Center, Bellevue Hospital, and Manhattan Veterans Administration
New York, New York

**NORMAN A. SCHNITZLEIN, PH.D.**
Professor, Anatomy and Radiology, University of South Florida College of Medicine
Consultant, James A. Haley Veterans Administration Hospital
Tampa, Florida

**THOMAS G. SEWARD, M.D.**
Clinical Instructor, University of Cincinnati, University Hospital
Staff Radiologist, Bethesda North Hospital
Cincinnati, Ohio

**JEROME J. SHELDON, M.D., F.A.C.R.**
Professor of Radiology, University of Miami School of Medicine
Attending Radiologist and Chief, Section of Neuroradiology, Computed Tomography, and Magnetic Resonance Imaging, Department of Radiology
Mt. Sinai Medical Center
Miami Beach, Florida

**KALEVI P. SOILA, M.D.**
Assistant Professor of Radiology, University of Miami School of Medicine
Attending Radiologist, Section of Neuroradiology, Computed Tomography, and Magnetic Resonance Imaging, Department of Radiology
Mount Sinai Medical Center
Miami, Beach, Florida

**CHARLES E. SPRITZER, M.D.**
Assistant Professor, Department of Radiology, Duke University Medical Center
Co-Director, Magnetic Resonance Imaging, Duke University Medical Center
Durham, North Carolina

**STEPHEN R. THOMAS, PH.D.**
Professor of Radiology, Division of Medical Physics, Department of Radiology, University of Cincinnati College of Medicine
Cincinnati, Ohio

**JEFFREY A. TOBIAS, M.D.**
Assistant Professor of Radiology, University of Miami School of Medicine
Staff Radiologist, Section of Neuroradiology, Computed Tomography, and Magnetic Resonance Imaging, Department of Radiology,
Mount Sinai Medical Center
Miami Beach, Florida

**RICHARD B. TOWBIN, M.D.**

Associate Professor, Radiology and Pediatrics, University of Cincinnati College of Medicine
Staff Radiologist, Children's Hospital
Attending Radiologist, University Hospital
Cincinnati, Ohio

**BUCKLEY TERPENNING, M.D.**

Radiology Resident, Department of Radiology
University Hospital
Cincinnati, Ohio

**SUSAN WEINBERG, M.D.**

Clinical Assistant, University of Cincinnati, University Hospital
Staff Radiologist, Bethesda North Hospital
Cincinnati, Ohio

# FOREWORD

Advances in equipment and knowledge related to radiology are occurring at an astonishingly rapid rate. On November 8, 1885, William Conrad Roentgen discovered x-rays. In 1972, Godfrey Hounsfield and George Ambrose introduced computed tomography at a meeting of the British Institute of Radiology. In the same year, Paul Lauterbur published the idea of spatially resolving nuclear magnetic resonance samples, naming it "zeugmatography." In 1977, Waldo Hinshaw and co-workers published a magnetic resonance image of a human hand and wrist, and by 1981 several centers were obtaining clinical magnetic resonance (MR) images.

In part because of thc ability to vary T1, T2, and spin-density weighting of images by varying radiofrequency pulse sequences and in part because of the differences in signal intensity caused by paramagnetic, magnetic susceptibility, preferential T2 relaxation enhancement, and flow effects, the interpretation of MR images is more difficult than was first anticipated. Our knowledge about magnetic resonance imaging (MRI) continues to increase at a rapid rate with increased clinical experience and with the contribution of new pulse techniques and paramagnetic agents.

At the present time, 85% to 90% of the images obtained with MRI systems are of the brain and spine. This book integrates our knowledge of magnetic resonance imaging with our knowledge of neuroradiology so that clinicians of every level of sophistication in the field, from medical students to experienced neuroradiologists, can better understand the applications of MRI for the diagnosis of lesions of the brain and spine. Each of the chapters includes state-of-the-art illustrations and is written by experts in the field. The book is comprehensive and well edited so that the reader will understand both how to perform and how to interpret MRI of the brain and spine. The multiple factors that alter signal intensity, the optimal technical factors to "tailor" the examination to the patient's signs and symptoms, and the various clues that can be used for differential diagnosis of lesions are clearly presented. The book is noteworthy for its up-to-date inclusion of relevant research material that has clinical utility.

Just as happened with computed tomography, magnetic resonance is currently changing from a "revolutionary" field to an "evolutionary" field. This well-referenced, coherent book will enable the clinician to be current in the concepts of magnetic resonance imaging in this highly dynamic field.

**MEREDITH A. WEINSTEIN, M.D.**

# PREFACE

The field of magnetic resonance (MR) imaging has changed dramatically since our initial experience with routine clinical imaging began five years ago at Mount Sinai Hospital in Miami Beach. At that time, a prototype 0.35 tesla unit was employed. Scanning times were lengthy (14 to 25 minutes), since the signal-to-noise scan characteristics were poor and many repetitions were required to generate images of diagnostic quality. Our unit was housed in an artificial building and set eccentrically on the hospital parking lot. All patients came with other correlating imaging studies, and if they didn't, studies were obtained. Spinal MR was accompanied by computed tomography (CT) and/or myelography. Brain MR was accompanied by CT in every case. With the persistence of many of my colleagues, pathology reports, operative reports, and clinical follow-ups were obtained so that we could enrich our understanding of this new modality.

Initially, we encountered some strange imaging phenomena since we were accustomed to anatomic interpretation and density characteristics of CT but not the complex behavior of MR hydrogen protons. Flow effects were the most difficult to comprehend. The effects of turbulence, time-of-flight, oblique in-plane and perpendicular plane flow phenomena were just being elucidated and published. Some of the first pediatric cases exhibited extreme signal hyperintensity in the pineal gland region on T2-weighted images (T2WI). These patients were thought to have pineal tumors; however, collectively, we soon realized that we had diagnosed six pediatric pineal region tumors in three weeks. Actually, these simply represented normal developmental cysts of the pineal gland. On other occasions, when patients were evaluated in the head and neck region, enlarged contour or increased signal of a pterygoid muscle were appreciated. An astute observer subsequently deduced that local anesthetic fluid injection by dentists with subsequent mild hemorrhage, not tumor, had produced these intramuscular signal and contour changes that resulted. One additional dilemma that proved quite frustrating was the occurrence of ferromagnetic effects at laminectomy and craniotomy sites when no metal was detectable with conventional radiographs. However, microscopic metallic fragments from the drill bits used at surgery proved to be the cause.

The total case experience of this editor has now exceeded eight thousand. All cases with positive findings were logged into our teaching file, and we have retained close clinicopathologic follow-up. Approximately 20% of these cases involve the body (neither brain nor spine). Experience has accrued on four field strengths, including 0.35, 0.5, 1.0, and 1.5 tesla. The debate rages as to what field strength is optimal for clinical MR imaging. It is true that imaging at lower field is more economical. Well-tuned and well-maintained low-field units provide images of excellent quality and produce fewer phase-dependent and chemical shift artifacts in body imaging. These effects are of little consequence when investigating the neural axis. However, with two-dimensional Fourier transform (2DFT) MR, high field (> 1.0 tesla) does provide superb quality, particularly with regard to improved image signal. This improved image signal affords one the luxury of thinner sections, since image noise with sections less than 4 or 5 mm can be prohibitive. In addition, many manufacturers have implemented various software "tricks" to reduce the phase-dependent, motion-related artifacts of flowing blood or respiratory motion that are more pronounced at high field strengths. Thus, image quality in the body at high field has markedly improved. A third variable governing image appearance is the quality and versatility of the surface coil. The selection, design, and quality of these coils varies with the manufacturer; in fact, some companies make surface coils only. Many of these coils interface well with some MR scanners but not with scanners of other manufacturers. In addition, these coils often cannot be used interchangeably with different scanners, particularly those of differing field strengths.

Even with all these obstacles, the technological progress of MR has been rapid. Initially, images were postprocessed for 30 minutes to 1 hour before they could be filmed with the desired spatial resolution and matrix. Sections of 5 mm were the thinnest obtainable, and field-of-view or zoom factor selections were not possible. We have just recently passed the age of 3-mm sections, with virtually instantaneous reconstruction in the desired matrix and field of view. Prescan, center-frequency, and other parameters required for setup are automatic and not often performed manually. Electrocardiographic gating, respiratory compensation, flow compensation, and other forms of motion reduction are flourishing. Perhaps these, too, will go the way of the great dinosaurs, and the Cretaceous period of MR will end. Newer pulsing sequences than spin-echo may dominate the scene. We are entering the age of cine MR, three-dimensional MR, 1-mm images, and contrast-enhanced MR (CEMR). CEMR should markedly improve the specificity of the modality and, in time, should revise the indications for CT versus MR in all parts of the body. It will be particularly helpful in evaluation of the supratentorial brain and in the differentiation of white matter lesions due to aging, microinfarction and neurodegeneration from metastasis and other disease entities.

This text is aimed at practicing radiologic clinicians in both the private and university setting. We have geared the physics and technical sections for both the beginning and the advanced MR practitioner. Always, we have kept in mind that this text is a clinical reference for those actually engaged in MR imaging, rather than a guide for those in research. Since formal MR training is not yet widespread, we believed it important to include as many protocols, appendices, and tables as are applicable. We also wanted this text to stand on its own with regard to discussions of individual disease states and hope we have done so.

Hopefully, the technology will change, but not too rapidly. With the advent of new supraconductive materials, the threat of having to replace the main magnet does exist. While this possibility may be costly, it can make millisecond MR imaging a reality, and there is no doubt that MR will be faster than CT. Meanwhile, our duty as radiologists is to continue to explore the applications of this modality and to utilize it to the fullest where appropriate.

There are still many disease states and body parts for which CEMR and MR are preferable as the sole imaging modality, and these are still being evaluated. Perseverance, dedication to detail, and the excitement of uncovering something new will likely spur on our colleagues to continue investigating this unique clinical tool.

**STEPHEN J. POMERANZ, M.D.**

# ACKNOWLEDGEMENTS

This text could not have been completed without the able technical assistance of Betsy Eicher, Cindy Hehman, Hollie Halloran, Sharon Burgraph, Maricarol Glaze and Jessie Johnson; the photographic expertise of Norton Photography & Associates; and the support of the Christ Hospital, its Medical Education Department (June Hosick, Director), its radiologists (Owen Brown, M.D., Radiology Chairman), and radiologic staff.

We are deeply indebted to General Electric Medical Systems for their commitment to excellence and to the future of imaging in medicine and for their continued support. We are also grateful to Siemen's, Inc., for their support.

Last, I would like to acknowledge several leaders in the subspecialty of radiology: my father-in-law, Dr. James Kereiakes, whose encouragement led me to this endeavor; his quiet leadership and dedication are what all young men strive for; Dr. Benjamin Felson, who first interested me in radiographic interpretation; Dr. Jerome Wiot, whose dedication to the education of young radiologists is unsurpassed; Dr. Manuel Viamonte, who gave me carte blanche support as a fellow and afforded me the luxury of exploring magnetic resonance imaging when it first became available in this country; and Dr. Anthony Proto, who kindled my wanting to know and understand, to the best of my ability, the discipline that we call radiology.

# CONTENTS

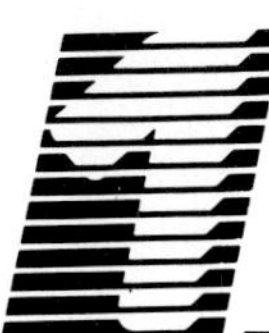

James G. Kereiakes, Ph.D.

# MAGNETIC RESONANCE IMAGING PHYSICS

Magnetic resonance imaging (MRI) is a rapidly evolving technology that within a relatively short period of time has become a well-accepted modality. The MRI parameters under the operator's control are many and can at times be bewildering. It is of extreme importance, however, that proper imaging techniques be used, since pathology can be masked or missed when they are not. It is therefore essential that the user of this sophisticated and complex modality have a basic understanding of the principles underlying MR imaging.

## MAGNETIC RESONANCE IMAGING EQUIPMENT

A vertical cross-section through an MRI system is illustrated in Figure 1–1.

### Magnet

Magnets as currently configured for MRI are of three general types: resistive, superconducting, and permanent. They result in significant differences in possible field strength, stability, uniformity, and cost.

Resistive magnets provide good field uniformity, are relatively inexpensive, require no cryogens, and provide transverse field possibilities. However, field strength is limited and unstable, a fringe-field problem exists (for longitudinal fields), and electrical costs are higher.

Very high field strengths are possible with superconducting magnets. Also, they usually have uniform and stable fields, cost more to buy and maintain, and require more expensive site preparation. Because of the potentially higher field strength, there is a fringe-field problem. In addition, cryogens, with a possible problem of quenching, are needed.

Permanent magnets are relatively inexpensive to maintain, have a low fringe-field, and require no cryogens. They also offer transverse field possibilities. However, field strength is limited, and they are both relatively heavy and temperature sensitive.

For all magnets, a relatively strong, uniform, and temporally stable magnetic field must be present. To achieve magnetic field uniformity and to compensate for alteration of structures in the environment by the magnetic field, coils (called shim coils) are usually incorporated into the magnet. A summary of the various coils used in MR imaging are listed in Table 1–1.

### Gradient Coils

Gradients in each of three directions must be available to perform MR imaging. These gradient coils provide a linearly rising magnetic field superimposed upon the uniform magnetic field. The magnitude of this gradient field is usually between 0.6 and 1 G/cm. A Maxwell coil pair provides the linear gradient in the magnetic field direction. The other two gradients are produced using opposing coil loops with parallel sides wrapped around a gantry. These coils provide gradients for the two remaining directions.

It is important that these gradients be linear and uniform to within a few percentage points. Their strength should ride above

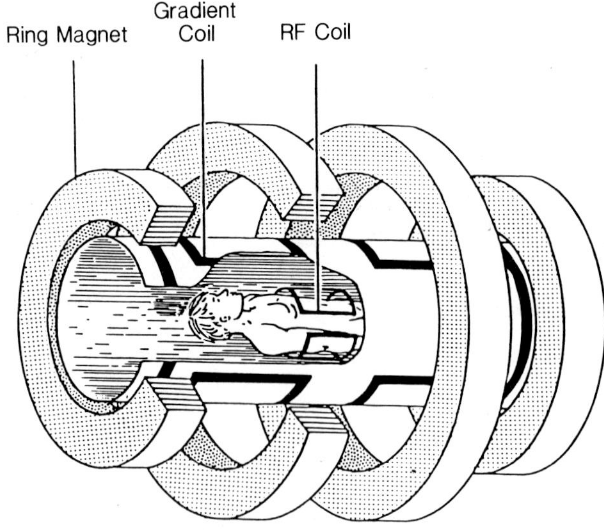


**Figure 1–1.** Cross-section through an MRI system with the ring magnets mounted in the vertical direction and the magnetic field horizontal. (From Kean DM, Smith MA. Magnetic Resonance Imaging: Principles and Applications. C1986, The Williams & Wilkins Company, Baltimore, p 63, with permission.)

any inhomogeneities in the main field magnets. The gradients define the slice thickness, resultant spatial resolution, and contrast sensitivity of the system.

## Radio Frequency (RF) Coil

RF waves excite the nuclear spin in the patient. RF coils are the so-called head and body coils in which the patient is placed. The coils serve as both the transmitters and the receivers of the MRI signal. The design of these coils is either saddle-shaped or solenoid type. In the case of the transverse magnetic field, solenoid coils are used, whereas saddle-shaped coils are used in the longitudinal magnetic field. The signal-to-noise ratio (SNR) for the solenoid RF coil is approximately twice that of a saddle-shaped coil of comparable size.

A significant increase of the SNR and the

**Table 1–1.** SUMMARY OF COILS USED IN MRI

| Main Field | Configuration |
|---|---|
| Resistive coils | |
| Air core | Either 1 pair (2 coils) or 2 pairs (4 coils) the diameters of which describe the surface of a sphere; the resulting field is either longitudinal or transverse |
| Iron core | Coil winding is directly around poles of the electromagnet (in either a C or an H configuration); the resulting field is always transverse |
| Superconducting coils | Winding are solenoid (around a gantry); conductors are of NbTi filaments in a copper matrix; the resulting fields are always longitudinal |
| Radio frequency (RF) coils | |
| For transverse field | Solenoid configuration; approximately two times the SNR advantage over a saddle-shaped coil of comparable size |
| For longitudinal field | Saddle-shaped coil |
| Surface coil | Circular loop coils placed directly over the anatomic region of interest serve as the RF signal receiver |
| Gradient coils | |
| Maxwell pair | Pair of coils with current flowing in opposite directions; used for the slice-selection gradient in the direction of the main field axis |
| Golay coils | Opposing, parallel-side coil, curved over the cylindrical surface of the gantry bore. There are two sets arranged at a 90° rotation to each other in order to define the x and y gradient axes |
| Shim coils | Additional small coils incorporated within a gantry to make the magnetic field more uniform |

*Source:* Lee SH, Rao KCVG. Cranial Computed Tomography and MRI. New York, McGraw-Hill Book Co., 1987, p. 63, with permission.

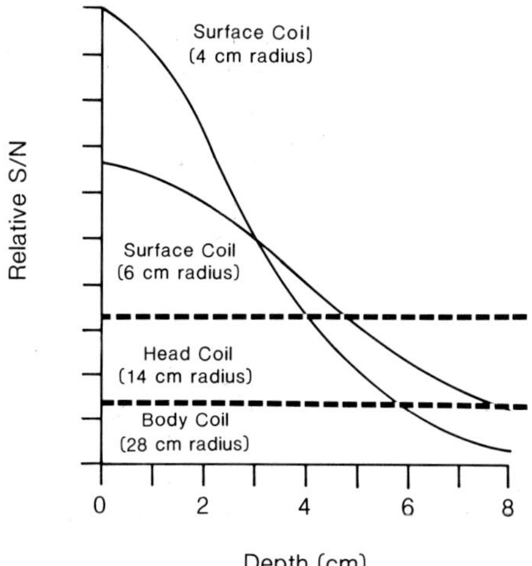


**Figure 1–2.** Comparison of surface coils versus body and head coils in terms of signal-noise ratio. (From Schenck JF. Signa System Operator Manual. Schenectady, N.Y., General Electric Co. OMS2 Rev. 11, 1986, with permission.)

consequent enhancement of spatial resolution and contrast sensitivity can be obtained by using surface coils. A surface coil is placed directly on the anatomical area to be imaged. The increased SNR of such a surface coil is due to both its small size and its proximity to the region of interest. The higher SNR permits more effective imaging through the use of smaller fields of view and thinner slices. Figure 1–2 illustrates the increased SNR for a surface coil relative to body or head coil, particularly for depths up to 5 to 6 cm. One disadvantage of surface coils is this possibly limited depth response.

### Environmental Considerations

In any installation of an MRI system, consideration must be given to possible field effects between the imager and its environment. The strength of the magnetic field would determine the distance at which an effect may be seen. Magnetic fields from the imaging system may interfere with electrical equipment such as electron microscopes and gamma cameras and may have effects on patients wearing cardiac pacemakers.

Homogeneity achieved in the magnet may be limited by static ferromagnetic material in the immediate environment. Moving ferromagnetic material, such as elevators, seriously interferes with the imager. It is possible, at increased cost, to use large ferromagnetic sheets around the magnet. To avoid possible interference from external RF radiation, the magnet can be shielded with aluminum sheets. In some cases, a slight change in the field strength of the main magnet can move the resonance frequency to a region where there is no interference with an external specific RF frequency.

Approximate fringe field values and corresponding distances for various magnetic field strengths are listed in Table 1–2. Specific objects that may be affected by the MRI system are noted.

## MAGNETIZATION

The most abundant element in the body is hydrogen, and the nucleus of the hydrogen atom possesses a property known as spin. When a hydrogen-containing body is placed in a magnetic field, equal numbers of protons point north (parallel, or spin-up) and south (antiparallel, or spin-down), corresponding to low and high energy states, respectively (Fig. 1–3). Initially, the individual magnetic moments cancel, giving zero magnetization. However, a redistribution occurs shortly thereafter in which a slightly greater number of hydrogen nuclei align parallel to the field, resulting in the body's being "magnetized." Substances with unpaired electrons (i.e., paramagnetic and ferromagnetic materials) have a greater "magnetic susceptibility" to the applied magnetic field.

The magnetization can be represented by a longitudinal component (which is along the z axis, aligned with the main magnetic field $B_o$) and a transverse component (which is along the x-y plane) (Fig. 1–4).

For transverse magnetization, the proton precesses about the z axis at a particular frequency, called the Larmor frequency. The Larmor relationship states that the angular frequency, $\omega$, of the precession is given by

$$\omega = \gamma B_o$$

in which $\gamma$ = gyromagnetic ratio (which is constant for a particular nucleus) and $B_o$ = external magnetic field.

The magnetic susceptibilities and gyromagnetic ratios for a few diagnostically relevant nuclei are listed in Table 1–3.

The net magnetization is the summation of the magnetic moments of the individual

**Table 1–2.** DISTANCE (IN METERS) OF THE FRINGE MAGNETIC FIELD STRENGTH FROM MRI SYSTEMS WITH MAGNETIC FIELD VALUES RANGING FROM 0.08 TO 1.5 T

| | | | Magnetic Field Strength (T) | | | | |
|---|---|---|---|---|---|---|---|
| | | | ***0.08*** | ***0.15*** | ***0.3*** | ***0.5*** | ***1.5*** |
| ***Devices Affected by MRI Systems*** | ***Objects Affecting MRI Systems*** | ***Fringe Magnetic Field Strength*** | ***Distance from Magnet (m)*** | | | | |
| Cathode ray tubes<br>X-ray tubes<br>MRI computer<br>Magnetic tape and disks<br>Credit cards<br>Analog watches | Large static ferromagnetic objects | 1 mT | 3.8 | 4.9 | 6.2 | 7.4 | 10.6 |
| Cardiac pacemakers | | 500 μT (5G) | 4.6 | 6.0 | 7.5 | 9.0 | 12.9 |
| | Large moving ferromagnetic objects, such as cars, lifts, etc.<br>Power transformers | 250 μT | 5.8 | 7.6 | 9.4 | 11.3 | 16.2 |
| Gamma cameras<br>Image intensifiers<br>CT scanners<br>Photomultipliers<br>Ultrasound systems | | 100 μT | 7.9 | 10.3 | 12.9 | 15.5 | 22.1 |

*Source:* Kean DM, Smith MA. Magnetic Resonance Imaging: Principals and Applications. © 1986, The Williams & Wilkins Company, Baltimore, 1986, p. 68, with permission.

hydrogen nuclei in both the z and the x-y directions. The net magnetization has a considerable z component since the x and y components of the individual nuclei cancel and become zero.

Transverse magnetization results from application of short bursts of radio frequency (RF) energy (i.e., radio waves) called RF pulses. The magnetization of the proton by the RF pulse results in the relaxation process illustrated in Figure 1–4. Longitudinal relaxation is illustrated by progressive elongation of the z component. Transverse relaxation is illustrated by the progressive decrease of the transverse component in the x-y plane.

Two types of MR signals can be produced by transverse magnetization. Immediately following a 90° pulse, the freely rotating transverse magnetization results in a signal called free induction decay, or FID (Fig. 1–5). This free induction decay signal has the following characteristics: it oscillates with components at the Larmor frequencies of the excited nuclei at the measuring site, and it

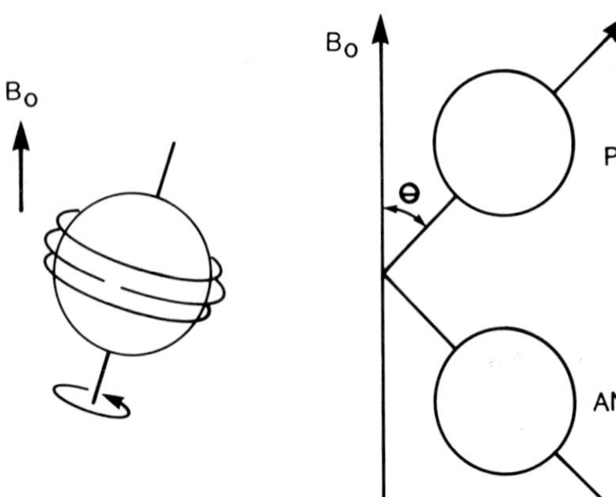


**Figure 1–3.** Representation of a spinning proton in a magnetic field, $B_o$.

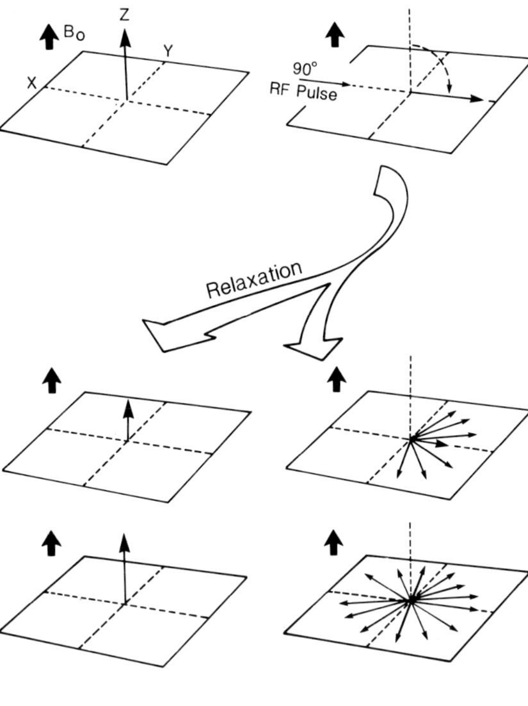


**Figure 1–4.** Images illustrating excitation and relaxation processes resulting from magnetic field and RF pulse. (From Dwyer AJ, Frank JA. In McCarthy S, Haseltine F, eds. Magnetic Resonance of the Reproductive System. Thorofare, N.J., Slack, Inc., 1987, p. 4, with permission.)

decreases in amplitude with time, mainly as a function of the transverse relaxation process. Nonuniformities in the main magnetic field will cause the protons to resonate out of phase.

Transverse magnetization (and induced signal) is lost at an exponential rate T2* (Fig. 1–6). A 180° pulse can be used intermittently to "refocus" the phase of the protons, causing them to recover transverse magnetization. However, complete rephasing is not possible, owing to the randomly fluctuating magnetic field. Thus the maximum intensity of the signal is limited by an exponentially decaying curve, the time constant being the second magnetic relaxation time, T2.

Relaxation comprises loss of the x and y components and increase of the z component. These processes occur simultaneously with a separate time constant. The $M_z$ component is referred to as longitudinal, or spin-lattice, relaxation, with a time constant T1 (Fig. 1–7). The $M_{xy}$ component is referred to as transverse, or spin-spin, relaxation, with a time constant T2 (Fig. 1–7). The longitudinal and transverse magnetizations should not be viewed simply as component vectors during the relaxation phase. If they were components, there would be a simple correlation between the decay of one and the growth of the other. In fact, it is observed that the transverse magnetization can disappear long before the full value of the longitudinal magnetization is restored. This difference between relaxation times of different tissues is of primary importance in MRI contrast.

**Table 1–3.** MAGNETIC PROPERTIES OF ELEMENTS OF BIOLOGIC INTEREST

| Isotope (with spin) | Effective Molar Concentration (mol/L) | Gyro-magnetic Ratio (mHz/T) | Magnetic Susceptibility (relative to $^1$H) |
|---|---|---|---|
| $^1$H | 99.0 | 42.58 | 1.0 |
| $^{13}$C | 0.10 | 10.71 | 0.016 |
| $^{17}$O | 0.031 | 5.77 | 0.029 |
| $^{19}$F | 0.0066 | 40.05 | 0.830 |
| $^{23}$Na | 0.078 | 11.26 | 0.093 |
| $^{31}$P | 0.35 | 17.24 | 0.066 |

## Physical Basis for T1 and T2

T1 (called the longitudinal, thermal, or spin-lattice relaxation time) is the time re-

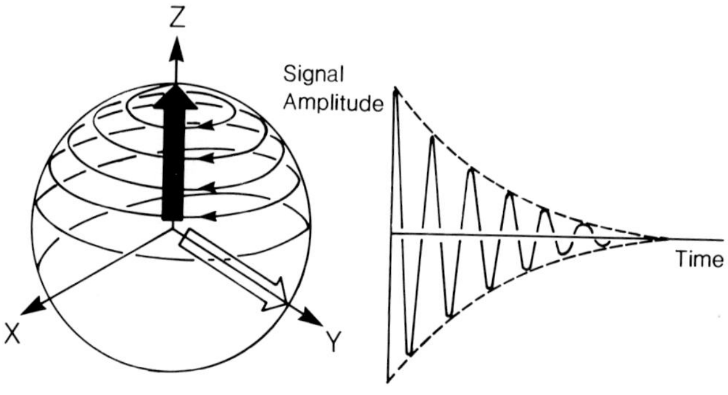


**Figure 1–5.** Free induction decay signal: the net magnetization is shown pictorially to spiral into the transverse plane of excitation, the graph depicts the decay of the MR response signal detected during relaxation. (From Principles of MR Imaging. Netherlands, Philips Medical Systems, 1984, p. 24, with permission.)

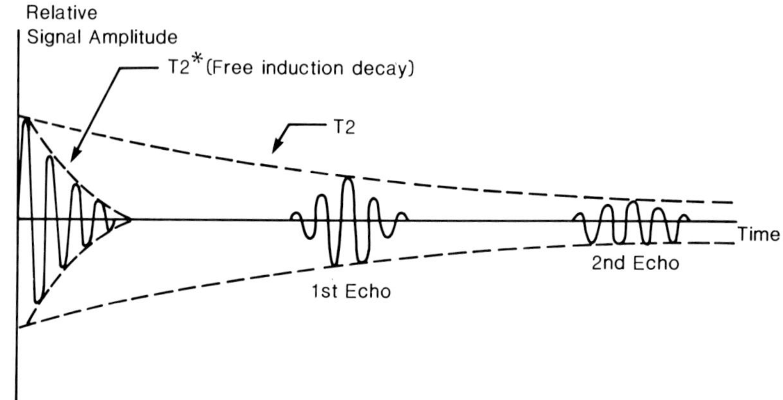


**Figure 1–6.** Representation of the MR response signal decaying at a rate given by T2*, with echoes decaying in peak amplitudes at a rate of T2*. (From Principles of MR Imaging. Netherlands, Philips Medical Systems, 1984, p. 22, with permission.)

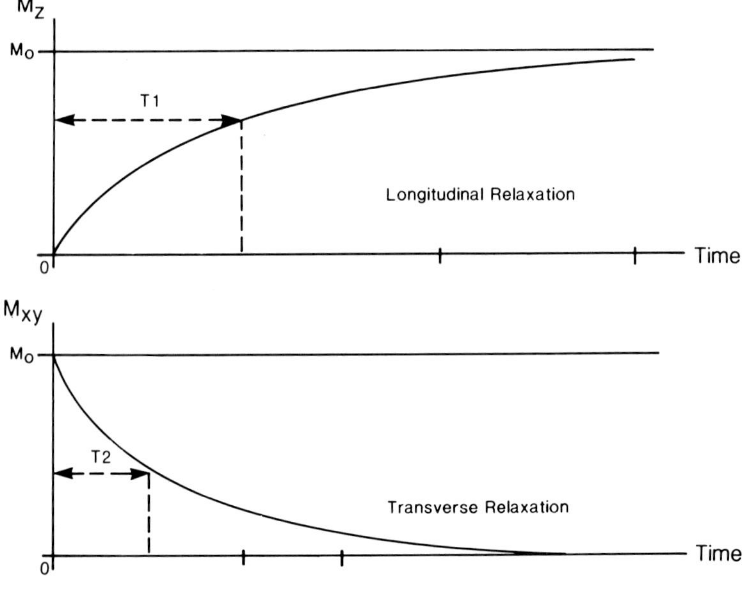


**Figure 1–7.** The longitudinal magnetization, $M_z$, returns gradually and reaches its initial value, $M_o$, when equilibrium is restored; the transverse magnetization, $M_{xy}$, will gradually diminish to zero. (From Principles of MR Imaging. Netherlands, Philips Medical Systems, 1984, p. 19, with permission.)

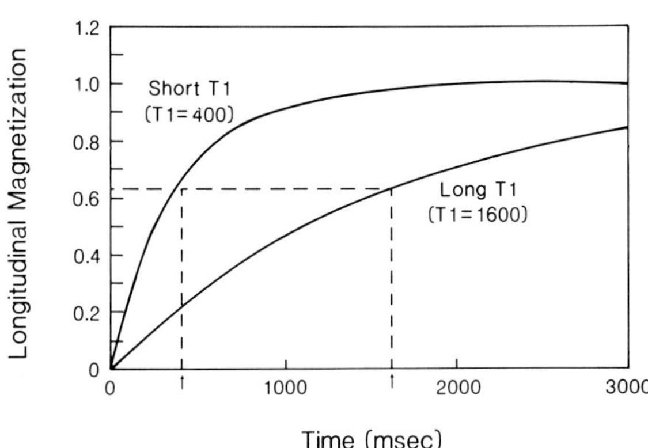


**Figure 1–8.** The T1 relaxation time describes the regrowth of longitudinal magnetization after it is reduced to zero by a 90° RF pulse. (From Ehman RL. In Berquist TH, ed. Magnetic Resonance of the Musculoskeletal System. New York, Raven Press, 1987, p. 25, with permission.)

quired to regain longitudinal magnetization following a 90° RF pulse (Fig. 1–8). T1 results from thermal interactions between the resonating protons and other magnetic nuclei in the magnetic environment, or lattice. All molecules have natural motions owing to vibration, rotation, and translation. The T1 relaxation time reflects the relationship between the frequency of these molecular motions and the resonant Larmor frequency. The water molecule is small and moves rapidly, whereas large proteins move slowly. Both have natural frequencies significantly different from the Larmor frequency and thus have long T1 relaxation times.

T2 (called the transverse, or spin-spin, relaxation time) reflects how long the resonating protons remain coherent or precess "in phase" following a 90° RF pulse (Fig. 1–9). T2 decay is due to magnetic interactions that occur between spinning protons and results only in a change in phase, leading to loss of coherence.

It should be apparent that an environment that is efficient for one form of relaxation may not be efficient for another. Typical tissue relaxation coefficients for two magnetic field strengths are given in Table 1–4.

## PULSE SEQUENCES

In MRI the difference in relaxation times of tissue components is most important because it is responsible for the contrast in the MR images. Image contrast can be manipulated by the choice of specific pulse sequences.

The principal pulse sequences are saturation recovery (SR), inversion recovery (IR), and spin echo (SE), derived from these basic sequences (Fig. 1–10). Fast-scan pulse sequences are described in a later section.

The simplest pulse sequence is called saturation recovery (also partial saturation, or repeated FID). Here, repetitive 90° RF pulses are applied to the sample, and the MRI signal is measured after each RF pulse. The repetition time, or time between pulses, is referred to as TR.

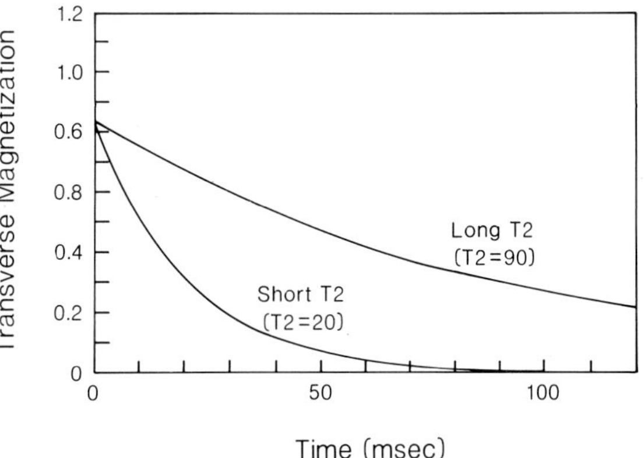


**Figure 1–9.** The T2 relaxation time describes the exponential decay of magnetization in the transverse plane after it is placed there by a 90° RF pulse. (From Ehman RL. In Berquist TH, ed. Magnetic Resonance of the Musculoskeletal System. New York, Raven Press, 1987, p. 26, with permission.)

**Table 1–4.** TISSUE RELAXATION CHARACTERISTICS

| | 0.5 T | | | 1.0 T | | |
|---|---|---|---|---|---|---|
| **Tissue** | ***T1* (*ms*)** | ***T2* (*ms*)** | ***T1*/*T2*** | ***T1* (*ms*)** | ***T2* (*ms*)** | ***T1*/*T2*** |
| Brain | 600 | 70 | 8.6 | 860 | 70 | 12.3 |
| Muscle | 540 | 50 | 10.8 | 750 | 55 | 13.6 |
| Fat | 220 | 60 | 3.7 | 220 | 60 | 3.7 |
| CSF | 3000 | 2000 | 1.5 | 3000 | 2000 | 1.5 |
| Blood | 850 | 200 | 4.3 | 900 | 200 | 4.5 |
| Aqueous humor | 3000 | 2000 | 1.5 | 3000 | 2000 | 1.5 |

*Source:* Fullerton GD. Radiographics 7:591, 1987, with permission.

Commonly used pulse sequences are SE and IR. The spin-echo sequence consists of a 90° pulse, followed by an echo delay time TE, after which the signal is sampled. TR indicates the total time of the sequence between 90° repetitive pulses. By choice of TR and TE, the spin-echo pulse sequence may be made either T1 weighted (short TR and TE) or T2 weighted (long TR and TE).

The inversion recovery pulse sequence consists of a 180° pulse followed by a delay of duration TI, a 90° pulse, and another delay time, TE, after which the signal is sampled. TR indicates the total time of the cycle. Inversion recovery pulse sequences are usually T1 weighted and provide good contrast of anatomy, since T1 values for normal tissues vary considerably (Table 1–4).

## MR IMAGE GENERATION

The generation of an image from the MR signals requires the spatial localization of these signals. A gradient magnetic field is superimposed upon the external magnetic field. Each point in the image precesses at its own particular frequency, which then corresponds to a particular spatial position. The signals along a gradient represent the sum of all the frequencies present. The amplitude of the signal originating from each particular point along that gradient is then determined from the various detected frequencies. The use of Fourier analysis transforms the frequency data into spatial position data. In earlier reconstruction approaches, one gradient was provided to de-

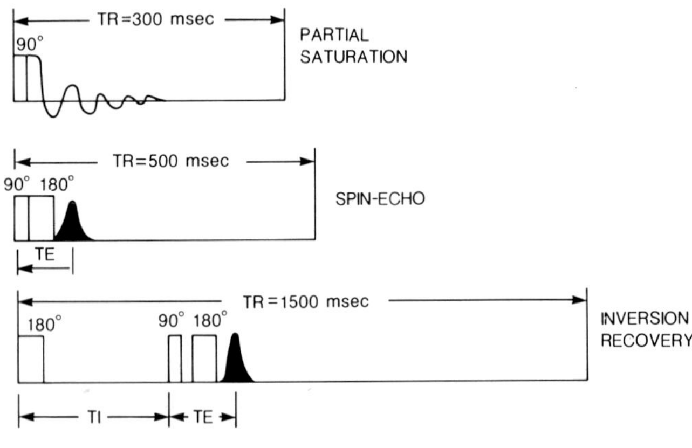


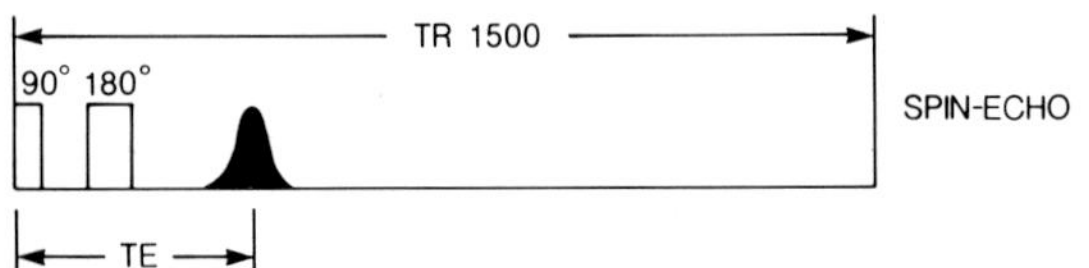


**Figure 1–10.** Schematic illustration of several commonly used pulse sequences for MR imaging in terms of a time axis. Specifically, the order and interval between the excitation pulses (indicated as rectangles) and sample times (dark peaks) are indicated by their positions along the horizontal axis. (From Dwyer AJ, Frank JA. In McCarthy S, Haseltine F, eds. Magnetic Resonance of the Reproductive System. Thorofare, N.J., Slack, Inc., 1987, p. 6, with permission.)

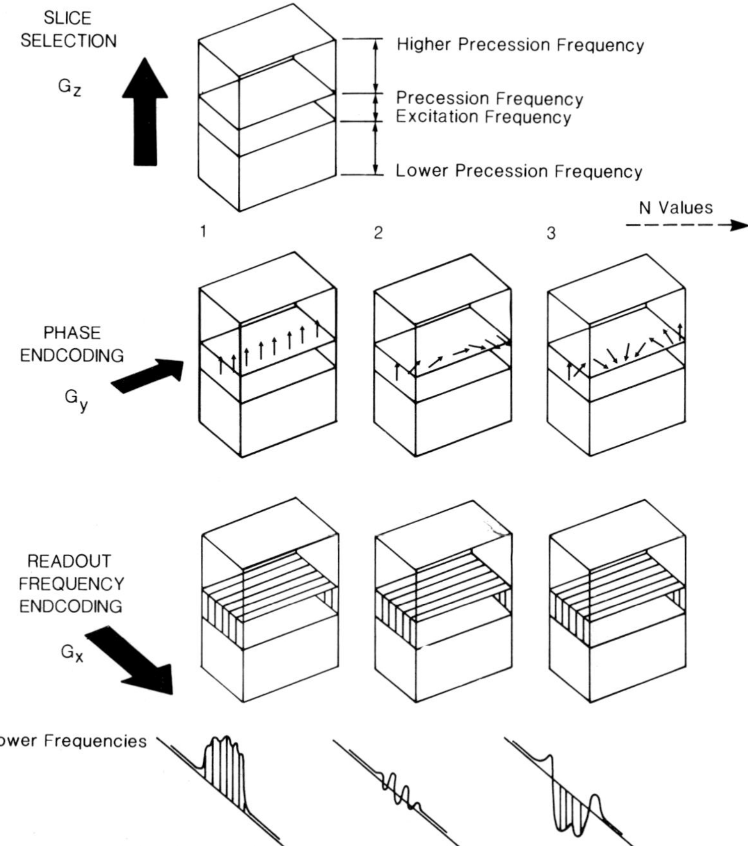


**Figure 1–11.** The slice is first selectively excited under gradient $G_z$; successive values of phase-encoding gradient $G_y$ are applied prior to the frequency gradient $G_x$. Each value of $G_y$ imposes a different amount of "twist," producing a different spectrum. (From Principles of MR Imaging. Netherlands, Philips Medical Systems, 1984, p. 44, with permission.)

fine a slice, and the second gradient was rotated at 1°-intervals to obtain 180 projections around the patient. Conventional back-projection algorithms were then used, as in the computed tomography (CT) approach. An approach less susceptible to motion artifacts and magnetic inhomogeneities and having more favorable signal-to-noise characteristics is the two-dimensional Fourier transform (2DFT) approach.

MR imaging by 2DFT requires activation of three gradients: slice selection, phase encoding, and readout (Fig. 1–11).

### Slice-Selection Gradient

The slice-selection gradient, $G_z$, sets the variation of frequency across the magnetic field (call it the z direction) to define a slice. Only spin in a particular slice, corresponding to the specific range of RF frequencies used, is excited. The slice-selection gradient can be oriented to yield transverse, coronal, or sagittal views. Increasing the range frequencies (band width) has the effect of increasing slice thickness. Slice thickness can also be varied by increasing the magnitude (or slope) of the gradient.

### Phase-Encoding Gradient

The excitation of the spins of the z slice is followed by selectively exciting spins to define the x-y coordinates. Rather than varying frequency in all three axes, a phase variation in the y direction has proved more advantageous. The phase gradient ($G_y$) alters the phase slightly along each y direction. When the phase gradient is turned off, each y position reverts to precessing at its original frequency, and each has a slightly different phase angle. The phase gradient must be repeated for each x position in the matrix array, e.g., 256 times for a 256 × 256 matrix.

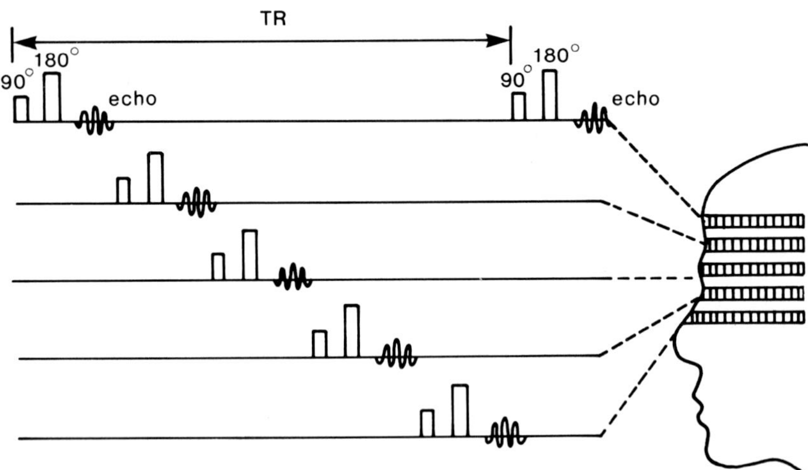


**Figure 1–12.** Multislice technique: in the time TR required to equilibrium by the first excited slice, other slices are measured in a suitable order. (From Principles of MR Imaging. Netherlands, Philips Medical Systems, 1984, p. 49, with permission.)

## Readout Gradient

After application of the z and simultaneously with y gradients, a final x-axis frequency gradient, $G_x$, is applied for reading out the signal and must be applied for each value of $G_y$. For each selected slice, the process interrogates each point defined by the x-y gradient combination until MR signals from the entire slice have been accumulated. Figure 1–11 summarizes the 2DF imaging sequence.

Three-dimensional Fourier transformations (3DFT) techniques are now being considered. For this case, a broad (nonselective) band of frequencies is used essentially to excite the entire volume. Two variable phase–encoding gradients are then applied simultaneously. Three Fourier transformations (FT) are performed, first along the readout gradient and then along the other two directions. These data are reformatted to yield any combination of slices, including oblique ones.

## Multislice Imaging Acquisition

The relatively long T1 relaxation time limits the shortness of the TR that can be used. The required interpulse delay times (TI or TE) can also be considerable for repeated sequences. For efficient use of TR and delay times, a multislice approach can be used. The TR interval can be utilized to excite other slices. The result is the acquisition of a multiple number of slice images at the end of the pulse sequence (Fig. 1–12). The slices are usually acquired in interleaved fashion to avoid crosstalk effects between slices, thus also allowing a little more time for recovery before giving the readout pulse.

The multislice technique allows not only acquisition of multiple slices but also use of different pulse-timing sequences. In a particular sequence, two separate and different TE-weighted images can be obtained, thus providing additional clinical information to allow differentiation between disease states.

## Chemical Shift Artifact

Although the majority of the MRI signal comes from the hydrogen nuclei of water molecules, lipid protons in fatty tissues can also contribute to the signal. Fat protons resonate at a slightly higher frequency than water protons. The difference between these frequencies is usually described as a fraction of the resonant frequency, a very small difference in frequencies (or the "chemical shift") expressed as parts per million (ppm). Fat protons resonate at a frequency 3 ppm higher than that of water protons. The absolute frequency difference depends on the strength of the main magnetic field (which determines the Larmor frequency). Since frequency determines the x, or readout, dimension subtle frequency differences between fat and water produce pixel shifts.

Although chemical shift artifact may be more noticeable at high field, it is also increased when the strength of the gradient is reduced. With improvement in the uniformity of lower field magnets, weaker gradients can be used without sacrificing frequency discrimination. Weaker gradients narrow the bandwidth, which reduces the noise, increasing the signal-to-noise ratio. Thus an unwanted side effect of increasing the SNR by weakening the gradients is to increase the chemical shift artifact. When chemical shift artifact is present and bothersome, it can be eliminated by increasing the strength of the gradient field (at a cost in the SNR).

## Paramagnetic Contrast Agents

Paramagnetic agents are of primary importance in MR imaging.[8–10] Paramagnetic relaxation enhancers shorten T1 and T2 relaxation times of neighboring hydrogen nuclei. This dual effect creates complex changes in the MRI signal, which further depends on the RF pulse sequence chosen. T1 shortening by paramagnetic agents acts to increase signal intensity; T2 shortening acts to decrease intensity. Concentration of the paramagnetic agents also affects the relative changes in T1 and T2 shortening. At high concentrations, the shortening of T2 predominates, causing a rapid decrease of echo signal intensity. Paramagnetic agents will also allow visualization of lesions using sequences with shorter TR, thus decreasing scan time and increasing patient throughput.

Table 1–5 provides a summary of potential paramagnetic agents. These agents have been delivered to biologic systems in MRI by three routes: oral, intravenous, and inhalation.

Two major categories of intravenous paramagnetic agents are suitable in MRI: organic free radicals, in particular the nitroxide spin labels, and transition metal and rare earth complexes, such as iron, manganese, and gadolinium. Of all the paramagnetic cations in the atomic table, $Gd^{3+}$ has the strongest relaxation rate enhancement properties. $Gd^{3+}$ contains seven unpaired electrons. An important feature in the relaxation rate enhancement by $Gd^{3+}$ is the presence of a relatively long electron spin relaxation time. Since as a free ion gadolinium is toxic to the liver, spleen, and bone marrow, it is complexed with DTPA for detoxification (Table 1–5).

**Table 1–5.** POTENTIAL PARAMAGNETIC COMPLEXES[10]

| Paramagnetic Ions | Chelators (Complexed to a Paramagnetic Species) |
|---|---|
| Transition metals | |
| Titanium ($Ti^{3+}$) | Polycarboxylic acids (EDTA, DTPA) |
| Nickel ($Ni^{2+}$) | |
| Iron ($Fe^{3+}$) | Siderophores (desferroximine) |
| Vanadium ($V^{4+}$) | Sugar acids (glucoheptonate) |
| Cobalt ($Co^{3+}$) | |
| Chromium ($Cr^{3+}$) | |
| Manganese ($Mn^{2+}$) | |
| Copper ($Cu^{2+}$) | |
| Lanthanide series | |
| Praseodymium ($Pr^{3+}$) | |
| Gadolinium ($Gd^{3+}$) | |
| Europium ($Eu^{3+}$) | |
| Dysprosium ($Dy^{3+}$) | |
| Actinide series | |
| Protactinium ($Pa^{4+}$) | |
| Nitroxide-stable free radicals (NSFRs) | |
| pyrrolidine and Piperidine | |
| Molecular oxygen ($O_2$) | |

*Source:* Modified from Runge VMN, et al. Enhanced NMR Imaging: a Review. AJR 141:1211, 1983, with permission.

An important category of paramagnetic agents is gases, most notably molecular oxygen, which has potential use in both proton and fluorine-19 MRI. Proton MRI relaxation rate enhancement has been observed after inhalation of 100% oxygen by human volunteers. However, oxygen does not exhibit strong proton relaxation enhancement in water and blood. Greater enhancement of T1 relaxation rates is possible with use of strong paramagnetic agents such as gadolinium, as indicated above. Paramagnetic molecular oxygen also has potential biomedical applications in fluorine-19 MRI. T1 measurements of injected oxygenated perfluorocarbon emulsion pharmaceuticals (blood substitutes) may be a sensitive parameter for the in vivo measurement of oxygen tension in blood vessels.[11]

Of the several types of paramagnetic materials (Table 1–5), the insoluble particulate species (as oral agents) and the metal ion chelates/complexes (as intravenous contrast media) seem to have the greatest immediate promise. Gadolinium-DTPA (Gd-DTPA) affords the best combination of in vivo lesion relaxation-rate enhancement, with favorable toxicologic and pharmacokinetic behavior.

**Table 1–6.** PARAMETERS THAT CHARACTERIZE THE MR IMAGE

| Primary Parameters | Secondary Parameters |
|---|---|
| Field strength | Spatial resolution |
| Field of view (FOV) | Signal-to-noise ratio (SNR) |
| Imaging slice | Scan time |
| Slice thickness | Coverage |
| Phase-coded projections (N) | Image contrast |
| Number of excitations (n) | |
| Repetition time (TR) | |
| Echo delay time (TE) | |
| Inversion time (TI) | |

*Source:* Modified from Wong WS, et al. Practical Magnetic Resonance Imaging: a Case Study Approach. Rockville, Md., Aspen Publishers, Inc., 1987, p. 18, with permission.

## MR IMAGING CONSIDERATIONS

The parameters that characterize the MR image are listed in Table 1–6.[12] "Primary" parameters are specified directly with the "secondary" parameters then being indirectly determined. The secondary parameters include the variables that are often used to describe image quality: spatial resolution, signal-to-noise ratio (SNR), coverage, scan time, and image contrast. The MR image is then characterized by the interrelation between the primary and secondary parameters.

### Spatial Resolution

The ability to discriminate subtle disease is proportional to SNR squared multiplied by the image contrast squared. The spatial resolution, determined by field homogeneity and the steepness of the gradients employed, may be increased until the SNR becomes the limiting factor, requiring more excitations and a longer scan time. Presently, resolution in clinical MR imaging has reached the 1-mm range.

### Signal-to-Noise Ratio (SNR)

The signal-to-noise ratio is determined by the following:[9]

**Voxel Size and Detection Volume.** The signal increases linearly with voxel volume, whereas the noise is independent of voxel volume. Increasing the number of phase-encoding gradients, $N_y$, has the effect of (*a*) voxel volume decreasing with $1/N_y^2$, reducing the SNR with increasing $N_y$, and (*b*) the signal increasing linearly with $N_y$ and the noise with $\sqrt{N_y}$, i.e., SNR decreases with increasing $N_y$.

**Number of Excitations (n).** The signal increases linearly with n and the noise, with $\sqrt{n}$, resulting in an increase of SNR by $\sqrt{n}$. Increasing the number of excitations is not an extremely efficient way to improve signal-to-noise ratio.

**Pulse Sequence Employed.** A small signal can result when there is incomplete recovery; sampling is performed when the T1 magnetization curve approaches a null point in inversion recovery, and for delayed echoes. The SNR in a spin-echo sequence can be increased by increasing the repetition time, TR, or the number of excitations, n. The highest SNR from tissue surrounded by air or bone is obtained when the echo time, TE, is kept to a minimum and TR is chosen at an optimal value.

**Field Strength.** The signal is proportional to the square of the field strength. Taking into account the properties of the detection coil, electronic equipment, and losses in tissue, SNR increases roughly linearly with field strength for strengths used in clinical imaging.

### Scan Time

The scan time depends on the number of projections, repetition time (TR), and number of excitations (n) to increase the SNR.[9] Typical values are 128 or 256, 0.5 to 2.0 seconds, and 1, 2, or 4, respectively.[9] For example, an image pixel size of 256, TR of 2 seconds, and two excitations will require a scan time of 17 minutes.

In two-dimensional Fourier transform methods (2DFT), to obtain an x-y image matrix, y signals must be gathered with varying degrees of phase encoding. The scan time for one slice is approximately 8 minutes. However, as indicated earlier, multiple slice techniques can be used to advantage in this situation.

For volume imaging (3DFT), one more phase-encoding gradient is necessary for spatial localization in the third dimension (the z direction). For z slices, z degrees of phase encoding are required in addition to y degrees. The scan time for a chosen slice thickness of 0.5 cm in a volume of 15 cm may be as much as 2 hours.[9]

### Image Contrast

With MRI the clinical challenge is to manipulate the parameters (Table 1–6) that are under the control of the operator to optimize the display of image contrast for the depiction of both anatomy and pathology. The main determinants of intensity or brightness in the MR image are the proton spin density, the T1 relaxation characteristics of the tissue, and the T2 relaxation characteristics of the tissue. Most clinical protocols are designed to employ a combination of sequences that exploit both the T1 and T2 characteristics of the tissue so that a range of pathology may be identified and characterized. The main variables that are manipulated in affecting MRI contrast are TR and TE (Fig. 1–13).[13]

In general, when both short TR and short TE are used, the produced image is dominated by T1 effects. Short TE and long TR results in an image in which proton spin density contributes. For long TR and long TE, the influence of T2 on the image is maximized. Thus a T1-weighted image (T1WI) results from using a short TR, maximizing the T1 effects, and from using a short TE, minimizing the contribution of T2 effects.

Proton spin density images are obtained when a long TR and short TE are used. The use of a long TR minimizes the effects of T1, and a short TE minimizes the effects of T2. Contrast within soft tissue is primarily a manifestation of differences in proton density.

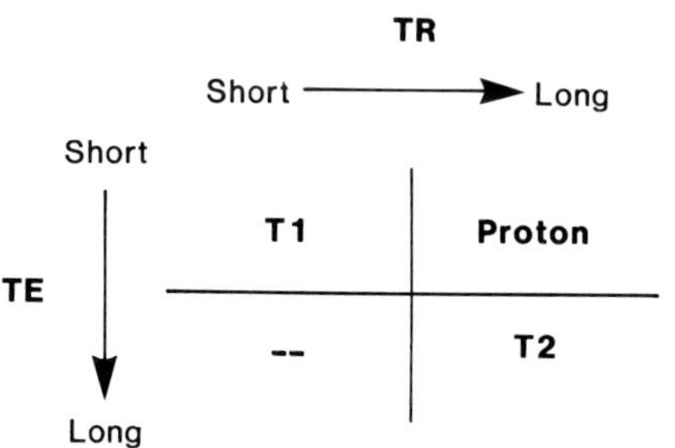


**Figure 1–13.** Manipulation of parameters that affect MRI contrast. (From Merritt CRB. In An Introduction to the Physics of Magnetic Resonance Imaging. Radiographics 7:1002, 1987, with permission.)

T2-weighted images are produced when long TR and long TE sequences are used. Effectively, long TR minimizes T1 contribution, and a long TE maximizes the T2 contribution to the image.

Most disease processes increase both T1 and T2 relaxation. A lesion has negative contrast (appears black) on T1-weighted images and positive contrast (appears relatively bright) on T2-weighted images if relaxation times are prolonged. Thus lesion conspicuity diminishes as T1 weighting is increased on a T2-weighted image. For the case where T1-weighted images may be preferred, increasing the T1 weighting increases contrast and enhances lesion conspicuousness.

## BIOLOGIC EFFECTS

Although questions have been raised about the long-term biologic effects of magnetic resonance imaging, there are still no published reports of harmful effects directly associated with the use of electromagnetic fields in clinical MRI.

Individuals undergoing MRI are exposed to three types of electromagnetic fields: static magnetic field, gradient (time-varying) magnetic field, and pulsed radio frequency (RF) magnetic field.[14, 15]

The Food and Drug Administration (FDA) issued guidelines in 1982 for the operation of MRI systems. These guidelines included whole- or partial-body exposures of 2 T for static magnetic fields and 3 T/second for gradient magnetic fields; RF electromagnetic fields are not to exceed a specific absorption rate of 0.4 W/kg averaged over the whole body or 2 W/kg averaged over 1 g of tissue.

### Static Magnetic Fields

An apparent physiologic effect of static fields is the augmentation of the T wave amplitude observed in electrocardiograms. The mechanism for this effect appears to be due to superimposition of low potentials on the normally occurring biopotential. These potentials result when the flow of a conductive fluid, such as blood, passes through a magnetic field. The effect appears to be linearly related to magnetic field strength.

In animal studies, no arrhythmias or alterations in heart rate are noted, with normal ECG resuming immediately after terminating the exposure to high magnetic fields. No change in blood chemistry or blood pressure is observed in the animals. At the field strengths employed in present MRI units, no notable changes in ECG tracings have been observed in volunteers undergoing imaging procedures.

### Gradient Magnetic Fields

Gradient magnetic fields can induce electric currents in body tissues. If the currents are intense enough, they can stimulate certain body tissues such as nerve cells and also skeletal and heart muscle fibers. However, the rate of change in magnetic field intensity required to produce observable effects such as heart fibrillation are far above those employed in MRI.

The most sensitive physiologic response to gradient magnetic fields is the sensation of visual light flashes owing to stimulation of magnetic retinal phosphenes. The biologic significance of this reaction is not known. It is felt that the threshold for this effect is not reached by the rates of change in magnetic fields used during clinical MRI.

### Radio Frequency (RF) Magnetic Fields

The primary biological effects of exposure to RF energy are associated with thermally induced changes. Athermal or "field-specific" changes have been described, although the mechanisms behind these changes are still controversial and not easily understood. The investigations available on thermoregulatory responses of humans exposed to radio frequency radiation do not directly apply because they involve either thermal sensations or therapeutic application of diathermy to localized regions of the body.

High field systems are more likely to cause measurable temperature elevations than low field systems. The rate at which RF energy is deposited in the patient involves several variables, including type of RF pulse (90° or 180°); number of RF pulses in a sequence (scan type and number of echoes); pulse width; repetition time (TR); patient size; anatomic region imaged; and type of coil used.[14] The actual increase in tissue temperature from exposure to RF radiation is also affected by the inherent physiologic aspects of the subject's thermoregulatory system: the ability to vasodilate, redistribution of blood flow, sweat, and so forth. Certain regions having reduced capabilities for heat dissipation (such as the testis and eye) are sites of potential harmful effects of excessive RF radiation exposures. Some detrimental effects on testicular function have been found by exposures sufficient to raise scrotal or testicular tissue temperatures or both between 37° and 42°C. Although it is highly unlikely that this temperature level will be approached during clinical MRI, studies are still needed.

Exposure of eyes of experimental animals to RF energy has revealed a possible cataractogenic effect as a result of thermal disruption of ocular tissues. However, even when MRI systems are operated above the recommended level for RF radiation, the resultant change in corneal temperatures is well below the threshold for thermal damage.

As indicated earlier, the FDA recommends limiting the RF power deposition during MRI to a whole body average specific absorption rate (SAR) of 0.4 W/kg and a local (1 g of tissue) SAR of 2 W/kg to avoid temperature-related effects.

### MRI During Pregnancy

There is no experimental evidence to suggest that the embryo or fetus is particularly sensitive to the magnetic fields employed in MRI. However, concern has been expressed over possible fetal effects; consequently, few installations have examined pregnant patients. MRI may be indicated for use in pregnant women if other non-ionizing forms of diagnostic imaging are inadequate or if MRI provides important information in patients who would otherwise require exposure to ionizing radiation.

### Ferromagnetic Hazards

Possible dangers associated with MRI procedures in patients with internal or external ferromagnetic devices include movement, induction of an electric current, and heating. Heating of ferromagnetic devices is not considered a significant hazard for small devices and low-strength systems. Increased heating possibilities for larger metallic devices needs further evaluation. Possible motion of a ferromagnetic foreign body can be injurious to an MRI patient. Artifacts that may degrade image quality or simulate pathology are possible in patients whose bodies contain ferromagnetic or nonferromagnetic materials.

MRI procedures should not be performed on patients with cardiac pacemakers owing to their possible movement, reed switch closure or damage, programming changes, and so forth. Procedures on patients with neurostimulators or other electrically activated biomedical systems should await studies on the effects of magnetic fields on these devices.

## References


1. Lee SH, Rao KCVG. Cranial Computed Tomography and MRI. New York, McGraw-Hill Book Co., 1987.
2. Kean DM, Smith MS. Magnetic Resonance Imaging: Principles and Applications. Baltimore, Williams & Wilkins, 1986.
3. Schenck JF. Signa System Operator Manual. Schenectady, N.Y., General Electric Company, OMS2 Rev. 11, 1986:6.
4. Dwyer AJ, Frank JA. Basic concepts of magnetic resonance imaging (MRI). In Magnetic Resonance of the Reproductive System. McCarthy S, Haseltine F, eds. Thorofare, N.J., Slack, Inc., 1987.
5. Principles of MR Imaging. The Netherlands, Philips Medical Systems, 1984.
6. Ehman RL. Interpretation of magnetic resonance images. In Berquist TH, ed. Magnetic Resonance of the Musculoskeletal System. New York, Raven Press, 1987.
7. Fullerton GD. Magnetic resonance imaging signal concepts. Radiographics 7:579–596, 1987.
8. Wesby GE. Paramagnetic pharmaceuticals in biomedical magnetic resonance. In Thomas SR, Dixon RL, eds. NMR in Medicine: the Instrumentation and Clinical Applications. AAPM Monograph No. 14, New York, American Institute of Physics, 1986.
9. Koops W. MR Imaging Compendium. Department of Radiology, University Hospital Dijkzigt, Rotterdam, The Netherlands, 1986.
10. Runge VMN, Clanton JA, Lukehart CM, et al. Enhanced NMR imaging: a review. AJR 141:1209, 1983.
11. Clark LC, Ackerman JL, Thomas SR, et al. Perfluorinated organic liquids and emulsions as biocompatible NMR imaging agents for fluorine 19 and dissolved oxygen. In Brulely D, Bicher HI, Reneau D, eds. Oxygen Transport to Tissue VI. New York, Plenum Press, 1985:385.
12. Wong WS, Tsuruda JS, Kortman KE, et al: Practical Magnetic Resonance Imaging: A Case Study Approach. Rockville, Md., Aspen Publishers, Inc., 1987.
13. Merritt CRB. MRI clinical image quality, safety, and risk management. Radiographics 7:1001–1016, 1987.
14. Shellock FG. Biological effects of MRI: a clean safety record so far. Diagn Imag Clin Med 9:96, 1987.
15. Morgan CJ, Hendee WR. Introduction to Magnetic Resonance Imaging. Denver, Multi-Media Publishing, Inc., 1986.

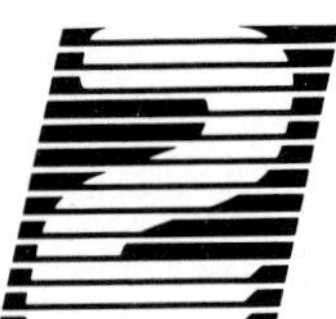

Stephen R. Thomas, Ph.D.
Stephen J. Pomeranz, M.D.

# FLOW EFFECTS IN MAGNETIC RESONANCE

In diagnostic imaging, subject motion generally introduces artifacts that degrade image quality. However, in magnetic resonance imaging (MRI), one important category of motion that can be exploited for diagnostic purposes is fluid flow. Flow phenomena, which include motion not only of blood but also of cerebrospinal fluid, are recognized as having a profound influence on the presentation of features within an MR image. Relatively early in the history of nuclear magnetic resonance (NMR), as analytical techniques were being developed, the basic effects of motion on the signal intensity were identified and described.[1-3] Applications monitoring flowing blood in vivo were attempted before the advent of MR imaging.[4,5] Observations of signal loss associated with high flow rates within vessels were noted on some of the first clinical MR images presented in the literature.[6] Theory, design, and applications of NMR blood flow instrumentation have been reported.[7] At the present time, most (although admittedly not all) aspects involving the contributions of fluid flow to magnetic resonance (MR) image contrast are relatively well understood. A significant number of papers including comprehensive review articles have been published on this topic.[8-22] The present chapter draws extensively from this body of literature to develop the conceptual basis of two major categories of flow phenomena in MRI: namely, (1) time-of-flight effects and (2) velocity-related phase shift phenomena. The discussion is limited to bulk flow geometries as found in (*a*) major vessels or compartments (arteries, veins, and cardiac chambers) and in (*b*) anatomic spaces (ventricles and subarachnoid space) as opposed to situations involving the microcirculation (tissue perfusion through capillaries[23]) and even smaller scale diffusion transport.

## GENERAL CONSIDERATIONS CONCERNING BLOOD AND CEREBROSPINAL FLUID FLOW

Blood flow through the larger vessels is characterized by various degrees of pulsatile motion that introduce temporally varying patterns and by spatial nonuniformities across the transverse luminal plane and along the flow direction. In arteries, the instantaneous maximum flow rates occur during the systolic portion of the cardiac cycle with peak aortic velocities in the range of 100 to 150 cm/sec. The average arterial flow velocities are considerably less (20 to 50 cm/sec) and decrease as these vessels progress into their branch configurations. Within the veins, flow rates will exhibit more uniform temporal properties with lower average velocities; however, fluctuations will be present from a number of sources, including pulsations transmitted from the right heart, respiration, and muscular motion.[13]

For fluid moving through a geometric, smooth-walled tube, velocity profiles representing the spatial distribution of flow within the lumen can be described as either laminar or turbulent. In general, laminar conditions are established at relatively low flow rates and are characterized by shells of increasing velocity as a function of distance from the wall. Ideally, this type of flow

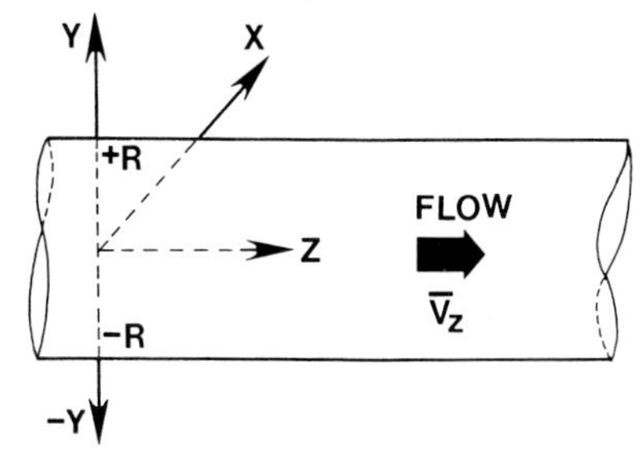


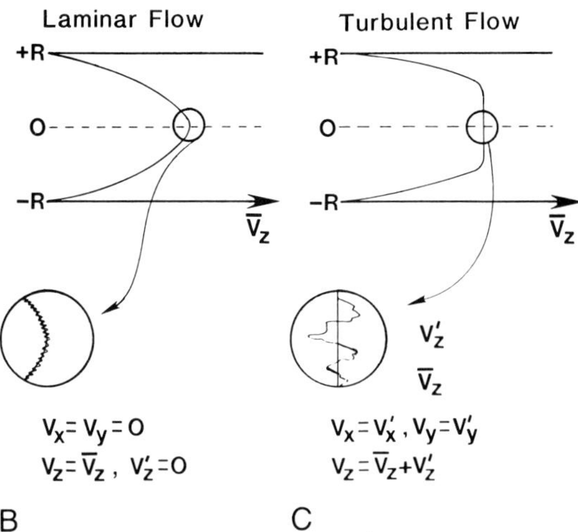


**Figure 2–1.** A schematic representation of concepts associated with laminar and turbulent flow. For laminar flow *(B)*, an average velocity $\bar{V}_z$ is established in the direction of flow with no transverse components being present ($V_x = V_y = 0$). The velocity profile assumes a more flattened shape for turbulent flow *(C)* with both transverse and axial fluctuations (indicated by a prime) around the average. (Modified from Bradley WG, Walach V, Lai K, et al. AJR 143:1167, 1984, with permission.)

exhibits a parabolic velocity profile (Poiseuille)—zero at the wall contact and maximum in the center, with an average velocity one half the maximum (Fig. 2–1). As the velocity increases further (for a given tube diameter), the profile assumes a more flattened shape. Ultimately, again in the idealized state, a point would be reached where all elemental fluid volumes would have the same velocity, producing a perfectly flat profile that represented the domain known as plug-flow. In laminar flow, the velocity component is entirely along the axial direction, whereas for turbulent flow there are transverse as well as axial components, with random fluctuations around the average values. As the flow rate increases, a transition zone occurs in which laminar flow persists in the boundary regions near the wall and turbulent conditions appear more interiorly. The velocity at which turbulence is initiated depends upon the fluid viscosity, and density and the tube diameter. Laminar flow may be maintained at higher velocities for liquids with greater viscosity. The onset of turbulence occurs at lower velocities as the diameter of the tube increases.[19, 22, 24]

The conceptual models just outlined apply to the specialized conditions of constant flow within a single-channel, smooth-walled tube. At best, they provide only an approximate description of the blood flow patterns expected in real anatomic vessels with pulsatile motions, irregular surfaces, tortuous pathways, and branching structures. Arterial pulsatile flow is characterized by components of both laminar and turbulent flow. Stenotic constrictions might establish laminar flow in the vicinity of the narrow opening with turbulent conditions appearing further downstream where the vessel diameter widens again. In addition, obstructive features such as plaques may set up recirculating swirling currents (eddies), where the local velocities may actually be reversed from the main current.[19, 22] Another aspect of the anatomic configuration that is important in interpreting the effects of blood flow within the MR image is the relationship of the vessel to the image plane. The vessel may be orthogonal to the plane, may intersect at an oblique angle, or may lie essentially within the plane. The influence of the orientation on blood flow image contrast is discussed in the following sections.

Motion of the cerebrospinal fluid (CSF) also has the capability of producing flow-related intensity variations in the MR image. Although bulk flow is associated with the production of approximately 500 ml of CSF per day within the choroid plexus of the lateral and third ventricles and its transit to the arachnoid villi, the dominant effects are caused by pulsatile motion established through cardiac rhythms and perhaps by contributions from generalized systolic cerebral expansion and the influence of nearby arteries, such as those at the base of the brain.[19] The net result is a relatively slow oscillatory motion that may influence the CSF intensity within the image.

## TIME-OF-FLIGHT EFFECTS

The bulk transit of individual (discrete) spin-volume elements known as isochromats through the image plane may result in (1) an increase in relative signal intensity within the flow channel (enhancement), (2) a decrease in the intensity (signal loss), or (3) no change at all. Within this all-encompassing range of options, the ultimate presentation will depend upon the interrelationship between multiple parameters, including flow velocity, orientation to the image plane, slice thickness, slice position within the multislice image volume, selective versus nonselective radio frequency pulses, repetition time (TR), and echo time (TE). Comparison of images among MRI systems additionally would have to take into account the magnetic field strength and specific software implementation, such as those providing velocity compensation or motion artifact suppression.[21] Time-of-flight (TOF) effects refer to aspects of image contrast or signal intensity that are influenced by both the physical motion of target nuclei and their magnetization history relative to the surrounding stationary tissue. The mechanisms that cause TOF effects must be distinguished from velocity-induced phase shift phenomena, which are discussed in another section.

### Flow-Related Enhancement

#### *Single-Slice, Selective Excitation Considerations*

Under steady application of the pulsing sequence, at the start of each new repetition, stationary nuclei within a slice defined by selective excitation may remain partially saturated, the degree of saturation dependent upon TR in relationship to T1. The signal intensity obtained is inversely related to the level of saturation present. The maximum signal occurs for unsaturated spin states that have been given time to return to full magnetic equilibrium (TR ≥ 5 T1). In general, this is not the case, and the steady state signal is reduced accordingly. If conditions of slow laminar flow exist, fully magnetized blood from outside the slice has the opportunity to move in and displace saturated blood during the repetition cycle. This unsaturated "new blood" exhibits a higher signal intensity per unit volume than blood remaining from the previous sequence. The fractional quantity of unsaturated blood introduced into the slice thickness D during the interval TR determines the magnitude of the signal increase. Thus if there is complete replacement (which would occur under conditions of $v \geq D/TR$), the enhancement reaches its maximum value and blood in the vessel appears bright relative to static blood and also possibly relative to the partially saturated adjacent tissues (depending upon the tissue T1 value).

Up to this point, for purposes of conceptual illustration, the discussion has tacitly assumed that 90° selective excitation pulses at a repetition period TR have been used, which would generate a free induction decay signal (i.e. saturation recovery, as opposed to the spin-echo techniques addressed later). In this case, the flow-dependent signal may be expressed analytically as[17]

$$S(v) = k\,[vTR/D + (1 - \sqrt{TR/D})\,(1 - e^{-TR/T1})] \quad \text{for } 0 \leq v \leq (D/TR) \qquad (1)$$

$$S(v) = k \text{ for } v \geq (D/TR)$$

in which the first term in the bracket represents the component resulting from the inflowing unsaturated blood and the second term is the contribution from the remaining partially saturated blood that has experienced at least two of the 90° pulses. The proportionality constant k is independent of flow and the relaxation time properties. As mentioned previously, the maximum signal occurs for complete replacement within the slice thickness, which establishes the relationship between the velocity, TR, and D ($v \geq D/TR$). Under the single-slice selective excitation conditions described, the signal would remain fixed at this value ($S_{max} = k$) for any further increase in flow velocity (Fig. 2–2). It should be recalled that idealized laminar flow is characterized by a parabolic profile, owing to a range of velocities with the maximum in the vessel center. Therefore the signal intensity varies over the luminal cross section. For maximum velocities in the range D/TR, the center portion appears brightest with a gradual fall-off in intensity toward the periphery (wall).

In most clinical MR imaging utilizing 2DFT techniques, spin-echo sequences are employed. Introduction of the 180° refocusing pulse and collection of an echo at time

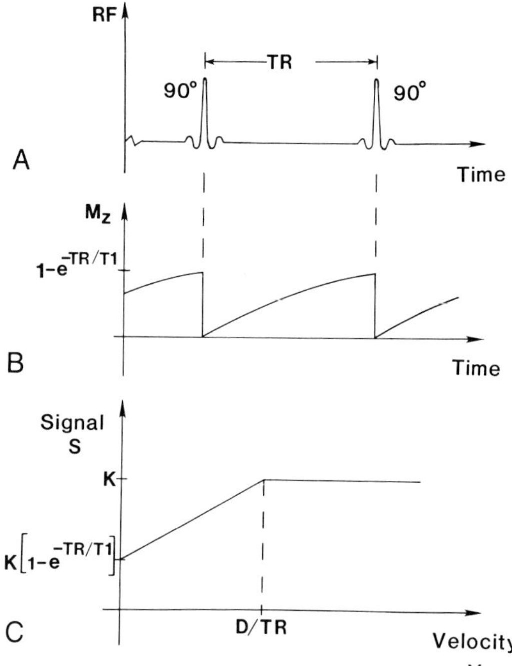


**Figure 2–2.** Single slice enhancement using selective 90° pulses (saturation recovery). *A* and *B* present the relationship between the selective 90° pulse and the magnetization of spins remaining within the single excited slice (of thickness D). The degree of recovery depends upon the repetition interval TR and T1 and is given by the expression $1-e^{-TR/T1}$. As shown in panel C (according to equation 1), the signal S will increase linearly with increasing velocity from a minimum of $k(1 - e^{-TR/T1})$ to a maximum of k for v = D/TR. At this point, complete washout has occurred during the interval TR, and fresh, unsaturated blood filling the slice thickness provides maximum signal. Further increase in flow velocity will not change the signal. (Modified from Axel L. AJR 143:1157, 1984, with permission.)

TE present a more complicated timing sequence for consideration when describing the effects of flow on signal intensity. Again, for this initial discussion, only single-slice selective excitation RF pulse sequences are considered. It is important to recognize that only those nuclei that receive both the 90° pulse and the 180° pulse within the interval TR contribute to the signal. Now, an additional signal-loss mechanism is present—those nuclei leaving the slice thickness during the period between the 90° and 180° pulses (namely, TE/2) are replaced by non–signal producing nuclei that have not been properly prepared (tagged) for the spin-echo sequence. For sufficiently low velocities, enhancement can still occur, however, because this lost component associated with flow during the interval TE/2 is more than offset by signal gain from unsaturated nuclei, which enter during the latter part of the TR repetition period and remain to receive both the 90° and 180° pulse within the next cycle (Fig. 2–3). Equation 1 may be modified to account for the reduction in signal ($T_o$ is defined in Fig. 2–3):[13, 17]

$$S_{SE}(v) \simeq k\,[v(TR/D) + (1 - vTR/D)(1 - e^{-(TR-T_o)/T1})]\,[(1 - vTE/(2D)]$$
$$\text{for } 0 \le v \le (D/TR)$$
$$S_{SE}(v) \simeq k[1 - vTE/(2D)]$$
$$\text{for } (D/TR) \le v \le (2D/TE)$$
$$S_{SE}(v) = 0 \quad \text{for} \quad v > (2D/TE) \qquad (2)$$

in which the expression in the second bracket represents the fractional reduction in intensity owing to flow exit over the period TE/2. Note that the degree of signal loss increases with the echo delay TE as well as with the flow velocity, v. (For simplicity, an additional signal reduction factor $e^{-TE/T2}$ not involving flow has been omitted from equation 2.) A schematic representation of the concepts associated with slow flow enhancement in spin-echo sequences is shown in Figure 2–4. Clinical examples of this effect are provided in Figure 2–5.

### *Multislice Selective Excitation Conditions*

Clinical MR imaging most often involves multislice, rather than single-slice, acquisition protocols. Under these conditions, an effective volume preparation of spin states is established, and the degree of flow-related enhancement present in an image depends upon its position within the slice sequence. Enhancement is greatest in the first slice, where the inflow of unsaturated blood is at a maximum and falls off in subsequent slices as a function of depth into the imaging volume. Figure 2–6 illustrates this phenomenon schematically under conditions of laminar flow. For multislice techniques employing a gap, the parameter D in Equation 2 becomes the distance represented by slice thickness plus gap. A clinical example is shown in Figure 2–7. Compensation for this enhancement phenomenon may be achieved through application of presaturation pulse sequences that apply RF power to regions outside the imaging volume (Fig. 2–8). Blood flowing into the first slice will now have the same degree of saturation as blood remaining

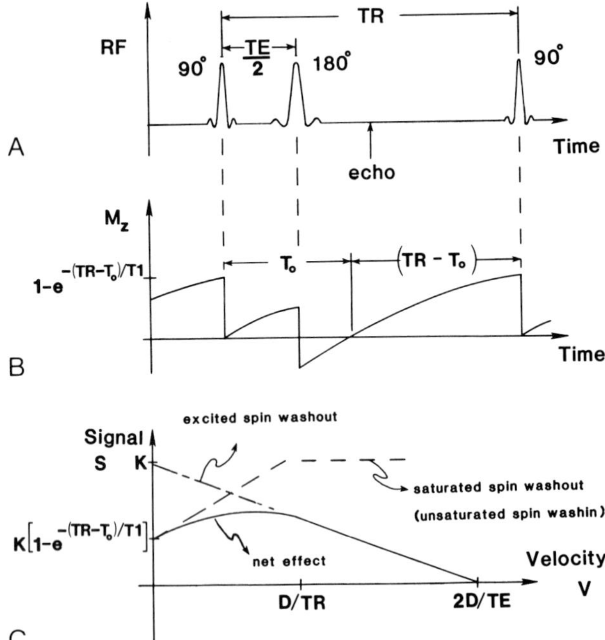


**Figure 2–3.** Combined effects contributing to the net flow signal for single slice, selective excitation spin-echo sequences. *A* and *B* present the relationship between the selective 90° and 180° RF pulses and the magnetization of spins remaining within the single excited slice (of thickness D). *C* shows the net signal resulting from washout of both excited spins that have not experienced the refocusing pulse and saturated spins. Enhancement appears at relatively low velocities, whereas complete signal loss occurs for v = 2D/TE. The interval $TR - T_o$ represents the time from zero crossing following the 180° pulse to the next 90° pulse. (Modified from Axel L. AJR 143:1157, 1984, with permission.)

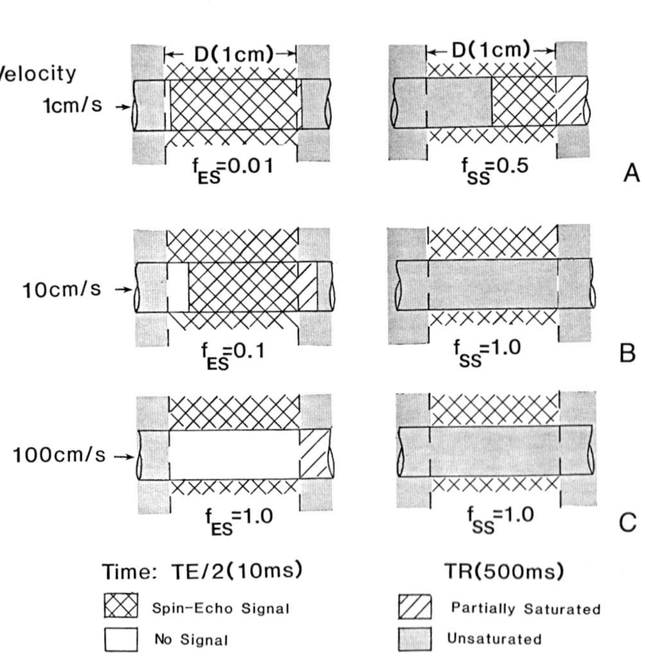


**Figure 2–4.** A schematic representation of spin-echo time-of-flight enhancement and high-velocity signal loss for the specific case of single-slice selective excitation with TE = 20 msec, TR = 500 msec, and slice thickness D = 1 cm. Two time points are shown (TE/2 and TR) for various flow velocities (illustrated here for simplicity as uniform velocity plug flow). Spins must receive both the 90° and 180° pulse in order to contribute to the spin-echo signal. The fraction of excited spins $f_{ES}$ removed (washed out) during the interval TE/2 before experiencing the 180° pulse (or equivalently, those that enter after the 90° pulse) represents the proportionate signal loss. At low velocities, $f_{ES}$ is small, and this loss effect may be overcome by the higher signal contribution of unsaturated spins that have entered during the repetition interval TR and receive both pulses ($f_{SS}$ is the fraction of saturated spins replaced by unsaturated spins during the TR interval). As seen in *A*, for v = 1 cm/sec $f_{ES}$ is much smaller than $f_{SS}$, thus slow flow enhancement within the vessel may occur, depending upon the relative T1 values of the fluid and the surrounding static tissue. For a velocity increase to 100 cm/sec (*C*), all excited spins are removed during the interval TE/2 ($f_{ES}$ = 1.0), producing complete signal void independent of the fact that unsaturated spins will fill the slice thickness ($f_{SS}$ = 1.0) by the time the sequence repeats. Note: (1) $f_{ES}$ = V TE/2D for $V < 2D/TE$, $f_{ES}$ = 1 for $V \geq 2D/TE$; (2) $f_{SS}$ = V TR/D for $V < D/TR$, $f_{SS}$ = 1 for $V \geq D/TR$.

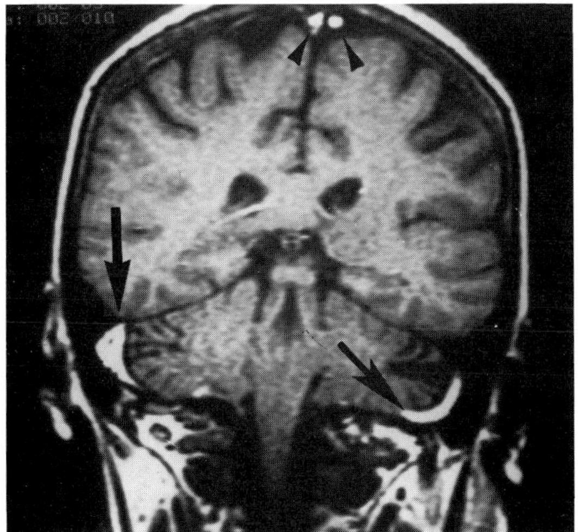

**Figure 2–5.** Time-of-flight enhancement in a spin-echo sequence. In-flow of unsaturated (fully magnetized) blood from outside the imaging volume produces a hyperintense signal within the transverse sinuses (arrows). Enhancement is also evident in the superior sagittal sinus and cortical vein (arrowheads). Imaging parameters: 1.5 T, TR 600/TE 20 3 mm, coronal.

within the slice and enhanced luminal signal will not occur.

### *High-Velocity Signal Loss*

For spin-echo sequences, as the flow velocity increases, the volume of blood replaced within the slice thickness during the period TE/2 increases. As described previously, this incoming blood has not been tagged with both the 90° and 180° pulses and thus will not contribute any signal. As indicated in Figure 2–3 and Equation 2, the flow-related signal loss becomes more significant at higher velocities according to the function $[1 - v(TE/2D)]$. When the velocity reaches a value of $v_m = 2D/TE$, the signal will be reduced to zero, and the vessel lumen will appear dark. This process for establishing total loss of signal is one of the principal mechanisms contributing to the phenomenon known as the flow void. The washout effect is represented schematically in Figure 2–9, and clinical illustrations are provided in Figures 2–7 and 2–10. The signal will remain zero for all velocities above $v_m$.

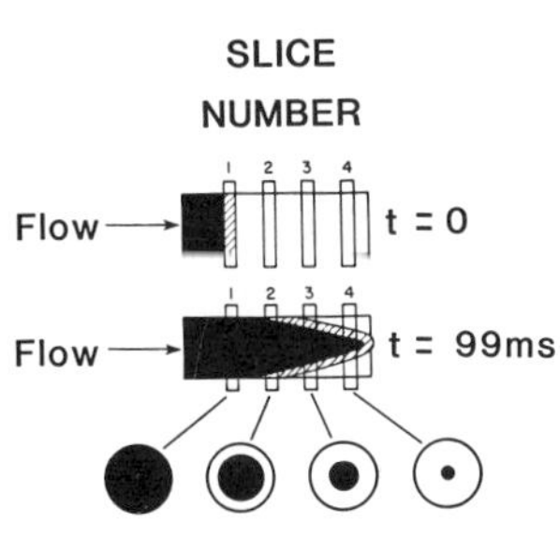


**Figure 2–6.** Multislice flow-related enhancement resulting from the parabolic profile of laminar flow. Higher velocity unsaturated isochromats entering the imaging volume toward the lumen center are able to move further into the slice series before experiencing their initial exciting 90° pulse. The transverse views indicate the pattern of decreasing cross section presented by the enhanced central region as a function of slice position. (From Bradley WG, Walach V, Lai K, et al. AJR 143:1167, 1984, with permission.)

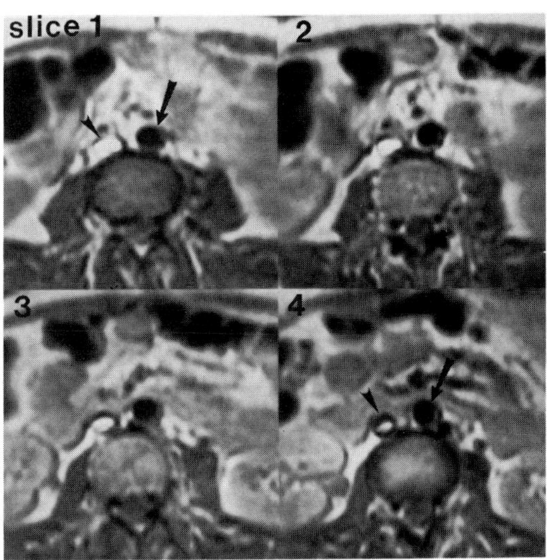


**Figure 2–7.** Multislice time-of-flight effects. Unsaturated (fully magnetized) blood entering the first slice produces enhancement within the vena cava (arrowhead). On subsequent images, proceeding deeper into the scan series, the enhanced luminal signal becomes progressively less pronounced, with hyperintensity confined to the central area in the fourth slice. This pattern is directly related to the laminar flow profile (see Fig. 2–6). The relatively higher velocity of the central isochromats allow them to proceed further into the series before experiencing their first saturating RF pulse (90°). The signal increase will disappear entirely from the vena cava lumen within the next several images of the series. In direct contrast, high-velocity washout along with a contribution due to turbulent dephasing produces complete loss of signal (flow void) in the aorta (arrow). Imaging parameters: 1.5 T, TR 1000/TE 20 5 mm, 2.5 mm gap, axial.

### *Oblique-Angle Effects*

For vessels inclined at an angle θ to the imaging plane (as opposed to the orthogonal

Flow Compensation Techniques

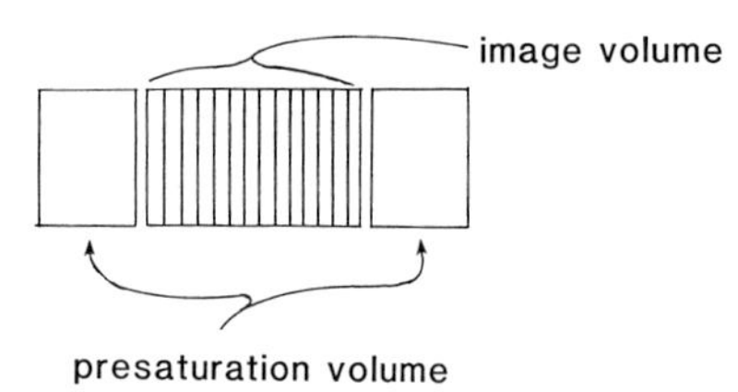


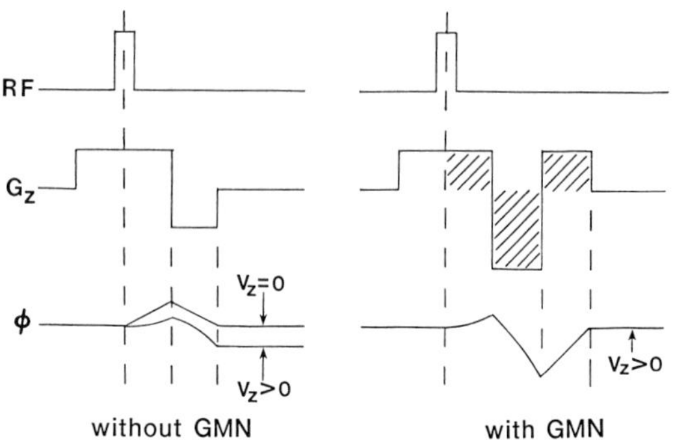


**Figure 2–8.** Flow compensation techniques. *A,* The presaturation method is designed to prevent time-of-flight slow flow enhancement through application of saturating RF pulses to regions outside of the imaging volume. Thus blood flowing into the first several slices of the imaging volume will already be saturated (or partially saturated), and the mechanism that leads to enhanced signal will not be present. *B,* Gradient moment nulling (GMN) compensates for velocity-related phase shifts. Additional lobes are added to the gradient pulse sequence to ensure that the net phase change of moving spins is zero. (General Electric Medical Systems, Milwaukee, Wis. product literature.)

orientation previously considered), additional effects may be present in the image. As illustrated in Figure 2–11, motion of the blood at an oblique angle provides a velocity component vcos(−) parallel to the slice plane. Those spins that experience both the 90° and 180° pulses move in the "downstream" direction and produce a displaced projection that appears as a flow signal in the image visualized outside the physical position of the vessel lumen (Fig. 2–12). Conversely, the flow signal will be reduced on the upstream side of the vessel.[13] Recognition of the geometric orgins of this artifact enables identification of the flow direction relative to the image plane in the case of oblique-angle transit.

### *Pseudogating*

Electronic cardiac gating to the ECG involves synchronization of the data acquisition sequence with the cardiac cycle. Under these circumstances, the blood flow signal is enhanced during the slower diastolic portion of the cycle and decreased during the faster, more turbulent conditions encountered in systole. A clinical example illustrating these effects is shown in Figure 2–13. Under conditions in which no gating is actually being employed, a phenomenon known as "pseudogating," which involves chance synchronization between the MR data acquisition for each slice and the cardiac cycle, may occur. This takes place if the repetition time TR is the same as or an integral multiple of the heartbeat interval.

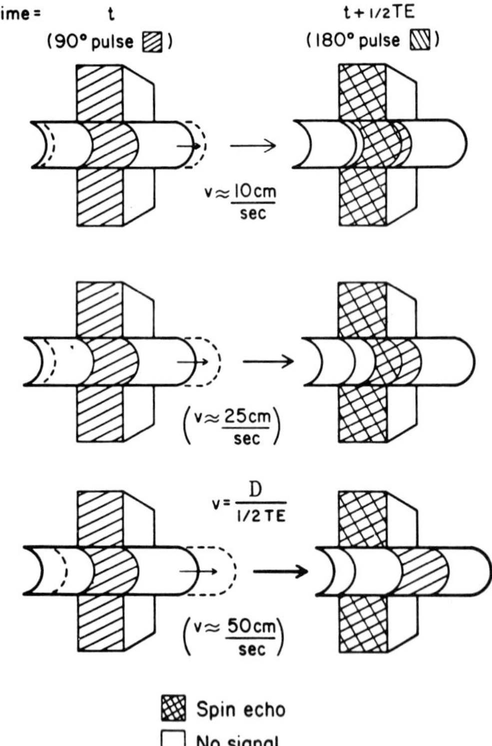


**Figure 2–9.** High-velocity signal loss (time-of-flight). Spins that leave the imaging section during the interval TE/2 do not contribute to the spin-echo signal. At sufficiently high velocities satisfying the condition v ≥ 2D/TE, all excited spins (those having received the 90° pulse) will have been washed out of the section before experiencing the 180° pulse resulting in complete loss of signal. (From Bradley WG, Walach V. Radiology 154:443–450, 1985, with permission.)

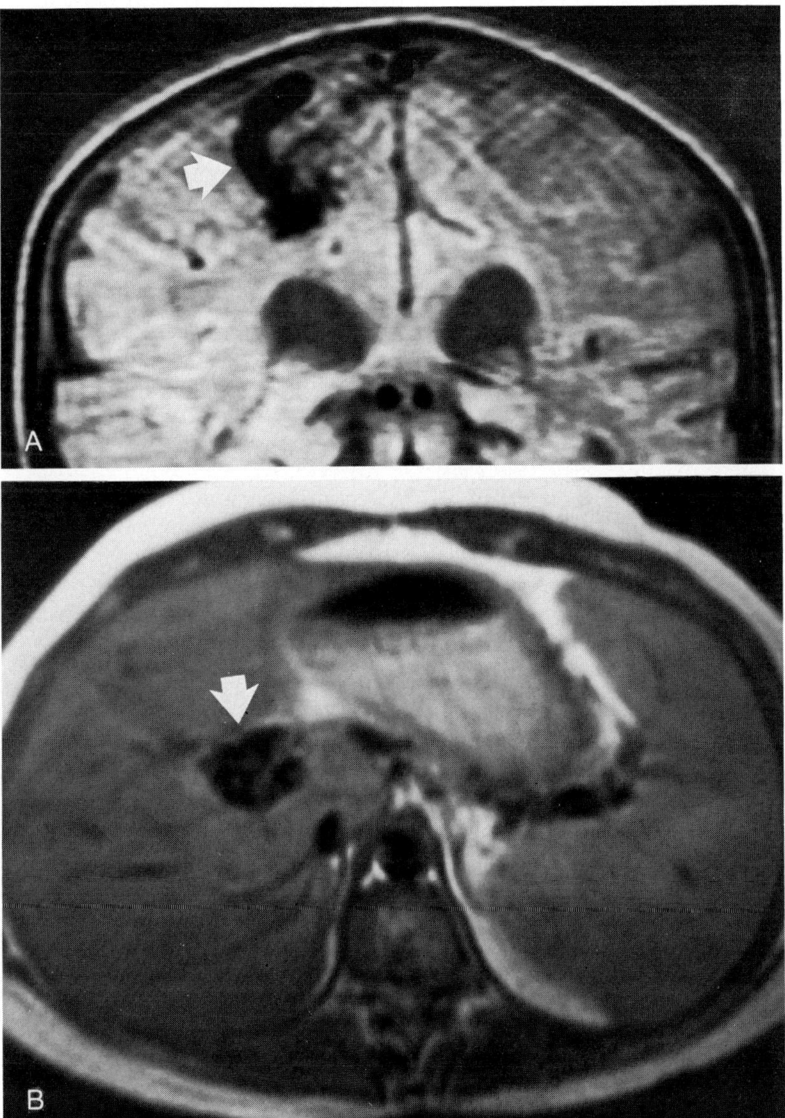


**Figure 2–10.** Time-of-flight flow void. *A,* Blood flow in the abnormal draining vein of an AVM (arrow) is of sufficiently high velocity that protons within the slice thickness do not receive both the 90° and 180° RF pulse necessary for spin-echo signal generation. Imaging parameters: 1.5 T, TR 1800/TE 20, 5 mm, coronal. *B,* Flow void present in cavernous portal vein transformation (arrow). Imaging parameters: 1.5 T, TR 1800/TE 20 10mm, axial.

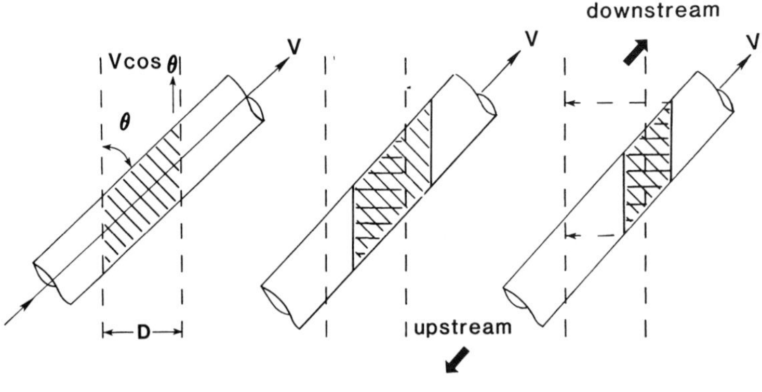


**Figure 2–11.** Effects of flow at an oblique angle to the imaging plane. *A,* Initial 90° pulse excitation. *B,* By the time of the 180° pulse, some of the excited spins have left the imaging plane, and only the cross-hatched portion receiving both pulses will contribute to the signal. *C,* By the time of echo formation, the group of prepared spins has moved partially out of the section. However, their apparent location within the image is given by the indicated projection back onto the plane, and displacement (i.e., misregistration) from the true position occurs in the downstream direction. (Modified from Axel L. AJR 143:1157, 1984, with permission.)

The image sequence exhibits enhanced signal within the lumen for slices acquired during diastole and signal loss for those associated with systole. This changing presentation as a function of slice position within a multislice image sequence has the potential for confusion when one is interpreting the cause of intraluminal signal intensity, and it may require that gating techniques be utilized to exclude pseudogating as the origin.[15]

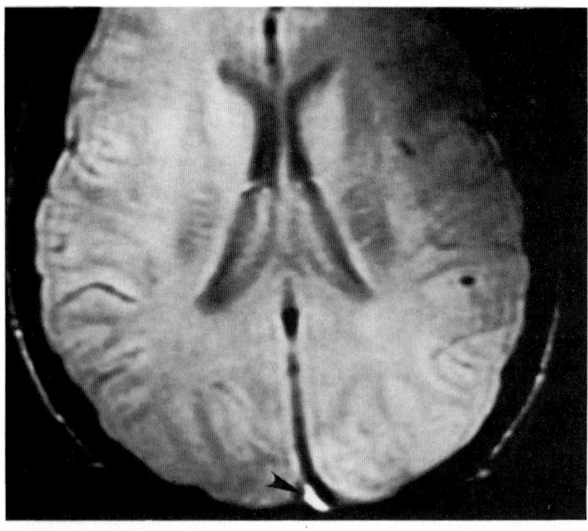

**Figure 2–12.** Time-of-flight oblique angle effect. Flow moving posteriorly within the superior sagittal sinus traverses obliquely to the image plane at the junction of the straight sinus. The signal is enhanced (arrowhead) owing to the in-flow of unsaturated blood, and at the same time, it is shifted in position as a result of the oblique angle phenomenon. Imaging parameters: 1.5 T, TR 1800/TE 20 5 mm, 2 mm gap, axial.

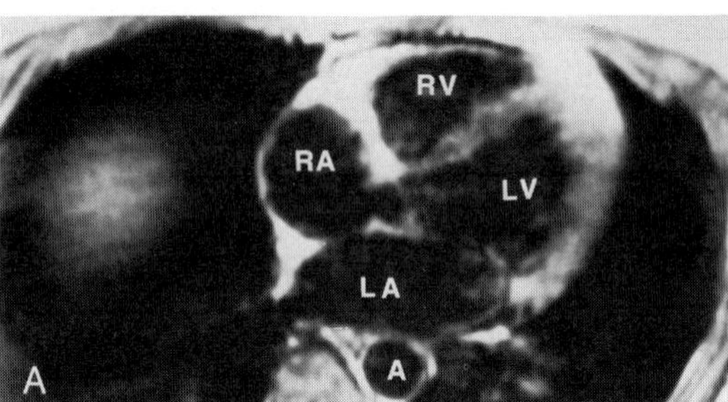


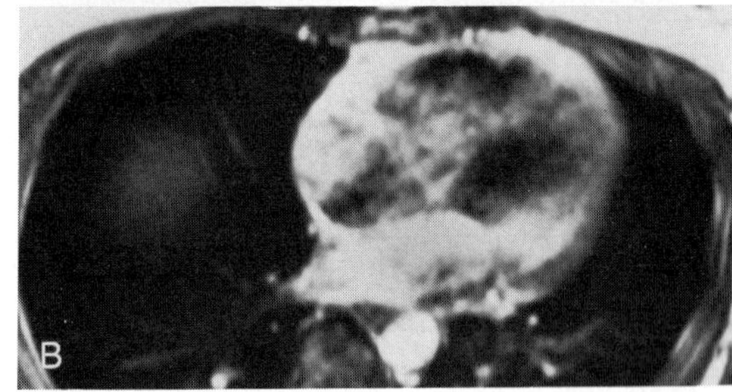


**Figure 2–13.** Systolic and diastolic ECG cardiac-gated images. *A,* Systolic image gated such that data acquisition occurs immediately following the R wave. Flow voids are evident in the aorta (A) and cardiac chambers (RA, LA [right and left atria]; RV, LV [right and left ventricles]) owing to high-velocity washout and turbulence. *B,* With a trigger delay of 650 msec after the R wave, acquisition occurs during diastole, and the slowly flowing blood exhibits time-of-flight. Imaging parameters: TR 1000/TE 20, 10 mm, axial.

### *Fast-Scan Effects*

Fast-scan techniques such as FLASH[25] and GRASS[26] make use of limited flip angles and gradient-recalled echoes. For these techniques, time-of-flight, flow-related enhancement may occur for both veins and arteries traversing the image plane and is not limited to slow venous flow evident only on the entry slice. Two aspects are responsible for these effects: (1) data acquisition involves sequential protocols in which all records are taken for the given slice before moving on to the next (as distinct from conventional interleaved multislice sequences); thus blood flowing into the imaging slice from adjacent regions is fully magnetized and contributes an enhanced signal relative to the partially saturated stationary spins; (2) the echo produced by gradient reversal is not subject to the timing constraints placed upon a radio frequency refocusing pulse–generated echo in which the flowing blood must receive both the 90° and 180° pulses within the slice in order to provide any signal. Figure 2–14 illustrates flow enhancement in a clinical fast-scan GRASS image.

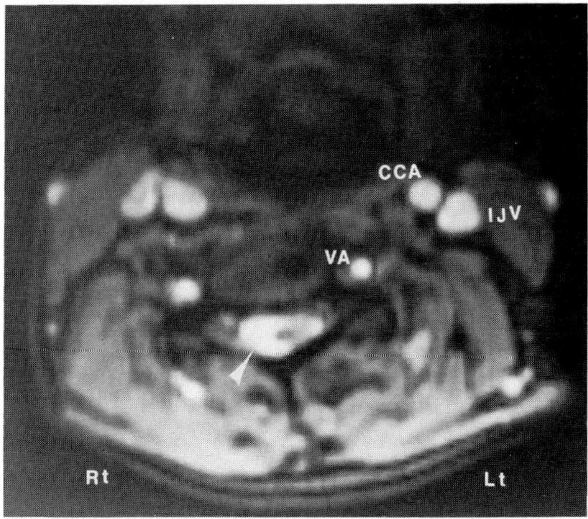


**Figure 2–14.** A transaxial GRASS scan at the level of the cervical spine in a patient with severe spinal cord atrophy due to congenital deformity. Flow-related enhancement is evident for blood within various vessels (VA, vertebral artery; CCA, common carotid artery; IJV, internal jugular vein) and for CSF in the subarachnoid space of the spinal canal (arrowhead). Image parameters: 1.5 T, TR 21/TE 12, flip angle 17°, 5 mm, axial.

## VELOCITY-RELATED PHASE SHIFT EFFECTS

The phase of a spatially localized group of spins (isochromats) is represented by the angle $\phi$ measured in the transverse plane relative to a chosen reference axis (Fig. 2–15). The rate of change of phase ($d\phi/dt$) as given by the Larmor equation is dependent upon the absolute magnetic field present at that location, which includes considerations of (1) the nominal applied static magnetic field $B_o$, (2) deviations from this owing to field inhomogeneities and molecular envi-

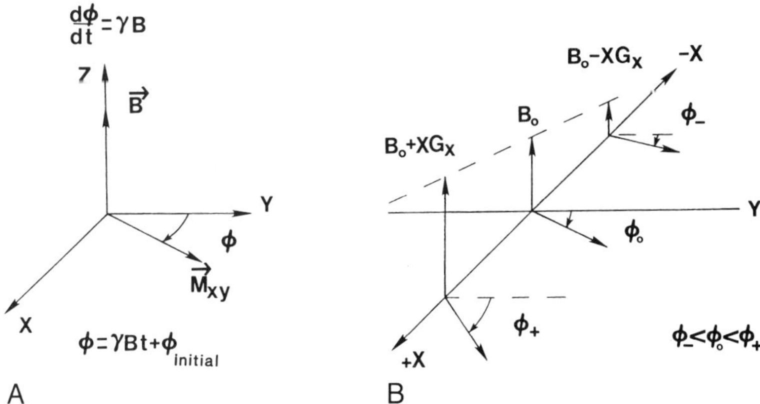


**Figure 2–15.** The concept of phase for spatially localized spins. *A,* Phase is represented by the angle between the transverse magnetization vector $\vec{M}_{xy}$ and the chosen reference axis (commonly the y axis). The rate of change of phase is given by the Larmor equation $d\phi/dt = \gamma B$. Integration provides the phase angle as a function of time, $\phi = \gamma Bt + \phi_{initial}$, in which B represents the absolute magnitude of the magnetic field present. *B,* With a gradient magnetic field $\vec{G}_x$ in the x direction superimposed upon the static field $B_o$, the magnitude of $\vec{B}$ will change as a function of x position. Thus at any point in time, the relative phase angle will depend upon position, as indicated by the examples $\phi_+$, $\phi_o$ and $\phi_-$. Spins (isochromats) moving along the gradient field would experience a net phase shift in a given time interval that would be directly related to their velocity.

ronment shielding (leading to the chemical shift effect), and (3) the gradient magnetic field strength at that position. Assuming a perfectly uniform main field, no chemical shift phenomena, and a linear gradient $\vec{G}(t)$, which may be a function of time, the rate of change of phase for isochromats undergoing generalized motion is

$$\omega = d\phi/dt = \gamma B = \gamma B_o + \gamma\vec{G}(t) \cdot \vec{r}(t) \quad (3)$$

The second term represents the phase-change contribution owing to the presence of the gradient [$\vec{r}(t)$ is the position vector of the isochromats at the time t]. For reasons of convenience in developing the concepts, motion will be taken parallel to the gradient direction and confined to the x axis (i.e., $\vec{r}(t) = x(t)\vec{i}$ and $\vec{G}(t) = Gx(t)\vec{i}$). The general expression for the gradient-induced phase shift is[27]

$$\Delta\phi = \gamma \int_0^t G_x(t)x(t)dt$$

$$= \gamma x(0) \int_0^t G_x(t)dt + \gamma \sum_1^\infty \frac{1}{n!} \int_0^t \frac{d^n x(0)}{dt^n} G_x(t)dt \quad (4)$$

The summation term provides for all categories of motion; for example, the first-order term (n = 1) represents velocity, the second-order term (n = 2) represents acceleration, the third-order term (n = 3) represents "jerk" or the rate of change of acceleration, and so forth. Thus it is seen that the net change in phase, or "phase accumulation," for the isochromats depends on a number of factors, including the gradient magnitude, gradient duration, and relative position within the gradient field as a function of time. These higher-order terms ($n \geq 2$) are mentioned here to provide sufficiently comprehensive background material necessary for understanding the practical phenomenon of phase shift–related signal loss owing to turbulent motion which is discussed below.

### *Uniform Velocity*

Under conditions of uniform velocity v, terms for $n \geq 2$ in Equation 4 will be zero. For a gradient of constant magnitude during the period under consideration, integration of Equation 4 gives

$$\Delta\phi = \gamma G_x x(0)t + \gamma G_x vt^2/2 \quad (5)$$

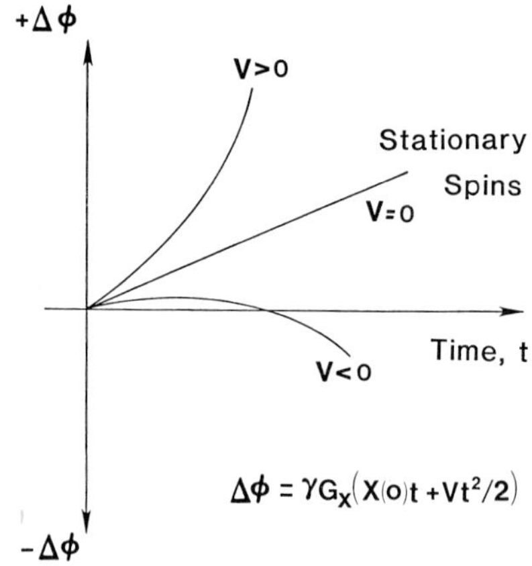


**Figure 2–16.** Phase change as a function of time for spins moving with uniform velocity in a gradient field of constant magnitude. Isochromats moving in the direction of increasing field gain phase relative to stationary spins, whereas those traveling against the gradient lose phase.

in which the expression is characterized by both a linear and a quadratic term in time. This means that isochromats moving along the direction of the gradient gain phase relative to stationary nuclei, whereas, conversely, those moving against the gradient will lose phase (Fig. 2–16). In order to understand the effect that flow-related phase changes will have on the intensity within an image created from either a spin echo or a gradient-recalled echo, it is necessary to describe the phase change existing at the time the echo is acquired. If coherence is reestablished and refocusing is complete ($\Delta\phi = 0$) for all isochromats within an imaging voxel independent of their velocity, the resultant signal will be larger than for the situation in which multiple phase values exist (i.e., the net transverse magnetization vector is reduced for multiple phase values).

## Spin-Echo Considerations—Even-Echo Rephasing

Figure 2–17 provides the schematic for a two spin–echo sequence under the application of a constant gradient. The resultant phase shift for isochromats having different velocities and different initial positions is illustrated. The 180° radio-frequency pulse reverses the sign of the phase angle but does not affect the rate of change of phase ($d\phi$/dt). As can be seen in Figure 2–17 and can be verified through integration of Equation 4 over properly designated time intervals

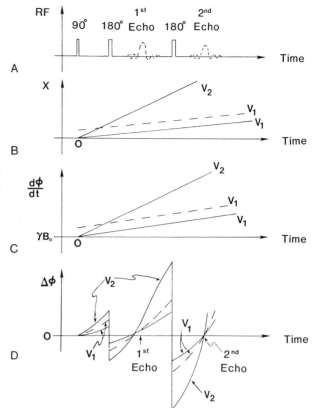

**Figure 2–17.** Even-echo rephasing under a constant, applied gradient field. *A,* The RF pulse sequence with the formation of first and second spin echo indicated. *B,* The position of spins as a function of time for two constant velocities $V_1$, and $V_2$. For $V_1$, two different initial positions are shown (solid and dashed lines). *C,* The corresponding rate of change of phase $d\phi/dt$ for uniform velocity in the direction of a constant magnetic field gradient. *D,* Net gradient-induced phase-shift accumulation $\Delta\phi$ for the moving spins. The 180° pulse reverses the sign of the phase. At the time of the first echo, the phase is independent of the initial position but proportional to velocity. For the second echo, phase is zero-independent of both position and velocity. (Modified from Axel L. AJR 143:1157, 1984, with permission.)

(TE/2) by paying attention to the phase reversal introduced by the 180° pulse, for the first echo the initial position dependence cancels for isochromats moving with the same velocity. However, the phase is generally nonzero and is dependent on velocity. This noncoherence will reduce the signal strength in that voxel relative to the second echo, where rephasing is complete and the phase shift is zero (independent of both velocity and initial position). This phenomenon, known as even-echo rephasing,[28] is the cause of second-echo relative enhancement and can be seen clinically in vessels or CSF spaces exhibiting slow laminar flow (Fig. 2–18). As the velocity increases to the point at which time-of-flight effects producing high-velocity signal loss take command, even-echo rephasing enhancement becomes less pronounced and eventually disappears altogether. Decreased signal strength for the first echo, as discussed above, has its origin in the fact that isochromats characterized by different velocities within the same voxel lose phase coherence, which is regained in the second echo. Thus, theroretically for modulus imaging, this phenomenon would

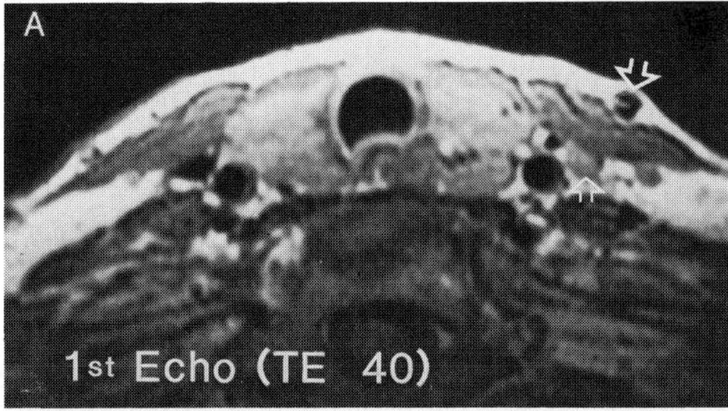


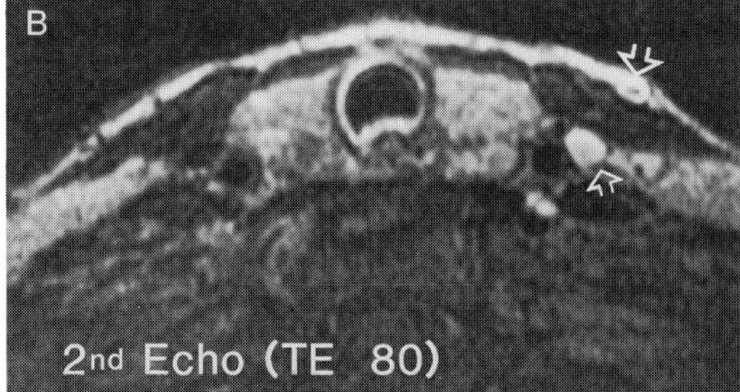


**Figure 2–18.** Even-echo rephasing. Multiecho neck images taken with a surface coil at the level of the thyroid. *A,* Reduced signal due to first echo dephasing is present in both the superficial and deep jugular veins (arrows). *B,* A signal increase is evident in both veins on the second (even) echo (TE 80). Image parameters: 1.5 T, TR 1800/TE 40/80 5 mm, axial.

not appear for situations involving plug flow, in which the velocity is constant over the lumen cross section. However, laminar flow, exhibiting a parabolic velocity distribution envelope across the lumen, provides a mechanism for varying velocities to be present within a given voxel.[16, 17] Figure 2–19 illustrates these concepts and demonstrates schematically why the even-echo image enhancement would be relatively stronger for the peripheral regions, where the distribution of velocities within a voxel is greatest.

In typical 2DFT imaging, three pulsed gradient sequences are employed: slice selection, phase encoding, and frequency encoding (read-out). The gradient pulses for slice selection and read-out are generally balanced. This means that they are applied symmetrically around the RF pulse, with polarity, magnitude, and duration adjusted appropriately for cancellation of phase shifts that otherwise would be introduced for stationary nuclei. This bipolarity will not cancel phase shifts resulting from motion. As discussed by Wedeen and colleagues, the net velocity-dependent phase shift for any voxel will be the sum of the shifts produced by each individual gradient.[29] Typically, the read-out gradient takes five to ten times longer than the slice-selection gradient, and its effect would be 25 to 100 times greater (for equal gradient magnitude) as a consequence of the time-squared dependence. (Positional shift artifacts resulting from motion in the direction of the slice-selection gradient are mentioned later.) The effect of the phase-encoding gradient on uniform velocity-induced phase shifts within the reconstructed image is not pronounced relative to stationary spins as a result of time-averaged location considerations in relationship to the phase-encoding pulses, which are not discussed here.

A schematic illustration depicting read-out gradient pulses symmetrically placed around refocusing 180° radio frequency pulses is shown in Figure 2–20. Similar to the situation for a constant gradient (see Fig. 2–17), the phase shift for the first echo is proportional to velocity, whereas complete refocusing independent of velocity occurs for the second echo, providing even-echo enhancement. A summary of the phase accumulation for various motional states as a function of velocity, time-to-echo (TE), gradient pulse duration, and magnitude is presented in Table 2–1.

A number of schemes have been devised to compensate for flow-induced phase shifts. These can be designed for the purpose of restoring the first-echo signal intensity lost

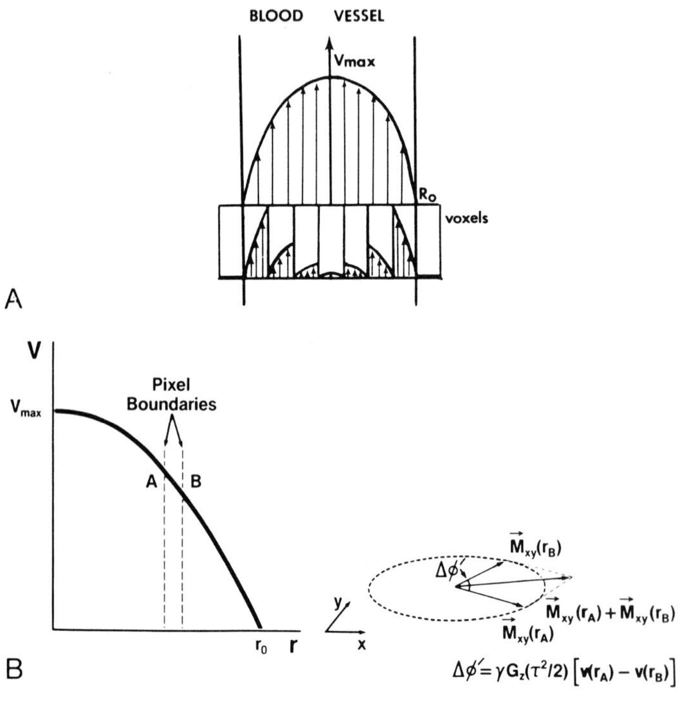


**Figure 2–19.** Relative phase shift within a voxel as a result of laminar flow parabolic velocity distribution. *A,* A schematic illustration of velocity variation within individual voxels. The greatest differences occur close to the vessel wall, producing the largest relative intravoxel phase shift. *B,* The relative phase shift $\Delta\phi'$ experienced by isochromats at the inner and outer pixel (voxel) boundaries is proportional to the difference in velocity at those positions. The resultant local transverse magnetization is reduced as a result of this phase-shift influence on the vector sum. (*A,* from von Schulthess GK, Higgins CB. Radiology 157:687, 1985, with permission; *B,* from Wehrli FW, Shimakawa A, MacFall JR, et al. J Comput Assist Tomogr 9:537, 1985, with permission.)

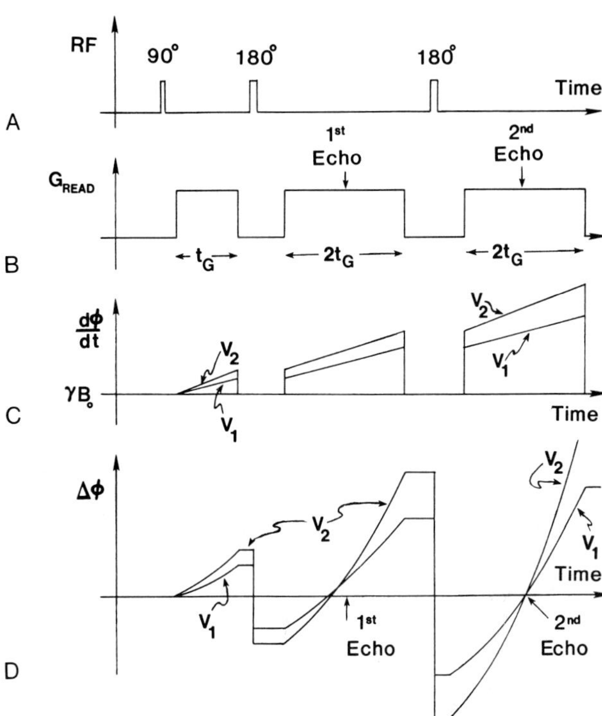


**Figure 2–20.** Even-echo rephasing with balanced readout gradient pulses placed symmetrically around the 180° RF pulses. *A*, Radio frequency pulse sequence. *B*, Balanced read-out gradient pulses with the position of the first and second spin echoes indicated. $t_G$ is the time interval during which the gradient following the 90° pulse is switched on. The gradient duration surrounding the echo is $2t_G$. *C*, The rate of change of phase, $d\phi/dt$ for two different velocities. *D*, Net gradient-induced phase-shift accumulation $\Delta\phi$ for the moving spins. Rephasing is complete with $\Delta\phi = 0$ at the time of the second echo.

due to velocity-dependent incomplete refocusing or for eliminating positional shift artifacts. One method, known as gradient moment nulling,[26, 30, 31] entails applying additional gradients fashioned in such a way that moving isochromats have the same phase as stationary ones at the time of the echo. This technique is illustrated in Figure 2–8*B* for the case of motion parallel to the slice-selection gradient. Flow along the slice-selection gradient direction perpendicular to the imaging plane is a common occurrence for axial scans. Phase shift accumulation for the moving isochromats causes them to be displaced in the phase-encoding direction, producing misregistration ghost artifacts in the image. Flow-compensation gradient techniques may be applied to eliminate phase shift–related artifacts. These concepts are illustrated in Figure 2–21.

## Gradient-Recalled Echoes

The recent fast-scan techniques mentioned previously use limited flip angles and gradient reversal instead of a 180° refocusing radio frequency pulse to generate the echo.[25, 26] Changing the polarity of the gradient switches the sign of the phase accumulation (i.e., from positive to negative) as a consequence of the direction of motion

**Table 2–1.** PHASE ANGLES FOR STATIONARY, CONSTANT VELOCITY, AND ACCELERATED ISOCHROMATS

| Time for 180° Pulse and Echoes | Stationary, $x_o$ $\phi/(\gamma G_x x_o)$ | Constant Velocity, $v_o$ $\phi/(\gamma G_x v_o/2)$ | Constant Acceleration, $a_o$ $\phi/(\gamma G_x a_o/6)$ |
|---|---|---|---|
| TE/2 (180°) | $t_G$ | $t_G^2$ | $t_G^3$ |
| TE (1st echo) | 0 | $2\,TEt_G - 2\,t_G^2$ | $3\,TE^2t_G - 3\,TEt_G^2/2$ |
| 3 TE/2 (180°) | $t_G$ | $4\,TEt_G - t_G^2$ | $6\,TE^2t_G + t_G^3$ |
| 2 TE (2nd echo) | 0 | 0 | $6\,TE^2t_G - 3\,TEt_G^2$ |
| 5 TE/2 (180°) | $t_G$ | $4\,TEt_G + t_G^2$ | $18\,TE^2t_G + t_3^3$ |
| 3 TE (3rd echo) | 0 | $2\,TEt_G - 2\,t_G^2$ | $9\,TE^2t_G - 9\,TEt_G^2/2$ |
| 7 TE/2 (180°) | $t_G$ | $8\,TEt_G - t_G^2$ | $36\,TE^2t_G + t_G^3$ |
| 4 TE (4th echo) | 0 | 0 | $12\,TE^2t_G - 6\,TEt_G^2$ |

*Source:* von Schulthess GK, Higgins CB. Radiology 157:687–695, 1985.
$t_G$ is defined in Figure 2–20 as the time interval during which the gradient following the 90° RF pulse is switched on.

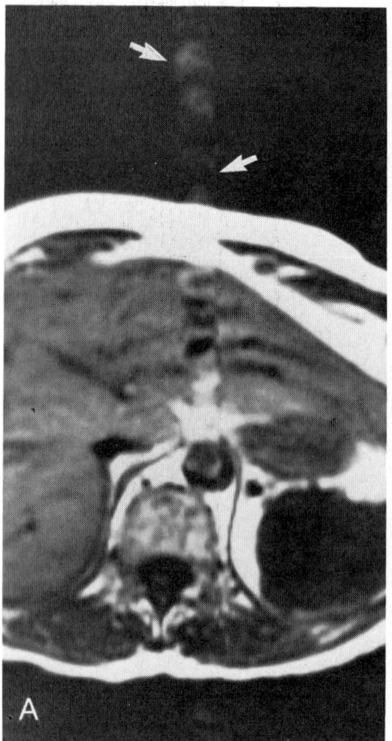


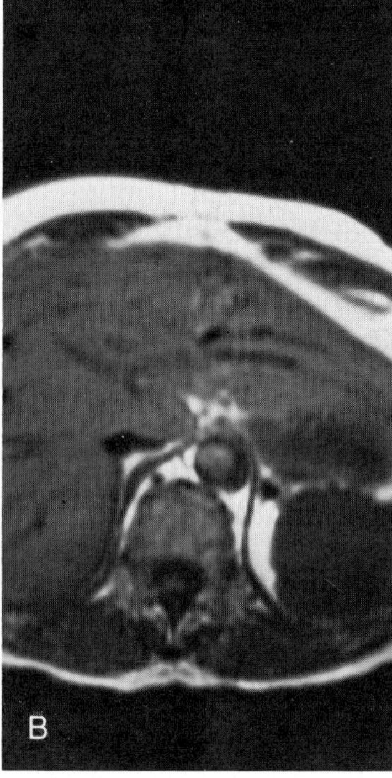


**Figure 2–21.** Flow compensation. *A,* Motion of blood within the aorta along the direction of the slice-selection gradient, perpendicular to the imaging plane, produces a net accumulated phase shift that causes ghost artifacts to be displaced in the phase-encoding direction (arrows). *B,* Application of flow-compensation gradients effectively eliminates the phase shift–related artifact.

relative to the gradient field. Figure 2–22 shows the example of a bipolar gradient pulse that will refocus stationary spins while producing a net (nonzero) velocity-dependent phase shift for moving isochromats. To eliminate this effect and desensitize gradient echo fast-scan images to phase-related flow intensities, it is common to introduce extra gradients similar in principle to gradient moment–nulling schemes. Note that both the bipolar gradient pair and two gradient pulses of equal magnitude, placed on either side of the first 180° refocusing radio frequency pulse, produce a velocity-dependent gradient-induced phase shift effect. (Compare Figs. 2–20 and 2–22.)

## Oblique, In-Plane Flow Misregistration

The significant mispositioning of vascular features within an image as a result of phase shift accumulation associated with the slice-selection gradient for flow orthogonal to the imaging plane has previously been discussed. As shown in Figure 2–21, vessel structures are displaced in the phase-encoding direction. Blood flowing within the imaging plane at an oblique angle relative to the phase-encoding and read-out directions experiences a phase shift that will also introduce spatial relocation of a somewhat more subtle nature.[16] Figure 2–23 provides a schematic that demonstrates this effect. The delay between phase encoding and read-out produces a misregistration such that flowing blood would appear outside the anatomic borders of the vessel. The degree of misregistration is dependent upon both velocity and angle. A clinical image illustrating the phenomenon is shown in Figure 2–24. The effect will be more pronounced on the second echo because of the longer delay between phase encoding and read-out. As indicated in Figure 2–23, a rough estimate of flow velocity may be calculated by using the measured displacement and angle.

## Nonuniform Velocity

The discussion up to this point has been directed toward flow exhibiting uniform velocity. However, cardiosynchronized pulsatile flow ("disturbed" flow), found in arteries, and turbulent flow, initiated by vascular junctions or obstructions, present different

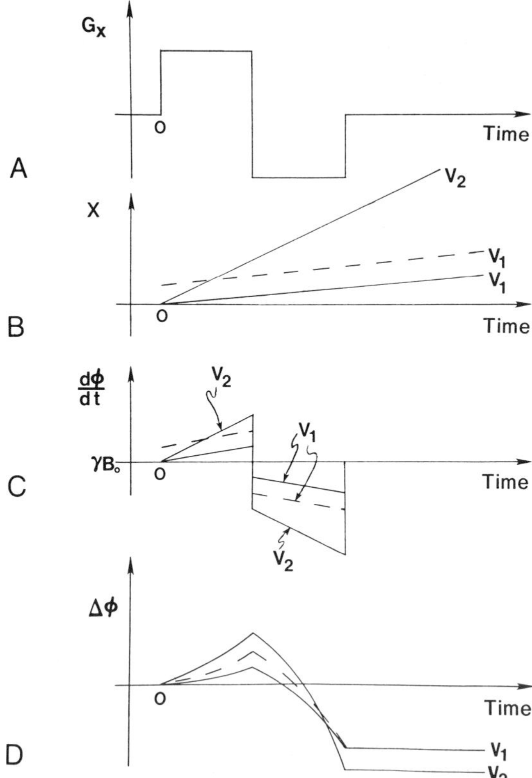


**Figure 2–22.** The effect of bipolar gradient pulses on the phase of moving spins. *A,* Bipolar gradient pulse sequence. *B,* The position of spins as a function of time for two constant velocities, $V_1$ and $V_2$. For $V_1$, two different initial positions are shown (solid and dashed lines). *C,* The corresponding rate of change of phase $d\phi/dt$ for uniform velocity in the direction of the magnetic field gradient. *D,* Net gradient-induced phase shift accumulation $\Delta\phi$ for the moving spins. Although gradient adjustments can be implemented so that phase is independent of initial position (producing a gradient-reversal echo), the phase is nonzero and is dependent upon velocity. (Modified from Axel L. AJR 143:1157–1166; 1984, with permission.)

models for analysis.[32] Motion associated with the higher-order terms in Equation 4, including acceleration (n = 2) and jerk (n = 3), produces a phase shift that is not refocused on even echoes. Table 2–1 compares the calculated phase angle at intervals of TE/2 for various motion states, including constant acceleration. The inability to restore coherence for any echo means that generalized signal loss will occur at all times under conditions of accelerated flow. Likewise, chaotic flow and turbulence appear as characteristic signal voids in the image. Additionally, artifacts manifested as intensity ghosting patterns (bright and dark bands parallel to the artery) have been associated with in-plane pulsatile motion.[33] This effect

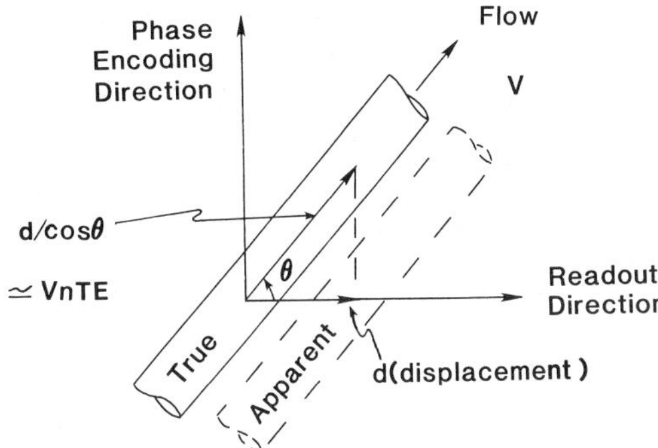


**Figure 2–23.** Spatial misregistration caused by in-plane flow oblique to the phase-encoding and read-out gradient directions. d represents the displacement of the vessel from its true position. Measurement of the angle $\theta$ and the displacement will allow a rough estimate of velocity (n is the echo number) as indicated under the condition that phase encoding occurs close to the 90° excitation pulse. (Modified from von Schulthess GK, Higgins CB. Radiology 157:687, 1985, with permission.)

has been attributed primarily to "accidental" velocity-sensitive phase encoding along the read-out gradient, which is present on the first echo but absent on even echos.

## Flow Imaging by Phase Display

The phase shift introduced by isochromats moving along a magnetic field gradient may

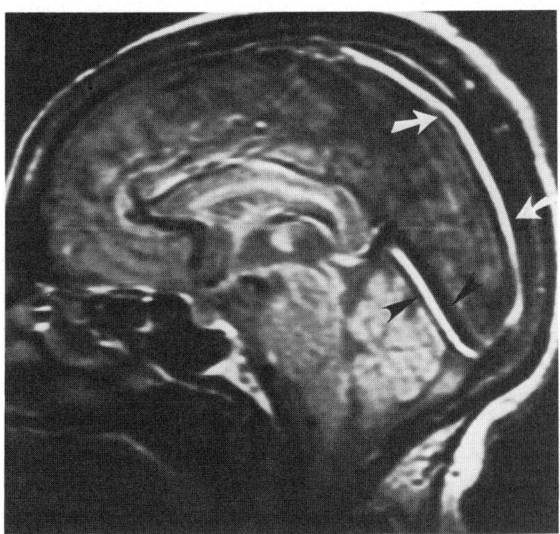

**Figure 2–24.** Oblique in-plane flow misregistration. Isochromats moving within the imaging plane oblique to the phase-encoding and read-out gradient directions exhibit a positional misregistration owing to phase-shift effects. This phenomenon is evident in both the superior sagittal sinus (arrows) and the straight sinus (arrowheads). The enhancement noted in these vessels is the result of even-echo rephasing. Image parameters: 1.5 T, TR 1700/TE 25/50 (second echo) 10 mm, sagittal.

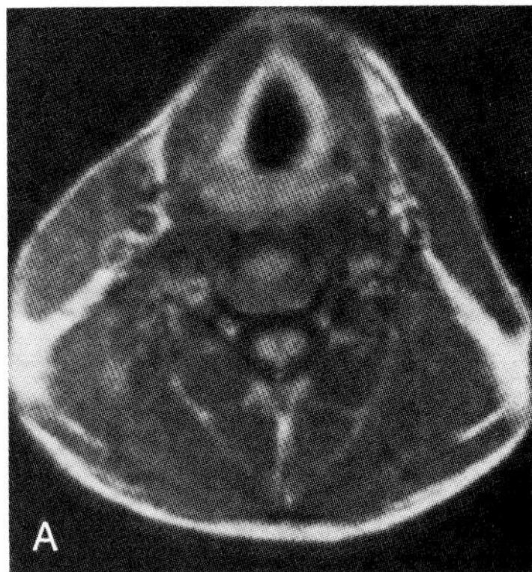


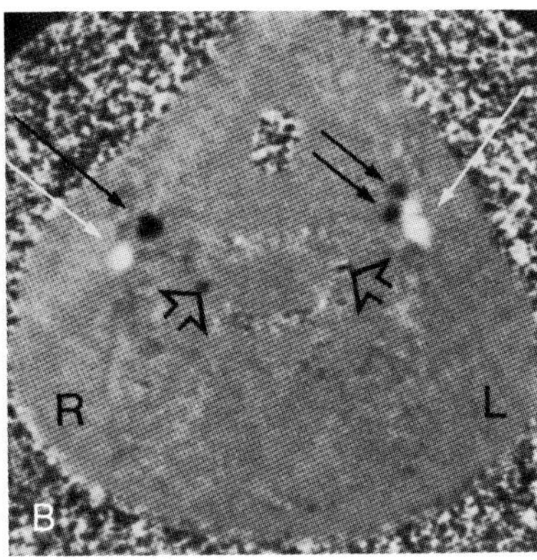


**Figure 2–25.** Normal anatomy for an $SE_{540/40}$ sequence *(A)* and phase map *(B)* at the same level of the neck 50 msec following the R wave. Blood flow is seen in right common carotid (long black arrow) and the left internal and external carotid arteries (short black arrows) as well as in the vertebral arteries (open black arrows). Venous flow is seen in the internal jugular veins (long white arrows). (From Bryant DJ, Payne JA, Firmin DN, et al. J Comput Assist Tomogr 8:588–593, 1984, with permission.)

be used directly as an indicator of flow. Gradient pulse sequences have been devised to facilitate phase accumulation or to accentuate phase differences produced by flow.[29, 34, 35] The quadrature nature of pulsed Fourier transform spectrometers establishes phase as an observable quantity that may be obtained from the real and the imaginary part of the image data. Calculation of phase for every pixel within the image and subsequent display provides a phase map (Fig. 2–25). Quantitation of phase shift would allow determination of the absolute velocity (subject to the assumptions involving uniform velocity).

### Magnetic Resonance Angiography

Projection techniques are capable of providing high-contrast angiographic presentation of vessels based on phase differences for flowing blood.[36] Wedeen and associates, one of the first groups to demonstrate this possibility, used cardiac-gated systole and diastole images with a conventional 2DFT spin–echo sequence set up to generate velocity-dependent phase shifts.[37] The gradient sequence involved setting $G_z$ to zero (no slice selection), phase encoding with $G_y$ in the normal fashion, and applying $G_x$ pulses as appropriate to achieve flow-related phase accumulation while at the same time providing the read-out gradient. The image obtained during the slow flow associated with diastole ($<$ 10 cm/sec) produces a relatively strong signal from blood on the first echo. However, during the fast flow of systole ($<$ 50 to 150 cm/sec) a greater degree of coherence loss is present owing to the increased velocity-dependent phase shifts. Subtraction of these two images removes the static proton signal (analogous to the process

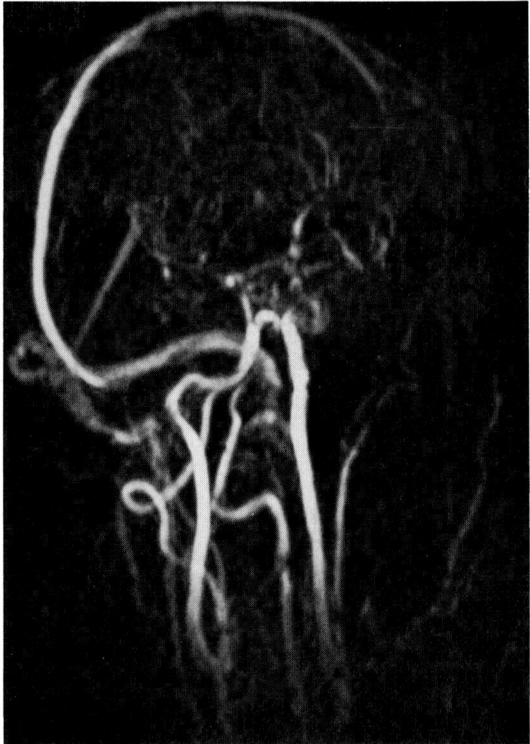

**Figure 2–26.** NMR angiographic image of the major blood vessels in the head. Flow is selectively detected by incorporating flow-encoding gradient pulses in the imaging sequence that induce a phase shift in the transverse spin magnetization which is directly proportional to velocity. (Courtesy of C.L. Dumoulin, General Electric Research and Development Center, Schenectady, N.Y.)

of x-ray digital subtraction angiography) and provides an image of pulsatile flow.

Disadvantages of this approach include (1) the dependence upon cardiac cycle pulsation for contrast and (2) the relatively long acquisition time required for the two sequential images, which introduces the practical problem of misregistration artifacts in the subtracted image owing to patient motion. These considerations are being addressed by two methods: the first is development of techniques that do not rely on the intrinsic pulsatile dynamics of the gated cardiac cycle but instead employ flow-encoding gradients to introduce a velocity-dependent phase shift. With this technique, veins as well as arteries can be visualized. Figure 2–26 provides an MR angiographic image of the major vessels in the head obtained by this method;[36, 38] the second uses a combination of phase-mapped angiography with fast-scan methodology (limited flip angle, short TR) to acquire subtracted images in 10 seconds or less.[36]

## PULSATILE CEREBROSPINAL FLUID AND ELECTROCARDIOGRAPHIC-GATED MR

The existence of cerebrospinal fluid (CSF) pulsation or movement (Fig. 2–27) and flow phenomena in the normal subarachnoid space[39] and in abnormal central nervous system cavities such as syringomyelia (Figs. 2–28 and 2–29) has been documented with MR.[40-44] The same factors that result in increased or decreased signal intensity of flowing blood alter the signal of pulsatile cerebrospinal fluid. Time-of-flight effects, first echo, and turbulent dephasing produce signal loss that is most pronounced when oscillatory flow rates are greatest—as in the narrow channels of the sylvian aqueduct (Fig. 2–30) or the foramen of Magendie. These same pulsatile flow effects are more common in the cervicothoracic CSF than in the lumbar spine. Since the subarachnoid

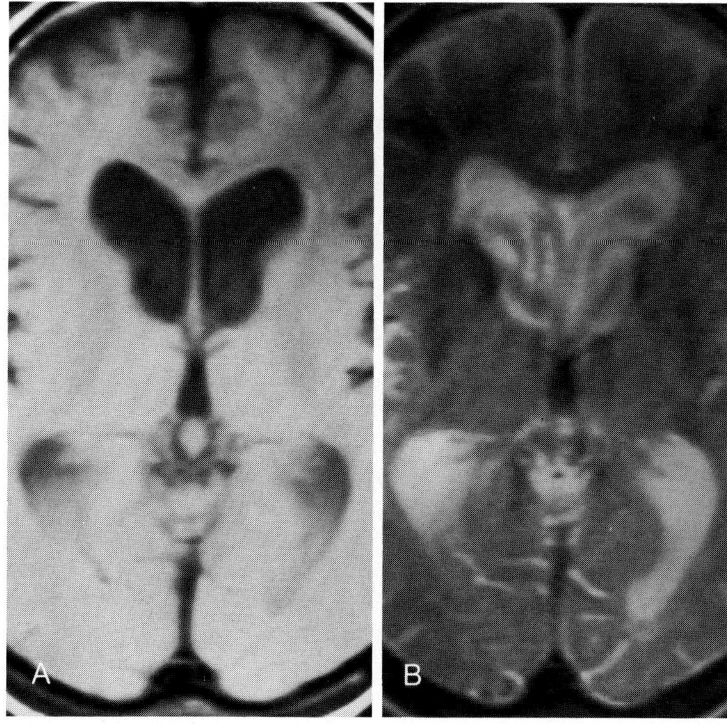


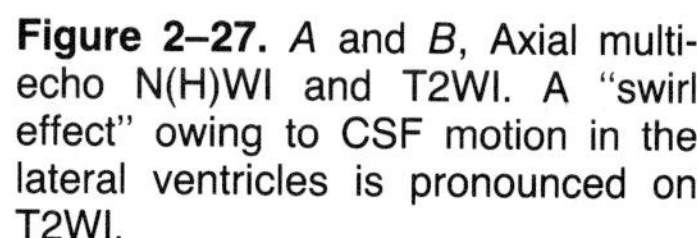

**Figure 2–27.** *A* and *B*, Axial multiecho N(H)WI and T2WI. A "swirl effect" owing to CSF motion in the lateral ventricles is pronounced on T2WI.

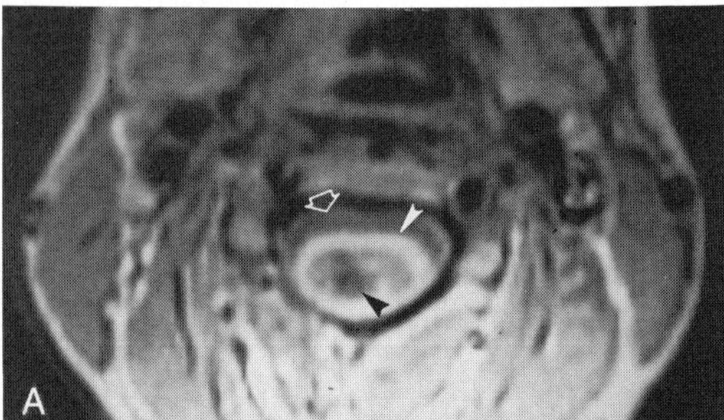

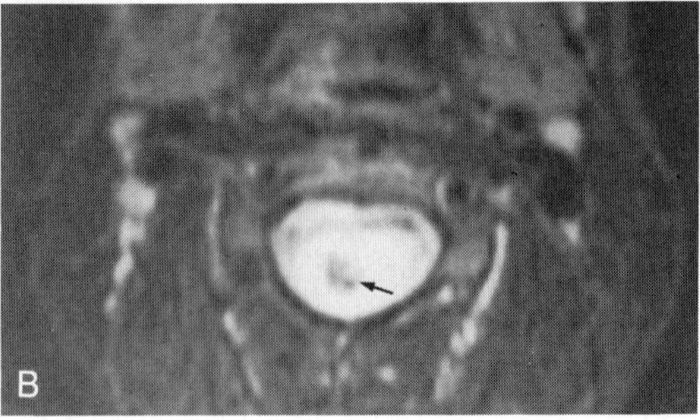

**Figure 2–28.** *A* and *B*, Axial multiecho N(H)WI and T2WI. On N(H)WI, the syrinx cavity contains central hypointensity (arrowhead) owing to pulsatile flow effect (flow void [FV]). Cord substance is hyperintense (white arrowhead), on N(H)WI and hypointense on T2WI. The thecal sac surrounds thinned cord; it is hypointense on N(H)WI (open arrow) and hyperintense on T2WI. FV in cyst persists on T2WI (arrow).

space is more capacious in the anterior cervical spine and posterior thoracic spine, harmonic modulation of proton precession by CSF pulsation predominates in these regions (Fig. 2–31). Normally, CSF in areas of minimal pulsation appears hyperintense on T2WI. Factors accentuating CSF flow-void signal loss include asymmetric pulse acquisition, heavy T2 weighting, and thin sections. Thin sections require steep gradients, a factor accentuating spin dephasing and CSF signal loss. Phase-related signal alterations along a magnetic gradient can be used to quantitate and map pulsatile CSF in-plane flow.[45] Areas of flow-related signal loss in the subarachnoid fluid of spine or brain may be so pronounced as to simulate aneurysm or vascular malformation (Fig. 2–32).

CSF signal increase may result from the slice entry phenomenon (first echo), even-echo rephasing (second echo), or chance synchronization with cardiac diastole. The resulting subarachnoid CSF signal alteration may be mistaken for a mass or an aneurysm with thrombus in the basal cisterns, spinal subarachnoid space, or ventricles (Fig. 2–32).

CSF oscillatory motion has several effects

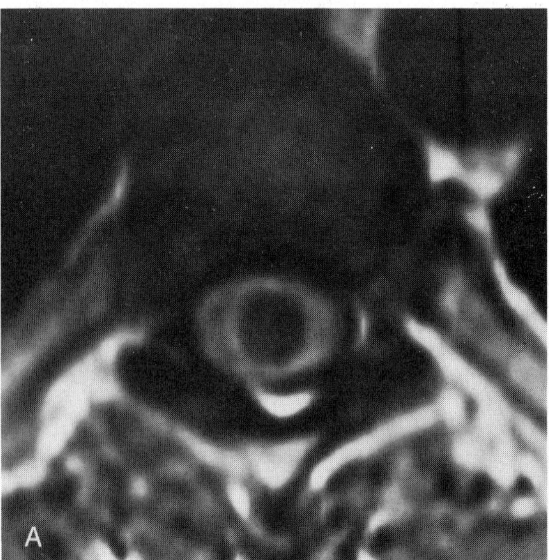

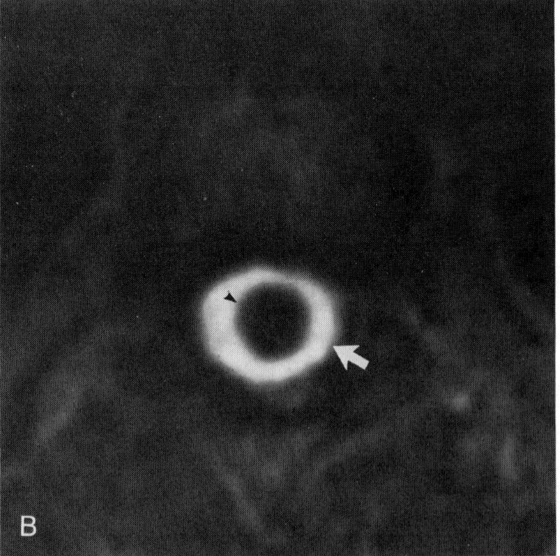

**Figure 2–29.** *A* and *B*, Axial (1.5 T) multiecho N(H)WI and T2WI. Cord syrinx exhibits flow-void (arrowhead) owing to CSF pulsation in cyst. Cord parenchyma is so attenuated that it is inseparable from the hyperintense thecal sac. Cord enlargement dampens pulsation in the surrounding thecal sac and promotes T2WI hyperintensity (arrow).

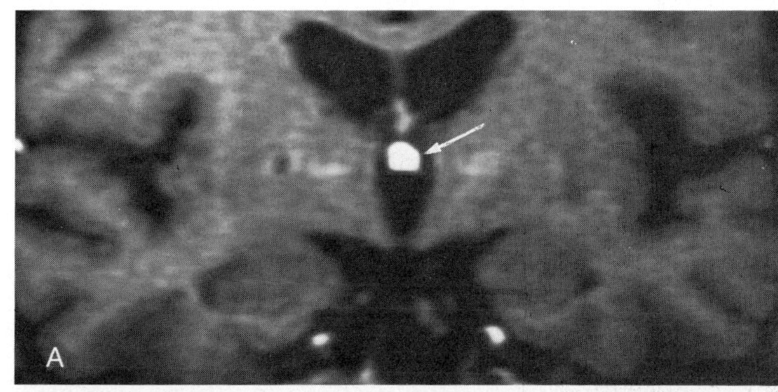


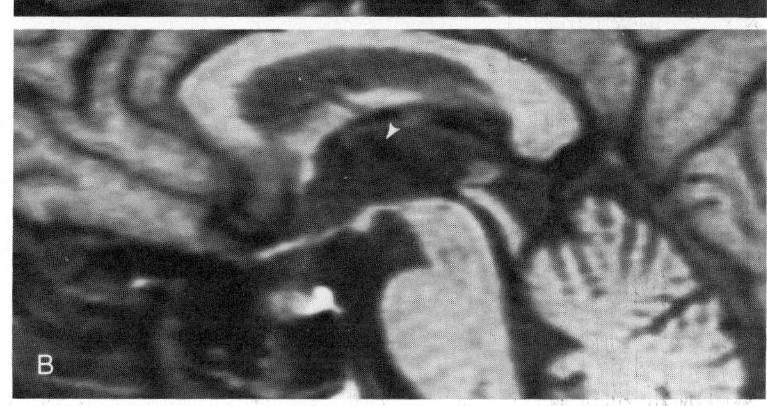


**Figure 2–30.** *A* and *B*, Coronal and sagittal T1WI (1.5 T). Signal hyperintensity in the anterosuperior third ventricle simulates lipoma (arrow). This flow-related signal increase represents a slice entry phenomenon of CSF. Flow void in the third ventricle (arrowhead) results from a CSF jet exiting the aqueduct in the sagittal projection.

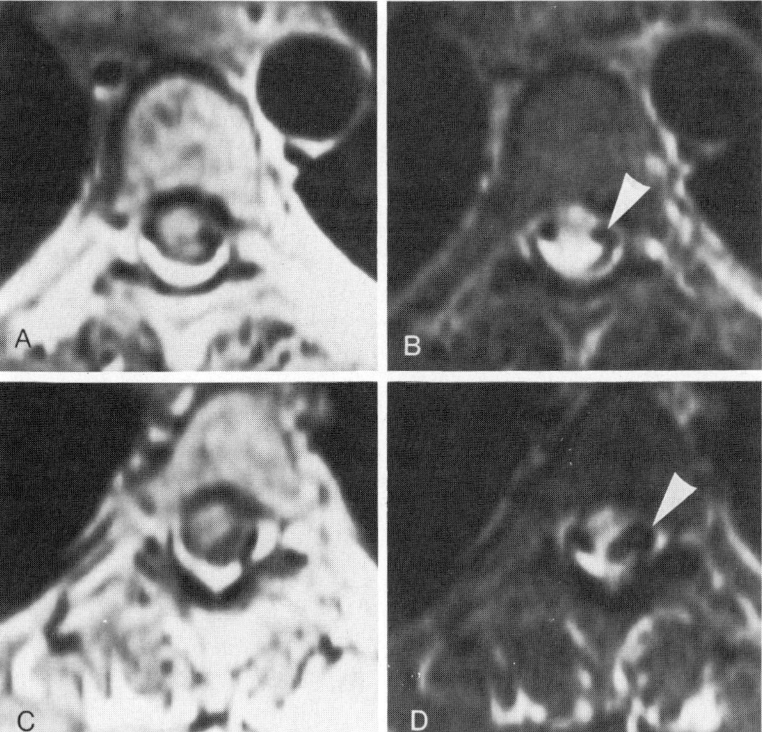


**Figure 2–31.** Axial (1.5 T) multiecho N(H)WI (*A* and *C*) and T2WI (*B* and *D*). CSF hypointensity (arrowheads) is present in the thecal sac owing to signal flow void [FV]. Normal septations and dentate ligaments predispose this region to flow effects that have been confused with vascular malformation. In *D*, hypointensity exists on T2WI but not on first echo N(H)WI in *C*. FV in vessels often exists on both echoes and in multiple-imaging planes.

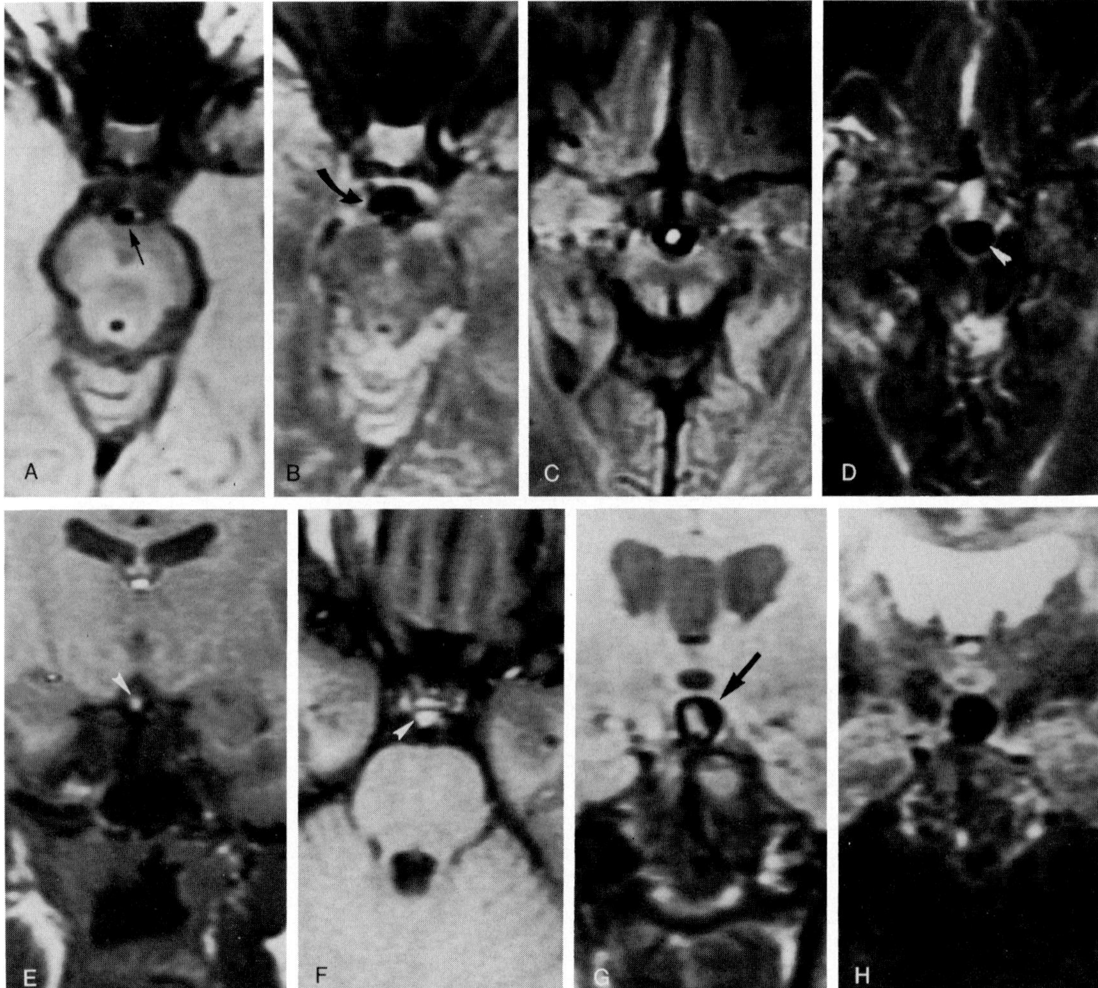


**Figure 2–32.** *A,* and *B,* Axial multiecho N(H)WI and T2WI at midbrain level. Hypointense flow void [FV] occurs in the basilar artery (arrow) on N(H)WI. The adjacent cistern is hypointense (curved arrow) owing to FV, unlike stationary fluid (hyperintense) on T2WI. Basilar artery aneurysm is simulated. *C* and *D,* Axial N(H)WI and T2WI from another patient show true basilar tip aneurysm (arrowhead) with first echo enhancement in aneurysm on N(H)WI. *E* and *F,* Coronal T1WI and axial N(H)WI. Slice entry phenomenon or enhancement of cisternal CSF (arrowheads) separate from and not contained by the hypointense normal basilar artery. *G* and *H,* Coronal N(H)WI and T2WI. True basilar tip aneurysm (arrow) exhibits first echo enhancement contained within aneurysm on N(H)WI only.

that alter the MR signal. They include (1) decreased CSF signal intensity; and (2) signal mismapping of moving CSF, the so-called "ghosting" artifact. Although these phase-sensitive ghosting artifacts can produce troublesome signal effects at the brain base (Fig. 2–33), some prove advantageous in clinical MR diagnosis. Noncommunicating cysts or cystic neoplasms may appear more hyperintense relative to CSF and therefore are more obvious owing to lack of motion-related signal loss (Fig. 2–34). In addition, foci of severe canal stenosis or block may appear more obvious in the sagittal plane resulting from dampened CSF pulsation caudad to the pathologic level. This circumstance results in more hyperintense CSF signal (less motion-related signal loss) and an exaggerated CSF myelographic effect.

Well recognized is the signal hypointensity of the sylvian aqueduct relative to intraventricular CSF.[46] The bulk CSF flow is craniocaudad, but higher rates of aqueductal CSF oscillatory or to-and-fro motion occur. The normal aqueductal flow–void signal (FVS) is absent when obstructive hydrocephalus exists (Fig. 2–35). The aqueductal FVS is more common and more prominent in patients with chronic communicating, or "normal pressure," hydrocephalus (NPH) than in patients with atrophy or acute communicating hydrocephalus or in normal volunteers. Therefore exaggerated FVS may be considered an ancillary sign of NPH,[47] one of the few treatable causes of dementia.[48] These aqueductal signal alterations in NPH are likely related to decreased ventricular compliance, which is most pronounced in chronic communicating hydrocephalus and internal obstructive hydrocephalus.[49] This decreased compliance increases CSF aqueductal outflow and exaggerates oscillatory CSF motion.

Disadvantages of oscillatory CSF motion are numerous. Because CSF pulsation alters its signal intensity, ventricular or subarachnoid fluid cannot always be used as a water standard of comparison for nonpulsatile cystic lesions. Areas of unusual and confusing signal intensity may be attributed to these phenomena. T2WI signal hyperintensity may occur in the thoracic spine as a result of stationary CSF in normal arachnoid loculations (Fig. 2–36). Similarly, loculated CSF in the internal auditory canal may simulate contour alterations of the seventh and

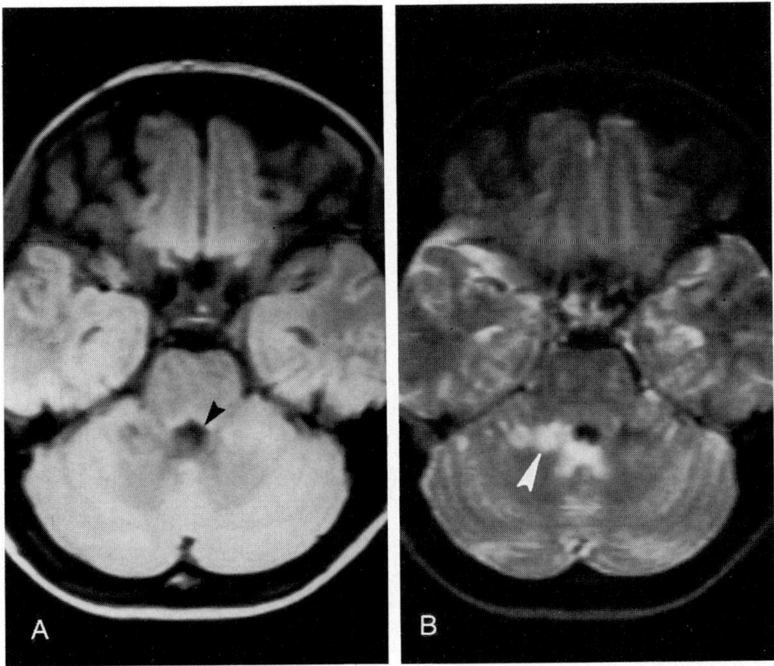


**Figure 2–33.** A 52-year-old woman with vertigo. *A* and *B*, Axial (1.5 T) multiecho N(H)WI and T2WI. Hyperintensity on T2WI (white arrowhead) projects over the brachium conjunctivum. This phase misregistration artifact is created by pulsation in the adjacent fourth ventricle (black arrowhead).

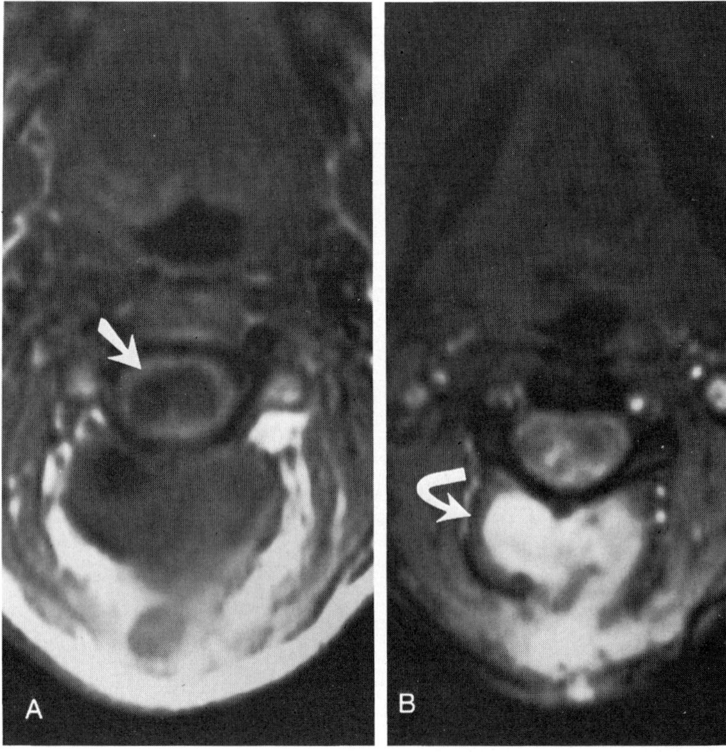

**Figure 2–34.** *A* and *B,* Axial T1WI and intermediate T2WI fast scan (TR 25/TE 12 msec, flip angle 11°). Cord syrinx (small arrow) and pseudomeningocele (curved arrow) are hypointense on T1WI. Flow effects in cyst on fast scan prevent expected T2 signal hyperintensity and could result in a false-negative diagnosis. Flow effects are minimal in pseudomeningocele.

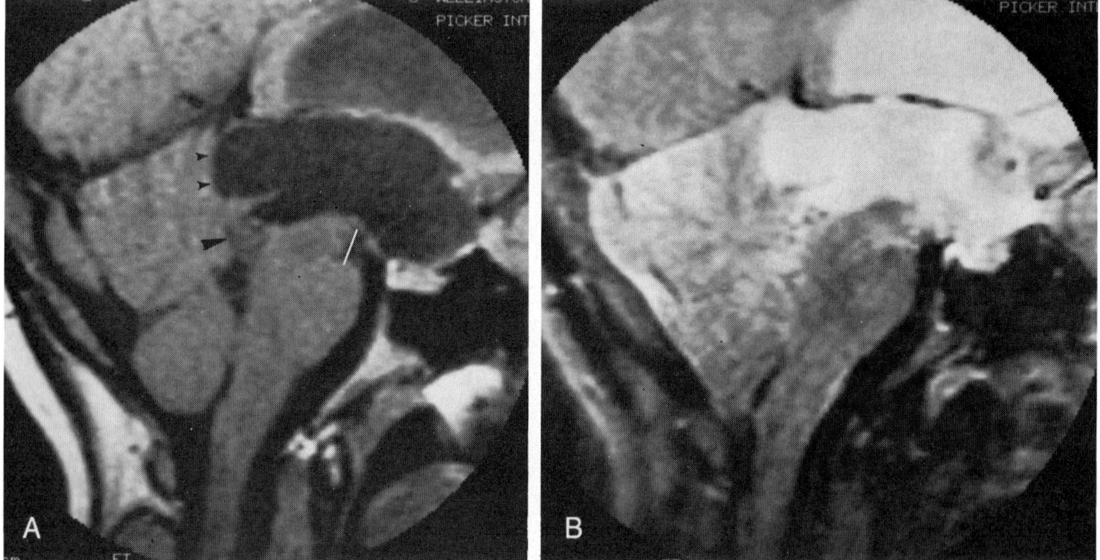


**Figure 2–35. Tectal glioma with aqueductal obstruction.** Progressive frontal headache. *A,* Sagittal T1WI (0.5 T). *B,* Sagittal T2WI. A tectal mass (arrowhead) obstructs the aqueduct of Sylvius and results in loss of the aqueductal flow void on T2WI. Other findings compatible with hydrocephalus include third ventricle pineal recess enlargement (arrowheads) and decreased (< 1 cm) mamillopontine distance (white line).

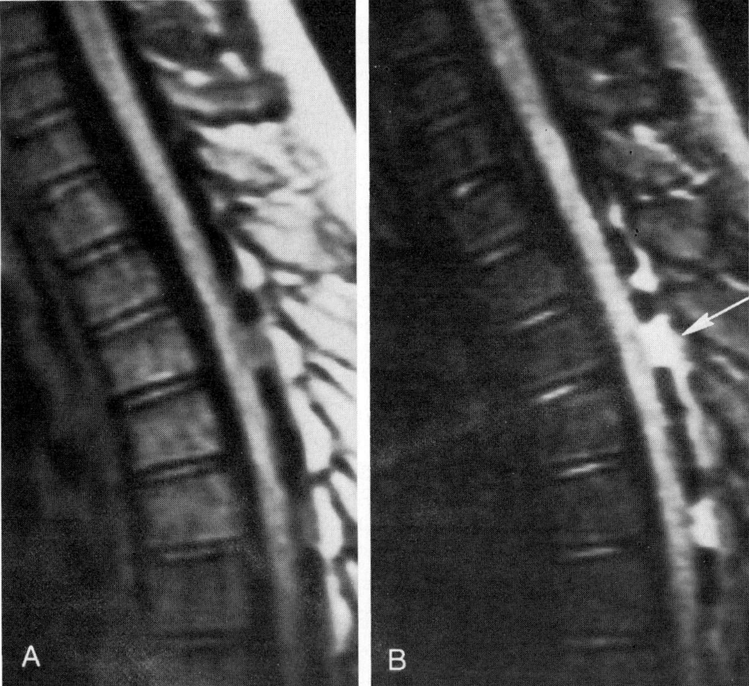


**Figure 2–36.** *A* and *B,* Sagittal multiecho N(H)WI and T2WI from a 12-year-old child. The thecal sac CSF is hypointense on both echoes owing to oscillatory movement. Ligaments and septations trap CSF foci and allow signal conversion to hyperintensity (arrow) on T2WI.

eighth nerve complexes, resulting in a "pseudoneuroma" appearance (Fig. 2–37). Bizarre CSF flow effects around arachnoidal septations can produce confounding signal intensities in patients with arachnoiditis. These effects are particularly prominent in the axial projection and are accentuated with long TR/TE pulse sequences as well as with thin sections.

When CSF-related oscillatory effects pro-

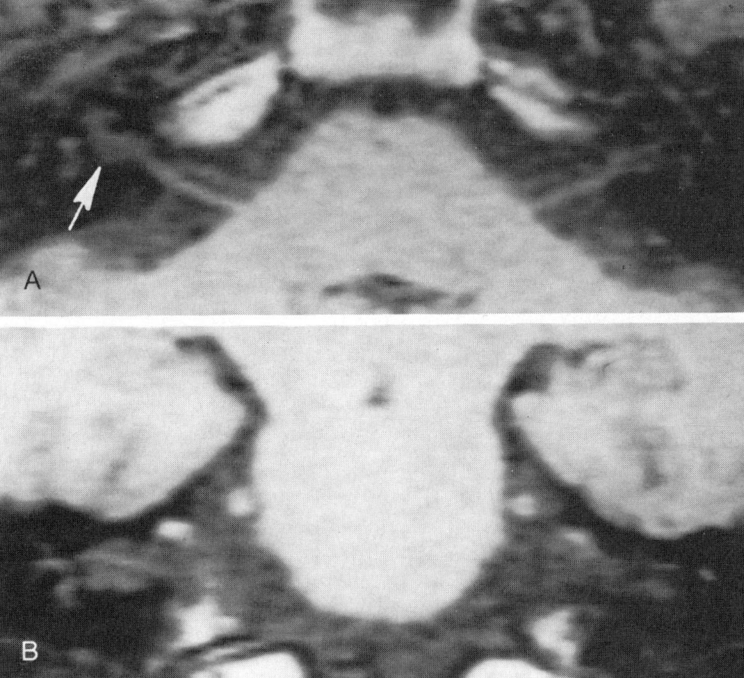


**Figure 2–37.** *A* and *B,* Axial and coronal 3-mm T1WI. Focal contour alteration at the eighth nerve–complex tip (arrow) is intermediate in signal intensity and simulates neuroma. Dampened CSF pulsation owing to loculation or adhesion likely accounts for this effect. Coronal view is normal. ECG-gated or Gd-DTPA MR may be useful in such difficult cases.

duce phase shift artifacts or bizarre signal alterations, several options exist: (1) orientation of the phase-encoding gradient can be "swapped" with the frequency gradient so that ghosting artifacts do not overlie an area of interest; (2) T1WI can be employed, since short TR/TE sequences minimize these effects; (3) slice thickness can be increased (an impractical alternative reducing spatial resolution); (4) electrocardiographic (ECG) or peripheral pulse gating can be employed;[50, 51] and (5) flow compensation (gradient moment nulling) can be employed. Gating at our institution is applied only when spinal cord or brain-stem neoplasm, ischemia, demyelination, or myelitis is sought and superior cord to CSF T2WI contrast is needed.[52] Gating minimizes phase-related artifacts projecting over vital areas of interest. Flow compensation appears to be an effective alternative method of utilizing CSF oscillatory effects to advantage and optimizing the "myelographic" effect of T2WI. Flow compensation is often used instead of gating on all sagittal multiecho sequences in the spine because it is faster and easier to implement than ECG–peripheral pulse gating.

Most ECG-gated acquisitions are obtained in the sagittal projection. Gating may be triggered by the R wave of the QRS complex or with commercially available systems linked to the peripheral finger pulse. The latter appears to be more effective in eliminating nonconductive cardiac electrical activity and is routinely used in spinal imaging at some centers instead of flow-compensation techniques. Since gating to the diastolic cardiac phase is most effective,[53] trigger delays of 500 msec from peripheral pulse (or QRS complex) may be selected. Image quality with diastolic gating improves most dramatically when asymmetric, widely spaced echoes are selected. When multislice technique is utilized, it is often impractical to image in the diastolic cardiac phase. However, little difference in cord visualization between diastolic and systolic gating occurs when symmetric echoes are employed, since the phenomenon of even-echo rephasing itself functions as a flow-compensation technique. Alternatively, a nongated symmetric 4- or 8-pulse echo train can yield the same effect. Gated T2WIs are generated by triggering or synchronizing to every other or every third heartbeat with one, or occasionally two, excitations. While other techniques, particularly fast-scan protocols, produce T2-appearing images by exploiting CSF oscillatory effects, these images must be viewed with caution since they enhance the cord/CSF interface but do not yield true intra-axial T2 cord or brain information.[54] In addition, flow phenomena and phase artifacts with fast-scanning techniques can result in altered CSF signal simulating pathologic disease or anatomy (Fig. 2–38). Gradient moment nulling (flow compensation) is rou-

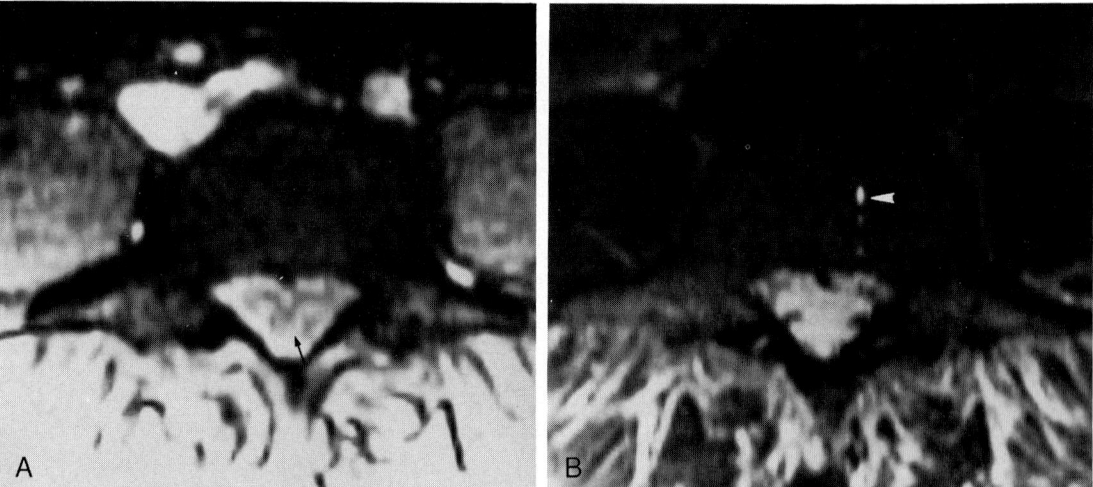


**Figure 2–38. A diagnosis of cord tethering is suggested.** A 32-year-old woman with back pain. *A,* Axial T2WI (gradient echo) fast scan at L5. Intermediate signal pseudoconus with anterior exiting nerve roots is simulated (arrow) by CSF-flow phenomenon. *B,* Axial T2WI (spin-echo) through L5. Normal hypointense nerve roots are present in the thecal sac but no actual conus is present. Incidentally noted is an artifact (arrowhead) produced by variation in the radio frequency (RF) power supply.

tinely used with fast-scan sequences. Fast-scan protocols are primarily employed in the evaluation of cervical disk disease and in differentiation of soft disk herniation from "hard disk" or spur.

## PITFALLS IN VASCULAR MR ASSESSMENT

At times, great difficulty arises when trying to distinguish flow effects producing signal increase (slice entry phenomena, even-echo rephasing, diastolic effects) from vascular occlusion or thrombosis. Summation of many of these effects with factors producing signal decrease may result in unusual and confusing intravascular signal alterations (Fig. 2–39). Methods used to differentiate flow effects from occlusion (negative T2-calculation value,[16] phase-display imaging,[29, 34, 35] MR angiography,[36–38] or fast scanning[25, 26]) are discussed earlier in this chapter. The most reliable sign of true occlusion is persistence of an intravascular signal alteration in all planes and all pulsing sequences (compare Figs. 2–39 and 2–40). Negative T2 calculation values may not always be accurate, but they suggest patency rather than vessel occlusion. Fast scanning may be quite helpful and sensitive in confirming the diagnosis of vascular occlusion.[55] Sequences employing larger flip angles and longer repetition times appear especially helpful in cases when flow is very slow since occlusion can sometimes be simulated, even with fast-scan techniques. In addition, certain pitfalls exist in the application of limited flip angle imaging when assessing vascular patency. Since thrombi frequently contain red blood cells, the signal of these red cell breakdown products (deoxyhemoglobin, methemoglobin, and hemosiderin) change with time[56] and may produce susceptibility effects. These subsequent intravascular signal changes are quite easily detected with gradient-refocused fast-scan techniques.[57] However, differentiation of signal alteration owing to deoxyhemoglobin in acute/subacute thrombosis and hemosiderin in chronic thrombosis may be difficult at high field. Attention to T1 and conventional spin-echo sequences will assist in dating thrombotic events.

As intravascular flow phenomena can mimic thrombosis, so too can true thrombosis masquerade as vessel patency, particularly at high field strengths. The signal evolution of venous occlusion roughly approximates that described for parenchymal intracranial hematoma at high field.[58] Al-

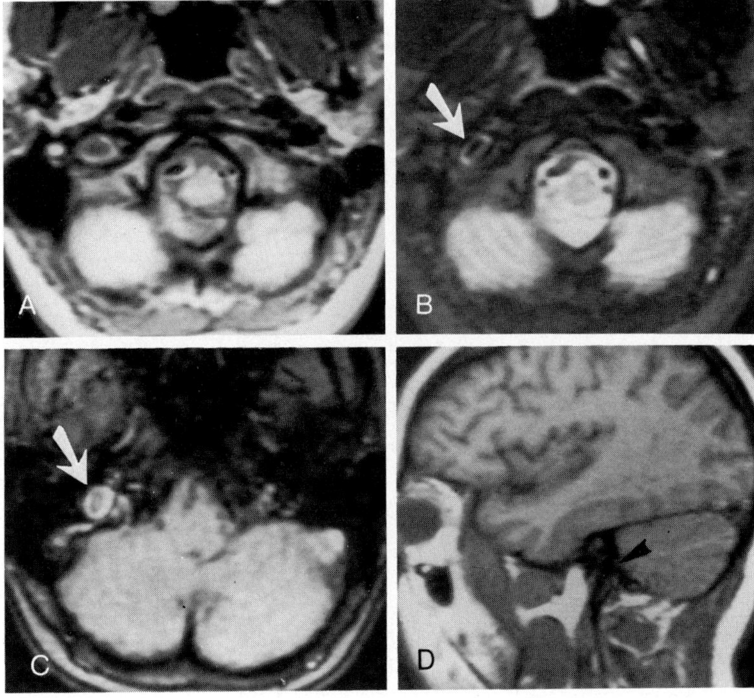


**Figure 2–39.** A 27-year-old woman with toxemia of pregnancy and seizures (1.5 T). *A* and *B*, Axial multiecho N(H)WI and T2WI (TR 1800/20/80). *C*, Axial fast scan (flip angle 20°/TR 25/TE 13) flow compensated. *D*, Sagittal T1WI (SE TR 600/TE 20). A ring of signal hyperintensity (arrow) circumscribes central intermediate signal on N(H)WI, T2WI, and fast-scan image suggesting subacute jugular venous occlusion. However, slow flow is actually present and normal flow void is apparent on sagittal T1WI (arrowhead), stressing the importance of multiplanar MR in vascular evaluation. Signal mimicking occlusion on fast scan will occur less frequently by employing longer TR and larger flip angles (see text).

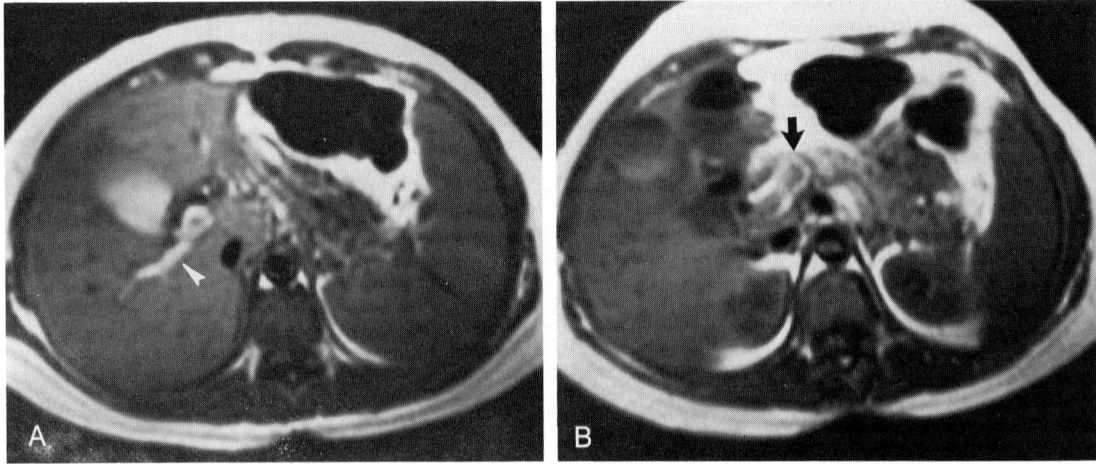

**Figure 2–40. Partial vein thrombosis.** A 29-year-old woman with abdominal pain. *A*, Axial T1WI (TR 800/TE 20 msec). Subacute (68 hours) occlusion of the right portal vein (arrowhead) shows signal hyperintensity on T1WI. *B,* A more caudal axial section better defines circumferential signal hyperintensity and central intermediate signal in the occluded main portal vein (arrow). This pattern is similar to that seen in the subacute phase of hematomas on T1WI.

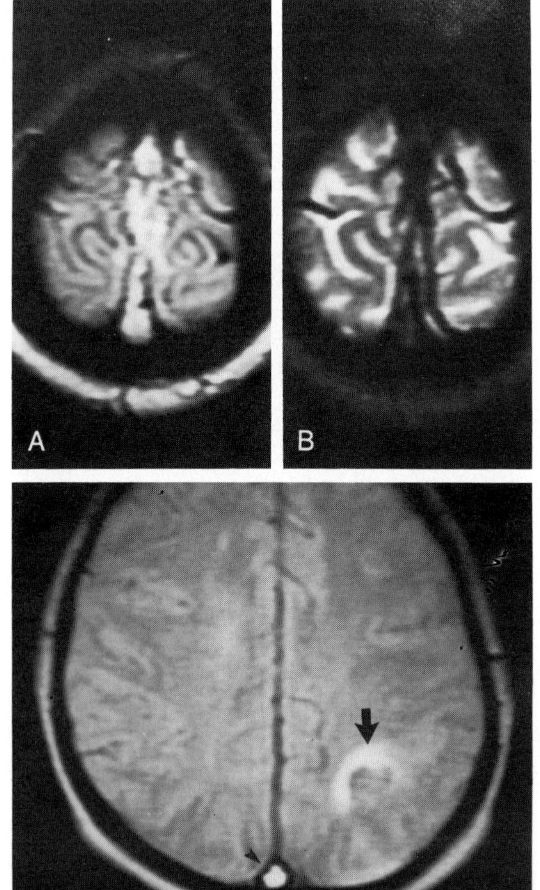

**Figure 2–41. Dural venous sinus thrombosis.** A 24-year-old woman on birth control pills (1.5 T). *A* and *B,* Axial multiecho N(H)WI and T2WI in early transition phase (62 hours) of acute to subacute sagittal sinus thrombosis. Susceptibility effect at high field strength produces thrombus hypointensity in T2WI, incorrectly suggesting vascular patency with first echo enhancement. *C,* Axial T2WI in chronic phase (15 days) shows venous infarct (black arrow) and hyperintensity (black arrowhead). Isointensity of thrombus may occur with occlusions on T2WI at 1.5 T during transition from acute (hypointense) to chronic (hyperintense) thrombosis.

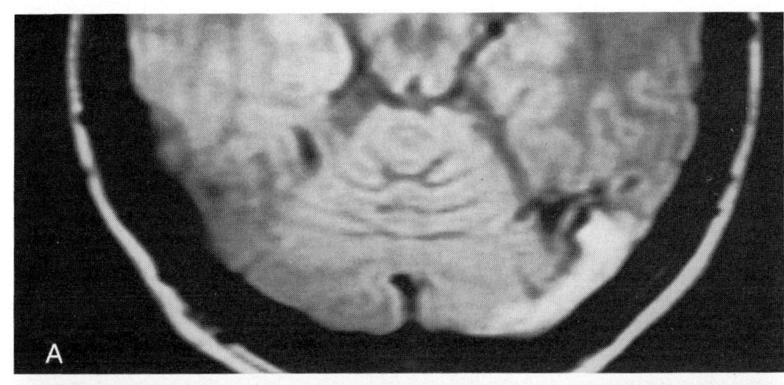


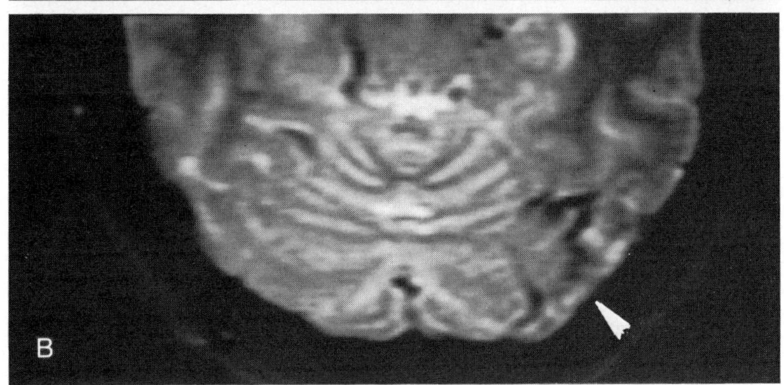


**Figure 2–42. Early subacute dural venous sinus thrombosis.** *A* and *B,* Axial (1.5 T) multiecho N(H)WI and T2WI (TR 2000/TE 20/80 msec). Late transition phase of acute to subacute left transverse sinus thrombosis (80 hours) is hyperintense on N(H)WI but isointense (arrowhead) on T2WI. Inability to recognize the abnormal isointense signal on T2WI may lead to false interpretation of N(H)WI as first echo enhancement rather than thrombosis.

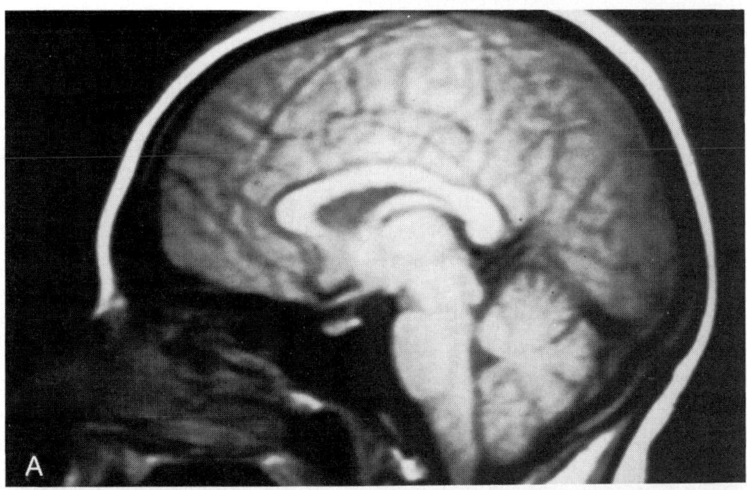


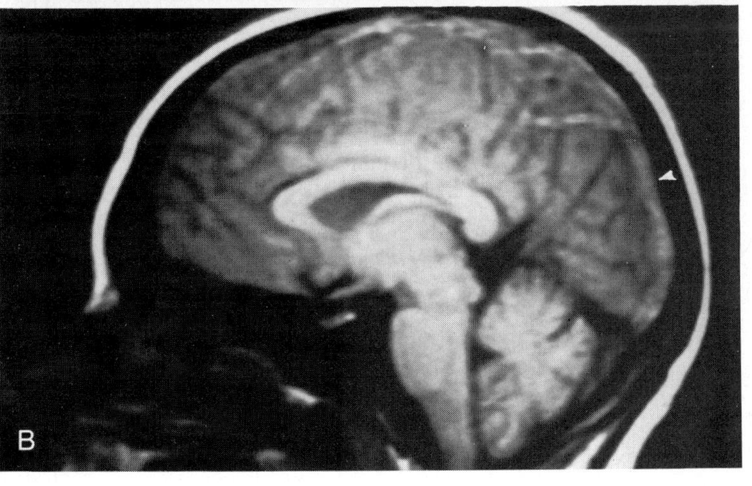


**Figure 2–43. A 20-year-old woman with sagittal sinus thrombosis.** *A* and *B,* Sagittal T1WI. At 3 hours postictus *(A)* thrombus is isointense with brain and virtually undetectable. The only clue is absence of cortical gyri and sulci peripherally at the brain's margin—the "faceless brain" sign. At four days *(B),* thrombus is now hyperintense (arrowhead) and visible.

though acute hematomas are hypointense at high field on T2WI, we have encountered many instances of acute thrombosis, quite hypointense on the second echo or T2WI of a multiecho sequence. This phenomenon likely is attributable to preferential T2-relaxation shortening effects of red blood cell paramagnetic breakdown products. As a result, signal hypointensity may be present on the first echo, but hypointense flow-void signal is simulated on the second-echo image. Therefore the signal increase on the first-echo image may be incorrectly attributed to a slice entry phenomenon or first-echo effect (Fig. 2–41).

As an intravascular clot evolves acutely from its hypointense signal to its chronic hyperintense signal intensity at 1.5 T on T2WI, isointensity with brain in the later subacute phase (8 to 10 days) may occur (Fig. 2–42). Such signal isointensity with adjacent brain could be easily overlooked on T2WI.

Since acute venous thrombosis on T2WI at high field may simulate vessel patency, one can turn to T1WI for assistance. It is important to keep in mind that acute thrombosis is either isointense or slightly hypointense with gray matter at many field strengths and can also be easily missed. When this occurs on sagittal T1 scout images in the sagittal sinus, the peripheral brain may appear "featureless," since the isointense clot blends with the signal of underlying brain parenchyma (Fig. 2–43).

Last, T1WI utilizing short TR and TE are prone to flow-related signal increase owing to time-of-flight or slice entry phenomena. These high-signal intravascular effects are accentuated at high field strengths and with partial saturation techniques. Because these flow effects are so frequent on T1W scout images, actual thromboses may be "written off" (compare Figs. 2–5 and 2–44) as flow phenomena while their true thrombotic etiology goes unrecognized.

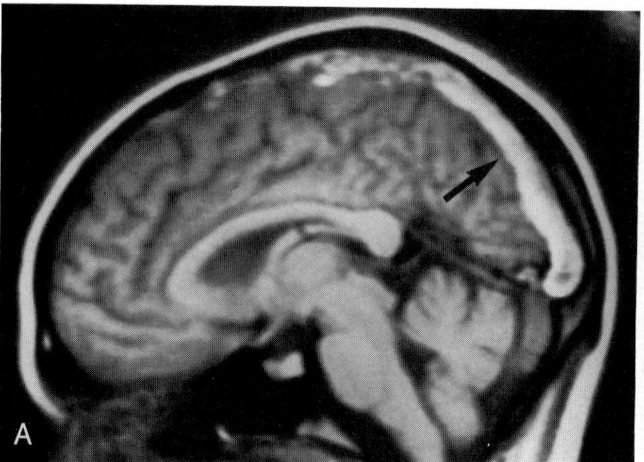


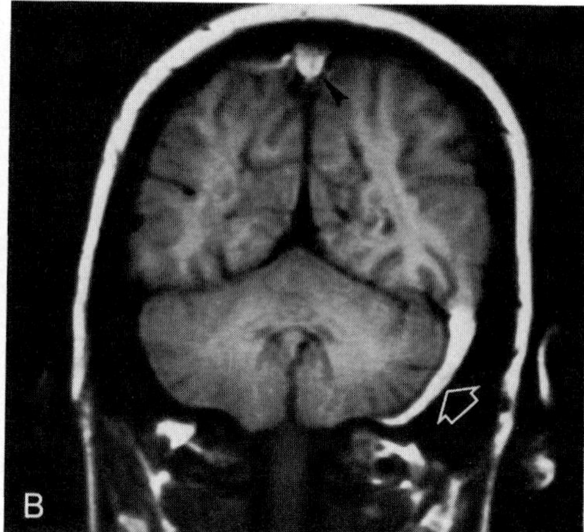


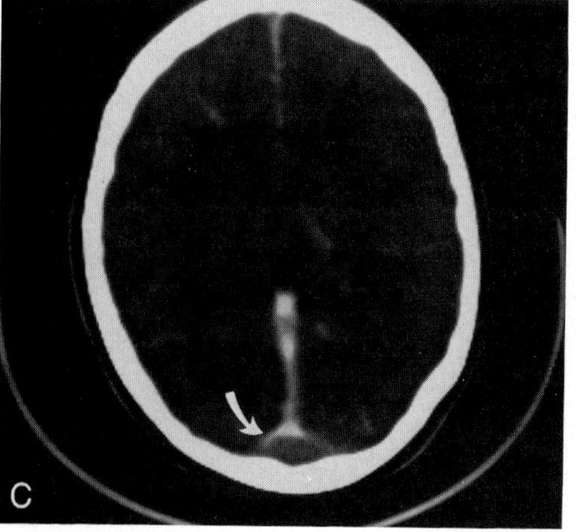


**Figure 2–44. Subacute dural venous sinus thrombosis.** An 18-year-old woman with headaches for seven days (1.5 T). *A,* Sagittal T1WI (SE TR 600/TE 20). *B,* Coronal T1WI. *C,* Axial CECT. Hyperintense T1WI signal (arrow) in the superior sagittal sinus (SSS) is confluent and expands the sinus but could be confused with in-plane flow phenomenon. Demonstration of signal alteration in another plane is the most reliable method of confirming this subacute thrombosis (arrowhead). The lateral sinus is also occluded (open arrow). CT "delta sign" of SSS thrombosis is present (curved arrow).

## References


1. Suryan G. Nuclear resonance in flowing liquids. Proc Indian Acad Sci (A)33:107, 1951.
2. Hahn EL. Spin echoes. Phys Rev 80:580–594, 1950.
3. Carr HY, Purcell EM. Effects of diffusion on free precession in nuclear magnetic resonance experiments. Phys Rev 94:630, 1954.
4. Singer JR. Blood flow rates by nuclear magnetic resonance measurements. Science 130:1652, 1959.
5. Morse OC, Singer JR. Blood velocity measurements in intact subjects. Science 170:440, 1970.
6. Hawkes RC, Holland GN, Moore WS, et al. Nuclear magnetic resonance (NMR) tomography of the brain: a preliminary clinical assessment with demonstration of pathology. J Comput Assist Tomogr 4:577, 1980.

7a. Battocletti JR, Halbach RE, Salles-Cunha SX, et al. The NMR blood flowmeter—theory and history. Med Phys 8:435, 1981.

7b. Halbach RE, Battocletti JR, Salles-Cunha SX, et al. The NMR blood flowmeter. Med Phys 8:444, 1981.

7c. Salles-Cunha SX, Halbach RE, Battocletti HJ, et al. The NMR blood flowmeter applications. Med Phys 8:452, 1981.

8. Garroway AN. Velocity measurements in flowing fluids by NMR. J Phys D 7:L159, 1974.
9. Singer JR. NMR Diffusion and flow measurements and an introduction to spin phase graphing. J Phys E 11:281, 1978.
10. Crooks LE, Mills CM, Davis PL, et al. Visualization of cerebral and vascular abnormalities by NMR imaging: the effects of imaging parameters on contrast. Radiology 144:843, 1982.
11. Kaufman L, Crooks LE, Sheldon PE, et al. Evaluation of NMR imaging for detection and quantification of obstructions in vessels. Invest Radiol 17:554, 1982.
12. Moran PR. A flow-velocity zeugmatographic interlace for NMR imaging in humans. Magn Reson Imag 1:197, 1982.
13. Axel L. Blood flow effects in magnetic resonance imaging (review). AJR 143:1157, 1984.
14. Wehrli FW, MacFall JR, Axel L, et al. Approaches to in-plane and out-of-plane flow imaging. Noninvas Med Imag 1:127, 1984.
15. Bradley WG, Waluch V. Blood flow: magnetic resonance imaging. Radiology 154:443, 1985.
16. von Schulthess GK, Higgins CB. Blood flow imaging with MR: spin-phase phenomena. Radiology 157:687, 1985.
17. Wehrli FW, Shimakawa A, MacFall JR, et al. MR imaging of venous and arterial flow by a selective saturation-recovery spin echo (SSRSE) method. J –545,Comput Assist Tomogr 9:537, 1985.
18. Axel L, Morton D. Flow effects in magnetic resonance imaging. In Thomas SR, Dixon RL, eds. NMR in Medicine: The Instrumentation and Clinical Applications. New York, American Institute of Physics, Inc., 1986:326.
19. Bradley WG. Magnetic resonance appearance of flowing blood and cerebrospinal fluid. In Brant-Zawadzki M, Norman D, eds. Magnetic Resonance Imaging of the Central Nervous System. New York, Raven Press, 1986:83.
20. Wedeen VJ. Flow MRI holds promise in vascular diagnosis. Diag Imag 84, May 1986.
21. Bradley WG. Sorting out the meaning of MRI flow phenomena. Diag Imag, 102, May 1987.
22. Bradley WG, Waluch V, Lai K, et al. The appearance of rapidly flowing blood on magnetic resonance imaging. AJR 143:1167, 1984.
23. Ahn CB, Lee SY, Nalcioglu O, et al. The effects of random directional distributed flow in nuclear magnetic resonance imaging. Med Phys 14:43, 1987.
24. Bird RB, Stewart WE, Lightfoot EN. Transport Phenomena. New York, Wiley Publishing Co., 1960:153.
25. Haase A, Frahm J, Matthaei D, et al. Flash imaging: rapid NMR imaging using low flip angle pulses. J Magn Reson 67:258, 1986.
26. Wehrli FW. Introduction to Fast-Scan Magnetic Resonance. General Electric Medical Systems. Brochure 7299, 1986.
27. Nayler GL, Firmin DN, Longmore DB. Blood flow imaging by cine magnetic resonance. J Comput Assist Tomogr 10:715, 1986.
28. Waluch V, Bradley WG. NMR even-echo rephasing in slow laminar flow. J Comput Assist Tomogr 8:594, 1984.
29. Wedeen VJ, Rosen BR, Chesler D, et al. MR velocity imaging by phase display. J Comput Assist Tomogr 9:530, 1985.
30. Glover GH. Flow Artifacts in MRI. Theory and Reduction by Gradient Moment Nulling. General Electric Medical Systems Applied Science Laboratory Technical Report, 1985.
31. Pattany PM, Marino R, McNally JM. Velocity and acceleration desensitization in 2DFT MR imaging (Abstract). Magn Reson Imag 4:154, 1986.
32. McDonald DA. Blood Flow in Arteries, 2nd ed. Baltimore, Williams & Wilkins, 1974.
33. Perman WH, Moran PR, Moran RA, et al. Artifacts from pulsatile flow in MR imaging. J Comput Assist Tomogr 10:473, 1986.
34. Bryant DJ, Payne JA, Firmin DN, et al. Measurement of flow with NMR imaging using a gradient pulse and phase difference technique. J Comput Assist Tomogr 8:588, 1984.
35. Young IR, Bydder GM, Payne JA. Flow measurement by the development of phase differences during slice formation in MR imaging. Magn Reson Med 3:175, 1986.
36. Pearce R. MR angiography measures, displays blood velocity. Diagn Imag 92, January 1987.
37. Weeden VJ, Meuli RA, Edelman RR, et al. Projective imaging of pulsatile flow with magnetic resonance. Science 230:946, 1985.
38. Dumoulin CL, Souza SP, Hart HR. Rapid scan magnetic resonance angiography. Magn Reson Med 5:238, 1987.
39. DuBoulay GH. Pulsatile movements in CSF pathways. Br J Radiol 39:255, 1966.
40. Sherman JL, Citrin CM. Magnetic resonance demonstration of normal CSF flow. AJNR 7:3, 1986.
41. Sherman JL, Citrin CM, Bowen BJ, et al. MR demonstration of altered cerebrospinal fluid flow by obstructive lesions. AJNR 7:571, 1986.
42. Sherman JL, Citrin CM, Gangarosa RE, et al. The MR appearance of CSF pulsations in the spinal canal. AJNR 7:879, 1986.
43. Rubin JB, Enzmann DR. Harmonic modulation of proton MR precessional phase by pulsatile motion: origin of spinal CSF flow phenomena. AJNR 8:307, 1987.

44. Rubin JB, Enzmann DR. Imaging of spinal CSF pulsation by 2DFT MR: significance during clinical imaging. AJNR 8:297, 1987.
45. Edelman RR, Wedeen VJ, Davis KR, et al. Multiphasic MR imaging: a new method for direct imaging of pulsatile CSF flow. Radiology 161:779, 1986.
46. Sherman JL, Citrin CM, Gangarosa RE, et al. The MR appearace of CSF flow in patients with ventriculomegaly. AJNR 7:1025, 1986.
47. Bradley WG, Kortman KE, Burgoyne B. Flowing cerebrospinal fluid in normal and hydrocephalic states: appearance on MR images. Radiology 159:611, 1986.
48. Greenberg JO, Shenkin HA, Adam R. Idiopathic normal pressure hydrocephalus: a report of 73 patients. J Neurol Neuro Psych 40:336, 1977.
49. Hakim S, Venegas JG, Burton JD. The physics of the cranial cavity hydrocephalus and normal pressure hydrocephalus: mechanical interpretation and mathematical model. Surg Neurol 5:187, 1976.
50. Citrin CM, Sherman JL, Gangarosa RE, et al. Physiology of the CSF flow-void sign: modification by cardiac gating. AJNR 7:1021, 1986.
51. Bergstrand G, Berstrom M, Nordell B, et al. Cardiac-gated MR imaging of cerebrospinal fluid flow. J Comput Assist Tomogr 9:1003, 1985.
52. Enzmann DR, Rubin JB, O'Donohue J, et al. Use of cerebrospinal fluid gating to improve T2-weighted images. Part II. Temporal lobes, basal ganglia, and brain stem. Radiology 162:768, 1987.
53. Enzmann DR, Rubin JB, Wright A. Use of cerebrospinal fluid gating to improve T2-weighted images. Part I. The spinal cord. Radiology 162:763, 1987.
54. Henning J, Friedburg H, Strobel B. Rapid nontomographic approach to MR myelography without contrast agents. J Comput Assist Tomogr 10:375, 1987.
55. Spritzer CE, Sussman SK, Blinder RA, et al. Deep venous thrombosis evaluation with limited-flip-angle, gradient-refocused MR imaging: preliminary experience. Radiology 166:371, 1988.
56. Macchi PJ, Grossman RI, Gomori JM, et al. High-field MRI of cerebral venous thrombosis. J Comput Assist Tomogr 10:10, 1985.
57. Gomori J, Grossman RI. Head and neck hemorrhage. In Kressel HY, ed. Magnetic Resonance Annual. New York, Raven Press, 1987:71–112.
58. Gomori JM, Grossman RI, Goldberg HI, et al. Intracranial hematomas: imaging by high-field MR. Radiology 156:99, 1985.

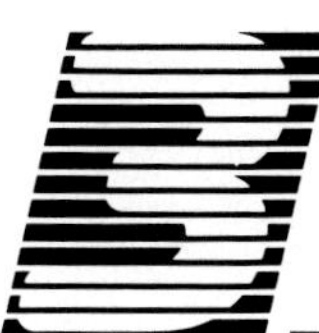

**Stephen J. Pomeranz, M.D.**

# INTRODUCTION TO CRANIOSPINAL MR

## INDICATIONS

The efficacy of magnetic resonance (MR) in the diagnosis of central nervous system (CNS) disease is well established. Many studies are being carried out to compare the sensitivity and specificity of MR with noncontrast computed tomography (NCCT) and contrast-enhanced computed tomography (CECT). A summary of examination preferences is provided in Appendix I. MR provides no ionizing radiation, yields direct multiplanar images, and usually requires no intravenous agent to improve contrast resolution. We believe that when sensitivity between CECT and MR is approximated, MR should be the favored modality for pediatric neurologic evaluation in patients who tolerate intravenous contrast poorly; for craniospinal diagnosis in pregnancy; and when disease in the posterior fossa, brain stem, temporal lobes, or upper cervical cord is clinically suspected. Recommended protocols for MR examination of these and other regions in the craniospinal axis are summarized in Appendix II.

## BASIC CLINICORADIOLOGIC PARAMETERS

An understanding of the basic operator-dependent variables that determine image contrast and quality are vital to proper MR evaluation (Table 3–1). The following section addresses these variables as they relate to daily clinical MR implementation. Let us begin with two important determinants of image contrast, T1 and T2 relaxation.

### Repetition Time

Repetition time (TR), a determinant of T1 relaxation, has been addressed in Chapter 1. It represents the time interval between successive 90° pulses in a spin-echo sequence. Short repetition times produce T1WI (Fig. 3–1*A*). Since longer repetition times decrease T1-dependent image contrast and increase the number of potential slice locations, signal-to-noise ratio (SNR), and imaging time in linear fashion, attention must be paid to all parameters selected.[1, 2] For instance, some imaging protocol options provide for either 3 (or 5)-mm sections and 20 (or 24)-cm field of view (FOV). One should not choose the higher spatial resolution (3-mm/20-cm) options if one plans to use 2 excitations (nex) and short TR (< 500), because these parameters all create unfavorable SNR. In another example, a T2WI protocol obtained with 6 nex would create intolerable imaging times. Choice of TR will depend on desired contrast, available scan time, patient cooperation, number of averages (av) or excitations, chosen slice thickness, and number of slice locations necessary for diagnosis.

### Echo Time

Echo time (TE) emphasizes differences in T2-dependent image contrast (Fig. 3–1*B*) as TE is prolonged.[3] Echo time represents one half the time interval between successive 90° and 180° pulses of a spin-echo sequence. The shortest echo times available maximize image signal but minimize differences in T2-

**Table 3–1.** EFFECT OF INCREASING OPERATOR-DEPENDENT MR IMAGING PARAMETERS

| Parameter | Option | Spatial Resolution | SNR | T1 | T2 | Imaging Time | ROI* | #Slices Length | Miscellaneous |
|---|---|---|---|---|---|---|---|---|---|
| TR | ↑ | NC† | ↑ | ↓ | ↑ | ↑ | NC | ↑ | ↓ time-of-flight effect (flow-related signal ↑) |
| TE | ↑ | NC | ↓ | ↓ | ↑ | NC | NC | ↓ | ↓ time-of-flight effect (signal increase); slice no. = TR/TE + K |
| Echo strategy | single | NC | NC | NC | NC | NC | NC | ↑ | minimal crosstalk effect, inc no. of slices for given TR |
| Echo strategy | multi | NC | NC | NC | NC | NC | NC | ↓ | ↑ crosstalk artifact; ↓ no. of slices for a given TR |
| Matrix size | ↑ | ↑ | ↓ | NC | NC | ↑ | NC | NC | Scan time ~ no. of y, or phase-encoding, views |
| Slice thickness | ↑ | ↓ | ↑ | NC | NC | NC | NC | ↑ | ↑ partial volume effect ↓ time-of-flight effect |
| FOV‡ | ↑ | ↓ | ↑ | NC | NC | NC | ↑ | NC | ↓ aliasing artifact; SNR ~ FOV squared |
| No. of averages, excitations, or data sets | ↑ | NC | ↑ | NC | NC | ↑ | NC | NC | §SNR ~ square root of the no. of averages; ↓ motion artifact owing to image-averaging effect |
| Scan type | fast | NC | ↓ | NC | NC | ↓ | NC | ↓ | Owing to ↓ SNR, thin slices and small FOV impractical; scan time ~ no. of slices |
| Scan type | spin-echo | NC | ↑ | NC | NC | ↑ | NC | ↑ | Longer scan times allow ↑ no. of slices per scan series |
| Coil | surface | ↑ | ↑ | NC | NC | NC | ↓ | NC | Signal fall-off with ↑ depth; ↓ motion artifact outside ROI; more obvious motion effects inside ROI; ↓ aliasing effect; narrow FOV range; spatial resolution improves over whole-volume coil only because of ability to select smaller FOV with better SNR |
| Coil | volume | ↓ | ↓ | NC | NC | NC | ↑ | NC | No signal fall-off with depth; better SNR deep; inferior SNR superficially; ↑ FOV range; ↑ aliasing effect; sensitive to motion effect in entire volume imaged; not position-sensitive |

*Table continued on opposite page*

dependent contrast.[4] The cost of scanning with prolonged echo times is twofold: (1) diminished SNR and (2) decreased number of obtainable sections per given TR. Since lengthened TE creates unfavorable signal characteristics, it is unwise to obtain thin sections with long TE unless one is prepared to utilize many averages or substantial repetition times or both.

## Voxel Size

Voxel size and spatial resolution are determined by section thickness (Fig. 3–2), FOV, and matrix size. The slice profile in MR is determined by the gradient strength, or shape of radio frequency (RF) excitation pulses (frequency range), which in turn depends on the duration of the RF pulse. A longer pulse results in a thinner section, because it produces a narrower frequency range for a particular gradient strength. Markedly prolonged RF pulse lengths are impractical, since the time until the first obtainable echo (TE) may be prolonged. Therefore each particular MR system has a limiting section thickness for the minimum desired TE.[5]

The slice selection width of a 180° pulse

**Table 3–1.** EFFECT OF INCREASING OPERATOR-DEPENDENT MR IMAGING PARAMETERS *Continued*

| Parameter | Option | Spatial Resolution | SNR | T1 | T2 | Imaging Time | ROI* | #Slices Length | Miscellaneous |
|---|---|---|---|---|---|---|---|---|---|
| Fourier | 3DFT | ↑ | ↑ | NC | NC | ↑ | ↓ | ↓ | SNR ~ to square root of the no. of slices; slice no. is independent of TR and is a determinant of scan time; therefore slice no. is limited by scan time; no cross-excitation artifact; motion sensitivity ↑ relative to 2DFT‖; no aliasing artifact |
| Fourier | 2DFT | ↓ | ↓ | NC | NC | ↓ | ↑ | ↑ | SNR ~ TR, FOV, data sets, and matrix, but is independent of slice nos.; dependent on TR cross-excitation effect; ↓ motion sensitivity relative to 3DFT**; aliasing artifact |
| Compensation | respiratory | NC | ↑ | NC | NC | NC | NC | ↓ | ↑ set-up time; scan time unaffected; ↓ phase-related motion artifacts; coherent noise reduction improves SNR |
| Compensation | flow | NC | ↑ | NC | NC | NC | NC | ↓ | SNR improved only by reduction in flow-related coherent noise |
| Gating | cardiac | NC | ↑ | ↓ | NC | ↑ | NC | ↓ | Scan time ↑; coherent noise reduction improves SNR; ↓ no. of slices per acquisition; ↑ set-up time; TR determined by heart rate therein governing T1 weighting |

*ROI = region of interest.
†NC = no change.
‡FOV = field of view.
§SNR = signal-to-noise ratio.
‖2DFT = two-dimensional Fourier transformation image.
**3DFT = three-dimensional Fourier transformation image.

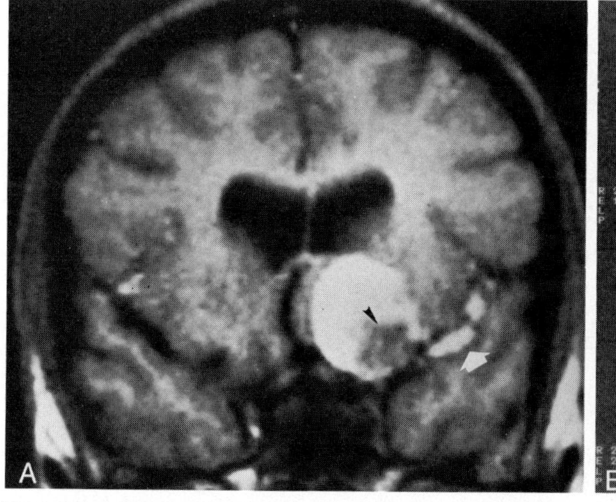


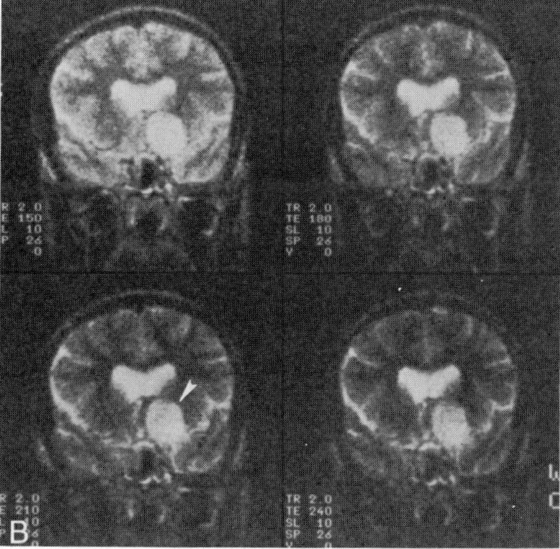


**Figure 3–1. Dermoid tumor with rupture and chemical meningitis.** A 23-year-old man with sudden onset of headaches and meningismus (0.35 tesla [T]). *A*, Coronal T1WI (TR 300/TR 35). Hyperintense mass (short T1 relaxation) with intermediate signal intensity nodule (black arrowhead) has a component extending into the sylvian fissure (white arrowhead). Notice that in this case T1WI is more sensitive in depicting intrasylvian disease. *B*, Coronal 8'-echo pulse train T2WI (only 4 echoes shown); the lesion is hyperintense on T2WI, compatible with its long T2 relaxation. The intrasylvian component is hidden.

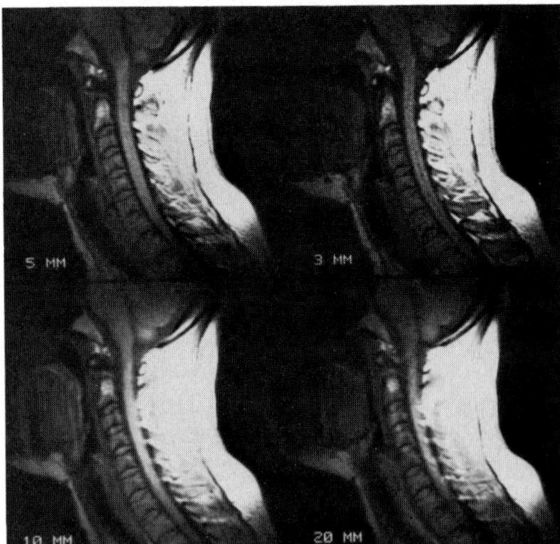


**Figure 3–2. The effect of varying slice thickness.** From a volunteer, sagittal cervical spine with all parameters held constant except voxel thickness (1.5 T). With thinner slices and decreased voxel size, image signal-to-noise ratio (SNR) decreases, whereas spatial resolution increases. Section thickness above 5 mm has resulted in volume averaging of posterior ligament and fat. The thin, 3-mm section appears grainy, or noisy.

is normally wider than the desired slice thickness, but the ultimate sharpness of a slice profile is determined by the quality of both the 90° and 180° RF synchronous pulses. Since even the infinitely long, or ideal, synchronous pulses result in partial excitation of tissue in adjacent sections on multiecho sequences, this "crosstalk" reduces the effective TR for a given slice, decreases image contrast, and produces inaccurate T1 weighting. For now, this problem is circumvented by selecting gaps of 20% to 50% of the nominal slice thickness. The amount of interslice gap will depend on the size of the pathology being sought and the distance requiring MR coverage. Marked reduction in slice gap will produce image degradation on multiecho images. Therefore two options are available when gapless imaging is desired: (1) utilize gap imaging and perform a section series of images to "fill in" the gapped slice locations [interleaving, or interlacing, technique], or (2) use a contiguous program that chooses section gaps equal to the slice thickness and automatically fills these in on a second scan series without requiring a repeat scan set-up. Both of these approaches at least double the scan time. Newer pulse sequences are being developed to obviate this problem.[6] When high-resolution anatomic information is desired (as in the sella or internal auditory canal [IAC]), we perform a high-resolution, truly gapless single-echo protocol in one or two planes, reserving multiecho T2WI for selected cases. Unlike their multiecho counterparts, single-echo gapless T1WI produce minimal image degradation owing to crosstalk.

When selecting a slice thickness, remember that a direct linear relationship exists between image signal and slice thickness. Therefore one would be ill-advised to choose a detailed matrix (256 × 256) and thin section (3 mm) if planning to use only a few excitations, small FOV, and short TR—all parameters minimizing image signal. These factors must be balanced against one another, the degree of patient cooperation, and the available scan time. Some suggestions for examination slice thickness may be found under imaging protocols in the appendices of this text (I and II).

## Matrix Size

Matrix size in MR (Fig. 3–3), unlike CT, is an important determinant of imaging time. However, like CT, it is a determinant of image SNR when other parameters are held constant. The MR read-only, or x, gradient may be changed without altering imaging time. The number of y, or phase-encoded, views affects scan time in direct linear fash-

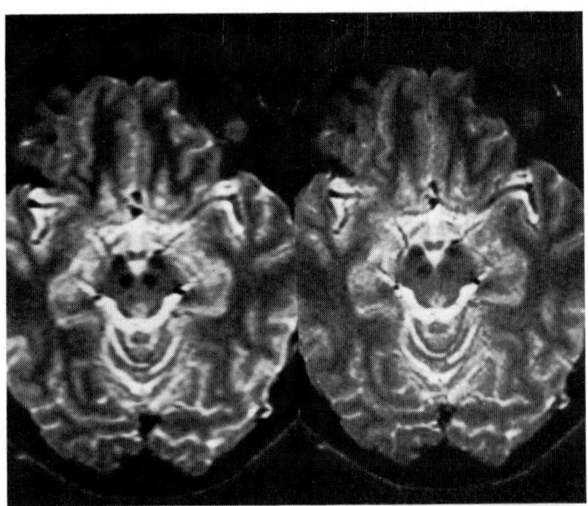

**Figure 3–3. The effect of varying image matrix.** Axial T2WI at 128 × 256 (reader's left) and 256 × 256 (right), with all other parameters held constant (1.5 T). Doubling the y matrix decreases pixel size and improves spatial resolution and image detail. Signal-to-noise ratio is decreased but not to a detrimental degree. Imaging time is doubled.

**Table 3–2.** EFFECT OF VARYING MATRIX SIZE ON PIXEL SIZE, SNR, AND SCAN TIME WITH CONSTANT FOV (16 cm) AND EXCITATIONS (2)

| Matrix (Phase × Frequency) | Pixel Volume ($mm^3$) | SNR | Scan Time (min) TR = 1 sec |
|---|---|---|---|
| 128 × 128 | 1.56 | 2.00 | 4.27 |
| 128 × 192 | 1.04 | 1.33 | 4.27 |
| 128 × 256 | 0.78 | 1.00 | 4.27 |
| 192 × 256 | 0.52 | 0.82 | 6.40 |
| 256 × 256 | 0.39 | 0.71 | 8.53 |

ion (Table 3–2). Therefore doubling the number of y views doubles scan time. Although this method improves spatial resolution and decreases pixel size, there is a penalty that occurs in the form of reduced SNR, whether the number of x or of y views is increased. Most vendors offer at least three matrix options: 128 × 128; 128 × 256 (y); and 256 × 256. Images are often interpolated and displayed in a 256 × 512 or a 512 × 512 format. The 256 × 256 matrix is reserved for (1) detailed, gapless, single-echo imaging of small regions of interest (the sella or IAC); (2) times when one is prepared to use many excitations; and (3) patients who are cooperative.

## Field of View

Field-of-view (FOV) selections (Fig. 3–4) depend on the desired spatial resolution (pixel) and the region-of-interest area (Tables 3–3 and 3–4). Since the effect of FOV reduction on image signal is not linear but exponential (squared), correct FOV selection is crucial. Selecting a small FOV, 256 × 256 matrix, and thin sections may not be optimal unless one utilizes factors that prolong aquisition but improve image signal, such as multiple excitations, longer repetition times, or both.

A further penalty of FOV reduction is image wraparound, or aliasing. This artifact occurs primarily in the phase, or y, direction when an excessively small FOV is selected. On most commercially available units, coronal sections are most prone to aliasing, followed by sagittal and then by axial orientations. Aliasing is easily minimized in the read, or x, direction by bandpass filters and their adjustment. Occasionally, when a small FOV is desired and wraparound obscures a vital anatomic structure, switching the phase (y) and frequency (x) gradient directions ameliorates this problem. In addition, off-center FOV is available on many units. A trick is employed to minimize aliasing, or wraparound, when high-resolution, small FOV MR is necessary: An FOV twice that selected by the operator is automatically implemented in the phase direction only (No-phase Wraparound from General Electric Medical Systems). Simultaneously, in the phase direction the matrix

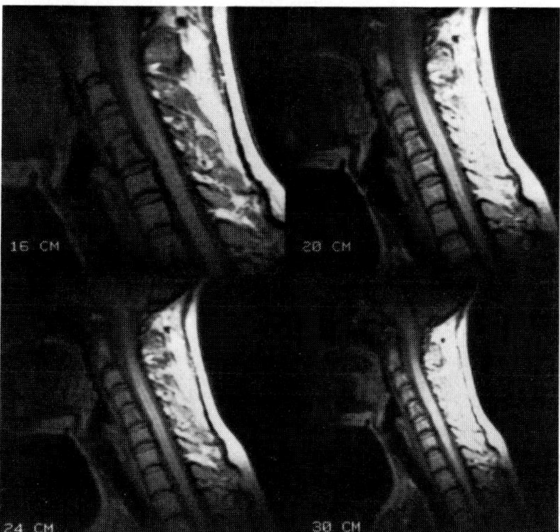


**Figure 3–4. Effect of varying field of view FOV) at 1.5 T.** Sagittal cervical spine T1WI from a volunteer. FOV is varied while all other parameters are held constant. With smaller FOV, spatial resolution improves, whereas image signal-to-noise ratio (CSNR) and region of interest area decrease. In this patient, FOV 16 to 20 cm seems the most appropriate balance of resolution and SNR. Notice the incidental C5-C6 disc herniation.

**Table 3–3.** SURFACE COIL PIXEL SIZE, FOV, AND MAGNIFICATION

| Field of View (cm) | Pixel Size (mm) for 128 × 256 Matrix | Pixel Size (mm) for 256 × 256 Matrix | Gradient Magnification |
|---|---|---|---|
| 25.5 | 1 × 2 | 1 × 1 | 0.0 |
| 20.4 | 0.8 × 1.6 | 0.8 × 0.8 | 1.25 |
| 19.7 | 0.77 × 1.54 | 0.77 × 0.77 | 1.30 |
| 18.2 | 0.71 × 1.42 | 0.71 × 0.71 | 1.40 |

**Table 3–4.** FOV VARIATION WITH 256 × 256 MATRIX AND 2 EXCITATIONS

| FOV (cm) | Pixel Volume ($mm^3$) | SNR | Scan Time (min) TR = 1 sec |
|---|---|---|---|
| 12 | 0.22 | 0.40 | 8.53 |
| 16 | 0.39 | 0.71 | 8.53 |
| 20 | 0.61 | 1.10 | 8.53 |
| 24 | 0.88 | 1.59 | 8.53 |

is doubled (from 256y × 256x to 512y × 256x). In this manner, the spatial resolution is held constant. However, by doubling the matrix, scan time would also be doubled. This is automatically counteracted by halving of the number of operator-selected excitations or averages. The bandpass filters that minimize aliasing in the frequency-encoded direction do not provide precise localization or encoding of signal. Therefore, the same trick may be employed in the frequency direction (No-frequency Wraparound) or in both phase and frequency orientations.

### Excitations and Averages

Excitations [nex] and averages [av] refer to the number of times a data set of a specified image series is repeated or averaged (Fig. 3–5). Repeated averaging of this data set improves the image signal-to-noise ratio (SNR) but at a cost of directly prolonging scan time (Table 3–5). SNR improvement does not rise linearly but is increased as the square root of the number of averages (1 average = 2 excitations). Images obtained with many excitations are further improved by the tendency to average out motion artifacts. The number of nex or av is chosen depending upon the other parameters selected. Since increased scanning time and SNR occur with long repetition times, the use of many excitations is not necessary in this instance. However, when factors that reduce image signal are chosen—short TR, long TE, thin sections, or small FOV—then more excitations or averages become a necessity.

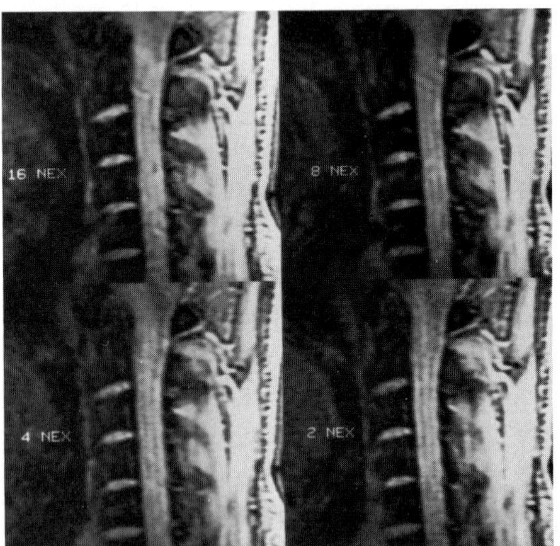


**Figure 3–5. Effect of varying excitations, averages, or repetitions, while holding all other parameters constant during sagittal fast-scan of the cervical spine.** When comparing signal-to-noise ratio (SNR) between 16 and 2 nex images, the 16 nex image appears "smoother" and demonstrates greater signal. However, signal increase is not as pronounced as expected, since signal gain is not linear but a square root function of the number of averages or repetitions.

**Table 3–5.** EFFECT OF VARYING EXCITATIONS OR AVERAGES ON SCAN TIME AND SNR AT 128 × 256 MATRIX/16-cm FOV

| Excitations | SNR | Scan Time (min) TR = 1 sec |
|---|---|---|
| 1 | 0.71 | 2.13 |
| 2 | 1.00 | 4.27 |
| 4 | 1.41 | 8.53 |
| 6 | 1.73 | 12.80 |

## ADVANCED CLINICORADIOLOGIC PARAMETERS

### Scout Images

Scout images are intended for localization of other slice orientations. Therefore the shortest TR, smallest matrix size, and fewest available excitations or averages are used to minimize examination setup time. The shortest TE is implemented, since it will provide the best SNR with a short TR and few excitations. Modification of the scout image may be indicated in several cases. For instance, if a sagittal T1-weighted image (T1WI) of a known chordoma is desired, the scout may be converted into a diagnostic image set. This is done by placing the center slice on the patient's nasion, doubling the excitations, and modestly increasing the TR. A scout image is not performed in our sellar protocol. Instead, initial sagittal 3-mm sections are performed with small FOV, 6 nex, and a central slice positioned over the nasion. The sella has yet to be missed with this method.

### T1-Weighted Images

T1-weighted images (T1WIs) employ short TR and TE (Fig. 3–6).[7] Their generation and physical properties are addressed elsewhere in the text. The clinical utility of such sequences is relevant to this section. Obvious

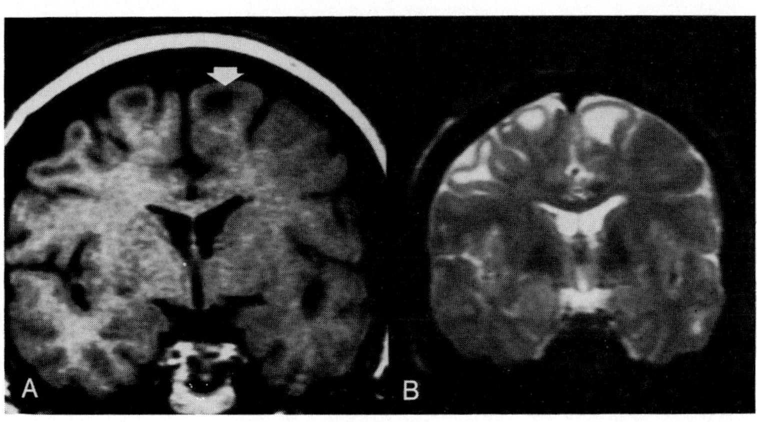


**Figure 3–6.** A 26-year-old woman with a seizure disorder. *A*, Coronal T1WI (TR 600/TE 20); *B*, coronal T2WI (TR 1800/TE 100). Examples of T1-weighted and T2-weighted images at 1.5 T. Weighting is properly identified by observing that on T1WI the white matter is white and the gray matter is gray; CSF-containing structures are hypointense; fat-containing structures are hyperintense; and many forms of pathology (cortical tubers [arrow]) are hypointense on T1WI spin echo pulsing sequences. T2-weighting is identified by noting that white matter is gray and gray matter is white, CSF-containing structures are hyperintense, fat-containing structures are hypointense, and many pathologic conditions are hyperintense.

uses of T1WI include characterization and staging of hemorrhagic phenomena (hyperintense), delineation of fat-containing lesions (hyperintense and exhibiting chemical-shift effect), and elucidation of cysts (hypointense and approximating CSF signal intensity).

T1WI are utilized on all scout sequences because of their speed and the fact that their SNR characteristics allow one or one-half excitation imaging. SNR characteristics of T1WI are innately superior to longer TR spin-echo sequences for several reasons: (1) shorter scan times reduce coherent motion-related image noise from flowing blood, swallowing, and so forth; (2) some manufacturers may utilize different T1 pulsing sequences (partial saturation); and (3) only single-echo images are usually obtained, minimizing "crosstalk" incongruities. Therefore when anatomic information is vital and contour alterations rather than contrast alterations allow diagnoses, examinations may be performed with only single-echo T1WI.

This approach is implemented in the following situations: (1) patients with normal T1WI sella and IAC; (2) clear-cut T1WI sellar microadenoma or macroadenoma; (3) patients being evaluated for suspected disk disease who have no conventional radiographic, clinical, or MR sagittal scout view evidence of spondylosis, myelopathy, or other non–disk related spine disease; (4) obvious disk herniations that correlate with clinically symptomatic sites and are visualized on sagittal T1WI; (5) evaluation of the larynx, oropharynx, and nasopharynx; and (6) screening for medullary bone disease or complete spinal block.

### T2-Weighted Images

T2-weighted images (T2WI) are used for detection of pathology when image contrast, not contour, is vital to diagnosis (Figs. 3–6*B* and 3–7*B*).[8] T2WI are often obtained with a multiecho protocol. The first echo utilizes a short TE (< 35 msec) and long TR (≥ 1000 msec) and is often referred to as a spin density, or proton density, N(H)WI (Fig. 3–7*A*). The second echo consists of both long TE and long TR and is more T2-weighted. Actually, heavily T2-weighted images require TR > 3000 and TE > 100, but this is often impractical. By convention, although it is not scientifically exact, T2WI in this section and under recommended protocols of the text refer to a multiecho sequence that includes both N(H)WI and the more T2-weighted second-echo images at each slice location.

T2WI are invaluable in screening and detection of intraxial pathology of the posterior fossa, supratentorial brain, and spine. T2WI often provide tissue contrast between pathology, brain or spinal cord, and hyperintense CSF (an "intrathecal-contrast" effect). However, T2WI signal intensity is also val-

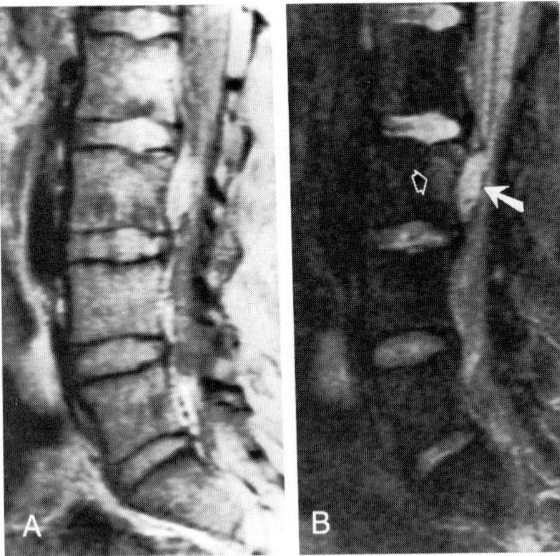


**Figure 3–7. Example of sagittal multiecho sequence (1.5 T).** *A*, N(H)WI (TR 800/TE 20). *B*, T2WI TR 1800/TE 80). The proton, or spin density–weighted, image N(H)WI minimizes the contribution of T1 and T2 relaxation. Therefore, only the density or concentration of hydrogen protons available to generate the MR signal is measured. However, T2WI accentuates differences in T2 proton relaxation between tissues. Both images demonstrate an extradural metastatic mass (arrow), but only T2WI shows adjacent skeletal signal alteration (clear arrow). Density-weighted images are identified by the following: (1) intermediate signal intensity of water-containing structures; (2) excellent image signal characteristics; (3) white matter appears gray, whereas gray matter appears white; and (4) fat-containing structures remain hyperintense. N(H)WI images are "anatomy" images and demonstrate contour but may "hide" contrast alterations.

uable in improving diagnostic specificity. At high, intermediate, and even low field strengths, hypointense, T2-dependent susceptibility effects allow diagnosis of acute hemorrhagic phenomena that may go undetected by CT. Comparison of abnormal signal intensities with known anatomic structures is often helpful on multiecho sequences. For example, a cyst (signal homogeneity, isointensity with CSF, and absence of T2WI edema) can be differentiated from epidermoid (inhomogeneously hyperintense relative to CSF) and cystic neoplasm (poorly matches CSF signal and circumferential, hyperintense T2WI edema). Similarly, the absence of circumferential T2WI edema on one margin of an isointense or hypointense mass suggests an extra-axial lesion, e.g., meningioma. T2WI MR is helpful in differentiating convexity or skull base meningiomas from gliomas or other extra-axial masses on axial CT. Some authors have recommended the acquisition of four or eight echoes for a given TR at each slice location of a multiecho T2WI. This procedure has been referred to as a pulse train, or an echo train (see Fig. 3–1*B*). It has been used to facilitate the T2-dependent contrast differences between cystic foci (hyperintense), tumor (intermediate), and edema (hyperintense). Similarly, the mere detection or absence of edema may be vital to a specific diagnosis, as in the differentiation of a calcified arteriovenous malformation from a low-grade glioma. This pulse-train strategy is only occasionally needed and can be used in body imaging to improve T2 calculation or signal intensity measurements. Many pathologists report a poor correlation between described CECT and MR glial tumor margins; therefore radiation ports are aimed at covering both tumor and edema imaging correlates. Multiplanar MR is superior to CECT in edema detection, localization, and radiation or surgical treatment planning.

## T1- and T2-Calculations and Calculated Images

T1 and T2 calculations and calculated images have application in body MR[9] but are not often used in craniospinal imaging owing to lack of specificity.[10–12] T2-relaxation ratios and signal intensity analyses are used to characterize liver lesions but provide little improvement in diagnostic specificity of CNS lesions or pathology.[13] A map of the relaxation times of a section are obtained by generating calculated images. A pixel-by-pixel representation of either T1 or T2 values of a tissue (T1 or T2 map) is converted to a gray or color scale. Unlike conventional acquired spin-echo images, increased signal intensity is assigned for prolonged T1 or T2 relaxation times. Therefore long T1 and T2 relaxations are assigned high signal intensities on calculated images, whereas in conventional images, short T1 and long T2 relaxations are assigned signal hyperintensity.[14] Occasionally, threshold levels may be set for structures that exhibit very long T1 and T2 relaxations (CSF) and may saturate the allotted gray scale. Thus such structures may be removed from the image and assigned absent signal. Slowly flowing blood that undergoes even-echo rephasing may appear quite hyperintense on conventional im-

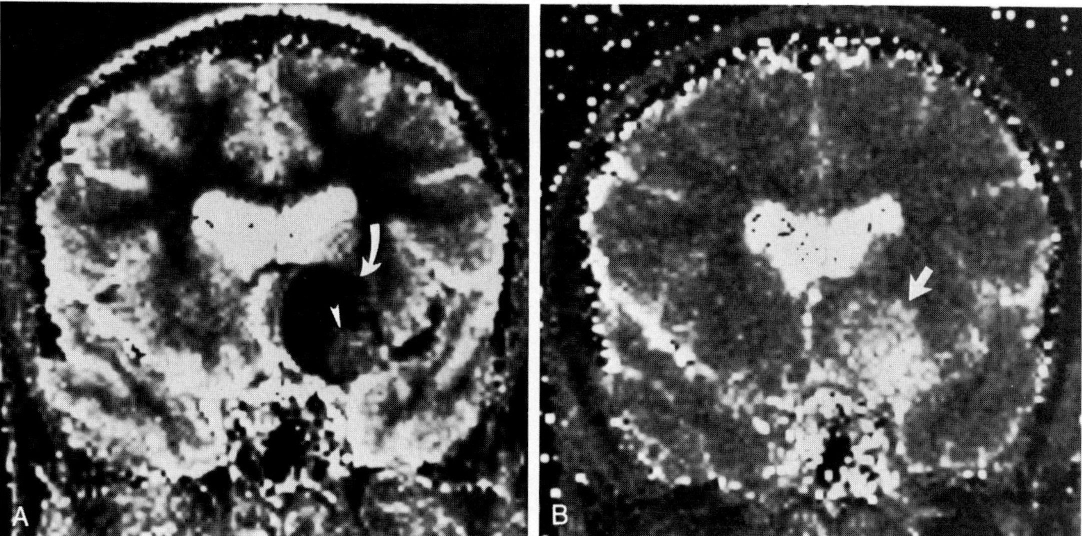


**Figure 3–8. Dermoid tumor with rupture and chemical meningitis (calculated images).** *A,* T1-calculated image. *B,* T2-calculated image. Pixel assignment in calculated images are made according to absolute relaxation values. Therefore, if T1 relaxation is short, pixel assignment is hypointense (curved arrow). If T2 relaxation is long or is a large value, pixel assignment is hyperintense (arrow). Visualization of intratumoral nodule (arrowhead) and intra-sylvian rupture are enhanced on T1-calculated image.

ages but is further highlighted in comparison with stationary tissue on calculated images. T2-calculated images may be useful in distinguishing flow phenomena (negative calculated values) from true vascular occlusion.[15, 16] This is discussed with greater detail in Chapter 2 of this text.

A T2 calculation and a T2-calculated image (Fig. 3–8*B*) is acquired by obtaining with at least two echoes in the same pulsing sequence, and constant TR with other parameters unchanged.[17, 18] In this manner, T2 calculation does not prolong imaging time but does involve postprocessing time. The accuracy of both T1 and T2 calculations is limited by the assumption that relaxation decays following an exponential curve.[19, 20] In fact, they are multiexponential, and accurate definition of such a curve requires at least a seven-point sample.[21] T2 calculation requires an eight-echo pulse train, which is available on some scanners. However, the acquisition of eight echoes limits the number of slices allotted in a given TR. T2-calculated images are occasionally used to evaluate vascular signal alterations[22] or to enhance contrast of lesions with short T2 relaxation (low signal intensity) when longer echoes are desired.[23] Such lesions yield poor SNR on heavily T2WI but may be more apparent when displayed in a T2-calculated fashion. T2-calculated images yield little additional information in the distinction of tumor and edema when compared with conventional spin-echo, multiecho images.

The acquisition of accurate T1 calculations and T1-calculated images (Fig. 3–8*A*) is extremely impractical. These images are obtained by varying the pulse-sequence interval or repetition time (TR), keeping all other parameters constant.[24, 25] Each TR requires a new image series or sequence; therefore accurate T1 measurements may require as many as eight different sequences, which is extremely time consuming.[26] Comparison of T1 relaxation times on different MR scanners is made more complex by the fact that T1 relaxation is frequency dependent and is prolonged at higher field strengths.[27]

## Extrapolated Images

Extrapolated images are a form of image synthesis[28, 29] in which construction from retrospective data allows rapid optimization of contrast by theoretically varying imaging parameters. First, source images with differing echo times and repetition times are acquired. Then computed images of tissue properties, including spin density and T1 and T2 relaxation, are formed using least square curve fit and the prior source images. Finally, synthesized images are generated with newly selected pulsing sequence parameters (new TR and TE). The computed images are formed, and the derived MR equations describe signal behavior.[30] In this manner, image contrast can be varied without the acquisition of an additional pulsing sequence. This time-saving technique has not met with widespread use and is accompanied by moderate SNR diminution. Conjugate image synthesis is discussed later, with fast-scan techniques (Chap. 4); it consists of acquisition of only one half of a data set and interpolation of the remaining portion. This technique attempts to symmetrize a data set, decreasing imaging time by one half but decreasing SNR.

### Multislice, Multiecho Techniques

Multislice, multiecho MR techniques (Fig. 3–7) have greatly improved the ability to image the craniospinal axis in reasonable time frames. The advantages and disadvantages of multiecho when compared with single-echo protocols have already been discussed. Multiple echoes allow both density and T2WI with differing contrasts to be obtained in one imaging sequence but with increased crosstalk artifact. Single-echo protocols allow acquisition of only one echo, but more slices are obtainable for a given TR in addition to minimal crosstalk artifact. Single-echo protocols are desirable when contour, not contrast, information is a prerequisite and long segments of anatomic coverage with gapless imaging are required.

We rarely limit our sequence acquisition to a single section in the craniospinal axis except when T2-calculated or electrocardiographic (ECG)-gated images are desired, an unusual occurrence. An important difference between single-section and multisection imaging is that both the 90° and 180° pulses are section selective in multislice protocols, whereas the 180° pulse stimulates the entire volume in single-section imaging.[31] This has several effects, not the least of which is alteration of T1 and T2 relaxation calculations and calculated images.[32]

It is important to understand that multisection acquisition actually takes place between successive 90° pulses at one section to stimulate subsequent sections. Thus TR, or repetition time, selection dictates the allowable number of sections using multislice technique. TR must exceed the number of sections desired times the longest echo time selected according to this formula:

$$TR > (\text{number of slices})\ (TEE' + \text{constant})$$

TEE′ represents E′ × TE1, in which E′ is the echo number and TE is the echo delay of the first echo chosen in milliseconds. The constant varies with each manufacturer and ranges from 13 to 16 milliseconds.

### Nonorthogonal Planes

Nonorthogonal, or oblique, planes with rotation around any one of these three orthogonal planes (Fig. 3–9) is possible with simultaneous application of any two of three orthogonal field gradients (slice selection, readout, or phase encoding).[33] Compound angulation is possible but complex, requiring simultaneous application of three gradient fields. Compound angulation and single imaging–plane offsets of greater value are accompanied by image degradation.[34] The methods of scan set-up for nonorthogonal imaging are available from each manufacturer. The clinical utility of this imaging option is now addressed.

Nonorthogonal imaging planes have been employed primarily in cardiovascular[35–39] or orthopedic[40] MR but have several craniospinal applications. Tangential visualization of obliquely oriented anatomic strucures, such as the orbits, eighth nerve complexes, carotid arteries, and sacrum, is possible. Nonorthogonal spine imaging has obvious advantages in eliminating partial volume effects in disk space evaluation.[41] A technique of multiple-angle, variable-interval, nonorthogonal MR (MAVIN)[42] had initially been developed, allowing selective angulation at each disk space level during the same acquisition series. We now routinely angle our axial spine sections through multiple disk space levels on our 1.5 T unit. Angled "paracoronal" sections may be useful in spinal cord or conus evaluation, particularly when pronounced scoliosis precludes long-segment sagittal cord visualization.[43] In addition, phase-related flow and swallowing artifacts are less likely to project over the cord in this plane.[44] Potential disadvantages of

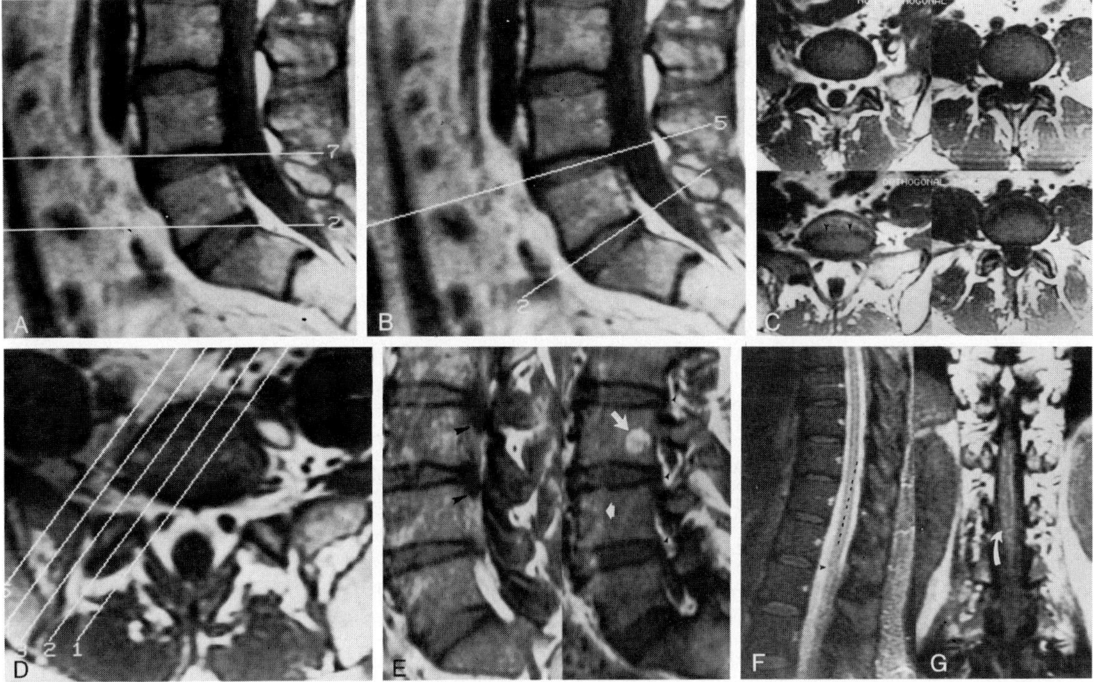

**Figure 3–9. Oblique (nonorthogonal) MR applications in the spine.** *A* and *B,* Sagittal T1WI scout images show levels and angle of axial *(A)* or para-axial *(B)* acquisition. With MR, unlike CT, any angle is possible, and multiple sections at three or four disk-space levels are obtainable on one imaging series. *C,* Comparison of nonorthogonal (top) and orthogonal (bottom) axial T1WI. Vertebral body and disk space are averaged (arrowheads) on orthogonal axial images. Artifact posteriorly on nonorthogonal MR results from crosstalk. *D,* Axial T1WI illustrates angle of foraminal parasagittal nonorthogonal sections. *E,* Oblique sagittal sections demonstrate nerve roots in the lateral recess (large arrowheads) and foramina (small arrowheads). The bright spot in vertebral body (arrow) is a normal variant. Phase artifact (short white arrow) from flow in the adjacent aorta projects parallel to the longitudinal spine axis. *F* and *G,* Conus (arrowhead) is identified on sagittal T2WI *(F).* Axis of the paracoronal section (black line) produces a frontal view of the conus on T1WI (curved arrow).

nonorthogonal sections include a predilection to wraparound artifact in the phase-encoding direction and crosstalk artifact.

## Three-Dimensional MR

Three-dimensional MR holds great promise in improving spatial resolution and providing thin and contiguous sections. Examinations and protocols described elsewhere primarily address two-dimensional (2D) Fourier transform multiecho images. Inner volume, or selective 3D, imaging excites a slab of tissue, and individual 3D slices are obtained by using additional phase encoding in the slice-selection direction. Since additional projections are necessary for slice definition, SNR improves with the square root of the number of slices.[45] Slices in the central portion of the slab do not experience the signal loss at the slice edge due to the RF pulse shape of 2D sections. Very thin (submillimeter) contiguous sections (Fig. 3–10) are achieved and can be reformatted in any orientation[46] since slice thickness is not limited by either the narrowness of RF bandwidth or the gradient strength, as in 2D methods. Therefore widened RF bandwidths allow very short TE scans despite thin slices. Since the slice number is independent of TR and SNR is maintained despite short TR in 3D imaging, very short TR T1WI, or fast-scan sequences, are well suited for this strategy.

Major 3D-imaging disadvantages include (1) scan time proportional to the slice number as well as to TR, number of y views, and excitation number and (2) increased motion sensitivity, resulting from two phase-encoded axes (y and slice selecting). The latter may be minimized with cardiac gating or flow-correction software. The former may be ameliorated by developing techniques such as hybrid echo planar[47] or multislab.[48] New fast-imaging pulse sequences such as

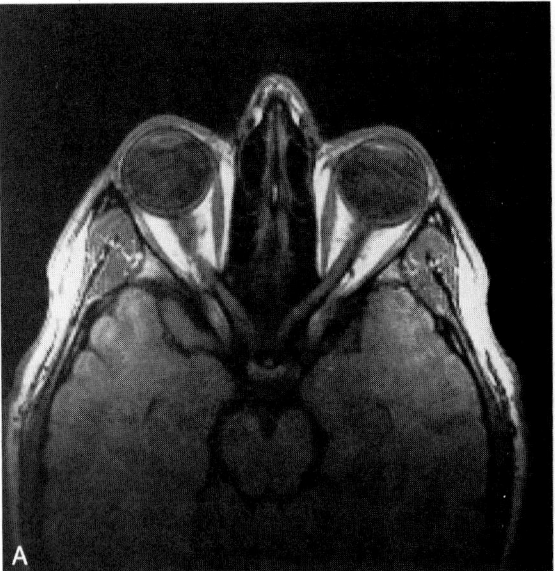


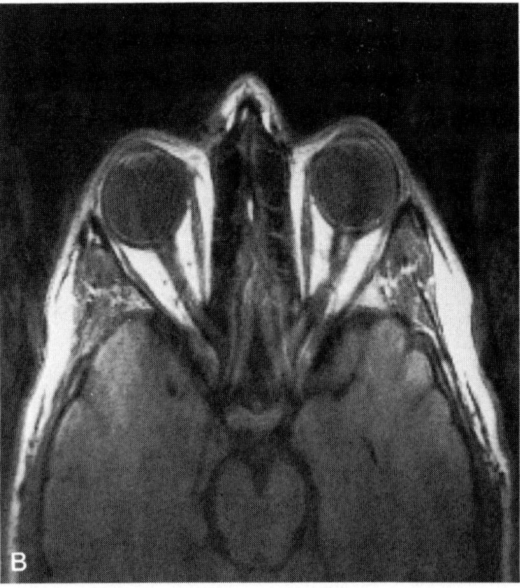


**Figure 3–10. Comparison of 3DFT and 2DFT MR.** *A,* 3D T1WI axial orbit: 1.6 mm gapless section; multislab selection. *B,* 2D T1WI axial orbit: 5-mm section with 2-mm gap. Although while the scanning times between these two techniques are approximated, both image sharpness and SNR are superior on the thinner section 3D image, proving that 3D imaging compensates for the loss in SNR of acquiring a very thin section. Furthermore, truly contiguous sections are possible with 3D without evident crosstalk or image degradation. (Courtesy of S. Harms, M.D.; Radiology Dept., Baylor University, Dallas, Texas.)

fast low-angle shot (FLASH),[49] stimulated echo acquisition mode (STEAM),[50] gradient-recalled acquisition steady state (GRASS), and rapid acquisition with relaxation enhancement (RARE)[51] take advantage of inherent 3D-image signal averaging. Since imaging time is prolonged when examining larger volumes, small FOV selections complement this technique and limit image noise from moving regions outside areas of interest. In addition, the problem of aliasing or wraparound is eliminated with the 3D strategy.

Areas of immediate craniospinal application for the 3D technique include the sella, internal auditory canal, pediatric spine,[52] and disk space evaluation.

### Surface Coils

Surface coils (SC) are radio frequency (RF) coils that demonstrate greater sensitivity to the tissue MR signal over a small specified volume. The RF coil, a loop of conducting material that acts as an inductive element in a resonance circuit, is commonly employed as a whole-volume coil (head or body). Whole-volume coils produce a homogeneous magnetic field over a large volume and are uniformly sensitive to tissue signal and noise in the excitation field. In contrast, the sensitivity of surface coils to both MR tissue signal and noise decreases in nonlinear fashion with increased distance or depth into a specified region.

The patient's thermal noise is the dominant noise source in coils used at field strengths less than 1 tesla (T). Since the body is a conducting medium, thermal noise is produced when randomly moving charge carriers in the body induce random coil currents. The body's conductivity, impedance, or both results in some dissipation of tissue MR signal as heat. At field strengths above 1 T, capacitance between the patient and coil becomes a greater noise determinant.[53] Dielectric losses occur when coil currents pass directly to ground through a patient, thus bypassing electronic detection. The impedance to current flowing via this path is inversely proportional to the current frequency and therefore to field strength. The noise explanations described above (patient conductivity, random charge carriers, and dielectric loss) help explain why some patients yield poor MR tissue signal regardless of patient size or body habitus.

Since surface coils that are used as both transmitter and receiver generate a nonuniform excitation field, most current designs employ a receive-only mode. The standard body coil functions as the transmitter. Decoupling the RF magnetic fields of body and surface coils is required to prevent transmission of RF power into the surface coil when the receive-only surface coil mode is employed.[54] This is achieved by orienting the coils (body and surface) so that their magnetic fields are orthogonal to one another or by electronic decoupling with crossed diodes. Coils that are not properly immobilized may lose their orthogonal orientation to the magnetic field with undesirable coupling to the body coil.

One measure of coil performance is the Q value, or quality factor. It describes the ratio of energy stored in the magnetic field induced by a coil to the thermal energy loss owing to resistance. Q is a measure of resistive dissipation in the coil circuit when a coil is empty or unloaded (uncoupled). Minimal energy is lost in the coil as heat when high unloaded Q exists. Therefore, high Q is often desirable but not always optimal. When a patient is placed within or under a coil, the Q falls as magnetic field energy is lost in the form of tissue resistance. This occurs when the MR signal from the patient "couples" with the coil (induces a current) and the induced field produced by current of a coil couples with the patient. The Q is now loaded.

Therefore coil Q is inversely proportional to power loss and diminishes with RF power dissipation in the conductive tissue examined (coupling). Coils with very high Q exhibit diminished coupling. A coil's quality factor is described by the equation

$$Q = (\text{frequency})/(a + b)\sqrt{\text{frequency}\ d\ (\text{frequency}^2)}$$

in which a is proportional to the coil material's (copper) DC resistivity, b is proportional to the coil's RF resistivity, and d corresponds to the degree of coil loading by the patient. SNR properties of a coil are proportional to the quality factor of the coil when loaded with a patient ($Q^L$).[55] Thus one can see that the frequency squared term (the effect of coil loading on the patient) dominates the above equation at higher frequencies ($>$ 0.3 T) and is a major determinant of both Q and SNR. The a and b terms in the above equation (representing noise due to coil materials) have been minimized by most manufacturers.

SNR properties of a coil are also directly proportional to coil-filling factor. Filling factor is the fraction of total RF magnetic flux falling within a volume of interest. Smaller surface coils possess higher filling factors.[56]

Surface coils couple strongly to specific regions of interest (ROI), so they are tuned and matched to body parts and individual patients. When large structures that fill its sensitive volume are imaged with a surface coil, tuning and matching each case is not essential, but a tuning "range" is established by the manufacturer. Conversely, when imaging small body parts where coupling is position sensitive, on-site tuning for each patient and body part is preferred.

Coil size selection depends on two variables: (1) size of a specified region to be covered and (2) its depth from the body's surface.[57] A general rule of thumb is that useful depth of tissue signal approximates 1 coil radius for planar shapes.[58–61] When objects are not inordinately deep, the smallest surface coil that can cover the area of interest should be used. Smaller coils may be designed with very high Q, reasonable coupling characteristics, and higher filling factors than large-diameter coils. More important, they are less sensitive to both thermal (incoherent) noise and coherent noise from vessel pulsation, respiration, or peristalsis.

Coil shape selection will depend on intrinsic coil characteristics, configuration of the area being evaluated, and its depth.[62] Coil characteristics are determined by the manufacturer. Since a planar coil's sensitive volume approximates the coil diameter or area in width and is one coil–radius deep,[63] structures with rectangular regions of interest such as the lumbar spine are imaged with rectangular coil geometry. Last, the depth of a specified area may dictate coil shape. Since small-radius planar configurations provide limited signal depth, planar coil configurations larger than the ROI may be required to attain these depths. This is contrary to one principle of surface coil imaging—that the smallest coil capable of imaging a specified ROI be employed. Large coils provide poorer coupling and SNR when attempting to image small regions of interest.[64] One potential compromise is the use of semicircular or

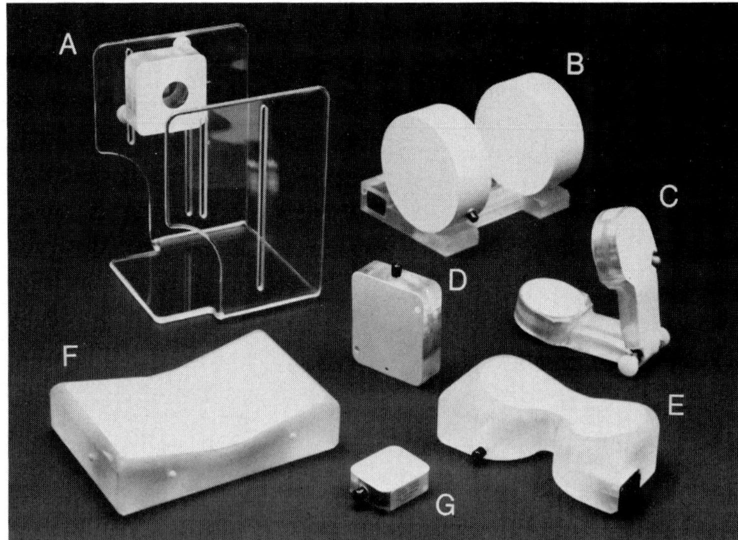


**Figure 3–11.** Several examples of surface (RF) coils. *A,* Head-holder with 3-inch temporomandibular joint coil; *B,* a tandem-pair coil for knee and face; *C,* an angled-pair for shoulder and extremities; *D,* an all-purpose 3-inch circular coil; *E,* a butterfly-shaped cervical spine coil; *F,* a butterfly-shaped lumbar spine coil; and *G,* 2-inch small parts, high Q coil. (Courtesy of L. Hutton, Medical Advances, Inc., Milwaukee, Wis.)

circumferential solenoid or loop gap resonator coils (Fig. 3–11).[65, 66] Since these configurations will elevate a patient above the scanning table, the size of the patient that will fit in the MR gantry is decreased. However, deep signal dropoff is minimized, especially when employing gradient magnification or small FOV with these designs.[67–69] Application in the neck and cervical spine is obvious.

Although phase-related motion artifacts are more apparent inside the FOV selected by a surface coil when compared with whole-volume counterparts, contribution of both coherent and incoherent noise outside the ROI is negligible. In contrast, whole-volume coils are sensitive to noise from the entire imaged planar volume. The superior SNR characteristics of surface coils allow selection of smaller FOV, reduced pixel sizes, and, therefore, higher spatial resolution. This may be implemented without the need for excessive numbers of averages, excitations, or repetitions. Furthermore, aliasing, or foldover, artifacts are minimized with surface coil receiving antennas. Last, phase-related or coherent noise effects projecting over an area of interest may be projected elsewhere or reduced by switching the orientations of phase and frequency gradient selection, flow or respiratory compensation technique, and ECG-gating.

## Chemical Shift Imaging

Chemical shift imaging has been extensively reviewed in the literature.[70] Different resonance frequencies between hydrogen protons in fat (methylene) and water are dependent on magnetic field strength. These different frequencies depend on the local chemical environment of each hydrogen proton. Chemical shifts are expressed in parts per million (ppm), since unlike resonance frequency, which is expressed in megahertz (MHz), this measurement does not depend on magnetic field strength.

Determination of the spatial distribution of nuclei with a specific resonance frequency, rather than imaging the entire resonance frequency spectrum (conventional MR acquisition), is called chemical shift imaging. Because the hydrogen MR spectrum of the human body consists of two major resonance peaks (fat and water), it is these two forms of hydrogen that are imaged most commonly. Through techniques that include selective saturation, selective excitation, image subtraction, and variation of time intervals between a 180° pulse and data acquisition, images displaying signal reflecting tissue hydrogen as only fat or only water (Fig. 3–12) can be obtained.[71–80]

Applications of this technique in the central nervous system are limited and may

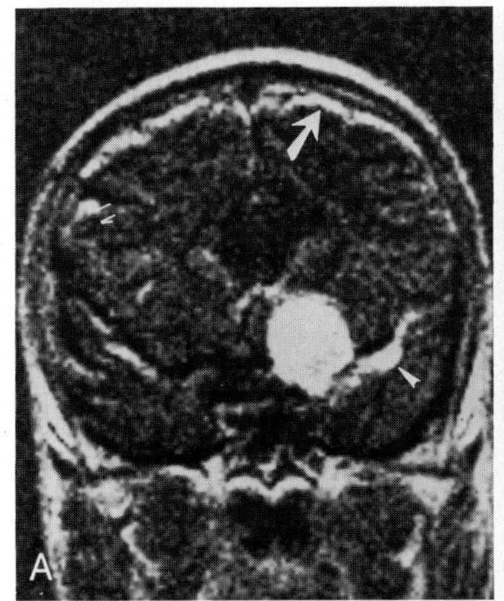

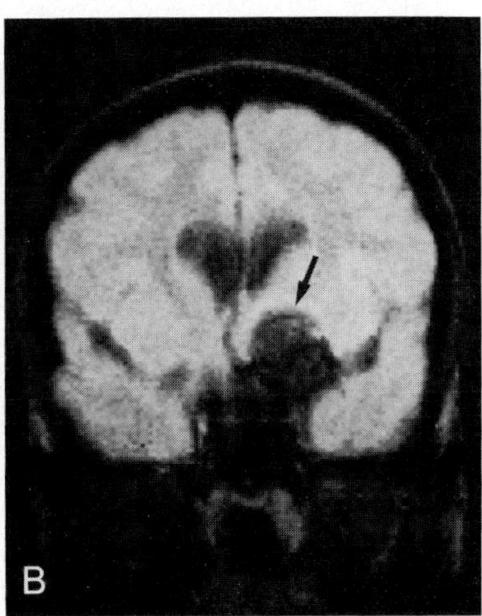


**Figure 3–12. A dermoid tumor with rupture and chemical meningitis (chemical shift images).** *A,* Coronal fat-only image. *B,* Coronal water-only image. Chemical shift images were performed at 0.35 T utilizing the method described by Dixon et al. (see text). Water image *(B)* shows lesion hypointensity (arrow) since "mobile" or bulk-phase water content is low. Fat-only image *(A)* makes the lesion, its Sylvian extension (arrowhead), and the hyperintense signal in the cerebral convexities (arrow) more conspicuous owing to chemical meningitis. Notice that on the water-only image, the CSF is not hyperintense, as would be expected. The bulk-phase water of CSF saturates the allotted gray scale and is thus incorrectly assigned a pixel intensity that is hypointense.

include selected cases of vertebral marrow evaluation for neoplasm.[81] Most uses have focused on detection of intrahepatic lesions and fatty liver replacement.[82–84] Rare intracranial cases in which chronic hemorrhagic lesions are difficult to distinguish from neoplasms with short T1 and long T2 relaxation (dermoid, craniopharyngioma) may be resolved with spectroscopic imaging.

Chemical shift imaging should not be confused with chemical shift artifact. Since the x, or read, gradient is frequency encoded, this gradient spreads frequencies according to position along the x gradient direction. Application of the read gradient to obtain a projection produces subtle separation of the fat and water proton components in the direction of the applied gradient. Depending upon pixel size, gradient strength, and field strength, two sets of image data may be formed that are shifted with respect to one another, resulting in edge artifacts.[85–87] Recognition of this chemical shift artifact on conventional spin-echo sequences in fat-containing lesions usually obviates performing actual chemical shift imaging and confirms the fat composition of a given lesion.

Magnetic susceptibility refers to the level of magnetization induced in a tissue by a polarizing field. The local field generated in a given tissue depends on this suceptibility as well as the experienced chemical shift effects and effects of intrinsic static polarizing field inhomogeneities. Contributions to susceptibility of a tissue may either enhance (paramagnetic effect) or decrease (diamagnetic effect) the local field. MR contrast agents take advantage of paramagnetic susceptibility effects (Fig. 3–13). Recently, frequency or phase maps that are corrected for polarizing field inhomogeneities have been constructed to view variations in tissue susceptibility with greater sensitivity.[88, 89] The shape of these maps and of the local field is altered by both chemical shift effect and tissue susceptibility. Therefore the brain is an ideal testing ground for such images since the contribution of lipid signal and brain metabolites are too low to affect image appearance.

Susceptibility mapping has focused on the paramagnetic contribution of species such as methemoglobin, deoxyhemoglobin, free $Fe^{3+}$, hemosiderin, and ferritin. Their paramagnetic contributions are governed by the formula

$$X_m = \frac{N m_o 2 u_o}{3kT}$$

in which $X_m$ is a tissue's molar susceptibility; $m_o$, its magnetic moment; N, the molecular unit volume concentration; and $u_o$, the magnetic permeability of free space. Close species apposition is required to initiate tissue susceptibility; therefore boundary effects between neighboring tissues dominate the appearance of a susceptibility map. Uncer-

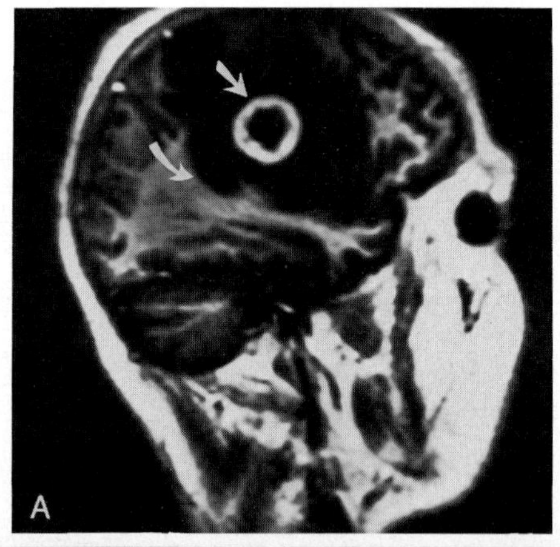


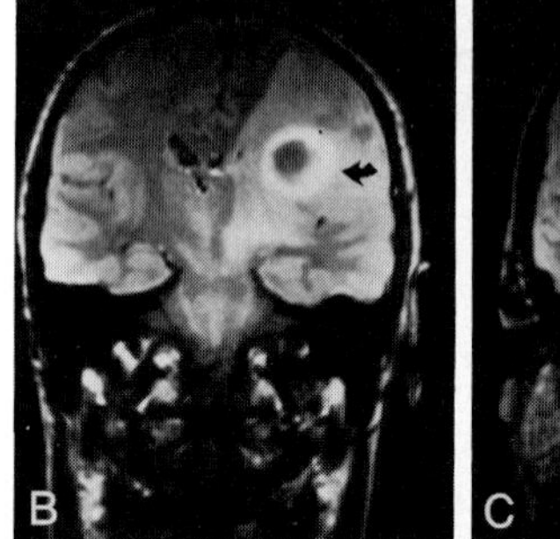


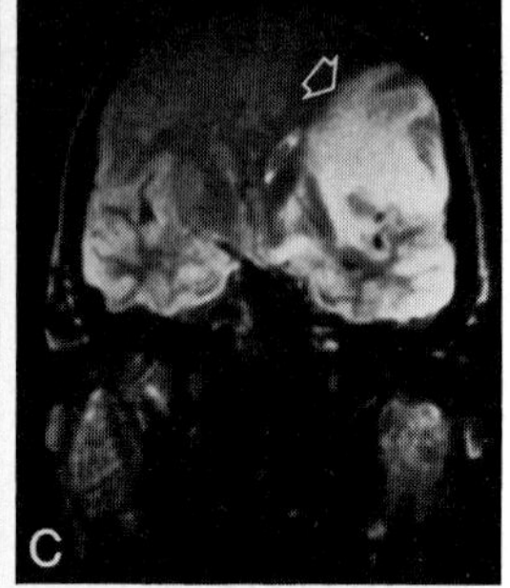


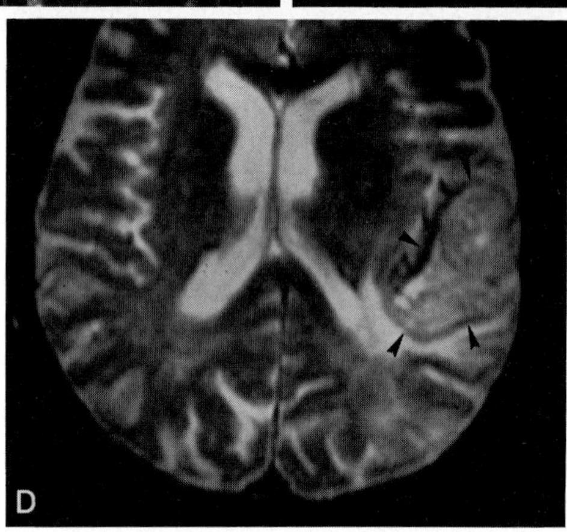


**Figure 3–13. Examples of inherent and iatrogenic paramagnetic susceptibility effects.** *A,* Sagittal inversion recovery T1WI (post-Gd-DTPA). *B,* Coronal N(H)WI (post–Gd-DTPA). *C,* Coronal N(H)WI (pre–Gd-DTPA). *D,* Axial noncontrast T2WI (1.5 T). Images *A–C* are performed on a patient with a brain abscess. T1 relaxation shortening and hyperintensity are apparent at the enhancing abscess rim (arrow) on sagittal T1WI. Edema is hypointense (curved arrow). Precontrast N(H)WI *(C)* demonstrates edema only (open arrow), but after contrast *(B),* wall enhancement is apparent (black arrow). Left temporal high-grade glioma from another patient *(D)* demonstrates circumferential T2* relaxation shortening, a field-dependent paramagnetic susceptibility effect due to peripheral hemosiderin deposition around the neoplasm (arrowheads). (A–C: Courtesy Runge V, M.D. New England Medical Center; Dept. of Radiology, Tufts University, Boston, Mass, with permission.)

tainty as to construction of the map is also due to the unpredictable shape of neighboring anatomic regions, their variable magnetic permeabilities, and the spatial distribution of paramagnetic species.

As expected, these paramagnetic components of hemorrhage are frequently observed in both the rim and central portion of hematomas. In addition, approximately one third of cerebral neoplasms (Fig. 3–13) may show circumferential rimlike susceptibility effects.[67] The clinical use of this technique is yet to be fully determined; however, distinction between "spontaneous intracerebral hematoma" and hemorrhagic neoplasm or early detection of hemorrhagic infarction and hematoma at lower field strengths is a potential application of susceptibility mapping.

## Motion Suppression

Respiratory, phase-related, and other forms of motion suppression have become an integral part of body MR and are useful in improving image quality in the spine (Fig. 3–14). Respiratory motion produces two types of image degradation: (1) ghosting and (2) blurring, or lack of sharpness owing to motion. Ghosting artifacts result when phase-encoding errors in the y direction produce spatial misregistration of signal acquired from moving structures. These coherent noise effects may occur in association with peristalsis, flowing blood, swallowing, or eye movement but are most prominent in the region of the anterior abdominal wall subcutaneous fat. Periodic phase-related signal smearing is accentuated at high field strengths, with increased TR, and with increased periodicity or depth of respiration. The periodicity of these effects is influenced by the ratio of repetition time to the respiratory cycle as well as the acquisition order of phase-encoding (y) views.

Actual gating to the respiratory cycle is impractical, since a twofold increase in imaging time does not decrease cardiovascular and peristaltic motion artifact. Currently, most scanners employ a technique that uses preliminary monitoring of the respiratory cycle. Subsequently, the proper order or direction of phase encoding (ROPE) that minimizes coherent noise effects is selected. No scan time prolongation occurs; however, a

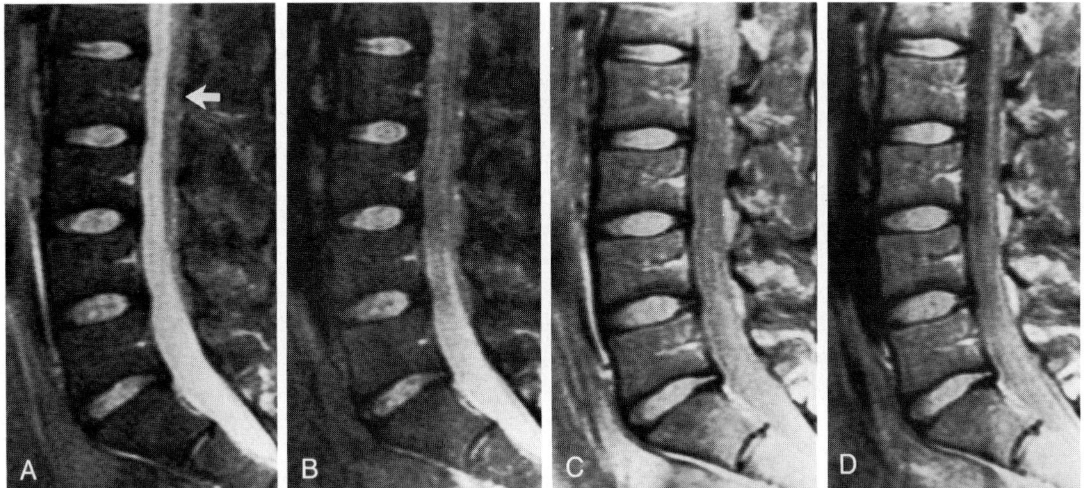


**Figure 3–14. Flow-compensation MR using gradient moment nulling.** *A,* Sagittal T2WI (flow-compensated). *B,* Sagittal T2WI (no flow-compensation). *C,* Sagittal N(H)WI (flow-compensated). *D,* Sagittal N(H)WI (no flow-compensation). With gradient moment nulling (flow compensation), the harmonic modulation, or oscillatory movement, of CSF is utilized to advantage. This rephasing event produces hyperintense CSF signal and accentuates differences between it and the cauda equina/conus medullaris (arrow). Note that on N(H)WI, the flow-compensated image has the opposite effect and minimizes contrast differences between nerve roots and CSF.

1-minute set-up time delay may be necessary. Another motion artifact suppression technique (MAST) involves modification of gradient fields during the evolution of the MR signal and may be used to improve craniospinal T2WI quality.

Other measures have been taken to minimize motion and phase-related artifacts. A simple solution involves a "phase-frequency swap." The phase and frequency planes of acquisition may be switched so that phase artifacts project in another direction from the specified area of interest. Another form of motion correction software is flow compensation. Flow compensation uses refocusing, or gradient moment nulling, and may produce intravascular signal hyperintensity but minimizes misregistration outside the vascular wall.[90, 91] Another method that compensates for flow and phase artifact relies on presaturation outside the area of interest utilizing 90° pulses.[92] This saturation technique is used in spine and body imaging in conjunction with respiratory compensation. Flow compensation may be used instead of saturation techniques, with or without ECG-gated MR when intramedullary cord disease is sought. Some centers routinely perform craniospinal imaging with MAST, ROPE, COPE, flow compensation, saturation techniques, cardiac and peripheral pulse gating, or combinations of these (see Appendix II). We routinely utilize flow compensation software on all our spine images, fast-scan sequences, and brain stem and foramen magnum evaluations when intravascular disease is not of primary concern. We now routinely use flow compensation on all our brain and posterior fossa T2WI examinations, provided that vasoarterial occlusive disease or venous thrombosis is not a diagnostic consideration. This markedly reduces coherent noise artifacts projecting over the brain stem and temporal lobes.

## Field Strength

Field strength considerations remain a subject of debate in the literature among manufacturers and radiologists. The biophysical aspects and potential hazards of scanning at high field strengths (>1.0 T) are subsequently addressed.

Magnetic field strength linearly increases the number of nuclei available for resonance; therefore the quantum energy emitted is also increased. The resulting MR signal (not SNR) is proportional to the magnetic field strength squared. Because of this fact, some have suggested superior cerebral lesion detection at high field as long as TR > T1 of a given tissue.[93] Ideally, for electrically lossy tissue samples, SNR increases linearly with mag-

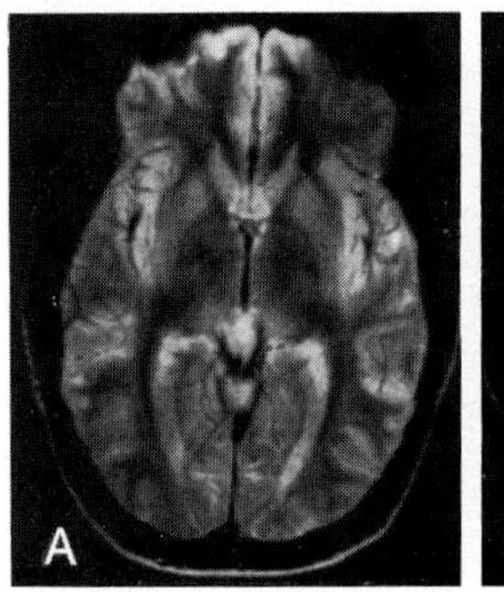

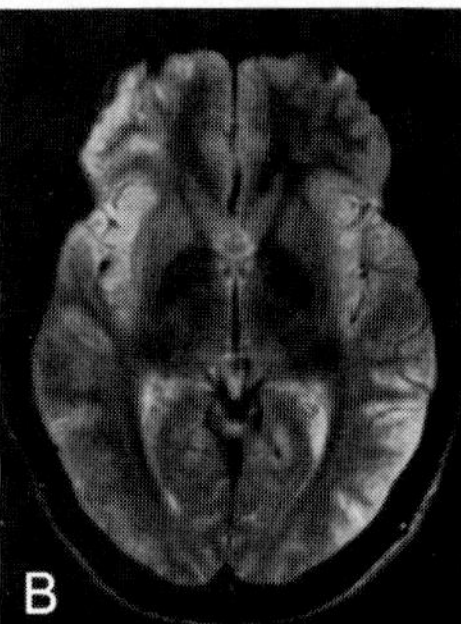

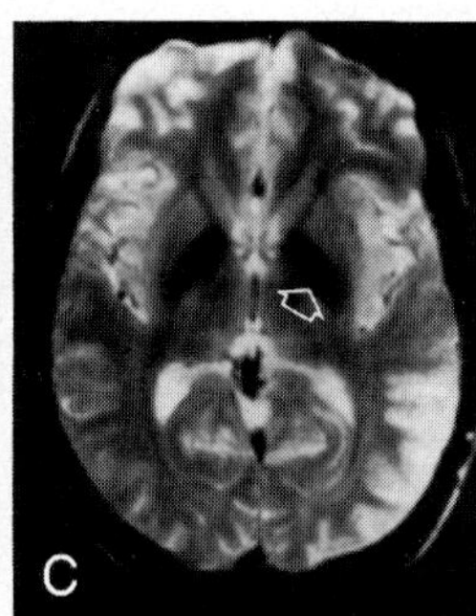


**Figure 3–15. A normal patient scanned at three field strengths.** *A,* T2WI (TR 2000/TE 80) (0.5 T). *B,* T2WI (TR 2000/TE 80) (1.0 T). *C,* T2WI (TR 2000/TE 80) (1.5 T). As the field strength increases, the image appears smoother and less noisy owing to improved signal-to-noise characteristics. Ferric iron, normally deposited in the globus pallidus with increasing age, becomes more apparent at high field strengths (arrow) owing to the T2-dependent proton relaxation enhancement that is accentuated at high field. This susceptibility effect is also normally seen in the reticular substantia nigra, the dentate nucleus of the cerebellum, and the red nucleus of adults.

netic field strength. Unfortunately, noise considerations are not always so predictable in vivo. As stated previously, thermal noise is the major noise determinant below 1 T, but above this level, capacitance between patient and coil allows currents to pass directly though a patient to ground, escaping electronic detection. This dielectric loss, patient conductivity, and random-charge carriers determine noise losses above 1 T. In addition, at higher resonance frequencies, RF antenna efficiency decreases. Still, there is a net SNR improvement at high field, but not as high as predicted experimentally. This SNR improvement does prove useful in the CNS when thin sections (< 3 mm) in the pituitary or cerebellopontine angle are desired.[94, 95] The ability of a scanner to obtain thin sections depends on magnetic gradient strength, not on the main magnetic field. The main magnetic field strength has no direct bearing on imaging time or patient throughput.[96]

The negative effect of increased field strength on scanner or operating costs and on shielding and site considerations is obvious. Three major factors adversely affect image appearance at increased field strengths: (1) exaggerated phase-shift artifacts, (2) chemical shift artifact, and (2) T1 relaxation time prolongation. Increased motion artifact in the phase-encoding direction owing to swallowing, blood flow, eye movement, or respiration can produce significant image degradation in the neck, spine, orbit, and, particularly, the abdomen. Chemical shift effect or pixel shift artifact is problematic in the abdomen[97] but not in the craniospinal axis, where signal from fat or methylene hydrogen is scant. However, relaxation time prolongation at high field is apparent in the CNS. For these reasons, lower field strengths appear better suited to abdominal MR imaging, while field strengths above 1 T provide equal or superior thin-section imaging in the CNS.

Those who perform MR examinations at multiple field strengths frequently observe diminished object and lesion contrast on T2WI at higher field strengths.[98] Although this does not actually obscure pathology, a tradeoff between diminished image contrast but improved SNR becomes a matter of individual preference. The reason for image contrast alterations[99] is partially explained by relaxation time effects.

At very low field strengths, T1 and T2 relaxations decrease with increased field. However, at magnetic strengths currently used for scanning (0.15 to 1.5 T), T1 relaxation increases and T2 relaxation is barely altered at progressively higher fields. In fact, T1 increases by 50% from 0.3 to 1.4 T,[100] and these T1 effects become more important for sequences in which TR is <2 T1. The resulting increase in T1 relaxation increases T1WI contrast. Since increased T1 relaxation decreases image signal intensity and there is still some T1 contribution on T2WI, image and lesion contrast is diminished on T2WI at higher fields.

An additional disadvantage of field-dependent T1-relaxation increase relates to the fact that optimal T1 tissue contrast occurs with longer TR at larger main magnetic fields.[101] Therefore the optimal T1 contrast images obtained with longer TR at high field strengths prolong scan time (TR ~ scan time).

### Health Effects and Hazards

Health effects and biophysical hazards of MR have been reviewed in the literature.[102, 103] Definitive adverse clinical effects of recurrent or chronic MR exposure are as yet unrecognized. Such MR effects may be subdivided into three categories, related to (1) static magnetic field, (2) gradient magnetic field, and (3) RF electromagnetic field. We initially address static field effects.

The Food and Drug Administration (FDA) has proposed a whole- or partial-body exposure of 2 T for static and 3 T/second for gradient magnetic fields. These recommendations are based on a lack of demonstrable mutagenic effect in mammalian cells, human cultured lymphocytes, and murine spermatogenesis.[104–108] However, at 2.5 T flowing blood in myocardial vessels generates potentials that approach the myocardial cellular depolarization threshold. One static field physiologic effect is the linear augmentation of T-wave amplitude on ECGs. This amplitude increase appears related to superimposition of low potentials on normal biopotentials. These low potentials are produced when a conductive fluid (blood) passes through a magnetic field.[109] No significant physiologic sequelae appear to occur with these T-wave alterations; however, they should not be confused with myocardial ischemia or potassium toxicity. These ECG changes revert to normal immediately upon cessation of field exposure. Since magnetic fields act on current paths, one might expect diminished nerve conduction velocity. Indeed, conduction velocity is decreased, but only by 10% at field strengths of 24 T.[110]

A potential adverse static field effect relates to cardiac pacemakers. At approximately 10 gauss (G), the pacemaker reed switch may be closed, resulting in conversion from a synchronous to an asynchronous mode.[111] Therefore this number has been divided by two (5-G line) as a safety factor for pacemaker wearers. At higher field strengths, complete pacemaker inhibition results. Other scan contraindications include implanted neurostimulators and ball-valve (pre-6000 Starr-Edwards) cardiac valvular prostheses. Some modern metallic and many porcine cardiac valve prostheses are safely scanned, even at 1.5 T.[112]

Concern that static field exposure may result in heating or deflection of implanted metal objects (hip prostheses, pessaries, metallic plates, intrauterine devices, Harrington's rods, tantalum mesh, and surgical wires or clips) is unfounded, even at 1.5 T.[113, 114] In fact, diagnostic images of disk spaces and spinal cord are obtainable in patients with Harrington's rod prostheses. We have successfully scanned patients with portacatheters, Swan-Ganz catheters, ventricular shunts, and metallic stapedectomy prostheses.[115] A more complete list of scannable and potentially harmful iatrogenic devices is presented in Tables 3–6 and 3–7.

When the safety of scanning a device is in question, the device is tested for ferromagnetic properties with a hand-held magnet or at the scanner gantry face. Ferromagnetic objects have a higher probability of experi-

**Table 3–6.** DEVICES SAFELY SCANNED WITH MR 1.5 TESLA

| |
|---|
| Surgical staples, metallic sutures—both in the acute and chronic postoperative state (clips include hemoclip tantalum and 316 L SS; Ligaclip tantalum and 316 L SS; Surgiclip M-9.5; SGIA SS) |
| Coronary artery washer/markers for bypass |
| Wires and wire sutures |
| Dentures |
| Portacatheters |
| Swan-Ganz catheters |
| Ventriculoatrial and ventriculoperitoneal shunts and Acc-Flow shunt connectors |
| Holter's shunt connector and valves |
| Holter-Rickham reservoir |
| Omaya reservoir |
| Central venous catheters |
| Harrington's rods |
| Some metallic cardiac valvular prostheses: Bjork-Shiley convexo-concave; Medtronic Hall; Starr-Edwards 2400 |
| Some porcine cardiac valvular prostheses: St. Jude's; Carpentier-Edwards |
| Silverstone carotid clamp |
| Dural venous metallic clips |
| Weck's clips |
| Orthopedic joint or extremity prostheses |
| Orthopedic nails, compression plates, screws |
| Dental amalgam and orthodontic braces |
| Stapedectomy prostheses (Xomed; Richards-McGee piston; Richards-Schuknecht; Richards Plasti-Pore; Richards Trapeze Platinum; Richards House-Type) |
| Tantalum and steel wire mesh |
| Metallic craniotomy plate |
| Pessaries and intrauterine devices (all types) |
| Radioactive seed implants and radium applicators |

**Table 3–7.** CONTRAINDICATIONS TO MR

Cardiac pacemaker
Neurostimulator (Tens unit)
Aneurysm clip circle of Willis
Insulin pump
Kimray-Greenfield filter or other metallic caval occlusive device
Metallic cardiac valve prostheses: Starr-Edwards 1260, 2320, 6000; Smelloff-Cutter; Bjork-Shiley universal spherical
Porcine cardiac valve prostheses: Hancock; Hall-Kaster; Lillehei-Kaster
Ball-valve type penile prostheses
Permanent hearing aid/cochlear implant 3M/House and 3M/Vienna
Unattachable Holter's monitor or defibrillator
Mandatory respiratory dependency
Imbedded shrapnel fragments or known metal worker
Persistent tremor or movement disorder (relative contraindication)
Inability to maintain supine or prone position (relative contraindication)
Mandatory continuous IVAC intravenous catheter system

**Table 3–8.** MAGNETIC INDUCED ANEURYSM CLIP TORQUE

| Undeflected | Moderate Deflection |
|---|---|
| Yasargil (all) | Mayfield (304 SS) |
| Sugita (Elgiloy) | Pivot (17-7PH) |
| Heifetz (Elgiloy) | Drake (301 SS) |
| Vari-angle Mcfadden (MP 35N) | **Marked Deflection** |
| **Minimal Deflection** | Heifetz (17-7PH) |
| | Vari-angle (17-7PH) |
| Scoville (EN58J) | Downs multipositional (17-7PH) |
| Drake (DR 20) | Sundt-Kees (17-7PH) |
| | Kapp (405 SS) |

*Source:* Adapted from Dujovny M, Kossowsky N, Kossowsky R, et al. Aneurysm clip motion during magnetic resonance imaging. Neurosurgery 17:543, 1985.

encing deflective forces and producing both geometric distortion and signal loss.[116] These effects are accentuated at higher field strengths and geometric distortion is exaggerated with fast-scanning techniques.

Ferromagnetic artifacts may occur at craniotomy or laminectomy sites in the absence of radiographically detectable metal density. This results from skeletal deposition of microscopic-sized drill bit fragments at the operative site. Nonferromagnetic metals may cause focal signal loss but not geometric distortion. Changing magnetic fields generating currents are the mechanism by which nonferromagnetic signal alterations occur. These alterations depend on gradient strength but not on the static magnetic field.

A group of patients in which caution is exercised when performing MR are those with shrapnel in their bodies or sheet metal workers. Occult intraocular ferromagnetic foreign bodies can produce blindness in this patient subset.[117] Similarly, subcutaneous shrapnel flakes or metal-containing eye makeup mixtures may produce pruritic erythematous reactions when patients are scanned.

Because of potential deflective forces, patients with intracranial aneurysm clips are not scanned. The deflection of these clips is directly related to their martensite content (Table 3–8). Although aneurysm clips containing no martensitic alloy exhibit no rotational force or ferromagnetic sensitivity and newer, nonradiopaque, nonmetallic clips are scannable,[18] we do not scan patients with any radiopaque intracranial aneurysm clips. Other metallic staples and clips not used for aneurysm clipping, even in the immediate postoperative period, have been scanned at our institution without complication. Patients with skin staples have been scanned at 1.5 T, and in one case, staple torque was visible. This deflective variability is likely related to staple bending and differing staple alloy contents. Therefore we recommend skin staple removal, if possible, before MR examination. The safety of filters, stents, and coils is less clear, but undeflected devices (Table 3–9) have been scanned safely at our institution at high field strengths (1.5 T) in vivo.

Gradient magnetic fields induce electrical currents according to Faraday's law. Electrical current in conductive biologic tissue could produce nerve, muscle, or cardiac depolarization.[119] Ventricular fibrillation may result from induced cardiac nerve currents. Fibrillation would depend on cell membrane sensitivity as well as the waveform, amplitude, repetition rate, and duration of the gradient field. The gradient field exposure limit assigned by the FDA (3 T/second) provides a wide safety margin. Skeletal muscle contraction or cutaneous sensory stimuli would certainly precede the occurrence of ventricular arrhythmia.[120] A sensitive physiologic response to gradient magnetic fields is the presence of visual light flashes due to magnetic retinal phosgene stimulation.[121] The threshold for this magnetophosgene effect is not reached with clinical MR.[122]

Owing to resistive effects, thermal tissue alterations are the most important sequelae of RF electromagnetic fields. We will not

**Table 3–9.** DEFLECTION OF INTRAVASCULAR STENTS, COILS, AND FILTERS AT LOW AND HIGH FIELD STRENGTHS

| |
|---|
| **Undeflected** |
| Greenfield filter (titanium) |
| Mobin-Uddin IVC umbrella/filter |
| Amplatz retrievable IVC filter |
| Cragg nitinol spiral IVC filter |
| Maass helical IVC filter |
| Maass helical endovascular stent |
| **Mildly Deflected (< 5 dynes × 10²)** |
| Greenfield filter (stainless steel) |
| Palmaz endovasdular stent |
| Gianturco embolization coil |
| **Markedly Deflected (> 15 dynes × 10²)** |
| Gunther retrievable ICV filter |
| Gianturco bird nest IVC filter |

*Source:* Adapted from Teitelbaum GP, Bradley WG, Klein BD. Radiology 166:657, 1988.

concern ourselves with athermal RF effects.[123] RF-related tissue heating is directly proportional to the square of the RF frequency. Since higher field strength increases this frequency, temperature elevations are more likely with more powerful static magnetic fields. The current FDA limitation of RF power deposition during MR corresponds to a whole-body average specific absorption rate (SAR) of 0.4 watt (W)/kg. A local (per gram of tissue) SAR of 2 W/kg was proposed by the National Radiological Protection Board (NRPB). The whole-body SAR limit was adopted from the American National Standards Institute (ANSI).[124] Their estimation was based on animal behavior alteration after 60 minutes of chronic 2450-MHz RF exposure, divided by a safety factor of 10.[125] Current peak whole-body SAR limitations imposed by the FDA approximate 8 W/kg.

Factors affecting the amount of RF thermal effect include (1) exposure duration, ambient conditions, and the patient's basic thermoregulatory system; (2) the type of RF-pulsing sequence employed; (3) the number of RF pulses in a sequence (scan type and number of echoes); (4) the pulse width; (5) TR; (6) patient size, or tissue mass; (7) the coil type (linear versus quadrature excitation); and (8) the size of the selected volume of interest as determined by FOV and slice thickness.[126] As expected, temperature elevation would be more apt to occur with small FOV, thin sections, long TR, and multiple RF-pulsed multiecho images, since this would deposit the most power in the smallest tissue volume.[127] Organs with the poorest heat dissipating capabilities are the orbit and the testes. Utilizing current operating parameters at 1.5 T, these systems are functioning well below the threshold of thermal damage in these organs.[128] In addition, only minimal systemic temperature alterations without significant heart rate, respiratory rate, or blood pressure alterations have been documented in vivo at 1.5 T.[129, 130] No clinical MR evaluations of patients with altered thermoregulatory physiology have been performed to date.

### *MR During Pregnancy*

MR during pregnancy has not yet been subject to any formal institutional recommendations. A review of 20 in vivo and in vitro studies has not shown any evidence of cytogenetic or developmental alteration.[131] Since the potential for thermal and athermal effects of chronic RF exposure exist, pregnant patients are not routinely scanned. However, if MR can solve the designated problem, any patient requiring a procedure that delivers ionizing radiation will undergo MR instead. This is particularly true in the craniospinal axis, where during pregnancy MR replaces CT.

## References


1. Wehrli FW, Macfall JR, Shutts D, et al. Mechanisms of contrast in MR imaging. J Comput Assist Tomogr 8:369, 1984.
2. Pykett IL, Buonanno FS, Brady TJ, et al. Techniques and approaches to proton NMR imaging of the head. Comput Radiol 7:1, 1983.
3. Ortendahl DA, Hylton N, Kaufman L, et al. Analytical tools for magnetic resonance imaging. Radiology 153:479, 1984.
4. Mitchell MR, Tarr RW, Conturo TE, et al. Spin echo technique selection: basic principles for choosing MRI pulse sequence timing intervals. Radiographics 6:245, 1986.
5. Crooks LE, Watts J, Hoenninger J, et al. Thin-section definition in magnetic resonance imaging. Radiology 154:463, 1985.
6. O'Donnell M, Adams WJ. Selective time-reversal pulses for NMR imaging. Magn Reson Imag 3:377, 1985.
7. James AE, Partain GL, Holland GN, et al. Nuclear magnetic resonance imaging: the current state. AJR 138:201, 1981.
8. Droege RF, Weiner SN, Rzeszotarski MS, et al. Nuclear magnetic resonance: a grey scale model for head images. Radiology 148:763, 1983.

9. Ferrucci JT. MR imaging of the liver. AJR 147:1103, 1983.
10. Darwin RH, Drayer BP, Riederer SJ, et al. T2 estimates in healthy and diseased brain tissue: A comparison using various MR pulse sequences. Radiology 160:375, 1986.
11. Araki T, Inouye T, Suzuki H, et al. Magnetic resonance imaging of brain tumors: measurement of T1. Radiology 150:95, 1984.
12. Bydder GM, Pennock JM, Steiner RE, et al. The NMR diagnosis of cerebral tumors. Magn Reson Med 1:5, 1984.
13. Komiyama M, Yagura H, Baba M, et al. MR imaging: possibility of tissue characterization of brain tumors using T1 and T2 values. AJNR 8:65, 1987.
14. Mills CM, Crooks LE, Kaufman L, et al. Cerebral abnormalities: use of calculated T1 and T2 magnetic resonance images for diagnosis. Radiology 150:87, 1984.
15. Kucharczyk W, Brant-Zawadski M, Lemme-Plaghos L, et al. MR technology: effect of even-echo rephasing on calculated T2 values and T2 images. Radiology 157:95, 1985.
16. von Schulthess GK, Augustiny N. Calculation of T2 values versus phase imaging for the distinction between flow and thrombus in MR imaging. Radiology 164:549, 1987.
17. Jackson JA, Schneiders NJ, Ford JJ, et al. Improvements in the clinical utility of calculated T2 images of the human brain. Magn Reson Imag 3:131, 1985.
18. Schneiders NJ, Post H, Brunner P, et al: Accurate T2 NMR images. Med Phys 10:642, 1983.
19. Kjos BO, Ehman RL, Brant-Zawadski, et al. Reproducibility of relaxation times and spin density calculated from routine MR imaging sequences: clinical study of the CNS. AJR 144:1165, 1985.
20. Kjos BO, Ehman RL, Brant-Zawadski M. Reproducibility of T1 and T2 relaxation times calculated from routine MR imaging sequences: phantom study. AJR 144:1157, 1985.
21. Pykett IL, Rosen BR, Buonanno FS, et al. Measurement of spin-lattice relaxation times in nuclear magnetic resonance imaging. Phys Med Biol 28:723, 1983.
22. Kaufman L, Crooks LE, Sheldon PE, et al. Evaluation of NMR imaging for detection and quantification of obstructions in vessels. Invest Radiol 17:554, 1982.
23. Feinberg DA, Mills CM, Posin JP, et al. Multiple spin-echo magnetic resonance imaging. Radiology 155:437, 1985.
24. Hardy CJ, Edelstein WA, Vatis D, et al. Calculated T1 images derived from a partial saturation-inversion recovery pulse sequence with adiabatic fast passage. Magn Reson Imag 3:107, 1985.
25. Inouye T, Araki T. A method for T1 relaxation time computed images. Magn Reson Med 1:179, 1984.
26. Evelhoch JL, Ackerman JJH. NMR T1 measurements in inhomogeneous $B_1$ with surface coils. J Magn Reson 53:52, 1983.
27. Ortendahl DA, Hylton N, Kaufman L, et al. Analytical tools for magnetic resonance imaging. Radiology 153:479, 1984.
28. Bobman SA, Riederer SJ, Lee JN, et al. Synthesized MR images: comparison with acquired images. Radiology 155:731, 1985.
29. Bobman SA, Riederer SJ, Lee JN, et al. Cerebral magnetic resonance image synthesis. AJNR 6:265, 1985.
30. Bobman SA, Riederer SJ, Lee JN, et al. Pulse sequence extrapolation with MR image synthesis. Radiology 159:253, 1986.
31. Kneeland JB, Knowles RJR, Cahill PT. Multi-section multi-echo pulse magnetic resonance techniques: optimization in a clinical setting. Radiology 155:159, 1985.
32. Rosen BR, Pykett IL, Brady TJ. Spin-lattice relaxation time measurements in two-dimensional nuclear magnetic resonance imaging: corrections for plane selection and pulse sequence. J Comput Assist Tomogr 8:195, 1984.
33. Huber DJ, Mueller E, Heubes P. Oblique magnetic resonance imaging of normal structures. AJR 145:843–846, 1985.
34. Slone RM, Buck LL, Fitzimmons JR. Varing gradient angles and offsets to optimize imaging planes in MR. Radiology 158:531, 1986.
35. Higgins CB, Stark D, McNamara M, et al. Multiplane magnetic resonance imaging of the heart and major vessels. AJR 142:661–667, 1984.
36. Dinsmore RE, Wismer GL, Levine RA, et al. Magnetic resonance imaging of the heart: positioning and gradient angle selection for optimal imaging planes. AJR 143:1135, 1984.
37. Murphy WA, Gutierrez FR, Levitt RG, et al. Oblique views of the heart by magnetic resonance imaging. Radiology 154:225, 1985.
38. Feiglin DH, George CR, MacIntyre WJ, et al. Gated cardiac magnetic resonance structural imaging: optimization by electronic structural axial rotation. Radiology 154:129, 1985.
39. Akins WE, Hill JA, Fitzsimmons JR, et al. Importance of imaging plane for magnetic resonance imaging of the normal left ventricle. Am J Cardiol 56:366, 1985.
40. King CL, Henkelman RM, Poon PY, et al. MR imaging of the normal knee. J Comput Assist Tomogr 8:1147, 1984.
41. Edelman RR, Shookimas GM, Stark DD, et al: High-resolution surface coil imaging of lumbar disk disease. AJR 144:1123, 1985.
42. Reicher MA, Lufkin RB, Smith S, et al. Multiple-angle variable-interval non-orthogonal MRI. AJR 147:363, 1986.
43. Gawehn J, Schroth G, Thron A. The value of paraxial slices in MR imaging of spinal cord disease. Neuroradiology 28:347, 1986.
44. Edelman RR, Stark DD, Saini S, et al. Oblique planes of section in MR imaging. Radiology 159:807, 1986.
45. Kumar A, Welti D, Ernst RR. NMR Fourier zeugmatography. J Magn Reson 18:69, 1975.
46. Totty WG, Vannier MW. Complex musculoskeletal anatomy: analysis using three-dimensional surface reconstruction. Radiology 150:173, 1984.
47. Haacke EM, Bearden FH, Clayton JR, et al. Reduction of MR imaging time by the hybrid fast-scan technique. Radiology 158:521, 1986.
48. Kramer DM, Compton RA, Yeung HN. A volume 3D analogues of 2D multislice or "multislab" MR imaging. In program of the Society of Magnetic Resonance in Medicine, London, Aug 19–23, 1985.

49. Frahm J, Haase A, Matthaei D. Technical note. Rapid three-dimensional MR imaging using the FLASH technique. J Comput Assist Tomogr 10:363, 1986.
50. Frahm J, Merboldt KD, Hanicke W, et al. Stimulated echo imaging. J Magn Reson 64:81, 1985.
51. Haase A, Frahm J. NMR imaging of spin-lattice relaxation using stimulated echoes. J Magn Reson 65:481, 1985.
52. Gallimore GW Jr, Harms SE. Selective three-dimensional MR imaging of the spine. J Comput Assist Tomogr 11:124, 1987.
53. Hoult DI, Lauterbaur PC. The sensitivity of the zeugmatographic experiment involving human samples. J Magn Reson 34:425, 1979.
54. Bendall MR, McKendry JM, Cresshull ID, et al. Active detune switch for complete sensitive volume localization in vivo spectroscopy using multiple RF coils and depth pulses. J Magn Reson 60:473, 1984.
55. Evelhoch JL, Crowley MG, Ackerman JH. Signal-to-noise optimization and observed volume localization with circular surface coils. J Magn Reson 56:110, 1984.
56. Haase A, Hanicke W, Frahn MJ. The influence of experimental parameters in surface coil NMR. J Magn Reson 56:401, 1984.
57. Bradley WG, Kortman KE, Crues JV. Central nervous system high resolution magnetic resonance imaging: effect of increasing spatial resolution on resolving power. Radiology 156:93, 1985.
58. Smyth WR. Static and Dynamic Electricity. New York, McGraw-Hill, 1968.
59. Edelman RR, McFarland E, Stark DD, et al. Surface coil MR imaging of abdominal viscera. Part I. Theory, technique, and initial results. Radiology 157:425, 1985.
60. Fitzsimmons JR, Thomas RG, Mancusco AA. Proton imaging with surface coils on a 0.15-T system. Magn Reson Med 2:180, 1985.
61. Schenck JF, Foster TH, Henkes JL, et al. High field surface coil MR imaging of localized anatomy. AJNR 6:181, 1985.
62. Bendall MR, Gordon RE. Depth and refocusing pulses designed for multiphase NMR with surface coils. J Magn Reson 53:565, 1983.
63. Fisher MR, Barker B, Amparo E, et al. MR imaging using specialized coils. Radiology 157:443, 1985.
64. Axel L. Surface coil magnetic resonance imaging. Comput Assist Tomogr 8:381, 1984.
65. Kneeland JB, Jesmanowicz A, Froncisz W, et al. High resolution MR imaging loop-gap resonators. Radiology 158:247, 1986.
66. Akins EW, Fitzsimmons JR, Mancuso AA, et al. Double loop receiver coil for MR imaging at 0.15 T. J Comput Assist Tomogr 10:1083, 1986.
67. Lufkin RB, Votruba J, Reicher M, et al. Solenoidal surface coils in magnetic resonance imaging. AJR 146:409, 1985.
68. Arakawa M, Cooks LE, McCarten B, et al. Comparison of saddle-shaped and solenoidal coils for magnetic resonance imaging. Radiology 154:227, 1985.
69. Kulkarni MV, Patton JA, Price RR. Technical considerations for the use of surface coils in MRI. AJR 147:373, 1986.
70. Brateman L. Chemical shift imaging: a review. AJR 146:971, 1986.
71. Bottomly PA, Foster TH, Leue TM. In vivo nuclear magnetic resonance chemical shift imaging by selective irradiation. Proc Natl Acad Sci USA 81:6856, 1984.
72. Rosen BR, Vedeen VJ, Brady TJ. Selective saturation NMR imaging. J Comput Assist Tomogr 8:813, 1984.
73. Dixon WT. Simple proton spectroscopic imaging. Radiology 153:189, 1984.
74. Hall LD, Sukumar S. A new image-processing method for NMR chemical microscopy. J Magn Reson 56:314, 1984.
75. Haase A, Frahm J. Multiple chemical-shift-selective NMR imaging using stimulated echoes. J Magn Reson 64:94, 1985.
76. Haase A, Frahm J, Hanicke W, et al. $^{1}$H NMR chemical shift selective (CHESS) imaging. Phys Med Biol 30:341, 1985.
77. Frahm J, Haase J, Hanicke W, et al. Chemical shift selective MR imaging using a whole-body magnet. Radiology 156:441, 1985.
78. Joeseph PM. A spin echo chemical shift MR imaging technique. J Comput Assist Tomogr 9:651, 1985.
79. Ordidge RJ, Van de Vyver FL. Re: separate water and fat MR images. Radiology 157:551, 1985.
80. Axel L, Glover G, Pelc N. Chemical-shift magnetic resonance imaging of two-line spectra by gradient reversal. Magn Reson Med 2:428, 1985.
81. Sepponen RE, Sipponen JT, Tanttu JI. A method for chemical shift imaging: demonstration of bone marrow involvement with proton chemical shift imaging. J Comput Assist Tomogr 8:585, 1984.
82. Lee JKT, Dixon WT, Ling D, et al. Fatty infiltration of the liver: demonstration by proton spectroscopic imaging. Radiology 153:195, 1984.
83. Rosen BR, Carter EA, Pykett IL, et al. Proton chemical shift imaging: an evaluation of its chemical potential using an in vivo fatty liver model. Radiology 154:469, 1985.
84. Heiken JP, Lee JKT, Dixon WT. Fatty infiltration of the liver: evaluation by proton spectroscopic imaging. Radiology 157:707, 1985.
85. Soila KP, Viamonte M Jr, Starewicz PM. Chemical shift misregistration effect in magnetic resonance imaging. Radiology 153:819, 1984.
86. Babcock EE, Brateman L, Weinreb JC, et al. Edge artifact in MR images: chemical shift effect. J Comput Assist Tomogr 9:252, 1985.
87. Dwyer AJ, Knop RH, Hoult DI. Frequency shift artifacts in MR imaging. J Comput Assist Tomogr 9:16, 1985.
88. Faul D, Arbart J, Margosian P. Quick measurement of magnetic field variations within the body. Radiology 153:303, 1984.
89. Young IR, Khenia S, Thomas DGT, et al. Clinical susceptibility mapping of the brain. J Comput Assist Tomogr 1:2, 1987.
90. Axel L, Morton D. MR flow imaging by velocity-compensated/uncompensated difference images. J Comput Assist Tomogr 11:31, 1987.
91. Gullberg GT, Wehri FW, Shimakawa A, Simons MA. MR vascular imaging with a fast gradient refocusing pulse sequence and reformatted images from transaxial sections. Radiology 165:241, 1987.
92. Felmlee JP, Ehman RL. Spatial presaturation: a method for suppressing flow artifacts and improving depiction of vascular anatomy in MR imaging. Radiology 164:559, 1987.

93. Bilaniuk LT, Zimmerman RA, Wehrli FW, et al. Cerebral magnetic resonance: comparison of high and low field strength imaging. Radiology 153:409, 1984.
94. Bilaniuk LT, Zimmerman RA, Wehrli FW, et al. High field MR imaging of pituitary lesions. Radiology 153:415, 1984.
95. Daniels DL, Herfkins R, Koehler PR, et al. Magnetic resonance imaging of the internal auditory canal. Radiology 151:105, 1984.
96. Crooks LE, Arakawa M, Hoenninger J, et al. Magnetic resonance imaging: effects on magnetic field strength. Radiology 151:127, 1984.
97. Barker B. Chemical shift artifact in nonspectroscopic NMR imaging (abstract). Presented at the third Annual Meeting of the Society of Magnetic Resonance in Medicine, New York, Aug 13–17, 1984.
98. Posin JP, Arakawa M, Crooks LE, et al. Hydrogen MR imaging of the head at 0.35 T and 0.7 T: effects of magnetic field strength. Radiology 157:679, 1985.
99. Kaufman L. NMR imaging techniques. Diagn Imag 4:28, 1982.
100. Wehrli FW, Macfall JR, Glover GH, et al. The dependence of nuclear magnetic resonance image contrast on intrinsic and pulse sequence timing parameters. Magn Reson Imag 2:3, 1983.
101. Ortendahl DA, Hylton NM, Kaufman L, et al. Analytical tools for magnetic resonance imaging. Radiology 153:479, 1984.
102. Budinger TF. Nuclear magnetic resonance (NMR) in vivo studies: Known thresholds for health effects. J Comput Assist Tomogr 5:800, 1981.
103. Adams DF. Biologic effects and potential hazards of nuclear magnetic imaging. Cardiovasc Intervent Radiol 8:260, 1986.
104. Schwartz JL, Crooks LE. NMR produces no observable mutations or cytotoxicity in mammalian cells. AJR 139:583, 1982.
105. Cooke P, Morris PG. The effects of NMR exposure on living organisms. II. A genetic study of human lymphocytes. Br J Radiol 54:622, 1984.
106. Wolff S, James TL, Young GB, et al. Magnetic resonance imaging: absence of in vitro cytogenetic damage. Radiology 155:163, 1985.
107. Withers HR, Mason KA, Davis CA. MR effect on murine spermatogenesis. Radiology 156:741, 1985.
108. Prasad N, Lotzova E, Thornby JI, et al. Effects of MR imaging on murine natural killer cell cytotoxicity. AJR 148:415, 1987.
109. Tenforde TS, Gaffey CT, Moer BR, et al. Cardiovascular alterations in *Macaca* monkeys exposed to stationary magnetic fields: experimental observations and theoretical analysis. Bioelectromagnetics 4:1, 1983.
110. Wikswo JP Jr, Barach JP. An estimate of the steady magnetic field strength required to influence nerve conduction. IEEE Trans Biomed Eng 27:722, 1980.
111. Pavlicek W, Geisinger M, Castle L, et al. The effects of nuclear magnetic resonance on patients with cardiac pacemaker. Radiology 147:149, 1983.
112. Soulen RL, Budinger TF, Higgins CB. Magnetic resonance imaging of prosthetic heart valves. Radiology 154:705, 1985.
113. Davis PL, Crooks L, Arakawa M, et al. Potential hazards in NMR imaging: heating effects of changing magnetic fields and RF fields on small metallic implants. AJR 137:857, 1981.
114. Laakman RW, Kaufman B, Han JS, et al. MR imaging in patients with metallic implants. Radiology 157:711, 1985.
115. Applebaum EL, Valvassori GE. Effects of magnetic resonance imaging fields on stapedectomy prostheses. Arch Otolaryngol 111:820, 1985.
116. New PFJ, Rosen BR, Brady TJ, et al. Potential hazards and artifacts of ferromagnetic and nonferromagnetic surgical and dental materials and devices in nucelar magnetic resonance. Radiology 147:139, 1983.
117. Kelly WM, Paglen PG, Pearson JA, et al. Ferromagnetism of intraocular foreign body causes unilateral blindness after MR study. AJNR 7:243, 1986.
118. Dujovny M, Kossowsky N, Kossowsky R, et al. Aneurysm clip motion during magnetic resonance imaging: in vivo experimental study with metallurgical factor analysis. Neurosurgery 17:543, 1985.
119. Bernhardt J. The direct influence of electromagnetic fields on nerve and muscle cells of man within the frequency range 1 Hz to 30 MHz. Radiat Environ Biophys 16:309, 1979.
120. Saunders RD, Smith H. Safety aspects of NMR clinical imaging. Br Med Bull 40:148, 1984.
121. Budinger TF. Thresholds for physiologic effects due to RF and magnetic fields used in NMR imaging. IEEE Trans Nucl Sci NS-26:2821, 1979.
122. Budinger TF. Nuclear magnetic resonance (NMR) in vivo studies: known thresholds for health effects. J Comput Assist Tomogr 5:800, 1981.
123. Adey WR. Tissue interactions with nonionizing electromagnetic fields. Physiol Rev 61:435, 1981.
124. American National Standards Institute (ANSI). Safety levels with respect to human exposures to radiofrequency electromagnetic fields. 300 HKz to 100 GKz. Silver Spring, Md., IEEE Press, 1982.
125. deLorge J. Disruption of behavior in mammals of three different sizes exposed to microwaves: extrapolation to larger mammals. In Proceedings of the 1978 Symposium on Electromagnetic Fields in Biological Systems. Ottawa, Canada, June 1978.
126. Glover GH, Hayes CE, Pelc NJ, et al. Comparison of linear and circular polarization of magnetic resonance imaging. J Magn Reson 64:255, 1985.
127. Bottomley PA, Redington RW, Edelstein WA, et al. Estimating radiofrequency power deposition in body NMR imaging. Magn Reson Med 2:336, 1985.
128. Shellock FG, Crues JV. Changes in corneal temperature produced by high-field magnetic resonance imaging: experience in 118 patients (abstract). Magn Reson Imag 4:95, 1986.
129. Shellock FG, Crues JV. Temperature, heart rate, and blood pressure changes associated with clinical MR imaging at 1.5 T. Radiology 163:259, 1987.
130. Kido DK, Morris TW, Erickson JL, et al. Physiologic changes during high field strength MR imaging. AJNR 8:263, 1987.
131. Shellock FG. Biological effects of MRI: a clean safety record so far. Diagn Imag Clin Med (February):96, 1987.

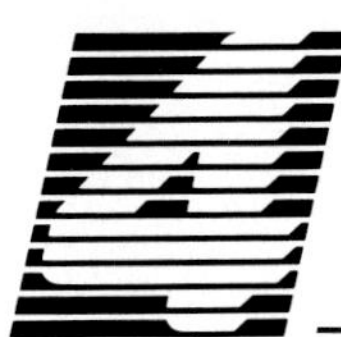

Charles E. Spritzer, M.D.
James MacFall, Ph.D.

# FAST-SCAN IMAGING

Magnetic resonance (MR) imaging, owing to its multiplanar capability and its high intrinsic contrast, is an excellent, noninvasive modality for evaluating the central nervous system. Unfortunately, MR imaging has several disadvantages. The initial capital outlay may be twice the cost of a state-of-the-art CT scanner, and long scanning times are necessary to adequately evaluate a patient. These deficiencies result in several secondary disadvantages, including poor throughput, lengthy patient backlogs, high cost per examination, patient discomfort as a result of long scanning times, and image degradation owing to both patient and physiologic motion.

Early, single-slice spin-echo techniques with a 2-second repetition time (TR), 256 phase encodings (NP), and two excitations per phase encoding (nex) yielded a T2-weighted image in 17 minutes. Incorporating a multislice acquisition and decreasing the nex to 1 improves the efficiency of the technique to about 25.6 seconds per slice, assuming that 20 slices are obtained. However, considering physiologic and patient motion, the total data collection interval is still long (approximately 8.5 minutes), resulting in respiratory, cardiac, and motion artifacts. If a single slice could be obtained within a few seconds, these artifacts would be reduced or eliminated.

Accordingly, to improve both image quality and patient throughput, patient scan time must be decreased. A large number of faster scanning techniques have been reported in the literature. This section provides a brief description of some of the more interesting ones.

## LIMITED FLIP ANGLE, GRADIENT REFOCUSED, PULSE SEQUENCES

The use of short repetition times reduces scanning time. For example, a single slice with a TR of 40 msec with nex of 1 and NP of 128 results in a 5-second scanning time. However, such a short TR in a typical spin-echo sequence results in a major signal loss due to saturation of the protons, since the flip angle for the excitation is usually fixed at 90°.

Limited flip angle (LFA) gradient refocused techniques address this problem by allowing the flip angle of the pulse sequence to be adjusted rather than fixed at 90°. This additional degree of freedom allows one to maximize the ratio of signal to background noise (SNR) for a given TR. In addition, it allows for adjustment of T1 and T2 weighting (tissue contrasts) without affecting scan time. Most LFA pulse sequences do not use a 180° radio frequency (RF) pulse to refocus the spins, as do spin-echo sequences. Elimination of that pulse may improve the SNR by allowing the selection of very short echo times and makes implementation of short repetition times possible. An additional benefit of using a small excitation pulse flip angle ($\alpha$) and eliminating the 180° RF pulse is reduced patient power deposition.

### Steady-State Free Precession

The idea of setting up a steady-state free precession (SSFP) is one of the earliest in NMR literature.[1] The concept naturally

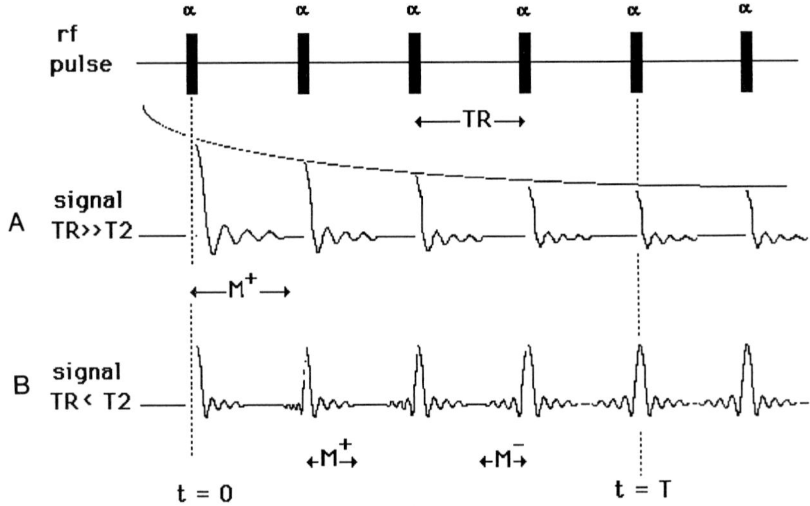


**Figure 4–1. A pulse sequence consisting of a series of RF pulses with flip angle alpha and a repetition time of TR.** The signal from one RF pulse to the next changes until steady state equilibrium is reached after a time T. *A,* For TR > T2, the signal $M^+$ is the free induction decay (FID) generated by the concomitant RF pulse. *B,* For TR < T2, both $M^+$ and $M^-$ signals are generated. The $M^-$ signal is a stimulated echo created by the two preceding alpha pulses.

arises when studying the signal from a sample that is subjected to a series of regularly spaced RF pulses that tilt the spins (protons) through angle α (Fig. 4–1*A*). Initially, the signal changes with each new RF pulse. After a time T > T1; however, the signals all appear to be identical. At this point, a steady state has been established. The term *free precession* refers to the fact that for the sequence in Figure 4–1, the signal is observed during a time in which no RF power is applied, i.e., the protons are free to precess only under the influence of the main magnetic field (and its inhomogeneities).

If the time between pulses (TR) is much longer than T2, it is relatively easy to show[2] that the amplitude of the signal just after the RF pulse is:

$$M^+(TR) = M_0 \frac{\sin(\alpha)\,(1 - \exp[-TR/T1])}{[1 - \cos(\alpha)\exp(-TR/T1)]} \qquad (1)$$

in which $M_0$ is the net magnetic moment vector at T = 0. Note that when α = 90°, Equation 1 reduces to the more familiar form:

$$M^+(TR) = M_0\,(1 - \exp[-TR/T1]) \qquad (2)$$

The value of α that gives the maximum signal in Equation 1 for a given T1 and TR is called the Ernst angle ($\alpha_E$). The Ernst angle, TR and T1, are related by the following:

$$\cos(\alpha_E) = \exp(-TR/T1) \qquad (3)$$

For very long pulse intervals (TR >> T1), the Ernst angle is 90°, which says that 90°

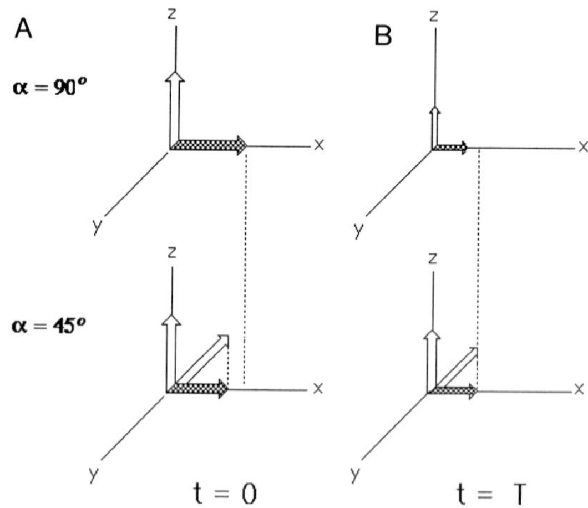


**Figure 4–2. Vector diagrams demonstrating how an SSFP partial flip angle may provide greater signal than a 90° flip angle.** *A,* At T = 0, the first 90° pulse produces a larger transverse magnetization and therefore more signal. *B,* At some time T, steady state is achieved, and for TR < TI, the longitudinal magnetization is greater for the 45° pulse than for the 90° pulse, because longitudinal recovery of magnetization is faster. This results in greater transverse magnetization.

pulses give the best SNR for long TR. For very rapid pulses (TR << T1), the Ernst angle tends toward small angles.

Figure 4–2 shows how the use of a small flip angle allows a larger value of longitudinal magnetization to exist than would be the case if the flip angle were 90° for TR < T1. With this large equilibrium value of the longitudinal magnetization, a small flip angle can produce a relatively large amount of transverse magnetization and detected signal.

When TR is less than or equal to T2, spin-spin relaxation effects cannot be ignored, because the SSFP signal is also influenced by the transverse magnetization precession rate during the interpulse interval. This rate of precession is dependent upon applied gradients, tissue chemical shift, and field inhomogeneities. If there is no precession (i.e., in the rotating frame of reference, $M^+$ (TR) always points along the x axis), the transverse magnetization reaches a steady-state value $M^+$, which is dependent upon $\alpha$, TR, T1, and T2. If there is 180° of precession between the $\alpha$ pulses, then the transverse magnetization alternates between some value $M^+$ on odd number pulses and 0 on even number pulses, yielding an average value of $M^+/2$ (Fig. 4–3). Other angles of precession result in values between these two extremes. Hence for flip angles smaller than the Ernst angle, small precession angles give larger signals. The situation is reversed for large flip angles since the protons not precessing become saturated, resulting in less longitudinal magnetization and therefore in less signal. The protons undergoing 180° precession do not become saturated since every other RF pulse restores longitudinal magnetization by driving the protons to the z axis.

Since both flip angle and the amount of precession that occurs between RF pulses

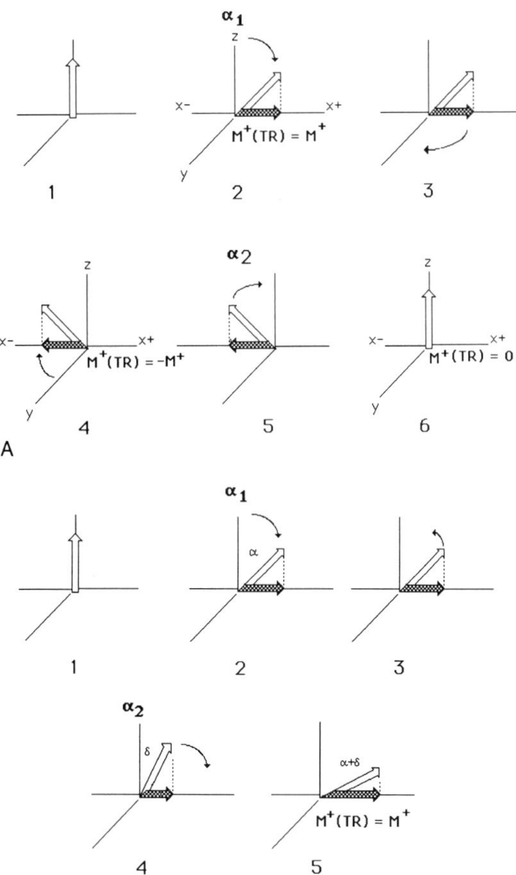


**Figure 4–3. Effect of precession on steady state signal as seen in the rotating frame of reference for small flip angles.** If protons are off resonance, there will be precession. *A*, 180° precession. Following the first RF pulse, transverse magnetization [$M^+$ (TR)] is oriented along the x axis and equals $M^+$ (2). The transverse magnetization then precesses 180° (4) and is oriented along the −x axis. The second RF pulse (5) then drives the magnetization to the longitudinal magnetization (z) axis, resulting in 0 transverse magnetization (6). This process repeats itself, with every odd pulse producing a net $M^+$ value and every even pulse producing 0 transverse magnetization, yielding an average value of $M^+/2$.

*B*, Zero = degree precession. The initial RF pulse rotates the net magnetization alpha degrees (2). During the interval between the first and second RF pulses, there is some recovery of longitudinal magnetization, so that the apparent angle between the magnetic moment vector and z axis is delta. The second RF pulse tilts the protons alpha degrees from their present position (4), so that the net magnetization vector is alpha plus delta degrees from the z axis (5). This process repeats itself until the amount of longitudinal recovery balances the effects of the RF pulse.

affect SSFP, two contrast regimes exist. One involves the steady state for the longitudinal magnetization, in which repetition times are long enough so that the transverse magnetization does not participate in the SSFP. This is thus a T1 and spin density regime. The other regime occurs with short repetition times and involves both the longitudinal and transverse magnetizations and depends on tissue T2 as well as T1 and spin density. Lengthening TE adds T2* information in either contrast regime.

## Imaging Considerations—FLASH, GRASS, FISP

Imaging with SSFP requires that magnetic field gradient pulses be incorporated into the pulse sequence. These gradients obviously can affect the amount of precession of a given spin between pulses since the gradient may be considered as a huge transient inhomogeneity in the main magnetic field. The major differences between fast-scan sequences such as fast low angle shot (FLASH),[2] gradient-recalled acquisition in the steady state (GRASS),[3] and fast imaging with steady precession (FISP)[4] are due to the details of the arrangement of the imaging gradients to affect the spin equilibrium.

Consider the effect of applying a single gradient pulse between the RF pulses of the SSFP sequence shown in Figure 4–1. With the gradient turned off, there is essentially no precession, and the signal is maximized at a small flip angle as previously described.

With the application of even very small gradients, the signal level drops rapidly for small flip angles, since the gradients cause precession, breaking up the SSFP. This is the reason such gradients are often called "spoiler" gradients. For larger flip angles, the opposite effect occurs. Signal can be increased with the presence of gradients, since some of the spins precess enough to create a large longitudinal equilibrium, whereas for small precession angles, the equilibrium signal is small, since the longitudinal magnetization steady state created is also small (Fig. 4–4).

One conclusion to be drawn from this discussion is that it is difficult to "spoil" the SSFP with the application of constant linear gradients. Such gradients simply create a new equilibrium that is optimized at a different flip angle. Since the equilibrium

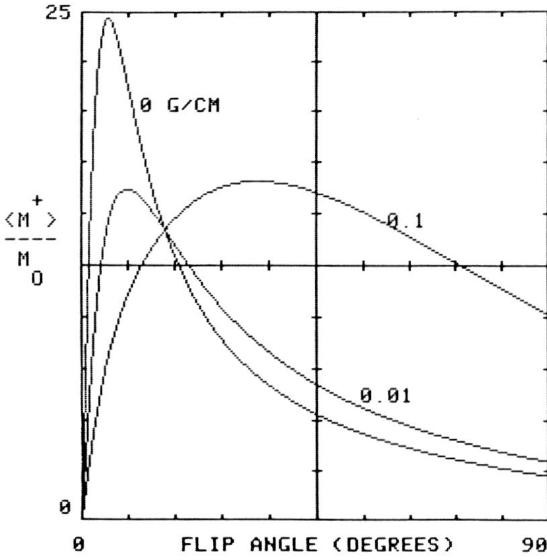


**Figure 4–4. Dependence of the signal $M^+$ on flip angle alpha.** Assuming no precession, signal is maximized for small flip angles when no gradients are applied. With larger flip angles, signal decreases due to saturation effects. With the application of a small gradient (0.01 G/cm), precession occurs, breaking up SSFP. This results in signal loss. The opposite is true with the application of larger gradients (0.1 G/cm). Signal is increased with larger flip angles, since precession results in a large longitudinal equilibrium.

value also depends on T1 and T2, the addition of various constant gradients to a sequence will alter the optimum flip angle and the image contrast, making it difficult to draw detailed conclusions about image contrast from the classic equations.[5-8]

The simplest such imaging sequence, FLASH, is shown in Figure 4–5A. The slice and read-out gradients are always the same, whereas the phase-encoding gradient varies throughout the sequence. The echo is refocused at the center of the read-out gradient, which means that the latter half of this gradient acts as a spoiler gradient. Also, the leading part of the slice selection gradient (before the start of the RF pulse) tends to act as a spoiler in the slice direction. Finally, the phase-encoding gradient acts as a variable spoiler gradient throughout the sequence. Hence FLASH attempts to spoil the SSFP on all of the gradient directions. This circumstance originally led to consideration of FLASH as a T1-weighted sequence since the T2 weighting owing to the SSFP should be disrupted by the spoiler gradients.

FLASH suffers from an artifact that appears as a narrow central band of higher signal (Fig. 4–6) for large flip angles when TR < T2. Application of only the read-out

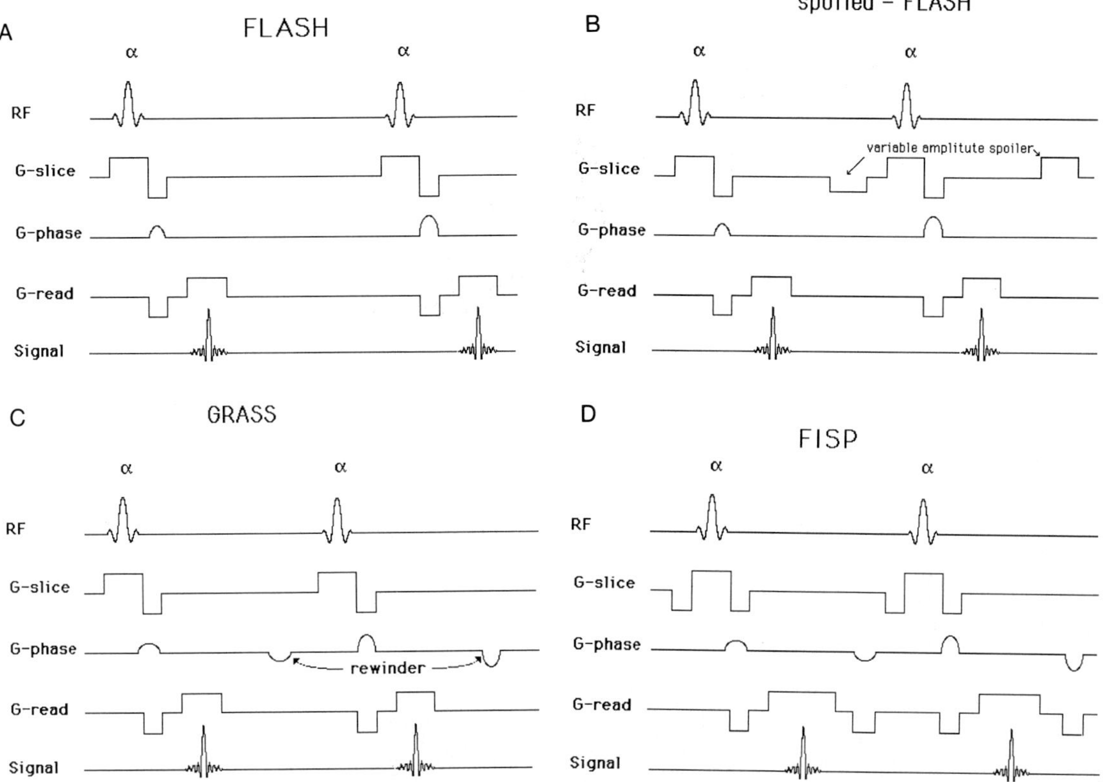


**Figure 4–5. *A*, FLASH, *B*, spoiled-FLASH, *C*, GRASS, and *D*, FISP pulse diagrams.** The variable phase–encoding gradient and the second half of the read-out gradient disrupt steady state free precession in the FLASH sequence. A variable amplitude spoiler further disrupts SSFP in the spoiled FLASH sequence. In the GRASS sequence, an additional gradient pulse in the phase-encoding direction reverses, or "rewinds," the disruption of SSFP caused by the phase-encoding gradient, making it more T2 weighted than the FLASH sequence for short TR. In the FISP sequence, rewinding gradient pulses are applied on all three axes in an attempt to maintain SSFP.

and slice-selection gradients would result in SSFP since these are constant linear gradients. However, the variation of the phase-encoding gradient necessary to produce position information disrupts the SSFP equilibrium in the peripheral regions of the slice, resulting in less signal. In the center of the image, the phase-encoding gradient strengths are small and do not disrupt the SSFP, resulting in more signal. Averaging appears to lessen the effect of this artifact.

A second broad central artifact associated with view-to-view phase differences of residual magnetization has also been described.[7] Although not as prominent as the artifacts already mentioned, it is relatively insensitive to averaging.

Haase and associates[9] modified the FLASH sequence by introducing a time-varying spoiler on the slice-selection axis in order to effectively break up the SSFP without creating effects that vary in the imaging plane. This sequence is termed *spoiled FLASH* (Fig. 4–5*B*).

GRASS is another technique developed at about the same time as FLASH (Fig. 4–5*C*).[3] The application of an additional gradient pulse in the phase-encoding direction distinguishes GRASS from FLASH. This pulse is known as a "rewinder," and its purpose is to reverse, or rewind, the disruption of SSFP caused by the phase-encoding gradient. Maintenance of the transverse steady state leads to GRASS being more T2 weighted than FLASH. In fact, the signal dependence reflects the ratio T1/T2.[3] The rewinder pulse also eliminates the central artifact seen on FLASH images.

Finally, a third approach is provided by the FISP pulse sequence (Fig. 4–5*D*).[4] FISP employs additional gradient pulses on all gradient axes to reverse the effects of all the imaging gradients. In this manner, an attempt is made to keep all of the magnetiza-

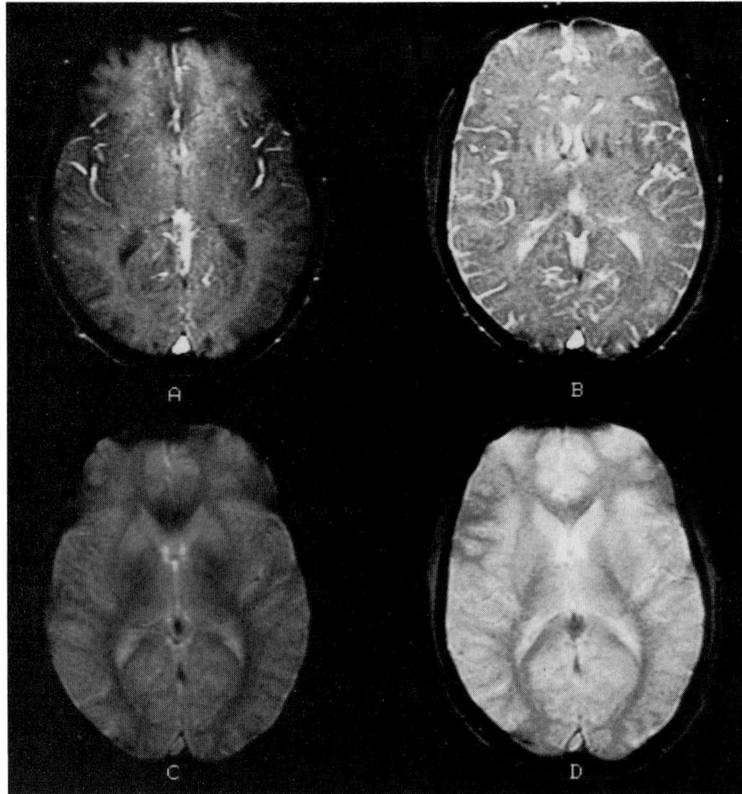


**Figure 4–6. FLASH and GRASS images of a normal volunteer.** In FLASH *(A)* and GRASS *(B)* images TR = 33 msec, TE = 14 msec, and alpha = 70°. CSF appears dark on the FLASH image owing to disruption of SSFP. The rewinder pulse on the GRASS image maintains SSFP, resulting in bright CSF signal. With TR = 200 msec, TE = 30 msec, and alpha = 10°, both the FLASH *(C)* and GRASS *(D)* images show CSF as high signal owing to T2* effects. Note the peripheral areas of decreased signal on the FLASH images, most apparent in *A*. Variation of the phase-encoding gradient disrupts SSFP equilibrium in these regions, resulting in less signal. Two nex, 256 × 128 matrix, 10-mm thickness.

tion aligned so that a "true" SSFP (presumably with no precession between RF pulses) is established. In practice there is enough inhomogeneity owing to the main magnetic field, the chemical shift (fat-water), or the gradient eddy currents, so that even with balanced gradients, the spins precess enough to change the SSFP away from that predicted by the classic equations.

### Gradient-Echo Effects

The use of a gradient echo introduces effects that are not usually observed with spin echoes. As the echo time increases, signal is lost at a rate characterized by T2*, rather than by T2. T2* is a combination of the actual tissue T2 and the dephasing effects of "local" static field inhomogeneities:[10]

$$1/T2^* = 1/T2 + \pi \Delta v$$

in which $\Delta v$ is the local magnetic field inhomogeneity in Hz. Note that the SSFP determining the longitudinal magnetization still depends on T2. It is only the echo amplitude that is reduced at a rate of T2* owing to the rapid dephasing in the local field inhomogeneity. For example, Equation 1 may be modified to include a T2* term:

$$M^+ (TR) = M_0 \frac{\sin(\alpha)\,(1 - \exp[-TR/T1])}{[1 - \cos(\alpha)\,\exp(-TR/T1)]} \exp(-TE/T2^*) \quad (4)$$

Since T2* is always shorter than T2, this effect leads to low signals and susceptibility effects near regions of high inhomogeneity such as metallic clips, tissue-air interfaces, and areas of hemosiderin deposition.

Another effect resulting from using a gradient echo is the appearance of a chemical shift artifact "of the second kind." The first type of chemical shift artifact is the familiar one in which pixels that contain fat are shifted from those that contain water by a spatial amount equivalent to the frequency difference of the fat and water. A second kind of chemical shift artifact results from the fact that the phase difference of fat and water changes constantly from the moment

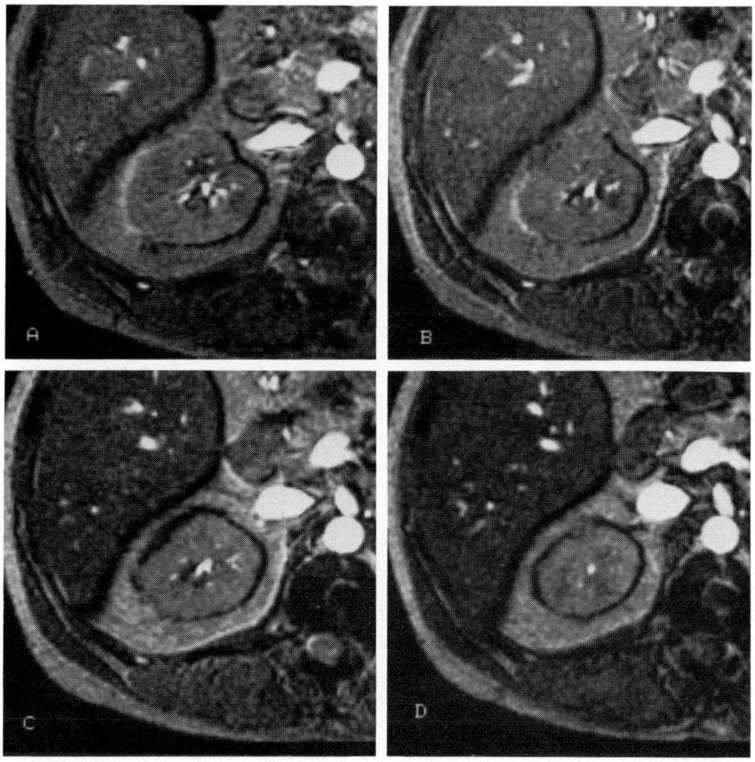

A B C D

**Figure 4–7. Chemical shift artifact "of the second kind."** GRASS images through the right kidney with TR = 33 msec, alpha = 30 degrees, and TE varying by one millisecond intervals from 13 msec *(A)* to 16 msec *(B)*. The chemical shift artifact is seen as a band of high signal to the right of the kidney on the in-phase image *(A)*. In the phase-opposed image *(D)*, this band turns dark, since fat and water are 180° out-of-phase, which cancels signal.

of excitation.[11] With spin-echo imaging, the RF-refocused echo causes the fat and water to be nearly "in phase" during the echo acquisition. With gradient echoes, however, the fat and water have a phase relation that is a function of TE. At 1.5 T, the fat and water are in phase at TE = 4.5 msec and every 4.5 msec thereafter. At other field strengths, the times differ, depending upon the actual fat-water frequency difference. It is therefore possible to make an image with the fat and water in phase or 180° out of phase (phase opposed), by imaging at TE = 13.5 msec (in phase) or at TE = 15.75 msec (phase opposed). Pixels that contain both fat and water have lower signals when phase opposed than when in phase (Fig. 4–7). This phenomenon may prove diagnostically useful in some cases and is analogous to the chemical shift imaging technique described by Dixon.[12]

## Contrast Guidelines

Clinically, it is important to know how to generate images that are T1, T2, or density weighted. Broadly speaking, T1-weighted images are useful for delineating anatomy, whereas T2-weighted images are useful for showing pathology and edema and for converting cerebrospinal fluid (CSF) to high signal, producing an "MRI myelogram".[13] Essentially, the parameters available to affect contrast for LFA are TR, TE, and $\alpha$. When TR is short enough that the transverse magnetization participates in the SSFP, the imaging gradients may also exert an influence on contrast.

Consider first the case in which TR >> T2: FLASH, FISP, and GRASS sequences have similar contrast behavior since the transverse magnetization does not participate in the SSFP. Practically, this happens when TR > 100 msec, since most normal T2 values are less than this. The exception is for CSF which has T2 values nearer 300 msec. In this event, the signals and contrasts can be modeled by using Equation 4. For large flip angles (from 60° to 90°), a T1-weighted image can be formed as long as TE is kept short (TE < 15 msec). The amount of T1 weighting can be varied by changing $\alpha$. Figure 4–8 shows the signal dependence

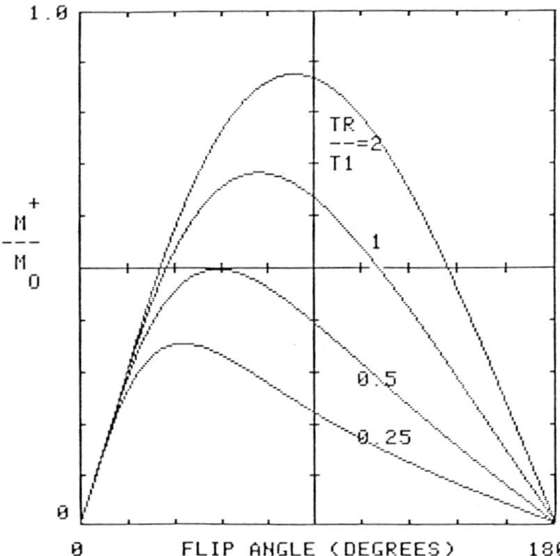


**Figure 4–8. Dependence of signal upon flip angles, alpha, TR, and T1.** For large values of TR relative to T1, signal is maximized at a 90° flip angle. As TR is decreased, the angle producing maximum signal also decreases. The flip angle at which signal is maximized is known as the Ernst angle.

for several values of TR/T1 as a function of α from Equation 4 (TR >> T2). For very small values of α, the signal is mostly density weighted and independent of T1. The T1 weighting is increased as α is increased toward 90° (Fig. 4–9).

Note that the ability to change T1 weighting by varying flip angle means that a T2*-weighted image can be created by using small values of α to minimize the T1 weighting and longer values of TE to increase the T2* weighting (Equation 4). Since T2 is a component of T2*, the contrast is similar to that of a T2-weighted spin-echo image. The drawback to this approach is reduced signal owing to the small flip angle and long echo time (Fig. 4–9).

For TR < T2, GRASS and FISP become significantly T2 weighted as the SSFP is affected by transverse equilibrium. Moderate to large flip angles also result in greater T2 weighting. To the extent that they successfully break up the transverse equilibrium, FLASH and spoiled FLASH remain T1 weighted. This is illustrated in Figure 4–6, which shows FLASH and GRASS images for TR = 33 msec, TE = 14 msec, and α = 70°. The FLASH image shows stronger T1 weighting, whereas the GRASS image shows a more T2-weighted appearance. Table 4–1 summarizes the contrast mechanisms described above.

**Table 4–1.** LIMITED FLIP ANGLE CONTRAST

| | TR | TE | Flip Angle |
|---|---|---|---|
| T1 weighted | Long (200 msec)[2] | Short (12 msec) | Large (60°) |
| Density weighted | Long (200 msec) | Short (12 msec) | Small (10°) |
| T2* weighted | Long (200 msec) | Long (50 msec) | Small (10°) |
| T2 weighted[1] | Short (30 msec) | Short (12 msec) | Moderate (30°) |

[1]GRASS, FISP, or other SSFP sequences.
[2]Numbers in parentheses are examples of long and short times and large and small degrees.

## Clinical Applications

Localization may be the most straightforward clinical application of limited flip angle, gradient refocused (LFA) images and other fast scan techniques. A solitary LFA image may be obtained in less than 5 seconds, providing the anatomic information necessary for more diagnostic runs.

### *Hemorrhage, Iron, and Calcification*

With the possible exception of acute subarachnoid bleeds, parenchymal and extra-axial hemorrhagic lesions are readily detected by MR imaging.[14] Using spin-echo pulse sequences, it has been suggested that high field strength units are more sensitive in detecting hemorrhage and may more uniquely characterize its temporal evolution from oxyhemoglobin to methemoglobin and finally to hemosiderin.[15, 16] This added sensitivity and specificity has been attributed to preferential T2 relaxation effects, which vary as the square of the magnetic field strength.

However, these preferential T2 relaxation effects are also dependent upon the square of magnetic susceptibility variations,[16] and LFA images have been shown to be extremely sensitive to such susceptibility changes.[17-19] Several studies have shown that utilization of these pulse sequences, typically with α = 15 to 25°, TE = 30 msec, and TR > 100 msec, increases the capability of both low and mid field strength units in detecting hemorrhage when compared with both long and short TR/TE spin-echo sequences.[18-20] The simultaneous implementation of phase-sensitive mapping further increases the sensitivity and specificity of these pulse sequences to detect hemorrhage

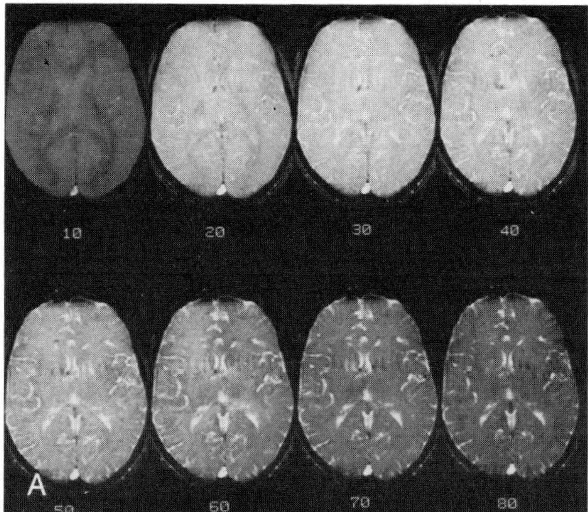


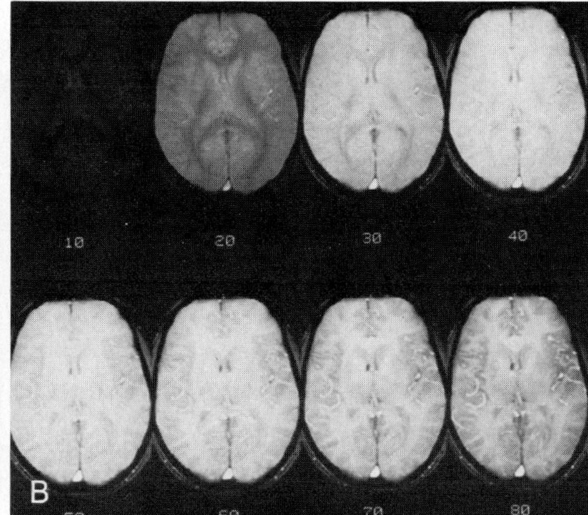


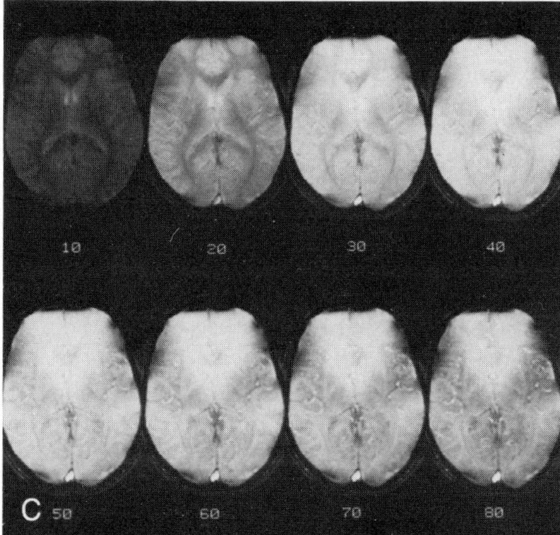


**Figure 4–9. Contrast dependence of GRASS imaging on flip angle (alpha), TR, and TE.** *A,* TR = 33 msec, TE = 14 msec, and alpha varies from 10° to 80°. With increasing flip angle, T2 weighting increases owing to steady-state free precession. *B,* TR = 200 msec, TE = 14 msec, and alpha varies from 10° to 80°. Contrast becomes less dependent upon proton density and more dependent upon Tl relaxation times as the flip angle is increased. At 80°, white matter is brighter than gray matter, owing to its shorter Tl value, while at a flip angle of 20°, gray matter is brighter than white matter owing to its greater density. *C,* TR = 200 msec, TE = 30 msec, and alpha varies from 10° to 80°. Longer echo times increase T2* contrast. CSF appears brighter than in *B* (compare alpha = 20° in both *B* and *C*). In *A,* that signal increases until alpha is somewhere between 30° and 40° (the Ernst angle) and decreases as alpha is further increased to 80°. Lengthening the repetition time results in the Ernst angle becoming larger. In *B* it approaches 50°, consistent with the information obtained in Figure 4–8.

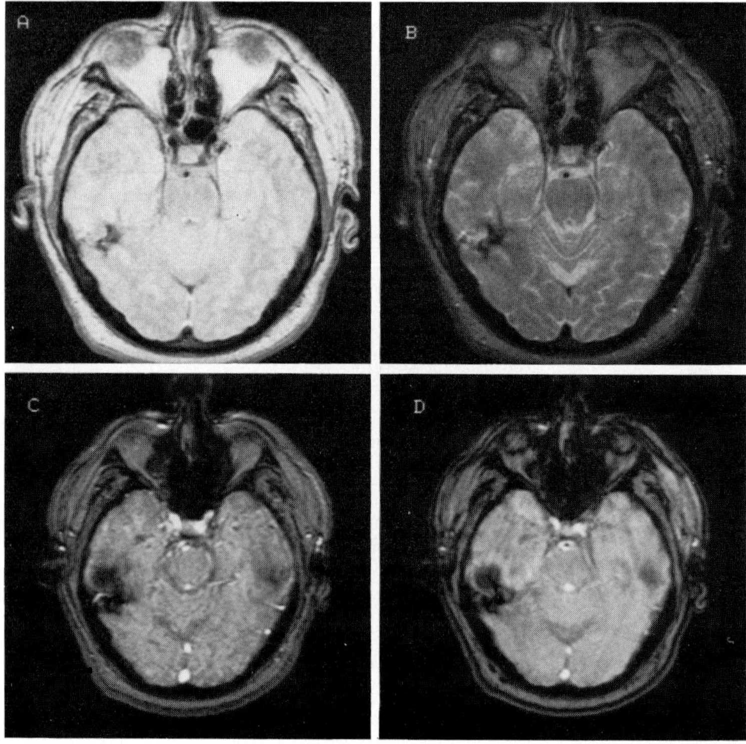


**Figure 4–10. A 46-year-old man with right temporal arteriovenous malformation.** The 500/20 msec *(A)* and 2800/70 msec *(B)* spin-echo sequence demonstrate the lesion. The area of decreased signal presumably represents an old bleed. The 33/14 msecs/30° *(C)* and 200/14 msec/20° *(D)* GRASS images show the area of old hemorrhage to be larger than suspected on the spin-echo sequences.

by displaying the associated susceptibility changes.[20]

Even at 1.5 T, LFA images have been shown to be more sensitive than spin-echo pulse sequences in the detection of hemorrhage (Fig. 4–10).[21, 22] However, it has been suggested that these images may be *too* sensitive in that the changing signal intensity patterns of evolving hematomas may be entirely obscured by the large susceptibility effect, which creates a hypointense signal for intracellular deoxyhemoglobin and methemoglobin and hemosiderin alike.[16]

It has been reported that LFA images are also a sensitive means of detecting parenchymal accumulations of ferritin.[23] The clinical importance of such observations has been described by Drayer and colleagues,[24] who observed that patients with Parkinson plus syndromes have abnormal concentrations of iron in the putamen and to a lesser extent in the caudate nucleus and the substantia nigra.

LFA images may also improve the sensitivity of identifying calcifications, an area in which MR is notoriously weak when compared with CT.[23, 25]

### *Nonhemorrhagic Lesions*

With the appropriate choice of flip angle, repetition, and echo times, an image with contrast similar to that of a T2-weighted spin-echo image may be generated with significant timesavings (see previous discussion) (Fig. 4–11).[17, 19, 20]

Apart from hemorrhagic lesions, the preliminary experience of multiple investigators using various LFA-imaging parameters is that conventional multiple-echo, spin-echo images with long repetition times are superior to the LFA pulse sequences for identifying intracranial masses and white matter diseases.[18, 20, 23, 26-28] Cited explanations for the poorer performance of the LFA images include the following:

1. Poor signal-to-noise ratio owing to short scanning times. Depending upon the particular imaging parameters chosen, there may be up to 58% less signal than conventional images.[18]

2. Susceptibility artifacts. The same factors that account for the heightened sensitivity to hemorrhage when compared with spin-echo images also result in greater sus-

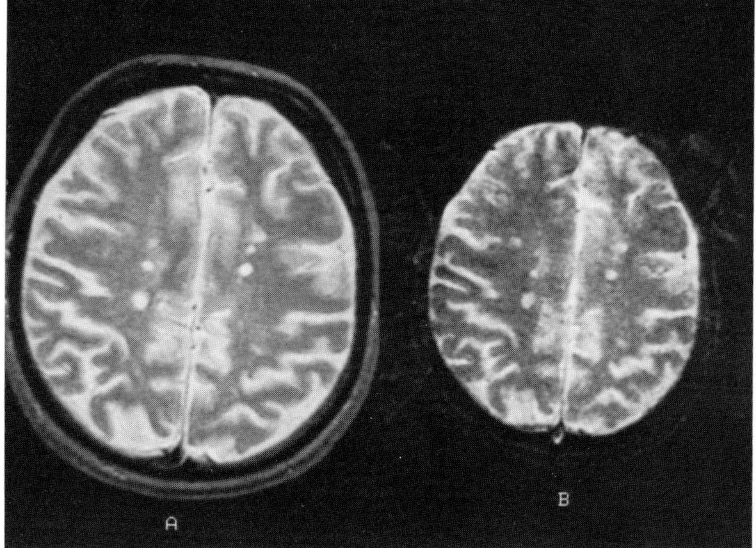


**Figure 4–11. A 42-year-old man with multiple sclerosis.** The 2800/70 msec spin-echo images *(A)* show multiple areas of abnormal signal within the white matter. The 200/50/10 degree GRASS image *(B)* shows similar findings.

ceptibility artifacts. Images of the frontal and temporal lobes, mastoid regions, and sella turcica are all degraded by susceptibility artifacts from adjacent air-filled structures.[18, 20, 27]

3. Periventricular abnormalities that are obscured by the high signal emanating from the CSF.[20]

4. Nonuniform RF pulse application across the desired image location.[20, 29] Protons within the center of the image receive more RF power, resulting in a larger flip angle than the protons at the edges of slices. Although this fact is more important for more T1-weighted LFA images owing to the larger flip angles, it still degrades image quality with smaller flip angles.

Some investigators have suggested that images utilizing extremely short echo times with small flip angles, so-called proton density or $M_0$ images, minimize susceptibility artifacts and still provide diagnostic information.[30, 31] Clearly, further experience is necessary to determine the precise clinical utility of LFA images in detecting intracerebral lesions.

### Flow

Since the NMR technique has been applied to clinical imaging, the signal void created by flowing blood on partial saturation, inversion recovery, and spin-echo images has provided investigators with a sensitive, noninvasive means of assessing vessel patency.[32-35] For example, Olson and coworkers[32] reported that magnetic resonance may be more sensitive than contrast-enhanced CT in diagnosing giant intracranial aneurysms. However, in 5 of 15 cases, it was unclear whether intraluminal signal represented thrombi or flow-related phenomena, a distinction felt to "have clinical implications." Numerous other investigators have characterized these flow phenomena and have noted that excluding thrombus can be difficult.[36-40]

Flowing blood appears bright on LFA images owing to the continuous inflow of fully magnetized protons, which produce more signal than the partially saturated protons in the adjacent stationary tissues. In contrast with spin-echo imaging, in which there may be reduced or absent intraluminal signal with rapidly flowing blood because of the slice-selective 180° radio-frequency pulse, blood with high velocities remains bright on LFA pulse sequences as a result of the nonselective gradient echo.[41]

If the protons of an object move while imaging gradients are applied, they experience a changing magnetic field, producing phase accumulations that are inconsistent with their positions at the time of signal detection. This creates image artifacts, so-called "ghost" images, of the object at incorrect spatial positions.[42] Since the blood signal is bright, the artifacts can be quite noticeable, making it important in LFA sequences to include extra gradients that serve to cancel the accumulated phase errors of flowing protons.[43] Such gradients can compensate for various kinds of motion as constant velocity (first order), velocity plus constant acceleration (second order), velocity plus linear acceleration (third order), and so on.[44] First order correction suffices for most artifacts; however, up to third order correction has been shown to be useful for some circumstances. A drawback of this technique is that each set of extra gradients can cause the minimum echo time to be increased, leading to loss of signal and less T1 or density weighting.

From the preceding discussion, one would expect flowing blood to appear bright and intraluminal thrombus to have decreased or absent intraluminal signal (Fig. 4–12).[45] However, several potential pitfalls exist. Slow venous flow may be difficult to distinguish from intraluminal thrombus (see Fig. 2–39). At high velocities, fully magnetized protons replace the partially saturated blood protons within the image slice. With decreasing velocity, the protons within the vessel remain in the voxel longer and become more saturated, resulting in less signal.

Although the contrast between flowing blood in the adjacent stationary tissues is dependent upon numerous factors, including tissue relaxation times and blood velocity, the judicious choice of imaging parameters can maximize the capability of LFA images to detect slow flow.[46] For a given velocity, decreasing slice thickness increases the proportion of unsaturated to saturated blood protons. This results in higher intraluminal signal.

One can also increase the flip angle, thereby producing more saturation of the stationary protons, resulting in greater contrast between the flowing blood and adjacent tissues. At least in the heart and extremities, maximum contrast appears to occur with flip angles ranging from 45° to 60°.[45, 47]

It is also important that the selected imaging plane be perpendicular to the vessel in question in order to maximize contrast. In-plane blood flow allows time for multiple excitations to the blood protons, resulting in partial saturation and decreased intraluminal signal. Additionally, partial volume averaging and its concomitant loss of signal is not an issue when vessels are examined in cross section.

A second potential limitation in assessing vessel patency by LFA images is the presence of intraluminal clot with high signal.[48] If thrombus has a very short T1 relaxation time, such as seen in methemoglobin, it may appear similar to flowing blood on LFA images. This limitation may necessitate the use of spin-echo images to entirely exclude

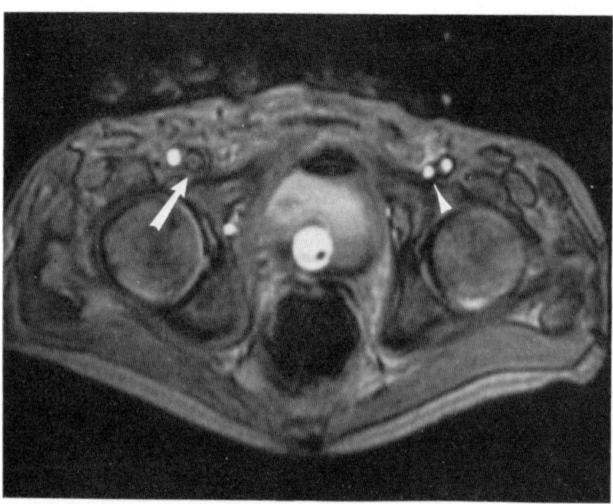

**Figure 4–12. A 70-year-old man with deep venous thrombosis.** Patent left femoral vein (arrowhead) shows high signal owing to flowing blood. Intraluminal thrombus causes decreased signal in the right femoral vein (arrow). TR 33 msec/TE 13 msec/alpha 45°.

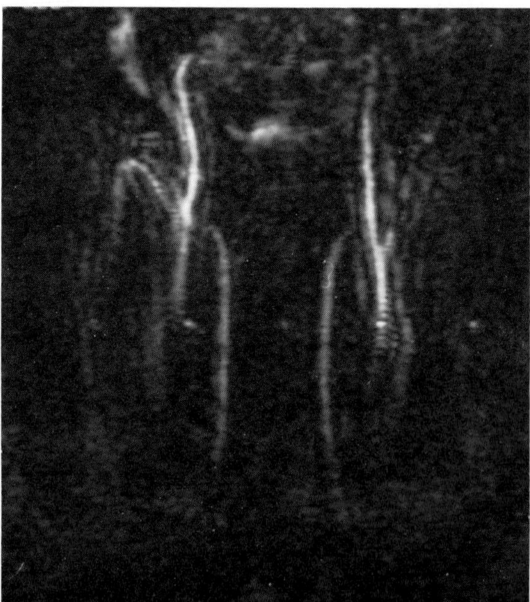

**Figure 4–13. Limited flip-angle MR subtraction angiogram of the carotid arteries.** Signal differences of flowing blood between systole and diastole were used to generate this image. Sixteen phase encodings were obtained. Total scanning time, 9 seconds. TR 33 msec, TE 13 msec alpha, 30°. (Courtesy of T. Tascyan, S. Riederer, Duke University, Durham, N.C.)

thrombus. An alternative approach may be to retain the phase information available with the LFA data acquisition and generate a phase map.[49]

Numerous MR imaging techniques have been developed in attempts both to quantify blood flow and to display the information in a fashion analogous to a true angiogram.[50-52] These techniques have been applied to LFA pulse sequences, resulting in images produced in well under one minute (Fig. 4–13).[53, 54] Like conventional two-dimensional LFA images, these "MR angiograms" are extremely sensitive to turbulent flow. Turbulent flow causes dephasing of blood protons, resulting in absent intraluminal signal.[55] This circumstance may represent a significant limitation, as nonvisualization of stenotic vessels by MR could represent either complete obstruction or simply severe vessel narrowing with marked turbulence. It remains to be seen if MR angiography will develop into an adjunct technique for evaluating vascular anatomy and pathology.

### Myelogram Effect

Magnetic resonance imaging is increasingly being used for evaluating the spinal cord and canal. On T2-weighted spin-echo images, the high signal from CSF noninvasively simulates the appearance of a myelogram; however, the lengthy scanning times predispose these images to numerous motion and flow artifacts.[56] Because of the long T2 and T2* relaxation times of CSF, LFA images are able to replicate this myelogram effect with significant timesavings over conventional spin-echo images (Fig. 4–14). As outlined previously, by using short TRs and TEs combined with moderate flip angles, the residual transverse magnetization of CSF provides additional signal, making the CSF appear bright in relation to other substances.

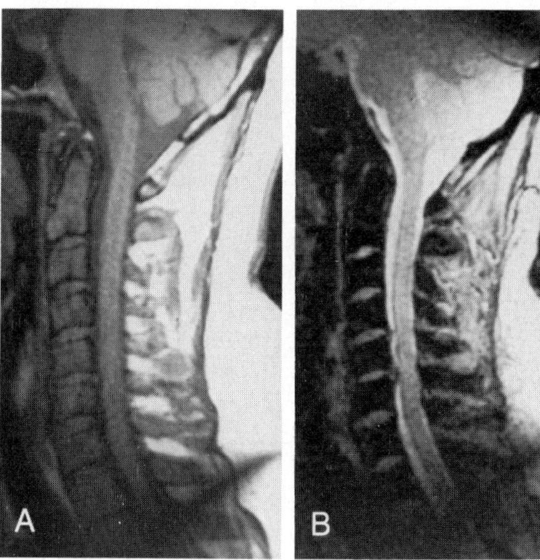


**Figure 4–14. A 45-year-old woman with C5-C6 disk herniation.** 500/20 msec spin-echo image *(A)* shows the disk herniation. The 67/20 msec, 10°-flip angle GRASS images *(B)* show impingement on the thecal sac at this level. Note the high signal from CSF.

Ghost artifacts created by the pulsatile flow of CSF can be reduced by the application of gradient compensation as described earlier.

Preliminary studies suggest that for extra-axial abnormalities, LFA images are as effective as more traditional pulse sequences.[13, 57, 58] However, as in the brain, LFA images appear less sensitive in depicting intra-axial abnormalities.[59] Additionally, the marked susceptibility changes caused by bone and fat may obscure the detection of vertebral body abnormalities on LFA images.[56, 59] LFA images can assist in differentiation of soft disk (intermediate signal) from calcified spur (hypointense signal).

### T1 Measurements

Although the measurement of T1 and T2 relaxation times has not reliably separated benign from malignant processes, these measurements can still be clinically useful. Although T2 measurements can be obtained in a single acquisition, in general, T1 measurements require multiple acquisitions. Using LFA images, T1 measurements have been obtained in one tenth the time of conventional techniques.[60]

### Volume Acquisition

When compared with two-dimensional Fourier transform acquisitions, three-dimensinal Fourier transform (3DFT) spin-echo techniques have several advantages, including (1) thin slices that are truly contiguous, (2) good signal-to-noise ratio per slice, and (3) the ability to reformat data in nonorthogonal planes. The major drawback to 3DFT spin-echo imaging has been the long data acquisition time. By using the three-dimensional LFA technique, volumes of tissue can be imaged in minutes instead of tens of minutes. Potential areas of application include the spine and preoperative localization of intracerebral neoplasms.[61, 62]

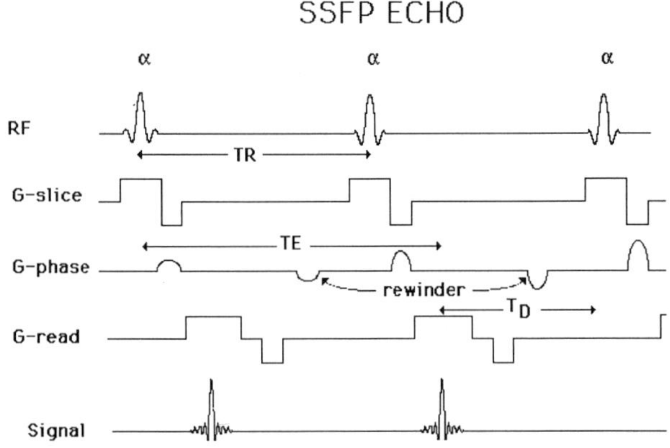


**Figure 4–15. SSFP echo.** Like the GRASS pulse sequence, the phase-encoding gradient contains a rewinder designed to maintain SSFP. Modification of the read-out gradient allows detection of the $M^-$ portion of the signal. This signal is generated by the prior two α pulses enabling TE to be larger than TR. This increases the T2 weighting of the pulse sequence. T2* effects are determined by the time between the read-out gradient and the application of the next alpha pulse ($T_d$).

## OTHER TECHNIQUES

### Acquisition of the SSFP Echo: Contrast-Enhanced–Fourier Acquisition in the Steady State

Two signals are generated when TR < T2 (Fig. 4–1*B*). The first signal, $M^+$, corresponds to a free-induction decay generated by the coinciding RF pulse. The second signal, $M^-$, is a stimulated echo created by the preceding two RF pulses. By only using the $M^-$ signal, it is possible to have an echo time that is longer than the repetition time, i.e., TE = 2TR − td where Td is the time between the application of the read-out gradient and the next RF pulse (Fig. 4–15).[63] Acquisition of this echo creates an image that is more heavily T2 weighted than is possible with a SSFP image based on the $M^+$ signal, i.e., GRASS or FISP. This sequence has also been described as contrast-enhanced–Fourier acquisition in the steady state (CE-FAST).[64] The heavier T2 weighting presumably improves the contrast accounting for the contrast-enhanced designation. Like the GRASS and FISP pulse sequences, the phase-encoding gradient is balanced in order that the SSFP not be "spoiled."

This technique produces a heavily T2-weighted image with fewer T2* effects than would be expected from a GRASS or FISP image using a similar echo time. This is because the T2* effects are determined by td, which can be kept short compared with TE. With slight modification of this sequence, both the $M^+$ and $M^-$ signals can be acquired. Thus a short and a long TE image can be acquired simultaneously. Some technical difficulties are realized when these pulse sequences are implemented on current imaging systems.

### Ernst Angle Spin Echo/FAST TE

It is possible to improve "conventional" spin-echo imaging by using an "α pulse" instead of a 90° initial pulse in a 90°–180° sequence. For a longer TR (i.e., TR >> T2), this method allows establishment of an improved longitudinal magnetization steady state over that obtained with a 90° pulse. In a 90°–180° spin-echo sequence, the 180° RF pulse inverts the longitudinal magnetization, lengthening the time for significant longitudinal magnetization to recover (Fig. 4–16*A*). If the longitudinal magnetization could be left oriented along the main magnetic field (+z axis), recovery of longitudinal magnetization would be quicker, allowing for a faster scan.

Two techniques have been proposed to do this. Ernst-angle spin echo (EASE) recognizes that in the spin-echo case there is an analog to the Ernst angle.[65] In fact, the optimum angle is $\alpha = 180° - \alpha_E$. Thus by using a flip angle that is greater than 90°, the longitudinal magnetization is still inverted by the time the 180° pulse occurs (TE << T1), which then replaces the spins along the +z axis (Fig. 4–16*B*). This allows the spins to recover more completely by the time of the next pulse, establishing a larger equilibrium value of the longitudinal magnetization. Although spins with very short T1 values can relax fast enough to defeat this scheme by re-aligning along the +z axis before the 180° pulse occurs, such spins are

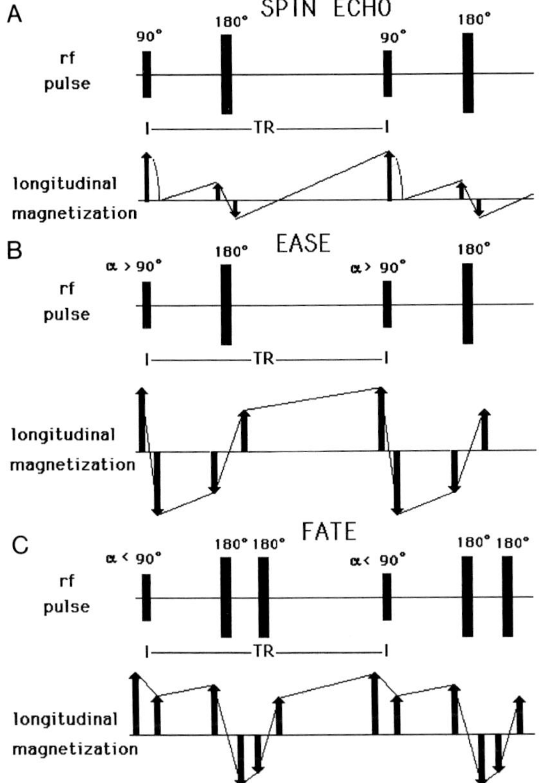


**Figure 4–16.** *A,* In a spin-echo sequence, the 180° RF pulse inverts the longitudinal magnetization, increasing the time to full recovery of these spins. *B,* The EASE sequence employs an initial flip angle greater than 90°, which inverts longitudinal magnetization along the −z axis. The 180° RF pulse then realigns the spins along +z, accelerating recovery of longitudinal magnetization. *C,* In the FATE sequence, small flip angle alpha maintains longitudinal magnetization while the two 180° RF pulses maintain its orientation in a positive direction, facilitating recovery.

also able to recover to a large equilibrium even after the inversion by the 180° pulse.

The FAST TE (FATE) sequence replaces the 90° RF pulse with a flip angle of less than 90° and employs a second 180° RF to restore longitudinal magnetization along the +z axis (Fig. 4–16C).[66] The second 180° pulse reduces efficiency and increases RF power deposition when compared with the EASE sequence. But if it is desirable to obtain two echoes for diagnostic purposes, the FATE sequence may show advantages over the conventional 90°, 180°, 180°, double spin-echo approach.

## Driven Equilibrium Sequences

Like SSFP, the driven equilibrium Fourier transform (DEFT) sequence attempts to maintain significant longitudinal magnetization by re-aligning transverse magnetization along the +z axis (Fig. 4–17).[67] In its simplest form, the DEFT sequence is a 90°, 180°, 90° RF pulse sequence. The acquired data is obtained in FID following the first 90° pulse. The 180° pulse then refocuses the dephasing transverse magnetization as in a conventional spin-echo sequence. As the protons refocus, a second 90° RF pulse drives the magnetization to the longitudinal axis. Thus the longitudinal magnetization is kept at a relatively large value that is nearly independent of TR. For imaging, in order to actually acquire a spin echo, second 180° and 90° pulses are used.[68]

The contrast developed by this sequence is similar to that of an FISP pulse sequence. DEFT imaging may produce contrast that agrees more closely with predicted SSFP values than FISP imaging since the 180° RF pulse refocuses protons before driving them back along the z axis.

For short repetition times, DEFT images are much more T2 weighted and have greater signal to noise than SE images. This technique may provide an additional means of generating "myelogramlike" spinal images. Since a 180° RF pulse is used, susceptibility artifacts are minimized. Disadvantages of DEFT include poor tissue contrast, large RF power deposition, and sensitivity to eddy currents.

## Fourier Space

Data acquisitions using conjugation techniques, echo planar imaging, hybrid scanning, and stimulated echo acquisition mode (STEAM) pulse sequences may be best understood by viewing the data collection in Fourier, or k, space. Modern imaging systems use the two-dimensional Fourier transform method for spatial encoding. The raw data produced by this method of spatial encoding is essentially a Fourier transform of the image. This Fourier transform can be thought of as a plot of signal amplitude as a function of the Fourier frequency (k) in the frequency direction ($k_x$) and the phase direction ($k_y$) of the imaged object that has been acquired over time. The frequency information is encoded by the read-out gradient. The phase encoding fills lines of Fourier, or k, space for each value of the phase-encoding gradient that is acquired.

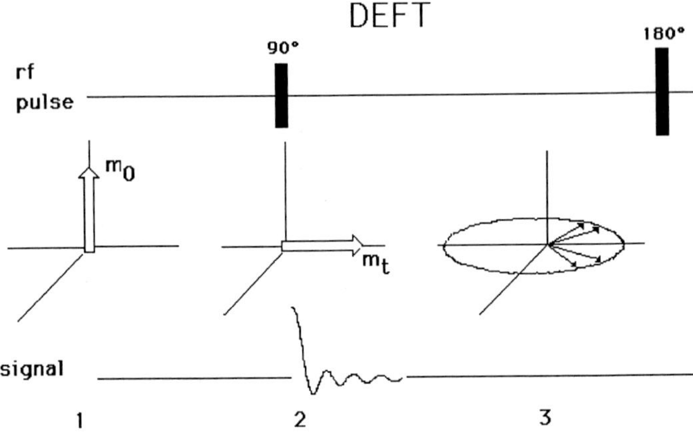


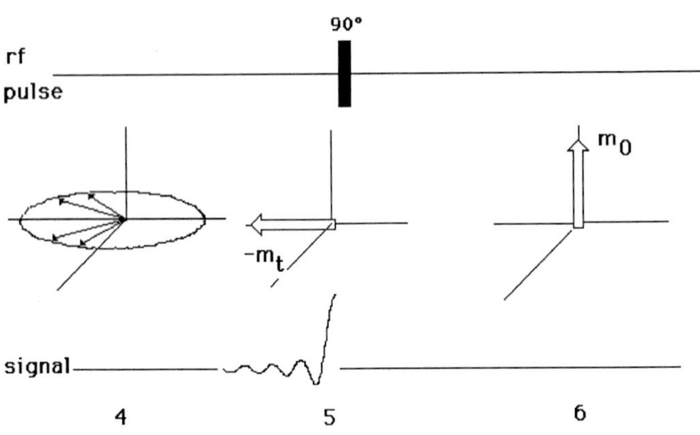


**Figure 4–17. DEFT pulse sequence.** The first 90° and the 180° RF pulse function as in a spin-echo sequence. The 90° pulse rotates the longitudinal magnetization into the transverse plane, and the 180° RF pulse rephases the transverse magnetization. At the time the protons refocus (5), the second 90° pulse drives the transverse magnetization back along the longitudinal (z) axis.

For spin-echo imaging, every time an echo is acquired, the frequency-encoding gradient maps signal into the $k_x$, or frequency axis, of Fourier space. The phase-encoding gradient determines which line of Fourier space along the phase encoding axis ($k_y$ axis) is being obtained. Spin-echo imaging steps through Fourier space, filling it line by line with each different phase encoding (Fig. 4–18*A*). Once Fourier space is entirely filled, an inverse Fourier transform produces an image from this data.

## Limited View Reconstruction/ Conjugation

Perhaps the simplest method of reducing scanning time is to decrease the number of sample points. For conventional spin-echo imaging, imaging time (T) is determined by the following equation:

$$T = TR \times nex \times NP$$

in which TR equals repetition time, nex equals the number of excitations, i.e., the number of times that the same phase-encoding echo is acquired, and NP equals the number of steps or views in the phase-encoding direction, i.e., matrix size. It can be seen that by decreasing any variable on the right hand side of the equation that total scanning time can be reduced. However, the consequences of such reductions may be unacceptable. For example, if the repetition time is shortened, there is loss of both signal relative to noise and T2 relaxation information. This loss of T2 contrast is generally considered unacceptable since many abnormalities in the central nervous system are best detected on more T2-weighted images. If the number of views in the phase-encoding direction is reduced, tissue contrast is maintained at the expense of spatial resolution, producing an unsatisfactory image.

Finally, one can reduce the number of excitations. Assuming a reduction from two to one excitation, scanner time is decreased

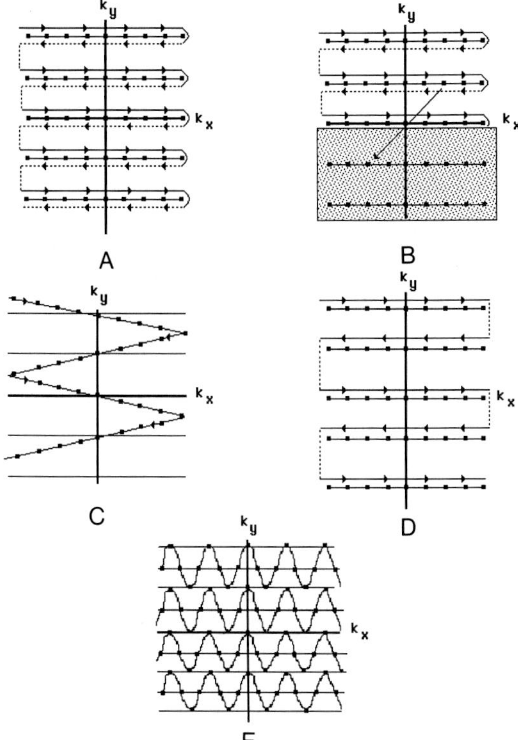


**Figure 4–18. K space representations of *A*, spin-echo imaging; *B*, conjugated spin-echo imaging; *C*, echo-planar imaging; *D*, modified echo-planar imaging; and *E*, hybrid scanning.** *A*, Each line in the $k_x$ direction represents one view or application of the read-out gradient. From view to view, the phase-encoding gradient is changed, resulting in the value of $k_y$ being changed. In this example, k space is filled after five views, or lines, are obtained. *B*, As in spin-echo imaging, data in the top half of k space is acquired in a line-by-line fashion. Because of the symmetry of k space, this data can be transposed to form the negative half of k space and phase corrections can be made.

*C*, In echo-planar imaging (EPI), k space is traversed in a single acquisition. The rapid modulation of the read-out gradient results in rapid traverses in the $k_x$ direction. The constant phase-encoding gradient causes a linear incremental change in the $k_y$ direction. The resulting pattern is a tilted rectilinear path. *D*, By modifying the phase-encoding gradient, a more rectangular path through k space can be traversed. *E*, By sinusoidally varying the phase-encoding gradient, k space is traversed by a series of sine waves Notice that each sine wave fills an entire line and one half of the lines above and below its center. Since two lines of data are acquired with each acquisition, scan time is reduced by a factor of two.

by one half, and spatial resolution and contrast remain unchanged. The penalty for such a change is a reduction in signal-to-noise ratio by a square root of two.

Much of the data in k space is redundant. If corrections are made for accumulated phase differences, then the upper and lower half of k space contain comparable information. Because of this symmetry in k space, conjugation allows the first N/2 + 1 views to be used in order that the other N/2 views may be synthesized (Fig. 4–18*B*). This technique has also been incorrectly called one-half nex imaging. However, it is not the number of excitations that is reduced, but rather the number of phase-encoding steps.[63, 69, 70]

This technique results in an image with the same contrast and resolution as a conventional scan, but one that is acquired in 50% of the imaging time. Feinberg and colleagues suggested that several additional views be acquired to more accurately define the center of k space.[69] For instance, they acquired 138 projections instead of 128, to create a 256-line image. This resulted in a 46% rather than a 50% reduction in scanning time.

Because only one half the data is collected, signal-to-noise ratio is reduced by a factor of a square root of two. It should be noted that conjugate imaging may be combined with LFA images, echo planar, hybrid imaging, and other fast-scan techniques.

## Echo Planar Imaging

Rectilinear paths through k space are convenient since the fast Fourier transform is defined on a grid of points. However, other paths are possible. The best known of such techniques is echo planar imaging (EPI), first described by Mansfield in the mid-1970s.[71, 72] This technique employs a train of echoes to encode position.

Following a 90° RF pulse, a train of echoes is created by modulating the read-out gradients while simultaneously applying the phase-encoding gradient (Fig. 4–19). Just as for spin-echo imaging, the rapid change in the read-out gradient maps a path along the $k_x$ (frequency) axis in k space. The concomitant application of the phase-encoding gradient causes the simultaneous motion along the $k_y$ (phase) axis. This results in a k space trajectory appearing as a tilted rectilinear path, with each pixel in the image uniquely defined in the Fourier space, allowing reconstruction of a two-dimensional image (Fig. 4–18C). Most important, the entire image is created with a single data acquisition lasting a fraction of a second.

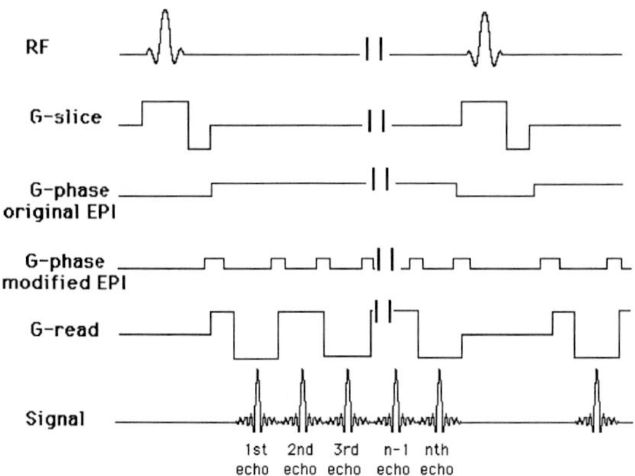


**Figure 4–19. Echo-planar imaging.** Rapid modulation of the read-out gradient in the presence of a constantly applied phase-encoding gradient (original EPI) creates a series of echoes that uniquely encode position information in Fourier space. The modified EPI sequence attempts to compensate for phase artifacts caused by T2 decay.

Both T1 and T2 contrast may be obtained in these images. By following the first echo train with a 180° RF pulse and a second modulation of the read-out gradient, T2 information can be acquired. Alternatively, varying the echo time of the first echo train will also change the T2 informational content.[73] By varying the delay (i.e., repetition time) between successive image acquisitions, spin-lattice contrast can be modified in a fashion analogous with spin-echo imaging. Accurate T1 and $M_0$ maps can be acquired using this technique, provided one accounts for partial nutation of protons at the edge of slices.[74]

The primary limitation of this technique is spin-spin decay during data acquisition. As the read-out gradient is modulated, there is simultaneous T2 decay which modifies the received signal creating artifacts. The EPI sequence can be made less susceptible to these artifacts by employing a phase-encoding gradient with multiple lobes (Fig. 4–18*D*).[75] A similar technique with improved gradients has recently been described.[76]

Disadvantages of the EPI sequence include the following: (1) Rapid modulation of read-out gradients is technically difficult in most commercial scanners. (2) A gradient echo renders these techniques sensitive to chemical shift artifacts and field inhomogeneity. (3) These sequences may suffer decreased signal to noise secondary to the large bandwidth necessary for short scanning times.

## RARE

An example of extreme T2 weighting is given by the sequence called rapid acquisition with relaxation enhancement (RARE).[77] In this sequence, a train of echoes are formed with 180° pulses. Thus most of the data is acquired for long echo times, leading to strong T2 weighting. The sequence has been found useful for producing images in which only CSF contributes, since the signal from all other tissues totally decays before the entire data train is acquired.

While RARE could theoretically proceed at a speed comparable to, for example, that of the echo planar sequence, it is limited by its much higher RF power deposition owing to the large number of 180° RF pulses. A low power version, fast low angle acquisition with relaxation enhancement (FLARE) has been proposed.[78] In this sequence, the nominal 180° pulses are reduced to 60°. This reduction results in a significant power-deposition reduction. However, the lower angle pulses produce many stimulated echoes, which change the echo weighting while still leaving the sequence heavily T2 weighted.

### STEAM and QUICK STEP

Stimulated echoes were first described by Hahn in the 1950s.[79] Current acronyms for stimulated echoes include stimulated echo acquisition mode (STEAM)[80] and quick stimulated echo progressive imaging (QUICK STEP).[81] This sequence employs a series of three 90° pulses that produce both a spin echo and a stimulated echo (Fig. 4–20).

The first 90° RF pulse tilts protons into the transverse plane. T2 relaxation occurs during the first TE/2 msec period. During this time, phase-encoding gradients are applied. The second 90° pulse will drive some of the protons to the longitudinal z axis, where they will retain the previously encoded phase information. The protons remaining in the transverse plane will give rise to a spin echo at time = TE, which occurs during the time period labeled TM. The third 90° pulse returns the stored spins from the longitudinal axis to the transverse

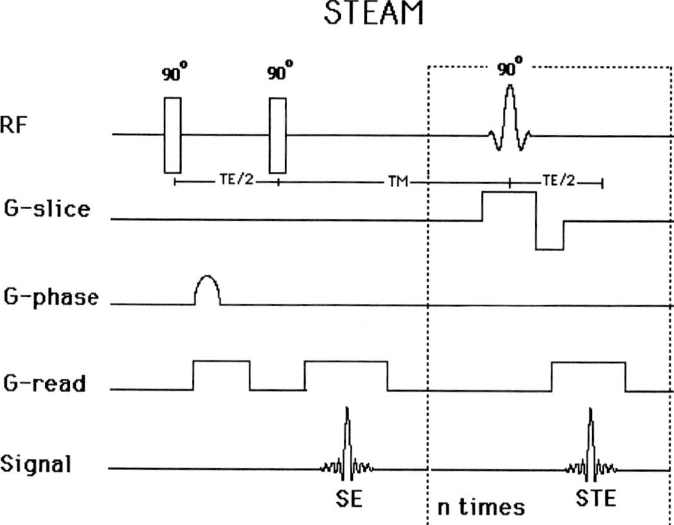


**Figure 4–20. STEAM pulse diagram.** Three 90° RF pulses create spin echo (SE) and a stimulated echo (STE). For a multiple-slice acquisition, the latter portion (dotted box) is repeated.

axis, creating a stimulated echo TE/2 milliseconds later. For the spins that are stored in the longitudinal axis, T2 relaxation occurs only during the time periods labeled TE/2, as dephasing occurs only while spins are in the transverse plane. During the time TM, T1 relaxation occurs, reducing signal intensity for the stimulated echo. Tissues with a short T1 lose signal intensity over the time marked TM, whereas tissues with a long T1 retain signal intensity.

Since most pathologic tissues have long T1 and T2 relaxation times, this pulse sequence simultaneously accentuates the difference between normal and abnormal tissues by both T1 and T2 relaxation mechanisms. This is in contradistinction to spin-echo imaging, in which a decreased signal associated with long T1 relaxation times tends to cancel the high signal resulting from long T2 relaxation values. The disadvantage of stimulated echo imaging is that the echoes have only approximately one half the intensity of an echo produced by a 180° RF pulse.

By modifying the basic pulse sequence, stimulated echoes can also be used to determine diffusion coefficients, to permit flow sensitive imaging, to allow for chemical shift selective imaging, and to generate T1 information more rapidly than can be performed with spin-echo imaging.[82-86]

Stimulated echo imaging has two separate mechanisms by which rapid scanning can be employed.[87] Because both the primary spin echo and the stimulated echo can be acquired, differential phase-encoding steps can be applied to the two echoes, reducing the number of repetitions needed for a given phase-encoded matrix by a factor of two. If the third 90° pulse in the sequence is replaced by a series of lower angle pulses, progressive phase encoding can be acquired for each additional pulse, further reducing the number of repetitions needed to produce an image. This mechanism can allow for single-shot real-time imaging.[80]

### Fast Fourier Imaging/Hybrid Scanning

The primary limitation of echo planar imaging is the necessity of acquiring the data faster than the T2 relaxation value of the tissues being examined. This requires some compromise in desired spatial resolution and in the rapidity with which the gradients are modulated. Several investigators have proposed schemes that combine elements of both echo planar imaging and spin-echo imaging.[88, 89] The advantage of these fast Fourier images or hybrid fast-scanning techniques is the ease with which they can be implemented on existing scanners while still resulting in a 50% greater decrease in scan time for a given repetition time. Just as in spin-echo imaging, a slice select gradient, 90° RF pulse, and 180° refocusing pulse are

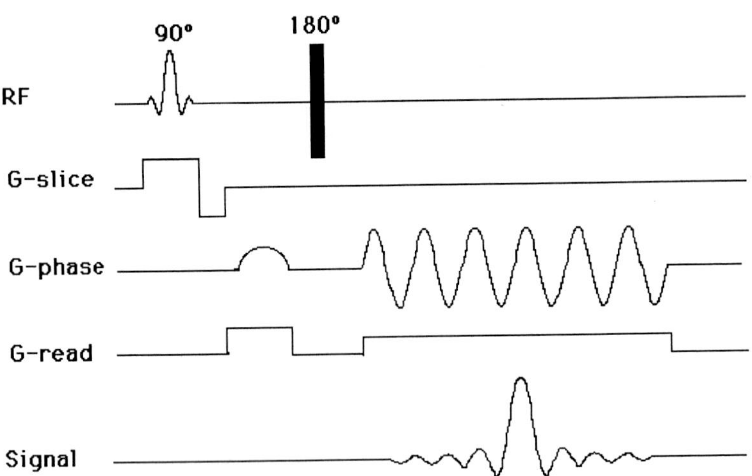


**Figure 4–21. Hybrid scan pulse diagram.** This technique employs elements of both spin-echo and echo-planar imaging. The pulse diagram is identical to a spin-echo sequence until the read-out gradient is applied. The interleaved sinusoidal variation of the phase-encoding gradient allows acquisition of several lines of k space.

applied (Fig. 4–21). The difference between the two pulse sequences occurs during readout. When the frequency encoding gradient is applied, the phase-encoding gradient is oscillated, enabling position information to be encoded in a fashion analogous to echo planar imaging. The difference is that in hybrid scanning the gradient oscillation and sampling rate are only fast enough to acquire information for several lines in k space instead of for the entire sample as an echo planar image (Fig. 4–18*E*). In order to generate an alias-free image, the reconstruction algorithm must correct for phase differences occurring from the multiple acquisitions. Compared with spin-echo images, the fast Fourier images are more sensitive to field inhomogeneity and susceptibility artifacts.

### Strip Scanning

This technique was first described by Mezrich and associates.[90] Like conjugated images, scanning time is decreased by reducing the number of acquired phase-encoding steps. The difference between the two techniques is that in strip scanning the physical dimension in the phase-encoding direction is reduced in proportion to the number of phase-encoding views deleted. A reduction in one half the total views results in an image acquired in one half the time. The image looks like a strip or a rectangle with the phase-encoding direction half as long as that in the frequency-encoding direction.

Implementation of this technique involves two simple modifications of the standard

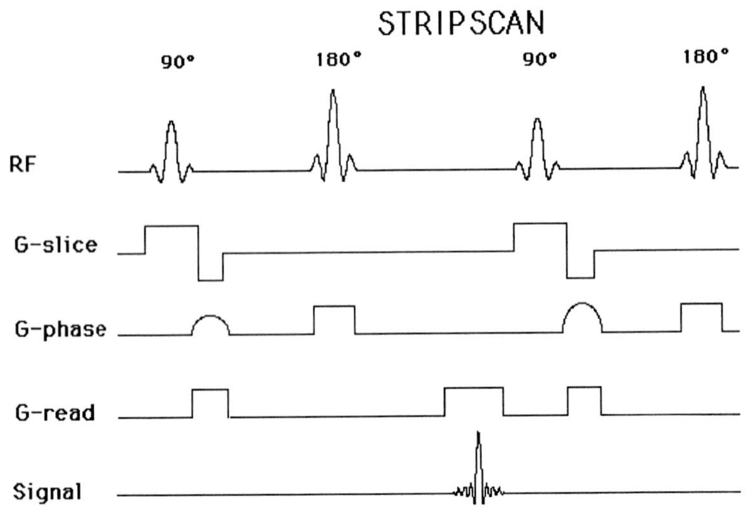


**Figure 4–22. Strip scan.** The second gradient lobe in the phase direction applied at the time of the 180° RF pulse limits the field of view imaged.

spin-echo pulse sequence (Fig. 4–22). First, the number of phase-encoding views is reduced, and, second, an additional pulse is applied along the phase-encoding gradient at the time of the 180° RF pulse. This additional lobe prevents aliasing in the phase-encoding direction and reduces the amount of tissue excited, thereby maintaining spatial resolution.

The advantage of this technique is that contrast and spatial resolution are maintained with significant time reduction assuming that a rectangular field of view images the area of concern, for example, the spine. As initially described, the technique is limited to single-slice acquisition, owing to the selective 180° RF pulse. Subsequent modification now allows a multislice acquisition. As with any technique that reduces imaging time, there is a concomitant decrease in signal-to-noise ratio.

## References


1. Ernst RR, Anderson WA. Application of Fourier transform spectroscopy to magnetic resonance. Rev Sci Instr 37:93, 1966.
2. Haase A, Frahm J, Matthaei D, et al. FLASH imaging: rapid NMR imaging using low flip angle pulses. J Magn Res 67:258, 1986.
3. Wehrli F. Fast scan magnetic resonance imaging: principles and contrast phenomenology. In Higgins C, Hricak H, eds. Magnetic resonance imaging of the body. New York, Raven Press, 1987.
4. Oppelt A, Graumann R, Barfuss H, et al. FISP—a new fast MRI sequence. Electromedica 54:15, 1986.
5. Mansfield P, Morris PG. NMR imaging in biomedicine. In Waugh JS, ed. Advances in magnetic resonance, Supplement 2. New York, Academic Press, 1982.
6. Freeman R, Hill HD. Phase and intensity anomalies in Fourier transform NMR. J Magn Reson 4:366, 1971.
7. Matsui S, Kuroda M, Kohno H. A new method of measuring T2 using steady-state free precession. J Magn Reson 62:12, 1985.
8. Sekihara K. Steady state magnetizations in rapid NMR imaging using small flip angles and short repetition intervals. IEEE Trans Med Imag 6:157, 1987.
9. Haase A, Hanicke W, Merboldt KD. Transverse coherence in rapid FLASH NMR imaging. J Magn Reson 72:307, 1987.
10. Farrar T, Becker T. Pulse and Fourier transform nuclear magnetic resonance. New York, Academic Press, 1971.
11. Wehrli F, Perkins T, Shimakawa A, et al. Chemical shift induced amplitude modulations in images obtained with gradient refocusing. Magn Reson Imag, 5:157, 1987.
12. Dixon WT. Simple proton spectroscopic imaging. Radiology 153:189, 1984.
13. Enzmann D, Rubin J, Wright A. Cervical spine MR imaging: generating high signal CSF in sagittal and axial images. Radiology 163:233, 1987.
14. Brant-Zawadzki M. MR imaging of the brain. Radiology 166:1, 1988.
15. Gomori JM, Grossman RI, Goldberg HI, et al. Intracranial hematomas: imaging by high-field MR. Radiology 157:87, 1985.
16. Gomori JM, Grossman RI. Head and neck hemorrhage. In Kressel HY, ed. Magnetic Resonance Annual: 1987. New York, Raven Press, 1987:71.
17. Winkler ML, Ortendahl DA, Mills TC, et al. Characteristics of partial flip angle and gradient reversal MR imaging. Radiology 166:17, 1988.
18. Winkler ML, Olsen WL, Mills TC, et al. Hemorrhagic and nonhemorrhagic brain lesions: evaluation with 0.35 T fast MR imaging. Radiology 165:203, 1987.
19. Edelman RR, Johnson K, Buxton R. MR of hemorrhage: a new approach. AJNR 7:751, 1986.
20. Bydder GM, Payne JA, Collins AG, et al. Clinical use of rapid T2-weighted partial saturation sequences in MR imaging. J Comput Assist Tomogr 11:17, 1987.
21. Atlas SW, Grossman RI, Gomori JM, et al. MR imaging characteristics of intracranial hemorrhage using gradient-echo signal acquisition at 1.5 T: comparison with spin-echo imaging and clinical applications. Radiology 165(P):217, 1987.
22. Drayer BP, Rigamonti D, Johnson PC, et al. Limited flip angle MR imaging: hemorrhagic applications. Radiology 165(P):216, 1987.
23. Drayer BP, Bird R, Hodak JA, et al. Limited flip angle MR imaging: nonhemorrhagic applications. Radiology 165(P):39, 1987.
24. Drayer BP, Olanow W, Burger P, et al. Parkinson plus syndrome: diagnosis using high field MR imaging of brain iron. Radiology 159:493, 1986.
25. Oot RF, New PF, Pile-Spellman J. The detection of intracranial calcifications by MR. AJNR 7:801, 1986.
26. Fink U, Bauer WM, Yousry T, et al. MR imaging of pituitary adenomas: optimization of the examination technique. Radiology 165(P):160, 1987.
27. Steinberg PM, Montanez J, Hueftle MG, et al. Fast-gradient-echo short echo time imaging sequences in the evaluation of brain pathology. Radiology 165(P):143, 1987.
28. Larson TC, Mark AS, Kelly W, et al. Comparison of multiplanar fast MR imaging of the head with conventional spin-warp methods. Radiology 165(P):79, 1987.
29. Wehrli FW, Perkins TG, Shimakawa A. Chemical shift–induced amplitude modulations in images obtained with gradient refocusing. Magn Reson Imag 5:157, 1987.
30. Albert S, Leeds NE, Silvergleid R, et al. Potential applications of small tip angle proton density imaging. Radiology 165(P):153, 1987.
31. Haacke EM, Lenz GW. Short echo time, fast gradient-echo imaging. Radiology 165(P):30, 1987.
32. Olsen WL, Brant-Zawadzki M, Hodes J, et al. Giant intracranial aneurysms: MR imaging. Radiology 163:431, 1987.
33. Ohtomo K, Itai Y, Furui S, et al. MR imaging of portal vein thrombus in hepatocellular carcinoma. J Comput Assist Tomogr 9:328, 1985.
34. Weinreb JC, Mootz A, Cohen JM. MRI evaluation of mediastinal and thoracic inlet venous obstruction. AJR 146:679, 1986.

35. Hricak H, Amparo E, Fisher MR, et al. Abdominal venous system: assessment using MR. Radiology 156:415, 1985.
36. Waluch V, Bradley WG. NMR even echo rephasing in slow laminar flow. J Comput Assist Tomogr 8:594, 1984.
37. Bradley WG Jr, Waluch V. Blood flow: magnetic resonance imaging. Radiology 154:443, 1985.
38. Bradley WG Jr, Waluch V, Lai K-S, et al. The appearance of rapidly flowing blood on magnetic resonance images. AJR 143:1167, 1984.
39. Axel L. Blood flow effects in magnetic resonance imaging. AJR 143:1157, 1984.
40. von Schulthess GK, Higgins CB. Blood flow imaging with MR: spin phase phenomena. Radiology 157:687, 1985.
41. Wehrli FW, Shimakawa A, Gullberg GT, et al. Time-of-flight MR flow imaging: selective saturation recovery with gradient refocusing. Radiology 160:781, 1986.
42. Perman W, Moran P, Moran R. Artifacts from pulsatile flow in MR imaging. J Comput Assist Tomogr 10:473, 1986.
43. Glover G, Pelc N. A rapid-gated CINE MRI technique. In Kressel H, ed. Magnetic Resonance Annual. New York, Raven Press, 1988.
44. Pattany P, Phillips JJ, Hiu LC, et al. Motion artifact suppression technique (MAST) for MR imaging. J Comput Assist Tomogr 11:369, 1987.
45. Spritzer CE, Sussman SK, Blinder RA, et al. Deep venous thrombosis evaluation by limited flip angle gradient refocused magnetic resonance imaging. Radiology 166:371, 1988.
46. Fram E. Parameters determining the signal of flowing fluid in gradient refocused imaging: flow velocity, TR and flip angle (in preparation).
47. Nayler GL, Firmin DN, Longmore DB. Blood flow imaging by CINE magnetic resonance. J Comput Assist Tomogr 10:715, 1986.
48. Atlas SW, Grossman RI, Hackney DB, et al. MR imaging of intracranial vascular lesions using fast imaging. Radiology 165(P):217, 1987.
49. von Schulthess GK, Augustiny N. Calculation of T2 values versus phase imaging for the distinction between flow and thrombus in MR imaging. Radiology 164:549, 1987.
50. Wedeen VJ, Rosen BR, Brady TJ. Magnetic resonance angiography. In Kressel HY, ed. Magnetic Resonance Annual: 1987. New York, Raven Press, 1987:113.
51. Gullberg GT, Wehrli FW, Shimakawa A, et al. MR vascular imaging with a fast gradient refocusing pulse sequence and reformatted images from transaxial sections. Radiology 165:241, 1987.
52. Dumoulin CL, Hart HR Jr. Magnetic resonance angiography. Radiology 161:717, 1986.
53. Lenz GW, Haacke EM. Topical Conference on Fast Magnetic Resonance Imaging Techniques, Cleveland, 1987.
54. Tasciyan T, Lee JN, Decastro JB, et al. Fast limited flip angle MR subtraction angiography. In press.
55. Evans AJ, Blinder RA, Herfkens RJ, et al. Effects of turbulence on signal intensity in gradient echo images. Invest Radiol, 1988, in press.
56. Enzmann DR, Rubin JB, Wright A. Use of cerebrospinal fluid gating to improve T2-weighted images. Part I. The spinal cord. Radiology 162:763, 1987.
57. Koschorek F, Brinkmann G, Gremmel H. Value of fast field echo imaging in recurrence of lumbar disk herniations. Radiology 165(P):251, 1987.
58. Enzmann D, Rubin JB. Evaluation of short repetition time, partial flip angle, gradient recalled echo pulse sequence in cervical spine imaging. Radiology 165(P):251, 1987.
59. Runge VM, Osborne MA, Wolpert SM, et al. The application of paraxial scanning to MRI of the CNS. Magn Reson Imag 5:87, 1987.
60. Fram EK, Herfkens RJ, Johnson GA, et al. Rapid calculation of T1 using variable flip angle gradient refocused imaging. Magn Reson Imag 5:201, 1987.
61. Runge VM, Wood ML, Kaufman DM, et al. MR study of intracranial disease with three-dimensional FLASH. Radiology 165(P):250, 1987.
62. Gallimore GW, Harms SE. Selective three-dimensional MR imaging of the spine. J Comput Assist Tomogr 1:124, 1987.
63. Hawkes RC, Patz S. Rapid Fourier imaging using steady state free precession. Magn Reson Med 4:9, 1987.
64. Gyngel M. Steady state free precession sequences (abstract). Fast MRI Topical Conference, Cleveland, May 15–17, 1987.
65. MacFall JR. Personal communication.
66. Tkach J, Haacke E. Fast low angle spin echo (FATE) imaging (abstract). Fast MRI Topical Conference, Cleveland, Ohio, May 15–17, 1987.
67. Becker E, Ferretti J, Farrar T. Driven equilibrium Fourier transform spectroscopy—a new method for NMR signal enhancement. J Amer Chem Soc 91:7784, 1969.
68. Iwaoka H, et al. A new pulse sequence for "fast recovery" fast scan NMR imaging. IEEE Trans Med Imag 3:41, 1984.
69. Feinberg DA, Hale JD, Watts JC, et al. Halving MR imaging time by conjugation: demonstration at 3.5 kG. Radiology 161:527, 1986.
70. MacFall JR, Pelk NJ, Vavrek R. Correction of spatially dependent phase shifts for partial Fourier imaging. Mag Reson Med. In press.
71. Mansfield P. Multi-planar image formation using NMR spin echoes. J Phys 10:155, 1977.
72. Mansfield P, Pykett IL. Biological and medical imaging by NMR. J Magn Reson 29:355, 1978.
73. Crooks LE, Arakawa M, Hylton NM, et al. Performance characteristics of an echo planar imager (abstract). Topical Conference on Fast Magnetic Resonance Imaging Techniques, Cleveland, May 15–17, 1987.
74. Mansfield P, Guilfoyle DN, Ordidge RJ, et al. Measurement of T1 by echo-planar imaging and construction of computer-generated images. Phys Med Biol 31:113, 1986.
75. Likes R. Moving gradient zeugmatography. US Patent No. 4,307,343, Dec 22, 1981.
76. Rzedzian R, Pykett I. Instant images of the human heart using a new whole-body MR imaging system. AJR 149:245, 1987.
77. Hennig J, Nauerth A, Friedburg H. RARE imaging: a fast imaging method for clinical MR. Magn Reson Med 3:823, 1986.
78. Hennig J. FLARE—a fast method for MR myelography and MR urography (abstract 231). Society of Magnetic Resonance in Medicine 6th Annual Meeting, Aug 17–21, 1987.

79. Hahn EL. Spin echoes. Phys Rev 80:580, 1950.
80. Frahm J, Merboldt KD, Hanicke W, et al. Stimulated echo imaging. J Magn Reson 64:81, 1985.
81. Sattin W. Abstracts of papers. P. 932. 5th Annual Meeting of the Society of Magnetic Resonance in Medicine, Montreal, August, 1986.
82. Matthaei D, Frahm J, Haase A, et al. Multipurpose NMR imaging using stimulated echoes. Magn Reson Med 3:554, 1986.
83. Sattin W, Mareci T, Scott K. Exploiting the stimulated echo in nuclear magnetic resonance imaging. I. Method. J Magn Reson 64:177, 1985.
84. Sattin W, Mareci T, Scott K. Exploiting the stimulated echo in nuclear magnetic resonance imaging. II. Applications. J Magn Reson 65:298, 1985.
85. Haase A, Frahm J, Matthaei D, et al. MR imaging using stimulated echoes (STEAM). Radiology 160:787, 1986.
86. Matthaei D, Haase A, Frahm J, et al. Multiple chemical shift selective (CHESS) MR imaging using stimulated echoes. Radiology 160:791, 1986.
87. Sattin W. Exploiting the stimulated echo in rapid NMR imaging (abstract). Topical Conference on Fast Magnetic Resonance Imaging Techniques, Cleveland, Ohio, May 15–17, 1987.
88. van Uijen CM, Den Boef JH, Verschuren FJ. Fast Fourier imaging. Magn Reson Med 2:203, 1985.
89. Haake EM, Bearden FH, Clayton JR, et al. Reduction of MR imaging time by the hybrid fast-scan technique. Radiology 158:521, 1986.
90. Mezrich RS, Axel L, Dougherty L, et al. Strip scan: a method for faster MR imaging. RadioGraphics 6:833, 1986.

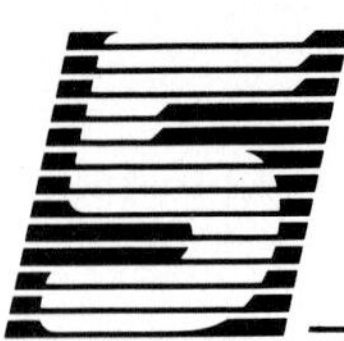

D. A. Kaffenberger, M.D.
H. N. Schnitzlein, Ph.D.
F. Reed Murtagh, M.D.

# MAGNETIC RESONANCE ANATOMY OF THE HEAD AND SPINE

An understanding of magnetic resonance imaging (MRI) of the central nervous system (CNS) must necessarily begin with a review of the anatomy of the region. MRI is capable of extremely accurate anatomic imaging of the CNS. It also affords excellent gray–white matter differentiation—as good, in fact, as seen in fixed-slice specimens.[1] The differentiation is mostly due to difference in water content of the two main types of brain matter: the neurons themselves in the gray matter, and the axons and supportive glial elements in the white matter. Lipid content in the axonal areas has been shown to contribute also to the overall scale of contrast between tissues.[2] Another important factor is the location of trace-element depositions in the brain matter; particularly important is iron deposition in the basal ganglia and other structures.[3]

Protons in moving materials such as blood or cerebrospinal fluid give off varying strengths of signals during recovery from excitational states.[4] If material is flowing fast enough through the plane of imaging slice, as with blood in the carotid arteries, no signal at all may be registered, giving a "flow-void" effect. Other tissues with tightly bound protons, such as bone, or areas with few or no protons, such as air in body cavities, also give a signal void. In the sections that follow, note particularly the regions around the base of the skull, in which rapidly flowing blood in the petrous portion of the carotid artery is indistinguishable from the sphenoid bone at the base of the skull, which in turn is indistinguishable from the air contained in the adjacent sphenoid sinus. The images in this section were generated on either a General Electric Signa model MR scaner operating at 1.5 tesla (T), or a Siemens Somation unit at 0.35T. Short TR and TE sequences were used to emphasize the anatomic aspects of each slice, and the images were copied on a 512 × 512 matrix. The images chosen were taken from routine scans performed on patients, rather than volunteers, and are representative of day-to-day imaging quality.

It is always difficult to limit detail with anatomic demonstrations. We have elected to be extensive in detail, partly as a means of emphasizing the anatomic sensitivity of this modality and partly because of a desire to be complete. We know from experience the frustration of attempting to identify the

*Text continued on page 130*

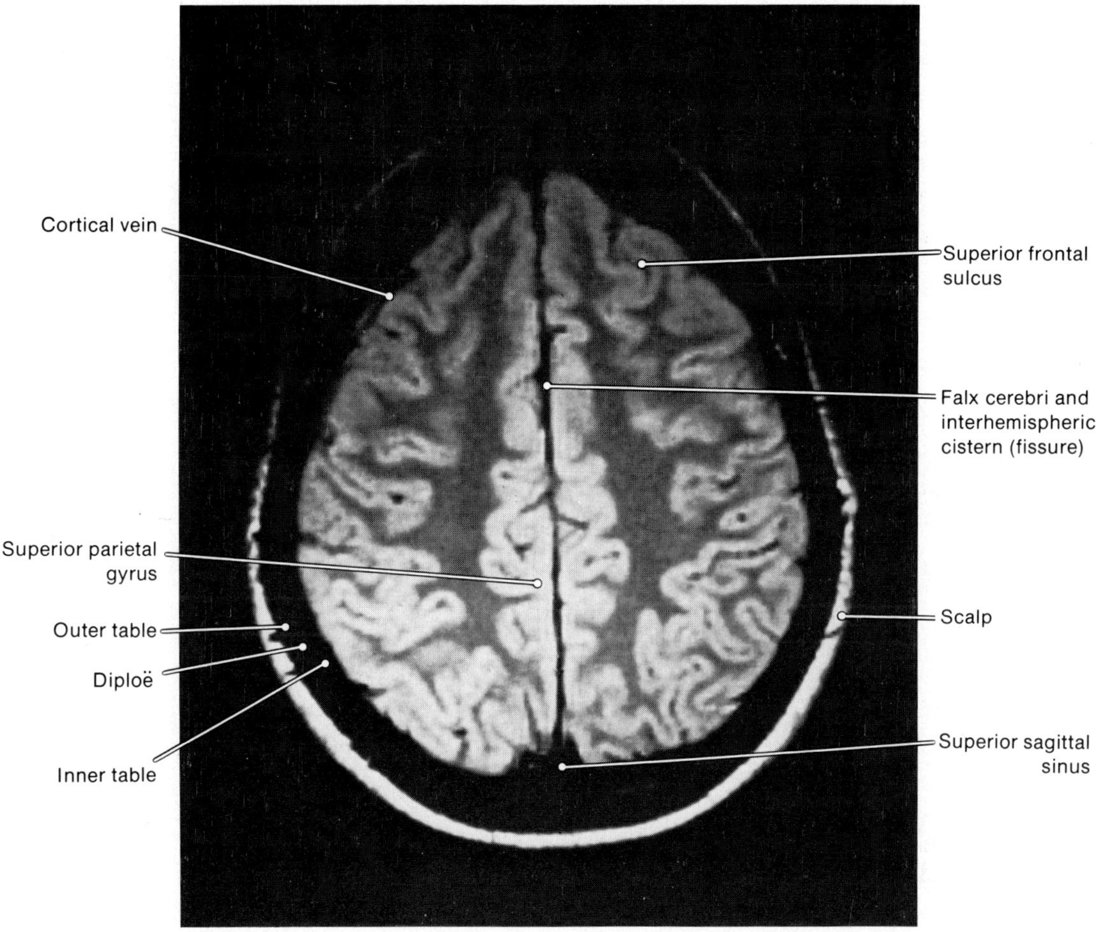

Cortical vein

Superior frontal sulcus

Falx cerebri and interhemispheric cistern (fissure)

Superior parietal gyrus

Outer table

Diploë

Inner table

Scalp

Superior sagittal sinus

**Field=1.5T TR=2.0s TE=35ms SL=4mm**

**Plane of Section**

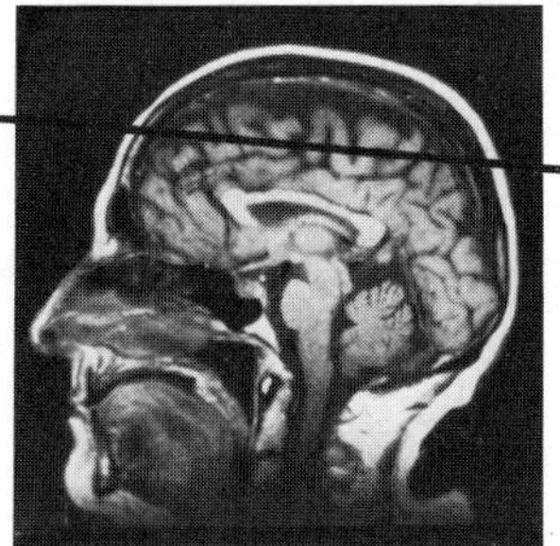

**Figure 5–1.** The upper head.

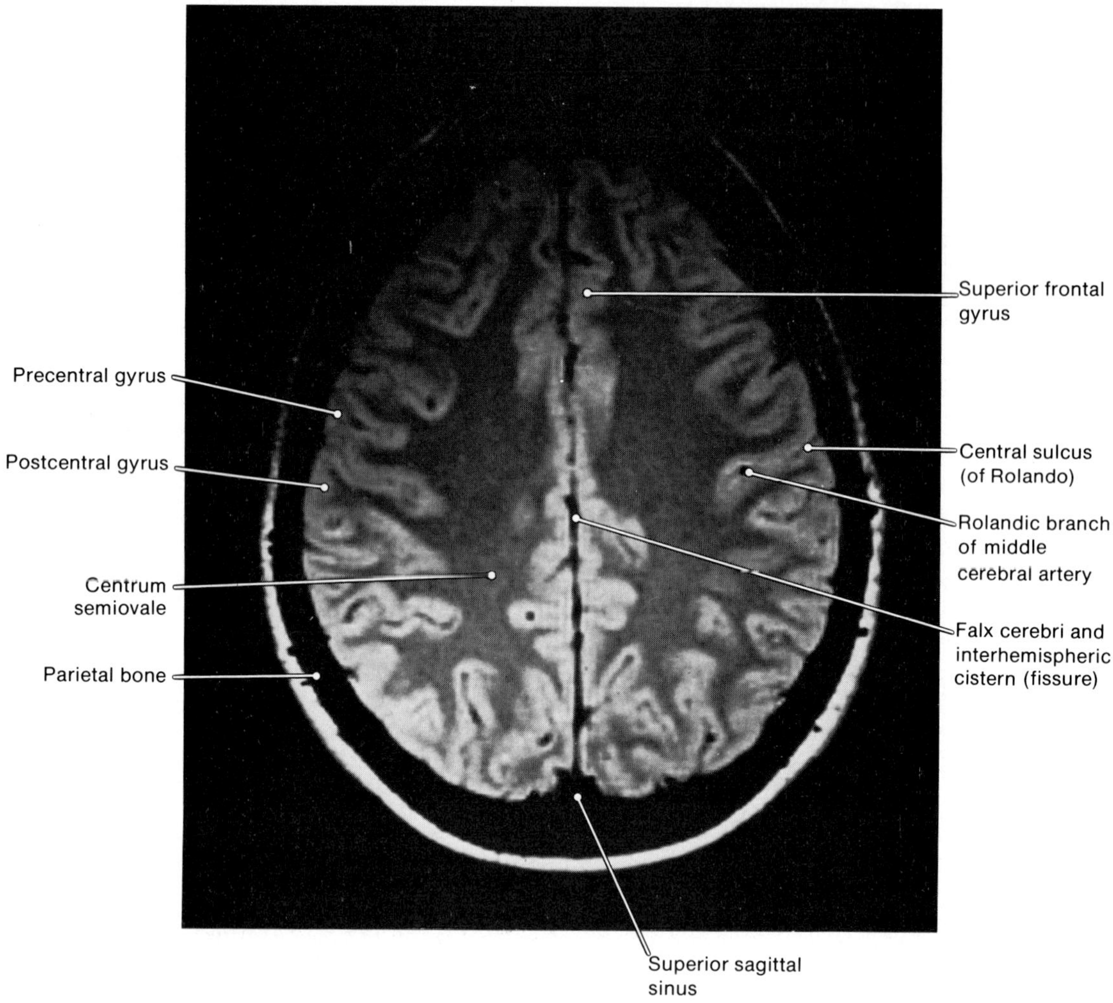

Superior frontal gyrus
Precentral gyrus
Central sulcus (of Rolando)
Postcentral gyrus
Rolandic branch of middle cerebral artery
Centrum semiovale
Falx cerebri and interhemispheric cistern (fissure)
Parietal bone
Superior sagittal sinus

**Field=1.5T TR=2.0s TE=35ms SL=4mm**

**Plane of Section**

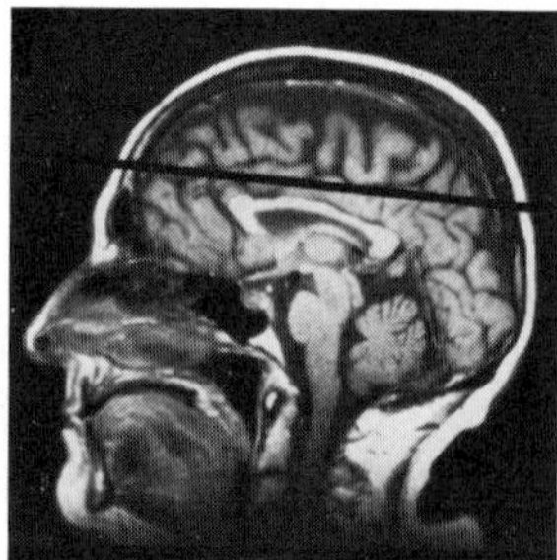

**Figure 5–2.** The centrum semiovale.

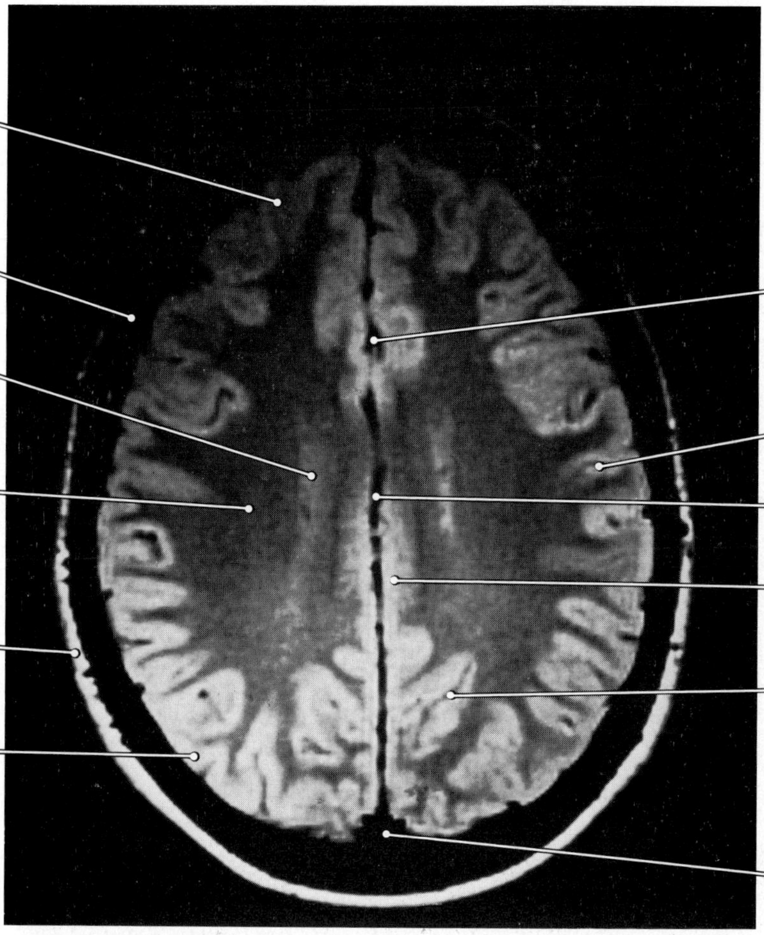

Superior frontal gyrus

Frontal bone

Body of caudate nucleus

Centrum semiovale

Scalp

Angular gyrus

Callosomarginal artery

Central sulcus (of Rolando)

Interhemispheric cistern (fissure)

Cingulate gyrus

Parieto-occipital fissure

Superior sagittal sinus

**Field=1.5T TR=2.0s TE=35ms SL=4mm**

**Plane of Section**

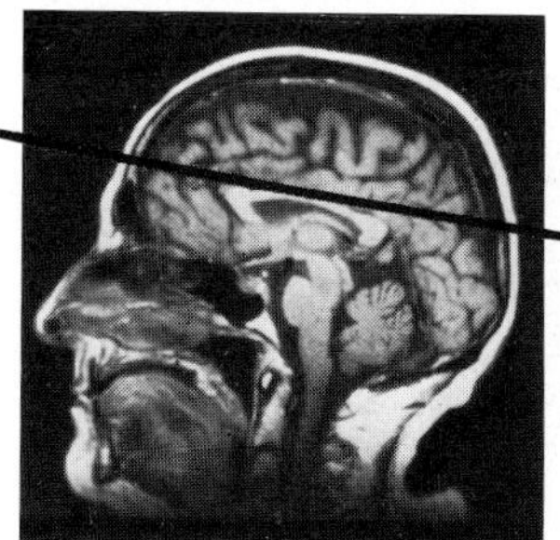

**Figure 5–3.** Above the corpus callosum.

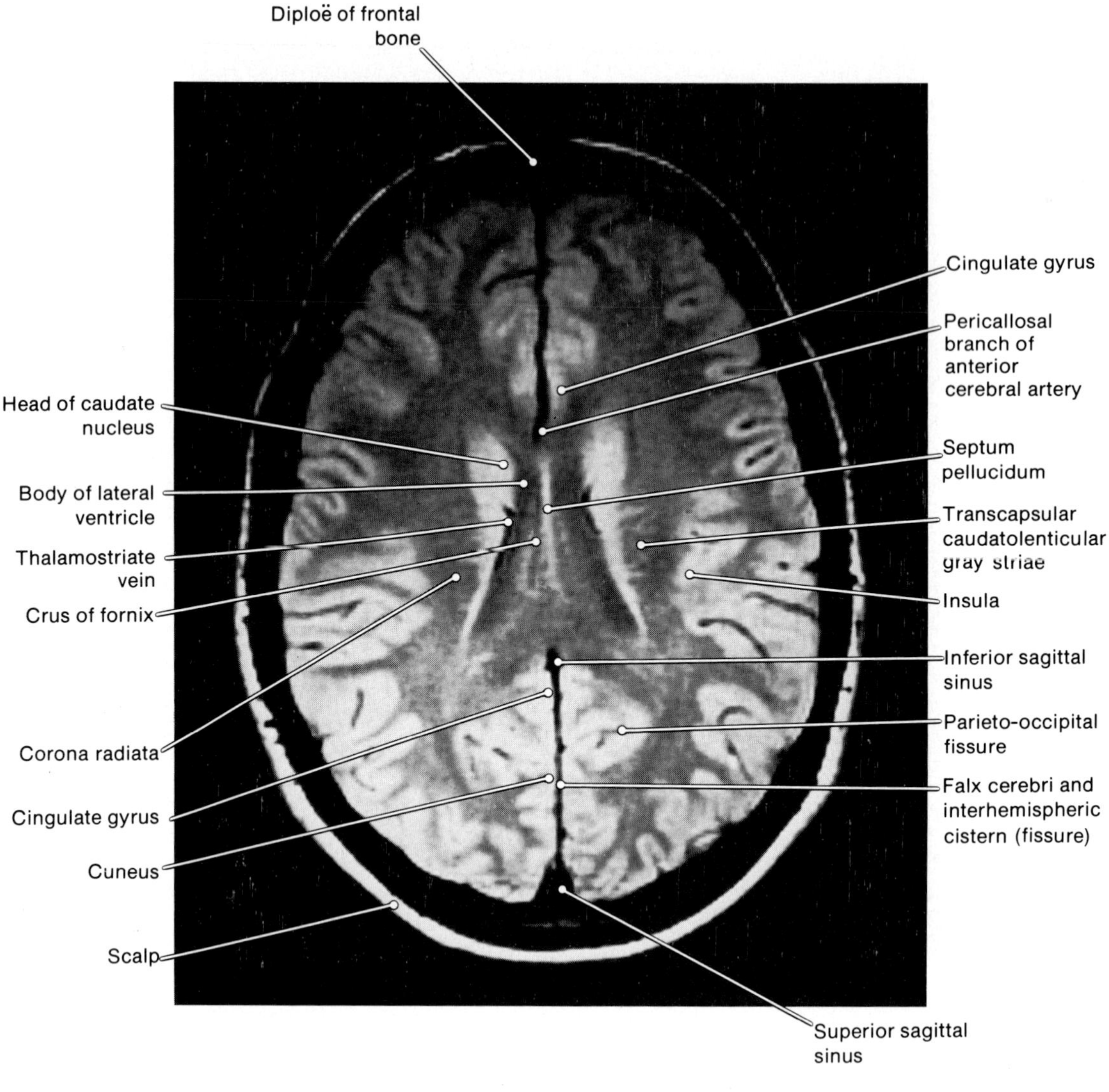

Diploë of frontal bone

Cingulate gyrus

Pericallosal branch of anterior cerebral artery

Head of caudate nucleus

Septum pellucidum

Body of lateral ventricle

Transcapsular caudatolenticular gray striae

Thalamostriate vein

Crus of fornix

Insula

Inferior sagittal sinus

Parieto-occipital fissure

Corona radiata

Cingulate gyrus

Falx cerebri and interhemispheric cistern (fissure)

Cuneus

Scalp

Superior sagittal sinus

**Field=1.5T TR=2.0s TE=35ms SL=4mm**

**Plane of Section**

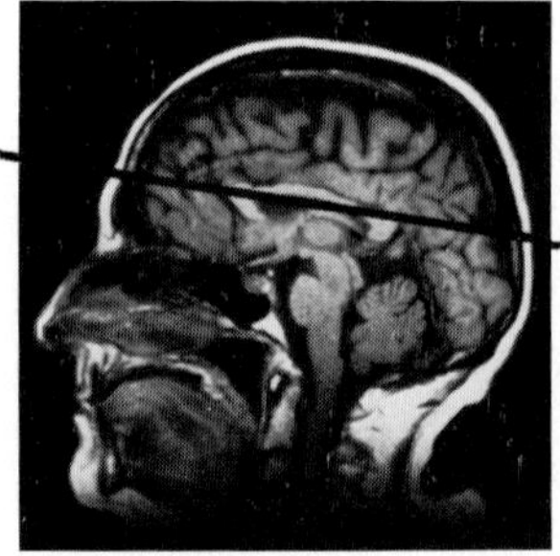

**Figure 5–4.** The corpus callosum.

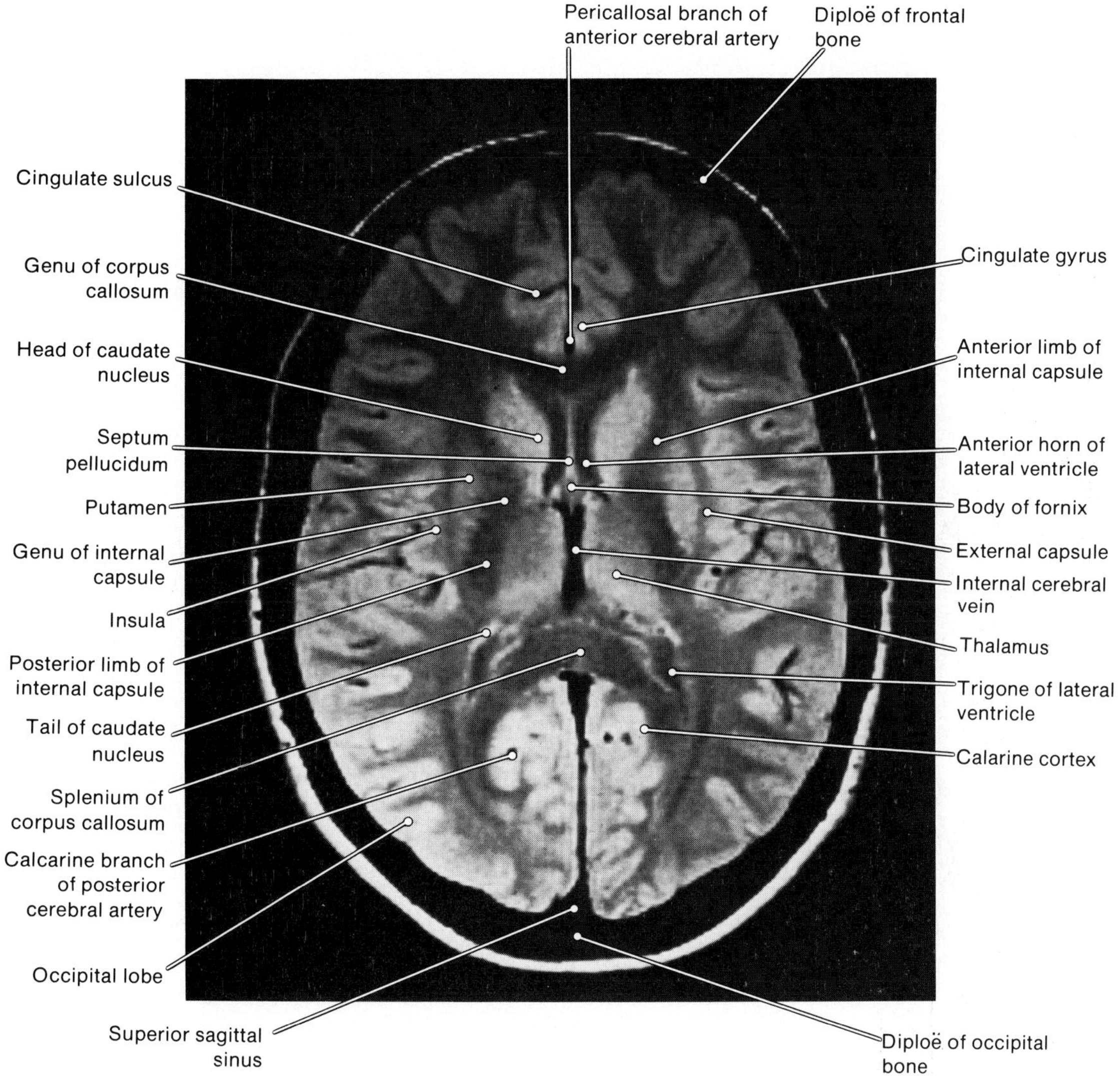

Pericallosal branch of anterior cerebral artery

Diploë of frontal bone

Cingulate sulcus

Genu of corpus callosum

Head of caudate nucleus

Septum pellucidum

Putamen

Genu of internal capsule

Insula

Posterior limb of internal capsule

Tail of caudate nucleus

Splenium of corpus callosum

Calcarine branch of posterior cerebral artery

Occipital lobe

Superior sagittal sinus

Cingulate gyrus

Anterior limb of internal capsule

Anterior horn of lateral ventricle

Body of fornix

External capsule

Internal cerebral vein

Thalamus

Trigone of lateral ventricle

Calarine cortex

Diploë of occipital bone

**Field=1.5T TR=2.0s TE=35ms SL=4mm**

**Plane of Section**

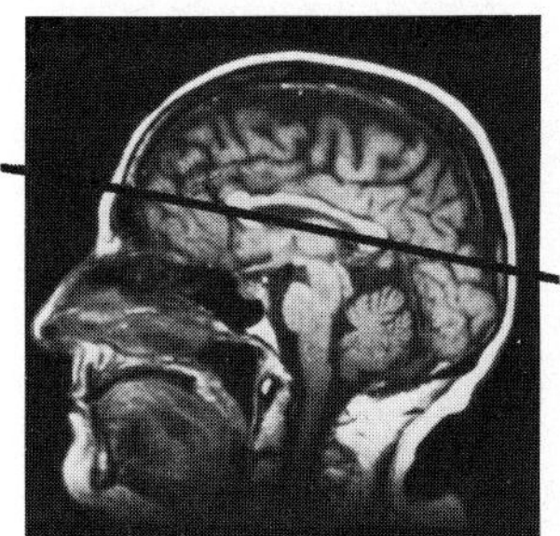

**Figure 5–5.** The superior thalamus.

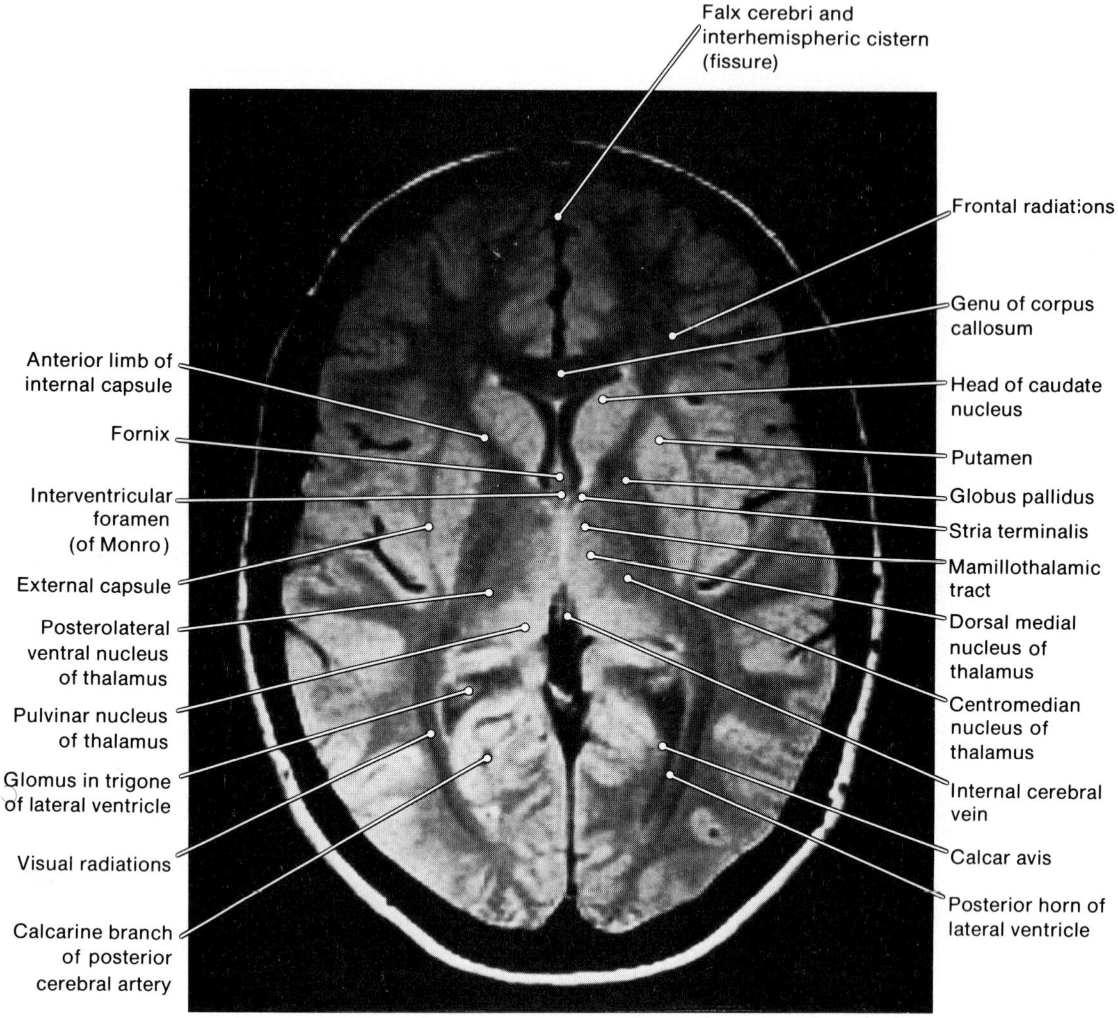

Falx cerebri and interhemispheric cistern (fissure)

Anterior limb of internal capsule

Fornix

Interventricular foramen (of Monro)

External capsule

Posterolateral ventral nucleus of thalamus

Pulvinar nucleus of thalamus

Glomus in trigone of lateral ventricle

Visual radiations

Calcarine branch of posterior cerebral artery

Frontal radiations

Genu of corpus callosum

Head of caudate nucleus

Putamen

Globus pallidus

Stria terminalis

Mamillothalamic tract

Dorsal medial nucleus of thalamus

Centromedian nucleus of thalamus

Internal cerebral vein

Calcar avis

Posterior horn of lateral ventricle

**Field=1.5T TR=2.0s TE=35ms SL=4mm**

**Plane of Section**

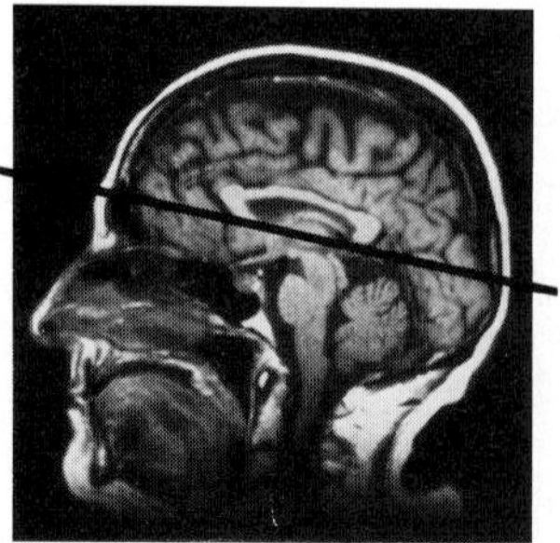

**Figure 5–6.** The midthalamus.

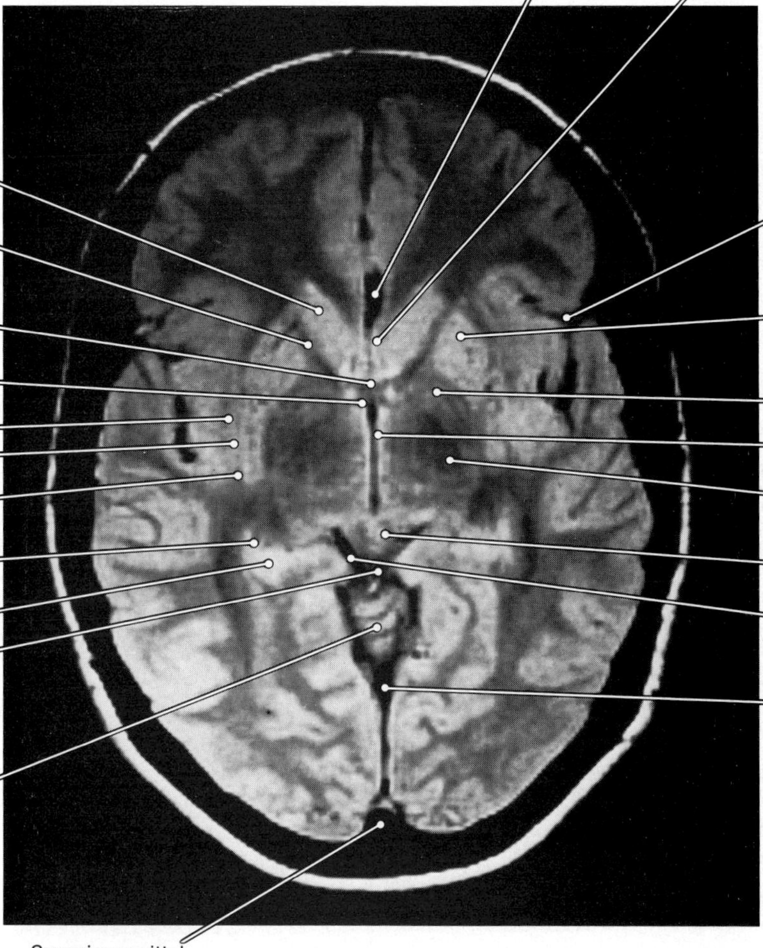

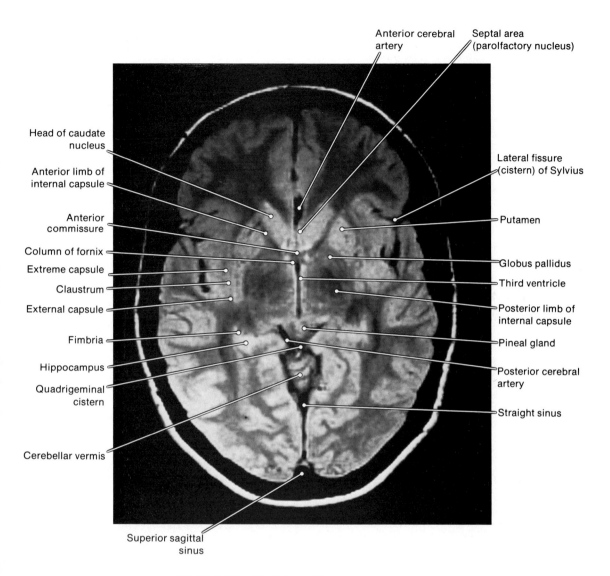

Anterior cerebral artery
Septal area (parolfactory nucleus)
Head of caudate nucleus
Lateral fissure (cistern) of Sylvius
Anterior limb of internal capsule
Anterior commissure
Putamen
Column of fornix
Globus pallidus
Extreme capsule
Third ventricle
Claustrum
External capsule
Posterior limb of internal capsule
Fimbria
Pineal gland
Hippocampus
Posterior cerebral artery
Quadrigeminal cistern
Straight sinus
Cerebellar vermis
Superior sagittal sinus

**Field=1.5T TR=2.0s TE=35ms SL=4mm**

**Plane of Section**

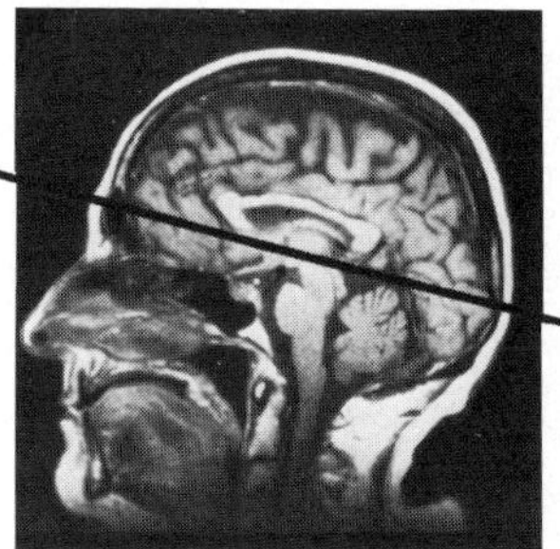

**Figure 5–7.** The pineal gland.

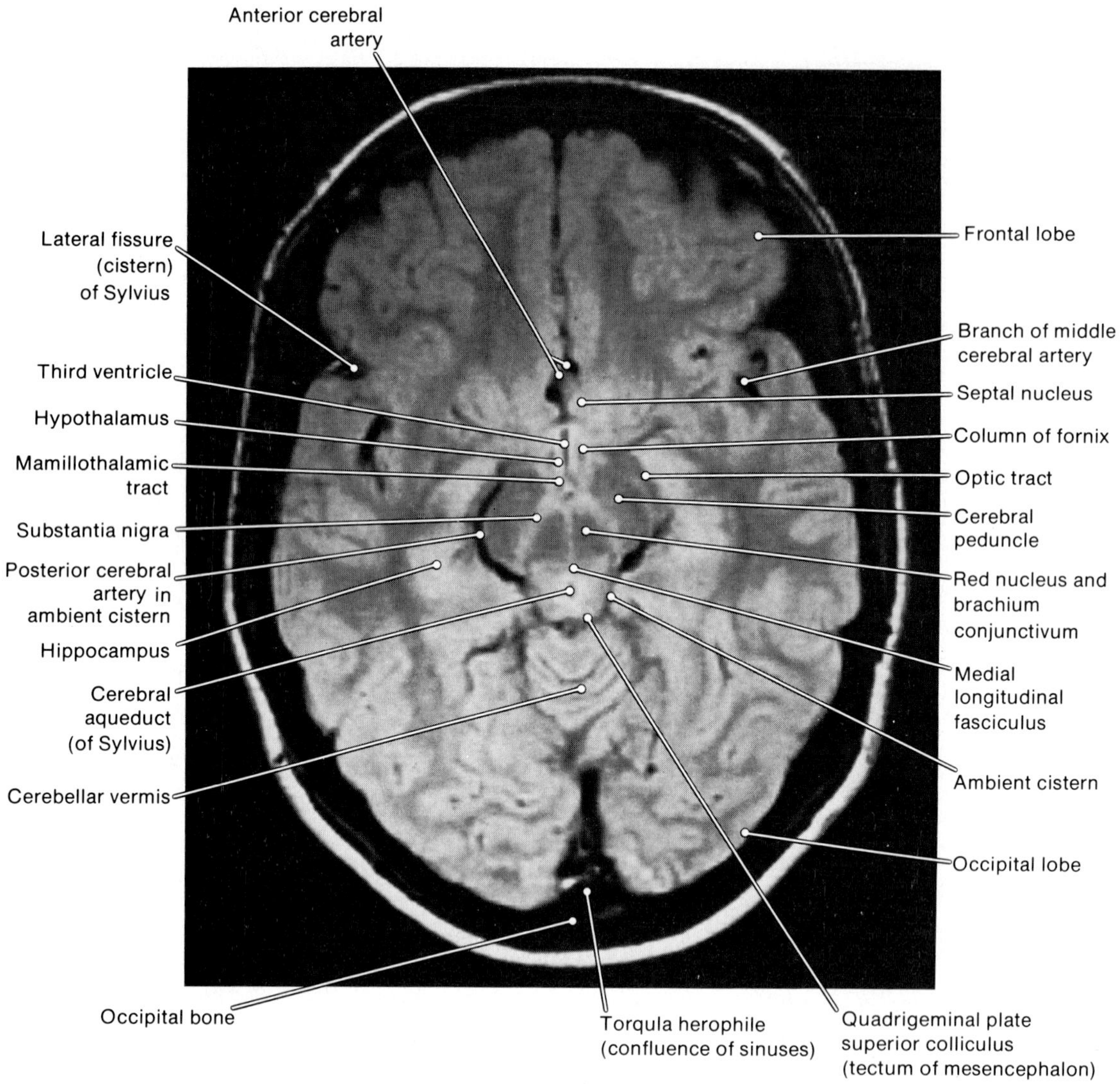

Anterior cerebral artery

Lateral fissure (cistern) of Sylvius

Third ventricle

Hypothalamus

Mamillothalamic tract

Substantia nigra

Posterior cerebral artery in ambient cistern

Hippocampus

Cerebral aqueduct (of Sylvius)

Cerebellar vermis

Frontal lobe

Branch of middle cerebral artery

Septal nucleus

Column of fornix

Optic tract

Cerebral peduncle

Red nucleus and brachium conjunctivum

Medial longitudinal fasciculus

Ambient cistern

Occipital lobe

Occipital bone

Torqula herophile (confluence of sinuses)

Quadrigeminal plate superior colliculus (tectum of mesencephalon)

**Field=1.5T TR=2.0s TE=35ms SL=4mm**

**Plane of Section**

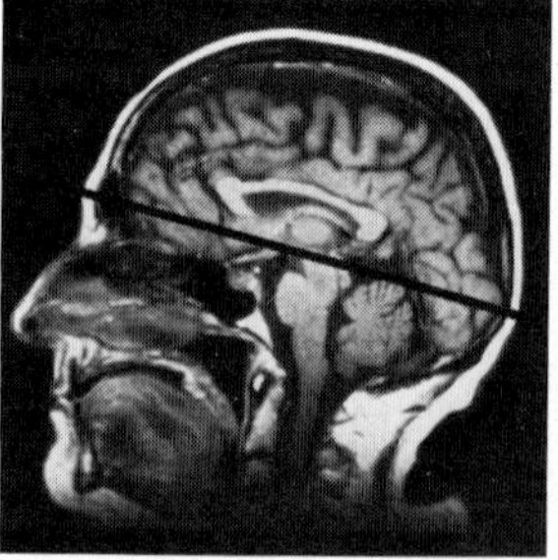

**Figure 5–8.** The superior colliculus.

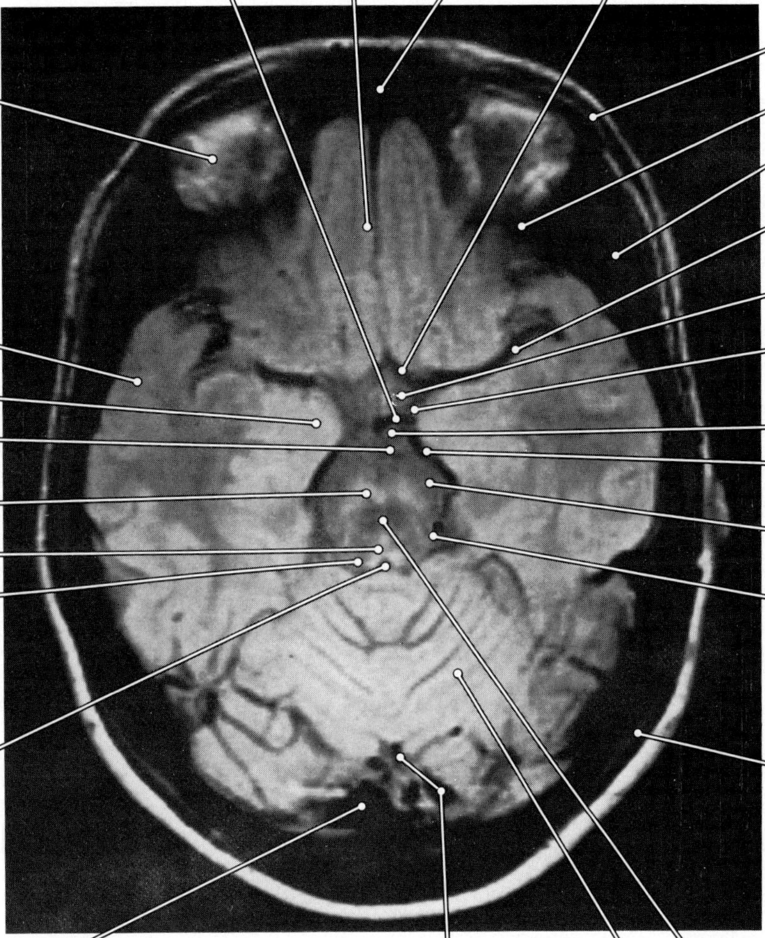

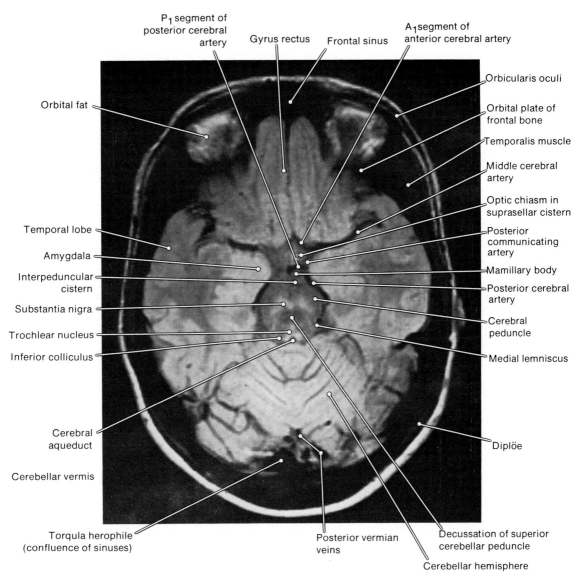

$P_1$ segment of posterior cerebral artery
Gyrus rectus
Frontal sinus
$A_1$ segment of anterior cerebral artery
Orbital fat
Orbicularis oculi
Orbital plate of frontal bone
Temporalis muscle
Middle cerebral artery
Optic chiasm in suprasellar cistern
Temporal lobe
Posterior communicating artery
Amygdala
Mamillary body
Interpeduncular cistern
Posterior cerebral artery
Substantia nigra
Cerebral peduncle
Trochlear nucleus
Inferior colliculus
Medial lemniscus
Cerebral aqueduct
Diplöe
Cerebellar vermis
Torqula herophile (confluence of sinuses)
Posterior vermian veins
Decussation of superior cerebellar peduncle
Cerebellar hemisphere

**Field=1.5T TR=2.0s TE=35ms SL=4mm**

**Plane of Section**

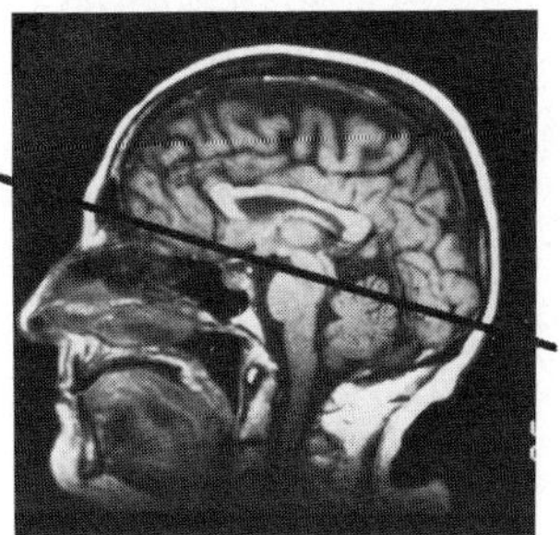

**Figure 5–9.** The inferior colliculus.

Perpendicular plate of the ethmoid bone
Ethmoid air cells
Temporalis muscle
Globe
Zygoma
Retrobulbar fat
Superior orbital fissure
Internal carotid artery (cavernous portion)
Infundibulum
Basilar artery
Superior cerebellar artery
Medial longitudinal fasciculus
Fourth ventricle
Falx cerebelli
Greater wing of the sphenoid bone
Opthalmic artery
Posterior communicating artery
Lateral dura of cavernous sinus (anterior petroclinoid ligament)
Basilar pons
Medial lemniscus
Cerebellar hemisphere
Cerebellar vermis
Superior cerebellar peduncle (brachium conjunctivum)

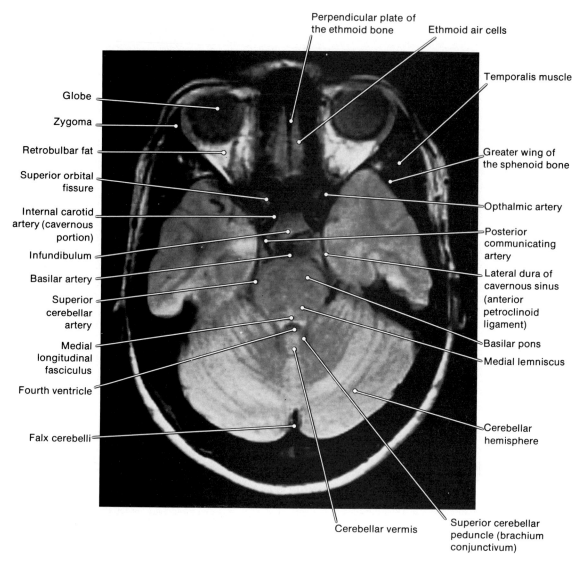

**Field=1.5T TR=2.0s TE=35ms SL=4mm**

**Plane of Section**

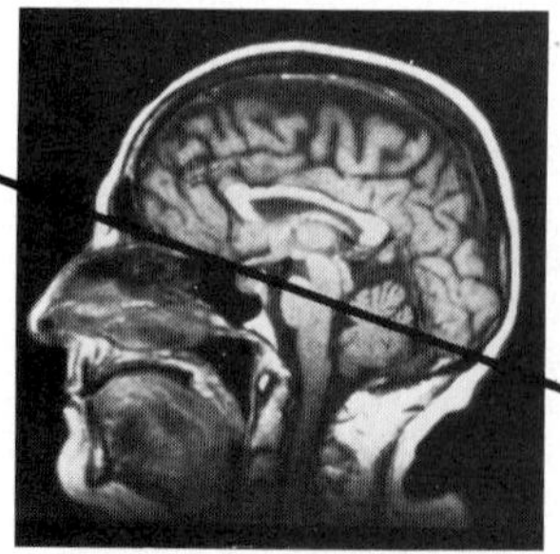

**Figure 5–10.** The basilar pons.

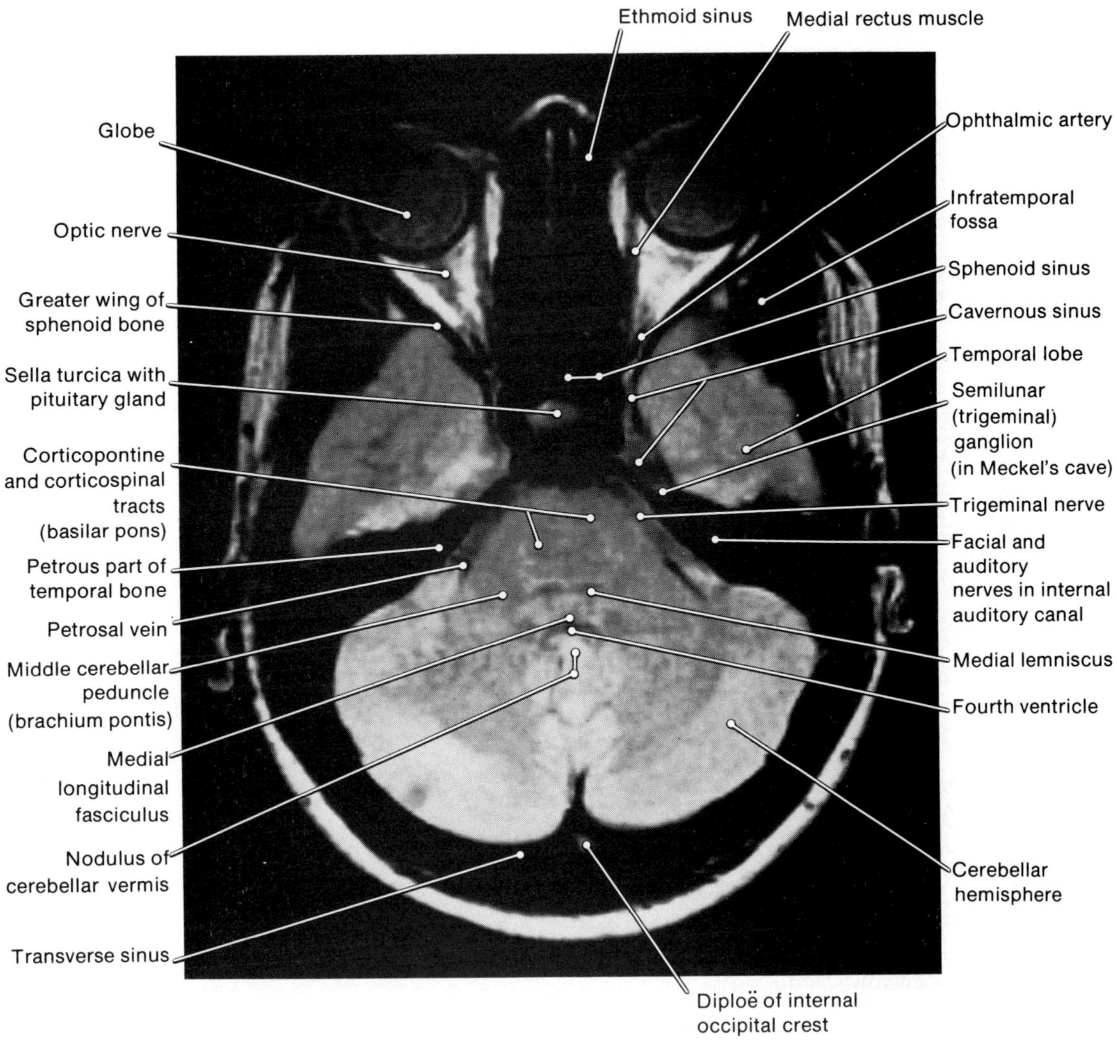

Ethmoid sinus
Medial rectus muscle
Globe
Optic nerve
Greater wing of sphenoid bone
Sella turcica with pituitary gland
Corticopontine and corticospinal tracts (basilar pons)
Petrous part of temporal bone
Petrosal vein
Middle cerebellar peduncle (brachium pontis)
Medial longitudinal fasciculus
Nodulus of cerebellar vermis
Transverse sinus
Ophthalmic artery
Infratemporal fossa
Sphenoid sinus
Cavernous sinus
Temporal lobe
Semilunar (trigeminal) ganglion (in Meckel's cave)
Trigeminal nerve
Facial and auditory nerves in internal auditory canal
Medial lemniscus
Fourth ventricle
Cerebellar hemisphere
Diploë of internal occipital crest

**Field=1.5T TR=2.0s TE=35ms SL=4mm**

**Plane of Section**

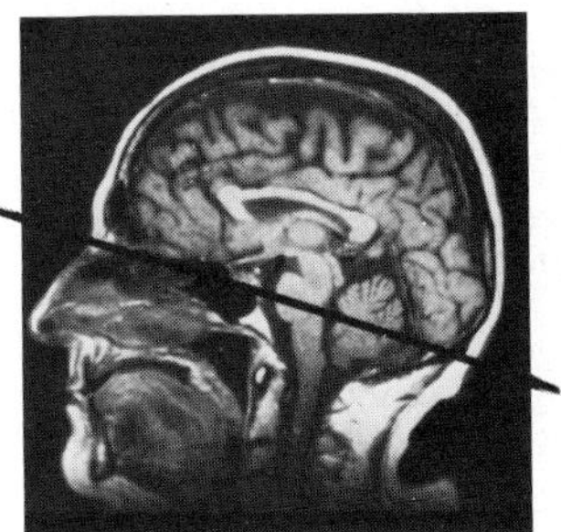

**Figure 5–11.** The sella turcica.

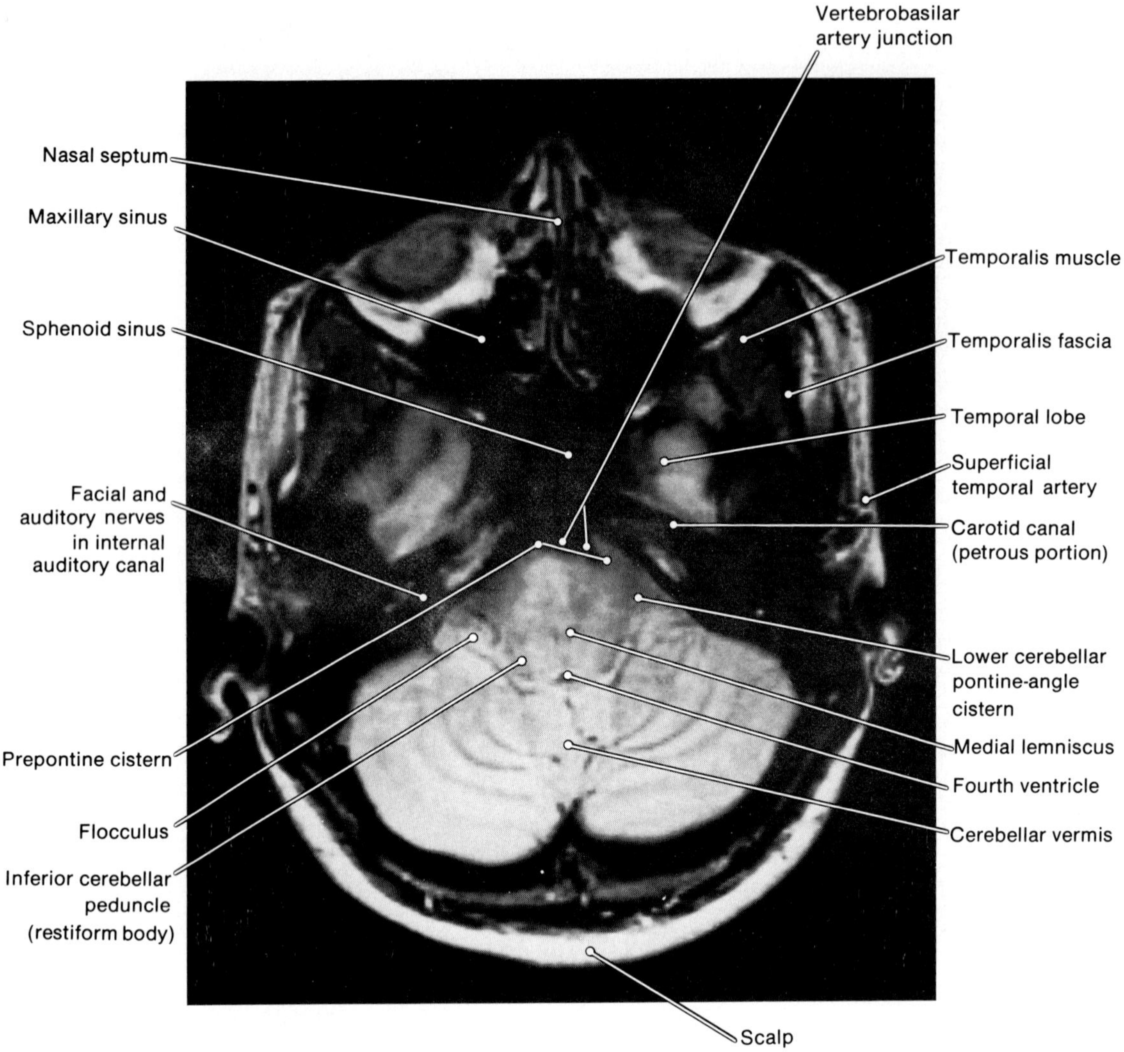

Vertebrobasilar artery junction

Nasal septum

Maxillary sinus

Sphenoid sinus

Facial and auditory nerves in internal auditory canal

Temporalis muscle

Temporalis fascia

Temporal lobe

Superficial temporal artery

Carotid canal (petrous portion)

Lower cerebellar pontine-angle cistern

Medial lemniscus

Fourth ventricle

Cerebellar vermis

Prepontine cistern

Flocculus

Inferior cerebellar peduncle (restiform body)

Scalp

**Field=1.5T TR=2.0s TE=35ms SL=4mm**

**Plane of Section**

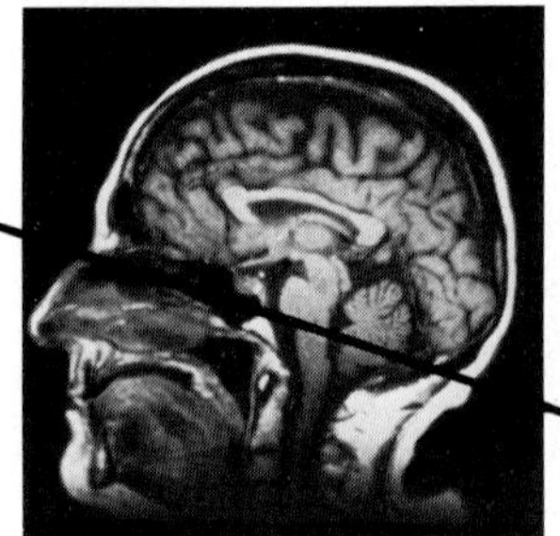

**Figure 5–12.** The pons-medulla junction.

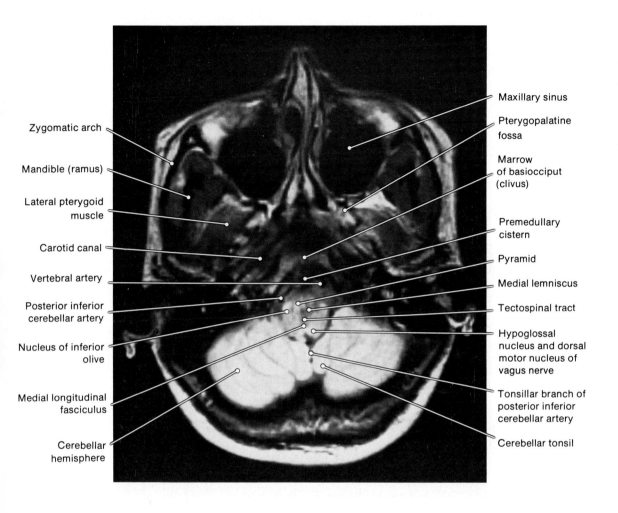

Zygomatic arch
Mandible (ramus)
Lateral pterygoid muscle
Carotid canal
Vertebral artery
Posterior inferior cerebellar artery
Nucleus of inferior olive
Medial longitudinal fasciculus
Cerebellar hemisphere
Maxillary sinus
Pterygopalatine fossa
Marrow of basiocciput (clivus)
Premedullary cistern
Pyramid
Medial lemniscus
Tectospinal tract
Hypoglossal nucleus and dorsal motor nucleus of vagus nerve
Tonsillar branch of posterior inferior cerebellar artery
Cerebellar tonsil

**Field**=**1.5T TR**=**2.0s TE**=**35ms SL**=**4mm**

**Plane of Section**

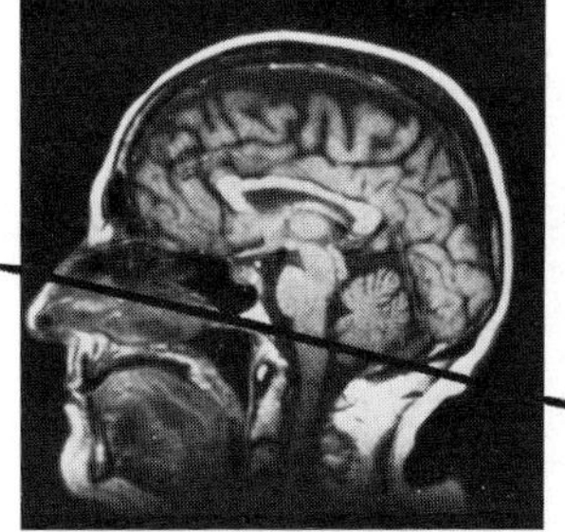

**Figure 5–13.** The pyramids.

Nasal Septum

Maxillary sinus

Medial pterygoid lamina

Lateral pterygoid lamina

Lateral pharyngeal recess (fossa of Rosenmüller)

Longus capitis muscle

Internal carotid artery

Jugular vein

Left vertebral artery

Marrow of occipital condyle

Right vertebral artery

Medulla

Cerebellar tonsil

Infraorbital nerve

Masseter muscle

Torus tubarius

Pharyngo-tympanic tube

Lateral pterygoid muscle

Medial pterygoid muscle

Mastoid process

Foramen magnum

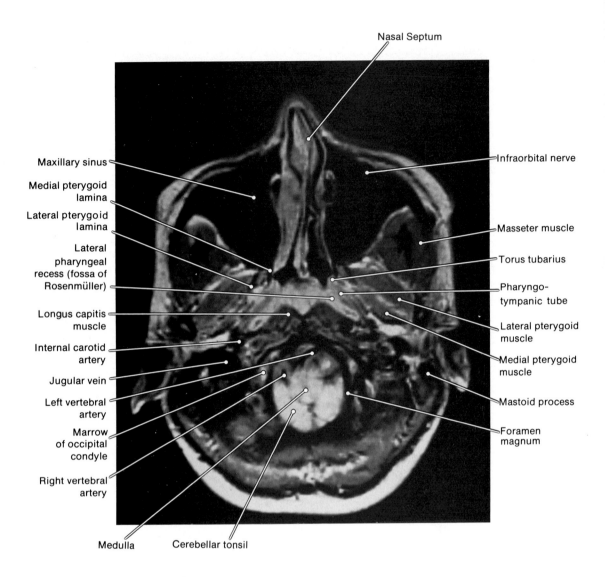

**Field=1.5T TR=2.0s TE=35ms SL=4mm**

**Plane of Section**

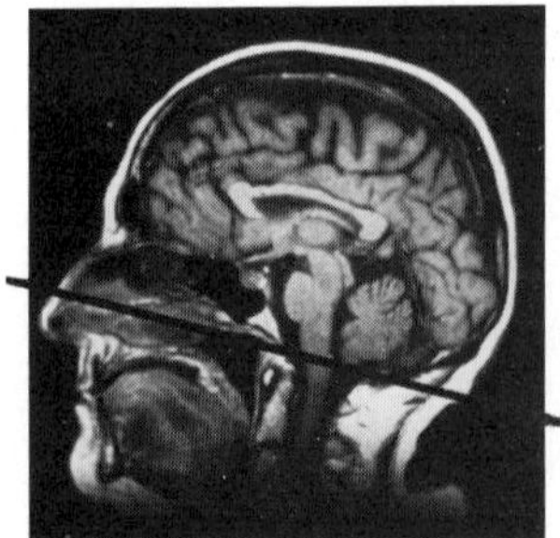

**Figure 5–14.** The atlanto-occipital joint.

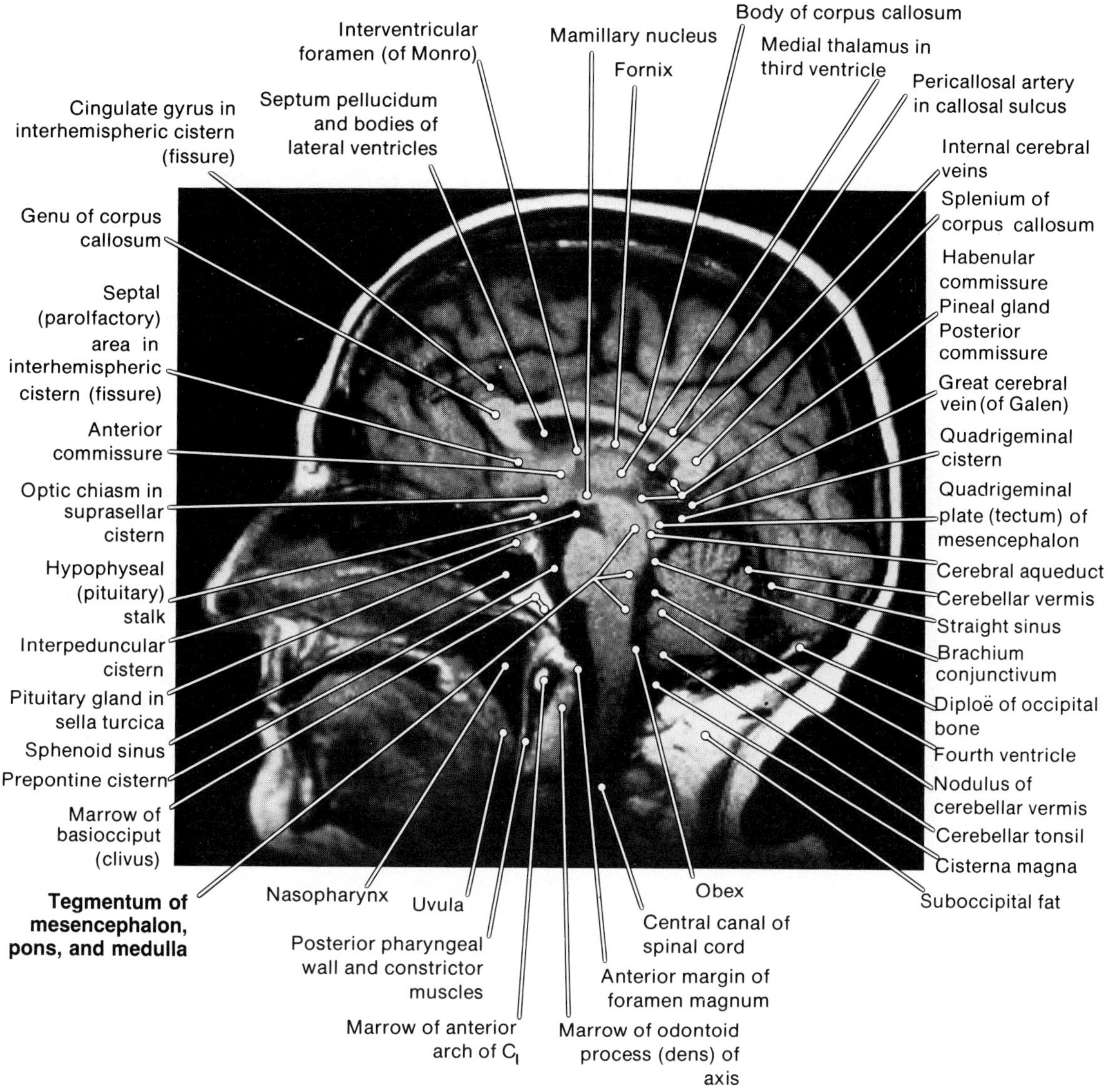

Interventricular foramen (of Monro)
Mamillary nucleus
Body of corpus callosum
Medial thalamus in third ventricle
Fornix
Pericallosal artery in callosal sulcus
Cingulate gyrus in interhemispheric cistern (fissure)
Septum pellucidum and bodies of lateral ventricles
Internal cerebral veins
Splenium of corpus callosum
Genu of corpus callosum
Habenular commissure
Septal (parolfactory) area in interhemispheric cistern (fissure)
Pineal gland
Posterior commissure
Great cerebral vein (of Galen)
Anterior commissure
Quadrigeminal cistern
Optic chiasm in suprasellar cistern
Quadrigeminal plate (tectum) of mesencephalon
Hypophyseal (pituitary) stalk
Cerebral aqueduct
Cerebellar vermis
Interpeduncular cistern
Straight sinus
Brachium conjunctivum
Pituitary gland in sella turcica
Diploë of occipital bone
Sphenoid sinus
Fourth ventricle
Prepontine cistern
Nodulus of cerebellar vermis
Marrow of basiocciput (clivus)
Cerebellar tonsil
Cisterna magna
Suboccipital fat

**Tegmentum of mesencephalon, pons, and medulla**

Nasopharynx
Uvula
Obex
Central canal of spinal cord
Posterior pharyngeal wall and constrictor muscles
Anterior margin of foramen magnum
Marrow of anterior arch of $C_1$
Marrow of odontoid process (dens) of axis

**Field=1.5T TR=0.5s TE=17ms SL=4mm**

**Plane of Section**

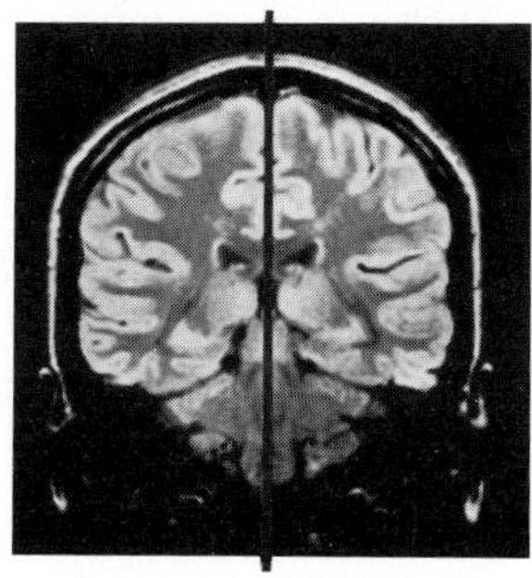

**Figure 5–15.** The midsagittal section: third ventricle.

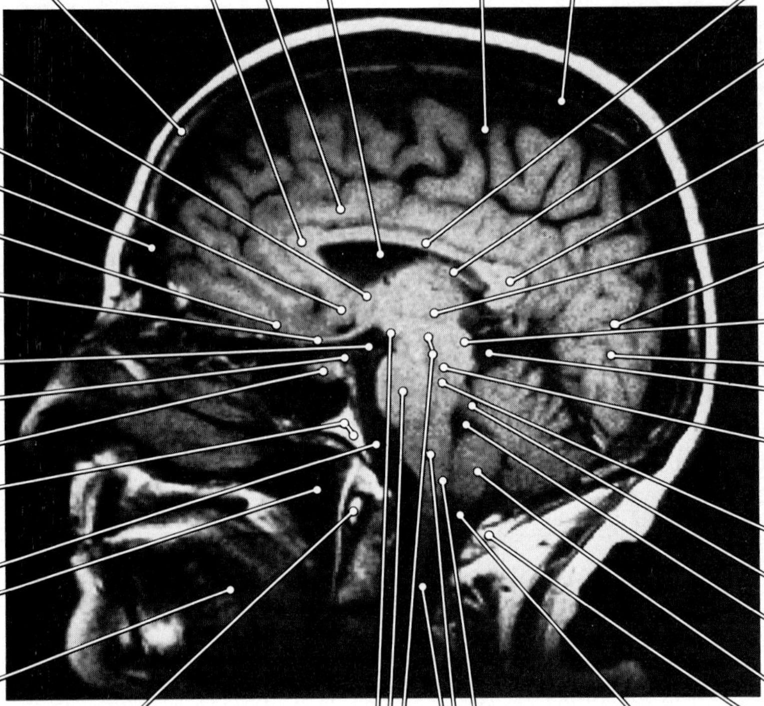

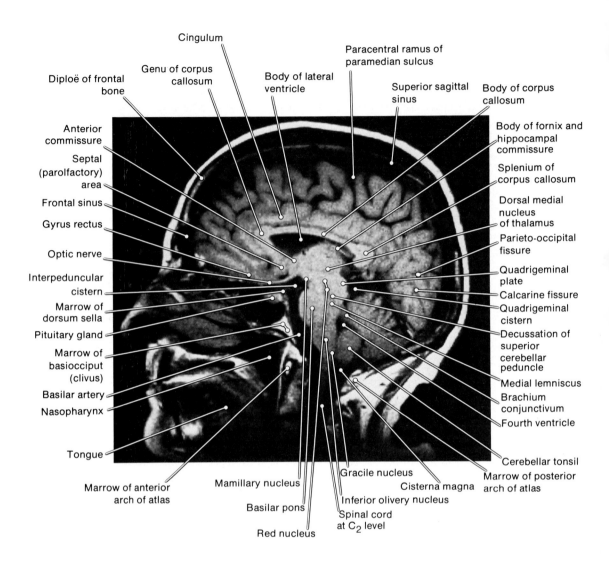

Cingulum
Paracentral ramus of paramedian sulcus
Genu of corpus callosum
Body of lateral ventricle
Diploë of frontal bone
Superior sagittal sinus
Body of corpus callosum
Anterior commissure
Body of fornix and hippocampal commissure
Septal (parolfactory) area
Splenium of corpus callosum
Frontal sinus
Dorsal medial nucleus of thalamus
Gyrus rectus
Parieto-occipital fissure
Optic nerve
Quadrigeminal plate
Interpeduncular cistern
Calcarine fissure
Marrow of dorsum sella
Quadrigeminal cistern
Pituitary gland
Decussation of superior cerebellar peduncle
Marrow of basiocciput (clivus)
Medial lemniscus
Basilar artery
Brachium conjunctivum
Nasopharynx
Fourth ventricle
Tongue
Cerebellar tonsil
Gracile nucleus
Marrow of posterior arch of atlas
Marrow of anterior arch of atlas
Mamillary nucleus
Cisterna magna
Inferior olivery nucleus
Basilar pons
Spinal cord at $C_2$ level
Red nucleus

**Field=1.5T TR=0.5s TE=17ms SL=4mm**

**Plane of Section**

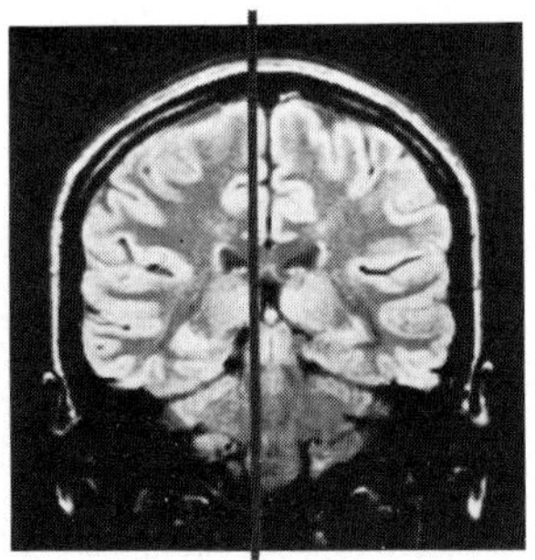

**Figure 5–16.** The paramedian plane.

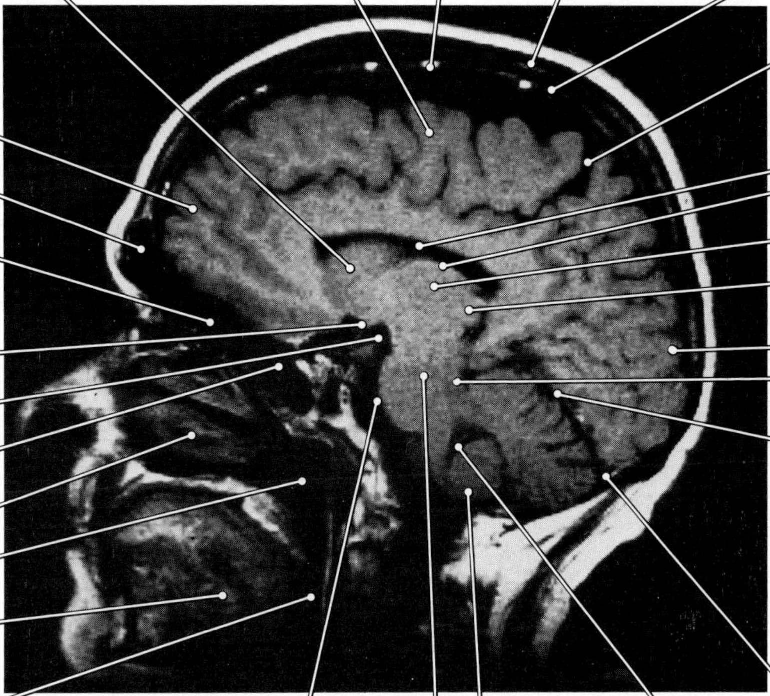

Superior cortical vein
Diploë of parietal bone
Parietal lobe
Caudate nucleus
Superior sagittal sinus
Marginal ramus of cingulate sulcus
Frontal lobe
Body of lateral ventricle
Frontal sinus
Body of fornix
Ethmoid sinuses
Thalamus
Pulvinar of thalamus
Optic tract
Occipital lobe
Oculomotor nerve
Tegmentum of pons
Sphenoid sinus
Superior cerebellar cistern and tentorium cerebelli
Inferior turbinate
Nasopharynx
Tongue
Oropharynx
Transverse sinus
Prepontine cistern
Basilar pons
Cerebellar tonsil
Fourth ventricle

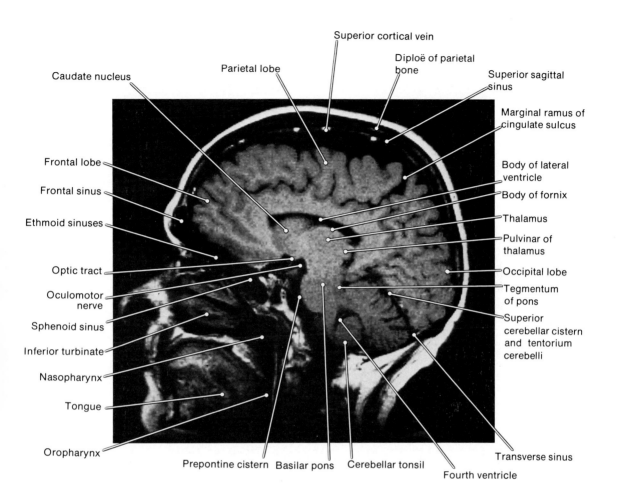

**Field=1.5T TR=0.5s TE=17ms SL=4mm**

**Plane of Section**

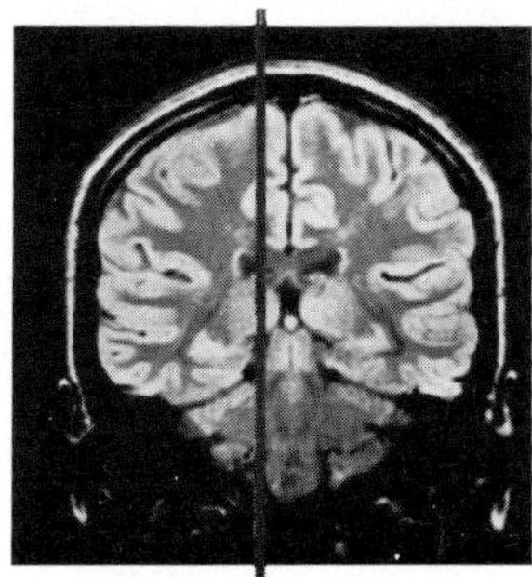

**Figure 5–17.** The right medial thalamus.

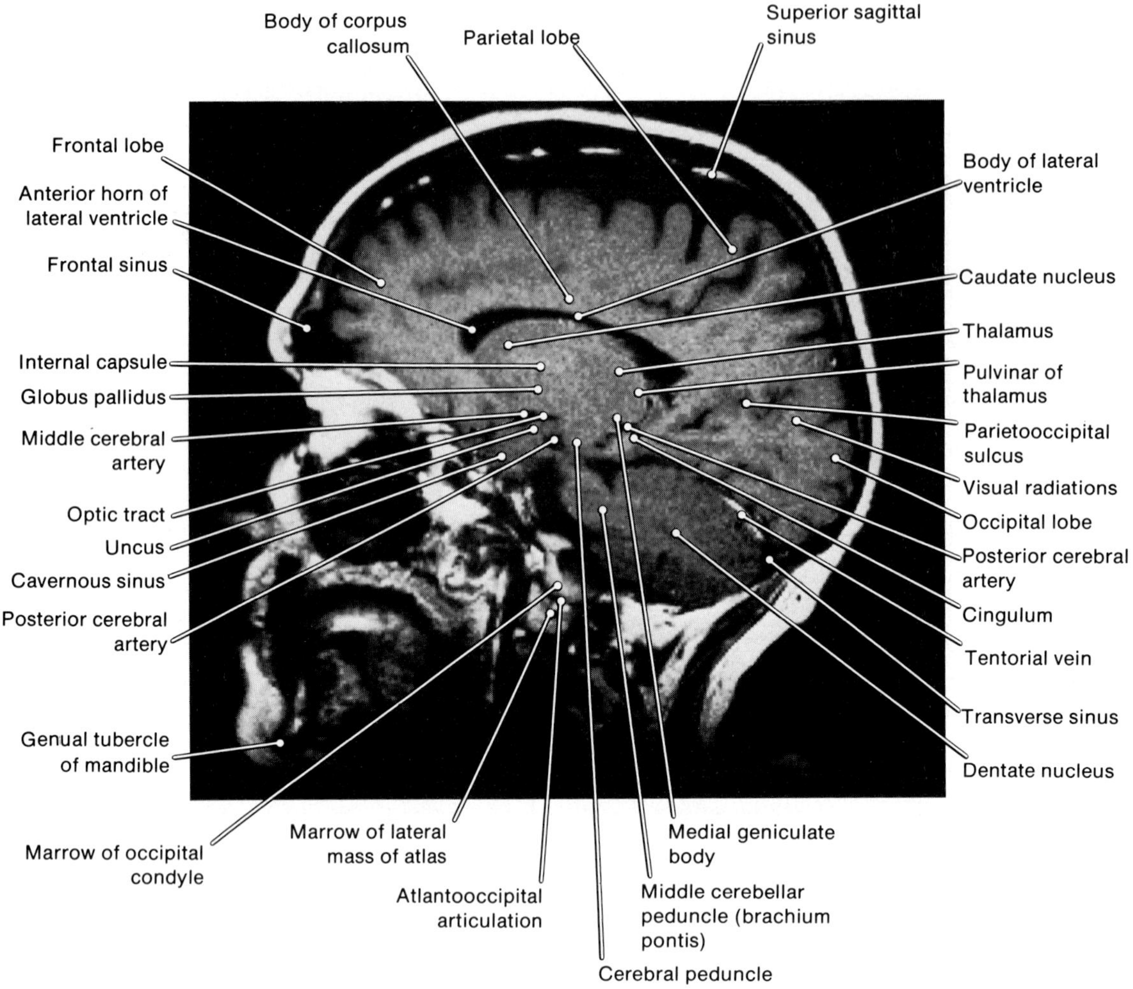

Body of corpus callosum
Parietal lobe
Superior sagittal sinus
Frontal lobe
Anterior horn of lateral ventricle
Frontal sinus
Internal capsule
Globus pallidus
Middle cerebral artery
Optic tract
Uncus
Cavernous sinus
Posterior cerebral artery
Genual tubercle of mandible
Marrow of occipital condyle
Marrow of lateral mass of atlas
Atlantooccipital articulation
Cerebral peduncle
Middle cerebellar peduncle (brachium pontis)
Medial geniculate body
Body of lateral ventricle
Caudate nucleus
Thalamus
Pulvinar of thalamus
Parietooccipital sulcus
Visual radiations
Occipital lobe
Posterior cerebral artery
Cingulum
Tentorial vein
Transverse sinus
Dentate nucleus

**Field=1.5T TR=0.5s TE=17ms SL=4mm**

**Plane of Section**

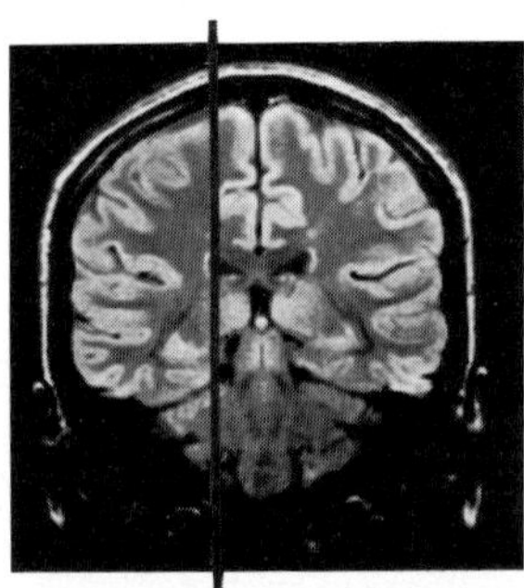

**Figure 5–18.** The right midthalamus.

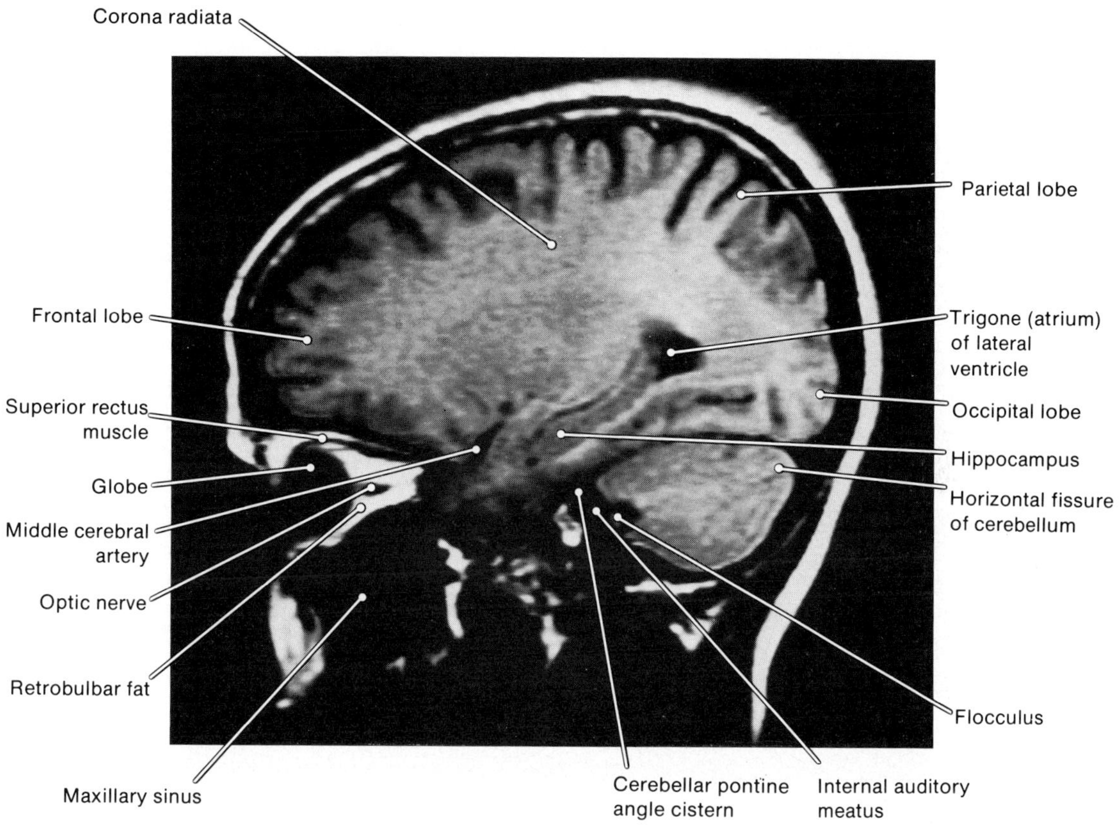

Corona radiata

Parietal lobe

Frontal lobe

Trigone (atrium) of lateral ventricle

Superior rectus muscle

Occipital lobe

Hippocampus

Globe

Horizontal fissure of cerebellum

Middle cerebral artery

Optic nerve

Retrobulbar fat

Flocculus

Maxillary sinus

Cerebellar pontine angle cistern

Internal auditory meatus

**Field=1.5T TR=0.5s TE=17ms SL=4mm**

**Plane of Section**

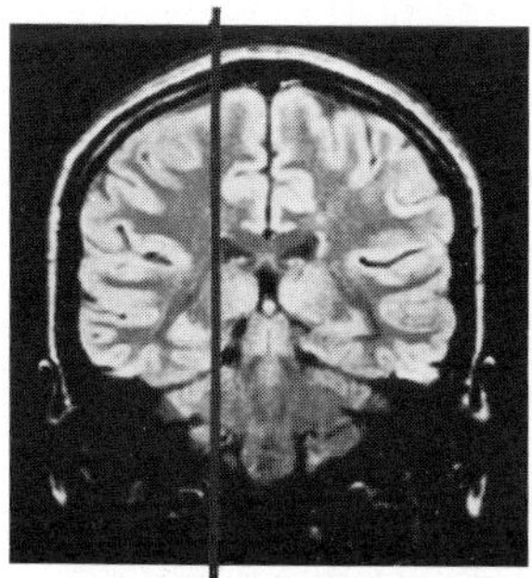

**Figure 5–19.** The internal auditory meatus.

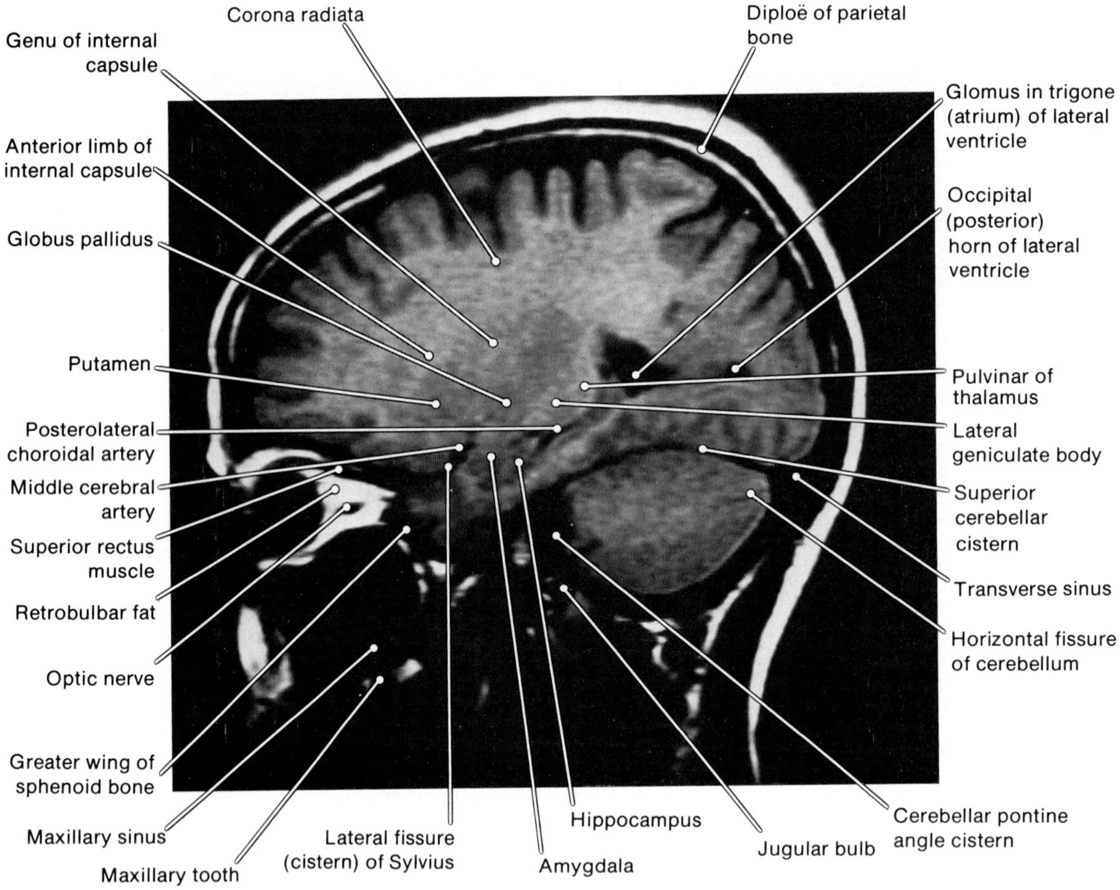

Corona radiata
Diploë of parietal bone
Genu of internal capsule
Glomus in trigone (atrium) of lateral ventricle
Anterior limb of internal capsule
Occipital (posterior) horn of lateral ventricle
Globus pallidus
Putamen
Pulvinar of thalamus
Posterolateral choroidal artery
Lateral geniculate body
Middle cerebral artery
Superior cerebellar cistern
Superior rectus muscle
Transverse sinus
Retrobulbar fat
Horizontal fissure of cerebellum
Optic nerve
Greater wing of sphenoid bone
Maxillary sinus
Maxillary tooth
Lateral fissure (cistern) of Sylvius
Hippocampus
Amygdala
Jugular bulb
Cerebellar pontine angle cistern

**Field=1.5T TR=0.5s TE=17ms SL=4mm**

**Plane of Section**

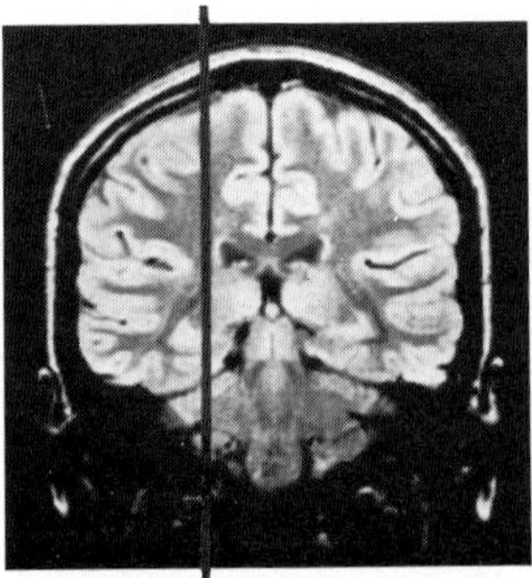

**Figure 5–20.** The right hippocampus.

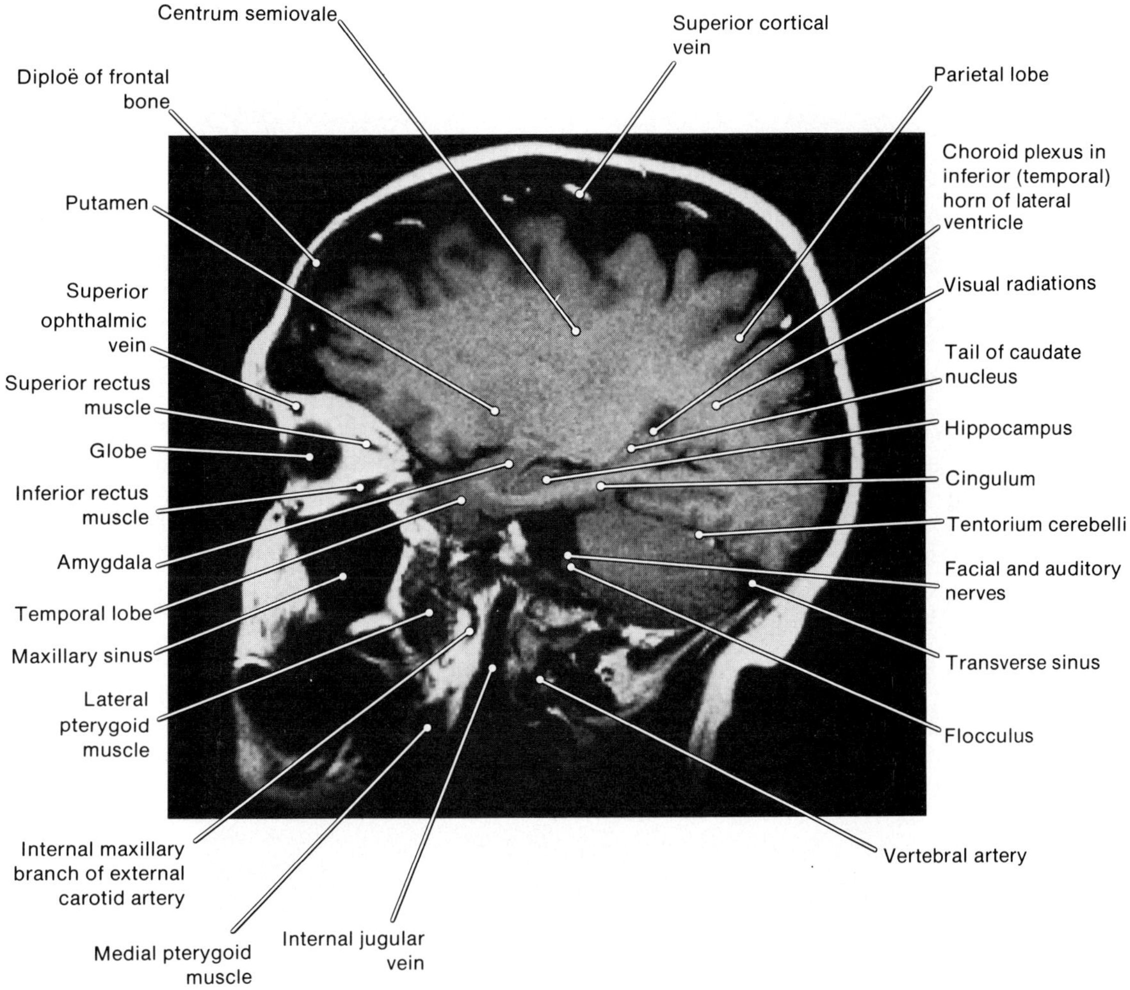

Centrum semiovale
Superior cortical vein
Diploë of frontal bone
Parietal lobe
Putamen
Choroid plexus in inferior (temporal) horn of lateral ventricle
Superior ophthalmic vein
Visual radiations
Superior rectus muscle
Tail of caudate nucleus
Globe
Hippocampus
Inferior rectus muscle
Cingulum
Tentorium cerebelli
Amygdala
Facial and auditory nerves
Temporal lobe
Maxillary sinus
Transverse sinus
Lateral pterygoid muscle
Flocculus
Internal maxillary branch of external carotid artery
Vertebral artery
Medial pterygoid muscle
Internal jugular vein

**Field=1.5T TR=0.5s TE=17ms SL=4mm**

**Plane of Section**

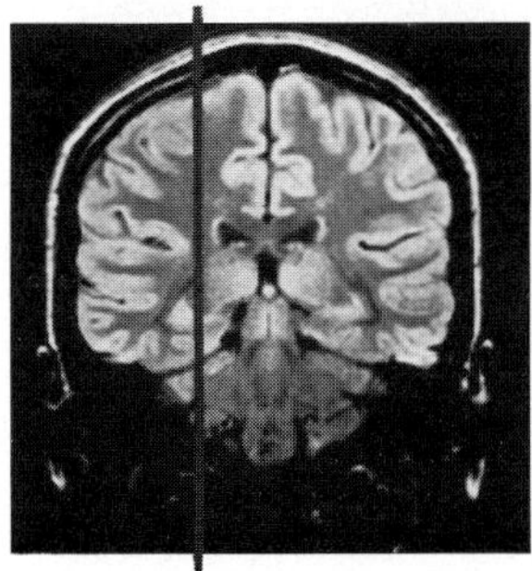

**Figure 5–21.** The right temporal horn of the lateral ventricle.

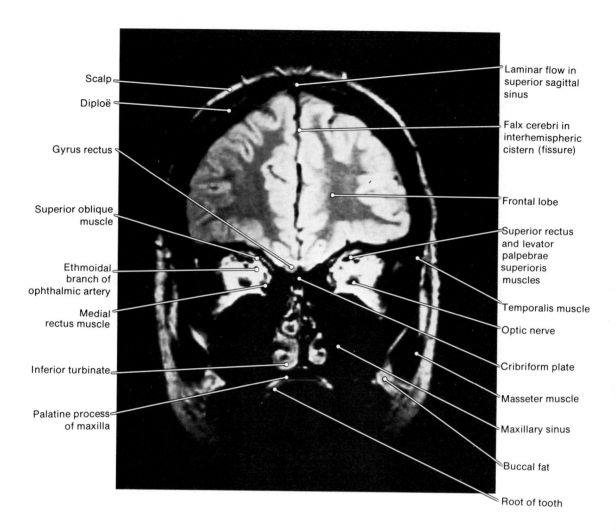

Scalp
Diploë
Gyrus rectus
Superior oblique muscle
Ethmoidal branch of ophthalmic artery
Medial rectus muscle
Inferior turbinate
Palatine process of maxilla

Laminar flow in superior sagittal sinus
Falx cerebri in interhemispheric cistern (fissure)
Frontal lobe
Superior rectus and levator palpebrae superioris muscles
Temporalis muscle
Optic nerve
Cribriform plate
Masseter muscle
Maxillary sinus
Buccal fat
Root of tooth

**Field=1.5T TR=2.0s TE=35ms SL=5mm**

**Plane of Section**

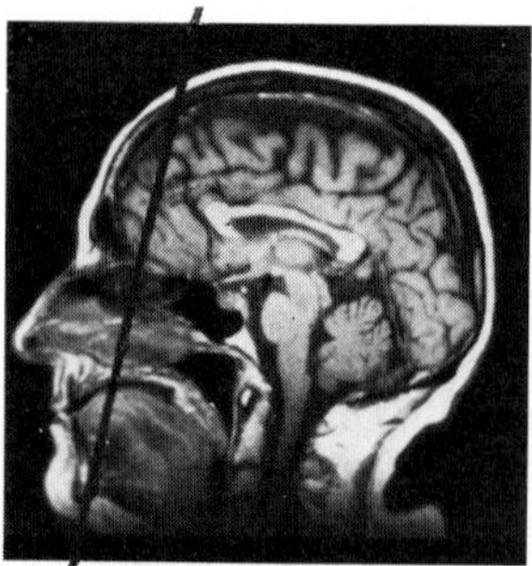

**Figure 5–22.** The orbit behind the globe.

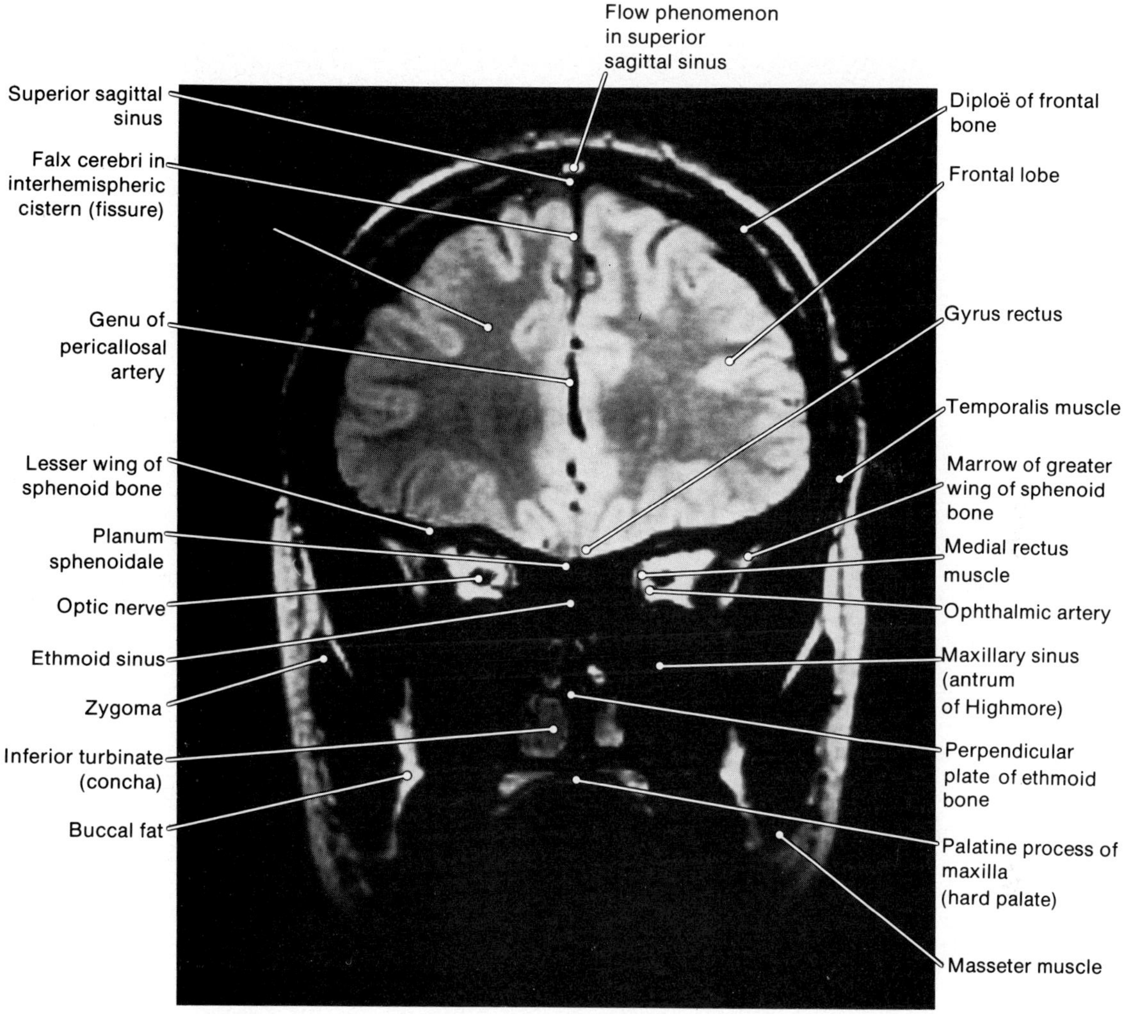

Flow phenomenon in superior sagittal sinus
Superior sagittal sinus
Falx cerebri in interhemispheric cistern (fissure)
Genu of pericallosal artery
Lesser wing of sphenoid bone
Planum sphenoidale
Optic nerve
Ethmoid sinus
Zygoma
Inferior turbinate (concha)
Buccal fat
Diploë of frontal bone
Frontal lobe
Gyrus rectus
Temporalis muscle
Marrow of greater wing of sphenoid bone
Medial rectus muscle
Ophthalmic artery
Maxillary sinus (antrum of Highmore)
Perpendicular plate of ethmoid bone
Palatine process of maxilla (hard palate)
Masseter muscle

**Field=1.5T TR=2.0s TE=35ms SL=5mm**

**Plane of Section**

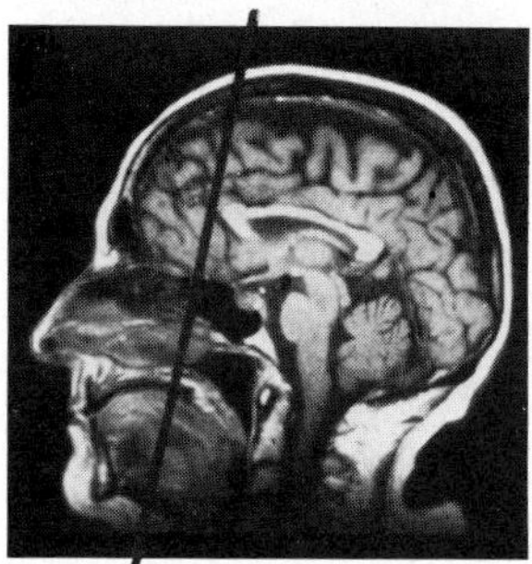

**Figure 5–23.** The posterior orbit.

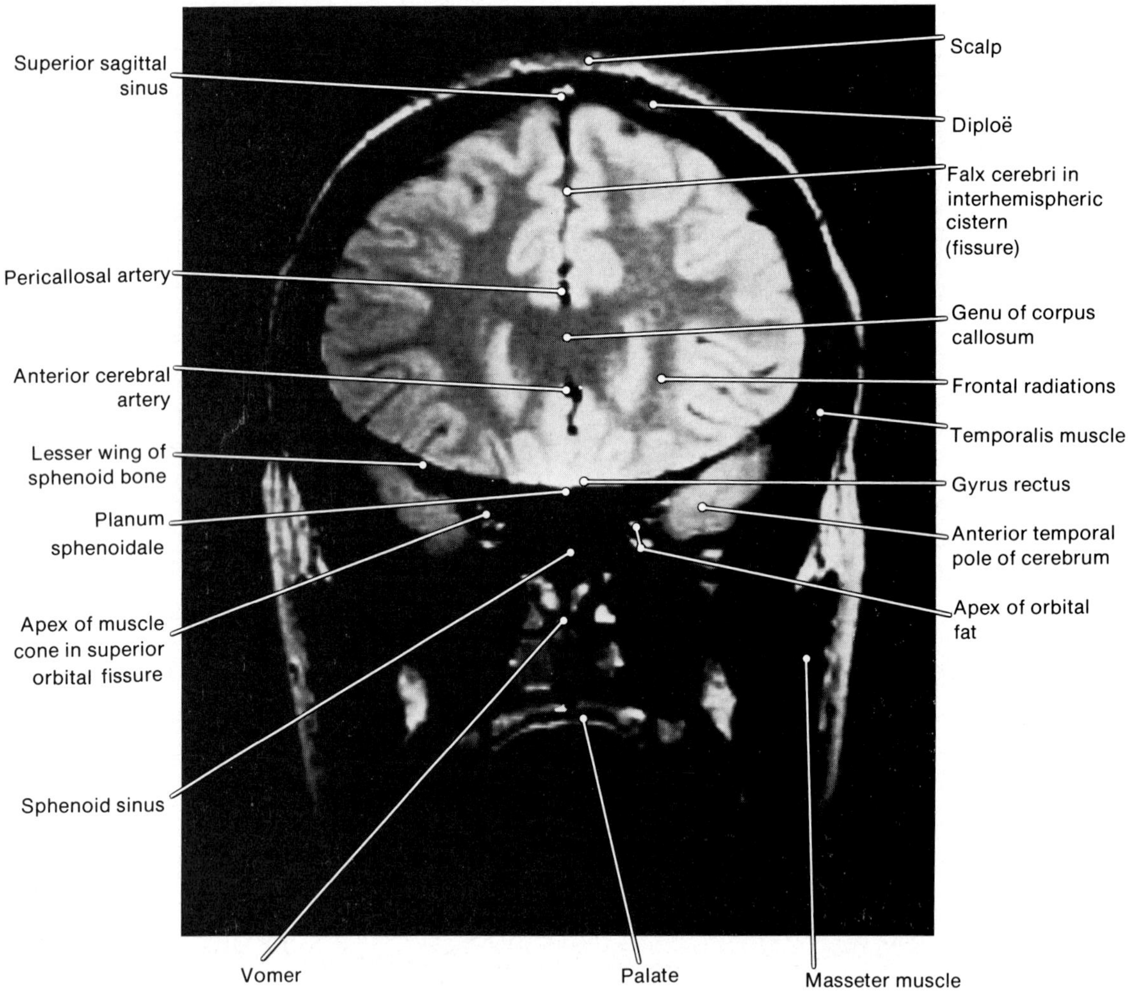

Superior sagittal sinus
Pericallosal artery
Anterior cerebral artery
Lesser wing of sphenoid bone
Planum sphenoidale
Apex of muscle cone in superior orbital fissure
Sphenoid sinus
Scalp
Diploë
Falx cerebri in interhemispheric cistern (fissure)
Genu of corpus callosum
Frontal radiations
Temporalis muscle
Gyrus rectus
Anterior temporal pole of cerebrum
Apex of orbital fat
Vomer
Palate
Masseter muscle

**Field=1.5T TR=2.0s TE=35ms SL=5mm**

**Plane of Section**

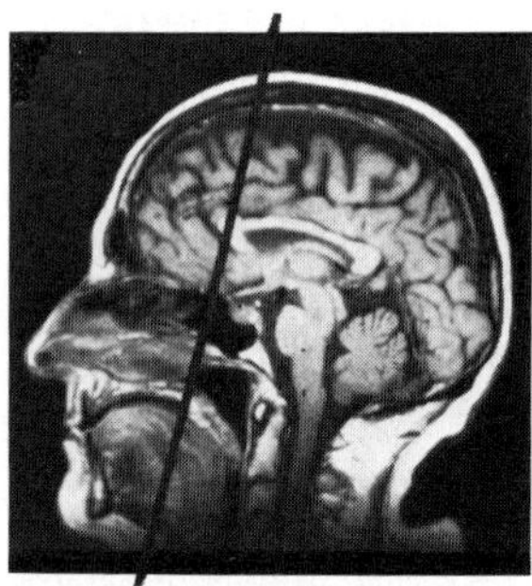

**Figure 5–24.** The apex of the orbit.

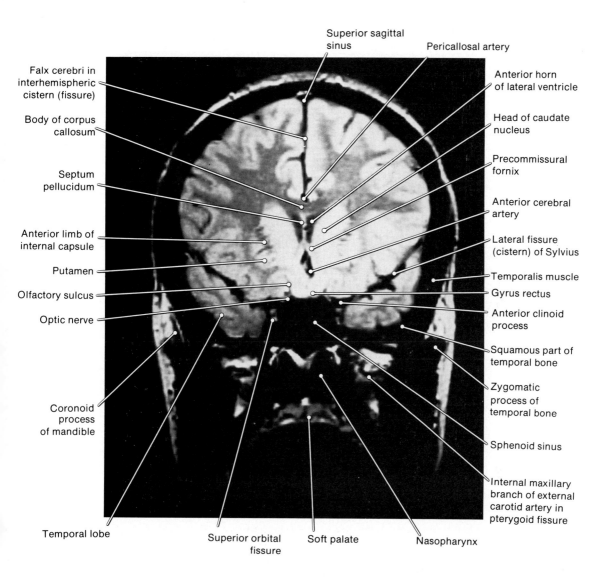

Superior sagittal sinus
Pericallosal artery
Falx cerebri in interhemispheric cistern (fissure)
Anterior horn of lateral ventricle
Body of corpus callosum
Head of caudate nucleus
Precommissural fornix
Septum pellucidum
Anterior cerebral artery
Anterior limb of internal capsule
Lateral fissure (cistern) of Sylvius
Putamen
Temporalis muscle
Olfactory sulcus
Gyrus rectus
Anterior clinoid process
Optic nerve
Squamous part of temporal bone
Zygomatic process of temporal bone
Coronoid process of mandible
Sphenoid sinus
Internal maxillary branch of external carotid artery in pterygoid fissure
Temporal lobe
Superior orbital fissure
Soft palate
Nasopharynx

**Field=1.5T TR=2.0s TE=35ms SL=5mm**

**Plane of Section**

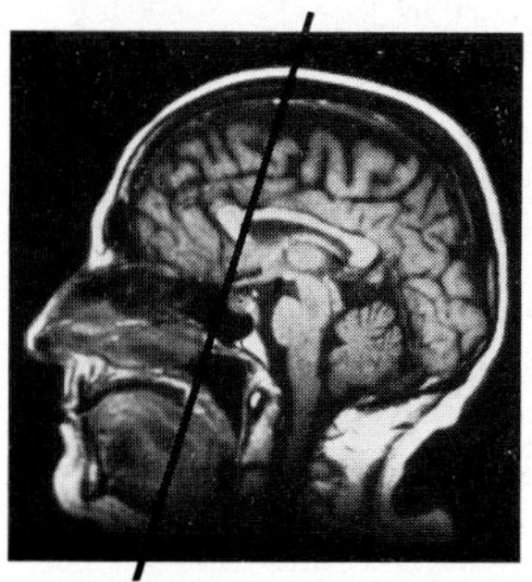

**Figure 5–25.** The superior orbital fissure.

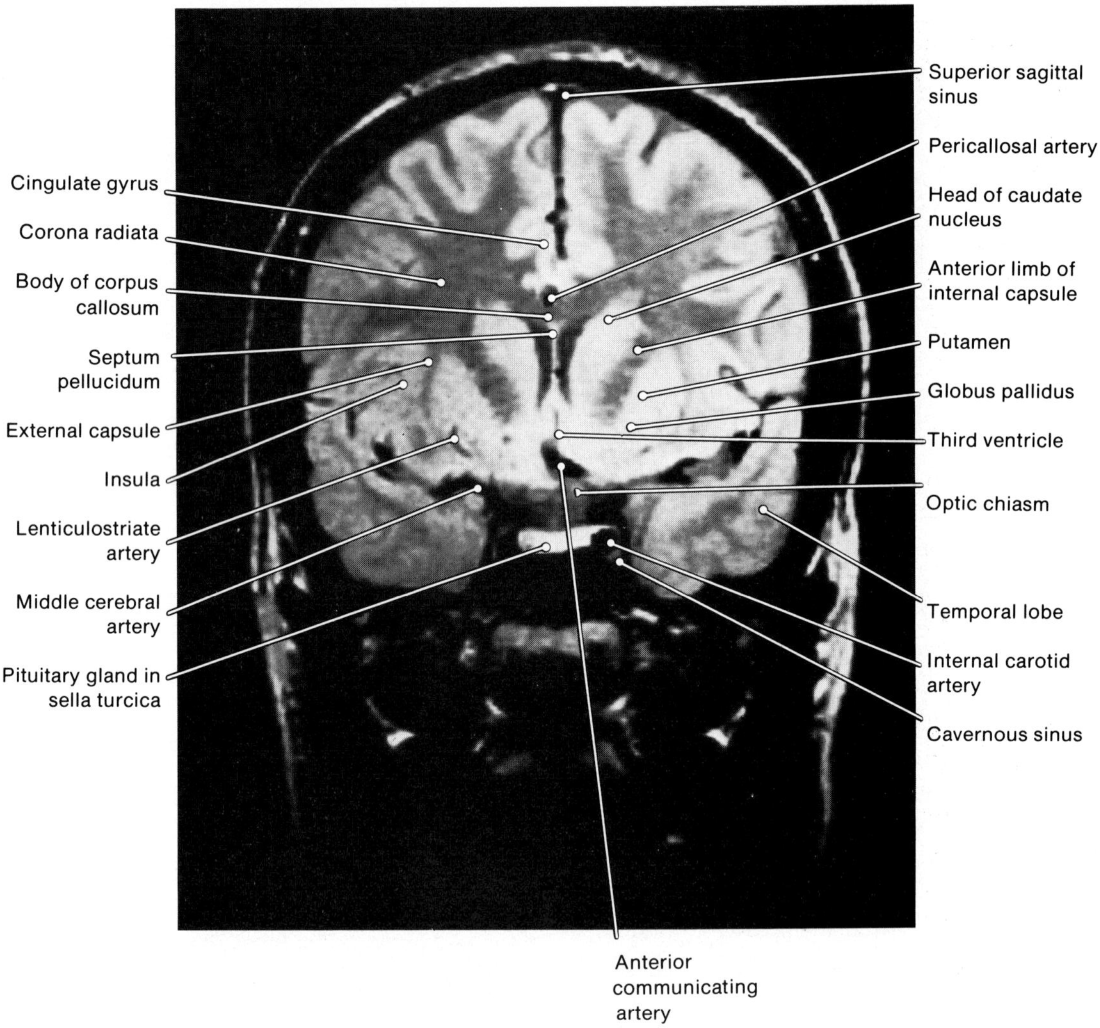

Superior sagittal sinus
Cingulate gyrus
Pericallosal artery
Corona radiata
Head of caudate nucleus
Body of corpus callosum
Anterior limb of internal capsule
Septum pellucidum
Putamen
External capsule
Globus pallidus
Insula
Third ventricle
Lenticulostriate artery
Optic chiasm
Middle cerebral artery
Temporal lobe
Pituitary gland in sella turcica
Internal carotid artery
Cavernous sinus
Anterior communicating artery

**Field=1.5T TR=2.0s TE=35ms SL=5mm**

**Plane of Section**

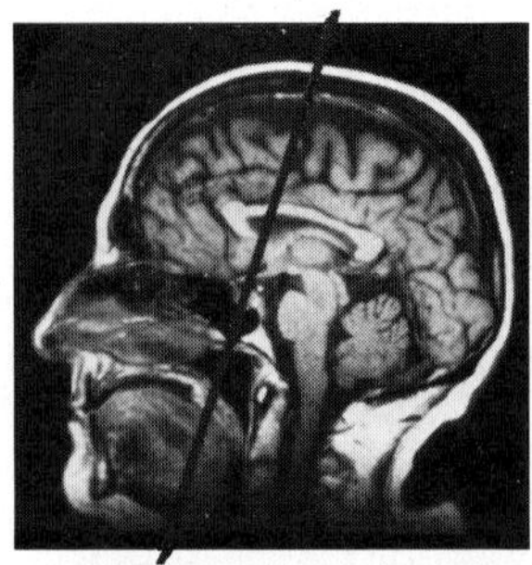

**Figure 5–26.** The sella turcica.

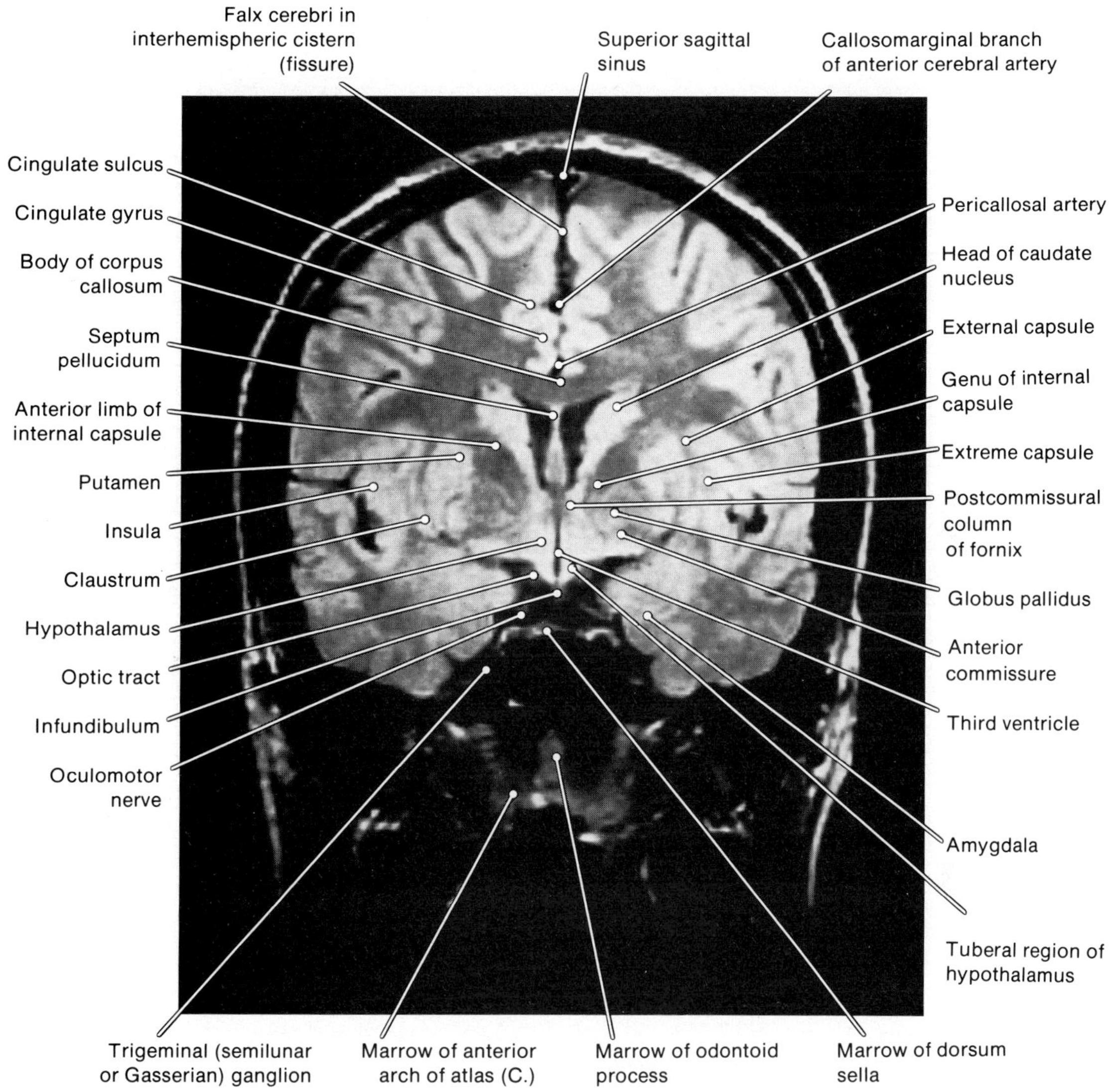

Falx cerebri in interhemispheric cistern (fissure)
Superior sagittal sinus
Callosomarginal branch of anterior cerebral artery
Cingulate sulcus
Cingulate gyrus
Body of corpus callosum
Septum pellucidum
Anterior limb of internal capsule
Putamen
Insula
Claustrum
Hypothalamus
Optic tract
Infundibulum
Oculomotor nerve
Pericallosal artery
Head of caudate nucleus
External capsule
Genu of internal capsule
Extreme capsule
Postcommissural column of fornix
Globus pallidus
Anterior commissure
Third ventricle
Amygdala
Tuberal region of hypothalamus
Trigeminal (semilunar or Gasserian) ganglion
Marrow of anterior arch of atlas (C.)
Marrow of odontoid process
Marrow of dorsum sella

**Field**=**1.5T TR**=**2.0s TE**=**35ms SL**=**5mm**

**Plane of Section**

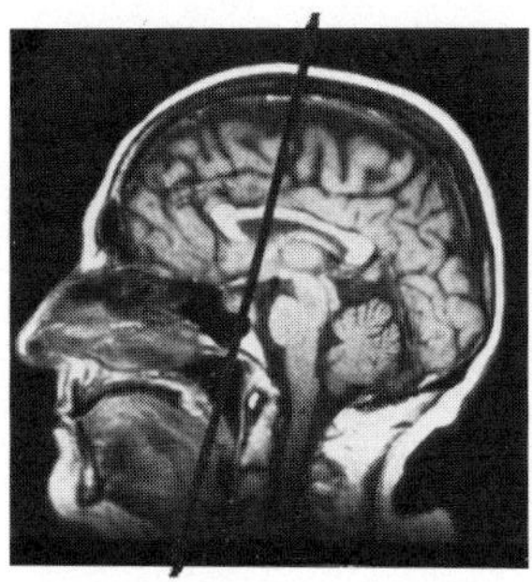

**Figure 5–27.** The infundibulum.

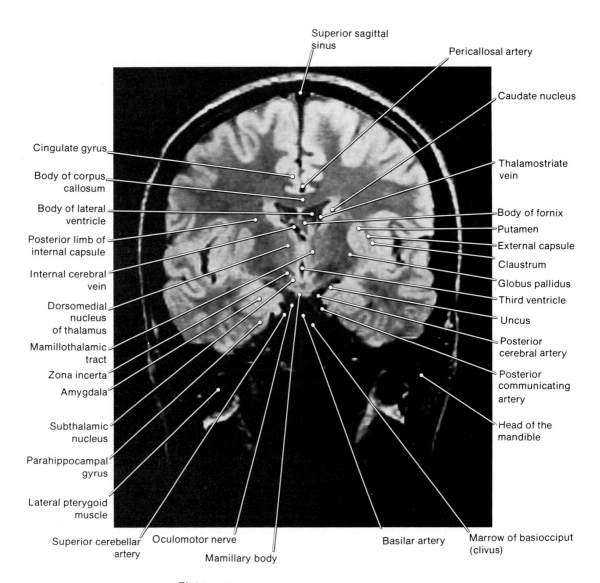

Superior sagittal sinus
Pericallosal artery
Caudate nucleus
Cingulate gyrus
Thalamostriate vein
Body of corpus callosum
Body of lateral ventricle
Body of fornix
Putamen
Posterior limb of internal capsule
External capsule
Claustrum
Internal cerebral vein
Globus pallidus
Third ventricle
Dorsomedial nucleus of thalamus
Uncus
Mamillothalamic tract
Posterior cerebral artery
Zona incerta
Posterior communicating artery
Amygdala
Subthalamic nucleus
Head of the mandible
Parahippocampal gyrus
Lateral pterygoid muscle
Superior cerebellar artery
Oculomotor nerve
Mamillary body
Basilar artery
Marrow of basiocciput (clivus)

**Field=1.5T TR=2.0s TE=35ms SL=5mm**

**Plane of Section**

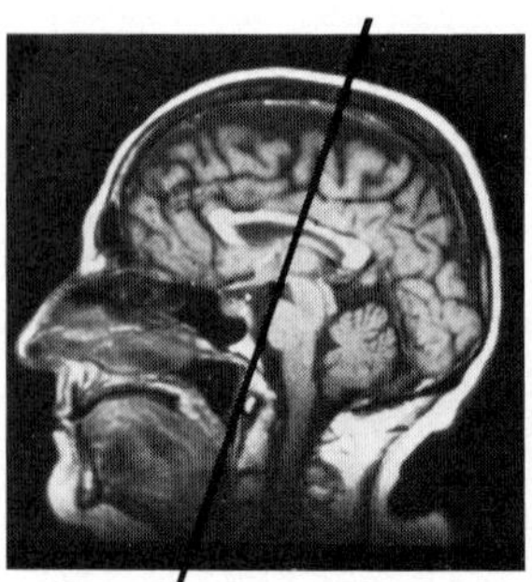

**Figure 5–28.** The mamillary body.

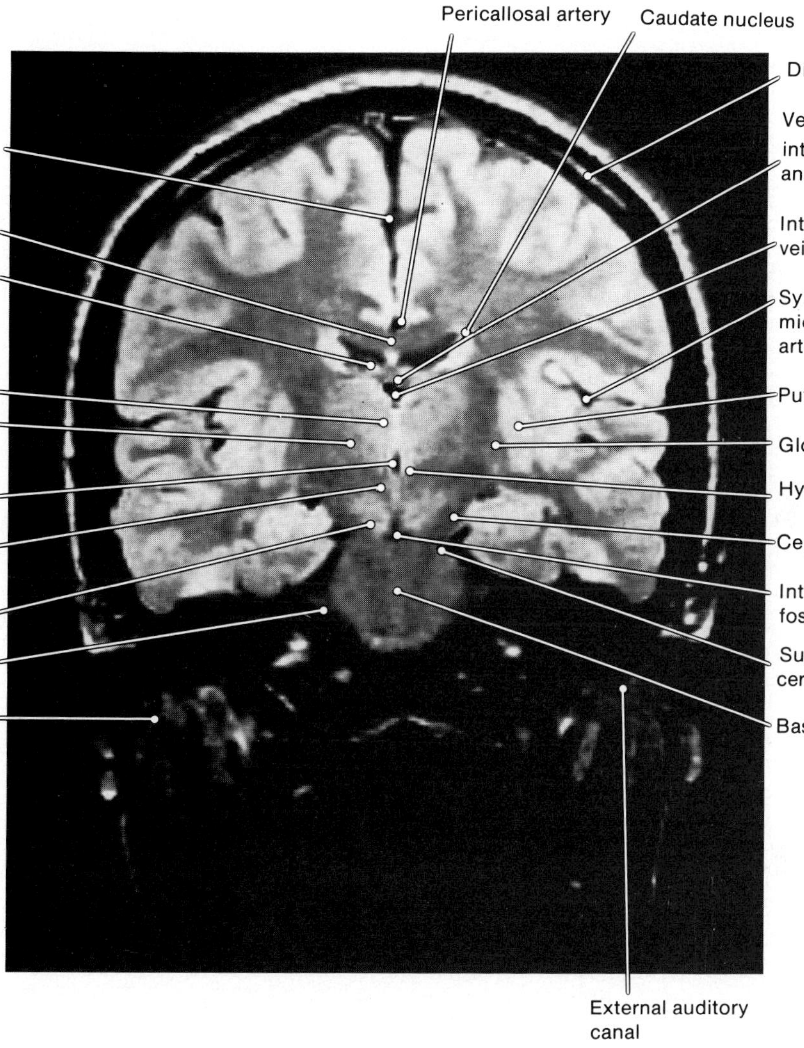

Pericallosal artery
Caudate nucleus
Diploë
Velum interpositum and tela choroidea
Internal cerebral veins
Sylvian branch of middle cerebral artery
Putamen
Globus pallidus
Hypothalamus
Cerebral peduncle
Interpeduncular fossa (cistern)
Superior cerebellar artery
Basilar pons
External auditory canal
Anterior cerebral artery
Corpus callosum
Choroid plexus in body of lateral ventricle
Thalamic nuclei: dorsal medial
posterolateral ventral
Third ventricle
Subthalamic nucleus
Substantia nigra
Trigeminal nerve
Superficial occipital artery

**Field=1.5T TR=2.0s TE=35ms SL=5mm**

**Plane of Section**

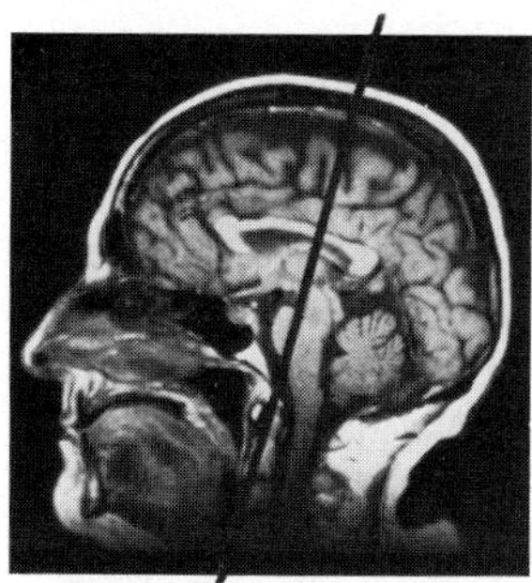

**Figure 5–29.** The cerebral peduncles.

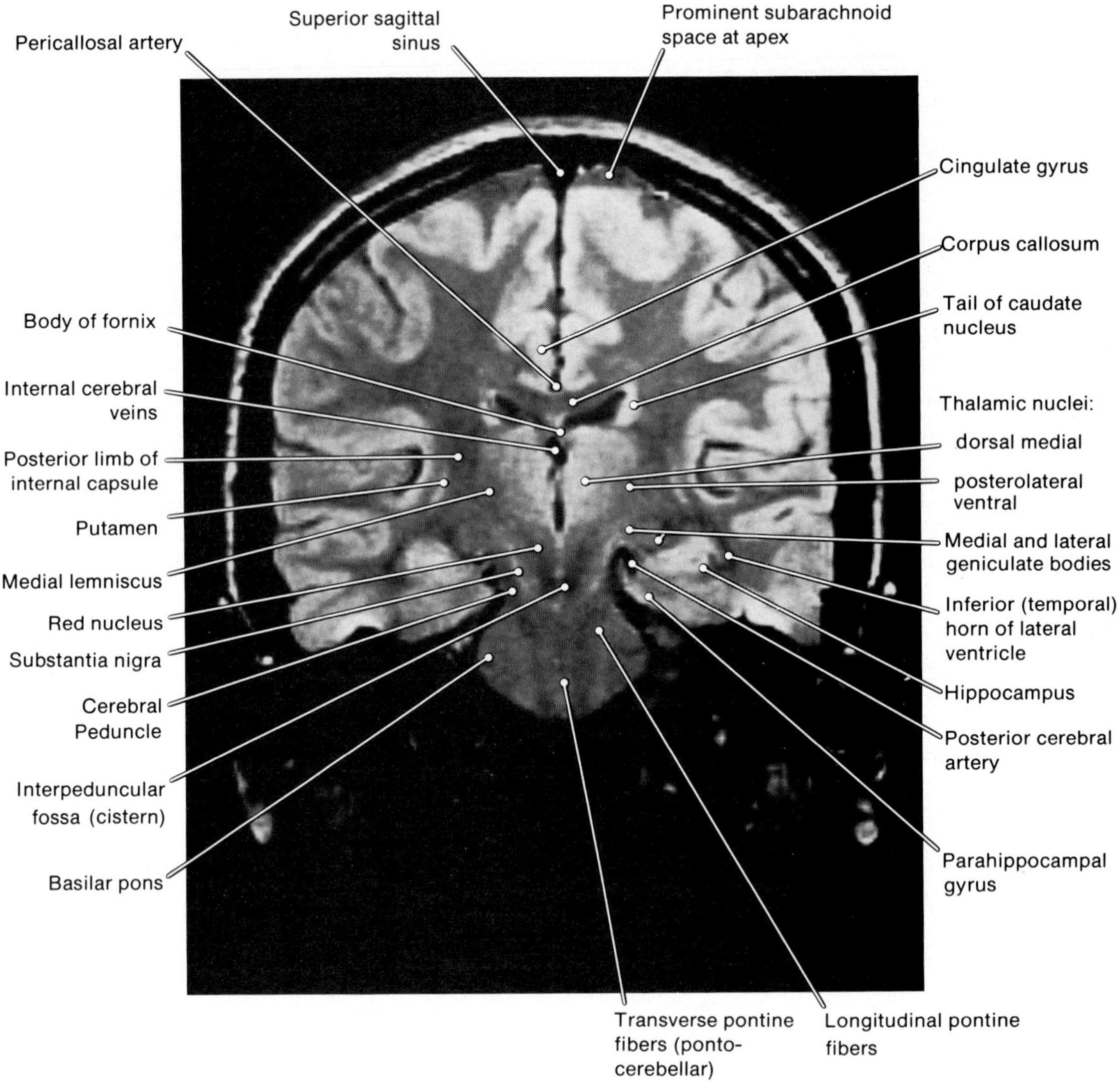

Pericallosal artery
Superior sagittal sinus
Prominent subarachnoid space at apex
Cingulate gyrus
Corpus callosum
Tail of caudate nucleus
Body of fornix
Internal cerebral veins
Thalamic nuclei:
dorsal medial
posterolateral ventral
Posterior limb of internal capsule
Putamen
Medial and lateral geniculate bodies
Medial lemniscus
Inferior (temporal) horn of lateral ventricle
Red nucleus
Substantia nigra
Hippocampus
Cerebral Peduncle
Posterior cerebral artery
Interpeduncular fossa (cistern)
Parahippocampal gyrus
Basilar pons
Transverse pontine fibers (ponto-cerebellar)
Longitudinal pontine fibers

**Field=1.5T TR=2.0s TE=35ms SL=5mm**

**Plane of Section**

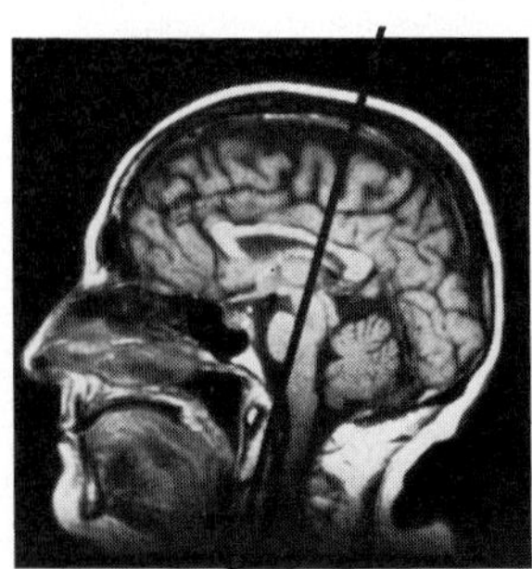

**Figure 5–30.** The red nucleus.

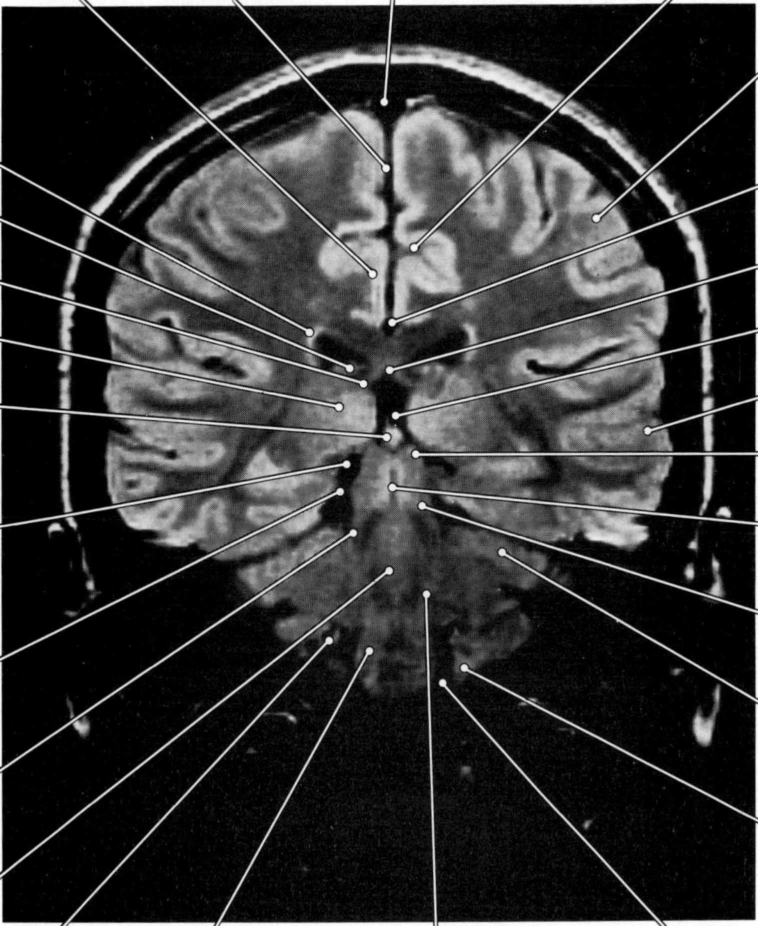

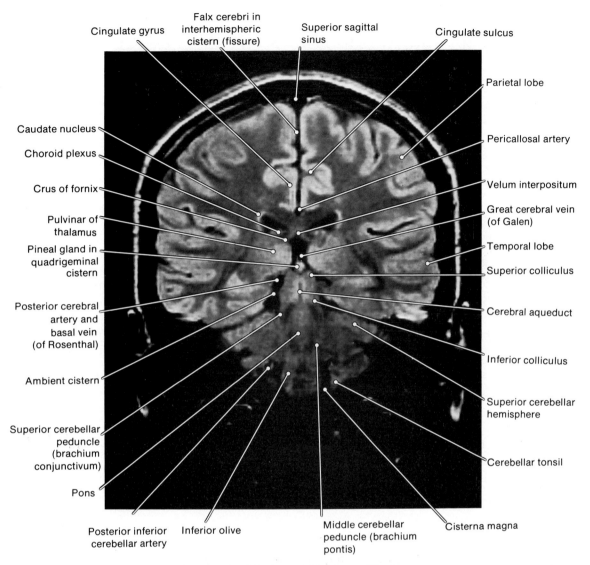

Cingulate gyrus
Falx cerebri in interhemispheric cistern (fissure)
Superior sagittal sinus
Cingulate sulcus
Parietal lobe
Pericallosal artery
Velum interpositum
Great cerebral vein (of Galen)
Temporal lobe
Superior colliculus
Cerebral aqueduct
Inferior colliculus
Superior cerebellar hemisphere
Cerebellar tonsil
Caudate nucleus
Choroid plexus
Crus of fornix
Pulvinar of thalamus
Pineal gland in quadrigeminal cistern
Posterior cerebral artery and basal vein (of Rosenthal)
Ambient cistern
Superior cerebellar peduncle (brachium conjunctivum)
Pons
Posterior inferior cerebellar artery
Inferior olive
Middle cerebellar peduncle (brachium pontis)
Cisterna magna

**Field=1.5T TR=2.0s TE=35ms SL=5mm**

**Plane of Section**

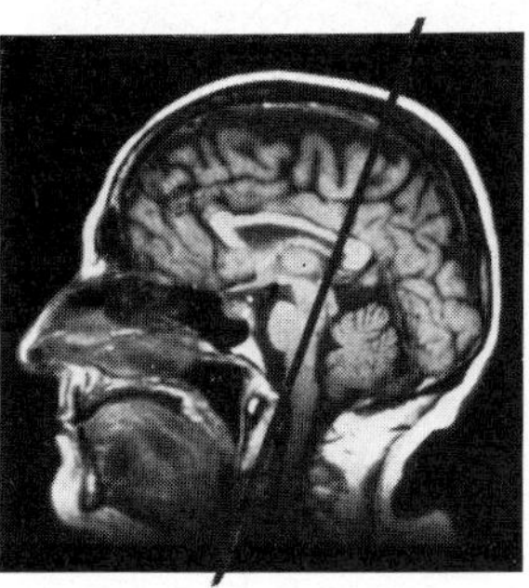

**Figure 5–31.** The pineal gland and the great cerebral vein.

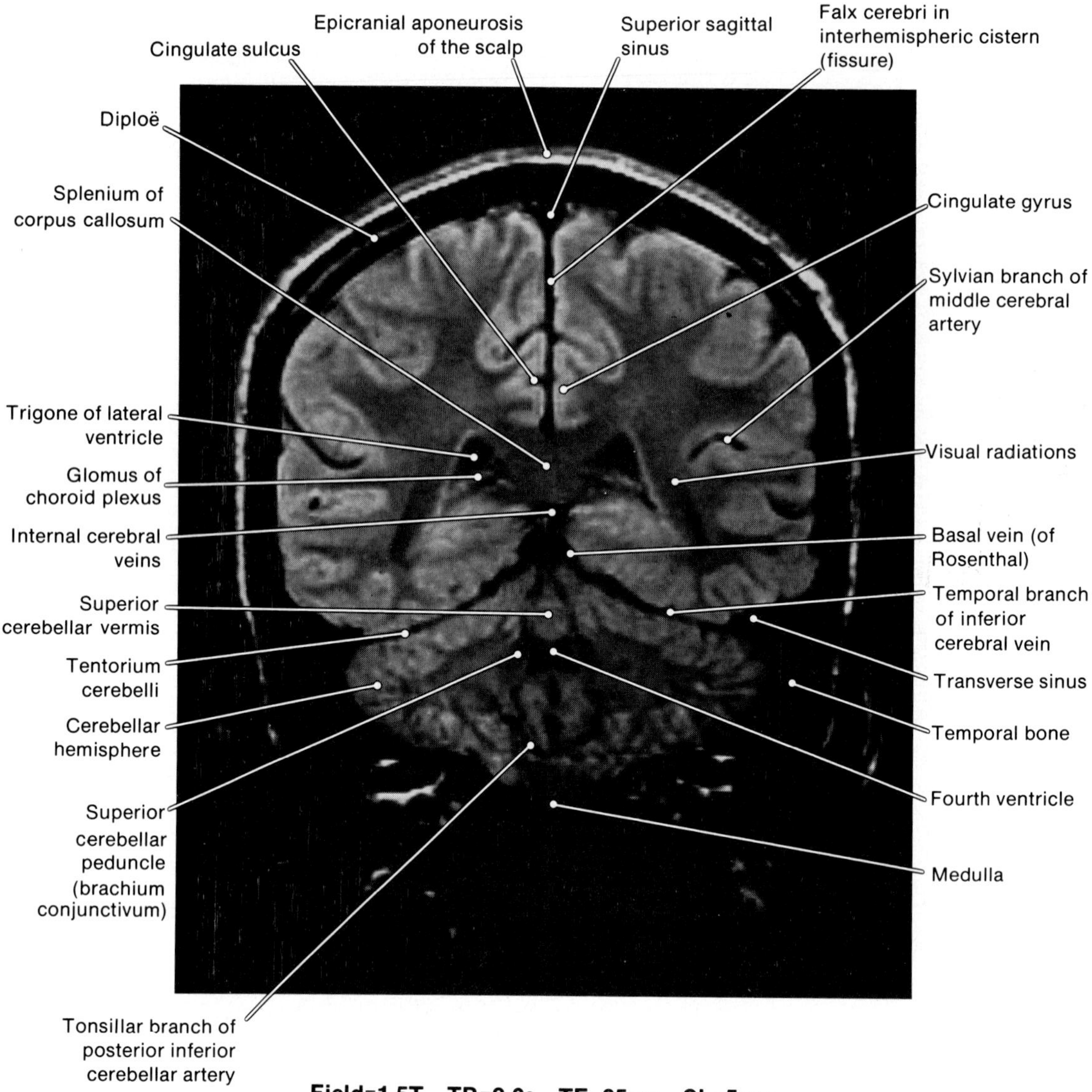

Cingulate sulcus

Epicranial aponeurosis of the scalp

Superior sagittal sinus

Falx cerebri in interhemispheric cistern (fissure)

Diploë

Splenium of corpus callosum

Cingulate gyrus

Sylvian branch of middle cerebral artery

Trigone of lateral ventricle

Glomus of choroid plexus

Visual radiations

Internal cerebral veins

Basal vein (of Rosenthal)

Superior cerebellar vermis

Temporal branch of inferior cerebral vein

Tentorium cerebelli

Transverse sinus

Cerebellar hemisphere

Temporal bone

Superior cerebellar peduncle (brachium conjunctivum)

Fourth ventricle

Medulla

Tonsillar branch of posterior inferior cerebellar artery

**Field=1.5T TR=2.0s TE=35ms SL=5mm**

**Plane of Section**

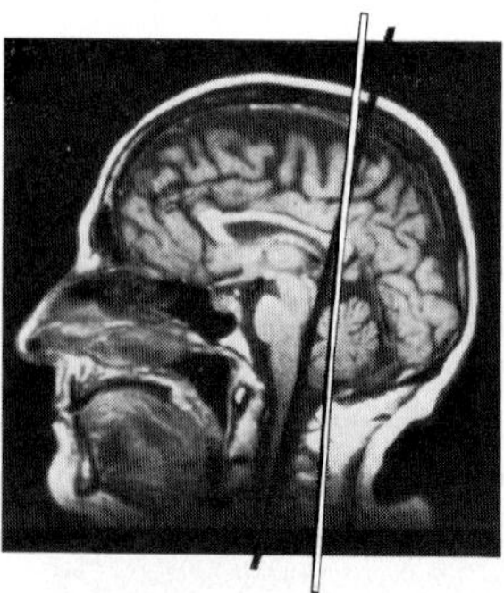

**Figure 5–32.** The splenium of the corpus callosum.

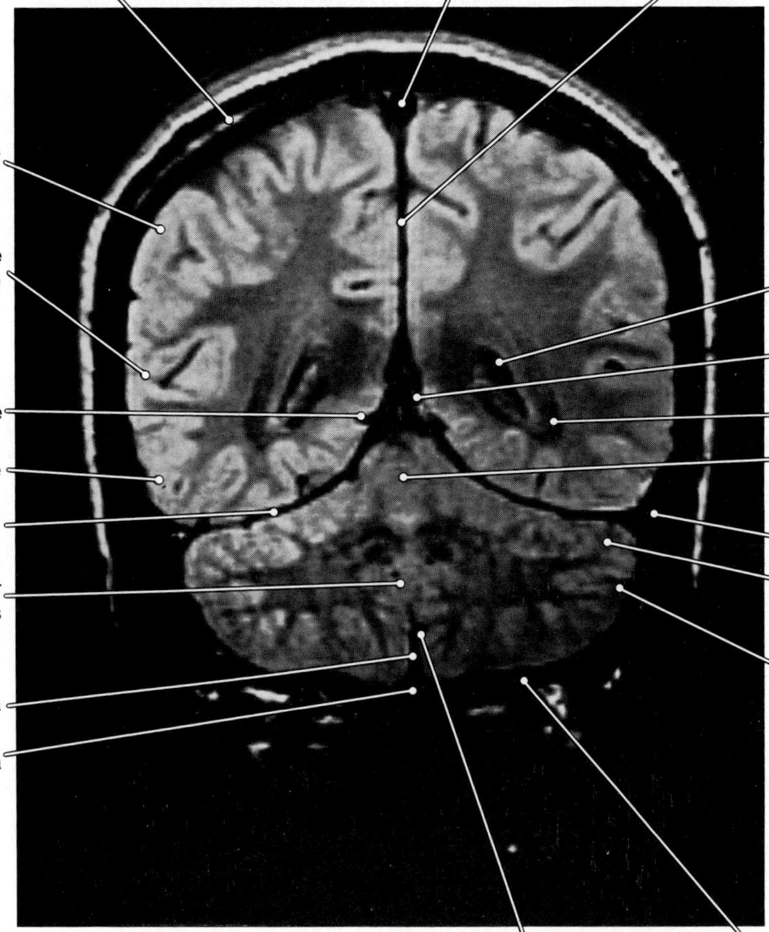

Diploë of parietal bone

Superior sagittal sinus

Falx cerebri in interhemispheric cistern (fissure)

Parietal lobe

Lateral fissure (of Sylvius)

Trigone of lateral ventricle

Basal vein (of Rosenthal)

Calcarine fissure

Visual radiations

Temporal lobe

Superior cerebellar vermis

Tentorium cerebelli

Transverse sinus

Inferior cerebellar vermis

Cerebellar hemisphere

Horizontal fissure of cerebellum

Vallecula

Cisterna magna

Retrotonsillar branch of posterior inferior cerebellar artery

Occipital bone

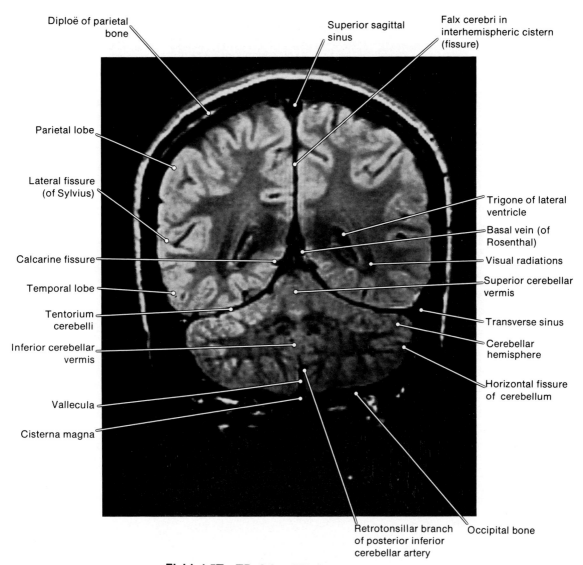

**Field**=**1.5T** **TR**=**2.0s** **TE**=**35ms** **SL**=**5mm**

**Plane of Section**

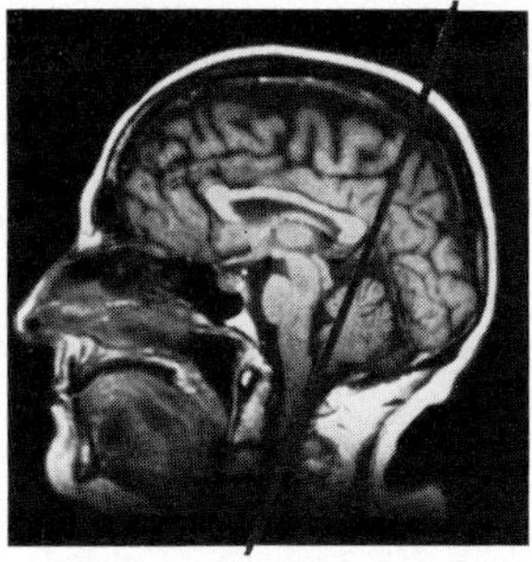

**Figure 5–33.** The apex of the tentorium.

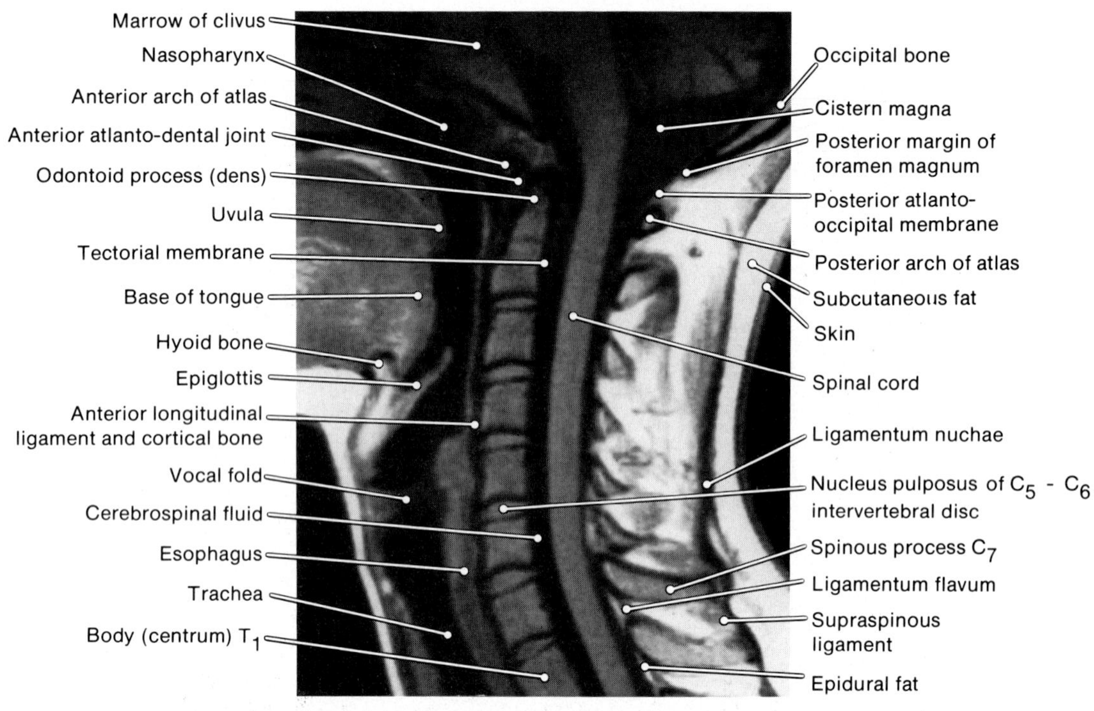
Marrow of clivus
Nasopharynx
Anterior arch of atlas
Anterior atlanto-dental joint
Odontoid process (dens)
Uvula
Tectorial membrane
Base of tongue
Hyoid bone
Epiglottis
Anterior longitudinal ligament and cortical bone
Vocal fold
Cerebrospinal fluid
Esophagus
Trachea
Body (centrum) $T_1$
Occipital bone
Cistern magna
Posterior margin of foramen magnum
Posterior atlanto-occipital membrane
Posterior arch of atlas
Subcutaneous fat
Skin
Spinal cord
Ligamentum nuchae
Nucleus pulposus of $C_5$ - $C_6$ intervertebral disc
Spinous process $C_7$
Ligamentum flavum
Supraspinous ligament
Epidural fat

**Field=1.OT TR=0.6s TE=17ms SL=5mm**

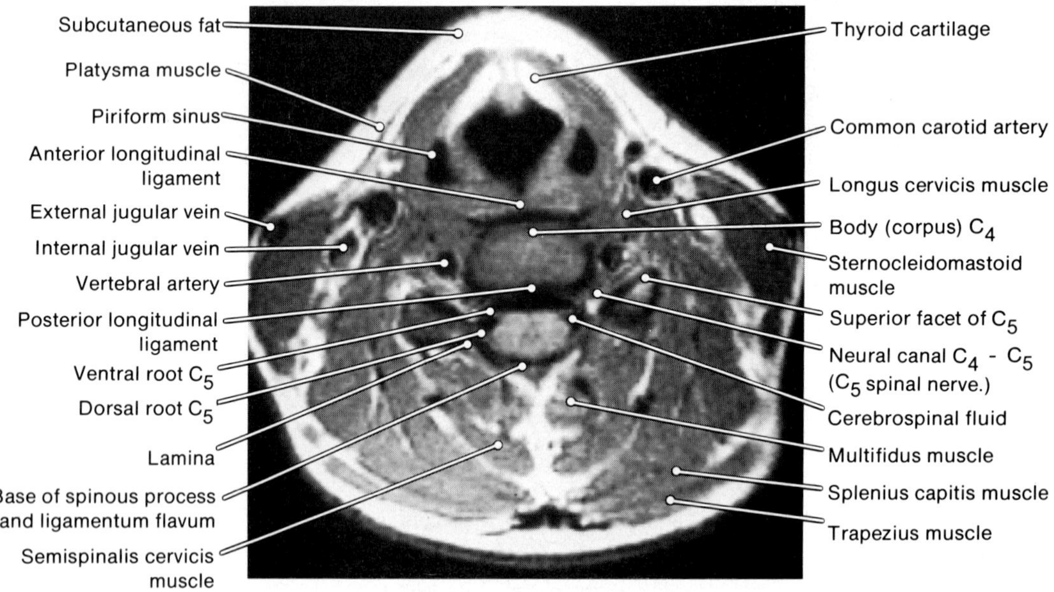
Subcutaneous fat
Platysma muscle
Piriform sinus
Anterior longitudinal ligament
External jugular vein
Internal jugular vein
Vertebral artery
Posterior longitudinal ligament
Ventral root $C_5$
Dorsal root $C_5$
Lamina
Base of spinous process and ligamentum flavum
Semispinalis cervicis muscle
Thyroid cartilage
Common carotid artery
Longus cervicis muscle
Body (corpus) $C_4$
Sternocleidomastoid muscle
Superior facet of $C_5$
Neural canal $C_4$ - $C_5$ ($C_5$ spinal nerve.)
Cerebrospinal fluid
Multifidus muscle
Splenius capitis muscle
Trapezius muscle

**Field=1.OT TR=0.6s TE=17ms SL=5mm**

**Figure 5–34.** The cervical spine.

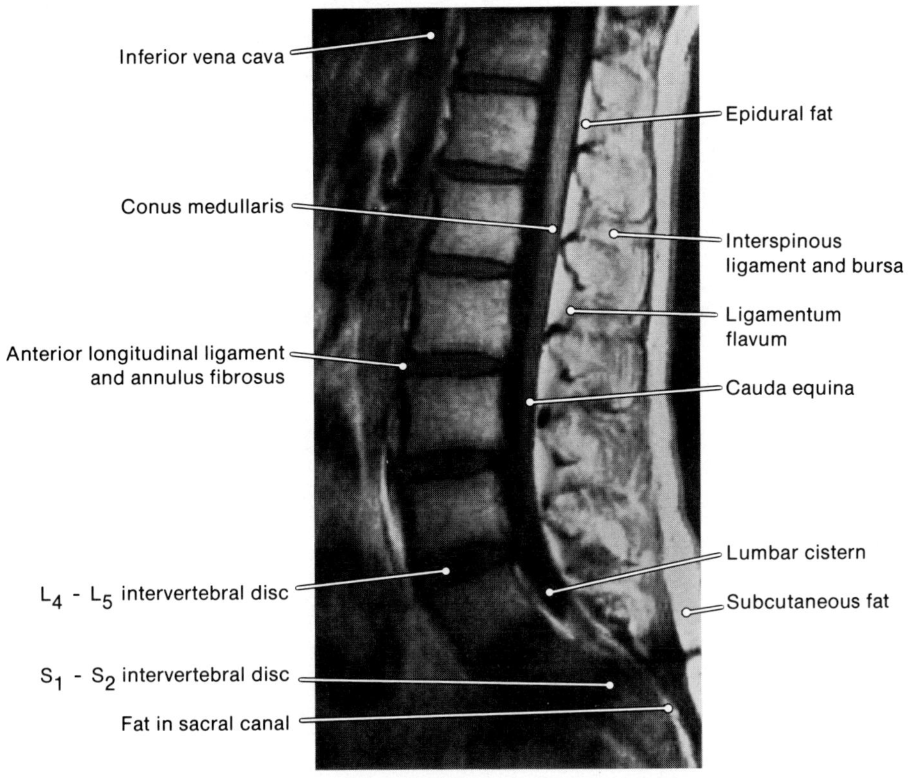


**Field=1.OT TR=0.40s TE=17ms SL=6.0mm**

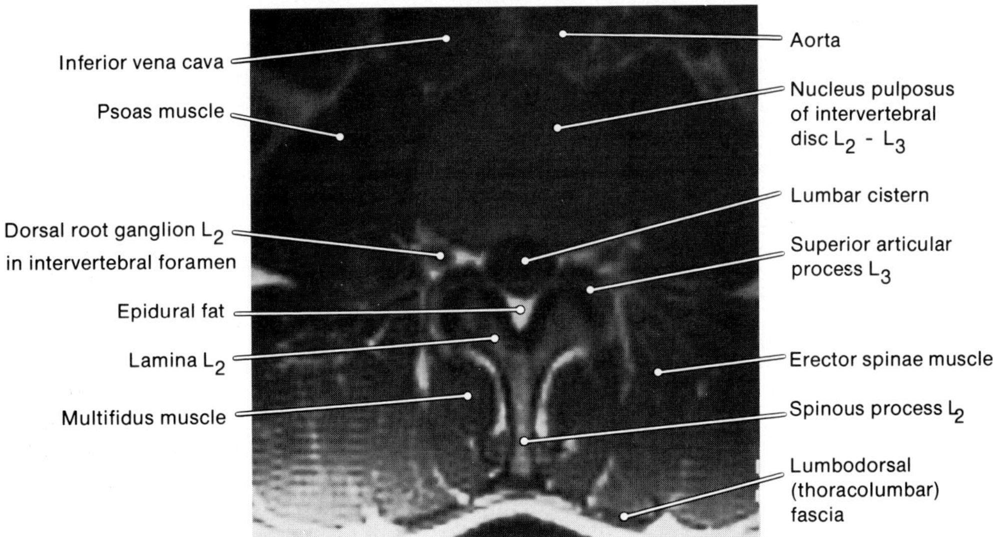


**Field=1.OT TR=0.40s TE=17ms SL=6.0mm**

**Figure 5–35.** The lumbar spine.

seemingly infinite minutiae that MRI is capable of displaying.

## References

1. Schnitzlein HN, Murtagh FR. Imaging anatomy of the head and spine. Munich, Urban and Schwartzenber, 1985.
2. Holland BA, Haas DK, Norman D, et al. MRI of normal brain maturation. AJNR 7:201, 1986.
3. Drayer BP, Burger P, Darwin R, et al. Magnetic resonance imaging of brain iron. AJNR 7:373, 1986.
4. Sherman JR, Citrin CM. Magnetic resonance demonstrations of normal CSF flow. AJNR 7:3, 1986.

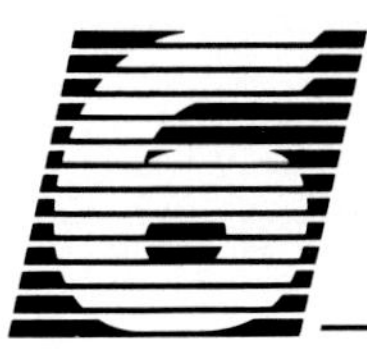

William S. Ball, Jr., M.D.
Richard B. Towbin, M.D.
Bokyung K. Han, M.D.

# CONGENITAL PEDIATRIC ANOMALIES OF THE BRAIN AND SPINE

Cross-sectional imaging represented by computed tomography (CT) and ultrasound (US) have reshaped our approach to the diagnosis of disorders of the central nervous system (CNS) in children. The ideal diagnostic cross-sectional imaging technique should provide us with optimal sensitivity and specificity in the detection of pathology, should accurately replicate anatomy in multiple projections at any age, should remain noninvasive, and should have no adverse biologic effect. Magnetic resonance imaging (MRI) holds great promise in satisfying many of these criteria. Its capability to image in multiple anatomic projections, separating normal from diseased tissue according to tissue signal characteristics, may enhance both our sensitivity and our specificity in the evaluation of the CNS. In addition, MRI is noninvasive, does not emit ionizing radiation, and is suitable for imaging at any age. Currently, at magnet strengths $< 2.0$ T, no adverse biologic effect has been detected in children. As in computed tomography (CT), both infants and young children require sedation for examination; nevertheless, MRI can be performed both safely and effectively in the younger age group through attention to the special needs of the pediatric patient. These special needs include careful control of the patient's environment, adequate yet safe sedation, careful monitoring of the child while in the scanner, and an understanding of parental concerns. Because of these qualities, MRI is rapidly becoming the preferred technique for imaging of the central nervous system in children.[1-4]

The cold surroundings of the scanner room must often be modified to provide a more acceptable environment to the younger patient. Since it is difficult to control the temperature within the scanning suite, a young infant must often be wrapped in blankets, plastic wrap, or both in order to prevent excessive heat loss. If artifical chemical heat or hot water bags are used, care must be taken to protect the skin from thermal injury. When a child is kept warm and comfortable, he or she is likely to require less sedation, thereby minimizing the risk. Allowing a parent to remain in the scanning suite during the examination does much to reassure an older child, and enhances cooperation between the family, the technologist, and the radiologist.

The spontaneous and incessant movements of a child constitute the single greatest barrier to quality MRI in the pediatric population. Patients under five years of age or older uncooperative patients require sedation for examination. Cooperative patients older than five years of age can often be successfully coached through long examinations. Claustrophobia is not as common in children as in adults but when present may require sedation. Chloral hydrate, 50 to 100 mg/kg/dose, is given orally for sedation in children under 24 months of age. Intravenous sedation is preferred for children older than 24 months. We use a combination of pentobarbital (Nembutal) 2 to 3 mg/kg/dose (maximum 5-6 mg/kg), and fentanyl (Sublimaze) 1 to 2 mcg/kg/dose (maximum 3-4 mcg/kg) for intravenous sedation. Fentanyl, when used in small amounts, potentiates the sedative effect of Nembutal without significant risk of respiratory depression. The intravenous route is preferred since it offers a more effective means of drug titration, is more comfortable for the child, and maintains vascular access if additional sedation or resuscitation is necessay. On the other hand, intramuscular sedation is uncomfortable, is slow in onset of action, often is ineffective owing to inconsistent absorption, and does not provide access for resedation if needed. Using these sedation protocols, we have not encountered any cardiorespiratory complications. All medications are administered by a registered nurse familiar with pediatric dosage regimens and with the radiologist in attendance.

Because of the potential risks from sedation, all patients are carefully monitored while in the scanner. Since the small patient is often lost from view within the gantry, monitoring is often difficult and challenging. Monitoring the patient by direct visualization alone is considered inadequate, especially for the sedated patient wrapped for warmth. We must therefore rely on monitoring of the heart and respiratory rate. Monitoring the respiratory rate by observing an object placed on the anterior surface of the chest is crude and unreliable. Monitoring of the heart rate is most easily accomplished using the CRT-ECG monitor provided for gated studies. A plastic anesthesia stethescope placed on the anterior chest wall allows direct auscultation of the heart if necessary. Oximeters, providing transcutaneous monitoring of $O_2$ saturation, offer a more sensitive means of evaluating the patient. All electronic monitoring devices require appropriate shielding from radio-frequency waves to prevent interference with image production and to prevent their dysfunction during scanning.[5]

The choice of appropriate scanning parameters, projection, and receiver coils must be tailored for each examination. Technical parameters may vary, depending upon the field strength of the magnet,[6, 7] the patient's age and size, and the available time. Often, imaging protocols are based on physician preference and experience in dealing with a particular clinical problem.

## TECHNICAL CONSIDERATIONS

### Pulse Sequence

In order to successfully evaluate complex congenital malformations of the CNS, MRI pulsing sequences are selected that provide the greatest anatomic resolution in the shortest amount of scanning time. With MRI still in its infancy, there has been little consensus as to which pulsing sequences are best. Controversy exists between the choice of inversion recovery (IR) versus spin-echo (SE) sequences and between TI- versus T2-weighted imaging.[1, 2, 4] IR sequences provide T1-weighted images with excellent contrast between white matter, gray matter, and CSF; however, IR is limited by its poor spatial resolution, decreased slice acquisition, and significant increase in scan time. Clinically, IR imaging can be useful in assessing brain maturation and the extent of myelinization in infants.[1, 8] For this purpose, we use a TR of 1000 to 1800 msec with a short TE of 20 to 30 msec. A T1 of approximately one third of the TR, with a range of 400 to 800 msec, is chosen. One to two excitations are usually sufficient for the purpose of myelin assessment (number of excitations, nex).

For the complete evaluation of the brain, we rely primarily on T1-weighted (T1WI) SE sequences, which provide the greatest anatomic detail. We begin each SE sequence with a sagittal localizer (TR 400-600 msec/TE 20 msec, matrix 256 × 128, 1 nex) from which additional projections and sequences are programmed. To improve resolution, a more detailed T1WI sagittal sequence (TR 600–800 msec/TE 20-30 msec, matrix 256 × 256, 2-4 nex) can be substituted to provide greater anatomic detail compared with the standard localizer scan. Currently, we continue to perform at least one sequence in the axial projection because of previous familiarity with this plane in CT. Further imaging planes are chosen, depending upon the anatomic area of interest. Since primary structural defects of the brain are often centered around the midline, they are best identified in the sagittal projection. The sagittal projection is especially helpful for visualization of midline structures such as the corpus callosum, the tectum, and the midbrain and the infratentorial structures, including the pons, brainstem, fourth ventricle, cerebellar vermis, and craniocervical junction. The coronal projection is of value in evaluating the interhemispheric fissure, the suprasellar and sellar structures, the hippocampal formation, and the middle cranial fossa. In the posterior fossa, coronal imaging is useful to assess the cerebellar peduncles and brainstem, and to detect inferior displacement of cerebellar and brainstem structures through the foramen magnum.

Two excitations are used routinely; although, four excitations (two averages) may be necessary to improve signal to noise. Resolution may also be improved by increasing the number of pixels within the matrix from 128 × 256 to 256 × 256 pixels. In either case, the tradeoff for improvement in resolution is a prolongation of the scan time. For T1WI sequences, the repetition time must be short enough to provide T1 weighting but long enough to provide adequate anatomic coverage (TR 400-1000 msec). The shortest TE possible (20-30 msec) is chosen.

Although we rely predominantly on T1WI, T2WI sequences are important in detecting white matter abnormalities, heterotopic gray matter, variations in vascularity, and alterations in cerebrospinal fluid flow. For each examination, we routinely include a T2WI sequence in the axial projection (TR 2000-3000 msec/TE 20-30/80-100, matrix 256 × 128, 2 nex). In the very young infant with increased brain water, we prefer a long TR of 2500 to 3000 msec and a longer TE of 100-120 msec, which provide optimal differentation of white and gray matter at this age.[9] Sampling of only two echoes at 20 to 30 msec and 80 to 100 msec is routine. In rare instances, four echoes (an echo train) may be sampled (TE 20-30 msec, 40-50 msec, 70-80 msec, 100-120 msec), to better separate abnormal areas of brain with increased signal from the surrounding CSF. In infants less than 12 months of age, the first echo of a multiecho sequence (TR 2000-2500 msec/TE 20-30 msec) often displays more CSF signal hypointensity and T1-weighting than expected for a proton density scan. In the future, T2–weighted gradient acquisition images (TR 200-400 msec/TE 20-30 msec/50-60 msec, flip = 10-20°) may prove satisfactory and may replace longer TR sequences for T2 weighting.

At the present time, all patients are scanned within the standard head coil (GE Signa, 1.5 T). McCardle has found benefit in using the wraparound extremity coil provided with the GE Signa system for cranial imaging in neonates and young infants with small calvariums (T1WI TR-1000 msec, TE 20 msec; T2WI TR-2500 msec, TE 80–160 msec, 1 nex).[10] Using this approach, he reports improved resolution and tissue signal differentiation in neonates with increased brain water (Fig. 6–1). We are currently evaluating use of a loop-gap resonator, tandem axial pair surface coil (MAI Inc., Milwaukee, Wis.)[11, 12] for examination of the neonatal cranium, the posterior fossa, and the craniocervical junction (Fig. 6–2). Our preliminary experience suggests for evaluating the posterior fossa and craniocervical junction, there is better resolution and an

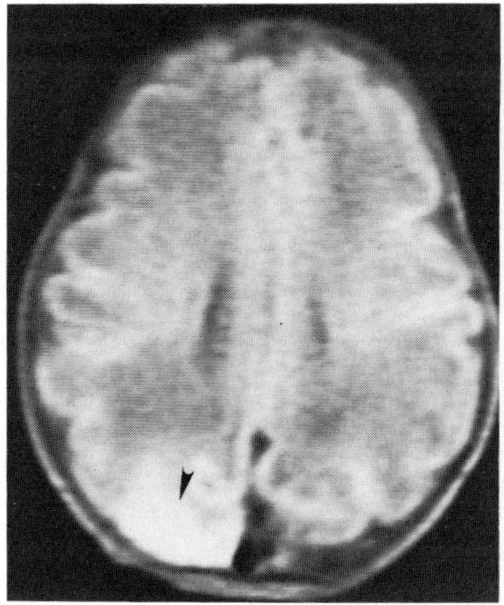

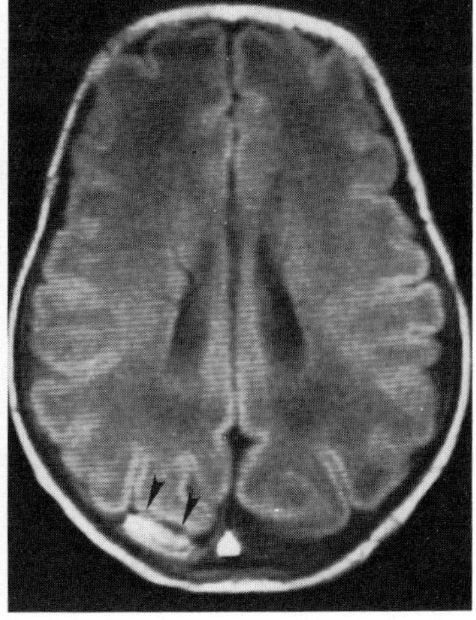

**Figure 6–1. Neonatal brain.** Axial T1WI (TR 800 msec/TE 20 msec) performed in *A* (the standard GE Signa head coil) and in *B* (the GE Signa extremity coil). Note improved resolution, improved differentiation between white and gray matter, and better visualization of a small posterior subdural hematoma (arrowheads). (Courtesy of C. McArdle, M.D., University Health Sciences Center, The University of Texas at Houston, Texas.)

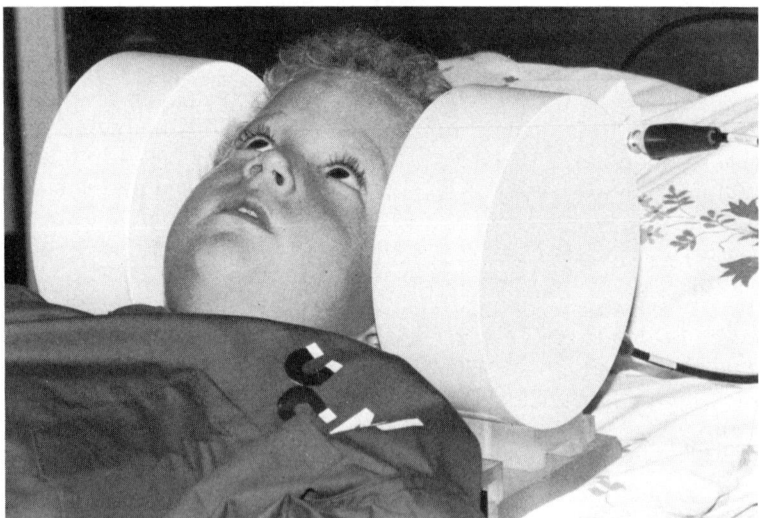

**Figure 6–2. Tandem axial planar pair, loop-gap resonator surface coil system.** Such coils allow improved visualization of the cervical spine, craniocervical junction, and posterior fossa in flexion and extension. (Courtesy of Medical Advances, Inc., Milwaukee, Wis.)

improved capability to image in flexion and extension, when compared with the standard head coil.

### Slice Acquisition

Both resolution and anatomic coverage depend in part on slice thickness. For T1WI and T2WI in any projection, a slice thickness of 5 mm is routinely used. In the cooperative or sedated patient, a 3 mm slice thickness can be chosen to cover smaller anatomic areas. For multiecho sequences, the interslice gap must be small enough to provide adequate coverage of the anatomic areas but must remain large enough to prevent image degradation by "crosstalk." For routine brain scanning, we prefer a gap of 1 to 2.5 mm. Gaps as small as 0.5 mm are now possible. Contiguous sections (0 gap) may be obtained with a single-echo technique. As an alternative, interleaved sections are obtained by alternating slice acquisition. Although interleaving reduces crosstalk and improves resolution, it does so at the expense of doubling scan time. Continuous or interleaved 3 mm thick sections are important in imaging small anatomic areas such as the sella or internal auditory canals. Resolution is also dependent on matrix size. By increasing the number of pixels within the matrix to 256 × 256, one can improve resolution. For T1WI, a doubling of scan time using a 256 × 256 matrix is acceptable without unreasonably prolonging the examination. In older children with larger head circumferences, increasing the matrix size often increases the noise to an unacceptable level. In this circumstance, we maintain a 256 × 128 matrix size but increase the number of excitations from 2 to 4. For routine scanning of the head, a 20- to 24-cm field of view is chosen. In infants with small biparietal diameters, the field of view may be reduced to 16 cm. Further decrease in the field of view in an attempt to improve resolution has an undesirable effect of decreasing signal, limiting coverage of the anatomic area of interest, increasing noise, and producing aliasing artifacts (wraparound).

Techniques are now available on most scanners that reduce pulsation artifact, especially prominent at the level of the lateral ventricles, the circle of Willis, and at the foramen magnum. Such techniques include cardiac gating or the use of refocused pulsations to reduce extravascular misregistration, and thereby improve visualization of the posterior fossa, the middle cranial fossa, and areas adjacent to the lateral ventricles. Readers are referred elsewhere within the text for a more detailed discussion of these modifications.

Most systems now incorporate a means of rapid data acquisition.[13, 14] The purpose of gradient acquisition is to provide relatively T1WI or T2WI with scan times of under 2 minutes. The technique of fast acquisition may differ from one scanner to another. Our experience is with the use of GRASS (Gradient Reversal Acquisition in the Steady

State) scanning with the GE Signa system (Fastscan). The physics of such data acquisition is beyond the scope of this chapter. Fast acquisition techniques are currently limited by poor signal to noise, decreased resolution, poor tissue contrast, and limitations in the number of slices that can be acquired in a single sequence. We use fast scan to provide additional information if time is limited, to produce a "myelographic" effect, to separate vascular flow void from the signal void of calcium, and to improve our recognition of calcification within the brain parenchyma. A myelographic effect can be achieved by using a TR 200 to 400 msec/TE 60 to 90 msec (flip 10°-20°). In order to improve tissue contrast differentiation between white and gray matter, a shorter TE, 10 to 20 msec, is chosen. This density-weighted sequence is effective in identifying heterotopic gray matter. Rapid data acquisition will not compensate for patient motion and therefore cannot be used to replace adequate sedation. It can however be used effectively if sedation time is limited. Excessive noise from the switching of the gradient coils in fast-scanning techniques may wake the sedated child. For this reason, ear putty is inserted before sedation if the use of fast-scanning techniques is anticipated.

## CEPHALOCELES

Congenital cephaloceles represent a herniation of meninges, neural tissue, or both beyond the confines of the cranial vault through a defect in the bony calvarium.[15-17] The terminology defining such herniations is often confusing but is best classified according to the contents of the herniated sac. Cranium bifidum refers to a group of conditions in which there is herniation of cranial contents through any midline bony defect. Craniomeningocele is an isolated herniation of meninges and cerebrospinal fluid (CSF). An encephalocele, or meningoencephalocele, represents herniation of both neural tissue and meninges. When ventricular herniation occurs as well, an encephalocystocele is present. In addition to occurring as congenital lesions, cephaloceles may be acquired. Acquired craniomeningoceles may be secondary to trauma (leptomeningeal cysts) or surgery (post surgical meningocele).[17]

Cephaloceles occur at a variety of sites.[15, 16] With rare exceptions, the defects are midline. Occipital defects are most common, followed by defects of the parietal calvarium, the frontoethmoidal region, and the basal skull in decreasing frequency of occurrence.[18] Frontoethmoidal encephaloceles are rare in North America but are common in Southeast Asia.[19] Female predominance is characteristic of occipital lesions; however, males tend to predominate in anterior defects.[20] The overall incidence of congenital cephaloceles is estimated at 1 in 10,000 live births.[21] Associated anomalies of the brain are often present and include agenesis of the corpus callosum, Chiari III malformation, holoprosencephaly, and Dandy-Walker deformity.[15, 17]

Occipital cephaloceles comprise three fourths of the congenital defects.[22] Encephaloceles are slightly more common than craniomeningoceles in the occiput.[23] With MRI, lesions of the occipital calvarium are best imaged in the sagittal and axial projections. The entire brain as well as the upper cervical spine should be surveyed for associated anomalies. Microcephaly is often present and may be severe in the presence of a large encephalocele. The bony defect is predominantly midline, occasionally asymmetric, and can vary in size. Very large defects often extend to the foramen magnum, or inferiorly to involve the posterior arch of the first cervical vertebrae (Fig. 6–3*A*). Visualization of the bony defect is difficult with MRI, but an estimation of its size can be obtained by measurement of the diameter of the neck of the herniated subarachnoid space (Fig. 6–3*B*). High-resolution T1WI sequences are of greatest benefit in defining the extent of the lesion and in determining its contents. The bulk of the herniated sac is low in signal on T1WI, owing to CSF. Neural tissue is identified by its shorter T1 values when compared with CSF. The signal emanating from the herniated neural tissue is usually similar in intensity to normal cerebellar gray matter. Varying amounts of cerebellar tissue may herniate into the sac. The hemispheric herniation is often asymmetrical, and the tissue is dysplastic in appearance. Rarely, the cerebellar hemispheres are completely absent. With large encephaloceles, the pons, medulla, and portions of the occipital lobes may also enter the sac. Whether or not it is herniated, the brain

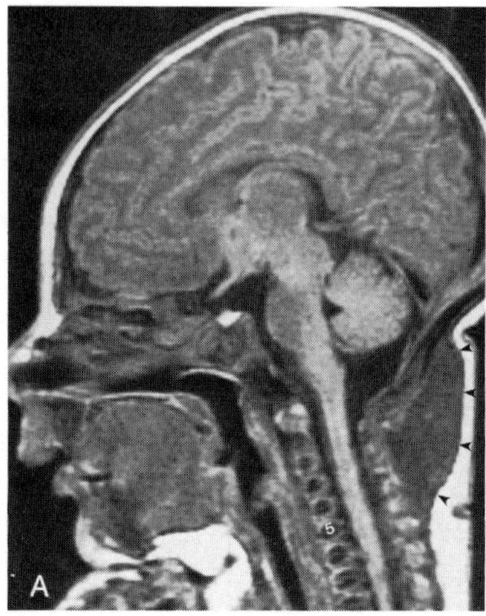


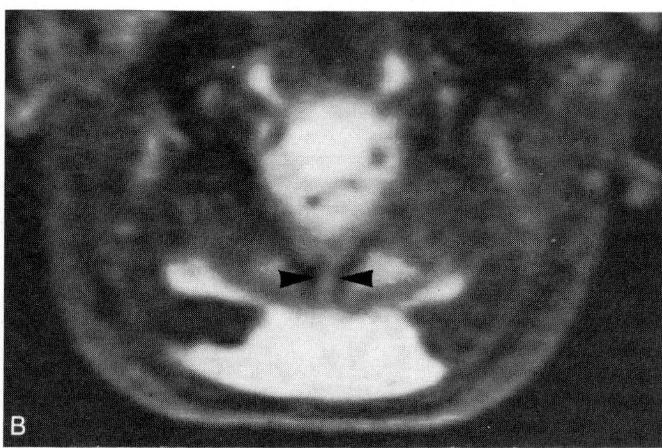


**Figure 6–3. Cervical craniomeningocele.** *A,* Sagittal T1WI (TR 600 msec/TE 20 msec) is seen. A well-defined occipital craniomeningocele extends from the base of the occiput to C5 arrowheads. No neural tissue within the herniated sac. *B,* Axial T2WI (TR 2500 msec/TE 100 msec). Small tract of CSF (arrowheads) provides communication between craniomeningocele and posterior fossa.

stem often appears hypoplastic, abnormal in shape, and inferiorly displaced. Herniation of the fourth ventricle into the sac with varying degrees of dilatation, is seen on occasion. The outside walls of the herniated sac are covered superficially with an uninterrupted layer of skin and high-signal subcutaneous fat. The skin and subcutaneous fat overlying the malformation are continuous with similar layers of the surrounding scalp.

MRI is also of value in identifying and localizing dural venous channels or aberrant dural venous sinuses that often rim the bony defect or, rarely, herniate along with brain into the hernia sac. Venous channels are recognized as peripheral tubular structures varying in signal, depending on their rate of flow. Their identification before surgical intervention is essential in order to prevent complications.

Parietal and occipital encephaloceles have similar features on MRI, differing only in the contents of the herniated sac. McLaurin[24] further categorized defects of the parietal region into (1) true encephaloceles, (2) ectopic glial tissue, (3) craniomeningoceles with and (4) without intracranial communication, and (5) craniomeningoceles with intracranial communication and a dermal sinus. The midline sagittal projection is best suited for the diagnosis and categorization of parietal cephaloceles. Central communication with the subarachnoid space is typically midline near the vertex (interhemispheric fissure). The straight sinus is often elevated in parieto-occipital cephaloceles and appears to insert at the base of the mass (Fig. 6–4). The sagittal sinus and surface cortical veins often rim the bony defect. Both the structural integrity of the sagittal sinus and its relationship to the dysraphic defect are best assessed in the coronal and sagittal projections. When the location of the venous sinuses is in doubt, the "angiographic" effect of a gradient acquisition image is useful. Because of the inability of MRI to adequately visualize bone, it is often difficult to detect a bony defect. Despite excellent anatomic detail, it may remain difficult on MRI to separate a dermoid from ectopic glial tissue or a craniomeningocele with an intact bony calvarium.[24] The diagnosis of dermoid is more likely when fat is present within the mass, which is bright in signal on T1WI and may decrease or increase in signal on T2WI. The presence of a lipomatous cord extending from the superficial mass to a deep cyst or a lipoma should also suggest the diagnosis of a dermoid sinus. With a dermoid, the sagittal sinus remains in normal location beneath the mass (Fig. 6–5).

The contents within the herniated sac of a frontoethmoidal or a basal encephalocele are difficult to evaluate by CT, cisternography, or both. The multiprojectional capability of MRI is not degraded by bone artifact, making it the ideal modality for the detec-

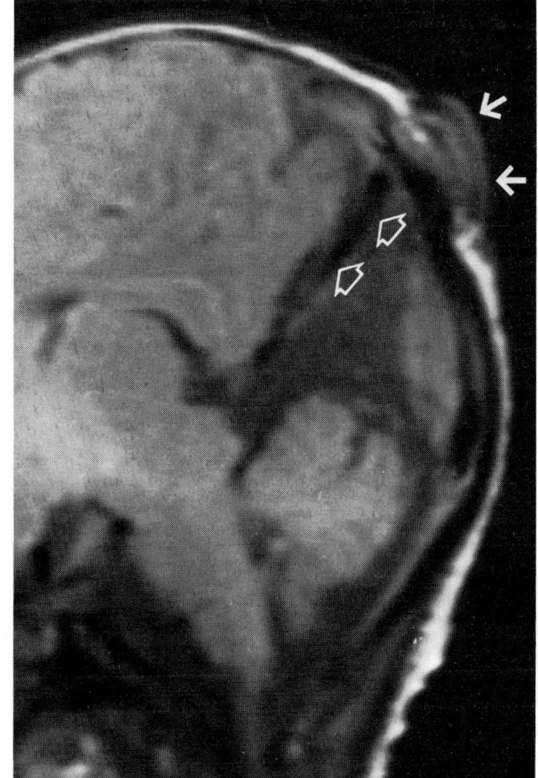

**Figure 6–4. Parietal encephalocele.** Sagittal T1WI (TR 2500 msec/TE 20 msec). Parieto-occipital encephalocele contains neural tissue (arrows), which is isointense to gray matter. Note elevation of the straight sinus (open arrows) and the transverse sinuses to the base of the defect.

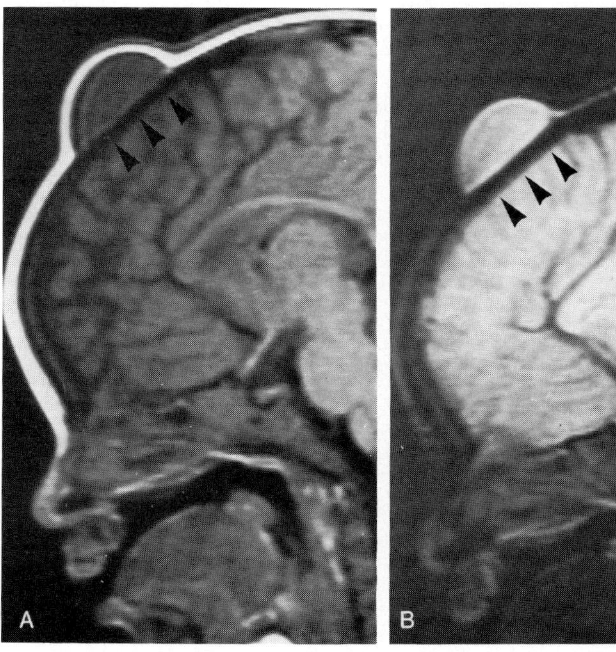


**Figure 6–5. Dermoid.** *A,* T1WI (TR 1000 msec/TE 20 msec). *B,* T2WI (TR 2500 msec/TE 100 msec). Well-demarcated scalp mass with a prolonged T1 and T2 relaxation. Note the nondisplaced sagittal sinus (arrows) beneath the mass. No communication exists between the scalp mass and the intracranial structures.

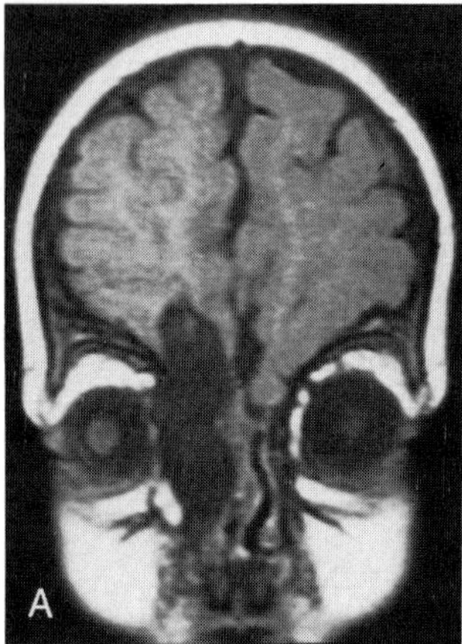


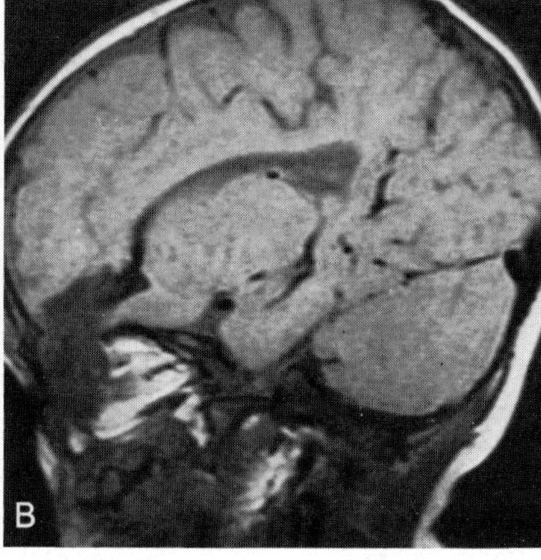


**Figure 6–6. Frontoethmoidal craniomeningocele.** *A,* Coronal T1WI (TR 720 msec/TE 20 msec); right defect with herniation of CSF into the frontoethmoidal region. *B,* Sagittal N(H)WI (TR 2500 msec/TE 20 msec). No neural tissue herniates into the cephalocele.

tion and categorization of encephaloceles in these regions (Fig. 6–6*A* and *B*). However, for both basal and frontoethmoidal encephaloceles, evaluation of bony detail remains essential. Often, such defects require extensive craniofacial reconstruction in addition to simple closure; therefore multiplanar CT is still considered a necessary adjunct to MRI in the evaluation of sincipital and basal lesions. Finally, MRI is also of benefit in searching for associated cranial malformations, such as agenesis of the corpus callosum and holoprosencephaly. Both conditions have an increased incidence in encephaloceles involving the frontoethmoidal and basal regions.[15]

## ARNOLD-CHIARI II MALFORMATION

The Chiari malformations comprise a complex group of anomalies that predominantly involve the midbrain, brain stem, cerebellum, and craniocervical junction.[25] In Chiari I malformation, cerebellar tonsillar herniation below the foramen magnum is combined with minimal elongation or kinking of the brain stem, hydrocephalus, and syringomyelia of the cervical cord.[26] Chiari III malformation is found in association with an occipitocervical encephalomeningocele into which are displaced a hypoplastic cerebellum and brain stem.[27] Chiari II malformation is most common and occurs in association with meningomyelocele. Rarely, isolated cases without meningomyelocele have been reported.[28] Chiari II malformation may present with progressive neurologic dysfunction as a result of hydrocephalus, brain stem or cerebellar compression, or from syringohydromyelia of the cord.

The extensive anatomic deformities characteristic of Chiari II malformation are well visualized using multiplanar MRI. High-resolution T1WI in the axial, coronal, and sagittal projections are often necessary to fully characterize this complex malformation. In Chiari II malformation, the degree of involvement of the midbrain, brain stem, cerebellum, and craniocervical junction varies in severity.[29] Characteristically, the medulla and fourth ventricle are displaced caudally into a widened foramen magnum and upper cervical canal (Fig. 6–7).[30] As seen best in the coronal and sagittal projections, herniation of the inferior vermis and cerebellar tonsils into the upper cervical canal occurs

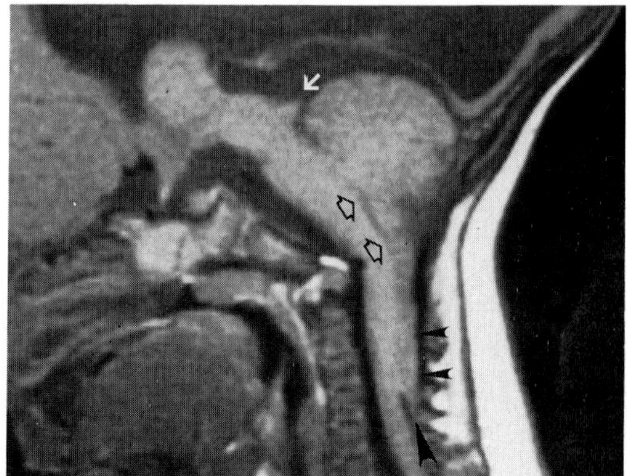

**Figure 6–7. Chiari II malformation.** Sagittal T1WI (TR 740 msec/TE 20 msec); herniation of the inferior vermis, cerebellar tonsils (arrowheads), and medulla into the upper cervical canal. In addition, tectal beaking (arrow), inferior displacement of a slitlike fourth ventricle (open arrows), and widening of the upper cervical canal are identified.

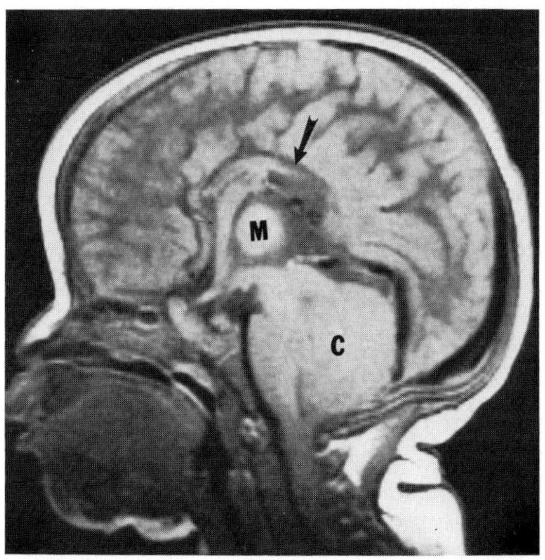


**Figure 6–8. Chiari II malformation.** Sagittal T1WI (TR 800 msec/TE 20 msec). There is low attachment of the tentorium cerebelli. The cerebellum (C) is elongated and extends superiorly through a hypoplastic incisura. Note enlargement of the massa intermedia (M) and partial absence of the posterior corpus callosum (arrow).

posterior to the displaced medulla and cervical cord. Herniation inferiorly as far as the upper thoracic spine has been reported.[31] The cerebellar tonsils may remain separate but not infrequently the tonsils may fuse, forming a posterior-inferior beak dorsal to the medulla. The medulla may fold or kink posteriorly within the upper cervical canal, below the tonsillar beak, to form a characteristic Z-bend deformity. Caudal displacement of the fourth ventricle is usually present. In 90% to 95% of cases, the fourth ventricle is small, deformed, and elongated; however, in 5% of cases it is enlarged.[30] The amount of deformity depends in part on the degree of inferior displacement of the brain stem.

The tentorium attaches in low position, in some cases just above the foramen magnum and is best visualized in the sagittal projection (Fig. 6–8). The cerebellum is usually elongated (towering), and projects superiorly through a hypoplastic tentorial incisura to form a pseudomass (Fig. 6–9). The cerebellum and its pseudomass are best demonstrated on a T1WI in the sagittal and axial projections. On axial scans, the cerebellar hemispheres may actually fold around the brainstem. The signal characteristics of the cerebellar hemispheres and brain stem in both T1WI and T2WI are normal despite the extensive deformity.

The occipital lobes often descend to a low position, lying posterior to the inferiorly displaced tentorium (Fig. 6–8). We speculate that in some instances this can result in further compression of the cerebellum, fourth ventricle, and brain stem and may be accentuated by the presence of hydrocephalus. The superior and inferior colliculi show varying degrees of fusion in both the axial and sagittal projections and appear as a posteriorly directed "tectal beak."

Ventricular enlargement is found in 98% of cases (Fig. 6–10).[30] With severe hydrocephalus, the corpus callosum is often thinned or absent. Ventricular dilatation is greatest at the level of the atria and occipital horns of the lateral ventricles. The frontal horns are characteristically squared laterally and beaked inferiorly (Fig. 6–11). Although the pathophysiology of hydrocephalus in Chiari II malformation is still unclear, it is

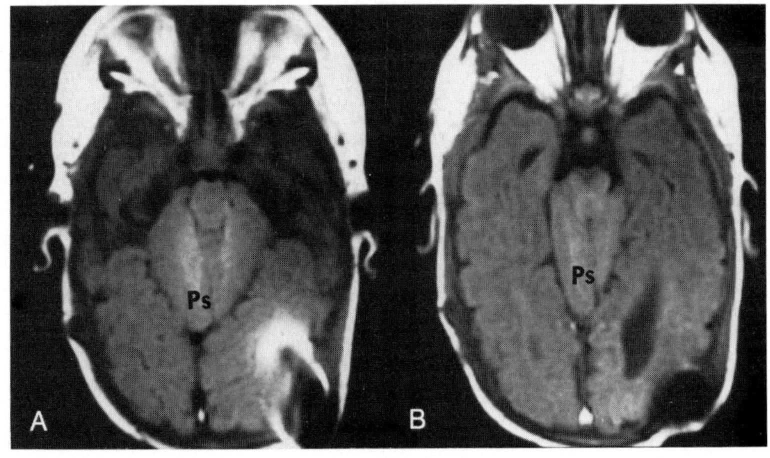


**Figure 6–9. Chiari II malformation.** Axial T1WI (TR 800 msec/TE 20 msec). *A* and *B,* An elongated cerebellum forms a pseudomass (Ps) at the tentorial incisura.

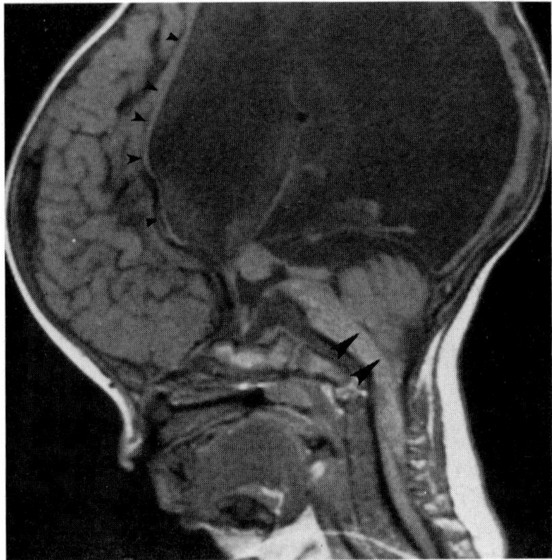

**Figure 6–10. Chiari II malformation.** Sagittal T1WI (TR 720 msec/TE 20 msec). Massive hydrocephalus due to obstruction at the aqueduct of Sylvius. Note slitlike, inferiorly displaced fourth ventricle (large arrowheads). The corpus callosum is hypoplastic with marked thinning (small arrowheads).

most likely secondary to obstruction at the aqueduct of Sylvius, at the outlet of the fourth ventricle, or at both places. With high-grade obstruction at the aqueduct, the typical CSF flow void sign (CFVS) seen on T2WI is often decreased or absent although the use of this sign as a reliable indicator of obstruction is inconclusive.[32, 33] With outlet obstruction of the fourth ventricle, the CFVS may be increased in the posterior aspect of the third ventricle, in the aqueduct, and in the upper fourth ventricle. When the third ventricle enlarges, the suprapineal and suprasellar recesses may become prominent. The massa intermedia, as seen best in the sagittal projection, is typically enlarged but displays normal signal characteristics (see Fig. 6–8). The falx cerebri is often hypoplastic or fenestrated, allowing interdigitation of medial gyri from both cerebral hemispheres. Migrational anomalies, including polymicrogyria and gray matter heterotopias, may accompany Chiari II malformation. Such migrational changes are best identified on a T2WI in the axial projection.

## HOLOPROSENCEPHALY

Holoprosencephaly occurs as a result of impaired cleavage of the developing midbrain and cerebral hemispheres. Roach reported the incidence of holoprosencephaly to be 1 in 16,000 live births.[33] Females predominate 3 to 1 in the alobar form, whereas the incidence of males and females is equal in the lobar variety.[33] Holoprosencephaly may be associated with various syndromes including trisomy 13, trisomy 15, trisomy 18, deletions 18p− and 13q—, and Meckel's syndrome.[34]

In its most severe form, the prosencephalon fails to undergo sagittal cleavage into separate cerebral hemispheres. In addition, the telencephalon and diencephalon fail to cleave transversely, resulting in midline fusion of the thalamic lobes. Finally, there is underdevelopment of both the olfactory and

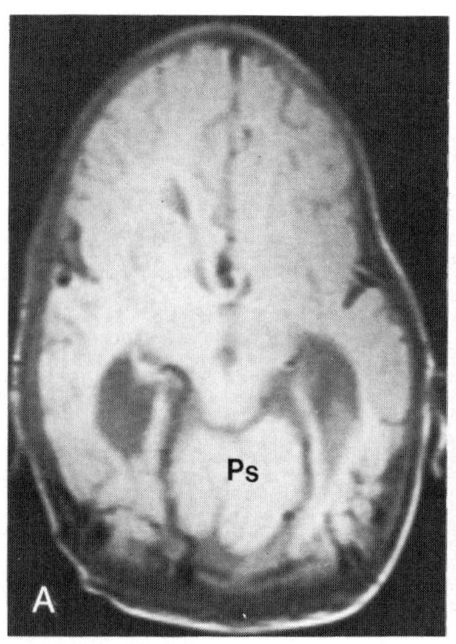


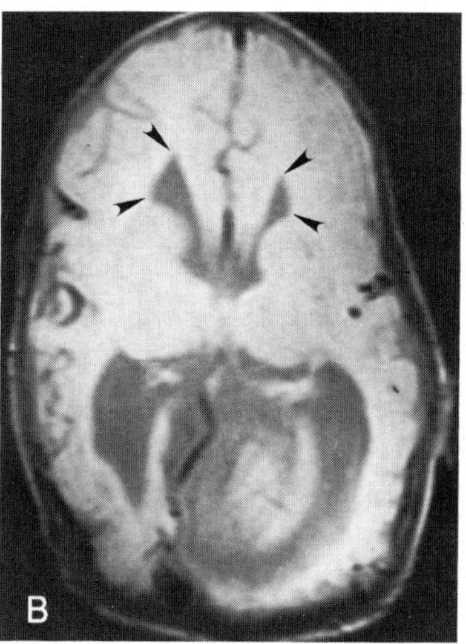


**Figure 6–11. Chiari II malformation.** *A* and *B*, N(H)WI (TR 2500 msec/TE 20 msec). Ventricular changes include mild dilatation of the atria and occipital horns of the lateral ventricles and lateral squaring with inferior beaking of the anterior horns (arrowheads). Ps = cerebellar pseudomass.

optic bulbs that can be complete, resulting in facial dysmorphism such as cyclopia, ethmocephaly, cebocephaly, premaxillary agenesis, and hypotelorism.[35] The malformation of facial features in some cases may be mild (autosomal dominant); however, the severity of facial dysmorphism often parallels the severity of the malformation.[33]

Holoprosencephaly can be subdivided into three types, depending on the severity of involvement.[36, 37] All three types are readily recognized on MRI. In the most severe form, alobar holoprosencephaly, a true monoventricular forebrain without an interhemispheric fissure is present. In the axial projection on T1WI, the low signal of the monoventricle (CSF) occupies the majority of the calvarium except for a thin rim of higher signal brain tissue, which may lie anteriorly or posteriorly. The shape of this rim is reminiscent of either a ball, a cup, or a saucer. Signal characteristics of the remaining cerebral tissue most closely resemble that of gray matter. The coronal projection is especially helpful in identifying the absent interhemispheric fissure and falx cerebri. This lack of division by a falx should not be termed a cerebral fusion; since it represents a failure of normal cleavage of the prosencephalon. In addition, the corpus callosum, septum pellucidum, and third ventricle are usually absent. Although fused, the thalamus maintains a normal signal intensity. The structures of the posterior fossa are surprisingly well preserved despite the degree of supratentorial involvement.

In the milder form known as semilobar holoprosencephaly, the developmental arrest occurs later, after the prosencephalon has undergone partial cleavage. Since cleavage proceeds from posterior to anterior, the posterior lateral ventricles and cerebral hemispheres appear well formed and are separated by a posterior interhemispheric fissure. The thalami have also undergone partial cleavage and are separated by a small hypoplastic third ventricle. As best seen in the coronal projection, the prosencephalic pattern persists in the anterior half of the brain. The corpus callosum may be absent or hypoplastic.

The mildest form is termed lobar holoprosencephaly. In this case, maturation has progressed to an almost complete separation of the cerebral hemispheres by a well-developed interhemispheric fissure and falx. Bridging cortical tissue may still remain anteriorly, indicating incomplete cleavage. The septum pellucidum is often absent.

Migrational abnormalities accompany disorders of telencephalization.[33] A T2WI may reveal areas of heterotopic gray matter and decreased white matter volume in the region of the centrum semiovale. Polymicrogyria is often present but is difficult to identify even on superficial surface sections.

## ABSENCE OF THE CORPUS CALLOSUM

Absence of the corpus callosum (ACC) represents a complex malformation of neural development. Most cases are sporadic; however, dominant, recessive, and X-linked recessive forms have been described.[38] Males and females are affected equally.[38] Often, focal neurologic deficit is not present; however, both seizures (60% to 70%) and developmental delay (70% to 80%) are common.[38] The corpus callosum develops as one of the neopallial commissures, which include the anterior and hippocampal commissures. Development begins near the end of the third month of gestation and is complete, including midline fusion, by the fifth month. Crossing of fiber tracts proceeds from the anterior commissure to the hippocampal commissure and, finally, to the corpus callosum itself. Decussation of fiber tracts within the corpus callosum proceeds from an anterior to posterior direction. The formation of the limbic system is also directly related to the development of the callosal commissure. The limbic formation includes the hippocampus, fornices, cingulate and parahippocampal gyri, the amygdala, hypothalamus, and portions of the thalami. Abnormalities in limbic formation often accompany deficiencies in formation of the corpus callosum.[39]

Absence of the corpus callosum arises either as a result of a developmental genetic defect or from an insult such as infection, anoxia, or vascular ischemia.[38] Absence of the corpus callosum is variable in severity, ranging from partial to complete. Malformations of the limbic system include enlargement and lateral displacement of the cingulate gyrus, hypoplasia and lateral displacement of the fornices, and deficient formation of the hippocampal gyrus. The septum pellucidum may be completely or partially absent. Because the system develops from anterior to posterior, partial absence usually involves the posterior portion; however, partial absence of the genu and rostrum, with an intact posterior segment, can occur.[38] Perhaps these cases are best explained by an encephaloclastic event rather than by a genetically determined defect in formation. White matter tracts that are unable to cross often course posteriorly within the medial walls of the lateral ventricles and are known as Probst's bundles.

The diagnosis of ACC on CT depends on the recognition of a constellation of secondary findings. On the other hand, sagittal MRI is capable of visualizing the corpus callosum directly.[39, 40] The corpus callosum is normally thin in the area of the rostrum and is thickest in the genu and midbody. The splenium represents the most posterior portion of the corpus callosum and appears bulbous. In the first six months of life, the corpus callosum is often difficult to identify on MRI (Fig. 6–12). At this age, it appears featureless, owing to its prolonged T1 relaxation time, which results from a lack of myelination. Visualization during this time may be improved with SE sequences using a TR of 2500 to 3500 msec. An IR sequence may also provide adequate visualization. With progressive myelinization, the T1 gradually shortens, allowing easier identification by the end of the first year of life.

With complete absence, only the anterior commissure and lamina terminalis remain. In the sagittal T1WI, the anterior commissure appears enlarged and elevated (Fig. 6–13). In partial absence, there is considerable variation in the shape of the corpus callosum. The rostrum, genu, body, or splenium are hypoplastic or absent to a varying degree. With absence of either the anterior or posterior corpus, the remaining portion of the body can appear pointed at either end (Fig. 6–14). With partial ACC, the signal characteristics of the remaining portion are normal, remaining isointense to white matter. In the axial projection, the anterior horns of the lateral ventricles appear slitlike, are

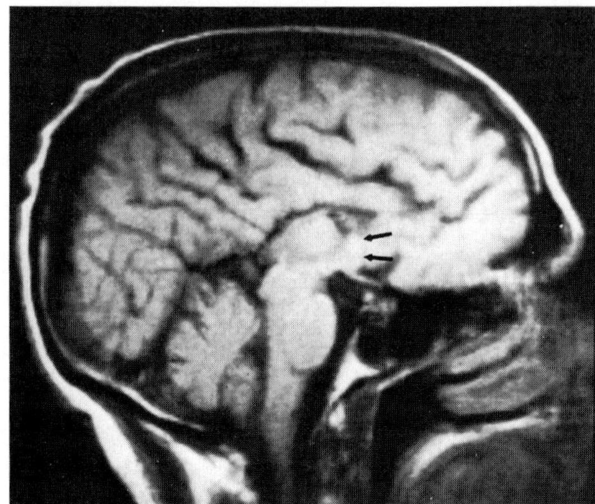

**Figure 6–13. Absence of the corpus callosum.** Sagittal T1WI (TR 500 msec/TE 30 msec). Only a vertically oriented anterior commissure and lamina terminalis remain (arrows). Note the "fanlike" radiation of the medial sulci toward the roof of the third ventricle.

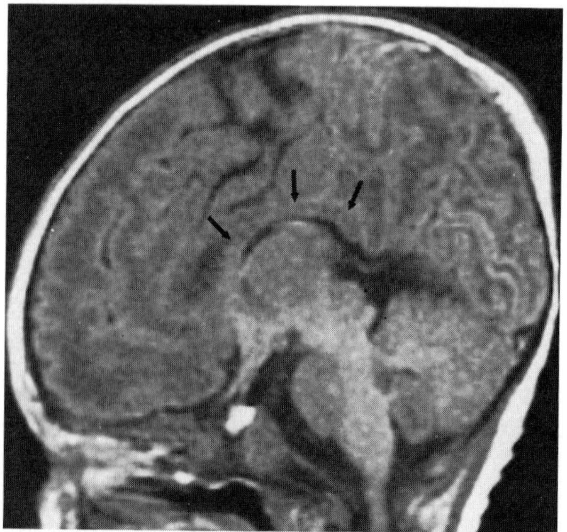

**Figure 6–12. Hypointense corpus callosum in a neonate.** Sagittal T1WI (TR 640 msec/TE 20 msec). A lack of myelination and an increase in water results in poor visualization of the corpus callosum (arrows).

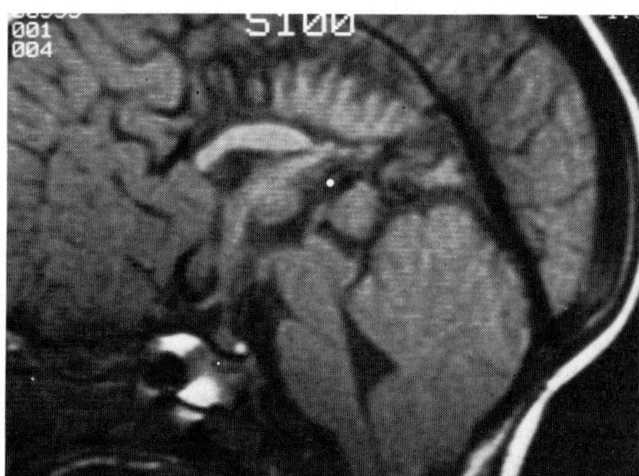

**Figure 6–14. Partial absence of the corpus callosum.** Sagittal T1WI (TR 600 msec/TE 20 msec). Absence of posterior body and splenium of the corpus callosum with dilatation and elevation of the suprapineal recess of third ventricle (dot).

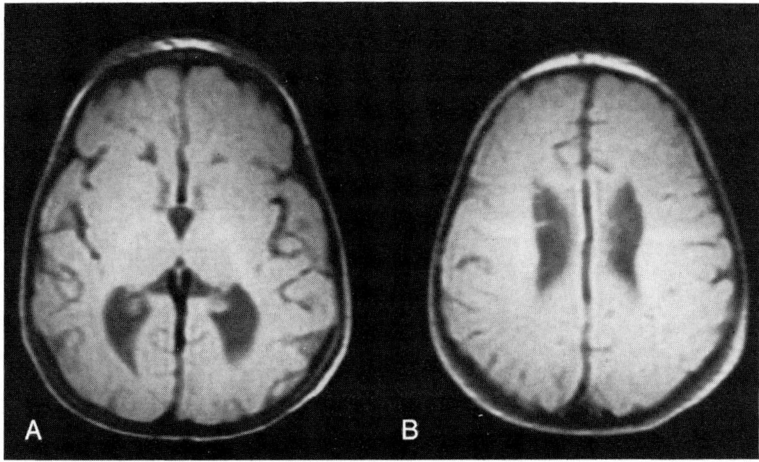


**Figure 6–15. Absence of the corpus callosum.** *A,* Axial N(H)WI (TR 2000 msec/TE 20 msec). The anterior horns are slit-like, beaked laterally, and concave medially. Culpocephaly is present posteriorly. Note the apposition of the third ventricle and the interhemispheric fissure. *B,* The lateral ventricles are parallel, rather than convergent anteriorly.

widely separated, and display prominent angulated lateral beaks, with concavity of their medial borders. Posteriorly, the lateral ventricular bodies are widely separated with dilatation of the atria and occipital horns (culpocephaly) (Fig. 6–15). Anteriorly, the long axes of the lateral ventricles are parallel, rather than convergent. Deficiencies in the hippocampal formation result in dilatation of the temporal horns (Fig. 6–16). The fornices, when identified, are hypoplastic and are laterally displaced. The medial cortical convolutions adjacent to the frontal horns and bodies of the lateral ventricles are often prominent owing to the presence of the uncrossed bundles of Probst (Fig. 6–17). These bundles are generally hypointense on a T2WI. Gray matter heterotopias may also

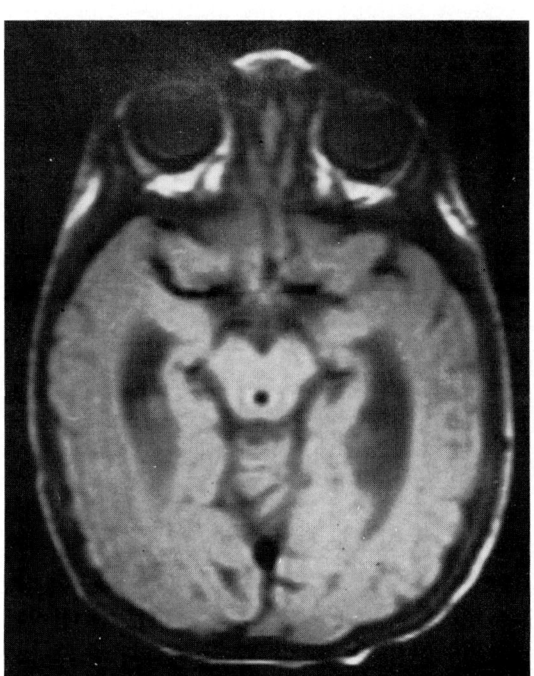

**Figure 6–16. Hypoplasia of the hippocampus.** Axial N(H)WI (TR 2000 msec/TE 20 msec). Dilatation and squaring of the temporal horns are due to deficiencies in the hippocampal formation.

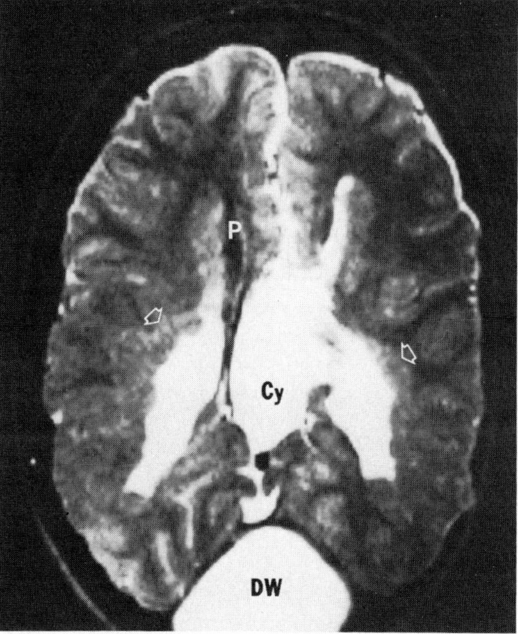


**Figure 6–17. Probst's bundles in absence of the corpus callosum.** Axial T2WI (TR 2500 msec/TE 100 msec). The uncrossed bundles of Probst are identified as linear areas of decreased signal (P) coursing in the medial walls of the lateral ventricles. Heterotopias of gray matter line the lateral ventricular wall (open arrows). Note the midline dorsal cyst (Cy) and the associated Dandy-Walker malformation (DW).

contribute to the lumpy appearance of the lateral ventricular walls.

With callosal absence, the third ventricle is often enlarged and extends anteriorly and superiorly into the interhemispheric fissure. A prominent suprapineal recess indicates absence of the posterior body and splenium.[41] Superior herniation of the third ventricle is best identified in the coronal projection. In callosal absence, the pericallosal arteries lie directly adjacent to the roof of the third ventricle as seen in the axial and sagittal projections. The paired internal cerebral veins and pericallosal arteries are splayed laterally, owing to interposition of the third ventricle and lateral separation of the hemispheres. A single, wandering anterior cerebral artery (azygos cerebral artery) is often present. On a midline sagittal section, the medial sulci of the hemisphere radiate centrally toward the roof of the third ventricle in a fanlike distribution (see Fig. 6–13). Atlas and colleagues also report identification of an acutely arched inferior margin of the cerebral hemisphere.[39]

The elevated third ventricle may or may not communicate with an interhemispheric cyst (Fig. 6–17). ACC has also been reported in association with other masses in the interhemispheric fissure, including lipoma;[42] arachnoid cyst;[43] and tumors such as astrocytoma, dermoid, or ependymoma.[44] A lipoma of the interhemispheric fissure is identified by its bright signal on a T1WI and decreasing signal on T2WI sequences. The lipoma lies adjacent to the region of the genu, which is often absent. A mass in the interhemispheric fissure of intermediate T1 weighting that increases in signal on a T2WI sequence should suggest the presence of a mass such as dermoid, ependymoma, or astrocytoma. An arachnoid cyst has similar T1 and T2 relaxation times to CSF.

ACC can be associated with migrational abnormalities (polymicrogyria and heterotopic gray matter)[38] that are best delineated on a T2WI sequence (Fig. 6–17). Alterations in the gyral pattern are best appreciated in the sagittal or coronal projections. In addition, ACC is not uncommonly associated with Chiari II and Dandy-Walker malformations, schizencephaly, or holoprosencephaly.[38, 39] In septo-optic dysplasia (de Morsier's syndrome), ACC is frequently present in addition to optic atrophy, absence of the septum pellucidum, and hypopituitarism (Fig. 6–18).[45, 46] This condition may actually represent the mildest form of holoprosencephaly. In Aicardi's syndrome, ACC can be present, along with infantile spasms, choanal atresia, and papillomas of the choroid plexus.

## LISSENCEPHALY

In lissencephaly, the normal migration of neuroblasts from the germinal matrix to the cortical surface is impaired. Morphologic expression is in two primary forms, agyria and pachygyria.[47–49] In agyria, the surface of the brain is smooth, being devoid of both convolutions and sulci. This is the most severe form of lissencephaly. In pachygyria, which some consider a milder form of lissencephaly, the gyri appear broad and flattened, with shallow sulci. For the purpose of this discussion, we will consider both

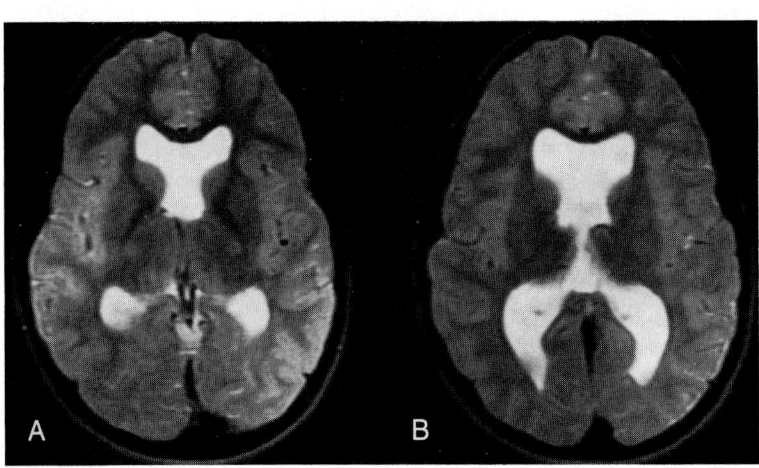


**Figure 6–18. Septo-optic dysplasia.** Axial T2WI (TR 2000 msec/TE 20 msec). *A* and *B*, Absence of the septum pellucidum and mild ventricular dysmorphism is present.

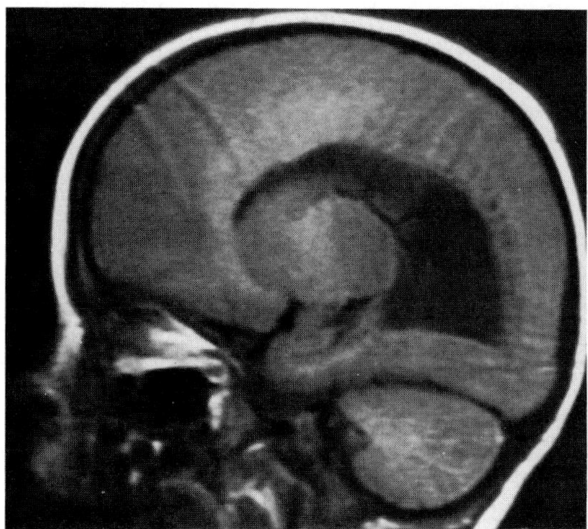

**Figure 6–19. Agyria.** Sagittal T1WI (TR 720 msec/TE 20 msec). The brain surface is smooth. Enlargement of the atrium and occipital horn of the lateral ventricle (culpocephaly) is common.

within the spectrum of migrational anomalies.[47, 49] The incidence of lissencephaly is not well documented, since milder forms go undiagnosed, even on CT. In its most severe form, clinical manifestations include intractable seizures, gross delay in motor development, mental retardation, and early death. Involvement of the brain is most commonly diffuse; however, asymmetrical, unilateral, lobular, and focal lissencephaly have been reported.[49] Although commonly considered an isolated anomaly, other associated malformations include various craniofacial dysplasias, encephalocele, Dandy-Walker malformation, holoprosencephaly, and schizencephaly.[49, 50] Both agyria and pachygyria are morphologically separate from polymicrogyria which is characterized by multiple abnormally small gyria and shallow sulci. Polymicrogyria is found in some cases of congenital porencephaly, schizencephaly, Arnold-Chiari malformation, and ACC.

MRI may well increase our capability to detect lissencephaly. Coronal and sagittal sections nicely demonstrate the smooth surface of the brain (Fig. 6–19). Both T1WI and T2WI sequences are useful in the evaluation of lissencephaly; however, we prefer high resolution T1WI for displaying the pathologic anatomy. Microcephaly is typically present, with reported brain weights less than the fiftieth percentile of the norm.[48] A sylvian fissure is present but appears shallow and broad. The fissure is often obliquely oriented and in severe cases appears almost vertical. The surrounding opercula is absent. These features give the brain a figure-eight appearance in the axial plane (Fig. 6–20).[47, 49]

On T2WI in the axial projection, the centrum semiovale generally appears decreased in volume. The ratio of gray to white matter normally is 1:3; however, in lissencephaly this ratio is often reversed (3:1).[47] In addition to being abnormal in volume, the centrum semiovale may persist in displaying a longer T2 relaxation similar to the immature pattern seen in infants less than three months of age (Fig. 6–20). This phenomenon is likely the result of delayed or abnormal myelination with an increase in the amount of free water within the white matter. Both the claustrum and the extreme capsule are absent. The corpus callosum may be hypoplastic or partially absent.

In pachygyria, the centrum semiovale is

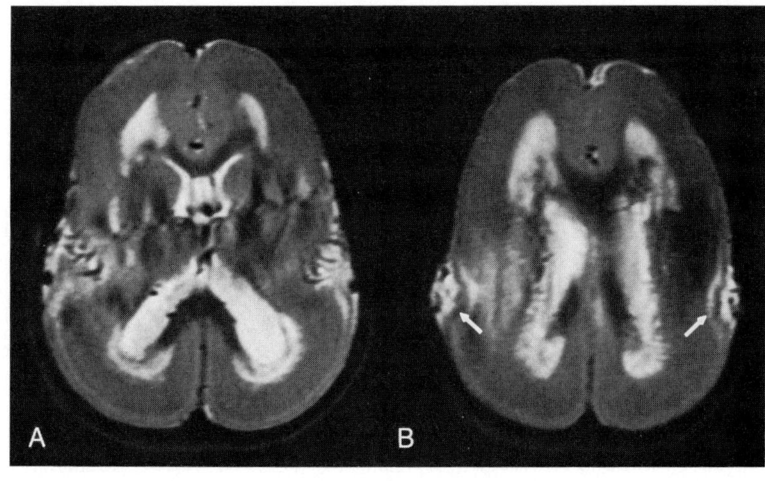


**Figure 6–20. Agyria.** Axial T2WI (TR 2500/TE 100 msec). *A* and *B*, The ratio of gray matter to white matter is approximately 3:1. An abnormal distribution of periventricular white matter with hyperintense signal is present. The sylvian fissures are prominent and vertically oriented owing to lack of operculization (arrows).

less severely involved and displays a more infantile pattern with a decreased number of peripheral interdigitations. This gives the centrum a coarse and thickened appearance. The signal emanating from the white matter on a T2WI may be normal or diffusely increased. Heterotopias of gray matter may also be present. As in agyria, both the body and occipital horns of the lateral ventricles are enlarged (culpocephaly), similar to the pattern found during the second midtrimester of development.

The distribution of agyria and pachygyria may be focal or unilateral. Isolated focal involvement should not be confused with the condition of hemimegaloencephaly, in which there appears to be overgrowth of brain tissue confined to a single cerebral hemisphere. Unlike lissencephaly, in hemimegaloencephaly the ratio of gray matter to white matter remains 1:3 or is equal with overgrowth of both layers.

Heterotopias of gray matter represent a third form of migrational abnormality.[49] The heterotopic collections usually lie adjacent to the lateral ventricular walls or within the anterior centrum semiovale. Heterotopic gray matter is isointense to normal gray matter on both T1WI and T2WI. Thinning of the gray matter in the peripheral cortex adjacent to the interhemispheric fissure is common.

## HEMIMEGALENCEPHALY

Recently, Kalifa and colleagues have refocused our attention on a rare anomaly of unilateral overgrowth of the cerebral hemisphere.[51] Clinically, these patients manifest intractable seizures, encephalopathy, or both.[51-54] We have now encountered four patients with features compatible with hemimegalencephaly. Pathologically, little is known of this disorder.[53, 55] Its main features include overgrowth of both gray and white matter with giant astrocytes[55] and it is most compatible with a hamartomatous malformation.[55]

In our experience, the frontal and parietal lobes are most commonly involved. The gyri appear broad and flat with shallow sulci (Fig. 6–21). Cortical gray matter is thickened but normal in signal on both T1WI and T2WI. The centrum semiovale also appears widened, with a decreased number of coarse interdigitations extending into the base of the gyri. On T2WI, white matter signal intensity may be normal or increased (Fig. 6–22).

The atrium, occipital horn, and temporal horn of the lateral ventricle are characteristically enlarged, whereas the anterior horn is frequently compressed (Fig. 6–23). The normal CFVS at the foramen of Monro is absent. Contrast ventriculography (CT) is helpful in confirming an obstruction at the foramen of Monro, likely owing to compression by the cerebral overgrowth (Fig. 6–24). On T2WI, despite proven obstruction, periventricular signal intensity remains normal.

## CONGENITAL PORENCEPHALY, SCHIZENCEPHALY

A focal loss of brain tissue resulting from an in utero encephaloclastic event is known as congenital porencephaly.[56, 57] In schizencephaly, the focal cortical defects are secondary to an arrest in normal brain devel-

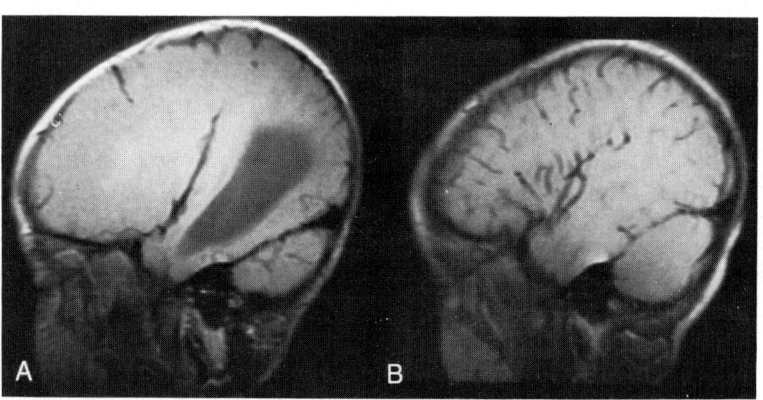


**Figure 6–21. Hemimegalencephaly.** Sagittal N(H)WI (TR 2000/TE 20 msec). *A*, There is marked overgrowth of the frontal and anterior parietal lobes on the right when compared with *B*, the normal left. Note the coarse gyral pattern anteriorly on the right.

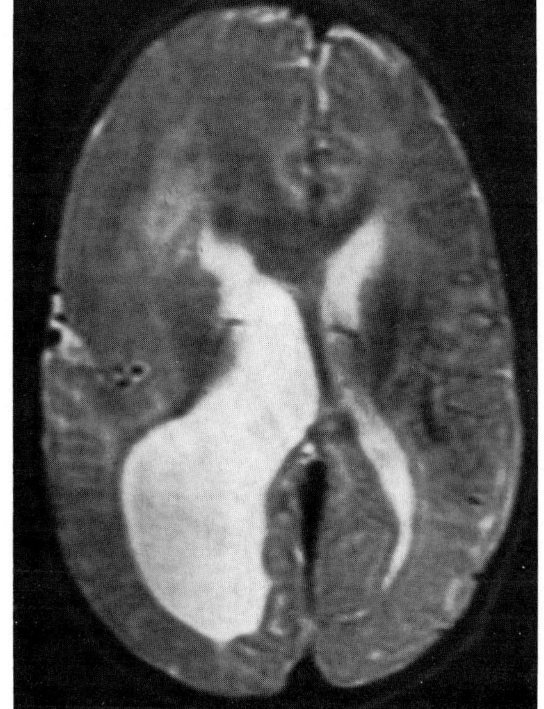

**Figure 6–22. Hemimegalencephaly.** Axial T2WI (TR 2500 msec/TE 100 msec). Abnormal right lateral ventricular enlargement. The white matter within the frontal and anterior parietal lobes is prominent, with a decreased number of interdigitations when compared with the left.

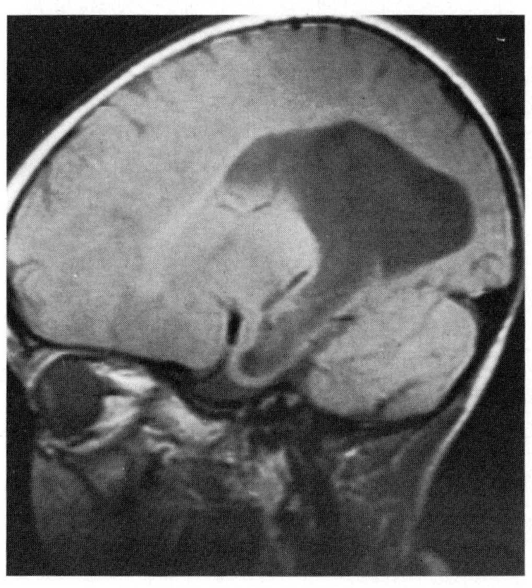

**Figure 6–23. Hemimegalencephaly.** Sagittal N(H)WI (TR 200 msec/TE 20 msec). Dilatation of the lateral ventricle to the level of foramen of Monro. The anterior horn appears compressed owing to overgrowth of the contiguous brain.

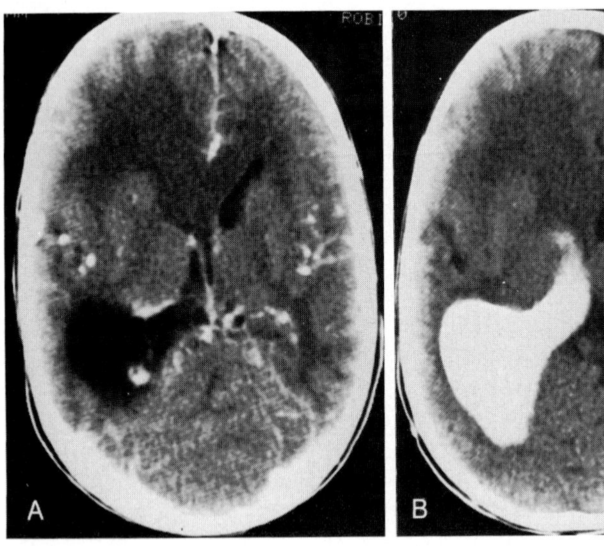

**Figure 6–24. Hemimegalencephaly.** *A,* Contrast-enhanced CT identifies the overgrowth of the brain and the prominence of the white matter centrally. Apparent obstruction of the right lateral ventricle at foramen of Monro, *B,* was confirmed by contrast ventriculography.

opment.[57] In reality, there is considerable overlap between these entities, which are often difficult to separate by means of imaging alone.[57]

Congenital encephaloclastic porencephaly is identified in 3% to 5% of patients presenting with focal motor neurologic deficit in the first year of life.[57] This condition results from an in utero insult such as trauma, infection, or vascular occlusion. Fifty to sixty percent of patients with congenital porencephaly present with symptoms before one year of age.[57, 58] Symptoms include spasticity, seizures, hemiparesis, cranial nerve deficit, and blindness. Coexistent defects such as agenesis of the corpus callosum and encephalocele have been reported.[57]

MRI can be helpful in separating congenital porencephaly from schizencephaly and in identifying the associated anomalies. Congenital porencephaly is best assessed on a T1WI in the axial and coronal projections. The defect is most frequently unilateral but can be bilateral and asymmetric. Although any area of the brain can be involved, the anterior parietal and posterior frontal cortices are most often affected (Fig. 6–25). Tissue loss involves both white and gray matter. In its classic presentation, a wedge-shaped defect communicates with the ventricular system and the overlying subarachnoid space. The signal characteristics within the cleft on T1WI and T2WI are similar to CSF. Adjacent gray and white matter are of normal signal but are decreased in thickness along the periphery of the cleft. Most often, the gray matter folds into the periphery of the cleft but does not line the entire defect as seen in schizencephaly.

Yakovlev and Wadsworth reported that schizencephaly is invariably bilateral and most often symmetric.[59] Several theories

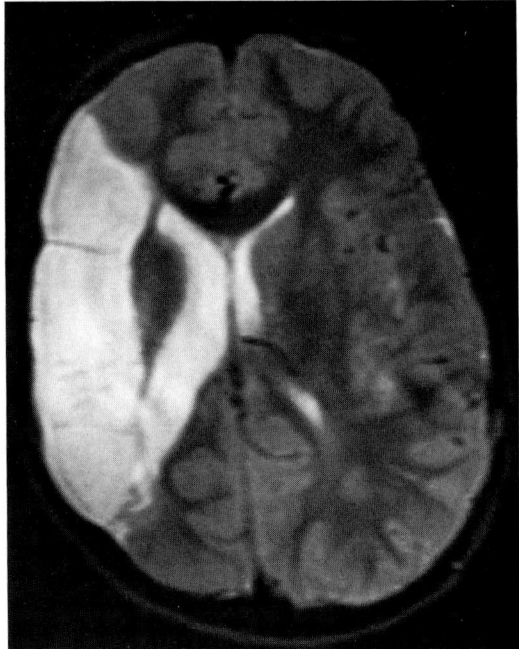

**Figure 6–25. Congenital porencephaly.** Axial T2WI (TR 2000 msec/TE 100 msec). A right porencephalic cyst is present. Volume loss is indicated by ipsilateral dilatation of the lateral ventricle and shift of the falx cerebri to the right.

have been proposed to explain the development of schizencephaly. The most tenable hypothesis is that the malformation results from a failure of neuroblast migration from the germinal matrix to the cortical surface. Histologically, the cleft is lined by ependyma and pia mater. In our experience, some degree of asymmetry is common. The clefts commonly involve the posterior frontal and anterior parietal cortices, including the region of the pre- and post-central gyri (Fig. 6–26).[60] Yakovlev and Wadsworth further divided schizencephaly into two groups, depending on whether the clefts were thin and fused (type I) or gaping (type II).[61, 62] We have not encountered type I patients on MRI.

In type II schizencephaly, the clefts are filled with CSF and therefore display signal characteristics similar to the ventricles. The cleft is characteristically lined by gray matter, which extends from the outer surface of the brain to the ventricular margin (Fig 6–27). Heterotopias may be found adjacent to the cleft, and focal polymicrogyria may be present at the periphery of the defect. Cortical surface veins with high signal intensity from slow flow lie on the surface of the gray matter and also line the cleft. Panventriculomegaly without obstruction is common. Despite their developmental differences, with MRI difficulty may still arise in separating schizencephaly from a bilaterally symmetric encephaloclastic defect.

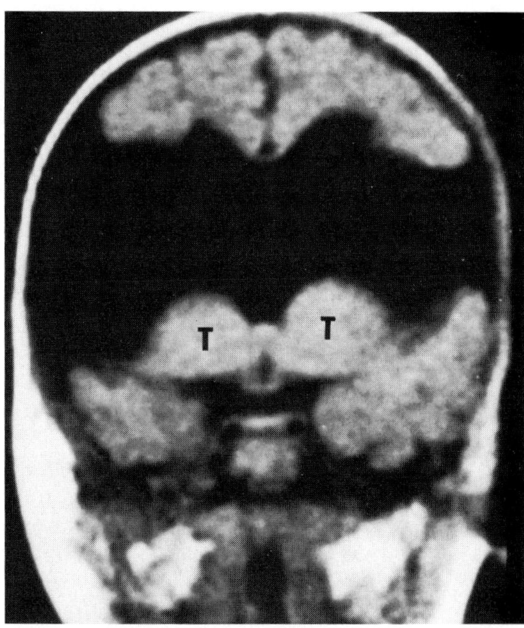


**Figure 6–27. Type II schizencephaly.** Coronal T1WI (TR 600 msec/TE 20 msec). Optimal demonstration of the bilateral symmetric clefts and absence of the corpus callosum. Partial midline fusion of the thalami (T) is present. (Courtesy S. J. Pomeranz, M.D., The Christ Hospital, Cincinnati, Ohio, and J. J. Sheldon, M.D., Mount Sinai Hospital, Miami Beach, Fla.)

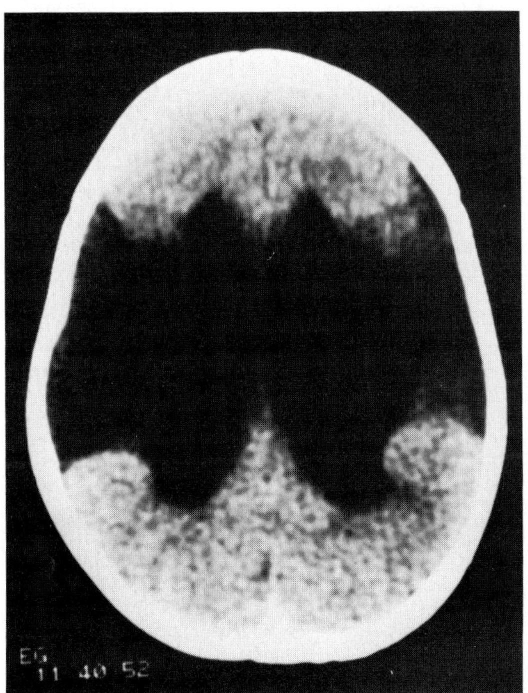

**Figure 6–26. Type II schizencephaly.** Axial unenhanced CT demonstrates bilateral symmetric clefts involving the posterior frontal and anterior parietal cortices. (Courtesy S. J. Pomeranz, M.D. The Christ Hospital, Cincinnati, Ohio, and J. J. Sheldon, M.D., Mount Sinai Hospital, Miami Beach, Fla.)

## AQUEDUCTAL STENOSIS

Obstruction of the ventricular system at the aqueduct of Sylvius is the most common cause of congenital hydrocephalus in children. Its incidence is estimated at approximately 0.9 to 1.5 cases per thousand live births.[63] Obstruction at the aqueduct is also associated with conditions such as Chiari II and Dandy-Walker malformations. We currently recognize four main pathologic types: (1) simple stenosis (inheritable as an X-linked hydrocephalus), (2) forking of the aqueduct (typical in Arnold-Chiari malformation), (3) congenital web or septum, and (4) periaqueductal gliosis (associated with von Recklinghausen's disease).[63] The most common cause of aqueductal obstruction is

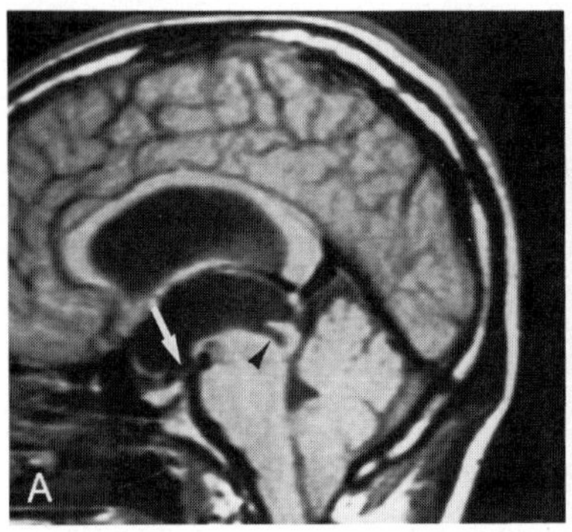


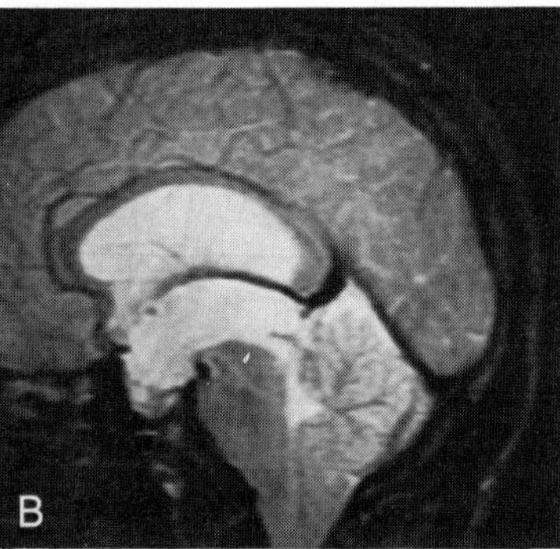


**Figure 6–28. Congenital aqueductal stenosis.** *A,* Sagittal T1WI (TR 600 msec/TE 20 msec). There is ballooning of the proximal aqueduct above a stenosis (arrowhead). The fourth ventricle is normal. Obstruction is indicated by ballooning of the anterior portion of the third ventricle (arrowhead) and a decrease in the pontomamillary distance (arrow). *B,* T2WI (TR 2000 msec/TE 80 msec). The CSFV is lacking in the anterior third ventricle and at the foramen of Monro. Note the difficulty in visualizing the narrowed aqueductal canal on T2WI.

simple stenosis with gliosis. Its etiology is unclear but is likely secondary to an in utero insult, such as vascular occlusion or inflammation. Rarely, an X-linked inheritable mode of transmission has been reported.[64] The second most frequent etiology is forking of the aqueduct, seen most commonly with Chiari II malformation. Aqueductal obstruction is found clinically with the signs and symptoms of increased intracranial pressure, including irritability, headaches, and increasing head circumference.

Obstruction secondary to aqueductal stenosis is readily identified on CT; however, MRI is capable of directly demonstrating the anatomic region of interest. MRI is also more sensitive than CT in the detection of periaqueductal lesions (tumor, arachnoid cyst), that can cause secondary obstruction. For direct visualization of the aqueduct, we rely primarily on high resolution T1WI in the direct sagittal projection (Fig. 6–28*A*). Thin sections at 0 gap or interleaved may be necessary to visualize the aqueductal area. T2WI are also of value in demonstrating the presence of increased transependymal flow and alterations in CSF dynamics. Increased transependymal resorption of CSF is identified by the presence of increased signal in the periventricular region proximal to the obstruction, resulting in an irregular (sawtooth) ventricular contour (Fig. 6–29).[33] The CFVS is often absent in the posterior aspect of the third ventricle and within the aqueduct itself (Fig. 6–28*B*) but may be increased in the anterior aspect of the third ventricle and in the region of foramen of Monro.[32, 33]

Obstruction at the outlet of the third ventricle produces elevation, stretching, and thinning of the corpus callosum. The pontomamillary distance is also decreased. Ballooning of the suprapineal and suprasellar-infundibular recesses are common and are best demonstrated in the midline sagittal

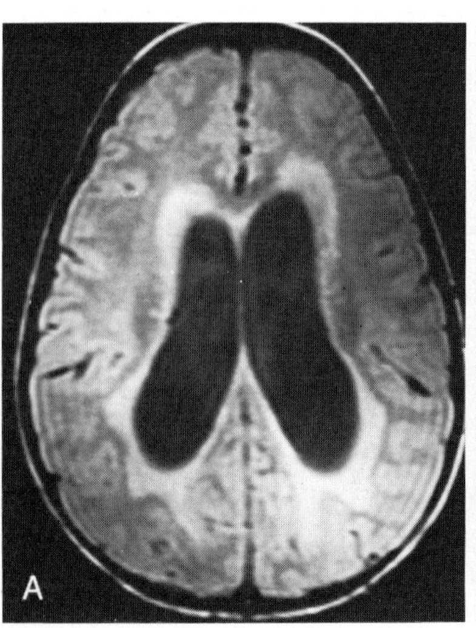


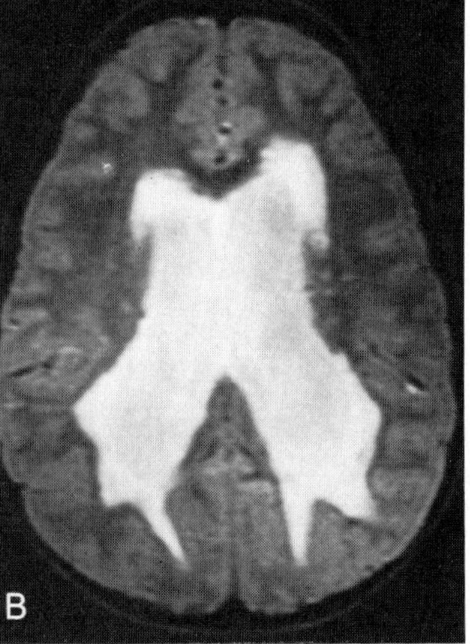


**Figure 6–29. Increased transependymal CSF flow with obstruction.** Axial, *A,* N(H)WI (TR 2000 msec/TE 20 msec), and *B,* T2WI (TR 2000 msec/TE 100 msec). Hydrocephalus present due to an obstruction at the aqueduct of Sylvius. Increased periventricular signal results from increased transependymal flow of CSF secondary to the obstruction.

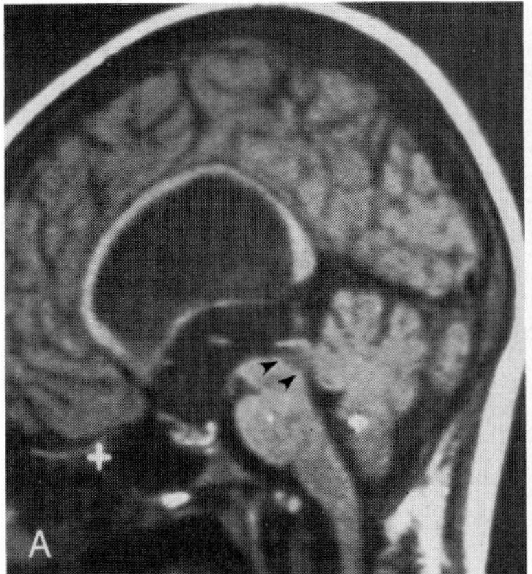


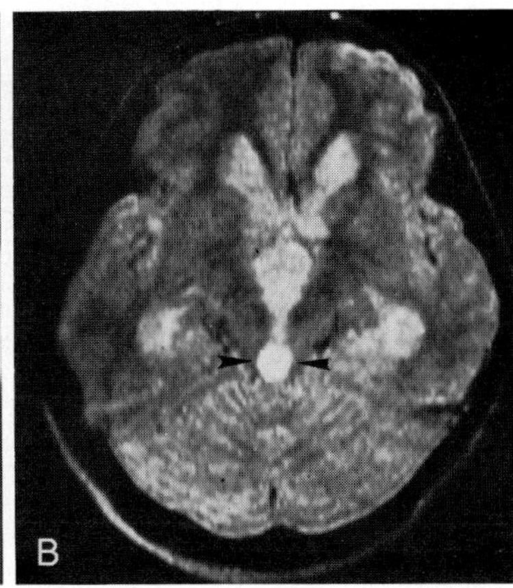


**Figure 6–30. Periaqueductal glioma.** *A,* Sagittal T1WI (TR 600 msec/TE 20 msec). Obstruction at the aqueduct of Sylvius. Subtle hypointensity surrounds the compressed aqueduct (small arrowheads). *B,* Axial T2WI (TR 2000 msec/TE 80 msec). The previously identified area of hypointensity around the aqueduct displays a very bright signal, even compared with the CSF (large arrowheads).

projection. MRI is an improvement over CT in separating a prominent suprasellar recess from an arachnoid cyst that may secondarily obstruct the aqueduct. Ballooning of the obstructed aqueduct can be occasionally demonstrated above a blind pouch, stenosis, or obstructed limb of a forked channel. The tissue surrounding the aqueduct may demonstrate hyperintensity on T2WI as a result either of local transependymal CSF flow[33] or from periaqueductal gliosis or glioma (neurofibromatosis) (Fig. 6–30). In aqueductal stenosis, the fourth ventricle is normal or small.

## MALFORMATIONS OF THE POSTERIOR FOSSA

A number of interesting and diagnostically challenging malformations arise within the posterior fossa. These conditions all comprise collections of CSF and varying degrees of hypoplasia of the cerebellum and brain stem. Included in this group is the Dandy-Walker malformation, Dandy-Walker variant, retrocerebellar arachnoid pouch (giant cisterna magna), and true arachnoid cyst. The Chiari malformations also predominantly involve the posterior fossa but are discussed elsewhere in this chapter.

### Dandy-Walker Malformation

This malformation was first described by Dandy and Blackfan in 1914.[65] It represents a complex structural malformation consisting of vermian agenesis, cystic dilatation of the fourth ventricle, agenesis of the foramina of Magendie and Luschka, and cerebellar hypoplasia.[66] Controversy exists as to whether the malformation arises as a result of agenesis of the outlet of the foramina of the fourth ventricle or as a dysraphic defect predominantly involving the cerebellum.[66] Dandy-Walker malformation is often associated with supratentorial midline and cortical malformations such as agenesis of the corpus callosum, aqueductal stenosis, holoprosencephaly, encephalocele, congenital porencephaly, and lissencephaly.[66]

Hydrocephalus is found in the majority of cases and is manifested clinically with prominence of the occiput, increasing head circumference, bulging of the anterior fontanelle, and other signs and symptoms of increased intracranial pressure. Ataxia, delayed motor development, and incoordination may result from dysplasia of the cerebellum and brain stem. Although occasional cases suggest an inheritable transmission, most are considered sporadic.

Multiplanar T1WI may be necessary to delineate the complex anatomic features of this malformation. Its hallmark is near-complete absence of the cerebellar vermis. Often the superior vermis is all that remains of this midline structure. The remaining vermis may be displaced superiorly and anteriorly by the cyst, occasionally appearing to fold over the quadrigeminal plate. Most of the expanded posterior fossa is filled by a large CSF space representing cystic dilatation of the fourth ventricle (Fig. 6–31). The cyst is lined by ependyma, and its roof is formed by the stretched and thinned roof of the fourth ventricle. The signal emanating from the cyst on T1WI and T2WI identifies it as CSF. Areas of CFVS are usually lacking

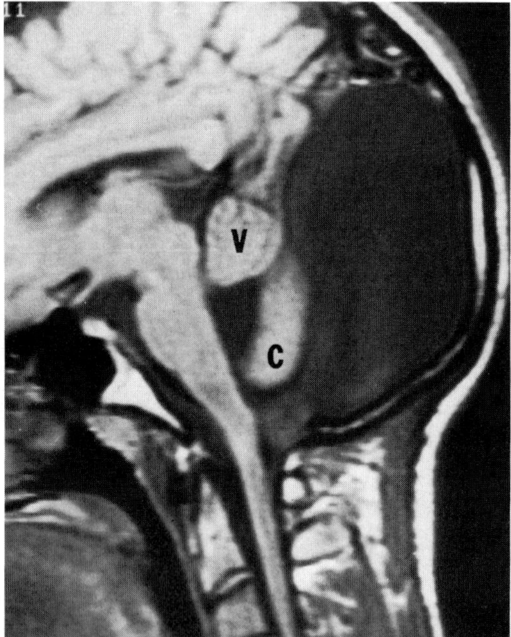


**Figure 6–31. Dandy-Walker malformation.** Sagittal T1WI (TR 650 msec/TE 20 msec). The superior vermis (V) is all that remains of this midline structure. A massive CSF cyst, representing a ballooned fourth ventricle, fills the posterior fossa, elevating and bowing the tentorium. Note infolding of the medial margin of a hypoplastic cerebellar hemisphere (C).

within the cyst and fourth ventricle but may be increased within the third ventricle. No communication exists between the cyst and the surrounding compressed subarachnoid space. The cyst occasionally herniates inferiorly through the foramen magnum to the level of C2, or superiorly through a hypoplastic incisura. Communication between the cyst and the fourth ventricle is best appreciated on axial and sagittal sections (Fig. 6–32).

Hypoplasia of the cerebellar hemispheres may or may not be symmetrical in appearance. The medial borders of the hemispheres appear to protrude into the walls of the cyst (see Fig. 6–31). When the hypoplasia is severe enough, all that remains of the cerebellum is nodules of tissue adjacent to the anterior wall of the cyst. Flattening of the brain stem against the clivus is frequently identified; however, the signal characteristics of both the brain stem and the cerebellum are usually normal. Sagittal MRI is particularly helpful in identifying the high insertion of the tentorium posteriorly above the lambda (torcula-lambda inversion) (see Fig. 6–31). The incisura of the tentorium may be widened. The transverse and straight sinuses, along the edge of the tentorium, may be hypoplastic. Unlike retrocerebellar arachnoid pouch and Dandy-Walker variant, the falx cerebelli is typically absent. When hydrocephalus is present, the aqueduct may appear enlarged, except in cases with associated aqueductal stenosis. The sagittal projection is also useful in identifying associated supratentorial anomalies.

## Dandy-Walker Variant

Dandy-Walker variant likely occurs more often than does Dandy-Walker malformation.[66] Controversy exists as to whether Dandy-Walker variant represents a milder form of the Dandy-Walker malformation. Dandy-Walker variant consists of absence of the inferior vermis and the presence of a retrocerebellar cyst, which communicates with the inferior aspect of the posterior fourth ventricle. The outlet foramina of the fourth ventricle are widely patent. Neuro-

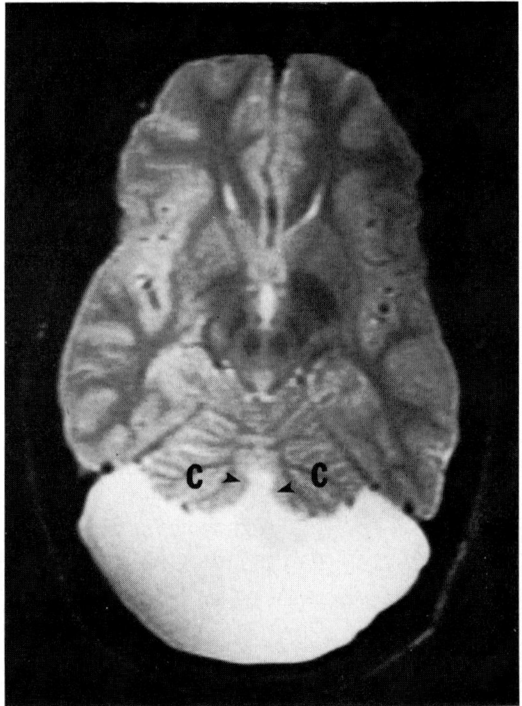


**Figure 6–32. Dandy-Walker malformation.** Axial T2WI (TR 2000 msec/TE 80 msec). The large posterior fossa cyst communicates directly with the fourth ventricle (arrowheads). Marked cerebral (C) hypoplasia is present.

logic dysfunction is generally milder, although Joubert has described a clinical presentation of mental retardation, respiratory rhythm abnormalities, and ataxia.[67] Other anomalies reported in association with Dandy-Walker variant include agenesis of the corpus callosum, holoprosencephaly, and lissencephaly.[66] The frequency of associated anomalies is less than in true Dandy-Walker malformation.

As in Dandy-Walker malformation, this anomaly is best assessed with a sagittal T1WI. The superior vermis and midvermis appear intact and are of normal signal intensity. The inferior vermis is typically absent, and the inferior surface of the remaining vermis appears flattened (Fig. 6–33). The cerebellar hemispheres can appear mildly hypoplastic; however, the adjacent CSF space does not extend laterally to the cerebellar hemispheres as in Dandy-Walker malformation. Except for its inferior aspect, where it communicates with the retrocerebellar cyst (Fig. 6–33), the fourth ventricle appears normal. A normal CFVS pattern was present within the aqueduct and upper fourth ventricle in our series. The retrocerebellar cyst is generally smaller than the cyst of Dandy-Walker malformation, but is larger in most cases than the CSF space found in retrocerebellar arachnoid pouch (giant cisterna magna). The tentorium is also elevated, but to a lesser degree than in Dandy-Walker malformation. A falx cerebelli is present in <10% of patients with Dandy-Walker variant.

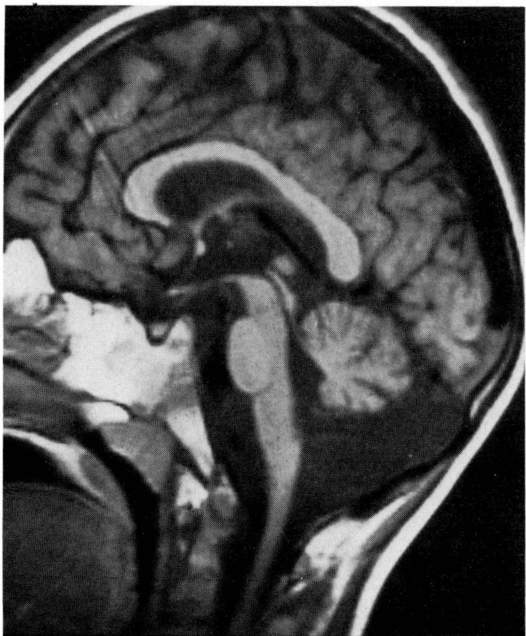

**Figure 6–33. Dandy-Walker variant.** Sagittal T1WI (TR 600 msec/TE 20 msec). There is partial absence of the inferior vermis. The inferior surface of the remaining vermis appears flattened. A posterior fossa CSF collection communicates directly with the lower one third of the fourth ventricle.

### Retrocerebellar Arachnoid Pouch

The retrocerebellar arachnoid pouch (Blake's cyst) is accompanied by a normal fourth ventricle, patent foramina of Luschka and Magendie, a prominent vallecula, and a retrocerebellar CSF collection with evagination of the tela choroidea of the fourth ventricle beneath an intact cerebellar vermis.[68] The literature is unclear as to whether the retrocerebellar arachnoid pouch is the same entity as a giant cisterna magna.[69, 70] Both entities are likely to have a similar appearance on MRI. A retrocerebellar arachnoid pouch is often an incidental observation and can be unassociated with any clinical abnormality. Morphologic anomalies of the brain are seen less frequently in this condition than in Dandy-Walker malformation and Dandy-Walker variant but have been reported to include hydrocephalus, agenesis of the corpus callosum, holoprosencephaly, and encephalocele.[66]

On sagittal T1WI, both the vermis and fourth ventricle appear normal (Fig. 6–34). The prominent vallecula, below the inferior vermis, is best seen in the axial projection. CFVS is normal within the fourth ventricle and in our cases was absent within the retrocerebellar CSF space. The CSF collection may appear to compress, but not to displace, the cerebellar hemispheres. The cerebellum displays normal T1- and T2-relaxation times. The tentorium can be normal or elevated. The tentorium is often bifid posteriorly, and through it the CSF space invaginates superiorly into a bifid posterior falx cerebri (Fig. 6–34). In the axial projection, a septum can be identified in 85% of cases, extending from the posterior surface of the calvarium into the CSF collection. This septum represents the falx cerebelli and its associated vascular structures.

### Arachnoid Cyst

Arachnoid cysts are isolated CSF collections arising as a result of duplication of the

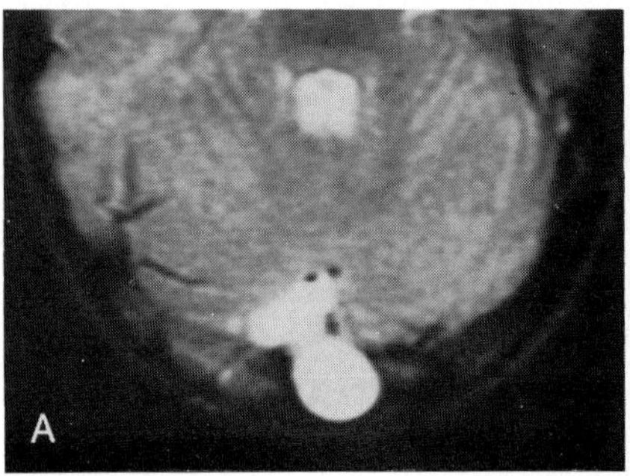


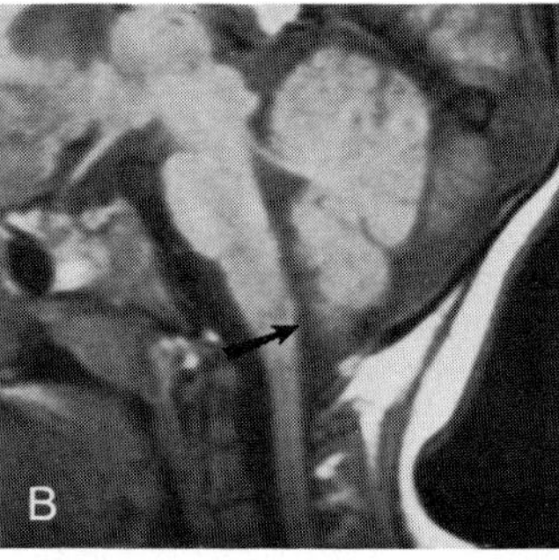


**Figure 6–34. Retrocerebellar arachnoid pouch.** *A,* Axial T2WI (TR 2500 msec/TE 100 msec). The prominent cisterna magna herniates superiorly through a bifid tentorial defect. *B,* Sagittal T1WI (TR 800 msec/TE 20 msec). The vermis is intact. The CSF collection communicates with the lower fourth ventricle in a normal fashion (arrow).

arachnoid membrane. Others speculate that an arachnoid cyst is due to an insult such as trauma, inflammation, or vascular occlusion.[71] Forty percent of arachnoid cysts are infratentorial.[72] In this location, they typically produce signs and symptoms of obstructive hydrocephalus and compression of the brain stem and cerebellum.[71] The patients present clinically with signs of increased intracranial pressure, ataxia, nystagmus, and abnormal gait. Why these cysts increase in size is not clear. Explanations for their growth include limited communication with the subarachnoid space, microtrauma with secondary bleeding, the presence of a semipermeable membrane, and ependyma within the lining of the cyst that produces CSF.[71] Within the posterior fossa, typical locations include posterolateral to the cerebellar hemispheres, the cerebellopontine angle cistern, and adjacent to the fourth ventricle.[72]

MRI is an excellent method for delineating the location, extent, and size of the cyst and in identifying complications of its presence, such as mass effect or obstruction of the fourth ventricle. Axial, coronal, and sagittal sections are often necessary to adequately examine the lesion and differentiate it from other posterior fossa CSF collections. In most cases, the fluid within the cyst parallels the signal characteristics of cerebrospinal fluid. Hemorrhage into the arachnoid cyst can alter both T1 and T2 signal characteristics, depending on the age of the blood. An increase in the protein content of the cyst could potentially alter the T1 and T2 relaxation as well. The inner surface of the cyst is smooth without evidence of mass. The adjacent brain may be displaced or indented but displays normal signal characteristics.[73] A loss of the normal architecture of the gray and white matter surrounding the cyst, marked irregularity of the margins of the cyst, or increased signal from the surrounding brain on a T2WI should suggest porencephaly, encephalomalacia secondary to a previous insult, or tumor.[73, 74]

An arachnoid cyst posterior to the cerebellar hemispheres can be difficult to differentiate from Dandy-Walker malformation, Dandy-Walker variant, or retrocerebellar pouch. In arachnoid cyst, unlike Dandy-Walker malformation and Dandy-Walker variant, the vermis remains complete, and there is no apparent communication between the cyst and the fourth ventricle. In arachnoid cyst, the CSF collection is usually eccentrically located and produces more lateral mass effect, especially on the CP angle cisterns. A falx cerebelli, if present, may be displaced by the cystic mass.

The remaining 60% of arachnoid cysts are supratentorial in location. Typical sites include the middle cranial fossa (Fig. 6–35), the suprasellar cistern, the cerebral convexity, the quadrigeminal plate cistern, and the interhemispheric fissure. The features and appearances of arachnoid cysts in these locations are generally similar to the infratentorial lesions. Even with MRI, some difficulty can arise in separating an arachnoid cyst from supratentorial cystic tumors or cystic porencephaly. Irregularity of the wall of the cyst, alteration in T1 and T2 values from typical CSF, the presence of a mass, or an abnormality in signal of the surrounding brain should suggest a diagnosis other than supratentorial arachnoid cyst.[73, 74]

## CRANIOCERVICAL JUNCTION

MRI has become the examination of choice for the evaluation of congenital anomalies of the cervical spine and craniocervical junc-

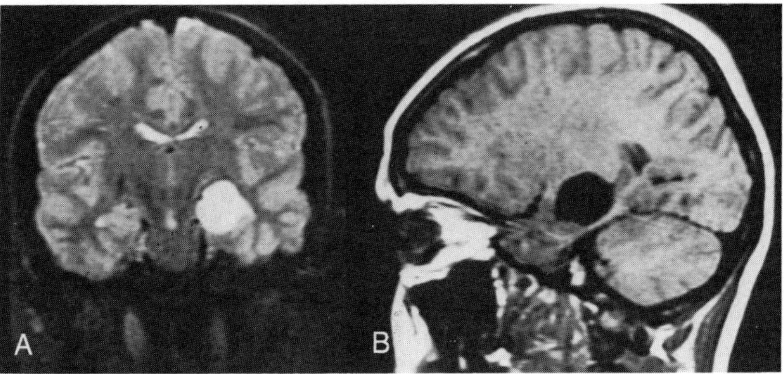


**Figure 6–35. Arachnoid cyst.** *A,* Coronal T2WI (TR 2000 msec/TE 100 msec). Well-demarcated cystic mass in the medial aspect of the left middle cranial fossa. The surrounding brain demonstrates normal signal characteristics. *B,* Sagittal T1WI (TR 600 msec/TE 20 msec). The long T1 relaxation time of the cyst is compatible with CSF.

tion, replacing both CT and CT myelography in most instances.[75, 76] A variety of malformations can affect the craniocervical junction and cervical spine in children. The Chiari I malformation is an anomaly of renewed interest, consisting of tonsillar herniation, compression of the medullocervical junction, syringobulbia (rarely), and syringohydromyelia in 50% of patients.[77] The clinical presentation is that of cerebellar dysfunction, including an unsteady gait, a peculiar downbeat nystagmus, pain, altered sensation, and sleep apnea. Signs of cord dysfunction such as spasticity, bulbar palsy, and weakness of the extremities are due to the presence of a syringomyelia or craniocervical compression. The frequency of hydrocephalus has been reported to be as high as 44% and likely is secondary to fourth ventricular outlet obstruction.[77] Basilar invagination, kinking of the medullocervical junction, and compression of the upper cervical cord may be present.[78-80] An important feature is that of herniation of the cerebellar tonsils into the upper cervical canal, commonly to the level of C1-C2 (Fig. 6–36). Barkovich and associates, in a review of 25 patients with the diagnosis of Chiari I malformation, noted that the mean position of the herniated tonsillar tissue was 13 mm below foramen magnum, with a range from 3 to 29 mm.[81] In a normal control group, the mean position for the tonsils was 1 mm below foramen magnum, with a range of 5 to 8 mm. Based on their findings, herniation of tonsillar tissue less than 2 mm is probably of no clinical significance. The herniated tonsillar tissue is not usually fused in the midline, and although they can maintain their rounded inferior margins, the tonsils tend to become inferiorly pointed or peg shaped. Asymmetric tonsillar herniation is common. The dysmorphic features of the tonsillar tissue and the extent of inferior herniation are best appreciated on a sagittal or coronal T1WI.[78, 79] The cisterna magna is frequently small or not visualized. Contraction of the subarachnoid space at the craniocervical junction suggests arachnoidal scarring or thickening at the foramen magnum, the upper cervical canal, or both (Fig. 6–37). These changes can be readily appreciated using the myelographic effect of a T2WI or a T2 gradient acquisition sequence. Since both the CSF and herniated tonsillar tissue increase in signal on T2WI, the herniated tonsillar tissue could go unrecognized on this sequence (Fig. 6–37).[79] Inferior displacement of the fourth ventricle is seen on oc-

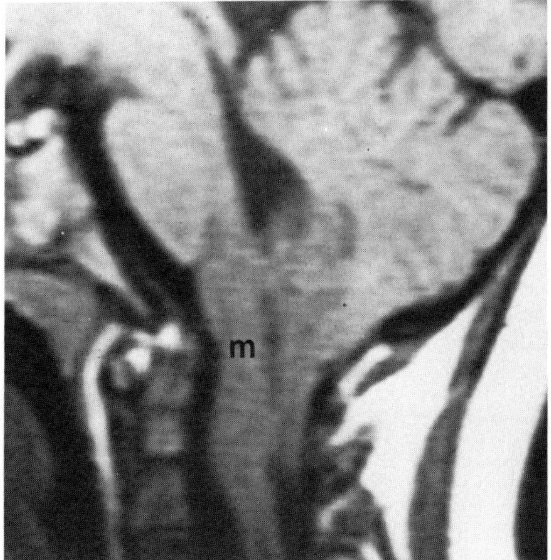


**Figure 6–36. Chiari I malformation.** Sagittal T1WI (TR 600 msec/TE 20 msec). Downward displacement of cerebellar tonsils to C2. The lower fourth ventricle and cisterna magna are compressed. The medulla is very minimally displaced inferiorly (m).

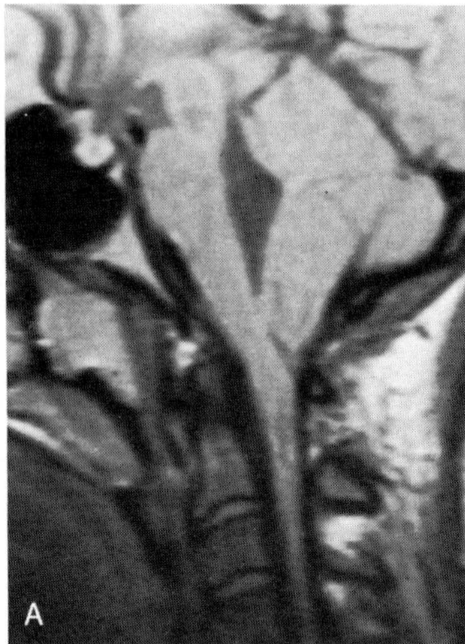


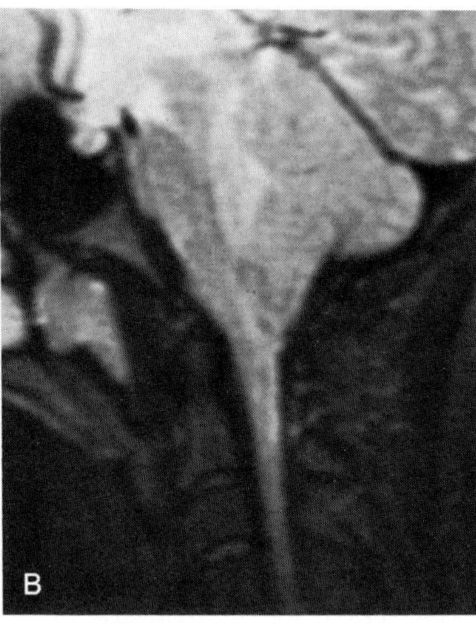


**Figure 6–37. Chiari I malformation.** *A,* Sagittal N(H)WI (TR 2000 msec/TE 20 msec), and *B,* Sagittal T2WI (TR 2000 msec/TE 80 msec). Herniation of peg-shaped tonsillar tissue is seen best on the N(H)WI. The myelographic effect of the T2WI shows contraction of the subarachnoid space at the foramen magnum and within the cisterna magna.

casion. With obstruction of the fourth ventricle, the CFVS within the fourth ventricle may be increased. On sagittal MRI, anterior kinking of the inferior medulla and upper cervical cord is well appreciated (Fig. 6–38). Kinking or compression may increase with flexion of the neck (Fig. 6–39) or in the presence of syringomyelia, basilar invagination, or hydrocephalus.[78, 79]

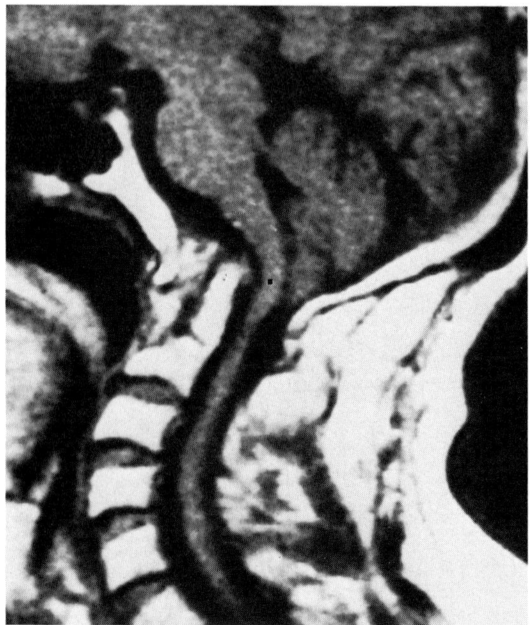

**Figure 6–38. Chiari I malformation.** Sagittal T1WI (TR 400 msec/TE 20/msec). Mild basilar invagination accentuates anterior kinking of the medullocervical junction. (Courtesy of S. J. Pomeranz, M.D., The Christ Hospital, Cincinnati, Ohio.)

Syringohydromyelia, syringobulbia, or both may involve the lower medulla and cervical cord (Fig. 6–40). Syringomyelia is reported to occur in 50% of patients with Chiari I malformation; however, improved recognition of this disorder with MRI will likely prove this figure to be higher.[82] The differentiation of syringomyelia from hydromyelia is generally not possible with MRI. Both T1WI, N(H)WI, and T2WI are necessary for complete analysis. With both syringomyelia and syringobulbia, the fluid within the cyst has signal characteristics similar to that of CSF.[78, 79] With T2 weighting, areas of CFVS are frequently seen within the cyst. In addition, increased signal may emanate from the cervical cord adjacent to the cyst cavity, representing gliosis within the cord. The overall width of the cord may be increased, normal, or decreased in the presence of a syrinx. The upper cervical canal may be widened in the presence of a larger syringohydromyelia.

MRI is equally valuable in evaluating other anomalies of the craniocervical junction in children. Craniocervical instability can be manifest in patients with an os odontoideum and assimilation, trisomy 21, spondyloepiphyseal dysplasia, basilar impression, and in the mucopolysaccharidoses.[82, 83] Dysfunction is often due to cord compression by a small foramen magnum or from subluxation and instability at the atlanto-occipital or the atlantoaxial level. Imaging in both flexion and extension should be performed to evaluate the dynamics of the compression (Fig. 6–41). In small infants,

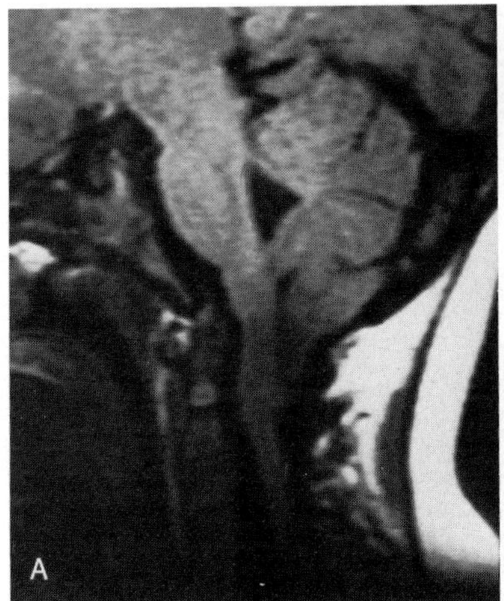


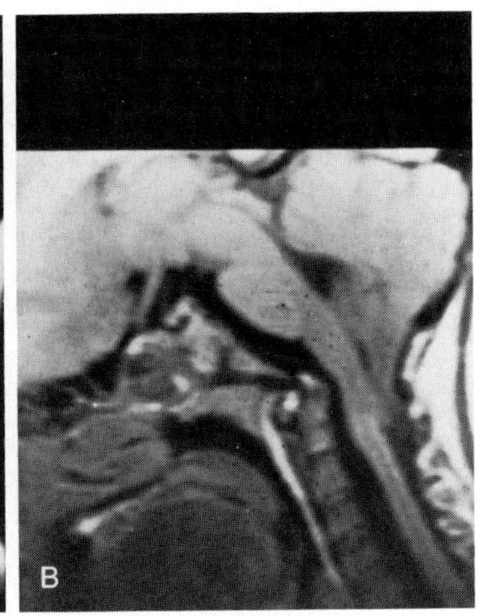


**Figure 6–39. Chiari I malformation.** *A,* Neutral sagittal T1WI (TR 600 msec/TE 20 msec) demonstrates typical tonsillar herniation to C2. *B,* Flexion sagittal T1WI (TR 600 msec/TE 20 msec). There is mild accentuation of the kinking and anterior compression of the medullocervical junction in flexion.

flexion and extension views are easily performed in the standard head coil. In older patients, similar views are best performed with a tandem pair of surface coils placed laterally, since flexion and extension views are often unsatisfactory with posteriorly placed surface coils.

The main limitation of MRI in the evaluation of the craniocervical junction is its inability to adequately image the bony architecture. For this reason, conventional or computed tomography remains an essential part of the evaluation. On MRI a small foramen magnum is suggested only by the amount of deformity, compression, or atrophy present at the cervicomedullary junction.

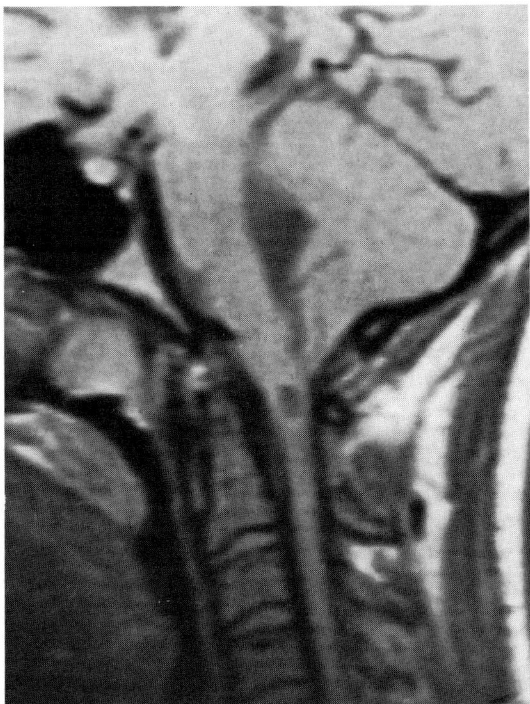

**Figure 6–40. Chiari I malformation.** Sagittal N(H)WI (TR 2000 msec/TE 20 msec). A focal syrinx is present at the craniocervical junction. Mild tonsillar herniation is present.

## NEUROCUTANEOUS SYNDROMES

The neurocutaneous syndrome comprises a group of disorders represented by abnormal proliferation of both mesenchymal and neuroectodermal tissue. The most characteristic manifestation is the development of hamartomas throughout the body. Included within this group are neurofibromatosis (von Recklinghausen's disease), tuberous sclerosis (Bourneville's disease), angiomatosis retini (von Hippel-Lindau disease), encephalotrigeminal angiomatosis (Sturge-Weber syndrome), and ataxia telangiectasia (Louis-Bar syndrome). Central nervous system disease is common in the neurocutaneous disorders. In only two of these disorders, tuberous sclerosis and Sturge-Weber syndrome, are the CT findings diagnostic. Recent evidence suggests that MRI may be a more sensitive means of identifying neurofibromatosis and the early changes of Sturge-Weber syndrome.[84-86] Questions still remain as to whether MRI is more sensitive than CT in the detection of tuberous sclerosis.[87]

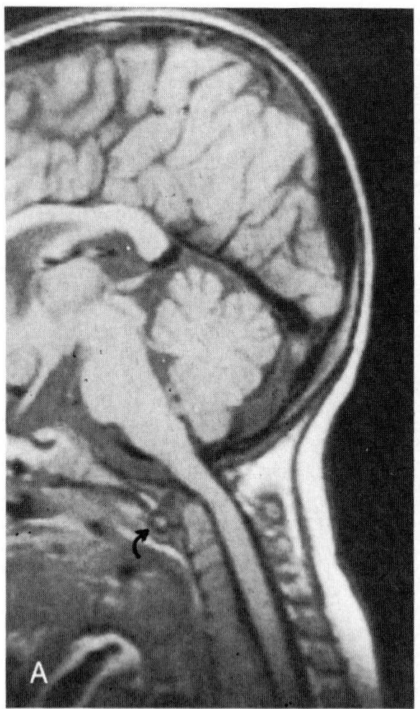


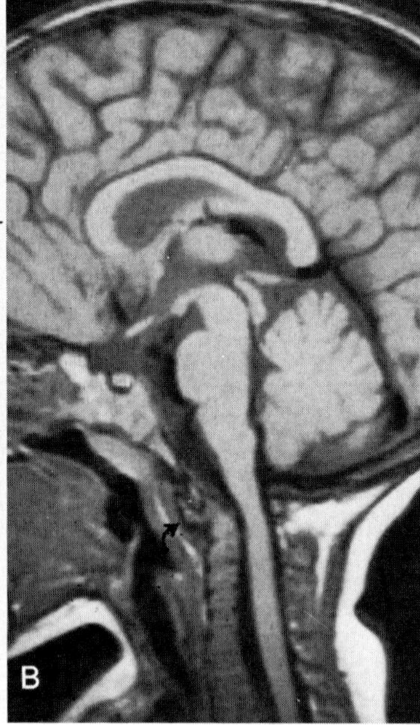


**Figure 6–41. Hurler's syndrome.** Sagittal T1WI (TR 1000 msec/TE 20 msec) in *A*, flexion, and *B*, neutral. The medullocervical junction is compressed by a tight foramen magnum. Compression and kinking of the cord is minimally accentuated in flexion. Note subtle anterior subluxation of C1 in flexion (arrows).

## Neurofibromatosis

Neurofibromatosis is an autosomal dominant disease with a high penetrance and is estimated to occur in 1 in 3000 live births.[88] Typical clinical features include subcutaneous hamartomas, café au lait spots, mental retardation, hypertension, and a propensity to develop tumors of the central nervous system.

Currently, neurofibromatosis has been divided into two specific patterns of presentation.[89] In peripheral, or von Recklinghausen's, neurofibromatosis (VRNF), manifestations include café au lait patches greater than 15 mm in diameter, dermal and peripheral nerve neurofibromas, plexiform neurofibromas, defects in the posterior orbital wall, pseudoarthroses of the tibia, kyphoscoliosis, and optic or chiasmatic gliomas. On the other hand, central or bilateral acoustic neurofibromatosis (BANF), is manifested by the presence of bilateral acoustic neuromas, neurofibromas of the spine roots, meningiomas, and gliomas. In BANF, dermal neurofibromas and café au lait spots are usually absent. Chromosomal analysis in BANF has revealed a deletion of genetic markers on chromosome 22.

Numerous manifestations within the CNS have been well documented in neurofibromatosis and include the development of intracranial tumors (benign and malignant), structural defects of the bony calvarium, arachnoid cyst, and vasculitis (moya moya disease).[90] Within the pediatric population, the most common intracranial neoplasm in neurofibromatosis is optic nerve glioma. This slowly progressive tumor may involve one or both optic nerves, the optic chiasm, or any portion of the optic tract. Schwannomas involving the acoustic nerve are not uncommon and are often bilateral. Meningomas, gliomas, ependymomas, oligodendrogliomas, and neurofibrosarcomas have all been reported in neurofibromatosis.[91] The appearance of these tumors on MRI are described elsewhere in this text.

Dysplasia of the sphenoid bone often occurs in neurofibromatosis. In its most severe form, there is absence of the greater wing of the sphenoid bone. Herniation of the temporal lobe or subarachnoid space into the back of the orbit results in a pulsating exophthalmos. Vascular involvement in neurofibromatosis is not infrequent. Fibromuscular disease commonly involves medium-sized vessels such as the renal and carotid arteries and can result in chronic occlusion at the carotid terminus with collateral flow through lenticulostriate and other small vessels.[92]

Multiplanar MRI has improved detection of structural defects of the calvarium, tu-

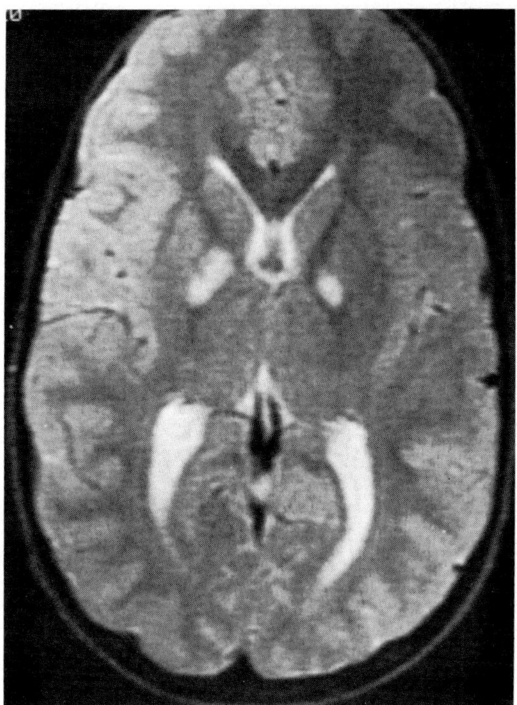

**Figure 6–42. Neurofibromatosis.** Axial T2WI (TR 2000 msec/TE 80 msec). Multiple focal areas of increased signal intensity are identified in the region of the internal capsule and globus pallidus.

mors, arachnoid cysts, and the early and late changes of vasculitis. There is growing evidence suggesting that MRI may be more sensitive than CT in the detection of parenchymal changes and suspected intracranial hamartomas in neurofibromatosis.[84] Recent reports have revealed multiple areas of increased signal on T2WI in patients not exhibiting clinical neurologic dysfunction.[84, 85] Common areas of involvement include the basal ganglia, posterior limb and genu of the internal capsule (Fig. 6–42), external capsule, corpus callosum (Fig. 6–43), thalami, cerebellar peduncles, and brain stem. The areas of increased signal are well demarcated from surrounding brain tissue and demonstrate a lack of mass effect or surrounding edema. On T1WI, they appear isointense to gray matter. At the present time, pathologic correlation is lacking; however, the possible etiologies include changes secondary to microangiopathic vasculitis, hamartoma formation, or focal demyelinization. Such areas are differentiated from neoplastic involvement by the lack of mass effect, surrounding edema, and clinical manifestations.

## Tuberous Sclerosis

The second most common of the phakomatoses is tuberous sclerosis. The classic clinical triad consists of adenoma sebaceum (75%), seizures (80%), and mental retardation (80%). Other manifestations are rhabdomyomas of the interventricular septum, renal angiomyolipomas, fibromuscular vascular disease, and hypopigmented patches, or nevi. The CT features of subependymal calcifications and cortical hamartomatous

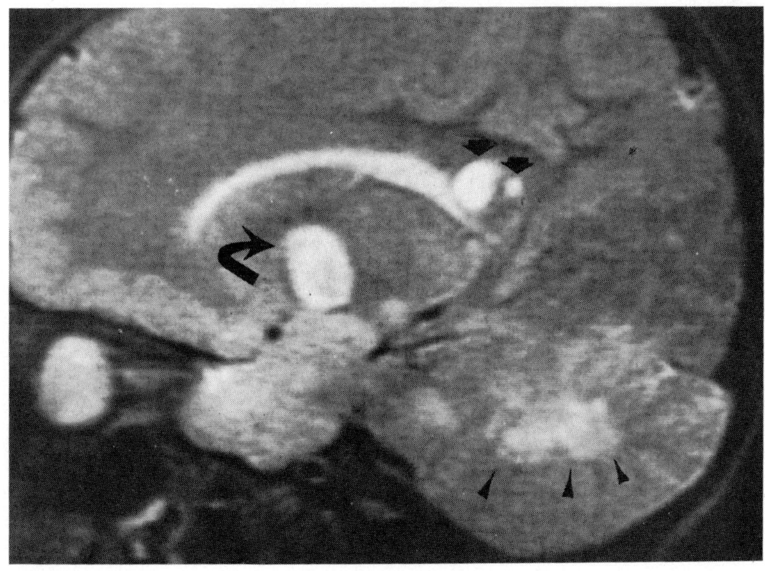

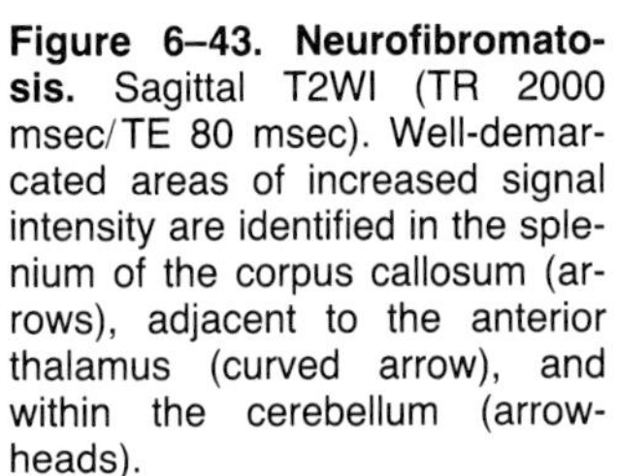

**Figure 6–43. Neurofibromatosis.** Sagittal T2WI (TR 2000 msec/TE 80 msec). Well-demarcated areas of increased signal intensity are identified in the splenium of the corpus callosum (arrows), adjacent to the anterior thalamus (curved arrow), and within the cerebellum (arrowheads).

hypodensities are considered pathognomonic for this disorder. Central nervous system involvement includes benign and malignant neoplastic processes, abnormal myelinization, and secondary changes from vasculitis. Multiple neoplasms occurring in tuberous sclerosis include benign hamartomas of the cortex, giant cell astrocytoma, ependymoma, and meningioma.

Hamartomatous involvement of the cortex and abnormalities of myelinization are readily identified on MRI in tuberous sclerosis.[87] Hamartomas are bright on T2WI, well demarcated from surrounding normal brain, and produce no mass effect or surrounding edema (Fig. 6–44). A more extensive pattern of increased signal emanating from the white matter suggests the presence of abnormal myelinization (Fig. 6–45). The classic subependymal calcified tubers are difficult to identify on MRI, and only large calcified tubers produce a signal void. Smaller calcified tubers are often isointense and go undetected. Because of its inability to consistently identify the subependymal calcifications, MRI has not replaced CT as a more sensitive examination in the diagnosis of tuberous sclerosis even though peripheral hamartomas are seen better with MRI. Detection of subependymal calcification can be improved with the use of gradient acquisition techniques (Fig. 6–46).

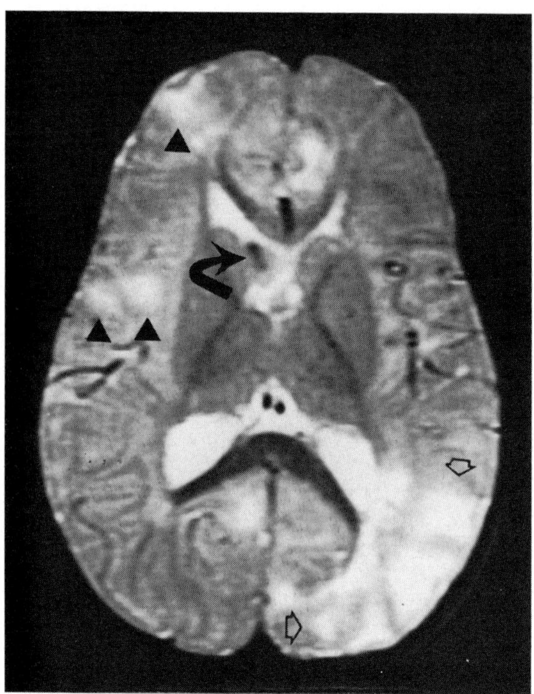

**Figure 6–45. Tuberous sclerosis.** Axial T2WI (TR 2500 msec/TE 80 msec). Multiple cortical areas of increased signal are compatible with hamartomas (arrowheads). Diffuse pattern of increased signal from white matter and gray matter in patient's left cerebral hemisphere (to reader's right) represents abnormal myelinization and hamartomas (open arrows). Absent signal at foramen of Monro identifies a subependymal calcification (curved arrow).

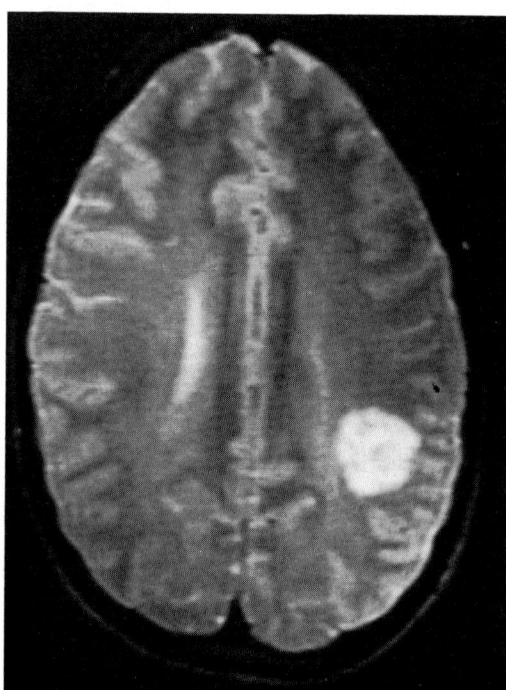

**Figure 6–44. Tuberous sclerosis.** Axial T2WI (TR 2500 msec/TE 80 msec). A hamartoma is identified in the patient's posterior left parietal lobe (to reader's right) as a well-demarcated area of increased signal without surrounding edema.

### Sturge-Weber Syndrome

Sturge-Weber syndrome consists of venous angiomas of the leptomeninges and ipsilateral cutaneous nevi, most commonly in the distribution of the ophthalmic division of the fifth nerve. Patients present clinically with mental retardation and intractable seizures, and they may develop hemiparesis. CT reveals enhancement of the leptomeningeal venous angioma, ipsilateral cerebral atrophy, and tramlike, or amorphous, calcifications within the cerebral cortex. Contralateral brain involvement is not uncommon.

MRI has similar sensitivity to CT in the detection of hemiatrophy, leptomeningeal

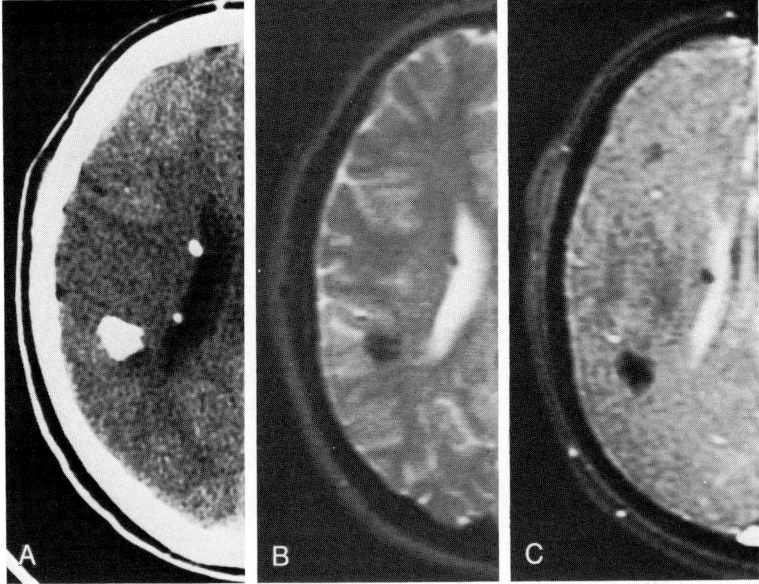

**Figure 6–46. Tuberous sclerosis.** *A,* Typical cortical and subependymal calcifications identified on unenhanced CT. *B,* Axial T2WI (TR 2500 msec/TE 80 msec). Areas of signal void demonstrate calcifications. Note calcium not well demonstrated on long TR-T2WI. *C,* Axial GRASS T2* (TR 24 msec/TE 13 msec/ϕ = 10°). Calcification more clearly defined owing to magnetic susceptibility.

angiomatosis, and angiomatous involvement of the ipsilateral choroid plexus (Fig. 6–47);[86, 93] however, it appears less sensitive in detecting the subcortical calcification. On T1WI, the vessels within the leptomeningeal angiomatosis appear bright and also as signal void, depending on their rate of flow. Stimac and colleagues have recently reported on angiomatous malformations within the choroid plexus as seen on MRI.[93] In their series on T2WI, the choroid plexus was enlarged and contained areas of both flow signal void and increased signal.

Recently, Jacoby and associates have reported on the MRI appearance of accelerated myelination in the ipsilateral involved cerebral hemisphere in early Sturge-Weber syndrome.[86] Inversion recovery sequences (TR 2050 msec/TI 500 msec) were used in demonstrating the pattern of myelinization of the cerebral hemispheres. Their observation indicates that the pattern of myelinization in the involved ipsilateral hemisphere is accelerated when compared with the contralateral uninvolved hemisphere. These authors observe that the pattern of accelerated myelination had similarities to the condition of status marmoratus seen following ischemic-hypoxic insult at birth. They speculate that perhaps the hypermyelination may

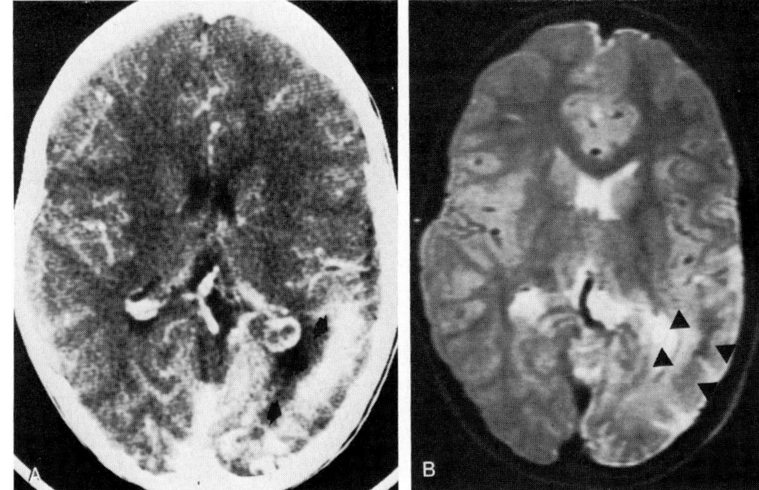

**Figure 6–47. Sturge-Weber syndrome.** *A,* Contrast-enhanced CT demonstrates angiomatous enhancement in patient's left parieto-occipital lobe (arrows; to reader's right). *B,* Axial T2WI (TR 2000 msec/TE 80 msec). Areas of signal void identify cortical calcification (arrowheads). Minimal volume loss of the left posterior hemisphere is present.

be secondary to chronic ischemia secondary to the leptomeningeal angioma.

## CONGENITAL MALFORMATIONS OF THE SPINE

As in the evaluation of congenital malformations of the brain, MRI has demonstrated considerable promise in the evaluation of congenital malformations of the spine.[94] The combination of conventional and CT myelography are currently the standards for evaluation of the spine. The disadvantages of myelography are its invasiveness and the use of ionizing radiation. MRI is a technique that is considered biologically safe, requires no ionizing radiation, is noninvasive, and provides the capability to directly visualize the cord and subarachnoid space in multiple projections. Techniques of sedation and monitoring for MRI of the spine are similar to those used for evaluation of the brain and are outlined in the previous section. Often when using surface coils for the spine, monitoring of a sedated patient is made easier by placing the child in the gantry feet first.

## TECHNICAL CONSIDERATIONS

### Pulse Sequence

Pulse sequences are chosen in order to provide optimum anatomic information in the shortest scanning time. We rely primarily on spin echo (SE) sequences for evaluation of the spine. Inversion recovery (IR) sequences can be used to identify the white and gray matter within the cord. Perhaps in the future such information may be of value in the detection of intrinsic diseases of the cord such as anterior-horn cell disorders. Currently, IR imaging of the spine is severely limited by image noise, decreased slice acquisition, and susceptibility to artifact produced by cardiac motion and intrinsic CSF pulsations.

T1WI SE sequences have distinct advantages for visualizing congenital anomalies of the spine. The combination of superb anatomic resolution, good tissue contrast, and the ability to identify fat as bright signal, are crucial elements in the assessment of spinal anomalies. T2WI are equally important in the evaluation of syringohydromyelia and intramedullary lesions, which often accompany congenital anomalies of the spine. The "myelographic effect" obtained with CSF on a T2WI or T2 gradient acquisition sequence can also be of benefit in identifying elements of a dysraphic defect.

The sagittal projection provides the greatest benefit in the examination of the spine; however, in the lower thoracic and upper lumbar spine, both coronal and sagittal sections are often necessary to identify the conus. We often use the axial projection to visualize the spinal contents in the presence of scoliosis, to evaluate the cord in cross-section, to search for a dermal sinus or tract, and to evaluate dysraphism with associated masses (i.e., lipomas, dermoids) that extend into the pelvis or subcutaneous tissue of the lower back. Visualization of spinal anomalies has significantly advanced with the use of orthagonal imaging of the cord in its long axis resulting in improved identification of the conus and other intrinsic cord anomalies.

An examination is begun with a T1WI localizer in the coronal projection (TR 400 msec/TE 20 msec, matrix 256 × 128, 1 nex), from which sagittal and axial sequences are planned. Additional T1 sequence parameters are chosen to optimize resolution and to reduce noise yet provide scans within a reasonable time (TR 400-600 msec/TE 20-30 msec, matrix 128 × 256, 2-4 nex). At the cost of increasing scan time, further improvement in resolution can be obtained by increasing the matrix size (256 × 256), or the number of excitations (4-6 nex). Routine T1WI are obtained with 5-mm thick sections and a gap of 0.5 to 1 mm. For improved visualization of the cord and subarachnoid space, 3-mm thick sections can be obtained at a 0.5- to 1-mm gap, with contiguous sections (0 gap), or with interleaving (obtaining alternate slices to prevent crosstalk). For T2WI, a slight improvement in resolution is possible by sampling a single, rather than multiple echoes (TR 1800-2000 msec/TE 80 msec, matrix 128 × 256, 2 nex). Our experience has shown that maximal contrast differentiation between the cord, the cauda equina, and the surrounding CSF is obtained at a TR of 1000 msec and a TE of 20 msec (Fig. 6–48). Use of this sequence often eliminates previous difficulties with identification of the conus in the sagittal projection.

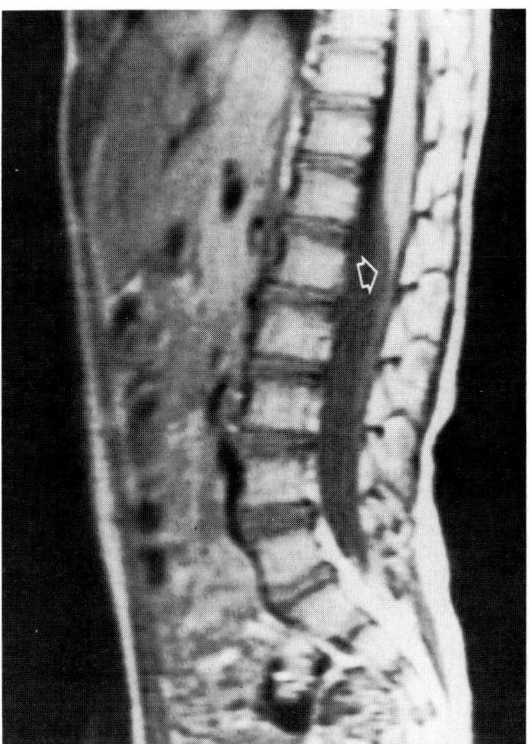

**Figure 6–48. Normal spine.** Sagittal T1WI (TR 1000 msec/TE 20 msec). Improved visualization of the conus (open arrow) with a TR of 1000 msec.

The presence of scoliosis, kyphosis, or both poses an additional problem in imaging the spine with MRI.[95] Difficulties with excessive curvatures can be minimized by attention to patient positioning and by imaging in the axial projection. Oblique imaging in the sagittal or coronal projection offers some improvement in the evaluation of the patient with complex curvatures.

Gating, flow compensation, and saturation (90° presaturation pulsing) are all useful techniques for reducing artifacts secondary to CSF pulsatile motion. They are especially helpful in the thoracic spine, where cardiac motion artifact is a problem. The use of gradient acquisition techniques has also gained in popularity. Such sequences are designed to provide T1WI and T2WI at a significantly reduced scanning time; however, their use is of limited benefit in the pediatric spine. Gradient acquisition images are useful in providing a T2 "myelographic effect" when a longer SE sequence is not feasible. It is also of benefit in obtaining rapid scans when assessing the effect of positional variation (flexion, extension) on the contents of the spinal canal.

### Surface Coils

Quality imaging of the spine is not possible without the use of surface coils. The standard head coil can be used for evaluating most craniocervical junctions and, in small infants, the entire spine. If visualization of the entire spine is necessary, the larger patient is placed on a series of coils to adequately cover the entire area of interest. Each coil can then be "plugged in" as needed to avoid moving a sedated child. To evaluate the craniocervical junction in flexion and extension, we prefer a pair of tandem axial planar coils placed lateral to the cervical spine and craniocervical junction. The advantages of this system design are ease of positional changes (flexion and extension), improved resolution, and artifact reduction.

## SPINAL DYSRAPHISM

The capabilities of MRI include noninvasive screening of the spine in the detection of dysraphic anomalies.[96-98] Spinal dysraphism results from an incomplete closure of the neural canal (neuralation) and deficient separation of neural elements from their surrounding investitures. The process of neuralation begins within the cervical spine and proceeds in both a cranial and caudad direction within the first trimester. The etiology of dysraphic states such as meningocele, myelocele, and myelomeningocele is best explained as a result of incomplete closure of this neural tube. Other lesions such as lipoma, lipomyelomeningocele, and dorsal dermal sinus are a result of incomplete separation and differentiation of the developing neural tube from its surrounding mesodermal and ectodermal elements.

### Spina Bifida Aperta

Spina bifida aperta, or cystica, is the term used to describe a group of dysraphic conditions characterized by the herniation of meninges, or neural elements, or both through a large posterior spinal defect. Meningocele refers to the herniation of meninges and CSF. In myelocele, the herniation consists predominantly of neural elements. The combination of both neural elements and subarachnoid space within the herniation is termed myelomeningocele. The common locations for such defects include the lumbar, lumbosacral, cervical, and thoracic spine, in decreasing order of frequency. In meningocele, the protrusion is usually covered with a full-thickness layer of skin that protects it from injury or leakage of cerebrospinal fluid. In patients with myelocele and myelomeningocele, the skin covering is lacking, thus increasing the risk of infection and leakage of CSF. In these cases, MRI is generally unnecessary before surgical intervention. In spina bifida aperta with an intact skin covering, a T1WI can delineate the extent of the defect, determine its contents, assess the relationship of the cord to the dysraphic defect, and document the presence of intramedullary abnormalities (syringohydromyelia, gliosis). It can also aid in differentiating these lesions from other dysraphic states with posterior masses (lipomyelomeningocele, dermal sinus) and is of benefit in assessing the craniocervical junction for the presence of Chiari II malformation and its complications.[99] Sequences with a short TR provide the greatest contrast differentiation between fat, CSF, and the neural elements. A T2WI is obtained to evaluate for potential intrinsic cord abnormalities such as gliosis, dermoid, epidermoid, or syringohydromyelia.

MRI is an excellent modality for evaluating the postoperative myelomeningocele patient with a progressive neurologic deficit. These deficiences may result from tethering of the cord by scar at the surgical site; from arachnoiditis, syringomyelia, or myelocystocele;[100] or from the development of masses within the cord (epidermoid, glioma). On T1WI, high-signal fat and low-signal fibrous tissue can be identified within the surgical defect. The subarachnoid space is often widened at the level of the bony defect (Fig. 6–49). The cord maintains a low position and often ends in a thin band as it approaches the surgical defect (Fig. 6–50). The signal from the cord is generally isointense but may be increased on T2WI in the presence of gliosis. Terminal dilatation of the central canal may be present and is called myelocystocele; however, a syringomyelia of the distal cord may have a similar appearance on MRI. On T1WI, both are characterized by low signal intensity that on T2WI increases to signal intensity typical of CSF (Fig. 6–51). Associated diastematomyelia can be present in 31% to 46% of patients with meningomyelocele.[101] The lesion may be

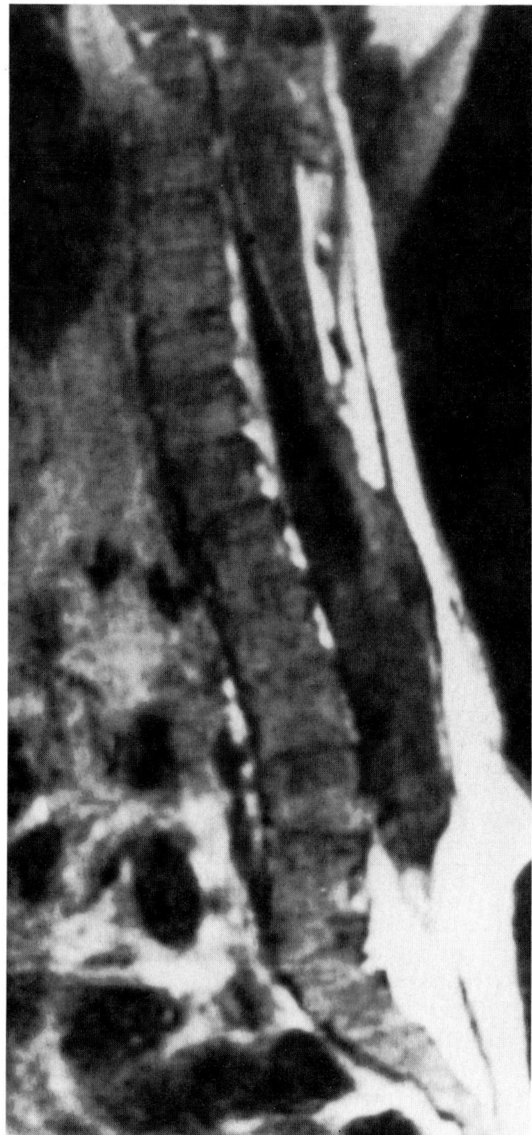

**Figure 6–49. Myelomeningocele, postoperative.** Sagittal T1WI (TR 800 msec/TR 20 msec). There is widening of the spinal cord and thecal sac at the level of the spinal dysraphism. Note the abundant fat about the surgical defect and surrounding the lower sacral thecal sac.

above, at, or below the level of the neural placode and often contributes to neurologic dysfunction. Diastematomyelia is optimally visualized in the coronal, oblique, and axial projections. High signal on a T1WI at the level of the cord, conus, filum terminale, or a diastematomyelia indicates the presence of a lipoma. A decrease in the subarachnoid space around the cord is indicative of arachnoiditis, which may occur following surgical repair (Fig. 6–52).

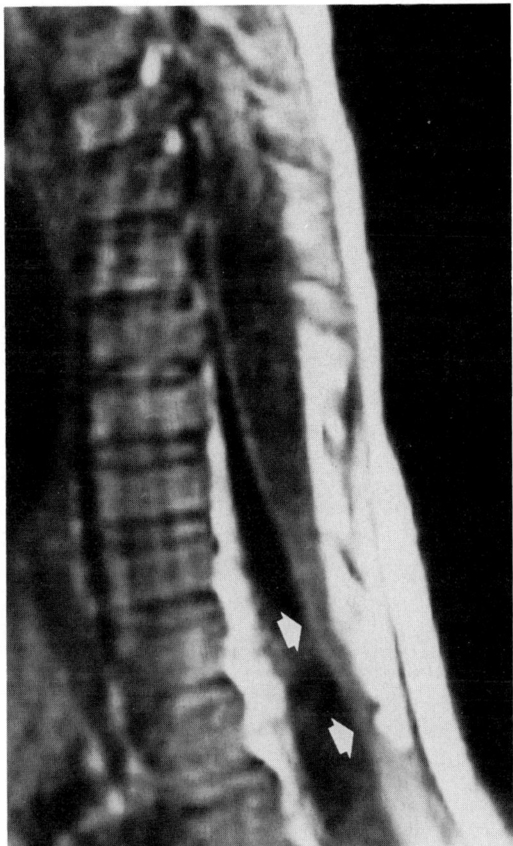

**Figure 6–50. Myelomeningocele, postoperative.** Sagittal T1WI (TR 800 msec/TE 20 msec). The cord is low in position and is tethered to the upper margin of the surgical defect by a thickened filum, or fibrous cord (arrows).

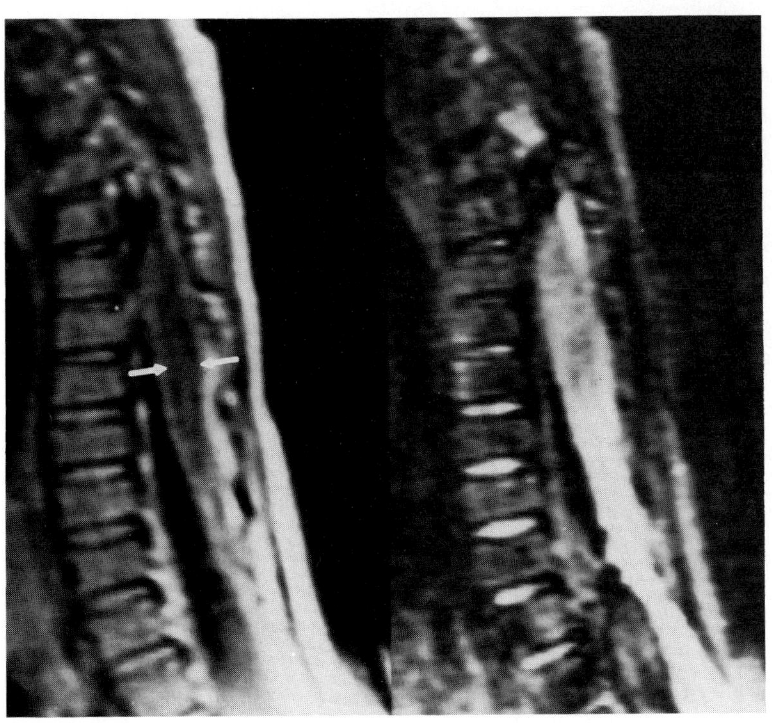

**Figure 6–51. Myelomeningocele, postoperative.** *A,* Sagittal N(H)WI (TR 2000 msec/TE 20 sec), and *B,* T2WI (TR 2000 msec/TE 80 msec). The distal cord is widened. The central canal is dilated (arrows) and hypointense and increases in signal intensity on a T2-weighted image. The presence of minimal pulsation signal void helps identify this as a syringomyelia.

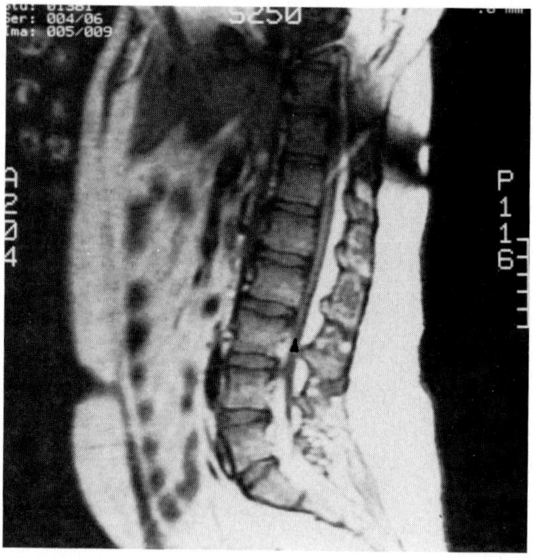


**Figure 6–52. Myelomeningocele, postsurgical arachnoiditis.** Sagittal T1WI (TR 600 msec/TE 20 msec). Marked decrease in the width of the subarachnoid space and a low-positioned cord (arrowhead). High-signal fat fills much of the spinal canal. Diffuse arachnoiditis was confirmed at surgery.

## Diastematomyelia

Sagittal clefting of the cord or filum terminale, often associated with a fibrous or osteocartilaginous partition, is known as diastematomyelia.[102] Diastematomyelia is divided into lesions with a single subarachnoid space and dural covering (group I) (Fig. 6–53) and those having separate arachnoidal and dural sheaths surrounding each hemicord (group II) (Fig. 6–54).[103] In either case, the cord splits into two hemicords that are often asymmetric and are separated by a cleft. Most often, the two hemicords reunite

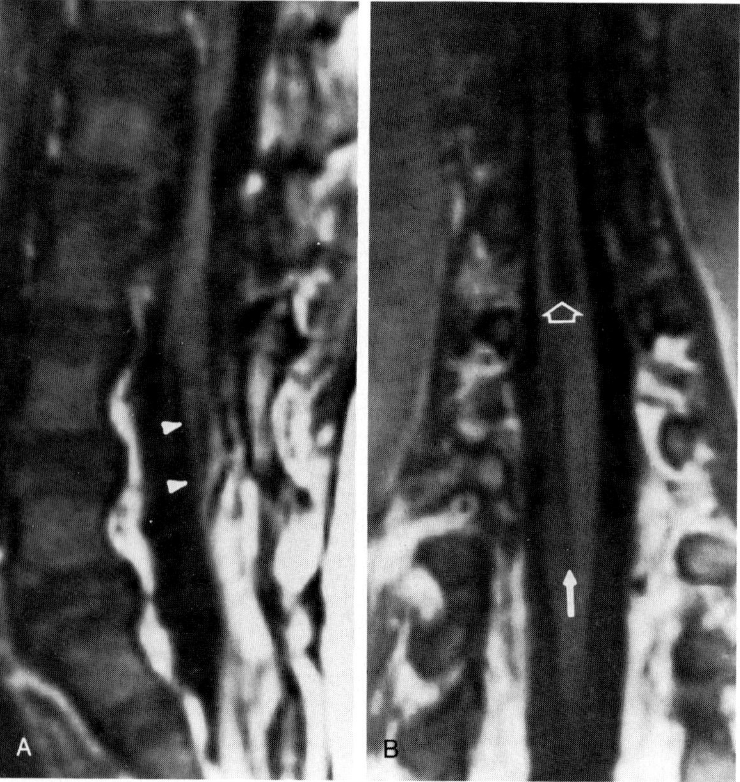


**Figure 6–53. Diastematomyelia.** *A,* Sagittal, and *B,* coronal T1WI (TR 600 msec/TE 20 msec). The cord is low in position and tethered posteriorly by a thickened filum terminale (arrowheads). The cord is split inferiorly (arrow), and a small syrinx is present proximally (open arrow). A single dural covering and subarachnoid space was found at surgery.

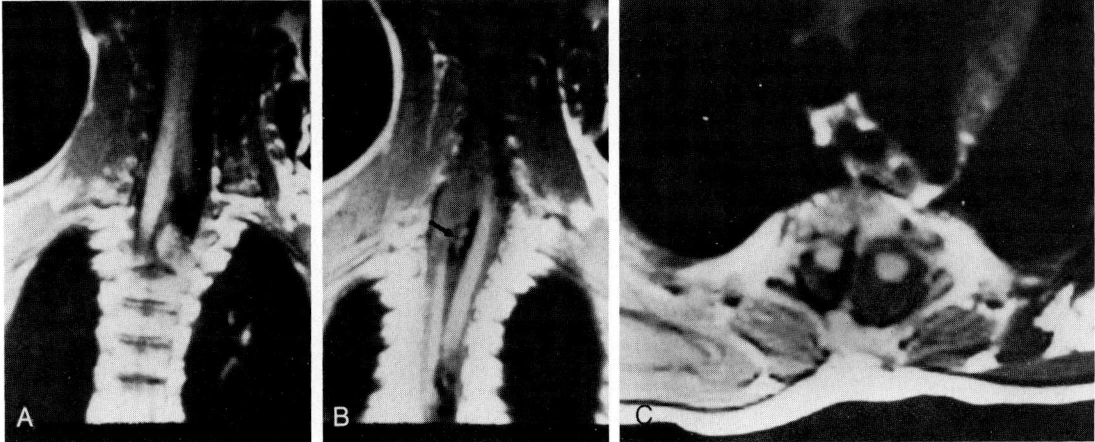


**Figure 6–54. Diastematomyelia.** *A* and *B*, Coronal T1WI (TR 800 msec/TE 20 msec). There is a complete division of the cord, which splits around a central bony spicule containing a small amount of fat (arrow). *C*, Axial T1WI (TR 800 msec/TE 20 msec). Each hemicord is surrounded by its own dural sheath. (Courtesy of A. Chambers, M.D., University Hospital, University of Cincinnati, Cincinnati, Ohio.)

inferiorly into a single structure (91%).[104] The length of splitting is variable, ranging from 2 to 14 vertebral segments. In those cases with a single arachnoid space and dural covering, the presence of a fibrous or osteocartilaginous septum is uncommon. In the presence of separate dural sheaths and subarachnoid spaces, a fibrous or osteocartilaginous septum often bisects the spinal canal and lies within the cleft formed by the two hemicords. The conus medullaris is found below L2 in three fourths of cases.[104] This anomaly is universally associated with focal segmental anomalies of the vertebral bodies and widening of the intrapedicular distance. The lesion may involve any level but is most common from the lower thoracic spine to the sacrum. Less common sites of involvement are the upper thoracic and the cervical spine. Associated anomalies include a thickened filum terminale, tethered cord, lipoma, epidermoid, dermoid cyst, aberrant dorsal nerve roots that often tether, and syringohydromyelia.[102]

The pathologic anatomy of diastematomyelia is best appreciated in the coronal and axial projections. In the presence of severe scoliosis and kyphosis, imaging is best accomplished in the coronal oblique or axial projection. On T1WI axial sections, the two hemicords are isointense and are surrounded by the hypointense CSF. Areas of bright signal may indicate the presence of a lipoma at the diastematomyelia, conus, or filum terminale. The axial projection is also best for documenting a thickened filum terminale (greater than 2 mm), which suggests tethering as well. The presence of a separate dural sheath around each hemicord is visualized in the axial projection as a horizontal figure eight with each circle representing the separate subarachnoid space (Fig. 6–54C). Han and co-workers reported limited success in identifying a fibrous or osteocartilaginous septum dividing the canal on MRI.[105] On T1WI, they were able to identify large bony spicules containing fatty marrow. Differentiation between a small bony spicule, a fibrocartilaginous septum, and normal extramedullary structures was not possible in their series. For this reason, computed tomography remains the modality of choice to delineate the bony changes before surgical intervention. With MRI, the remainder of the spinal canal can be surveyed for associated pathology such as a second diastematomyelia or a thickened filum terminale.

### Lipomyeloschisis

Lipomyeloschisis represents a group of disorders that have in common abnormalities of the cord and lipomatous masses within the spinal canal or dorsal subcutaneous tissue. Two common forms of myeloschisis are lipoma and lipomyelomeningocele.[106] Lipomas can occur at any level within the spine and can be either intradural or extradural.[103] Lipomas are readily identified on MRI and often appear in association with diastematomyelia, spina bifida aperta (cystica), dorsal dermal sinus, split notocord syndrome, tethered cord syndrome, and lipomyelomeningoceles. Isolated intradural lipomas occur with frequency at the level of the conus medullaris or filum terminale or are attached to the dorsal surface of the thoracic or cervical cord. In this situation, an extradural lipoma is usually not present; however, tethering of the cord by the lipoma to the dural surface can occur (Fig. 6–55).

Intradural and extradural lipomas are identified in more complex anomalies such as lipomyelomeningocele. In lipomyelomeningocele, the lipoma is often associated with a focal spina bifida aperta, a low-lying cord tethered by the lipoma, and an extradural fibrolipomatous mass that herniates through the spina bifida to form a dorsal subcutaneous mass covered by a thick layer of skin. Naidich and colleagues point to the fact that although variations exist, all lipomyelomeningoceles represent variations of this archetype.[106]

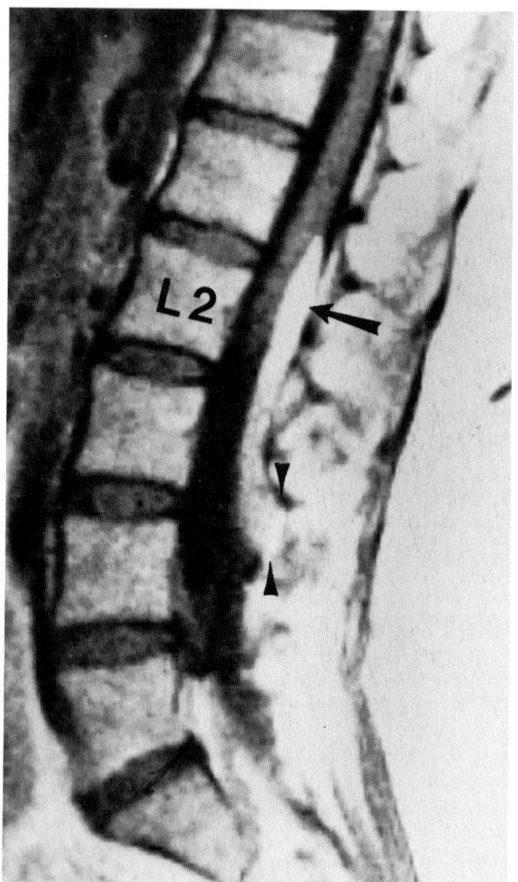


**Figure 6–55. Lipomyeloschisis.** Sagittal T1WI (TR 400 msec/TE 25 msec). The conus is normal at L2. An intradural lipoma (arrow) attaches to the distal conus and tethers the conus to an extradural lipoma posteriorly (arrowheads). (Courtesy of J. A. Tobias, M.D., Mount Sinai Hospital, Miami Beach, Fla., and S. J. Pomeranz, M.D., The Christ Hospital, Cincinnati, Ohio.)

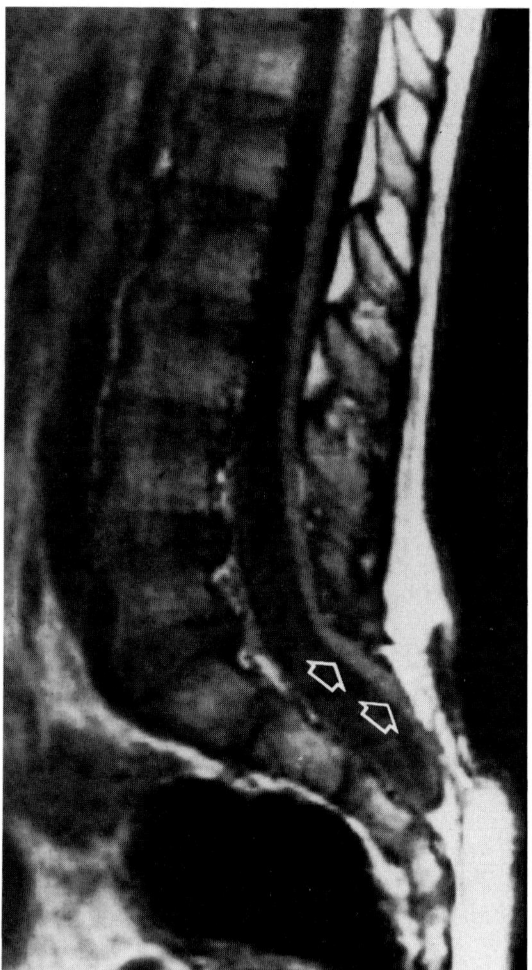

**Figure 6–56. Lipomyelomeningocele.** Sagittal T1WI (TR 800 msec/TE 20 msec). The cord is elongated and tethered posteriorly by a subcutaneous lipoma (open arrows). Note the widening of sacral subarachnoid space, which terminates posteriorly as a small meningocele.

The cord and conus are universally low in position (Fig. 6–56). The distal cord is open dorsally to form a neural placode, which is intimately related to the extradural lipoma. The lipomatous mass may extend cephalad to lie intradurally and attach to the cord at the level of the dorsal cleft. The lipoma may even extend into the central canal of the cord. The extent of the extradural lipoma is readily delineated on MRI. The subarachnoid space ventral to the placode is often widened and may actually appear to lift the placode and lipoma through the dysraphic defect and to form a meningocele (see Fig. 6–54). The dorsal surface of the meningocele is often bent at its cephalad margin by a prominent fibrovascular band. This fibrovascular band, according to Naidich and co-workers, may be the site of additional tethering.[106] The dorsal kinking of the subarachnoid space and cord is best identified in the sagittal projection and can be evaluated on both T1WI and T2WI. The neural placode is often seen as a plate of moderate signal intensity lying ventral to the bright signal of the extradural lipoma.

### Miscellaneous Spinal Dysraphism

Other dysraphic states can also be diagnosed by MRI. The primary tethered cord syndrome is manifest by a low-lying cord and thickened filum terminale without lipoma.[97, 106] Clinically, there is lower extremity weakness, gait disturbances, orthopedic deformities involving the lower extremities, and bladder or bowel dysfunction. Skin manifestations may be present, but are often unimpressive and include a dimple, angioma, or hypertrichosis. Lipomatous dorsal masses are rare. A spina bifida cystica is not present. The cord descends to a low position (< L3) with thickening of the filum terminale greater than 2 mm.[105] Thickening of the filum is best assessed in the axial projection utilizing 3 mm thin sections. The subarachnoid space in the lumbar canal may be normal or widened, and intradural lipomas of the conus of filum are uncommon. The cord is normal in signal intensity on both T1WI and T2WI.

Spinal dysraphism and a tethered cord are both manifestations of the dorsal dermal sinus. This condition includes a dorsal sinus tract that often connects the skin surface to neural tissue. The sinus tract may or may not be patent and can communicate with a dorsal dermoid cyst. If complete, the sinus tract will penetrate the dura and will connect with the dorsal surface of the lower cord, conus, or filum terminale, in which case the cord is tethered at this attachment. An intradural dermoid or epidermoid can rarely complicate this disorder. On MRI, the course of the dorsal dermal sinus is often identified as extending from the subcutaneous tissue to its intradural component, where it tethers the posterior cord (Fig. 6–57). The cord is often low and of normal signal intensity on both T1WI andT2WI. On T1WI, the dermal sinus itself is of low signal intensity but may contain high-signal fat.

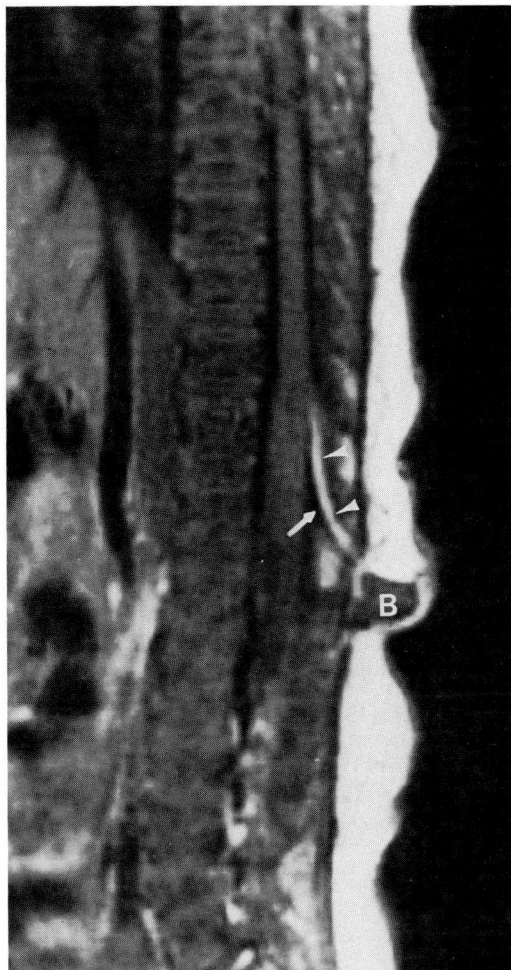


**Figure 6–57. Dorsal dermal sinus.** Sagittal T1WI (TR 400 msec/TE 20 msec). A lipoma (arrowheads) and a dorsal dermal sinus (arrow) extend from the subcutaneous tissue above an extra bony element (B) to perforate the dural space, where they attach to and tether the lower cord.

Malformations of the cord can also accompany the caudal regression syndrome.[107] Caudal regression is most commonly found in infants of diabetic mothers. The regression may be mild, with partial absence of the sacrum, or severe, with complete absence of the sacrum, lumbar spine, or lower thoracic spine (Fig. 6–58). The cord is often hypoplastic and shortened and may end

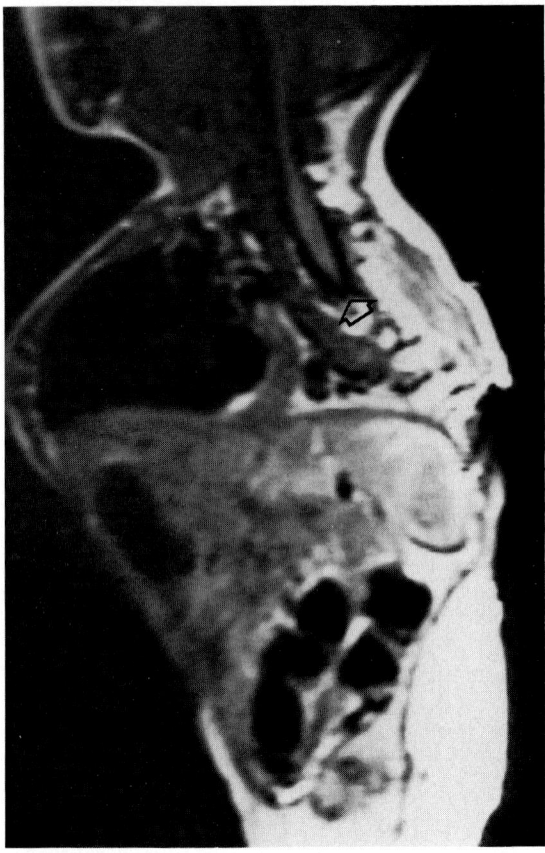

**Figure 6–58. Caudal regression syndrome.** Sagittal T1WI (TR 400 msec/TE 20 msec). Complete absence of the sacrum, lumbar spine, and lower half of the thoracic spine. The tip of the cord is well identified (open arrow) before surgical intervention.

with a bulbous glial tip. Tethering of the cord by a thickened filum terminale is not uncommon. Progressive neurologic dysfunction involving bladder and bowel control may result from tethering, syringomyelia, or an epidermoid. Because of scoliosis and kyphosis, evaluation is often best accomplished in the axial projection. MRI can eliminate the need of a technically difficult myelogram before orthopedic spinal surgery or when progressive neurologic dysfunction is present.

## SYRINGOHYDROMYELIA

Syringohydromyelia is defined as cystic cavitation of the cord, which may be congenital, may result from trauma or inflammation, or may be associated with intramedullary tumors, such as astrocytoma and ependymoma. Hydromyelia specifically refers to the cystic enlargement of the central canal of the cord, whereas syringomyelia is believed to be eccentric cavitation. In reality, there is considerable overlap, both pathologically and radiographically, between the two conditions. Even on MRI, distinction between these two entities is often not possible.[110] We will therefore refer to these two entities collectively as syringomyelia.

Syringomyelia can be associated with many congenital anomalies of the spine, including (1) Chiari I and II malformations, (2) myelomeningocele, (3) lipomyelomeningocele, (4) diastematomyelia, and (5) rarely, caudal regression syndrome. Involvement of the medulla is termed syringobulbia and is most commonly found in association with the Chiari I malformation.[111] Syringomyelia may involve a portion or all of the spinal cord. Anatomically, syringomyelia may vary in appearance from a unilocular longitudinal cavity (Fig. 6–59) to multiple cystlike cavities with the appearance of a string of beads (Fig. 6–60). Williams[112] and Gardner[113] divided syringomyelia into two types. In communicating syringomyelia, the syrinx cavity communicates directly with the subarachnoid space at the craniocervical junction

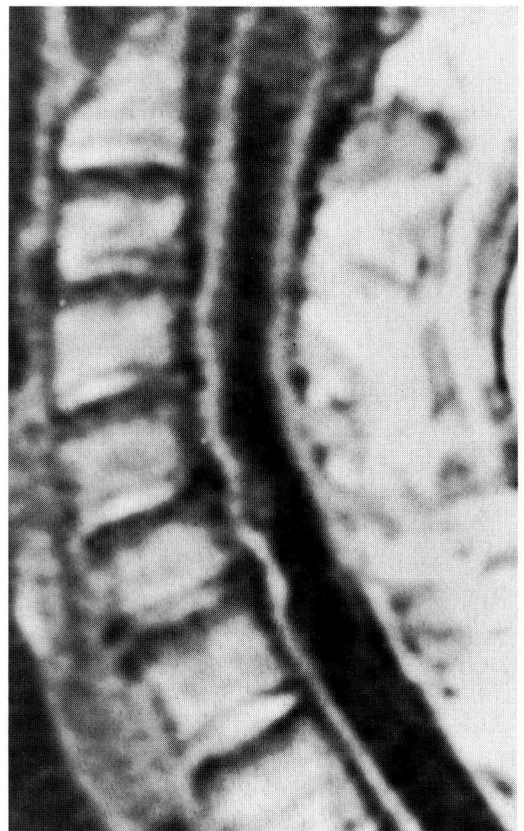

**Figure 6–59. Syringohydromyelia.** Sagittal T1WI (TR 500 msec/TE 20 msec). Extensive syringohydromyelia with a unilocular cavity.

through a gaping obex and is filled with cerebrospinal fluid. Noncommunicating syringomyelia, resulting from trauma or neoplasia, has no such communication. Although there is considerable overlap, congenital syringomyelia is best classified as the communicating type.

MRI has replaced conventional or CT myelography for the detection and evaluation of syringomyelia.[110, 111, 114] Both T1WI and T2WI sequences are necessary for characterization of the syrinx cavity. A T1WI provides optimal contrast between the cystic cavity and the surrounding cord. Yeats and associates suggest that T1 imaging with IR should be avoided, since contrast differentiation between gray and white matter within the normal cord might lead to the erroneous diagnosis of syringomyelia.[114] N(H)WI and T2WI are necessary to confirm the presence of CSF within the cavities. The pathology is best visualized in the sagittal and axial projections. We use the coronal projection for evaluation of a syrinx within the distal cord in order to determine its relationship to the conus medullaris.

On T1WI or N(H)WI sequences, the syrinx cavity is hypointense compared with the surrounding cord (Fig. 6–61*A*) The cord is often widened but may be normal or narrow in rare instances. The walls of the cord are paper thin in the presence of a large syrinx. As seen best in the axial projection, eccentric cavitation is often present.[110] The significance of these eccentric loculations is not completely clear; however, they can be seen in both a syrinx of congenital origin or one secondary to neoplasm. Sherman and colleagues have demonstrated that a T2WI is helpful for the detection of gliosis accompanying a syrinx cavity (Fig. 6–61*B*).[110] They point out that increased signal within the cord rostral to the cavity is common and likely represents changes secondary to gliosis, edema, or myelomalacia. The presence of gliosis with increased signal may be difficult to differentiate from a neoplastic process. The presence of the increased signal within a normal or small cord may be helpful in separating gliosis from neoplasm.

Sherman also demonstrated that on T2WI sequences a CFVS was present within the

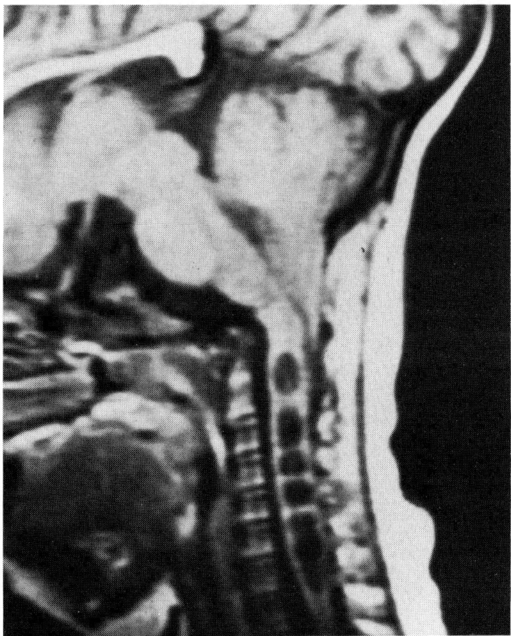

**Figure 6–60. Syringohydromyelia-Chiari I malformation.** Sagittal T1WI (TR 500 msec/TE 20 msec). Syringohydromelia with a string-of-beads appearance (multiple loculations).

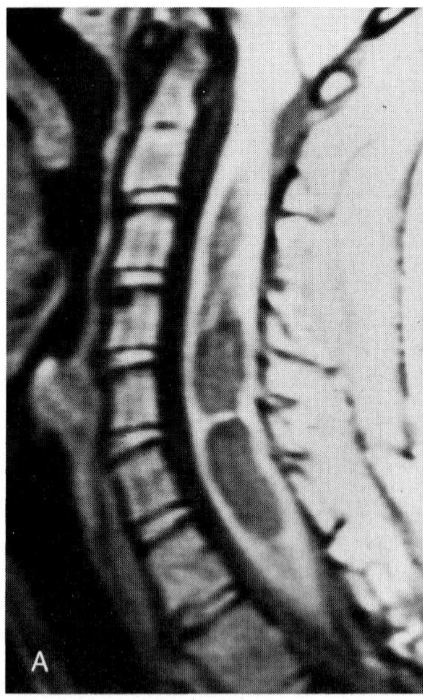


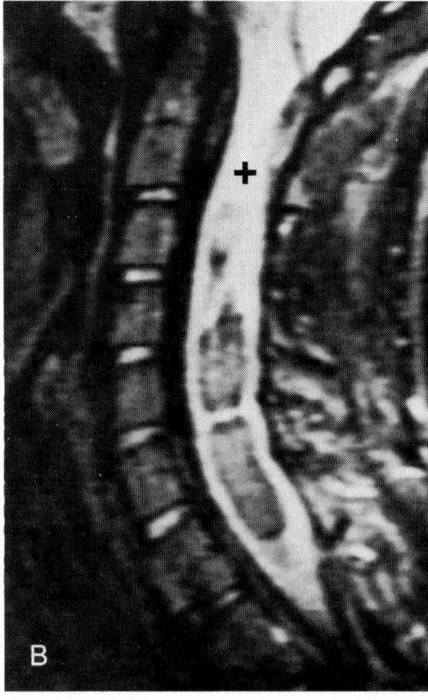


**Figure 6–61. Syringohydromyelia.** *A,* Sagittal N(H)WI (TR 1800 msec/TE 20 msec). A multiloculated syrinx of the cervical cord containing (low-signal) cerebrospinal fluid (CSF). *B,* Sagittal T2WI (TR 1800 msec/TE 20 msec). Persistent low signal within cystic cavities on a T2-weighted sequence represents signal void from CSF pulsations. Bright signal within cord above the syrinx is compatible with gliosis (+). (Courtesy of S. J. Pomeranz, M.D., The Christ Hospital, Cincinnati, Ohio.)

syrinx cavity in a high percentage of patients (Fig. 6–59*B*)[110] This CFVS was most frequently seen in the communicating type of syrinx (81%) and was indicative of pulsatile fluid shifts within the syrinx cavity made possible by external communication at the obex. They also inferred that the absence of CFVS may indicate the presence of septations arising from fibrous or glial scars that may make drainage of the syrinx cavity difficult. The presence or absence of CFVS was not helpful in differentiating a congenital syrinx from one associated with a tumor.

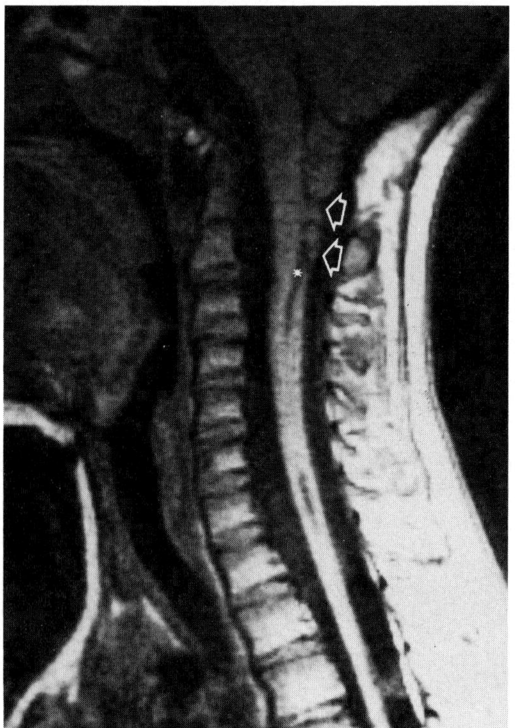

**Figure 6–62. Chiari II malformation with dilated central canal.** Sagittal T1WI (TR 800 msec/TE 20 msec). A gaping obex (asterisk) was identified just below the herniated tonsillar tissue (open arrows).

For syringomyelia involving the cervical cord, sagittal, T1-weighted 3-mm thick sections are preferred to identify a gaping obex (Fig. 6–62). This information may be helpful to the neurosurgeon before surgical intervention. MRI is also useful for the postoperative evaluation of the patient following drainage of the syrinx, to identify undrained loculations or cavities and to detect recurrent syringomyelia in the presence of an obstructed shunt.[115] Despite successful decompression, the syrinx cavity may not completely disappear, and small cavities or irregularity and prominence of the central canal may remain (Fig. 6–63).

Syringobulbia is best studied with MRI on sagittal and axial sections of the posterior fossa.[111] Syringobulbia is most commonly associated with Chiari I malformation but may be idiopathic. Sherman and colleagues identified two types.[111] The most common type was seen in association with Chiari I malformation and appeared as a slitlike cavity extending into the medulla above a syrinx of the cervical cord. The second type of syringobulbia was not associated with Chiari

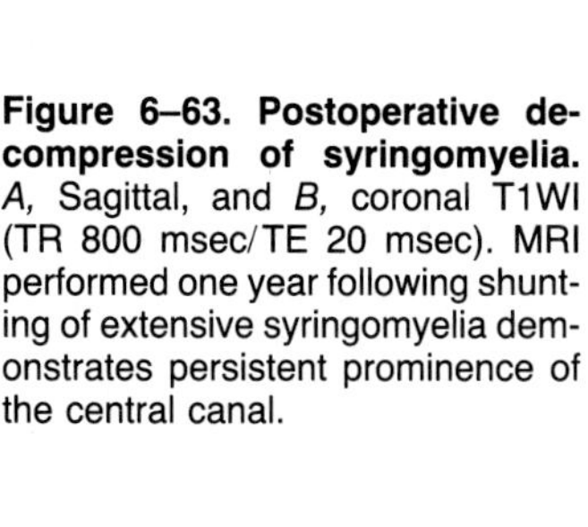

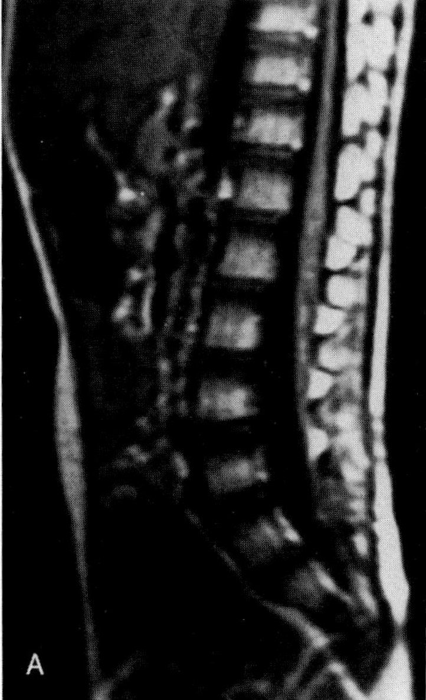


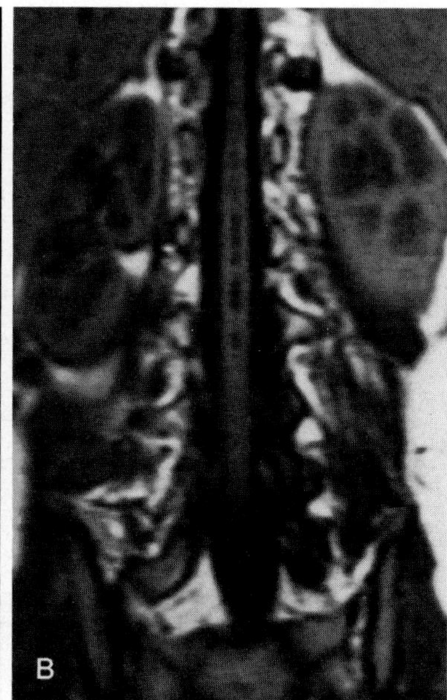


**Figure 6–63. Postoperative decompression of syringomyelia.** *A,* Sagittal, and *B,* coronal T1WI (TR 800 msec/TE 20 msec). MRI performed one year following shunting of extensive syringomyelia demonstrates persistent prominence of the central canal.

I malformation and had a saccular dilatation within the medulla rostral to a syringomyelia of the cervical cord. The signal characteristics of syringobulbia on MRI are similar to the findings of syringomyelia within the cervical cord.

## References


1. Levene MI, Whitelaw A, Dubowitz V, et al. Nuclear magnetic resonance imaging of the brain in children. Br Med J 285:774, 1982.
2. Dietrich RB, Lufkin RB, Kangarloo H, et al. Head and neck MR imaging in the pediatric patient. Radiology 159:769, 1986.
3. Han JS, Benson JE, Kaufman B, et al. MR imaging of pediatric cerebral anomalies. J Comput Assist Tomogr 9:103, 1985.
4. Johnson MA, Pennock JM, Bydeer GM, et al. Clinical NMR imaging of the brain in children: normal and neurologic disease. AJNR 4:1013, 1983.
5. McArdle CB, Nicholas DA, Richardson CJ, et al. Monitoring of the neonate undergoing MR imaging: technical considerations. Radiology 159:223, 1986.
6. Crooks LE, Arakawa M, Hoenninger J, et al. Magnetic resonance imaging: effects of magnetic field strength. Radiology 151:127, 1984.
7. Bilaniuk LT, Zimmerman RA, Wehrli FW, et al. Cerebral magnetic resonance: comparison of high and low field strength imaging. Radiology 153:409, 1984.
8. Smith FW. The value of NMR imaging in pediatric practice: a preliminary report. Pediatric Radiology 13:141, 1983.
9. Kuhn JP, Seidel FG, Narla LD. Techniques and strategies for MR of the neonatal brain. Presented at the Conjoint Meeting of the Society of Pediatric Radiology and European Society of Pediatric Radiology, May 30-June 4, 1987, Toronto.
10. McArdle CB. Personal communication, June 1987.
11. Kneeland JB, Jesmanowicz A, Froncisz W, et al. High resolution MR imaging using the loop-gap resonators. Work in progress. Radiology 158:247, 1986.
12. Hyde JS, Froncisz W, Jesmanowicz A, et al. Planar-pair local coils for high resolution magnetic resonance imaging, particularly of the temporomandibular joint. Med Phys 13:1, 1986.
13. Haacke EM, Bearden FH, Clayton JR, Linga NR. Reduction of MR imaging time by the hybrid fast scan technique. Radiology 158:521, 1986.
14. Haase A, Frahm J, Mathaei D, et al. FLASH imaging: rapid NMR imaging using low flip angle pulses. J Magn Reson 16:258, 1986.
15. McLaurin RL. Encephalocele and cranium bifidum. In Kalwars HL et al. eds. Handbook of Neurology. New York, Elsevier, 1987.
16. Diebler C, Dulac O. Cephaloceles: clinical and neuroradiological appearance. Associated cerebral malformations. Neuroradiology 25:199, 1983.
17. Byrd SE, Harwood-Nash DC, Fitz CR, et al. Computed tomography in the evaluation of encephaloceles in infants and children. J Comput Assist Tomogr 2:81, 1978.
18. Warkany J, Lemire RJ, Cohen MM. Encephaloceles. In Warkany J, Lemire RJ, Cohen MM, eds. Mental Retardation and Congenital Malformations of the Central Nervous System. Chicago, Year Book Medical Publishers, 1976:158.
19. Suwenwala S, Suwenwala N. A morphologic classification of sincipital encephalomeningoceles. J Neurosurg 36:201, 1972.
20. Simpson DA, David DJ, White J. Cephaloceles: treatment, outcome and antinatal diagnosis. Neurosurgery 15:14, 1984.
21. Leck I. Changes in the incidence of neural-tube defects. Lancet 2:791, 1966.

22. Barrow N, Simpson DA. Cranium bifidum. Investigation, prognosis and management. Aust Paediatr J 2:20, 1966.
23. Guthkelch AN. Occipital cranium bifidum. Arch Dis Child 45:105, 1970.
24. McLaurin RL. Parietal cephaloceles. Neurology 14:764, 1964.
25. Chiari H. Über der veränderungen des Kleinhirns, des Pons und der Medulla oblongata infolge von congenitaler Hydrocephalie des Grosshirns. Denkschriften der Akademie der Wissenschaften (Wien) 63:71, 1895.
26. Forbes W StC, Isherwood I. Computed tomography in syringomyelia and the associated Arnold-Chiari type I malformation. Neuroradiology 15:73, 1978.
27. Karch SB, Urich H. Occipital encephalocele: a morphological study. J Neurol Sci 15:89, 1972.
28. Teng P, Papatheodorou C. Arnold-Chiari malformation with normal spine and cranium. Arch Neurol 12:622, 1965.
29. Naidich TP, Pudlowski RM, Naidich JB. Computed tomographic signs of the Chiari II malformation. II. Midbrain and cerebellum. Radiology 134:391, 1980.
30. Naidich TP, McClone DG, Fulling KH. The Chiari II malformation. Part IV. The hindbrain deformity. Neuroradiology 25:179, 1983.
31. Peach B. Arnold-Chiari malformation: anatomic features of 20 cases. Arch Neurol 12:613, 1965B.
32. Sherman JL, Citrin CM, Bowen BJ, et al. MR demonstration of altered cerebrospinal fluid flow by obstructive lesions. AJNR 7:571, 1986.
33. El Gammal T, Allen MB, Brooks BS, et al. MR evaluation of hydrocephalus. AJNR 8:591, 1987.
34. Warkany J, Lemire RJ, Cohen MM. Holoprosencephaly: cyclopia series. In Warkany J, Lemire RJ, Cohen MM, eds. Mental Retardation and Congenital Malformations of the Central Nervous System. Chicago, Year Book Medical Publishers, 1981:176.
35. Lazjuk GI, Lurie IW, Nedzved MK. Further studies on the genetic heterogeneity of cebocephaly. J Med Genet 13:314, 1976.
36. Byrd SE, Harwood-Nash DC, Fitz CR, et al. Computed tomography evaluation of holoprosencephaly in infants and children. J Comput Assist Tomogr 1:456, 1977.
37. Hayashi T, Yoshida M, Kuramoto S, et al. Radiological features of holoprosencephaly. Surg Neurol 12:261, 1979.
38. Warkany J, Lemire RJ, Cohen MM. Agenesis of the corpus callosum. In Warkany J, Lemire RJ, Cohen MM, eds. Mental Retardation and Congenital Malformation of the Central Nervous System. Chicago, Year Book Medical Publishers, 1981:224.
39. Atlas SW, Zimmerman RA, Bilaniuk LT, et al. Corpus callosum and limbic system: neuroanatomic MR evaluation of developmental anomalies. Radiology 160:355, 1986.
40. Davidson HD, Abraham R, Steiner RE. Agenesis of the corpus callosum: magnetic resonance imaging. Radiology 155:371, 1985.
41. Byrd SE, Harwood-Nash DC, Fitz CR. Absence of the corpus callosum: computed tomographic evaluation in infants and children. Journal Assoc Can Radiol 29:108, 1978.
42. Dignan P StJ, Warkany J. Congenital malformations: the corpus callosum. In Wortis J, ed. Mental Retardation and Developmental Disabilities. New York, Brounner-Mazel 1977:106.
43. Probst FP. Congenital defects of the corpus callosum. Acta Radiol (Suppl) 331:1, 1973.
44. Cooney JF, Baker GS. Tumors involving the corpus callosum. Mayo Clin Proc 28:299, 1953.
45. Krause-Brucker W, Gardner DW. Optic nerve hypoplasia associated with absent septum pellucidum and hypopituitarism. Am J Ophthalmol 89:113, 1980.
46. Manelfe C, Rochiccioli P. CT of septo-optic dysplasia. AJR 133:1157, 1979.
47. Dobyns WB, McCluggage CW. Computed tomographic appearance of lissencephaly syndromes. AJNR 6:545, 1985.
48. Josephy H. Congenital agyria and defects of the corpus callosum. J Neuropathol Exp Neurol 3:63, 1944.
49. Warkany J, Lemire RJ, Cohen MM. Lissencephaly: agyria and pachygyria. In Warkany J, Lemire RJ, Cohen MM, eds. Mental Retardation and Congenital Malformations of the Central Nervous System. Chicago, Year Book Medical Publishers, 1981:200.
50. Byrd SE, Bohan T, Osborn RE, et al. CT and MRI detection of lissencephaly. Presented at the Twenty-fifth Annual Meeting, American Society of Neuroradiology, New York, May 10-15, 1987.
51. Kalifa G, Sellier N, Demange P, et al. MR imaging of hemimegalencephaly in children. Presented at the Seventy-second Scientific Assembly and Annual Meeting, Radiological Society of North America, Chicago, November 30-December 5, 1986.
52. Zimmerman RA, Bilaniuk LT, Grossman RI. Computed tomography and migratory disorders of human brain development. Neuroradiology 25:257, 1983.
53. Townsend JJ, Nielson SL, Malamud N. Unilateral megalencephaly: hamartoma or neoplasm? Neurology 25:448, 1975.
54. Mikhael MA, Mattar AG. Malformation of the cerebral cortex with heterotopia of the gray matter. J Comput Assist Tomogr 2:291, 1978.
55. Bignami A, Palladini G, Zappella M. Unilateral megalencephaly with nerve cell hypertrophy: an anatomical and quantitative histochemical study. Brain Res 9:103, 1968.
56. Nixon GW, Johns RE, Myers GG. Congenital porencephaly. Pediatrics 54:43, 1974.
57. Warkany J, Lemire RJ, Cohen MM. Porencephaly. In Warkany J, Lemire RJ, Cohen MM, eds. Mental Retardation and Congenital Malformations of the Central Nervous System. Chicago, Year Book Medical Publishers, 1981:191.
58. Naef RW. Clinical features of porencephaly. A review of 32 cases. Arch Neurol Psychiatry 80:133, 1958.
59. Yakovlev PI, Wadsworth RC. Double symmetrical porencephalies (schizencephalies). Trans Am Neurol Assoc 67:24, 1941.
60. Miller GM, Stears JC, Guggenheim MA, et al. Schizencephaly: a clinical and CT study. Neurology 34:997, 1984.
61. Yakovlev PI, Wadsworth RC. Schizencephalies: a study of the congenital clefts in the cerebral mantle. I. Clefts with fused lips. J Neuropathol Exp Neurol 5:116, 1946.
62. Yakovlev PI, Wadsworth RC. Schizencephalies. A

study of the congenital clefts in the cerebral mantle. II. Clefts with hydrocephalus and lip separated. J Neuropathol Exp Neurol 5:169, 1946.
63. Milhorat TH. Hydrocephalus. In Milhorat TH, ed. Pediatric Neurosurgery. Philadelphia, F.A. Davis Co., 1979:91.
64. Bickers DS, Adams RD. Hereditary stenosis of the aqueduct of Sylvius as a cause of congenital hydrocephalus. Brain 72:246, 1949.
65. Dandy WE, Blackfan KD. Internal hydrocephalus: an experimental, clinical and pathological study. Am J Dis Child 8:406, 1914.
66. Raybaud C. Cystic malformations of the posterior fossa: abnormalities associated with the development of the roof of the fourth ventricle and adjacent meningeal structures. J Neuroradiol 9:103, 1982.
67. Joubert M, Eisenring JJ, Robb JP, et al. Familial agenesis of the cerebellar vermis. A syndrome of episodic hyperpnea, abnormal eye movements, ataxia, and retardation. Neurology 19:513, 1969.
68. Gilles FH, Rockett FX. Infantile hydrocephalus: retrocerebellar "arachnoidal" cyst. J Pediatr 79:436, 1971.
69. Adam R, Greenberg JO. The megacisterna magna. J Neurosurg 48:190, 1978.
70. Archer CR, Darwish H, Smith K. Enlarged cisternae magnae and posterior fossa cyst simulating Dandy-Walker syndrome on computed tomography. Radiology 127:681, 1978.
71. Milhorat TH. Benign intracranial cyst. In Milhorat TH, ed. Pediatric Neurosurgery. Philadelphia, F.A. Davis Co., 1979:191
72. diRocco C, Caldarelli M, DiTrapani G. Infratentorial arachnoid cyst in children. Child's Brain 8:119, 1981.
73. Weiner SN, Pearlstein AE, Eiber A. MR imaging of intracranial arachnoid cyst. J Comput Assist Tomogr 11:236, 1987.
74. Kjos BO, Brandt-Zawadzki M, Kucharczyk W, et al. Cystic intracranial lesions: magnetic resonance imaging. Radiology 155:363, 1985.
75. Packer RJ, Zimmerman RA, Bilaniuk LT, et al. Magnetic resonance imaging of lesions of the posterior fossa and upper cervical cord in childhood. Pediatrics 76:84, 1985.
76. Lee BCP, Deck MDF, Kneeland JB, Cahill PT. MR imaging of the craniocervical junction. AJNR 6:209, 1985.
77. Forbes W StC, Isherwood I. Computed tomography in syringomyelia and the associated Arnold-Chiari type I malformation. Neuroradiology 15:73, 1978.
78. Spinos E, Laster DW, Moody DM, et al. MR evaluation of Chiari I malformations at 0.15 T. AJNR 6:203, 1985.
79. DeLaPaz RL, Brady TJ, Buonanno FS, et al. Nuclear magnetic resonance (NMR) imaging of Arnold-Chiari type I malformation with hydromyelia. J Comput Assist Tomogr 7:126, 1983.
80. Bloch S, Van Rensburg MJ, Danziger J. The Arnold-Chiari malformation. Clinical Radiology 25:335, 1974.
81. Barkovich AJ, Wippold FJ, Sherman JL, et al. Significance of cerebellar tonsillar position on MR. AJNR 7:795, 1986.
82. Logue V, Edwards MR. Syringomyelia and its surgical treatment—an analysis of 75 patients. J Neurol Neurosurg Psychiatr 44:273, 1981.
83. Bewermeyer H, Dreesbach HA, Hunermann B, et al. MR imaging of familial basilar impression. J Comput Assist Tomogr 8:953, 1984.
84. Kuhn JP, Cohen ML, Duffner PK, et al. MR imaging of the brain in neurofibromatosis. Presented at the Seventy-second Scientific Assembly and Annual Meeting, Radiological Society of North America. Chicago, November 30-December 5, 1986.
85. Zanella FE, et al. Neurofibromatosis of the central nervous system: demonstration by MRI. Presented at the Conjoint Meeting of the Society of Pediatric Radiology and European Society of Pediatric Radiology, Toronto, May 30-June 4, 1987.
86. Jacoby CG, Yuh WT, Afifi AK, et al. Accelerated myelination in early Sturge-Weber syndrome demonstrated by MR imaging. J Comput Assist Tomogr 11:226, 1987.
87. Vaghi M, Visciani A, Testa D, et al. Cerebral MR findings in tuberous sclerosis. J Comput Assist Tomogr 11:403, 1987.
88. Riccardi VM, Kleiner B. Neurofibromatosis: a neoplastic birth defect with two H peaks of severe problems. Birth Defects 13:131, 1977.
89. Neurofibromatosis. LINK, The Neurofibromatosis Association. Lancet, March 21, 1987:663.
90. Holt JF. Neurofibromatosis in children. AJR 130:615, 1978.
91. Pearce J. The central nervous system pathology in multiple neurofibromatosis. Neurology 17:691, 1967.
92. Brooks BS, El-Gammal T, Adams RJ, et al. MRI imaging of Moya-Moya in neurofibromatosis. AJNR 8:178, 1987.
93. Stimac GK, Solomon MA, Newton TH. CT and MR of angiomatous malformations of the choroid plexus in patients with Sturge-Weber disease. AJNR 7:623, 1986.
94. Han JS, Kaufman B, ElYousef SJ, et al. NMR imaging of the spine. AJNR 4:1151, 1983.
95. Samuelsson L, Bergstrom K, Thuomas KA, et al. MR imaging of syringohydromyelia and Chiari malformations in meningomyelocele patients with scoliosis. AJNR 8:539, 1987.
96. Barnes PD, Lester PD, Yamanashi WS, et al. MRI in infants and children with spinal dysraphism. AJR 147:339, 1986.
97. Altman NR, Altman DH. MR imaging of spinal dysraphism. AJNR 8:533, 1987.
98. Modic MT, Weinstein MA, Pavlicek W, et al. Magnetic resonance imaging of the cervical spine: technical and clinical observations. AJNR 5:15, 1984.
99. Cameron AH. The Arnold-Chiari and other neuroanatomical malformations associated with spina bifida. J Pathol Bacteriol 73:195, 1957.
100. Stanley P, Senac MO, Segall HD, et al. Syringohydromyelia following meningomyelocele surgery—role of metrizamide myelography and computed tomography. Pediatr Radiol 14:278, 1984.
101. Emery JL, Lendon RG. The local cord lesion in neurospinal dysraphism (meningomyelocele). J Pathol 110:83, 1973.
102. Naidich TP, McClone DG, Harwood-Nash DC. Spinal dysraphism. In Newton TH, Potts DG, eds. Computed Tomography of the Spine and Spinal Cord. San Anselmo, Calif, Clavadel Press, 1983:229.
103. James CCM, Lassman LP. Diastematomyelia: a

critical survey of 24 cases submitted to laminectomy. Arch Dis Child 39:125, 1964.
104. Hilal SK, Marton D, Pollack E. Diastematomyelia in children: radiographic study of 34 cases. Radiology 112:609, 1974.
105. Han JS, Benson JE, Kaufman B, et al. Demonstration of diastematomyelia and associated abnormalities with MR imaging. AJNR 6:215, 1985.
106. Naidich TP, McClone DG, Mutluer S. A new understanding of dorsal dysraphism with lipoma (lipomyeloschisis): radiographic evaluation and surgical correction. AJNR 4:103, 1983.
107. Emery JL, Lendon RG. Lipomas of the cauda equina and other fatty tumours related to neurospinal dysraphism. Dev Med Child Neurol (Suppl) 11:62, 1969.
108. Harwood-Nash DC, Fitz CR. Myelography. In Harwood-Nash DC, Fitz CR, eds. Neuroradiology in Infants and Children. St. Louis, CV Mosby Co., 1976:1125.
109. Campbell JB. Neurosurgical treatment of bladder and bowel dysfunction resulting from anomalous development of the sacral neural axis. Clin Neurosurg 8:133, 1962.
110. Sherman JL, Barkovich AJ, Citrin CM. The MR appearance of syringomyelia: new observations. AJNR 7:985, 1986.
111. Sherman JL, Citrin CM, Barkovich AJ. MR imaging of syringobulbia. J Comput Assist Tomogr 11:407, 1987.
112. Williams B. Current concepts of syringomyelia. Br J Hosp Med 4:331, 1970.
113. Gardner W, Angel J. The mechanism of syringomyelia and its surgical correction. Clin Neurosurg 6:131, 1975.
114. Yeats A, Brant-Zawadzki M, Norman D, et al. Nuclear magnetic resonance imaging of syringomyelia. AJNR 4:234, 1983.
115. Barkovich AJ, Sherman JL, Citrin CM, et al. MR of post-operative syringomyelia. AJNR 8:319, 1987.

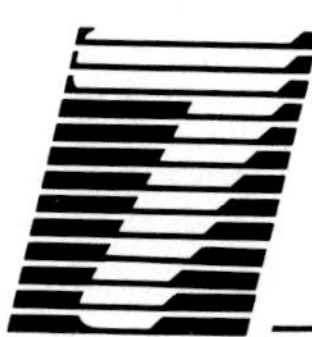

William S. Ball, Jr., M.D.
Richard B. Towbin, M.D.

# MRI OF PEDIATRIC CENTRAL NERVOUS SYSTEM NEOPLASMS

Brain tumors are the second most common solid tumor arising in childhood, with a reported incidence of 21 cases per million.[1] Ninety-eight percent of lesions are primary, unlike in adults, in whom a significant proportion of intracranial neoplasms are metastatic. Most series report a 66% incidence of childhood brain tumors originating infratentorially;[2] however, Naidich reports the incidence of infratentorial and supratentorial tumors to be about equal.[3] The overall prognosis of malignant intracranial tumors continues to be poor. Recent surgical advances, including laser and microsurgical techniques, offer the potential means of improving survival.[4] Such new techniques have again focused our attention on early detection. As a means of improving their results, neurosurgeons are once again turning to the neuroradiologists to provide a more sensitive means of early detection of central nervous system (CNS) neoplasia.

Magnetic resonance imaging (MRI) is a proven safe and effective modality for imaging the CNS in children.[5–7] How successful it will be in evaluating pediatric CNS neoplasia has not been proved. Preliminary reports suggest excellent sensitivity in identifying brain tumors, especially within the posterior fossa;[8, 9] however, data concerning its specificity are insufficient. Therefore the question of whether or not MRI will replace computed tomography (CT) in the diagnosis of pediatric tumors of the brain and spine goes unanswered. Perhaps time will reveal a complementary role for the two modalities. On the other hand, because of its multiplanar capability, superb anatomic visualization, capacity to differentiate tissues according to relaxation characteristics, and lack of ionizing radiation, MRI may eventually become the imaging method of choice.

Several authors have already reported their experience with MRI in pediatric CNS neoplasia.[10–12] They cite improvements over computed tomography in the detection of benign tumors, tumors within the middle and posterior fossas, and masses at the craniocervical junction. The disadvantages of MRI most often cited include cost, availability, greater demands for patient cooperation, relative insensitivity in detecting tumoral calcification, and difficulty in separating tumor from adjacent hemorrhage or peritumoral edema. Despite its shortcomings, MRI is an attractive alternative that may overcome many of the shortcomings of CT. In this chapter, we review the MRI features of the more common pediatric brain and spine tumors, and present our technical approach designed to obtain consistent, high quality images in children of all ages.

## TECHNICAL CONSIDERATIONS

Patient preparation, sedation, and monitoring during the MRI examination are discussed in Chapter 6. The technical parameters necessary for scanning change as we shift our emphasis from structural anomalies to the diagnosis and categorization of tumors of the brain and spine.

### Pulsing Sequence

MRI is a valuable tool for the early detection of CNS tumors. This is due primarily to its superb delineation of both normal and pathologic anatomy and its ability to distinguish between tissues, based on their T1 relaxation, T2 relaxation, and proton density. Since both anatomic detail and tissue characterization are important, we rely primarily on spin-echo (SE), T1-weighted imaging (T1WI), T2-weighted imaging (T2WI), and intermediate-weighted imaging (N[H]WI) for a complete evaluation. An inversion recovery (IR) sequence (TR = 1600-1800 msec/TE 20 msec/TI 500-600 msec, matrix 256 × 128, 1-2 nex) can be used to provide heavily T1-weighted images (i.e., for lesions isointense on an SE/T1WI) but are not used routinely in evaluating tumors of the brain. Each examination is begun with a low-resolution sagittal T1WI localizer sequence (TR 400–600 msec/TE 20 msec, matrix 256 × 128, 1 nex) from which additional sequences are programmed. We next proceed with a multiecho axial T2WI sequence (TR 2000–2500 msec/TE 20/80–100 msec, matrix 256 × 128, 2 nex), which is followed by a coronal sequence using the same parameters. Although a single axial T2WI sequence usually suffices, the coronal projection is especially helpful in evaluating tumors in the middle cranial fossa, lying near the vertex and within the posterior fossa. For higher resolution T2WI sequences, the number of excitations either can be increased from 2 to 4 nex, or a smaller matrix size of 256 × 256 can be used. We prefer to first increase the number of excitations, which improves signal-to-noise.

If an area of abnormality suggesting a neoplastic process is identified on the T2WI sequence, a high resolution T1WI sequence is performed through the area of pathology in the same projection. For this purpose, we use a T1WI sequence that provides optimal resolution and signal-to-noise (TR 400–600 msec/TE 20 msec, matrix 256 × 128 or 256 × 256, 2–4 nex). One then has the option of performing a contrast-enhanced MR (CEMR) using T1WI.

Gradient echo imaging, providing T2-weighted images, is an attractive alternative to the standard SE/T2WI sequence because of its rapid acquisition. The technique currently used by General Electric to obtain rapid images is gradient acquisition at a steady state (GRASS). A relatively T2-weighted sequence, containing 4 to 6 slices, can be obtained in under 4 minutes with a short TR (TR 20–30 msec/TE 10–15 msec, flip 20°–30°). A more heavily T2-weighted gradient acquisition image can be obtained by using a longer TR sequence (TR 200–400 msec/TE 30–50 msec, flip 10°–15°) but at a cost of increasing acquisition time, especially if one uses a 256 × 256 matrix and 4 nex to improve resolution. Although such imaging sequences are conceived in terms of T2-weighting, they do, in fact, produce images based on a tissue characterization known as T2*, which is always less than true T2 relaxation. The current limitations of gradient echo imaging include limited inherent contrast differentiation between normal and pathologic tissues (Fig. 7–1), decreased signal-to-noise, and increased magnetic susceptibility, which often degrades the image. Improved T2-related contrast between normal and pathologic tissues and between gray and white matter can be obtained by using gradient acquisition imaging with a shorter TE and flip angle (TR 200–400 msec/TE 20 msec, flip 20°). Decreases in signal-to-noise are compensated by increasing the number of excitations from 2 to 4 or 6 while still maintaining an acceptable scanning time. Further improvements in resolution can be obtained by extension of the matrix by 256 × 256. In the future, single-slice acquisition will be replaced by multiple-slice acquisition, improving the utilization of these techniques.

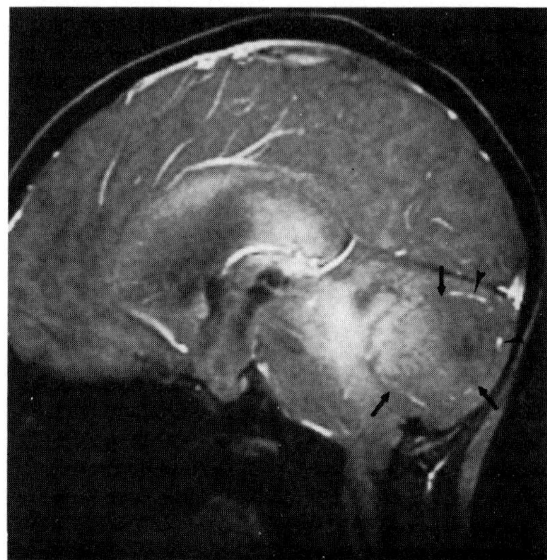

**Figure 7–1. Cystic cerebellar astrocytoma.** Sagittal GRASS T2*I (TR 24 msec/TE 13 msec/ϕ-30°). Note poor contrast differentiation between the macrocyst (arrows) and the surrounding brain. Prominent vessels were identified in the wall of the cyst as areas of hyperintense signal (arrowheads).

Magnetic susceptibility works both to the advantage and to the disadvantage of gradient echo imaging. This susceptibility results in unwanted artifact at the skull base, near the interface of paranasal sinus air and brain. This same phenomenon, however, improves visualization of both calcium and hemosiderin, compensating in part for the limitations of spin-echo imaging. Gradient acquisition imaging with or without flow compensation is helpful in evaluating vascular flow to the tumor and in differentiating calcification and hemosiderin from rapid vascular flow as a cause of reduced signal intensity in or around a tumor. Despite its potential advantages, we do not currently substitute the gradient echo T2*I sequence for the spin-echo T2WI sequence, since the longer TR images of T2WI provide optimal contrast differentiation.

Imaging of the brain with two-dimensional Fourier transformation (2DFT) is susceptible to artifacts produced by physiologic motion from vascular and CSF pulsations. "Ghosting" artifacts are produced in the phase direction adjacent to areas of high flow or extremes in pulsation (sella/suprasella, brain stem, foramen magnum). A significant reduction in this artifact can be achieved by several means. The simplest method is cardiac gating, in which data acquisition is obtained at the same point in the cardiac cycle, thus negating the effects of pusatile motion. A second, more effective technique is designed to refocus pulses that cause the "ghosting" artifact and thus decrease extravascular misregistration. We use gradient moment nulling (Flow compensation, GE, Milwaukee) routinely in the coronal and axial projections in order to eliminate the pulsation artifact from the middle cranial fossa, posterior fossa, and suprasellar cistern. A decrease in the number of obtainable slices results when using this technique; however, this generally does not prevent a complete survey of the brain in children.

For examination of the brain, all children are scanned in the standard head coil. Improved resolution and signal characteristics can be obtained by imaging the neonatal head in the wrap-around extremity coil provided with the GE Signa scanner. For evaluation of the spine, posteriorly placed surface coils are used routinely; however, in the craniocervical junction, we have found improved visualization with the use of a laterally placed, tandem, axial pair loop-gap resonator coil system, which allows for greater positional variation in scanning. This coil system has been further described in Chapter 6.

### Slice Acquisition

For routine scanning of the brain in any projection, a slice thickness of 5 mm is chosen. In the cooperative or sedated patient, smaller regions of interest are imaged with 3-mm thick sections. The benefits of improved resolution from thinner sections is negated by an increase in noise, unless there is a proportionate increase in data acquisition (i.e., increasing the number of averages). For T1- or T2-weighted sequences using 5 mm thick slices, a gap of 1 to 2.5 mm is adequate. For multiecho T2-weighted sequences, we use a minimum gap of 1 mm. For 3 mm thick sections, a gap of .5 mm can be obtained with insignificant image degradation.

## FURTHER TECHNICAL CONSIDERATIONS

Preoperative angiography is performed to assess tumor vascularity and to determine its relationship to major vascular structures. This is especially true for suprasellar tumors, which may involve the circle of Willis or directly invade the cavernous sinus. MRI is capable of delineating these relationships and can eliminate the need for angiography. The vascularity is best assessed on a T2WI, in which flowing blood produces signal hypointensity owing to a time-of-flight effect and phase shifts with respect to stationary spins. A similar appearance that is less conspicuous is produced on a T1WI. On a T1WI, high intravascular signal (without flow compensation) within an artery may indicate occlusion or slow flow within the vessel. With flow compensation, the appearance of signal, based on flow within the vessel, is reversed. Flowing blood may now appear bright in signal, producing an "angiographic" effect. With gradient acquisition, the washout of excited spins and fast flowing blood does not result in as much signal loss since 180° refocusing pulses are not utilized and unsaturated fully magnetized protons constantly wash in to the desired section; therefore flowing blood in both arteries and veins can appear bright in signal.

In the evaluation of CNS neoplasia, there are two notable disadvantages of MRI. First is its relative lack of sensitivity in identifying intratumoral calcification. Based on our experience with CT, the presence of calcification helps in establishing a diagnosis of tumor and aids in the differential diagnosis between tumors of various histologic types. Therefore the inability of MRI to readily identify calcification could compromise the sensitivity and specificity of this modality. In addition, the signal hypointensity produced by calcification is not easily differentiated from loss of signal produced by flowing blood or hemosiderin. Gradient acquisition imaging may solve part of this problem. Both long TR and short TR gradient echo sequences may improve identification of calcification within the tumor owing to its increased magnetic susceptibility. Magnetic susceptibility also explains the enhanced visualization of hemosiderin. Unfortunately, differentiation of calcification from hemosiderin resulting from previous hemorrhage is not possible on a gradient echo image. Fast-scanning techniques can be used to differentiate calcification from hypointensity secondary to flowing blood. In this sequence, flowing blood will produce a bright signal, as opposed to calcification, which will continue to display signal hypointensity. In a similar fashion, flow compensation can be helpful in separating rapidly flowing blood from calcification. As experience accumulates, perhaps there will be less reliance on the identification of calcium for diagnosis and categorization of tumors and perhaps other features of MR (e.g., signal characteristics) that might provide improved specificity can be explored.

The second disadvantage of MRI is in separating a tumor from surrounding CSF and peritumoral edema. Sampling of multiple echoes in a T2WI sequence may be effective in differentiating tumor from surrounding edema, based on subtle differences in T2 relaxation. This technique is called an echo-train sequence. In children older than one year of age, a sequence utilizing echo delays of 25, 50, 75, and 100 msec will suffice; however, in infants less than one year old, owing to increased brain water content, a longer TR and longer echo delays are performed (TR 2500–3000 msec/TE 30/60/90/120 msec). Such sequences are also invaluable for assessing tumors involving the brain stem, suprasellar region, and pineal region, where differentiation of tumor from surrounding CSF is often difficult. We continue to rely primarily on T1WI and N(H)WI to provide the optimal sensitivity in separating tumor from surrouding CSF. Despite these efforts, separation of the two may be difficult. In the future, MR contrast agents may improve our separation of tumor, CSF, and peritumoral edema.[13]

## INFRATENTORIAL NEOPLASMS

Infratentorial tumors are a histologically diverse group of neoplasms arising from the brain stem, cellular hemispheres, or adjacent structures. The most common tumors of the posterior fossa include cerebellar astrocytoma, medulloblastoma, brain stem glioma, and ependymoma. Rarely, hemangioblastomas, meningiomas, neural crest tumors, choroid plexus papillomas, chordomas, epidermoids, or undifferentiated sarcomas can involve the posterior fossa.[14] Although rare in children, acoustic neuromas are not uncommon in young adults with neurofibromatosis and are usually bilateral.[15, 16] The MR characteristics of acoustic neuromas in children are identical with those in adults and are described elsewhere in this text.

Tumors of the infratentorial region most often present between the ages of 3 and 8 years. Male and female incidence varies with each tumor type. Although the mode of clinical presentation may vary, cranial nerve involvement, gait disturbances, nystagmus, and signs and symptoms of increased intracranial pressure predominate.

### Cerebellar Astrocytoma

The incidence of cerebellar astrocytoma is similar to that of medulloblastoma, with a peak frequency between the ages of 3 and 8 years. Males and females are equally affected. This slow-growing tumor typically manifests by hypotonia, incoordination, truncal ataxia, and the signs and symptoms of increased intracranial pressure secondary to obstructive hydrocephalus. Clinical features of obstruction include morning headache and vomiting unassociated with nausea. As with other posterior fossa tumors, gait disturbances, nystagmus, and the signs of cerebellar dysfunction are common. On CT, two patterns of tumor can be identified.[17]

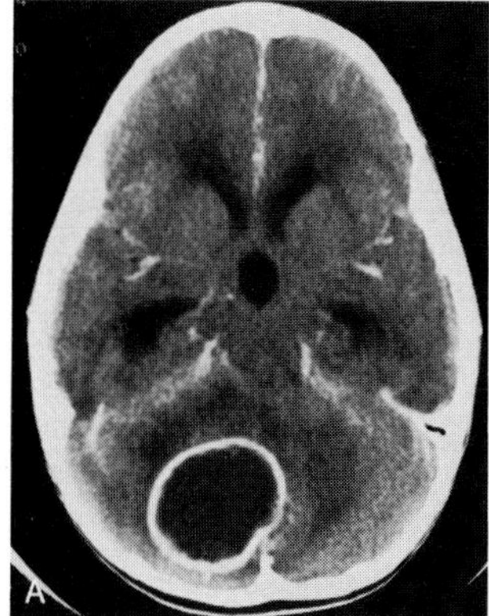

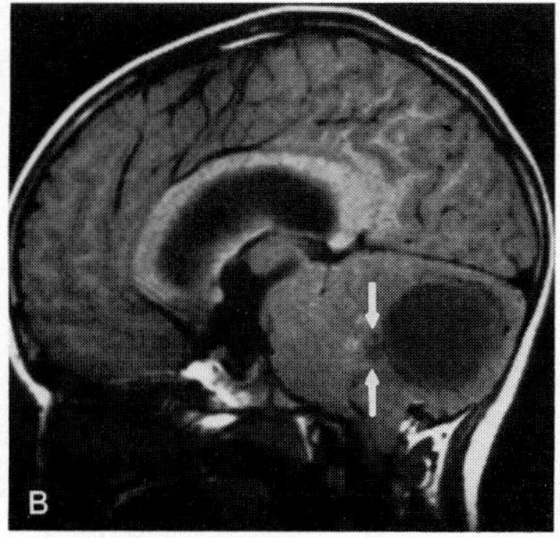

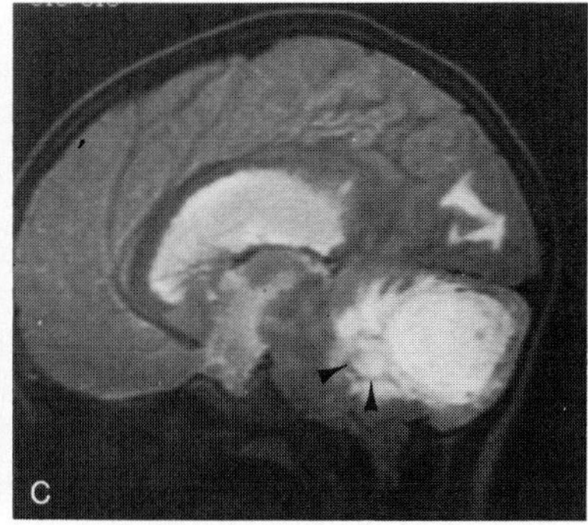


**Figure 7–2. Cystic cerebellar astrocytoma.** *A,* Enhanced CT reveals a low-attenuation macrocyst with a thick enhancing rim, characteristic of a cystic cerebellar astrocytoma. *B,* Sagittal T1WI (TR 600 msec/TE 20 msec). The macrocyst appears hypodense. A hypointense mural nodule is present anteriorly (arrows). *C,* Sagittal T2WI (TR 2500 msec/TE 100 msec). The macrocyst and mural nodule are both hyperintense; however, the cyst appears brighter. Note the isointense rim separating the nodule from the surrounding edema (arrowheads).

The most common type is the cystic astrocytoma, which appears as a single- or multilobulated, well-defined macrocyst, associated with a mass or containing a mural nodule within its wall. These tumors are usually eccentrically located within the cerebellar hemisphere and displace the fourth ventricle anteriorly and contralaterally. On unenhanced CT, the mural nodule is isodense and difficult to identify. The cyst is generally low in attenuation. Following contrast administration, the solid tumor or mural nodule will intensely enhance. The wall of the cyst may or may not enhance, with enhancement usually indicating its infiltration by tumor (Fig. 7–2*A*). Calcification is found in 20% of cerebellar astrocytomas.[18] The second type of cerebellar astrocytoma is generally solid, midline, and arises either within the vermis or from the medial cerebellar hemisphere. Although predominantly solid, smaller, variable-sized cysts can be identified within the tumor and represent cystic degeneration, necrosis, or areas of previous hemorrhage. On an unenhanced CT, the solid astrocytoma may be hypodense, isodense, or, rarely, hyperdense. Following the administration of contrast, moderate homogeneous enhancement is frequent; however, rarely, the enhancement may be minimal and inhomogeneous. The brain stem and midbrain may be the site either of origin or of secondary extension of an astrocytoma.

On a T1WI, the tumor, whether cystic or solid, overall is low in signal intensity and inhomogeneous.[10] Infrequently, the solid tumor or mural nodule may be isointense (Fig. 7–3*A*). The cysts appear lower in signal intensity compared with the hypointense solid tumor (Fig. 7–2*B*) but are slightly greater in intensity compared with CSF owing to the protein content of the cystic fluid. Differentiation of a tumor cyst from a benign

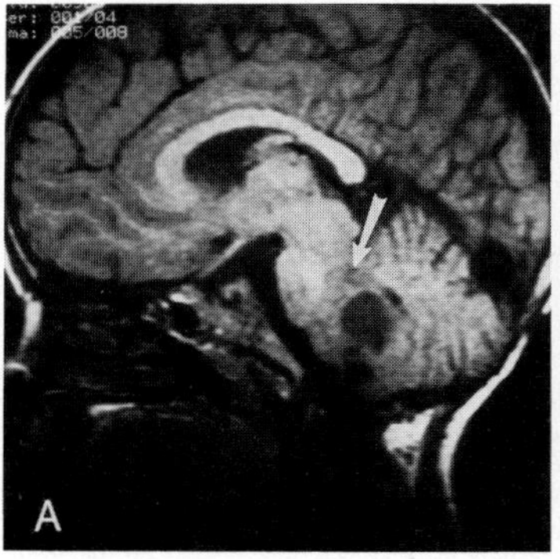

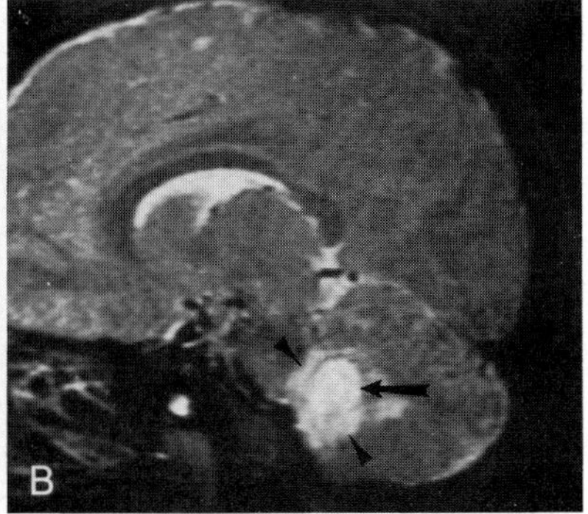


**Figure 7–3. Vermian cerebellar astrocytoma.** *A,* Sagittal T1WI (TR 600 msec/TE 20 msec). The vermian mass is predominantly isointense (arrows) but contains hypointense areas representing cystic necrosis. *B,* Sagittal T2WI (TR 2000 msec/TE 100 msec). The solid tumor (arrowheads) and cyst (arrow) are equally hyperintense.

collection of CSF (e.g., arachnoid cyst) requires a complete evaluation of the signal characteristics on T1-weighted, intermediate-weighted, and T2-weighted images.

On a T2WI, both the tumoral cyst and the solid tumor have a prolonged T2 relaxation and are therefore bright in signal (Fig. 7–2C).[10] The signal intensity of the cyst is often equal to and occasionally, greater than the signal intensity of the mural nodule. Differentiating the solid tumor from the surrounding edema or macrocyst may be difficult. The macrocyst can usually be separated by the presence of a low–signal intensity wall. On a T2WI, solid cerebellar astrocytomas also display hyperintensity that is often inhomogeneous owing to previous hemorrhage or necrosis (Fig. 7–3*B*). The signal characteristics of the solid astrocytoma are similar to ependymoma, making their differentiation by MRI difficult. Rarely, cystic ependymomas mimick the MRI pattern of a cystic astrocytoma. The location of the tumor, the lack of a macrocyst, and the more homogeneous pattern of signal distribution can be helpful in differentiating medulloblastoma from a cerebellar astrocytoma.

## Medulloblastoma

Medulloblastoma is a common midline neoplasm arising in the posterior fossa in children, with a peak incidence between 3 and 5 years of age. It is a highly malignant embryonic tumor and has sheets of small cells originating from the primitive medullary epithelium.[18, 19] It typically arises within the roof of the fourth ventricle and involves the vermis. Less commonly, medulloblastoma is found lateral to the vermis and fourth ventricle. Because of its location, the tumor may grow into the fourth ventricle or seed the subarachnoid space.[18] With obstruction of the fourth ventricle, the initial presentation is that of secondary hydrocephalus. On unenhanced CT, the tumor most often appears as a homogeneous, hyperdense, midline mass (Fig. 7–4*A*).[19] Gross calcification is uncommon, but microscopic calcification may contribute to its hyperdense appearance. Marked homogeneous enhancement results following contrast administration (Fig. 7–4*B*).[19] Small areas of low attenuation, representing areas of cystic degeneration or tumoral necrosis, may persist following enhancement.

On MRI, the tumor extent is best visualized in the sagittal and axial projections. In the axial projection, the tumor appears well demarcated from the surrounding cerebellum. It is, however, the sagittal projection that best demonstrates the relationship of the tumor to the fourth ventricle. The tumor arises within the roof of the fourth ventricle and lies posterior to the superior medullary velum. The ventricle is often identified as a crescent-shaped CSF collection anterior and superior, but not posterior, to the mass (Fig. 7–5*A* and 5*B*). This relationship is important in differentiating medulloblastoma from ependymoma, which is intraventricular and

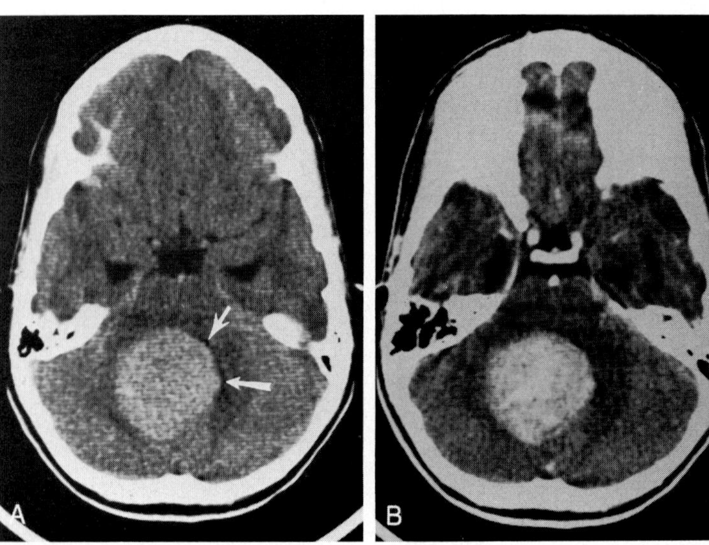


**Figure 7–4. Medulloblastoma.** *A,* A well-demarcated hyperdense midline mass lies posterior to the fourth ventricle (arrows). *B,* Intense homogeneous enhancement follows contrast administration.

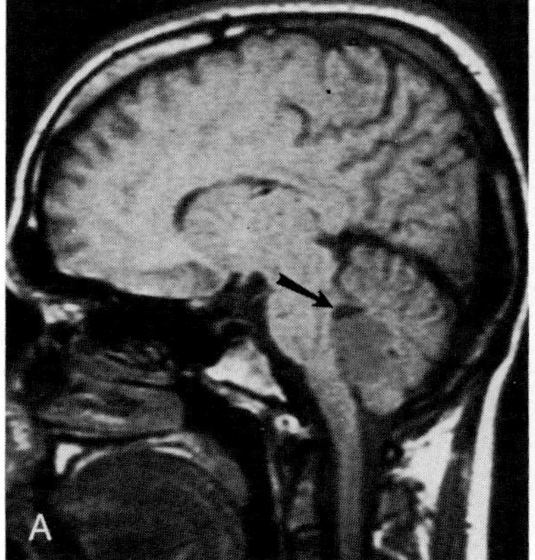


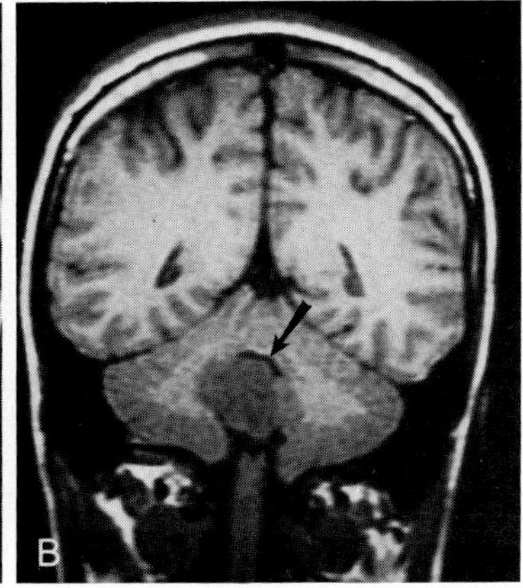


**Figure 7–5. Medulloblastoma.** *A* and *B*, Sagittal and coronal T1WI (TR 600 msec/TE 20 msec). In *A*, a homogeneous hypointense mass lies inferior and posterior to the fourth ventricle (arrow). *B*, On coronal section the relationship of the mass to the fourth ventricle is again identified (arrow). See CT in Fig. 7–4.

from brain stem glioma, which is anterior to the fourth ventricle. Coronal sections are occasionally necessary to detect supratentorial leptomeningeal metastasis, or inferior extension through foramen magnum.

On a T1WI, the tumor is hypointense, but has a T1 relaxation that is generally shorter than that of CSF (Fig. 7–6*A*). Although the pattern of signal within the tumor is usually homogeneous,[3] minor variations in hypointensity may exist. With medulloblastoma, the signal homogeneity is greater than that seen in ependymoma and cerebellar astrocytoma. On density-weighted images, N(H)WI, in two of three cases we have noted a higher signal, capsulelike rim in the margin of the tumor, which was not seen in patients with ependymoma or cerebellar astrocytoma (Fig. 7–6*B*). The etiology of this "pseudocapsule" is unclear, but it may prove to be an MR feature of medulloblastoma. On T2WI, the tumor displays a long T2 relaxation with homogeneous bright signal (Fig. 7–6*C*). The increase in tumor signal is variable, but areas of hypointensity are usually lacking, except in the presence of calcification or prominent tumor vascularity (without flow compensation) (Fig. 7–6*C*). Areas of necrosis or intratumoral microcyst display a more hyperintense signal than does solid tumor.

Ventricular obstruction secondary to tumor is clearly demonstrated. Increased transependymal flow is identified by its sawtooth pattern of bright signal intensity surrounding the dilated ventricular system on a T2WI. Areas of cerebrospinal fluid flow void (CSFV) may be lacking in the third ventricle

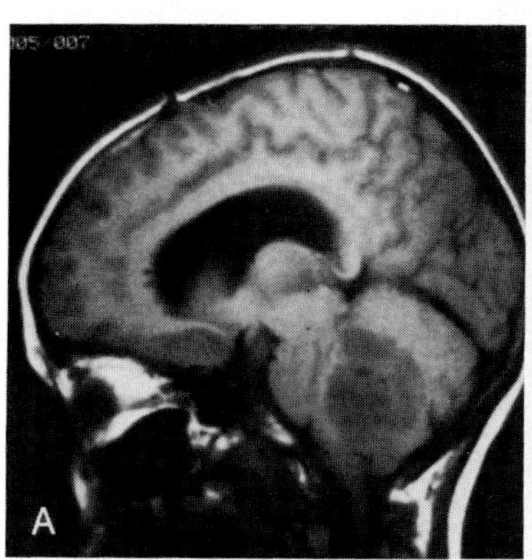


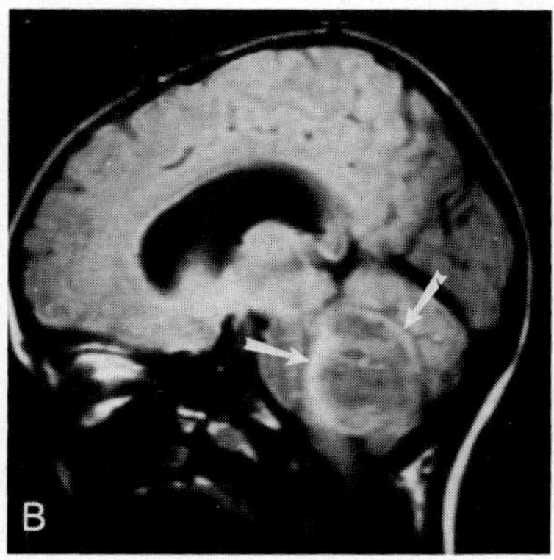


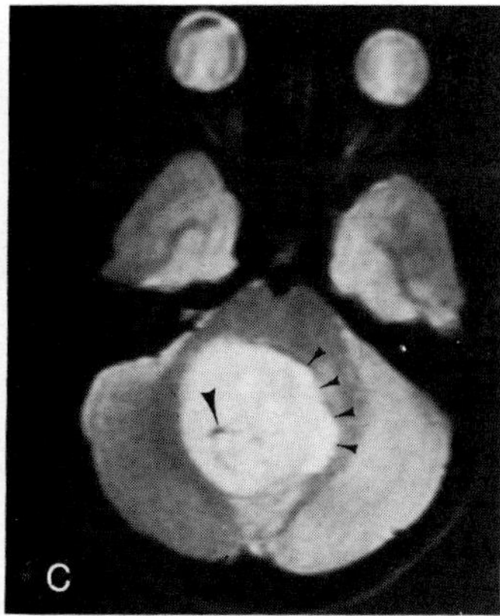


**Figure 7–6. Medulloblastoma.** *A*, Sagittal T1WI (TR 600 msec/TE 20 msec). The tumor is hypointense, relatively homogeneous, and lies posterior to the pons and medulla. *B*, Sagittal N(H)WI (TR 2000 msec/TE 20 msec). Note the presence of a hyperintense capsulelike rim in the margin of the tumor (arrows). *C*, Axial T2WI (TR 2000 msec/TE 100 msec). The tumor is homogeneous and hyperintense. A prominent vessel is identified deep within the tumor (large arrowhead). The fourth ventricle appears as a bright rim anterior and lateral to the tumor (small arrowheads).

if high-grade obstruction is present but remain prominent in the upper fourth ventricle or in the ventricle surrounding the tumor, owing to increased CSF pulsation in these areas.

## Brain Stem Gliomas

Brain stem glioma is a neuroectodermal tumor arising in the brain stem or the midbrain and may involve the posterior thalamus or upper cervical cord. These gliomas usually occur between the ages of 6 and 8 years, with an equal incidence in males and females.[20] The typical clinical presentation includes cranial nerve deficits, gait abnormalities, long-tract signs, and nystagmus. Hydrocephalus occurs less frequently and later than with other posterior fossa masses.[21] When hydrocephalus is present, the initial clinical features are often the result of the signs and symptoms of increased intracranial pressure. Rarely, patients may present with seizures alone.[22]

In the past, we have relied primarily on CT to diagnose brain stem glioma; however, visualization of the tumor has often been difficult owing to the presence of beam-hardening intrapetrous artifact. On an unenhanced scan, the involved brain stem is usually enlarged and can be either hypodense or isodense (Fig. 7–7*A*).[23, 24] Enlargement is indicated by posterior displacement of the fourth ventricle and compression of the surrounding cisterns.[23, 24] The basilar artery is often displaced anteriorly and laterally and is rarely encased. If greater than 50% of the basilar artery is covered by brain stem tissue, a brain stem mass is suggested. Alterations in the shape of the brain stem can also indicate the presence of tumor. Calcification within the tumor is rare and when present does not necessarily indicate a more benign process.[25] On occasion, extra-axial (exophytic) tumor, cyst, or both may extend from the brain stem. On a contrast-enhanced examination, the tumor enhances to varying degrees. In general, intra-axial tumors remain hypodense or isodense; however, portions of the mass, including exophytic tumor, may variably enhance. Although the size of the tumor may decrease following therapy, the enhancement pattern may remain unaltered.[26]

MRI is not susceptible to beam-hardening artifacts. Superb anatomic detail, combined with the ability to differentiate tissues, based on T1 and T2 characteristics, make MRI a superior modality for evaluating lesions of the brain stem. The sagittal and coronal projections are best for delineating the extent of involvement, especially inferior extension through foramen magnum (Fig. 7–8). The axial projection is helpful in detecting brain stem aysmmetry, alterations in brain stem size, and exophytic tumor extension into the lateral cisterns (e.g., cerebellopontine angle cistern). Occasionally, exophytic tumor may grow posterior to the fourth ventricle into the cisterna magna (Fig. 7–9). Sagittal MRI is likely superior to CT in differentiating

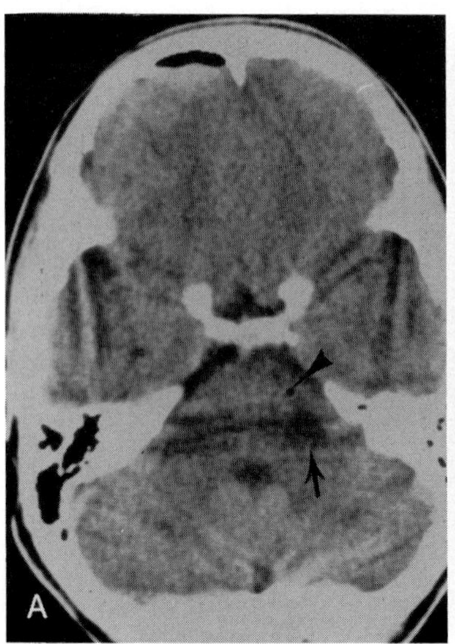


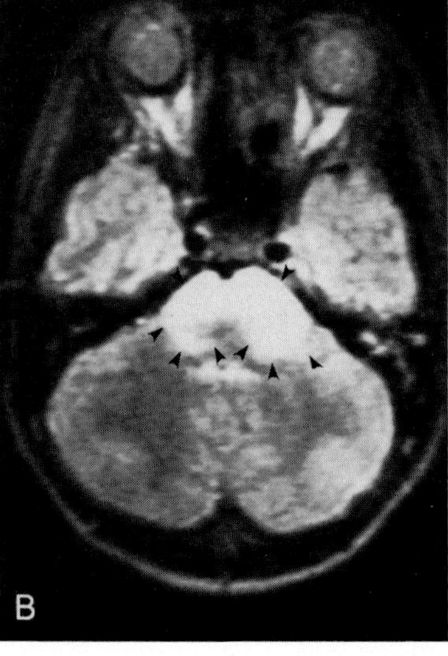


**Figure 7–7. Brain stem glioma.** *A,* Beam-hardening artifact partially obscures the brain stem, which is normal in density except for a hypodense area on the left (arrow). A stereotactic biopsy revealed a brain stem glioma (arrowhead). *B,* Axial T2WI (TR 2000 msec/TE 100 msec). The tumor is homogeneous and markedly hyperintense (arrowheads). The extent of tumor identified on MRI includes areas normal on the CT.

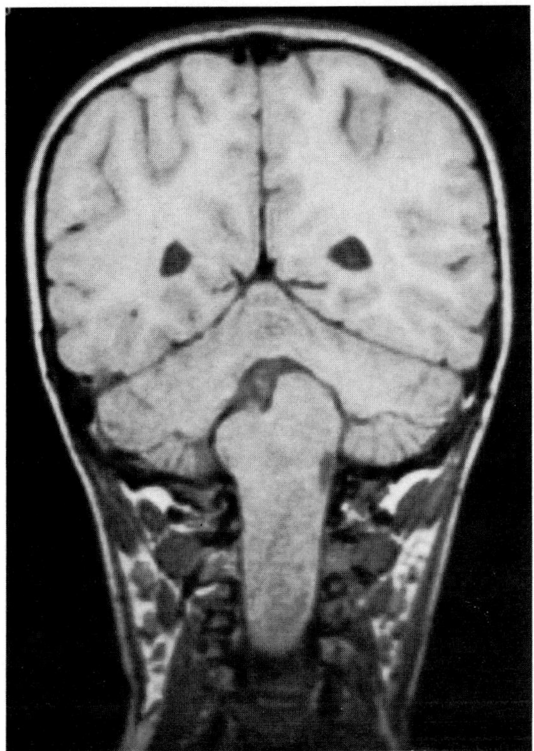

**Figure 7–8. Brain stem glioma.** Coronal T1WI (TR 800 msec/TE 20 msec). This projection provides optimal visualization of the isointense brain stem glioma, which extends below the foramen magnum to involve the upper cervical cord.

brain stem glioma from intraventricular ependymomas and midline vermian astrocytomas, both of which may secondarily involve the brain stem.

On a T1WI, brain stem gliomas are homogeneous, hypointense, and appear well demarcated from normal adjacent brain.[27] Because of its prolonged T1 relaxation, visualization can be improved with IR imaging; however, this is generally unnecessary unless the tumor is isointense on an SE/T1WI. Rarely, hemorrhage into the tumor produces focal areas of high signal on T1WI. Tumoral cysts are identified by their longer T1 relaxation when compared with the solid tumor (Fig. 7–10). Exophytic tumor is hypointense but also displays a shorter T1 relaxation compared with the surrounding CSF. On T2WI, the tumor is typically homogeneous and hyperintense in signal (Fig. 7–7*B*).[5, 27] Rarely, small focal areas within the tumor may remain isointense. Whether these areas represent variations in tumor cellularity or areas of normal brain adjacent to tumor is unclear. As might be expected, the T2 relaxation of the tumoral cyst can be greater than or equal to that of solid tumor.[3] Exophytic tumor also appears bright on a T2WI. Problems can arise in separating exophytic tumor from surrounding CSF (Fig. 7–9C); however, because of subtle differences in T2 relaxation, they can usually be separated on intermediate-weighted images.

MRI is clearly superior to CT in demonstrating the extent of involvement of brain stem gliomas for purposes of radiation treatment planning (Fig. 7–11).[28] In a series reported by Zimmerman and co-workers, 82% of brain stem gliomas involved the pons and medulla, followed by the midbrain, 59%; the

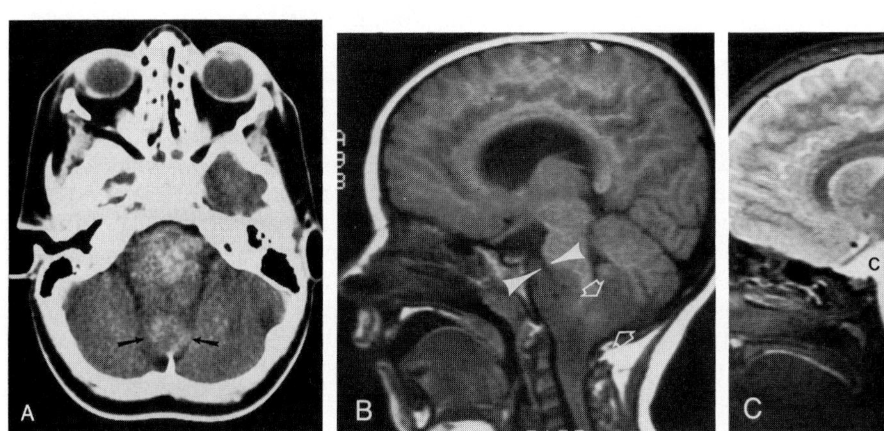


**Figure 7–9. Exophytic brain stem glioma.** *A,* On CECT the brain stem is enlarged, irregular, and minimally enhances owing to tumor infiltration. A second mass lies posterior to the brain stem (arrows), suggesting the presence of exophytic tumor. *B,* Sagittal T1WI (TR 800 msec/TE 20 msec). The tumor is hypointense. Hypointense exophytic tumor envelops the basilar artery anteriorly (arrowheads), with posterior extension (open arrows) into the cisterna magna. *C,* Sagittal T2WI (TR 2000 msec/TE 100 msec). Both exophytic and intra-axial tumor are hyperintense. Difficulty arises in separating exophytic tumor anteriorly (T) from surrounding CSF (C).

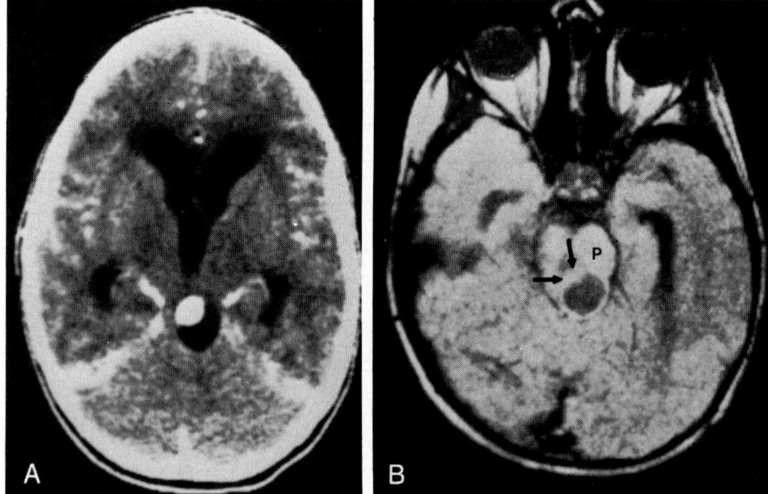


**Figure 7–10. Cystic brain stem glioma.** *A,* A well-demarcated cyst lies adjacent to an enhancing mural nodule of the upper brain stem and lower midbrain. *B,* Axial N(H)WI (TR 2000 msec/TE 30 msec). The left pons (P) is enlarged and mildly hyperintense, indicating the presence of tumor. Note that the mural nodule is relatively isointense (arrows). The cyst displays a prolonged T1-relaxation compared with solid tumor.

cerebellum, 41%; the upper cervical cord, 35%; and the posterior thalamus 29%.[29] Bradac and associates reported a reduction in tumor mass and a tendency to normalize signal within the tumor following therapy, findings they believed correlated well with clinical improvement.[27] Calcification may also develop within the brain stem following radiation therapy, and may be large enough to produce areas of signal hypointensity. We now consider MRI the modality of choice for long-term follow-up of brain stem tumors for which new chemotherapeutic and radiation treatment regimens offer potential improvement in long-term survival.[28]

## Ependymoma

Ependymomas account for approximately 6% to 12% of intracranial neoplasms in children and have a peak incidence between 4 and 5 years of age. Males are more often affected than females. Ependymomas arise within rests of ependymal cells and therefore can occur anywhere within the craniospinal axis.[30, 31] In practice, ependymomas arise as intraventricular tumors of the posterior fossa, supratentorially or within the spinal canal, in decreasing order of frequency.[30] Ependymomas of the third or fourth ventricle are more common in children under the age of 10 years.[31] In older children and adults, lateral ventricular, hemispheric, and spinal cord tumors predominate. The clinical presentation depends on tumor location. Tumors within the posterior fossa usually are manifested by nuchal pain, rigidity, headache, nausea, vomiting, gait disturbances, cranial nerve palsies, and nystagmus. There are no clinical features that differentiate this tumor from other posterior fossa masses.

The typical appearance on CT is that of a midline or slightly eccentric mass that lies within and obstructs the fourth ventricle.[32] Not infrequently, the tumor grows out of the fourth ventricle into the vermis, surrounding cisterns, brain stem, or cerebellar hemisphere. On an unenhanced CT, calcification or ossification is present in approximately 50% of patients (Fig. 7–12).[32, 33] The tumor may be hypodense or isodense. Rarely, as in medulloblastoma, it is hyperdense. Following intravenous contrast, there is moderate, inhomogeneous enhancement. Within the lesion, areas representing tissue necrosis or cyst formation may fail to enhance. The tumor often appears surrounded by a "halo" of low attenuation (CSF and peritumoral edema). The low attenuation of the "halo" indicates its intraventricular location (Fig. 7–12); however, this finding is nonspecific and is seen infrequently with intraventricular extension of medulloblastoma or cerebellar astrocytoma.

On MRI, the sagittal and axial projections provide the most accurate anatomic repre-

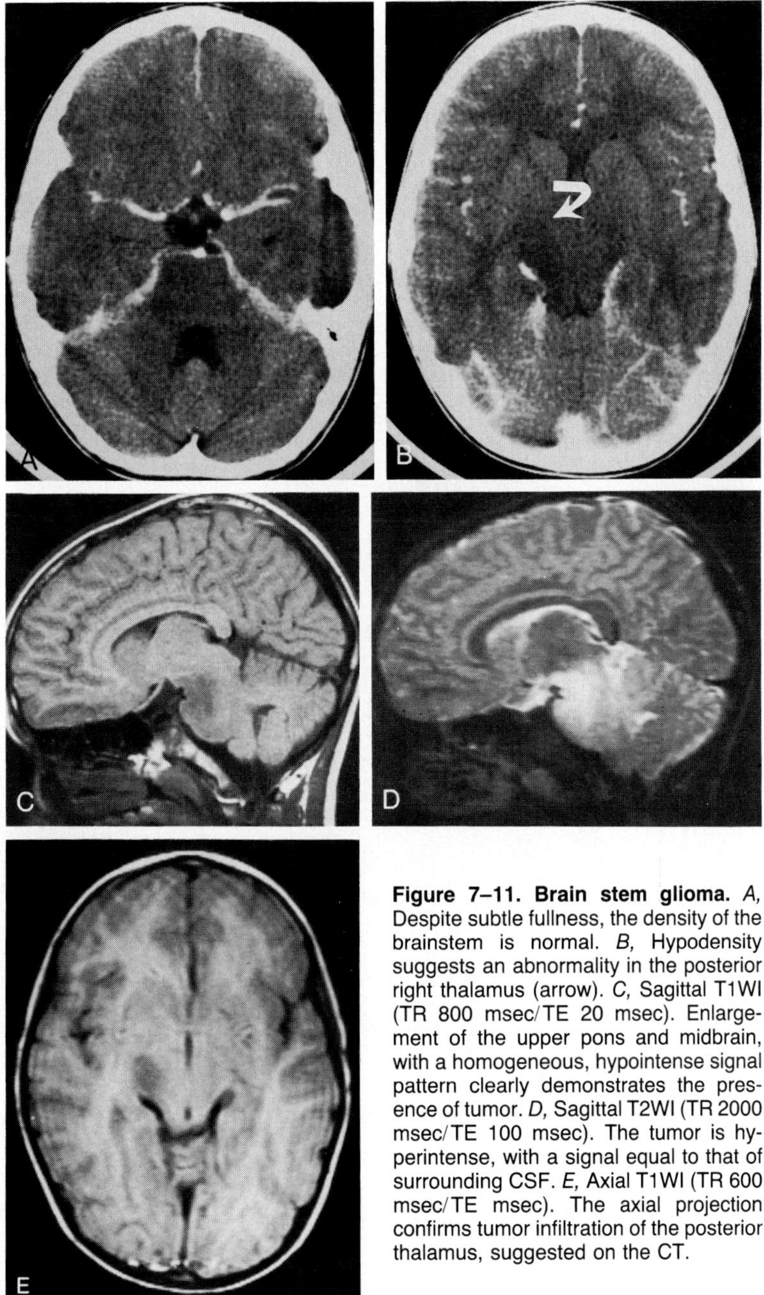


**Figure 7–11. Brain stem glioma.** *A,* Despite subtle fullness, the density of the brainstem is normal. *B,* Hypodensity suggests an abnormality in the posterior right thalamus (arrow). *C,* Sagittal T1WI (TR 800 msec/TE 20 msec). Enlargement of the upper pons and midbrain, with a homogeneous, hypointense signal pattern clearly demonstrates the presence of tumor. *D,* Sagittal T2WI (TR 2000 msec/TE 100 msec). The tumor is hyperintense, with a signal equal to that of surrounding CSF. *E,* Axial T1WI (TR 600 msec/TE msec). The axial projection confirms tumor infiltration of the posterior thalamus, suggested on the CT.

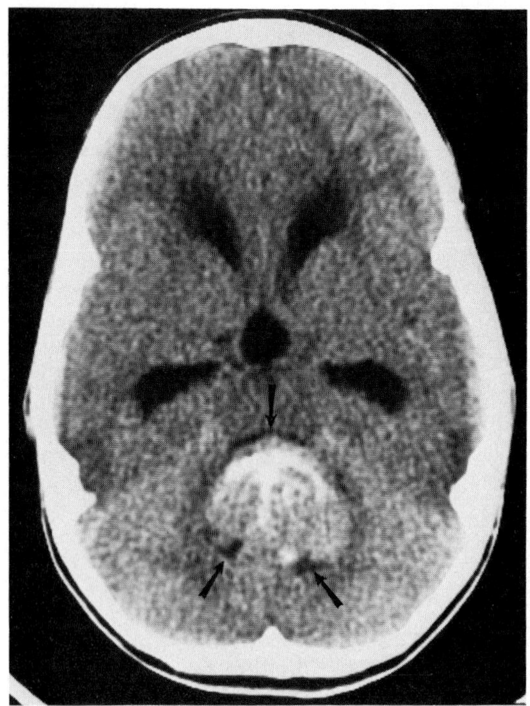

**Figure 7–12. Ependymoma.** A heavily calcified midline mass is identified in the posterior fossa. CSF anterior and posterior to the mass (arrows) indicates its intraventricular location. Moderate obstructive hydrocephalus is present.

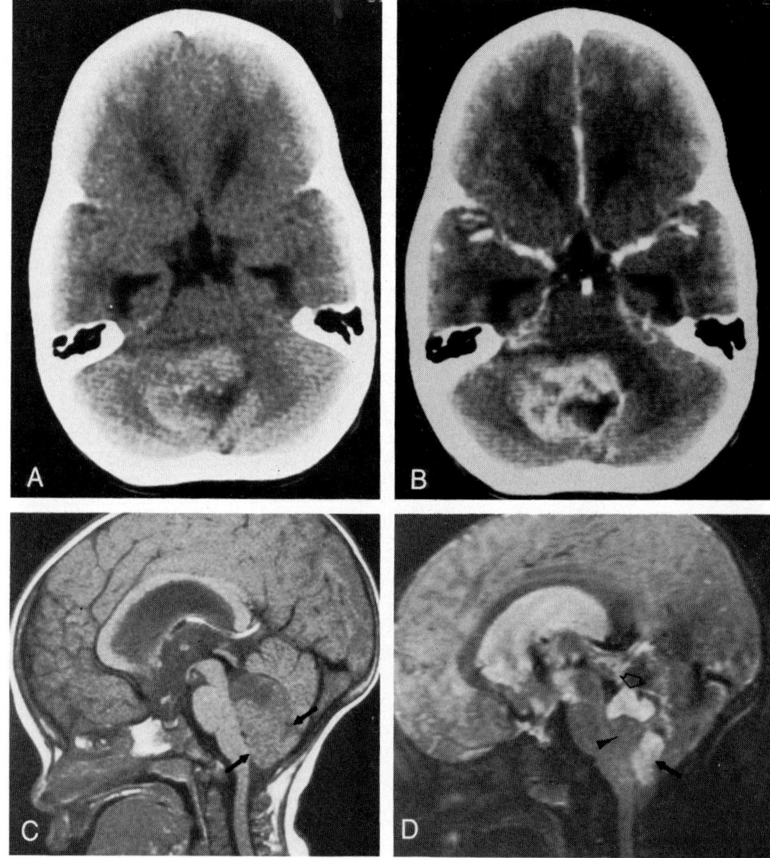


**Figure 7–13. Ependymoma.** *A,* The midline posterior fossa mass is mixed in attenuation, displays moderate inhomogeneous enhancement following contrast administration, *B.* *C,* Sagittal T1WI (TR 800 msec/TE 20 msec). The tumor has a mixture of hypointensity and isointensity. Note extension of the intraventricular tumor from the fourth ventricle into the cisterna magna (arrows). *D,* Sagittal T2WI (TR 2000 msec/TE 100 msec). The areas having the lowest signal intensity in *C* display the brightest signal intensity here (open arrow). Areas isointense in *C* appear both isotense (arrowhead) and moderately hyperintense (arrow) on this second echo image.

sentation of tumor. In addition, the coronal projection is helpful in evaluating extraventricular extension into cisterna magna or through the foramen magnum. On T1WI, the tumor is of mixed low signal intensity (Fig. 7–13). Areas of high signal on T1WI represent intratumoral hemorrhage (Fig. 7–14). The fourth ventricle can be identified as a thin rim of hypointense signal surrounding the tumor (Fig. 7–15). In general, the tumor is hyperintense on a T2WI; however, the degree of hyperintensity varies, depending on whether the tumor is cystic or solid (Fig. 7–16). Isointense areas may remain interspersed between areas of prolonged T2-relaxation. One such tumor that remained predominantly isointense in our series contained extensive calcification and ossification, which may account in part for its shorter T2 relaxation (Fig. 7–17). In our limited experience, exophytic tumor is of moderate hyperintensity and may require intermediate-weighted images to differentiate it from surrounding CSF. Overall, the amount of signal inhomogeneity within ependymomas was greater than that seen with medulloblastoma or brain stem glioma but was similar to that of cerebellar astrocytoma.

Gradient echo imaging aids in the identification of calcification within the tumor and helps identify engorged tumor vascularity in or around the periphery of the tumor before surgical intervention. The upper fourth ventricle and portions of the fourth ventricle draped around the tumor display prominent signal hypointensity owing to increased pulsatile flow adjacent to the tumor.

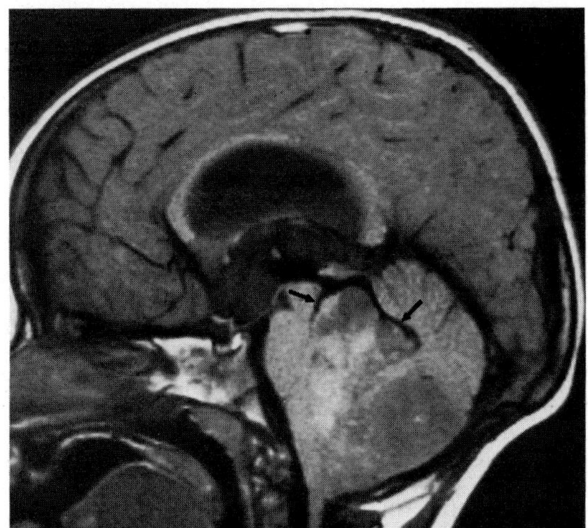

**Figure 7–14. Hemorrhagic ependymoma.** Sagittal T1WI (TR 600 msec/TE 20 msec). A large intraventricular mass is present with the fourth ventricle lying both anterior and posterior to the mass (arrows). High signal within the mass indicates previous hemorrhage.

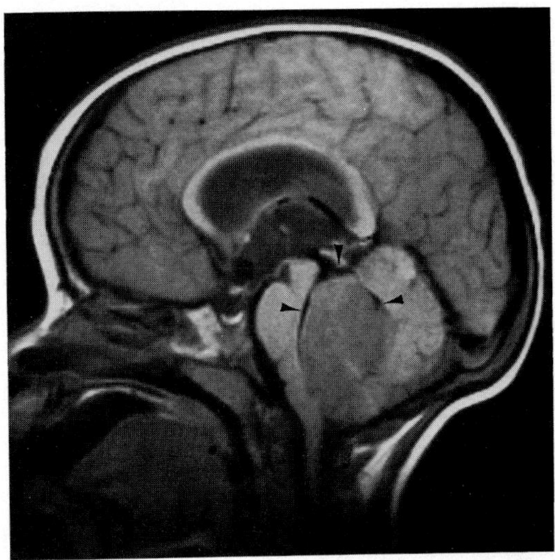

**Figure 7–15. Ependymoma.** Sagittal N(H)WI (TR 2000 msec/TE 20 msec). The fourth ventricle lies anterior, superior, and posterior (arrowheads), indicating the mass is intraventricular.

In our experience, tumors classified as primitive neuroectodermal tumors of the posterior fossa have features on MRI similar to ependymoma or astrocytoma, from which they were indistinguishable.

### Other

As previously stated, a variety of less common tumors arise in the posterior fossa in children. Hemangioblastoma, epidermoid, acoustic neuroma, and meningioma all have been reported.[14] Their features on MRI are similar to those described in adults and are discussed elsewhere in the text.

Chordoma and chondrosarcoma may present as a posterior mass arising in the clivus or petrous ridge in children.[34] Chordomas arise from notocordal remnants and are most frequent in the sacrum or clivus. They typically occur in the second decade of life but have been reported in a 4-month-old infant.[35] Patients present with cranial nerve abnormalities in ways similar to brain stem glioma. The sixth nerve, because of its close proximity to the tumor, is invariably involved. CT usually reveals a soft tissue mass extending from the superior or posterior sur-

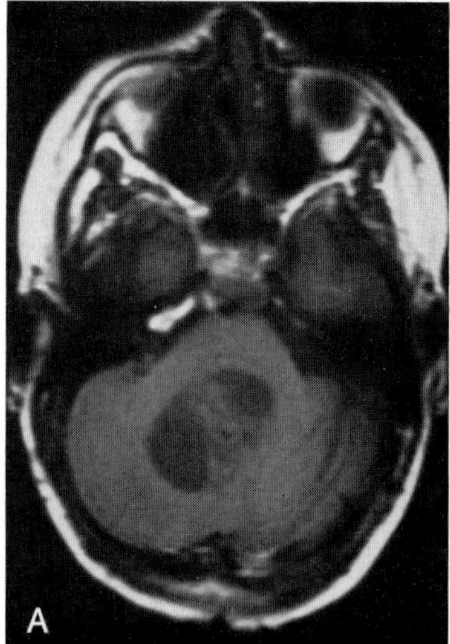


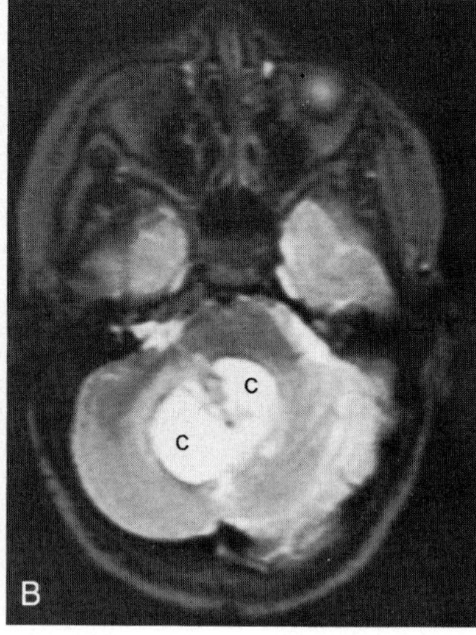


**Figure 7–16. Ependymoma.** *A,* Axial T1WI (TR 600 msec/TE 20 msec). Well-demarcated areas of marked hypointensity (tumor cyst) surround an isointense area of solid tumor. *B,* Axial T2WI (TR 2000 msec/TE 100 msec). The tumoral cysts (C) are markedly hyperintense, whereas the solid component remains isointense.

face of the clivus that is associated with gross bone destruction. Calcification is present in approximately half of these tumors. The mass is inhomogeneous with low attenuation; however, acute hemorrhage may produce areas of high attenuation within the tumor. Following intravenous contrast, the mass moderately enhances; however, a pattern of septated enhancement around areas of low attenuation (tumor necrosis or hemorrhage) has been reported.[36]

Chordomas or chondrosarcomas of the clivus are best imaged on MR in the sagittal projection. Imaging in the axial or coronal projections may be necessary to evaluate for anterior extension into the cavernous sinus, the sella turcica, or the suprasellar cistern. Posteriorly, the tumor may extend into the posterior fossa and displace or compress the brain stem (Fig. 7–18). Inferior extension into the nasopharynx through the body of the clivus can also occur. The tumors are generally of mixed signal intensity on a T1WI. In general, the tumor is mildly hypointense or isointense. Portions of the tumor that have undergone tissue necrosis have a more prolonged T1 relaxation. Areas of short T1-relaxation may indicate the presence of previous hemorrhage (Fig. 7–18). Calcification is identified as areas of marked

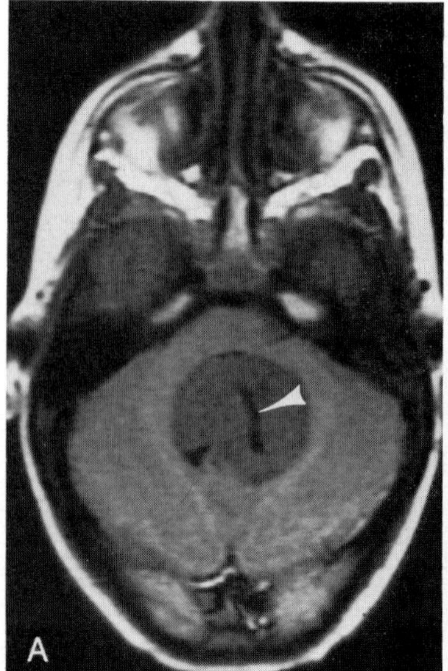


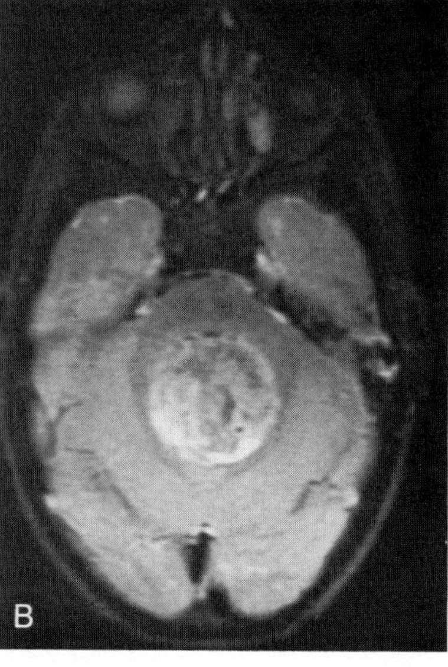


**Figure 7–17. Ependymoma.** *A,* Axial N(H)WI (TR 2000 msec/TE 20 msec). A prominent vessel courses through the mass (arrowhead). *B,* Axial T2WI (TR 2000 msec/TE 80 msec). The tumor remains predominantly isointense on the second echo. Pathologic sections revealed a large amount of punctate calcification and ossification throughout the tumor, which may have contributed to a shorter T2-relaxation time.

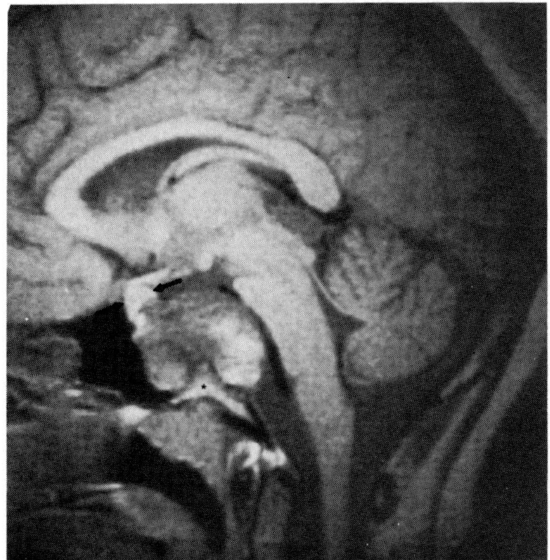

**Figure 7–18. Chordoma.** Sagittal T1WI (TR 800 msec/TE 20 msec). A well-circumscribed mass drapes over a partially destroyed clivus (asterisk). The pons is flattened, and the pituitary gland is displaced anteriorly (arrows). High signal in the posterior half of the mass represents hemorrhage, confirmed at surgery.

signal loss. An inhomogeneous pattern of variable hyperintensity occurs on the T2WI, and some areas may remain isointense. If a prolonged T2 relaxation is present within the chordoma, this may help separate it from meningioma, which is generally isointense on a T2-weighted sequence. The location of the tumor, the lack of a cyst, and the mixed inhomogeneous signal of the tumor, can help differentiate a chordoma from a craniopharyngioma growing posteriorly over the clivus.

## SUPRATENTORIAL TUMORS

Primary supratentorial tumors are a diverse group of neoplasms that vary widely in site of origin and cell type. Numerous classifications have been devised for categorizing supratentorial tumors by histology, tissue of origin, location, and response to therapy. We have found that identifying tumors by location is best suited to cross-sectional imaging. For the purpose of discussion, we have divided the supratentorial tumors into three primary regions of interest: the sella-suprasellar region, the pineal region, and the cerebral hemispheres. Within each region, there is a predilection for certain tumor types, although considerable overlap exists.

### Sella-Suprasellar Region

In children, the most common tumors arising within the sella-suprasellar area include craniopharyngioma, optic nerve glioma, hypothalamic glioma, pituitary adenoma, germinoma, teratoma, and Rathke's cleft cyst. Masses arising within this region may produce a variety of clinical signs and symptoms that are neurologic, visual, or secondary to endocrine dysfunction. Hydrocephalus secondary to obstruction of the posterior third ventricle or aqueduct of Sylvius results in increased intracranial pressure. Symptoms are nonspecific and include nausea, vomiting, headache, and irritability. Visual deficits arise from direct tumor involvement of the optic nerves and chiasm (e.g., optic nerve glioma) or are secondary to compression of the chiasm via local expansion. In the growing child, endocrinologic dysfunction is a frequent presentation. Dysfunction arises from neoplastic involvement of the hypothalamus, pituitary stalk, or pituitary gland. Diabetes insipidus, growth delay or advancement, amenorrhea, precocious puberty, and hypoprolactinemia all result from compression or infiltration by tumor of the hypothalamic-pituitary axis.

The pathologic features of the sella-suprasellar tumors are as diverse as the clinical features they produce. In the pediatric age group, a mass arising within the sella is most likely a craniopharyngioma, a Rathke's cleft cyst, or a pituitary adenoma. In the suprasellar cistern, craniopharyngiomas are most common, followed by chiasmatic gliomas, hypothalamic gliomas, germinomas, and teratomas.

### Craniopharyngioma

Craniopharyngiomas are epithelial tumors arising from squamous cell rests within the pars tuberalis of Rathke's pouch.[37] Their peak incidence lies between the ages of 5 and 10 years. The histologic features of craniopharyngioma vary, but they are generally benign, slow-growing neoplasms that compress but do not invade contiguous structures. The three primary features of craniopharyngioma are location (sella only: 4% to

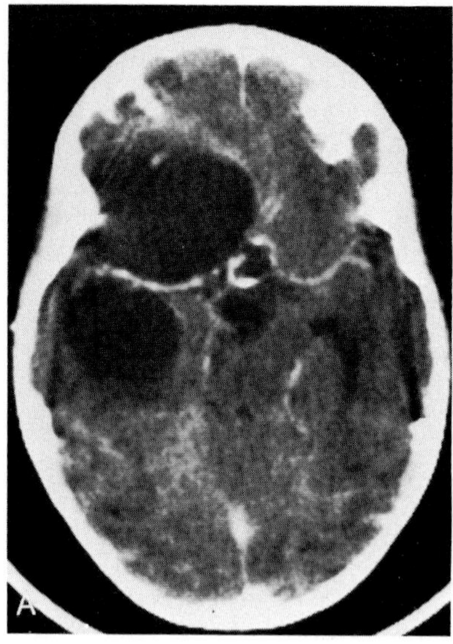


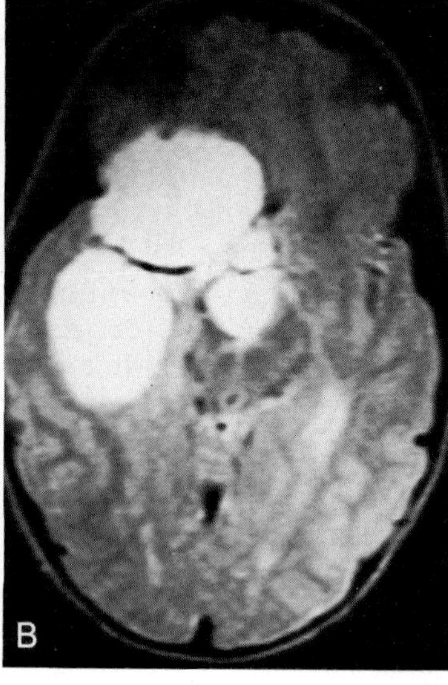


**Figure 7–19. Cystic craniopharyngioma.** *A,* Multilobulated cysts arising from a suprasellar tumor involve the suprasellar region and the anterior and middle cranial fossae. *B,* Axial T2WI (TR 2000 msec/TE 100 msec). The cysts are hyperintense, consistent with their proteinaceous contents. The middle cerebral artery is represented by a signal void as a result of flowing blood.

5%; sella and suprasellar region: 15%; suprasellar region only: 80%), presence of a suprasellar cyst (85%), and calcification (75%), most frequently found within the wall of the cyst.[38]

The location and extent of the tumor is best assessed in the sagittal and coronal projections. This predominantly suprasellar lesion may grow inferiorly into the sella, anteriorly into the anterior cranial fossa, laterally into the middle cranial fossa, superiorly into the hypothalamus and floor of the third ventricle, and posteriorly over the clivus. MRI is superior to CT in defining the extent of tumor before surgical intervention and in determining the most appropriate surgical approach. The tumor is defined by its relationship to the optic chiasm as being prechiasmatic (anterior), postchiasmatic (posterior), or both. In addition, T1WI and T2WI sequences are helpful in demonstrating the relationship of the tumor to adjacent vessels, obviating the need for a preoperative angiogram.

A tumoral cyst is present in 85% of craniopharyngiomas.[39] The cyst may grow rapidly and become quite large, expanding into the anterior and middle cranial fossas (Fig. 7–19). In one case, we have witnessed the development of a large tumoral cyst adjacent to a solid craniopharyngioma in a span of only two weeks. Often, the cyst appears to drape around or be indented by contiguous structures that help identify it as being fluid filled (Fig. 17–20). The contents of the cyst contain varying amounts of cholesterol and protein-rich keratin debris. Zimmerman has pointed out that the relative proportions of cholesterol (short T1 relaxation, short T2 relaxation) (Fig. 7–21), and keratin debris (intermediate T1 relaxation, long T2 relaxation) will determine the appearance of the tumor cyst on MRI.[40] This likely explains the wide variety of appearances reported

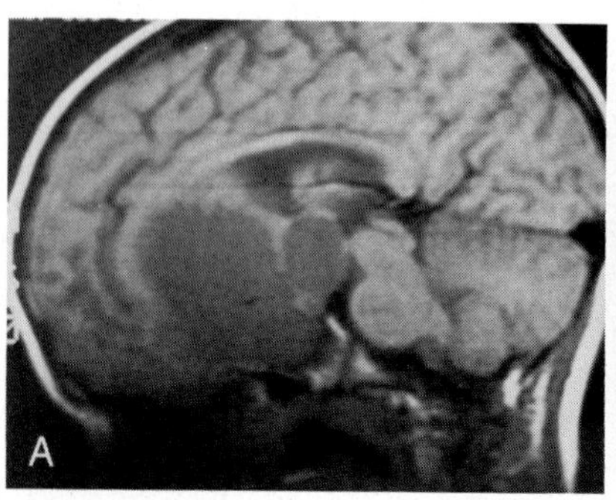


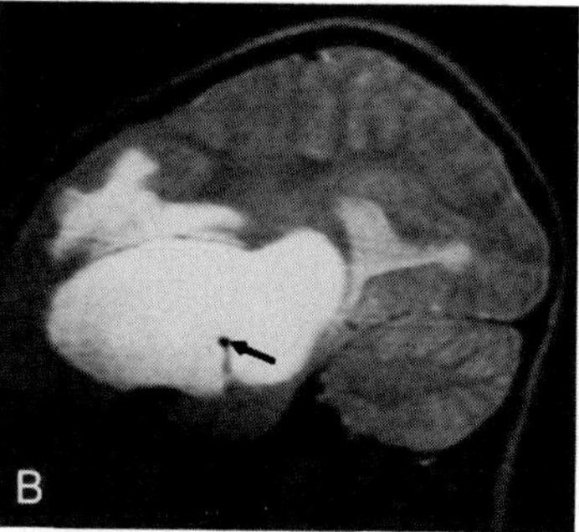


**Figure 7–20. Cystic craniopharyngioma.** *A,* Sagittal N(H)WI (TR 2000 msec/TE 20 msec). A multilobulated cystic mass extends from the suprasellar region anteriorly into the anterior cranial fossa and superiorly into the floor of the third ventricle. *B,* Sagittal T2WI (TR 2000 msec/TE 100 msec). The cyst drapes around the middle cerebral artery like a water bag (arrow).

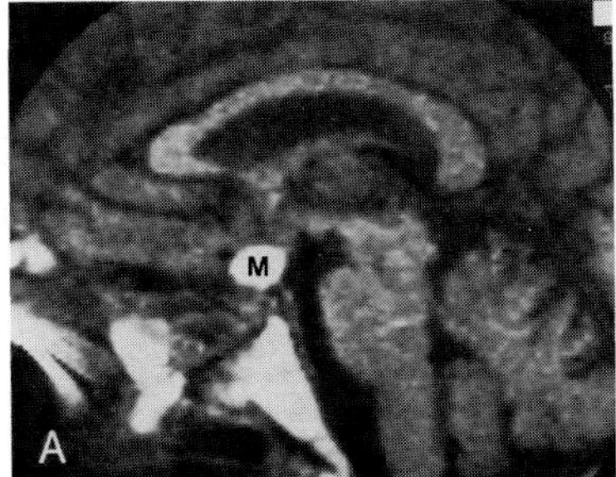


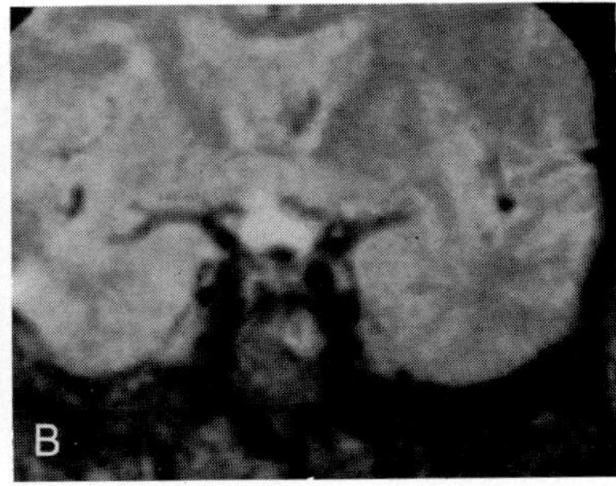


**Figure 7–21. Craniopharyngioma.** *A,* Sagittal T1WI (TR 600 msec/TE 20 msec). A well-demarcated hyperintense mass (M) is identified in the suprasellar cistern. *B,* Coronal N(H)WI (TR 2000 msec/TE 20 msec). The cyst appears to minimally decrease in signal intensity on the intermediate-weighted image. This appearance is best explained by the presence of cholesterol or previous hemorrhage within the cyst.

with craniopharyngioma on MRI. Further confusion arises if there is hemorrhage into the cyst.[41] Solid tumor is differentiated from the cystic component by its shorter T1 relaxation. Not infrequently, the solid component is often isointense or slightly hyperintense on a T1WI (Fig. 7–22).[41, 42] Although both the cyst and the solid tumor can be hyperintense on T2WI, the longer T2 relaxation of the proteinaceous cyst is helpful in differentiating the two.

Identification of calcium within the tumor has been a problem on MRI.[11] The use of gradient echo imaging (GRASS) with a short TR sequence improves the detection of calcification because of greater magnetic susceptibility. The detection of calcification is often unnecessary in the presence of other criteria, such as location and a tumoral cyst; however, similar signal characteristics on MRI may prevent differentiation of craniopharyngioma from a suprasellar dermoid tumor or teratoma. Suprasellar chiasmatic or hypothalamic gliomas may contain cystic areas and can mimic a craniopharyngioma. Finally, differentiation of an intrasellar craniopharyngioma from a Rathke's cleft cyst may not be possible on MRI alone.[43]

## Rathke's Cleft Cyst

A Rathke's cleft cyst represents a remnant of the cephalad invagination of Rathke's pouch.[43] The cyst is lined by a single layer of columnar or cuboidal epithelium that secretes mucus or colloid material.[44] The cyst rarely is symptomatic; however, when it is large, compression of surrounding structures may result in headaches, visual disturbances, or hypopituitarism.[44, 45] Rathke's cysts are predominantly intrasellar, but larger lesions can expand into the suprasellar space. Rarely, the cyst is completely suprasellar. The walls of the cyst are smooth, well defined, and do not contain calcium.

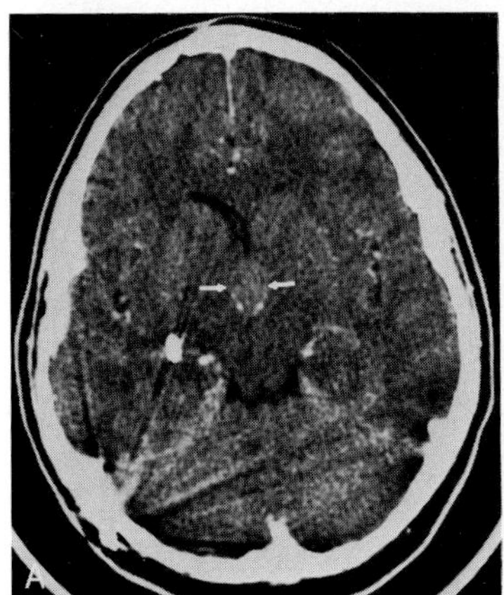

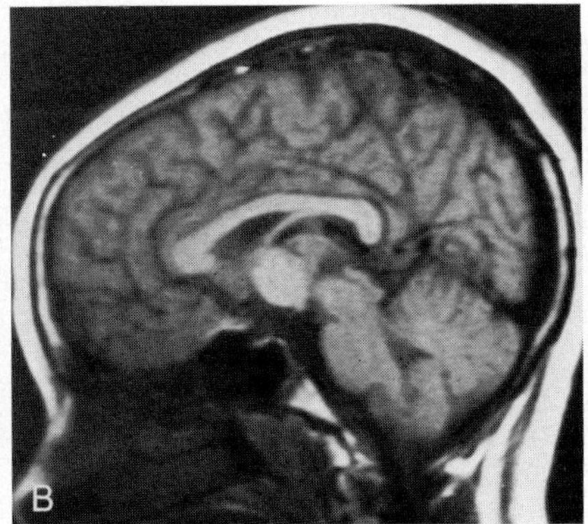


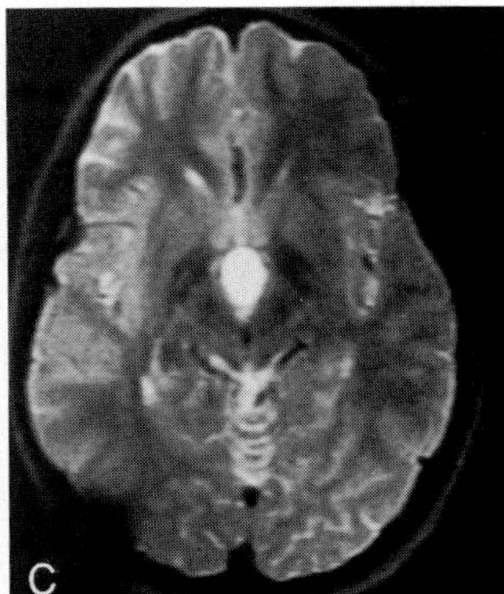


**Figure 7–22. Recurrent solid craniopharyngioma.** *A,* A solid midline mass occupies the region of the third ventricle (arrows). *B,* Sagittal T1WI (TR 800 msec/TE 20 msec). The mass appears slightly hyperintense. Its relationship to the third ventricle and suprasellar cistern is clearly demonstrated. *C,* Axial T2WI (TR 2000 msec/TE 100 msec). Marked signal hyperintensity emanates from the mass on this second echo image.

Because both Rathke's cleft cyst and craniopharyngioma arise from remnants of Rathke's pouch, it is not surprising that they demonstrate similar variations in signal intensity.

Kucharczyk reported two patterns in signal intensity eminating from Rathke's cleft cyst on MRI.[46] In the first type, the signal intensity was similar to that of CSF, with long T1 and T2 relaxations. He suggested that this pattern was best explained by the presence of serous fluid within the cyst. Such lesions are difficult to distinguish from suprasellar or intrasellar arachnoid cysts. In the second type, hyperintense signal was present on both T1WI and T2WI; Kucharczyk believed this circumstance was due to the presence of mucoid material. Hemorrhage into the cyst may have been partially responsible for this pattern. We have encountered a third pattern that was hyperintense on a T1WI (short T1 relaxation), and hypointense on the T2WI (very short T2 relaxation) (Fig. 7–23). On pathologic examination, hemosiderin was found within the fluid and the wall of the cyst. The short T1 relaxation was similar in appearance to that seen with craniopharyngiomas containing high amounts of cholesterol; however, the presence of cholesterol would not explain the appearance on T2WI. Perhaps this appearance is best interpreted as resulting from a combination of old hemorrhage (hemosiderin), cholesterol, and mucoid material.

Because of the similarities in location and signal intensity between craniopharyngioma and Rathke's cleft cyst, differentiation of the two on MRI may prove difficult. The presence of an isointense solid mass adjacent to the cyst on a T1WI or N(H)WI suggests the diagnosis of craniopharyngioma. On CT a lack of calcification and a low-attenuation cystic sellar lesion displaying minimal rim enhancement would favor the diagnosis of a Rathke's cleft cyst.

Pituitary adenomas in children are rare.[47] When present, their MR appearances are similar to those seen and reported in adults; therefore the reader is referred to Chapter 10 for their description.

## Optic Nerve Glioma

Optic nerve glioma may present as either a unilateral or a bilateral orbital mass. When bilateral optic nerve gliomas are present, the diagnosis of neurofibromatosis is suggested.[48] The slow-growing tumor can arise anywhere along the optic tracts, from the orbit to the occipital lobes. Ninety-five percent of children will present in the first two decades of life, 80% under 10 years of age.[49] Typically, they present clinically with visual loss, although, rarely, visual acuity is normal. Orbital tumors can also present with proptosis. Chiasmatic gliomas and tumors involving the optic radiations manifest with

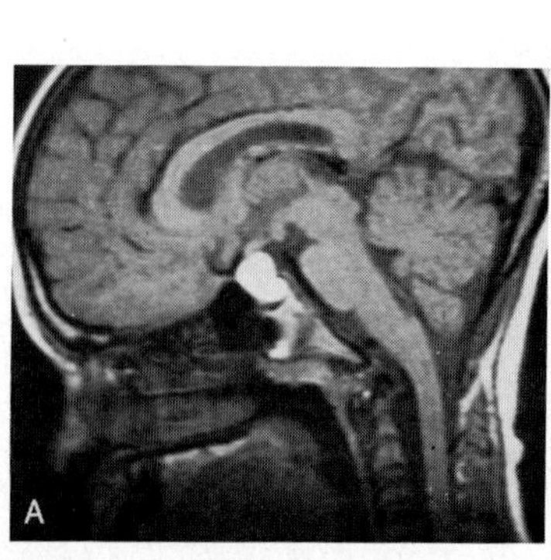


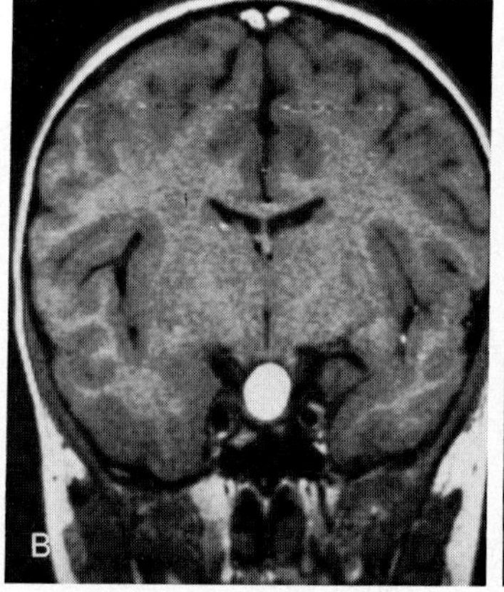


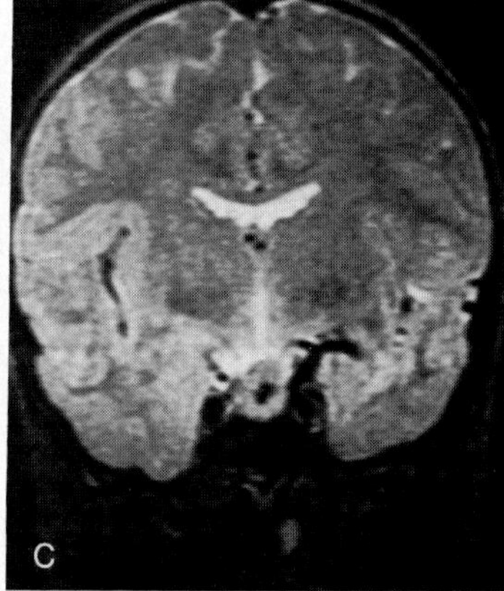


**Figure 7–23. Rathke's cleft cyst.** *A,* Sagittal T1WI (TR 600 msec/TE 20 msec). A well-defined cyst fills and expands the sella, and extends into the suprasellar cistern. The mass is markedly hyperintense and homogeneous in signal. *B,* Coronal T1WI (TR 600 msec/TE 20 msec). The mass is clearly separate from the chiasm and hypothalamus. *C,* Coronal T2WI (TR 2000/TE 100 msec). The mass decreases in signal intensity on the second echo image and contains an isointense outer layer and a hypointense inner layer. The presence of cholesterol, hemosiderin, from previous hemorrhage, or both accounts for this pattern.

visual loss and symptoms secondary to compression of adjacent structures. Savoiardo reported that in the presence of intraorbital tumor, intracanalicular and intracranial involvement is common.[50] In our experience, simultaneous intracranial involvement is uncommon. In the group of patients with neurofibromatosis, dural ectasia may also cause enlargement of the optic nerve sheaths. This enlargement can lead to the erroneous diagnosis of optic nerve glioma on CT. MRI is more sensitive than CT in differentiating optic nerve glioma from dural ectasia, which is identified as a prominent dilated subarachnoid space surrounding a normal or small optic nerve.

Within the orbit, the coronal and axial projections best demonstrate involvement of the optic nerves, whereas involvement of the chiasm may require imaging in the sagittal projection as well. Optic radiation involvement is clearly identified in the axial projection. Within the orbit, the signal intensity of an optic nerve tumor is variable on T1- and T2-weighted sequences. Cystic areas have a more prolonged T1- and T-2 relaxation when compared with solid tumor; however, the majority of tumors are solid and mildly hypointense or isointense on T1WI. On a T2-weighted sequence, the solid tumor is moderately hyperintense. Chiasmatic tumors are predominantly solid and display either hypointense or isointense signal on T1WI.[42] On T2WI the tumor is moderately hyperintense, making differentiation of tumor and surrounding CSF difficult at times. Chiasmatic tumoral cysts are more hyperintense in signal compared with solid tumor (Fig. 7–24). Infiltrative involvement of the optic radiations results in focal or diffuse high signal intensity in the distribution of the optic tracts. MRI appears to be more sensitive than CT in detecting posterior optic tract infiltration.[51]

Following radiation therapy, the appearance of both orbital and chiasmatic tumor may change. Cystic necrosis results in a more prolonged T1 and T2 relaxation in areas previously composed of isointense solid tumor. Perhaps the greatest benefit of MRI is its capability for long-term follow-up without ionizing radiation, since optic nerve gliomas must often be followed over many years in order to assess for progression and response to radiation or chemotherapy.

## Hypothalamic Glioma

The hypothalamus frequently is a site of gliomas in children.[52] Differentiation of this tumor from a chiasmatic glioma is often difficult on CT.[52] On unenhanced CT, hypothalamic gliomas appear as large amorphous masses in the floor of the third ventricle and suprasellar cistern that are low in

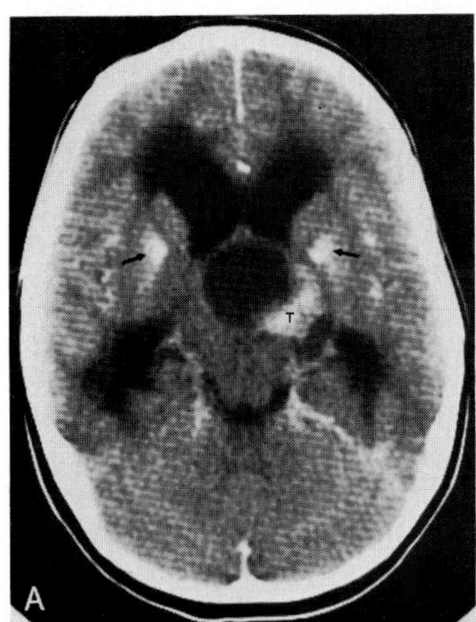


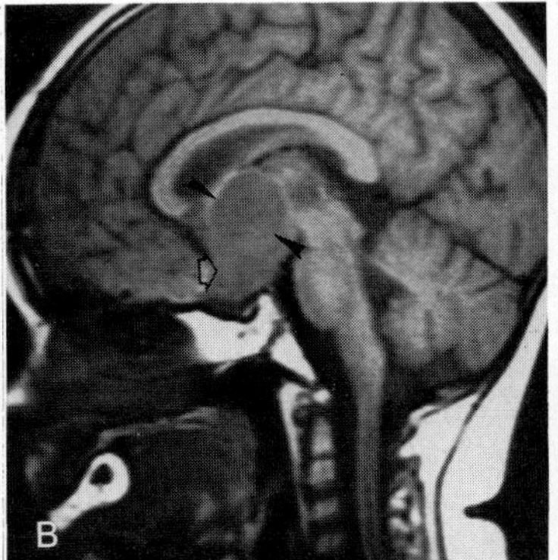


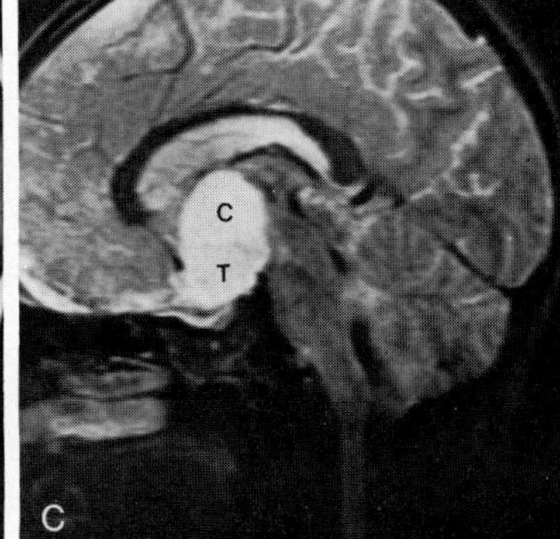


**Figure 7–24. Cystic optic nerve glioma.** *A,* Axial CECT. A large, predominantly cystic midline mass obliterates the third ventricle. Enhancement of tumor (T) is identified in the left, optic radiation. Obstructive hydrocephalus and radiation induced calcification (arrows) is present. *B,* Sagittal T1WI (TR 800 msec/TE msec). The combined solid (open arrow) and cystic (arrowheads) mass extends from the suprasellar region into the floor of the third ventricle. *C,* Sagittal T2WI (TR 2000 msec/TE 100 msec). The cystic component (C) has a brighter signal intensity compared to the solid tumor (T).

attenuation and rarely contain calcification. Intense, often homogeneous enhancement follows contrast administration. On MRI, the tissue characteristics of a hypothalamic glioma are similar to those of a chiasmatic glioma, having a prolonged T1 and T2 relaxation. Demonstration of a normal, uninvolved chiasm suggests the diagnosis of hypothalamic glioma. Involvement of the optic radiations is not a feature of hypothalamic glioma. In the presence of chiasmatic infiltration by a hypothalamic glioma, separation of the two on MRI is not possible unless orbital or optic tract tumor is also present.

### Other

Suprasellar germinomas and teratomas are rare lesions and have infrequently been reported on MRI.[53, 54] Brandt-Zawadski and Kelly described a single case of suprasellar germinoma that was isointense to gray matter on both T1WI and T2WI.[55] Germinoma may involve the hypothalamus or may appear as a mass within the pituitary stalk.[56] Teratomas and epidermoids arising in the suprasellar region have been reported. On MRI, this group may be confused with a suprasellar craniopharyngioma or cystic glioma. Teratomatous masses are categorized primarily by their mixed signal characteristics on both a T1- and T2-weighted sequence. The wide variation in signal intensity is due to the spectrum of tissue types present within these masses. Areas of fat (short T1 relaxation) may be interspersed between areas of solid tumor (isointense T1 relaxation) and proteinaceous fluid (hypointense to intermediate T1 relaxation). Epidermoid tumors do not usually contain calcium, whereas calcification is often present within a teratoma. Calcification can be identified as an area of signal loss within the tumor.

Rarely, hamartomas may develop in the tuber cinereum, resulting in precocious puberty.[57, 58] These tumors are benign, slow-growing lesions that either are hormonally active or produce endocrinologic symptoms by compressing the hypothalamus, pituitary stalk, or pituitary gland. Anatomically, the hamartoma grows from the tuber cinereum of the hypothalamus into the suprasellar cistern as a pedunculated mass lying posterior to the pituitary stalk and anterior to the mamillary bodies. The signal is slightly hypointense or isointense on a T1WI or N(H)WI (Fig. 7–25).[12] They are in general homogeneous; however, rarely mixed signal intensity is found in large tumors. On a T2WI, the hamartoma has a prolonged T2 relaxation.[12] Small tumors may be lost in the surrounding hyperintense CSF; therefore they are best demonstrated on a T1WI or N(H)WI in the sagittal or coronal projection or both. Not infrequently, the hamartoma can become quite large, resulting in displacement of the pituitary stalk anteriorly, the floor of the third ventricle superiorly, and the cerebral peduncles posteriorly. Even with significant displacement of contiguous structures, peritumoral edema is not present.

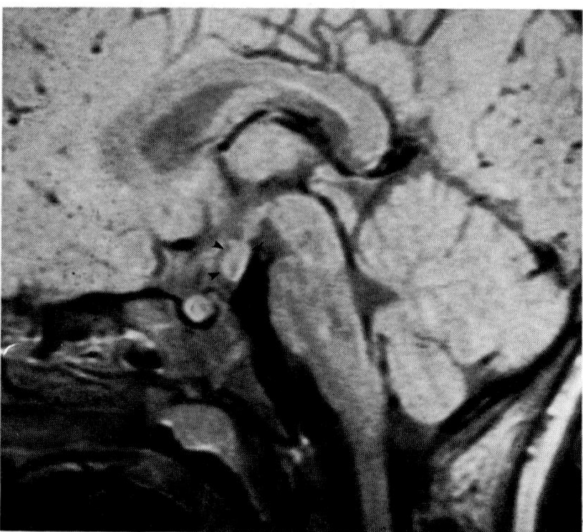

**Figure 7–25. Hamartoma of the tuber cinereum.** Sagittal N(H)WI (TR 2000 msec/TE 20 msec). An isointense pedunculated mass extends from the tuber cinereum into the suprasellar cistern (arrows). The appearance, location, and signal characteristics are consistent with a hamartoma.

### Pineal Region Lesions

The pineal region is an uncommon site for masses in childhood. The anatomy of this area is complex and functionally diverse. It includes the posterior third ventricle, the pineal gland, the tectum, the splenium of the corpus callosum, and the posterior midbrain. It is surrounded in part by the quadrigeminal cistern. The diversity of lesions occurring in this area include benign and malignant neoplasms, arachnoid cysts, and metastatic disease.[59, 60] Included in the list of benign or slow-growing tumors are hamartomas and periaqueductal gliomas, most frequently associated with neurofibromatosis. Unfortunately, the list of lesions displaying more rapid growth potential in this area is longer and consists of germ cell tumors, primary pineal cell tumors, primitive neuroectodermal tumors, gangliogliomas, and astrocytomas.[60] Astrocytomas typically arise in the posterior aspect of the corpus callosum, from the adjacent medial cortex, or from the posterior midbrain. Their appearance on MRI is similar to astrocytomas arising elsewhere within the cerebral hemispheres. Occasionally, gangliogliomas originate in the posterior floor of the third ventricle. MRI is especially helpful in separating tumors from congenital anomalies as a cause of obstruction of the sylvian aqueduct. Arachnoid cysts in the quadrigeminal cistern are rare, but when present, have features on MRI similar to arachnoid cysts arising elsewhere in the calvarium.

Advances in microsurgical techniques offer the potential for improved survival in patients with primary pineal region tumors.[60] Vorkapic and Pendl have brought to our attention the importance of accurately mapping tumors of the pineal region before surgical resection.[60] They stress the importance of cross-sectional imaging for demonstrating the relationship of the tumor to deep vascular structures. Until recently, imaging of mass lesions in the pineal region required the combination of contrast-enhanced CT and cerebral angiography. With its multiplanar capabilities, MRI is likely superior to CT for defining the extent of tumor. In addition, the ability of MRI to visualize the vascular anatomy will likely eliminate the need for cerebral angiography. Whether MRI is more sensitive than CT in determining the histologic type of tumor remains unclear.

In children, primary tumors arising within the pineal region are most likely germ cell tumors (germinoma, teratoma),[61] especially if the patient is male. Primary pineal cell tumors (pineoblastoma), are less frequent, but are the most common tumor arising within the pineal gland in young females. In our experience, pineoblastomas were most often associated with bilateral familial retinoblastoma.[62–65] Both tumors of pineal cell origin and germ cell origin arise posterior to the third ventricle in the midline. This is in contradistinction to astrocytomas and gangliogliomas that originate in structures adjacent to the pineal region and are therefore frequently eccentric in location. Germ cell tumors appear as predominantly solid masses that often are hyperdense before administration of contrast. Marked contrast enhancement is typical. Teratomas are identified by the presence of fat, ossification, calcification, and soft tissue densities. Dermoid tumors may have a similar appearance; however, epidermoids are predominantly cystic and are of CSF density. Primary pineal cell tumors are usually solid tumors but may contain cystic elements. Dense calcification arises frequently within the tumor.

The MRI characteristics of primary pineal cell tumors and germ cell tumors can overlap considerably, such that their differentiation on MRI may not be possible. On a T1WI, the presence of a hypointense cyst and hyperintense fat suggests the diagnosis of a teratoma. A predominantly cystic lesion with a T1 relaxation similar to CSF may indicate the presence of an epidermoid or arachnoid cyst. Solid pineoblastoma and germinoma both appear inhomogeneous and predominantly hypointense (Fig. 7–26). Areas of marked signal hypointensity may indicate the presence of globular calcification within the tumor, which is more consistent with a primary pineal cell tumor. On a T2-weighted sequence, both germ cell tumors and primary pineal cell tumors may appear hyperintense; however, germ cell tumors often remain isointense on the second echo.

Primitive neuroectodermal tumors, astrocytomas (Fig. 7–27), and gangliogliomas occurring in this region have a prolonged T1 and T2 relaxation and are therefore inseparable based on their MRI characteristics. Sagittal and coronal imaging may be essential in identifying their site of origin. Computed tomography still remains an important modality in assessing mass lesions of the pineal region for identification of the presence of fat, ossification, or calcification within the tumor.

## NEOPLASMS OF THE CEREBRAL HEMISPHERES

In children, the cerebral hemispheres are often the site of origin of both benign and malignant growths. Hamartomas are most often found in association with the neurocutaneous syndromes of tuberous sclerosis and neurofibromatosis. Rarely, hamartoma-like lesions such as meningoangiomatosis may involve the temporal lobe as well (Fig.

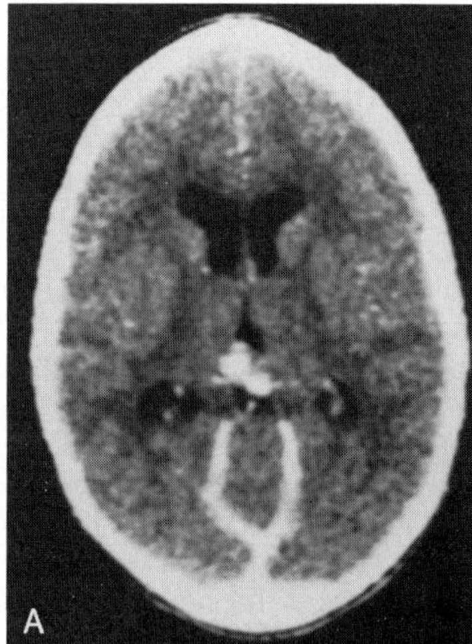


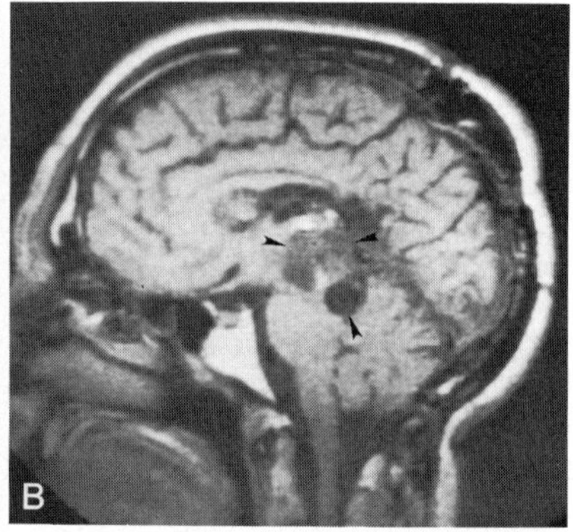


**Figure 7–26. Pinealoma.** *A,* A multilobulated enhancing mass occupies the pineal region. *B,* Sagittal T1WI (TR 600 msec/TE 20 msec). The sagittal projection optimally defines this mass of mixed signal intensity in the pineal region (arrowheads). (Courtesy of S. J. Pomeranz, M.D., The Christ Hospital, Cincinnati, Ohio.)

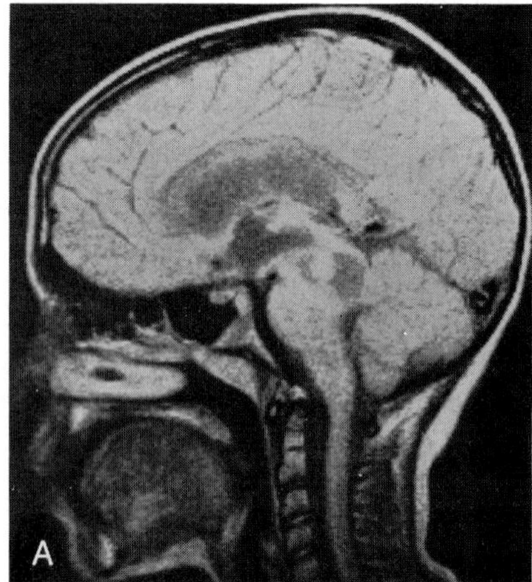


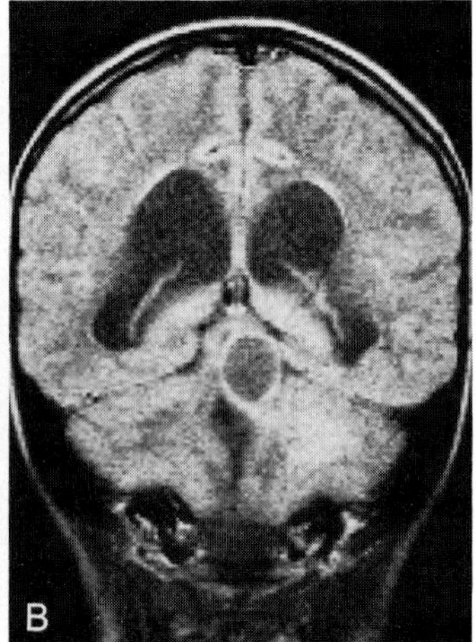


**Figure 7–27. Cystic midbrain glioma.** *A,* Sagittal T1WI (TR 800 msec/TE 20 msec). A mixed cystic mass with solid nodule originates in the posterior midbrain and extends into the pineal region. *B,* Coronal T1WI (TR 600 msec/TE 20 msec). The hypointense cystic component is well demarcated from surrounding structures by an isointense rim. (Courtesy of S. J. Pomeranz, M.D., The Christ Hospital, Cincinnati, Ohio.)

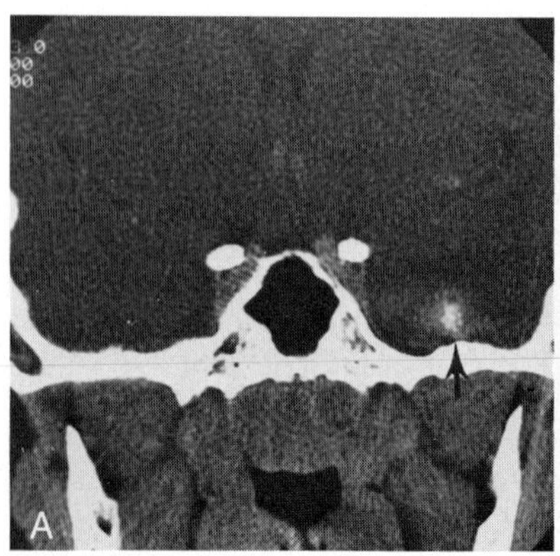


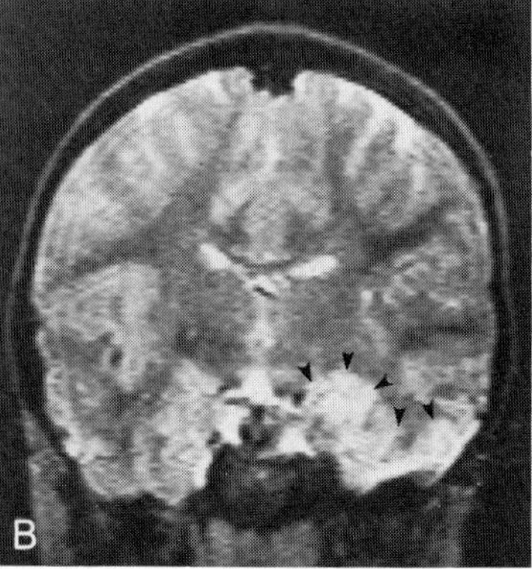


**Figure 7–28. Meningoangiomatosis of the left temporal lobe.** *A,* A partially calcified enhancing mass is present in the inferior aspect of the left temporal lobe (arrow). *B,* Coronal T2WI (TR 2000 msec/TE 100 msec). Hyperintense signal clearly demonstrates medial and lateral involvement of the temporal lobe (arrowheads), not seen on CT.

7–28). Hamartomatous lesions in the neurocutaneous syndromes are readily identified on MRI, and have been discussed in the section on congenital anomalies.

Unfortunately, malignant neoplasms of the cerebral hemispheres are all too frequent in children, despite their lower incidence when compared with adults. The majority of these malignancies are astrocytomas.[66] Less common tumors include oligodendrogliomas, primitive neuroectodermal tumor, ependymoma, and tumor of the choroid plexus (carcinoma). As in the adult, cerebral astrocytomas vary in grade from more benign lesions (grades I and II) to the aggressive and highly malignant glioblastoma multiforme (grade IV). The most frequent clinical presentation includes seizures, focal motor deficits, and signs and symptoms of increased intracranial pressure. The incidence in males and females is approximately equal.

Unlike with tumors in the posterior fossa, where MRI is clearly superior to CT, the value of MRI for evaluating supratentorial tumors is yet unproven. On the basis of MRI appearance, the abilities to differentiate histologic types of tumors and to evaluate their degree of aggressiveness are limited. Multiplanar MRI is superior to CT in defining the extent of pathology. We rely upon the T1WI and N(H)WI to elaborate on the pathologic anatomy, and to define the extent of the mass. The majority of hemispheric lesions are hypointense when compared with normal brain tissue, but they have a shorter T1 relaxation when compared with CSF.[67] Tumoral cysts likewise display hypointensity, but they remain slightly hyperintense compared with CSF. Tumoral cysts are differentiated from arachnoid cysts by their irregular outer margins, thick capsule, mural nodules, and surrounding edema.[67] Increased signal within the tumor on a T1WI suggests the presence of fat (e.g., teratoma), or hemorrhage. Several authors have indicated that benign lesions can be separated from more aggressive lesions on the basis of their T1 characteristics.[68] Benign processes appear isointense, whereas more aggressive lesions tend to be hypointense.[68] Although this generally is true, there is considerable variability, and many relatively benign processes may appear hypointense on a T1WI (Fig. 7–29).[11]

On a T2WI, cerebral neoplasms are bright in signal (prolonged T2 relaxation) (Fig. 7–30). Perilesional edema also appears bright, reflecting a breakdown in the blood-brain barrier. The T2 relaxation of edema is often longer than the T2 relaxation of solid tumor; however, in many cases separation of the two is often difficult. Histologic evidence indicates that tumor infiltration is often found within the areas of peritumoral edema;[69] therefore for the purpose of radiation treatment planning, separation of tumor and surrounding edema is often unnecessary. If separation of these two becomes necessary, intermediate-weighted images of an echo train T2-weighted sequence may be of help. In the future, contrast-enhanced MR may play an important role in identifying the tumor nidus. Areas of marked signal void on a T2WI often reveal the presence of cal-

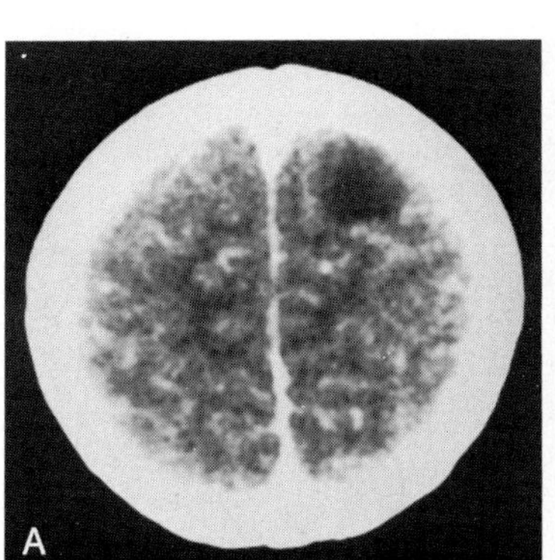

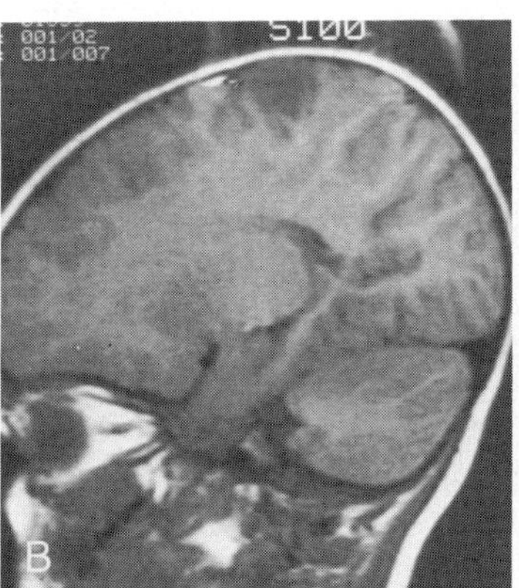

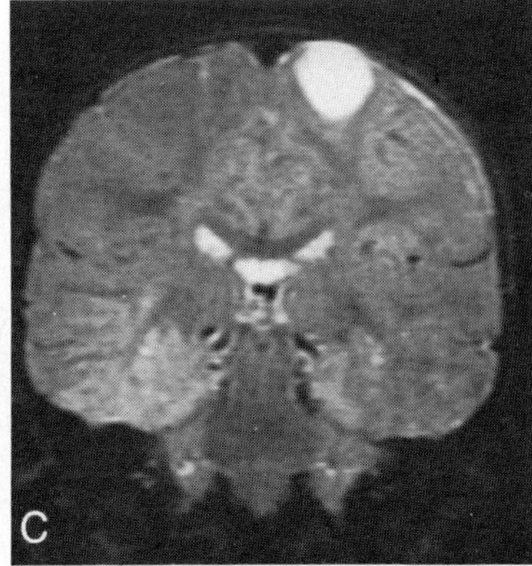


**Figure 7–29. Grade I astrocytoma.** *A,* A well-defined hypodense mass without enhancement is present in the patient's left superior parietal lobe. *B,* Sagittal T1WI (TR 600 msec/TE 20 msec). Although low in signal intensity, the mass has a shorter T1 relaxation compared with ventricular CSF. *C,* Coronal T2WI (TR 2000 msec/TE 100 msec). The tumor itself is hyperintense without peritumoral edema.

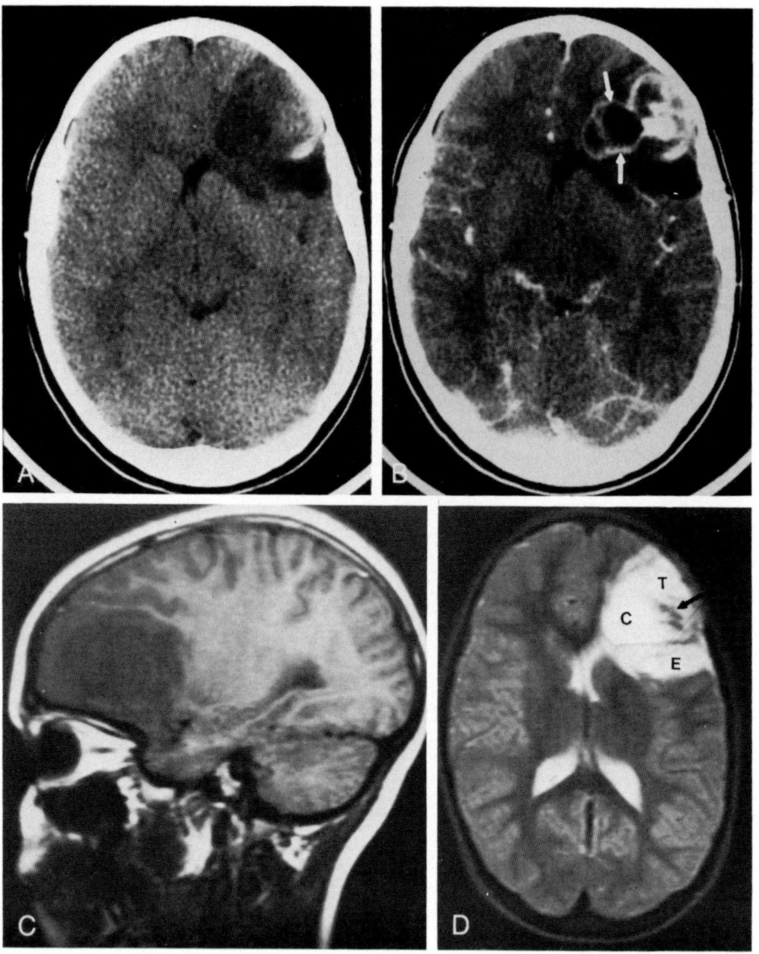


**Figure 7–30. Grade IV astrocytoma.** *A,* Unenhanced, and *B,* enhanced computed tomography. There is an ill-defined, hypodense mass at the patient's left frontoparietal junction. Calcification is seen in the periphery of the mass. Enhancement is present in the lateral solid component of tumor and in the wall of a medially located cyst (arrows). *C,* Sagittal T1WI (TR 600 msec/TE 20 msec). The mass is predominantly hypointense. Separation of tumoral cyst, solid tumor, and peritumoral edema is not possible. *D,* Axial T2WI (TR 2000 msec/TE 100 msec). The medial cyst (C) is brighter in signal when compared with the solid tumor (T) and the posterior peritumoral edema (E). Hypointensity (arrow) corresponds to the calcium seen on CT.

cification (Fig. 7–30*D*), hemosiderin from previous hemorrhage, or flowing blood in engorged tumoral vessels.

## SPINE

Primary and metastatic tumors of the spine are occasionally found in the pediatric age group.[70] As in adults, these lesions are categorized as intramedullary, extramedullary-intradural, and extradural. The types of tumors arising in children differ somewhat from those found in the adult population.[70] Familiarity with the type of lesions affecting children, the mode of presentation, and the natural history is important to the neuroradiologist faced with their diagnosis. Currently, myelography and CT myelography are relied on for the detailed assessment of spinal pathology. As for congenital lesions of the spine, use of MRI is making rapid advancement and may in the future replace myelography and CT myelography.

## TECHNICAL FACTORS

### Pulsing Sequence

For evaluation of the spinal axis, spin-echo (SE), T1WI and T2WI sequences are primarily used. Inversion recovery sequences, because of increase in noise, long scan times, and susceptibility to motion are not routinely performed. Such heavily weighted T1 images have not proved useful for the evaluation of masses in the spinal axis. Typically, we begin with a coronal localizer SE, T1-weighted sequence (TR 400–600 msec/TE 20 msec, matrix 256 × 128, 1 nex), from which a sagittal sequence is then prescribed. Our first sagittal examination is a high-resolution T1-weighted sequence (TR 400–600 msec/TE 20 msec, matrix 256 × 256, 4 nex). For evaluation of the spine, we use a combination of flow compensation and cardiac gating in order to eliminate pulsation artifacts. The sagittal examination can be followed by a single- or dual-echo sagittal T2WI sequence (TR 1800–2000 msec/TE 90 msec or 30/90 msec, matrix 256 × 128, 2–4 nex). If additional intermediate-weighted echoes are necessary to better identify cord pathology or to separate it from surrounding CSF, an "echo train" sequence is performed (TR 1800–2500 msec/TE 25/50/75/100 msec, matrix 256 × 128, 2 nex). In addition, the intermediate-weighted echoes are of value in the cord in differentiating cystic changes from solid tumor, both of which have a prolonged T2 relaxation. Coronal imaging, whether T1 or T2 weighted, is performed using oblique scanning through the long axis of the canal. The axial projection is of value for assessing extradural masses that extend into the paraspinous tissue and for intra-axial imaging in the presence of significant scoliosis.

Gradient echo-imaging (GRASS, fast scan) is a useful tool for imaging the spine in certain circumstances. The "myelographic" effect of the CSF can be useful in defining the relationship of ths subarachnoid space to an intramedullary or extradural mass. In the future, such sequences will become more practical once interleaved acquisition, providing multiple slices, becomes more practical.

### Slice Acquisition

Because the region of interest is smaller in the spine, 3-mm thick sections are routinely selected except for localizer sequences, in which 5-mm thicknesses suffice. With 3-mm thick sections, an interslice gap of 0.5 to 1 mm is used. All imaging of the spine is performed with posteriorly placed surface coils. Their size is chosen to balance resolution with adequate anatomic coverage. As in the evaluation of congenital anomalies, we often use a laterally placed, tandem, axial pair loop-gap resonator surface coil system for the evaluation of the craniocervical junction. For very small infants, the entire spine can be examined by placing the child longitudinally within the head coil from which the pads have been removed.

### Intramedullary Masses

Spinal cord tumors represent 6% to 8% of CNS neoplasms in children.[71] The incidence is equal in males and females. The peak age incidence is in the second decade of life, although tumors arising in patients less than 10 years old are not uncommon.[72] The majority of childhood intramedullary masses are astrocytomas, followed by ependymomas, and dermoid-epidermoid tumors, in decreasing order of frequency.[71] In the adult population, ependymoma is most common, followed by astrocytoma, and metastatic disease. The clinical presentation is often subtle and consists of local or radiating pain, paraspinous muscle spasm, and extremity weakness. The mode of presentation varies, depending on the level of involvement. Any portion of the cord can be involved; however, there is a predilection for the cervical cord and the cervicothoracic regions in children.

On T1WI the cord may be normal in size but is likely to be enlarged by the presence of the tumor. The enlargement is usually fusiform (Fig. 7–31) and may involve several vertebral segments or the entire cord. The signal characteristics can remain isointense on T1WI; however, in the majority of patients, the T1 relaxation is prolonged, resulting in signal hypointensity. On T2WI the signal intensity increases, so that the tumor appears bright in signal compared with the normal cord. Unfortunately, the tumor may not be appreciated on T2WI because of similar bright signal from the surrounding CSF. In this case, the tumor is more readily appreciated on T1 or intermediate scans with shorter TE (20–60 msec) (Fig. 7–32).

At times, differentiating congenital or post-traumatic syringohydromyelia from a cystic tumor of the cord can be difficult, since both display prolonged T1 or T2-relaxation.[73] Differentiation is further complicated by the fact that tumor and syrinx can coexist and also by the presence of gliosis, which can accompany congenital or acquired syringohydromyelia and can produce within the cord bright signal similar to that from a tumor.[74, 75] Several features help distinguish an idiopathic syringohydromyelia from a tumoral cyst. The signal characteristics of the fluid within a syrinx generally parallel that of CSF. Although tumoral cysts often display rather significant hypointens-

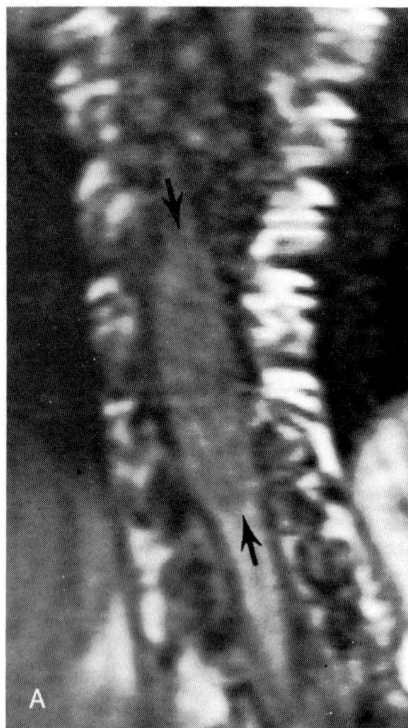

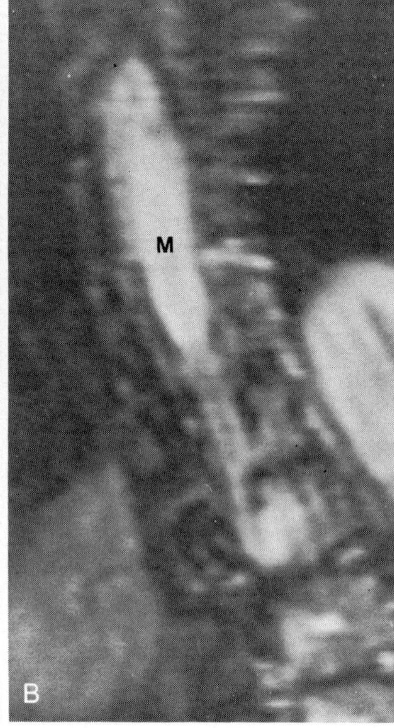


**Figure 7–31. Ganglioglioma of the thoracic cord.** *A,* Coronal T1WI (TR 600 msec/TE 20 msec). There is fusiform enlargement of the midthoracic cord (arrows). The tumor is hypointense but has a T1 relaxation shorter than that of CSF. *B,* Coronal T2WI (TR 1800 msec/TE 90 msec). The mass (M) appears bright in signal on the second echo.

ity, when compared with CSF, their fluid is slightly greater in signal owing to the presence of protein within the fluid and/or differing degrees of transmitted CSF pulsation. Also, because of the protein within the fluid, the T2 relaxation of a tumoral cyst is often greater when compared with an idiopathic syrinx. Areas of CSFV are often present in a communicating syringohydromyelia but are usually lacking in a tumoral cyst.[75] The presence of a CSFV is not helpful, however, in differentiating idiopathic syrinx from a syringomyelia associated with a tumor.[75] Despite these differences, the variability of both idiopathic syringomyelia and tumoral cyst may result in diagnostic difficulty on MRI. Rubin and colleagues points out that on occasion such difficulty may require CT myelography or intraoperative ultrasound to differentiate the two.[73] Rarely, difficulty may arise in differentiating a syringomyelia with gliosis from a solid tumor. Solid tumors usually display a shorter T1 relaxation and a longer T2-relaxation than the CSF located within an idiopathic syringomyelia. Gliosis associated with a syrinx typically is proximal to the cyst cavity and does not appear to expand the cord. In tumor, an associated syrinx may lie proximal or distal to the mass; however, the cord is usually enlarged.

## Extramedullary Masses

Extramedullary masses are more common than intramedullary tumor in children.[76] Extramedullary/intradural masses found in the pediatric population include "drop" metastases, dermoid-epidermoid tumors, teratomas, and lipomas. Metastatic spread of

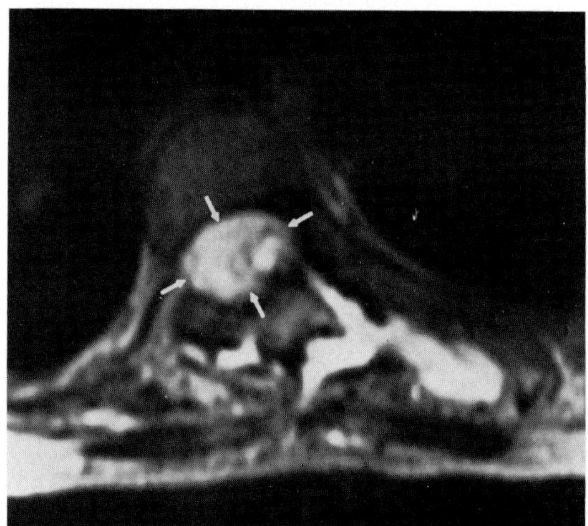

**Figure 7–32. Astrocytoma of the thoracic cord.** Axial N(H)WI (TR 1800 msec/TE 30 msec). The tumor fills the entire spinal canal (arrows) and is mixed in signal intensity (varying hyperintensity).

cranial or spinal neoplasms occurs with medulloblastoma, ependymoma, other primitive neuroectodermal tumors, astrocytomas, pineal tumors, and choroid plexus carcinomas.

Dermoid and epidermoid tumors, lipomas, and teratomas are usually associated with spinal dysraphism.[77] Neural elements give rise to most extradural masses in children. Epidural involvement is found with neuroblastoma, ganglioneuroblastoma, ganglioneuroma, leukemia, and lymphoma. Neurofibromas, which frequently involve the canal as "dumb-bell" lesions in children, are infrequent in young children. Rarely, the extradural space may be involved by hemangioma, lymphangioma, or both, spreading into the canal from the paravertebral space. For both intradural and extradural masses, the clinical presentation consists of pain and cord dysfunction secondary to compression. Presentation of signs and symptoms may be subtle and slowly progressive over a long period of time.

Both T1- and T2-weighted sequences are necessary for complete evaluation of extramedullary masses; however, we rely predominantly on T1WI to identify the mass and determine its extent of involvement (Fig. 7–33). Any extramedullary mass is first identified by its anatomic presence and extent, rather than by its abnormal signal characteristics. Multiplanar imaging may be necessary to adequately define the tumor. Coronal and axial imaging are especially helpful in defining lateral extension of mass. T2-weighted images have significant limitations in evaluating extramedullary-intradural masses. The problem lies in the simultaneous increase in signal within both the tumor and the surrounding CSF on a long TR/T2-weighted sequence (Fig. 7–34). Either failure to identify the tumor or understanding its size results. This difficulty can be overcome in part by use of T1- and intermediate-weighted images. Extradural masses, on the other hand, do not pose a similar problem. Their increased signal on T2WI is helpful in demonstrating lateral extension into the paravertebral tissues which remain isotense. The majority of extramedullary-intradural and extradural masses demonstrates a prolonged T2 relaxation time of moderate signal intensity. On T1WI the signal intensity of extramedullary tumors varies from hypointense to isointense. The presence of bright signal on a T1-weighted sequence suggests either the presence of fat (lipoma, teratoma) or previous hemorrhage into the tumor.

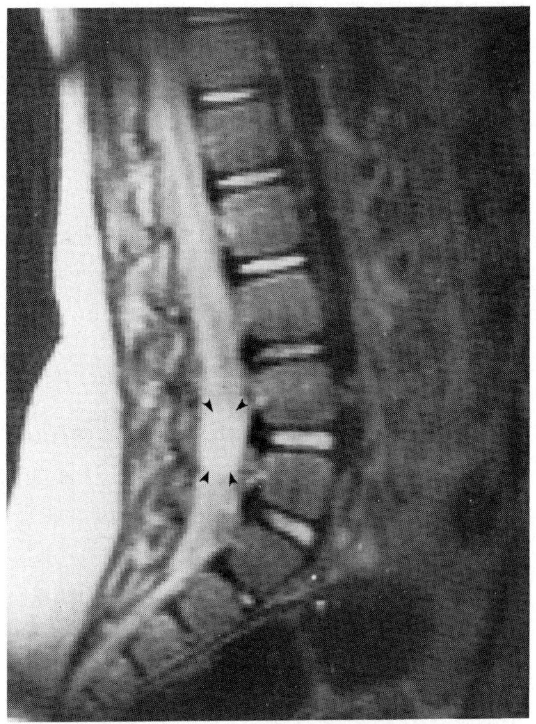

**Figure 7–34. Intraspinal dermoid cyst.** Sagittal T1WI (TR 2000 msec/TE 100 msec). The higher signal intensity of the dermoid cyst (arrowheads) is barely discernible from the surrounding CSF.

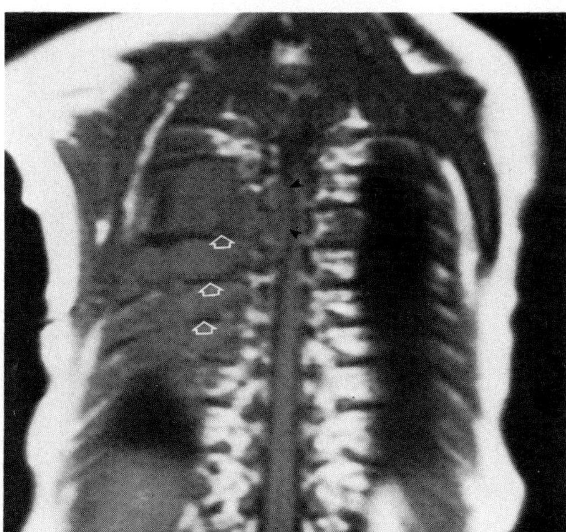

**Figure 7–33. Neuroblastoma.** Coronal T1WI (TR 600 msec/TE 20 msec). The tumor extends through the lateral foramina into the spinal canal (arrowheads), compressing the dural sac and cord. Note extensive extrathoracic involvement (open arrows).

Drop metastases pose an additional diag-

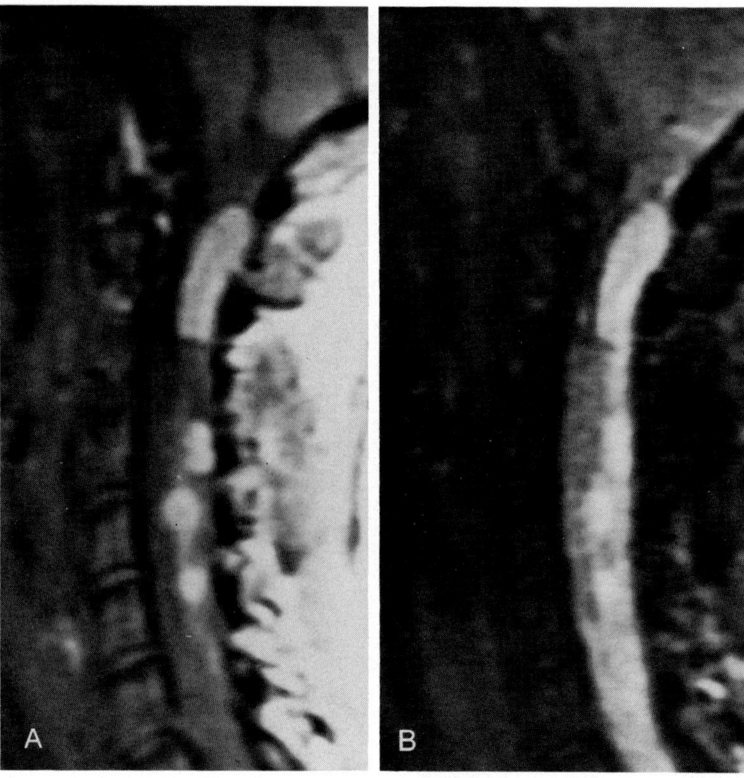


**Figure 7–35. Metastatic ependymoma.** *A,* Sagittal N(H)WI (TR 1800 msec/TE 20 msec). The metastatic deposits appear hyperintense compared with the cord and CSF. *B,* Sagittal T2WI (TR 1800 msec/TE 100 msec). The larger metastatic deposit in the upper cervical canal is clearly identified; however, the smaller deposits inferiorly are poorly demarcated from surrounding CSF and are better seen on N(H)WI. (Courtesy of S. J. Pomeranz, M.D., The Christ Hospital, Cincinnati, Ohio.)

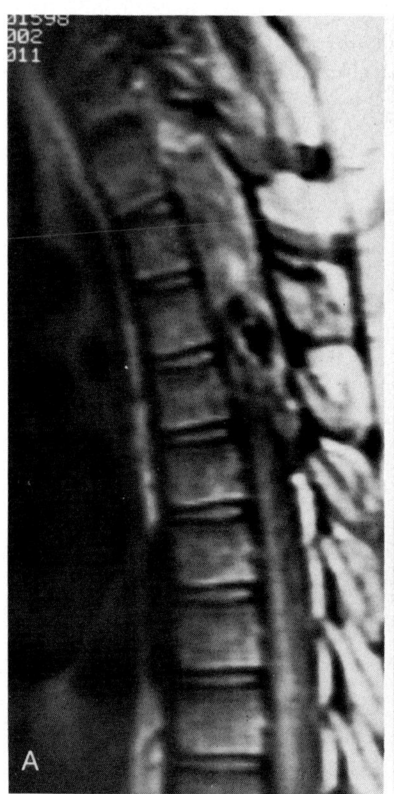


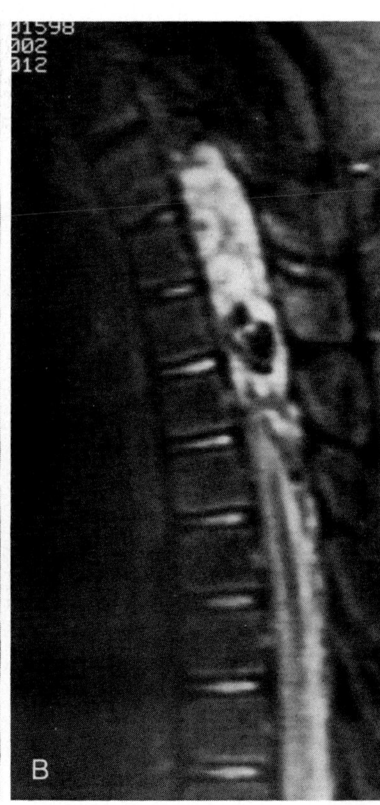


**Figure 7–36. Lymphangioma.** *A,* Sagittal N(H)WI (TR 1800 msec/TE 20 msec). An oblong mass fills a portion of the thoracic canal. The mass demonstrates marked variation in signal intensity. *B,* Sagittal T2WI (TR 1800 msec/TE 100 msec). Overall there is an increase in signal on the second echo image. Hypointense areas represent areas of previous hemorrhage (hemosiderin), prominent vascularity, or both.

nostic problem on MRI. The majority of drop metastases will be manifested as small nodules adherent to the cauda equina, spinal cord, or dural surface or free within the subarachnoid space (Fig. 7–35). Metastatic nodules can be as small as 1 to 3 mm. Involvement of the cauda equina produces a matted appearance of the spinal nerve roots that resembles arachnoiditis. A lack of inherent resolution combined with flow-related artifact makes visualization of the filum terminale and individual nerve roots within the cauda equina difficult on MRI. MRI therefore lacks the inherent sensitivity of CT myelography in identifying small metastatic foci. In this application, CT myelography is still the modality of choice. However, in the presence of an acute cord syndrome secondary to a high-grade partial or complete block by an intradural or extradural mass, MRI is the initial modality of choice and may spare the patient unnecessary pain and risk from lumbar or C1–C2 myelography.

When spinal dysraphism is present, a dermoid-epidermoid tumor or lipoma are the most likely causes of an extramedullary intradural mass.[77] The MRI characteristics may overlap considerably between such tumors, although the presence of fat strongly suggests the diagnosis of lipoma or teratoma. A dermoid tumor may be predominantly cystic, displaying prolonged T1 and T2 relaxation.

Epidural tumors in children are rare, neuroblastoma and lymphoma representing the most common causes.[78] Rarely, primary bone tumor of the vertebral elements is manifest as an epidural mass. The MRI appearance of both neuroblastoma and lymphoma are similar and appear as hypointense or isointense on T1WI (Fig. 7–33). Their signals may be isointense or only moderately hyperintense on a T2WI. Differentiation is based primarily on the patient's age and other associated features of the tumor (e.g., calcification in neuroblastoma). Rarely, hemangioma or lymphangioma may occur as an epidural mass.[79] In this case, the MRI appearance is more specific. On T1WI variations in signal intensity within the tumor are commonly the result of a mixture of hygromatous and solid elements (Fig. 7–36). On T2WI the cystic hygroma displays brighter signal when compared with the hyperintense signal intensity found in the more solid components. Areas of previous hemorrhage may appear bright on both T1- and T2-weighted sequences. In addition, the presence of large serpiginous vessels of low signal intensity secondary to increased flow are found interspersed within or around the periphery of the mass. This combination of marked variation in T1 and T2 characteristics, in addition to cystic elements, previous hemorrhage, and hypervascularity are virtually diagnostic of lymphangioma, hemangioma, or both.

## References


1. Silverberg E. Cancer statistics 1980. Cancer 30:23, 1980.
2. Bruno L, Schut L. Survey of pediatric brain tumors. In McLaurin RL, ed. Pediatric Neurosurgery: Surgery of the Developing Nervous System. New York, Grune & Stratton, 1982:361.
3. Naidich TP, Zimmerman RA. Primary brain tumors in children. Semin Roentgenol 19(2):100, 1984.
4. Crone K. Personal communication. March 1987.
5. Pennock JM, Bydder GM, Dubowitz LM, et al. Magnetic resonance imaging of the brain in children. Magn Reson Imag 4:1, 1986.
6. Johnson MA, Pennock JM, Bydder GM, et al. Clinical NMR imaging of the brain in children: normal and neurologic disease. AJR 141:1005, 1983.
7. Han JS, Benson J, Kaufman B, et al. MR imaging of pediatric cerebral abnormalities. J Comput Assist Tomogr 9:103, 1985.
8. Randell CP, Collins AG, Young IR, et al. Nuclear magnetic resonance imaging of posterior fossa tumors. AJR 141:489, 1983.
9. Lee BCP, Kneeland JB, Deck MDF, et al. Posterior fossa lesions: magnetic resonance imaging. Radiology 153:137, 1984.
10. Barnes PD, Lester PD, Yamanashi WS, et al. Magnetic resonance imaging in childhood intracranial masses. Magn Reson Imag 4:41, 1986.
11. Zimmerman RA. Magnetic resonance imaging of midline pediatric cerebral neoplasms. Acta Neurochir (Suppl.) 35:60, 1985.
12. Peterman SB, Steiner RE, Bydder GM. Magnetic resonance imaging of intracranial tumors in children and adolescents. AJNR 5:703, 1984.
13. Felix R, Schorner W, Laniado M, et al. Brain tumors: MR imaging with gadolinium-DTPA. Radiology 156:681, 1985.
14. O'Brien MS, Tindall SC. Posterior fossa tumors in childhood: unusual types. In McLaurin RL, ed. Pediatric Neurosurgery: Surgery of the Developing Nervous System. New York, Grune & Stratton, 1982:395.
15. Young DF, Eldridge R, Nager GE, et al. Hereditary bilateral acoustic neuroma (central neurofibromatosis). Birth Defects 7:73, 1971.
16. Alliez J, Masse JL, Alliez B. Bilateral tumors of the acoustic nerve and Recklinghausen's disease observed in several generations. Considerations on hereditary acoustic nerve tumors. Rev Neurol (Paris) 131:545, 1975.

17. Winston K, Gilles FH, Levitona A, et al. Cerebellar gliomas in children. J Nat Cancer Inst 58:833, 1977.
18. Miller JH, Fishman LS. Brain tumors. In Miller JH, ed. Imaging in Pediatric Oncology. Baltimore, Williams & Wilkins, 1985:74.
19. Kida Y, Kobayashi T, Yamada H, et al. CT findings of medulloblastomas: correlation of histological type. (abstract) Child's Brain 6:164, 1980.
20. Shin KH, Fisher G, Webster JH. Brainstem tumors in children. J Can Assoc Radiol 30:77, 1979.
21. Lassman LP. Pontile gliomas of childhood. Lancet 1:913, 1967.
22. Walker AE, Hopple TL. Brain tumors in children. J Pediatr 35:671, 1949.
23. Bilaniuk LT, Zimmerman RA, Littman P, et al. Computed tomography of brainstem gliomas in children. Radiology 134:89, 1980.
24. Weisberg LA. Computed tomography in the diagnosis of brainstem gliomas. CT 3:145, 1979.
25. Duffner PK, Klein DM, Cohen ME. Calcification in brainstem gliomas. Neurology 28:832, 1978.
26. McLaurin RL, Towbin RB, Aron BS. Brainstem gliomas: observations on CT appearance before and after treatment. In Concepts Pediatric Neurosurgery, Vol. 5. Basel, S. Karger, 1985:165.
27. Bradac GB, Schorner W, Bender A, et al. NMR in the diagnosis of intrinsic tumors of the brainstem. J Neuroradiol 12:223, 1985.
28. Fasano VA, Urciuoli R, Ponzio RM, et al. The effect of new technologies on the surgical management of brainstem tumors. Surg Neurol 25:219, 1986.
29. Zimmerman RA, Bilaniuk LT, Grossman RI, et al. Resistive NMR of brain stem gliomas. Neuroradiology 27:21, 1985.
30. Dohrmann GJ, Farwell JR, Flannery JT. Ependymomas and ependymoblastomas in children. J Neurosurg 45:273, 1976.
31. Coulon RA, Till K. Intracranial ependymomas in children. Child's Brain 3:154, 1977.
32. Oi S, Raimondi AJ. Ependymoma. In McLaurin RL, ed. Pediatric Neurosurgery: Surgery of the Developing Nervous System. New York, Grune & Stratton, 1982:419.
33. Yamada H. Brain tumors. In Yamada H, ed. Pediatric Cranial Computed Tomography. Tokyo, 1983:237.
34. Sassin JF, Chutorian AM. Intracranial chordoma in children. Arch Neurol 17:89, 1967.
35. Schroeder BA, Wells RG, Starshak RJ, et al. Clivus chordoma in a child with tuberous sclerosis: CT and MR demonstration. J Comput Assist Tomogr 11:195, 1987.
36. Dubois PJ. Brain tumors. In Rosenberg RN, et al., eds. The Clinical Neurosciences: Neuroradiology. New York, Churchill Livingstone, 1984:361.
37. Russell DS, Rubenstein LJ. Pathology of tumors of the nervous system, 4th ed. Baltimore, Williams & Wilkins, 1977:65.
38. Cabezudo JM, Vaquero J, Garcia de Sola R, et al. Computed tomography with craniopharyngiomas: a review. Surgical Neurology 15:422, 1980.
39. Petito CK, DeBirolami U, Earle KM. Craniopharyngiomas: clinical and pathological review. Cancer 37:1944, 1976.
40. Zimmerman RA. Magnetic resonance imaging of cerebral neoplasms. Magn Reson Annu 1985:113.
41. Pusey E, Kortman KE, Flannigan BD, et al. MR of craniopharyngiomas: tumor delineation and characterization. AJR 149:383, 1987.
42. Lee BCP, Deck MDF. Sella and juxtasellar lesion detection with MR. Radiology 157:143, 1985.
43. Maggio WW, Cail WS, Brookeman JR, et al. Rathke's cleft cyst: computed tomographic and magnetic resonance imaging appearances. Neurosurgery 21:60, 1987.
44. Yoshida J, Kobayashi T, Kageyama N, et al. Symptomatic Rathke's cleft cyst. Morphologic study with light and electronmicroscopy and tissue culture. J Neurosurg 47:451, 1977.
45. Trokoudes KM, Walfish PG, Holgate RC, et al. Sellar enlargement with hyperprolactinemia in a Rathke's pouch cyst. JAMA 240:471, 1978.
46. Kucharczyk W. The pituitary gland and sella turcica. In: Brandt-Zawadzki M, Norman D, eds. Magnetic Resonance Imaging of the Central Nervous System. New York, NY: Raven Press, 1987:202.
47. Farwell JR, Dohrmann GJ, Flannery JT. Central nervous system tumors in children. Cancer 40:3123, 1977.
48. Stern J, DiGiacinto GV, Houseplan EM. Neurofibromatosis and optic glioma: Clinical and morphological correlations. Neurosurgery 4:524, 1979.
49. Fog J, Seedorff HH, Vaernet K. Optic glioma, clinical features and treatment. Acta Ophthalmologica 48:644, 1970.
50. Savoiardo M, Harwood-Nash DC, Tadmor R, et al. Gliomas of the intracranial anterior optic pathways in children. Radiology 138:601, 1981.
51. Albert A, Lee BCP, Saint-Louis L, et al. MRI of optic chiasm and optic pathways. AJNR 7:255, 1986.
52. Miller JH, Pena AM, Segall HD. Radiological investigation of sellar region masses in children. Radiology 134:81, 1980.
53. Jenkin RDT, Simpson JK, Keen CW. Pineal and suprasellar germinomas. J Neurosurg 48:99, 1978.
54. Takeuchi J, Handa H, Nagata I. Supraselllar germinoma. J Neurosurg 49:41, 1978.
55. Brandt-Zawadzki M, Kelly W. Brain tumors. In Brandt-Zawadzki M, Norman D, eds. Magnetic Resonance Imaging of the Central Nervous System. New York, Raven Press, 1987:172.
56. Johnson MA, Pennock JM, Bydder GM, et al. Clinical NMR imaging of the brain in children: normal and neurologic disease. AJNR 4:1013, 1983.
57. Takeuchi J, Handa H, Miki Y, et al. Precocious puberty due to a hypothalamic hamartoma. Surg Neurol 11:456, 1979.
58. Kammer KS, Perlman K, Humphreys RP, et al. Clinical and surgical aspects of hypothalamic hamartoma associated with precocious puberty in a 15-month-old boy. Child's Brain 6:150, 1980.
59. Abay EO, Laws ER, Grado GL, et al. Pineal tumors in children and adolescents. J Neurosurg 55:889, 1981.
60. Vorkapic P, Pendl G. Neuroimaging of mass lesions of the pineal region in infancy and childhood. Acta Neurochir (Suppl.) 35:65, 1985.
61. Miller JH, Fishman LS. Brain tumors. In Miller JH, ed. Imaging in Pediatric Oncology. Baltimore. Williams & Wilkins, 1985:70.
62. Bullit E, Crain BJ. Retinoblastoma as a possible primary intracranial tumor. Neurosurgery 9:706, 1981.
63. Futrell NN, Osborn AG, Cheson BD. Pineal region tumors: computed tomographic-pathologic spectrum. AJR 137:951, 1981.
64. Zimmerman RA, Bilaniuk LT, Wood JH, et al. Com-

puted tomography of pineal, parapineal, and histologically related tumors. Radiology 137:669, 1980.
65. Naidich TP, Cacayorin ED, Stewart WA, et al. Germinal cell tumor of the pineal gland. AJR 146:1246, 1986.
66. Heiskanen O. Intracranial tumors of children. Child's Brain 3:69, 1977.
67. Kjos BO, Brandt-Zawadzki M, Kucharczyk W, et al. Cystic intracranial lesions: magnetic resonance imaging. Radiology 155:363, 1985.
68. Mills CM, Crooks LE, Kaufman L, et al. Cerebral abnormalities: use of calculated T1 and T2 MRI for diagnosis. Radiology 150:87, 1984.
69. Davis RL, Erlich SS. Neuroepithelial tumors of the CNS. In Rosenberg RN, et al., eds. The Clinical Neurosciences: Neuropathology. New York, Churchill Livingstone, 1983:85.
70. Desousa AL, Kalseech JE, Mealey J, et al. Intraspinal tumors in children. A review of 81 cases. J Neurosurg 51:437, 1979.
71. Epstein F, Epstein N. Intramedullary tumors of the spinal cord. In McLaurin RL, ed., Pediatric Neurosurgery: Surgery of the Developing Nervous System. New York, Grune & Stratton; 1982:529.
72. Banna M, Gryspaceral GL. Intraspinal tumors in children (excluding dysraphism). (Review.) Radiology 22:17, 1971.
73. Rubin JM, Aisen AM, DiPetro J. Ambiguities in MR imaging of tumoral cyst in the spinal cord. J Comput Assist Tomogr 10:395, 1986.
74. Gebarski SS, Maynard FW, Gabrielsen TO, et al. Posttraumatic progressive myelopathy. Radiology 157:379, 1985.
75. Sherman JL, Barkovich AJ, Citrin CM. The MR appearance of syringomyelia: new observations. AJNR 7:985, 1986.
76. McLaurin RL. Extramedullary spinal tumors. In McLaurin RL, ed. Pediatric Neurosurgery: Surgery of the Developing Nervous System. New York, Grune & Stratton; 1982:541.
77. Naidich TP, McClone DG, Harwood-Nash DC. Spinal dysraphism. In Newton TH, Potts DG, eds. Computed Tomography of the Spine and Spinal Cord. San Anselmo CA: Clavadel Press; 1983:299.
78. Baten M. Vannucci RC. Intraspinal metastatic disease in childhood cancer. J Pediatr 90:207, 1977.
79. Pia HW, Djindjian R. Spinal angiomas: advances in diagnosis and therapy. New York, Springer-Verlag, 1978.

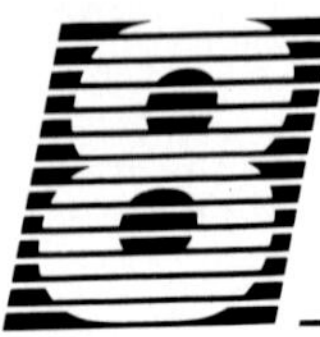

Stephen J. Pomeranz, M.D.

# MR OF SUPRATENTORIAL NEOPLASIA

## MR SIGNAL ALTERATIONS

### Signal Intensity

Although the attenuation values in computed tomography (CT) depend on electron density, magnetic resonance (MR) pixel signal intensity depends upon proton density, flow, and T1 and T2 relaxation according to the following formula:

$$\text{Intensity} = N(H)\, f(v) e^{-TE/T2} (1\text{-}e^{-TR/T1})$$

N(H) represents proton density, f(v) a function of flow, and TR and TE represent programmable sequence parameters that control T1 and T2 relaxation. Tissue magnetic susceptibility, paramagnetism, and chemical shift effects indirectly affect the local tissue magnetic field; and thus, pixel signal values. Images that have short TR ($<$ 1000 msec) and short TE ($<$ 35 msec) are T1-weighted (T1WI) images. These are recognized as such, since white matter is hyperintense relative to gray matter and cerebrospinal fluid (CSF) or ocular vitreous is hypointense relative to neural parenchyma. When echo time (TE) is held constant and TR is prolonged ($>$ 1000 msec), T1 recovery of most tissues is permitted, and images reflect differences in proton density. These images are recognized by a slight hypointensity of CSF relative to brain parenchyma and only subtle intensity differences between gray and white matter. Progressive TE prolongation ($>$ 50 msec) with long repetition times produces incremental T2-weighted (T2WI) images. The T2WI typically produce CSF or vitreous signal hyperintensity relative to neural parenchyma and white matter signal hypointensity relative to gray matter, using the spin-echo technique.

MR tissue appearance is dependent on T1 and T2 relaxation times to a greater extent than on mobile proton density. *Mobile* qualifies the degree of hydrogen proton binding. Lipid in the normal brain is not visible with conventional or chemical-shift MR.[1] This is because myelin lipid, though present, is tightly membrane-bound in the solid phase and possesses very short T2 relaxation.[2]

While proton hydrogen binding and phase (solid versus liquid) are determinants of proton relaxation, these effects may not lead to diagnoses that provide tissue specificity. The lack of MR T1- or T2-relaxation lesion characterization has been recognized by others (Table 8–1).[3] A tendency toward longer relaxation times occurs in glial neoplasms when compared with cerebral metastases. Cell-poor, fibrous meningiomas and acoustic neuromas have the least marked T1 and T2 relaxation prolongation.[4] Typically, the relaxation time prolongation that occurs in most cerebral neoplasms is not specific enough to make histologic diagnoses. Nevertheless, signal alterations of certain lesions allow specific diagnoses (Fig. 8–1). This is particularly true of lesions that exhibit shortened T1 relaxation, shortened T2 relaxation or both (Table 8–2).

Signal hyperintensity on T1WI may occur secondary to paramagnetic effects (hemorrhagic species, Gd-DTPA enhancement), fat-containing lesions or substances (Pantopaque), and flow-related (section entry or even-echo rephasing) phenomena. Therefore craniospinal lesions with shortened T1 re-

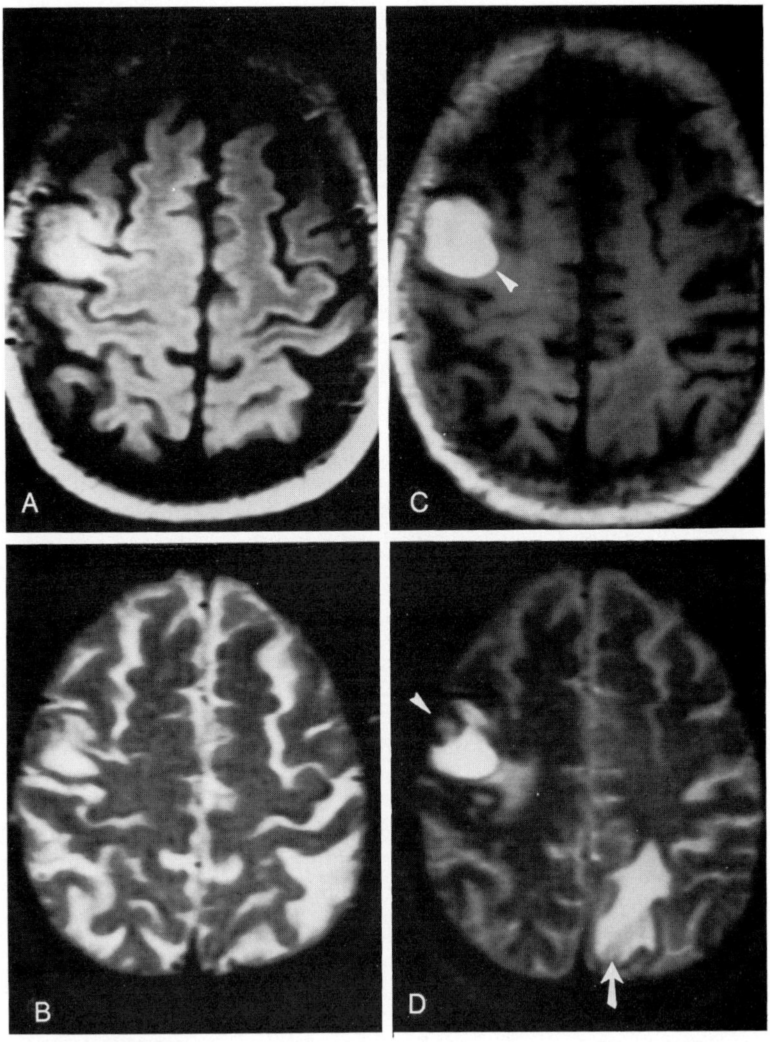

**Figure 8–26. Hemorrhagic melanoma metastases, postirradiation.** A 52-year-old woman with melanoma and headache (1.5 T). *A* and *C,* Axial N(H)WI and T2WI. *B* and *D,* Axial T1WI and T2WI, six weeks later. A right-sided perirolandic cortical mass is present initially. Lesions were hyperdense on NCCT (not shown). *B* and *D,* Images performed six weeks after irradiation and when the patient experienced sudden confusion and left extremity weakness. T1 hyperintensity (arrowhead, *B*) and lesion hypointensity (arrowhead) on T2WI are compatible with recent tumoral hemorrhage. New lesion on the patient's left (arrow) and all five lesions on earlier MR have hemorrhaged on other sections (not shown) in the interim.

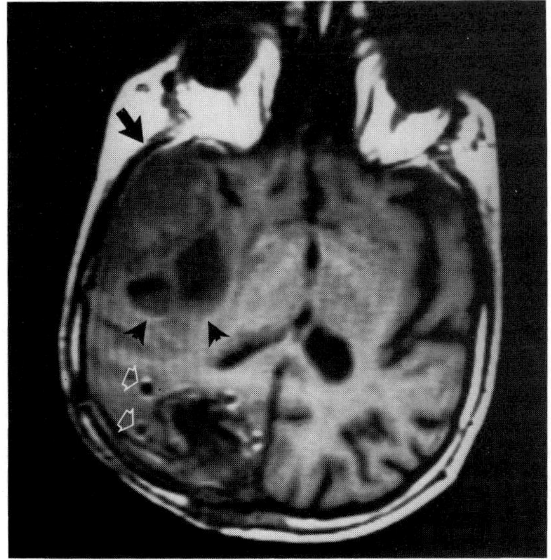

**Figure 8–27. Cystic metastases (oat cell carcinoma).** Axial T1WI. Dural temporal metastasis (black arrow) is not as hypointense as marginal macrocystic tumoral necrosis (arrowheads). Notice the subtle, increased signal of debris layering dependent in cysts (arrowheads). Signal hypointensity in patient's right occipital lobe represents postoperative encephalomalacia with nonferromagnetic effect of surrounding radioactive seed implants (open arrows).

little or no edema;[28] cyst formation is frequent.[104] Cyst formation appears as homogeneous T1- and T2-relaxation prolongation. Some metastases (lung) may simulate non-neoplastic cysts (Fig. 8–27).

The earlier detection of cerebral metastases and the superior detection of lesion multiplicity with MR is becoming more apparent.[105] The exquisite sensitivity of MR to white matter edema is fortuitous, since most lesions occur in white matter or at the gray-white junction. However, even T2WI are insensitive to pure gray matter lesions, subarachnoid, and leptomeningeal disease of any etiology. Melanoma may produce pure gray matter metastases. It is in these instances where CEMR is applicable and will dramatically improve MR sensitivity and specificity. CT is insensitive in the detection of small intrachoroidal metastases, and MR may be useful in these cases.[106]

### Pineal Region Tumors (TABLE 8–6)

Pineal region tumors can be divided into two major subtypes, pineal cell tumors (25%) and germ cell neoplasms (70%). The pineal cell group is slightly more frequent in women and includes pineocytoma, and pineoblastoma. The germ cell group predominates in men and includes germinoma (more than 50% of all pineal neoplasms), teratoma/teratocarcinoma, choriocarcinoma, embryonal cell carcinoma, and endodermal sinus tumors. Tumor-specific cell markers such as human chorionic gonadotropin (HCG) or alpha-fetoprotein (AFP) may elevate in the serum with germ cell neoplasm or teratoma, respectively. A propensity for CSF spread allows cytologic evaluation to improve diagnostic specificity. Endocrine dysfunction, including hypogonadism, precocious puberty, and diabetes insipidus may occur with any of these lesions. Aqueductal obstruction is not uncommon, and close tectal proximity may produce a vertical case palsy, Parinaud's syndrome. Miscellaneous peripineal neoplasms involving this region include lipoma, glioma, ganglioglioma, ganglioneuroma, metastasis, and neuroblastoma/neuro-ectodermal tumors. Pineal meningioma actually arises from the falx-tentorial junction. Peripineal cysts include

**Table 8–6.** PINEAL REGION NEOPLASMS

| Neoplasm | Sex | HCG | AFP | Relaxation T1 | Relaxation T2 | Contrast Uptake | Ca+ | Margin | CSF Seeding Cytodiagnosis | RT* Sens | Other |
|---|---|---|---|---|---|---|---|---|---|---|---|
| ***Germ Cell Origin*** | | | | | | | | | | | |
| *Germinoma* | M | + | – | +/= | ++ | ++ | – | Sharp | ++++ | +++ | may occur in supracistern w endocrine dysfunction; hydrocephalus common |
| *Teratoma* | M | – | – | –/+ | –/+ | –/+ | + | Sharp | – | – | cyst formation |
| *Teratocarcinoma* | M | –/+ | ++ | –/+ | ++ | + | – | Irregular | + | ++ | mild hemorrhagic tendency |
| *Choriocarcinoma* | | ++ | –/+ | +/– | ++ | ++ | – | Irregular | ++ | ++ | marked hemorrhagic tendency |
| *Embryonal Cell Carcinoma* | | + | – | ++ | ++ | ++ | – | Irregular | ++ | ++ | |
| ***Pineal Cell Origin*** | | | | | | | | | | | |
| *Pineocytoma* | F | – | – | +/= | +/= | ++ | + | Sharp | + | + | |
| *Pineoblastoma* | F | – | – | ++ | ++ | ++ | – | Irregular | + | + | larger size than pineocytoma |

*RT Sens = radiation sensitivity.

T1 and T2 refer to relaxation, not signal intensity; therefore + refers to T1 and T2 relaxation prolongation (hypointense and hyperintense, respectively), and – refers to shorter T1 and T2 relaxations (hyperintense and hypointense, respectively).

Equals sign: isointense.

M = male predominance

F = female predominance

the developmental group of dermoid and epidermoid cysts and arachnoid or ependymal cysts.

Sensitivity of MR in evaluation of pineal neoplasms is variable and depends on lesion type and calcification. Poor delineation of abnormal gland calcification impairs detection and diagnostic specificity. Pineal calcification should not be seen in a gland of normal size in children under six years old and in only 11% of 11- to 14-year-olds.[107] This weakness of MR is critical. For these reasons, we prefer CT as the initial modality in evaluation of these lesions, and CT and MR findings are discussed together.

The normal pineal gland is faintly visualized on T1WI and appears as an inhomogeneous focus of moderate signal intensity on T2WI. Normal-sized pineal glands may demonstrate marked increase in T2 signal intensity (4% to 10%) as an incidental finding.[108] This phenomenon may be manifested as small cysts that result from congenital variations in the third ventricular roof closure, as larger ependymal-lined cysts (Fig. 8–28) arising from primitive cells that differentiate into neuroglia, or as cysts that result from pineal parenchymal necrosis. These lesions are seen in 20% to 40% of autopsy series[109] and are poorly recognized on CT since attenuation of cyst and peripineal cistern is similar. They are rarely symtomatic,[110] range in size from 5 to 15 mm, have thin (2-mm) walls,[111] and exhibit fluid-fluid levels on MR owing to differences in protein concentration.

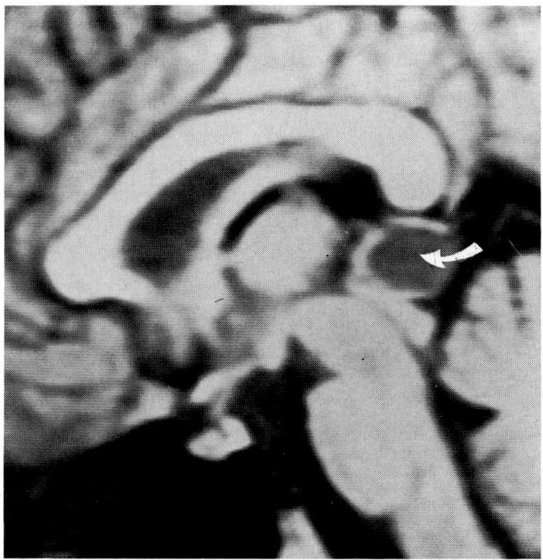

**Figure 8–28. Pineal cyst.** Sagittal (1.5 T) T1WI demonstrates hypointense cystic mass slightly more intense than CSF. Signal difference is likely related to CSF pulsations and cyst protein. (Courtesy of A. Chambers, M.D., Dept. of Neuroradiology, University Hospital, Cincinnati, Ohio.)

Germinoma is the most common pineal region tumor and histologically is identical to seminoma of the testes and ovarian dysgerminoma. This radio-sensitive, low-grade malignant lesion (except the suprasellar type), predominates in men, is noncalcified, is isodense or hyperdense on noncontrast CT, and moderately enhances. CSF tumor seeding and hydrocephalus are common. Suprasellar location ("ectopic pinealoma") may occur, producing endocrine or pituitary dysfunction, and rare germinomas of the basal ganglia or thalmus have been reported.[112] It has been suggested that germinomas exhibit isointensity on T1 and T2 images, germinoma with embryonal cell elements demonstrate long T1 and T2 relaxations, whereas pineoblastoma may have long T1 relaxation and isointense signal on T2-weighted images.[113] We have not found MR signal useful in improving diagnostic specificity in this region, with the exception of lipoma or teratoma (short T1) and choriocarcinoma (hemorrhagic signal on MR, hyperdense CT). Germinomas may be isointense or hyperintense relative (Fig. 8–29) to gray matter on T2WI. Our four cases of pineoblastoma were all hyperintense on T2WI. Specific MR applications of the pineal region include assessment of the vein of Galen, extension into adjacent brain parenchyma, and relationship to the mesencephalon or tectum since primary midbrain gliomas may masquerade as true pineal neoplasm. The sagittal orientation is particularly useful in these instances. Coronal MR may be helpful in distinguishing falco-tentorial meningioma from other peripineal lesions.

Other pineal germ cell neoplasms include teratoma/teratocarcinoma and choriocarcinoma, embryonal cell, and yolk sac carcinomas. The pineal gland is the most common site of intracranial teratoma. Calcification and sharp margins are frequent. On CT, cyst formation may be indistinguishable from fat since low attenuation measurements can overlap. MR makes this distinction, since fat exhibits signal hyperintensity and cysts have diminished signal on T1WI. Contrast enhancement of such lesions on CT or MR suggests malignancy. Teratocarcinomas are noncalcified and poorly defined, have a hemorrhagic tendency, occasionally contain

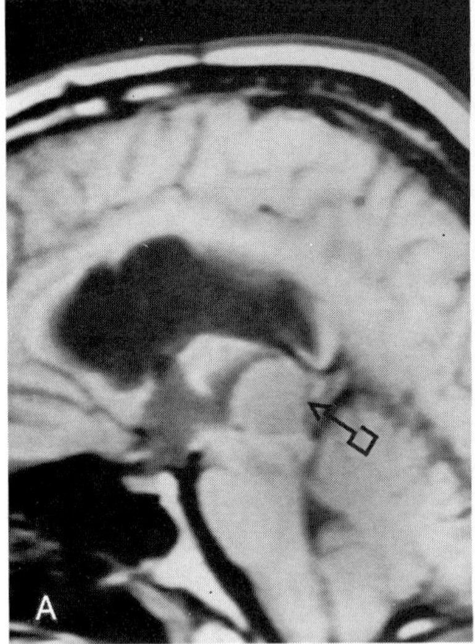


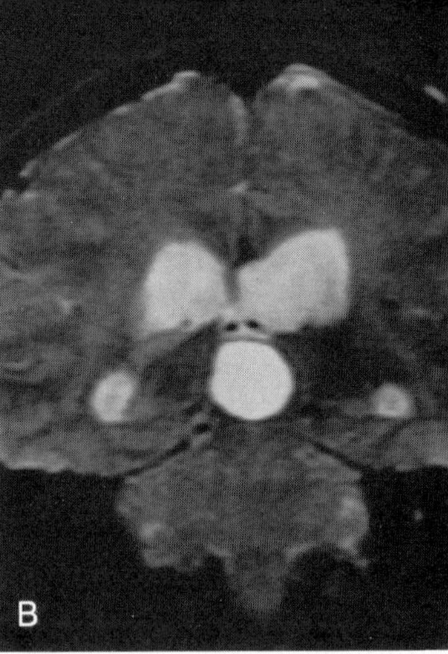


**Figure 8–29. Pineal germinoma.** A 32-year-old man with Parinaud's syndrome (1.5 T). *A,* Sagittal T1WI (TR 600/TE 20 msec). Isointense mass (arrow) displaces midbrain caudally. *B,* Coronal T2WI (TR 2000/TE 100 msec). Hyperintense mass lies on the brachium of superior colliculus.

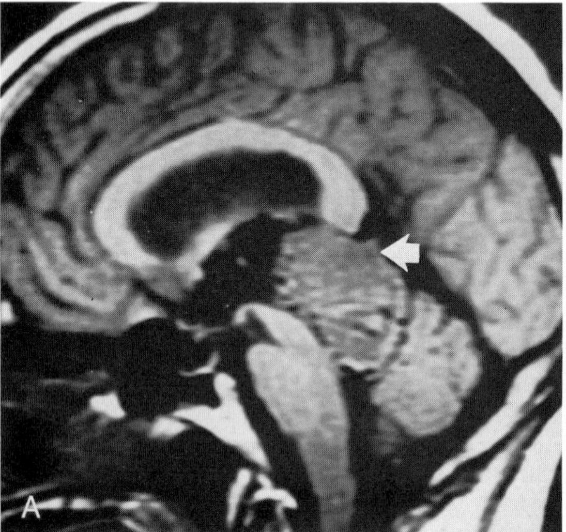


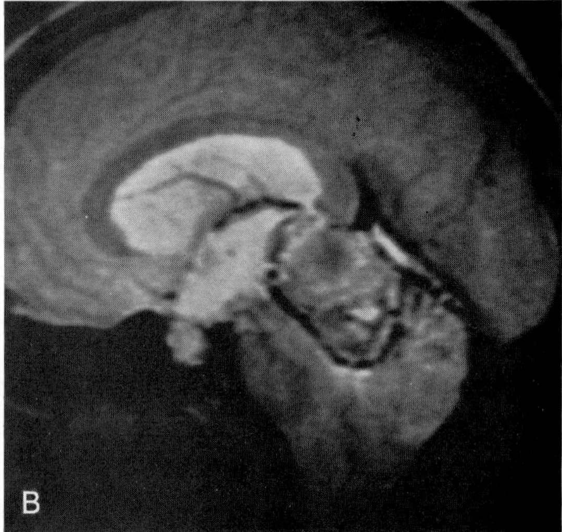


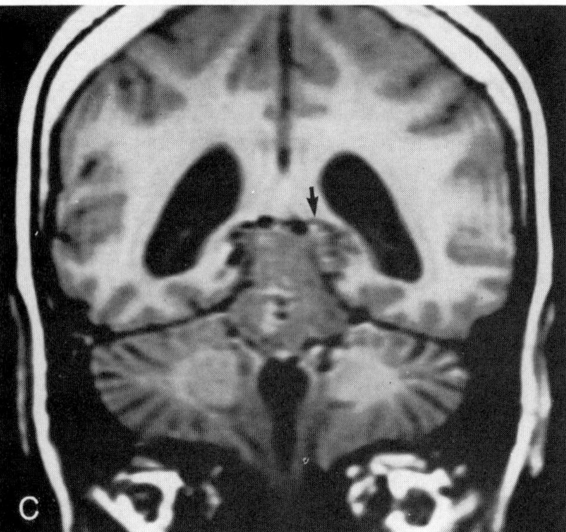


**Figure 8–30. Pineoblastoma.** A woman with headaches and mild gaze palsy (1.5 T). *A* and *B,* Sagittal N(H)WI and T2WI (TR 2000/TE 20/100 msec). Large pineal region mass (arrow) is isointense, containing foci of signal inhomogeneity on T2WI. *C,* Coronal T1WI. Mass is isointense with gray matter, contains hypointense foci (necrosis) and invades leftward brain parenchyma (arrow). (Courtesy of A. Chambers, M.D., Dept. of Neuroradiology, University Hospital, Cincinnati, Ohio.)

foci of fat, and may invade surrounding parenchyma. Choriocarcinomas have a marked hemorrhagic tendency.[114] Embryonal cell tumors also exhibit unsharp margins, irregular contrast enhancement, and prolonged relaxation times on MR.[38]

Like germinomas, pineal cell neoplasms are radiosensitive and may exhibit subarachnoid extension. Heavy pineal calcification in a female patient suggests the diagnosis of pineocytoma. Pineoblastomas are often large, hyperdense on noncontrast CT, homogeneously enhancing, and poorly circumscribed, and they yield signal hyperintensity on T2WI (Fig. 8–30). Focal calcification is more frequent in less aggressive pineal cell tumors, and isointensity or low spin density is more common in germinoma and pineocytoma. Hypodensity on CT is infrequent in germinoma or pineal cell lesions and suggests the diagnosis of teratoma/teratocarcinoma or pineal cyst.

In summary, CT is the modality of choice for initial pineal region evaluation, although specific applications of MR have been discussed. CSF seeding occurs in either pineal or germ cell neoplasm. Therefore, cytology is useful in diagnosis. Noncalcified lesions in a male patient are usually of germ cell origin, particularly germinoma, whereas calcified lesions in a female patient are of pineal cell origin, frequently pineocytoma. Negative CT numbers and short T1 relaxation on MR suggest a teratoid lesion. Malignant lesions have poorly defined margins and irregular, marked contrast enhancement on CT or MR. Sharp margins are seen in teratoma and pineocytoma. Hypodensity on CT makes pineal cell origin unlikely, and isointensity on multiple MR sequences favors germinoma or pineocytoma but is infrequent in more aggressive lesions. Calcification is rare in germinoma, teratocarcinoma, and metastasis. Contrast enhancement, CSF seeding, and homogeneous T1 prolongation on MR exclude teratoma.

## Epidermoidomas

Epidermoidomas, or congenital cholesteatomas, account for less than 1% of intracranial neoplasms. Most occur in the intradiploic calvarium, middle fossa/temporal lobe, petrous bone or cerebellopontine angle, suprasellar region, fourth ventricle, and intraspinal subarachnoid space. These lesions consist of a squamous epithelial lining with homogeneous, central, keratinaceous debris and lipid cholesterin. Unlike more midline dermoids and teratomas, these tumors lateralize, have thinner walls, may be serpiginous in shape and are often not associated with sinus tracts. Chemical meningitis and tumor rupture is most common with dermoid but may occur with epidermoid tumors. Hearing loss with cerebellopontine angle epidermoidomas is a late finding; however, trigeminal neuralgia and facial paralysis may occur.

Signal intensity of epidermoidomas on MR is extremely helpful in differentiating this lesion from cysts, cystic neoplasms, dermoids, teratomas, and lipomas (all low attenuation lesions on CT). Our series and those in the literature have shown that only 2 of 29 pathologically confirmed epidermoid tumors exhibited short T1 relaxation or bright signal on T1WI.[115, 116] Cholesterol granulomas of the petrous apex exhibit short T1 relaxation. Occasionally, this lesion has incorrectly been labeled as an epidermoidoma on CT or MR. Most epidermoids exhibit T1 and T2 prolongation (Fig. 8–31) and inhomogeneous signal.[41, 42, 117] Separation of an epidermoidoma from the fourth ventricle or eighth nerve complex is best achieved with MR. Serpiginous but sharp margins, inhomogeneous T1/T2 prolongation, absent edema, minimal mass effect, lateralized location, infrequent marginal calcification, and thin walls help differentiate this lesion from the following: (1) teratoma/dermoid (round, sharp margin; mixed or short T1 relaxation; midline location; associated sinus tract; thick walls; frequent calcification); (2) arachnoid or other cysts (sharp, round margins; homogeneous signal matches CSF; absent edema); (3) cystic neoplasm (T1/T2 prolongation, edema, mass effect). Most epidermoids are hypodense on CT (0 to −70 HU); however, high-density epidermoidomas may rarely be seen on CT owing to calcification or saponification of keratinized debris and may simulate meningiomas.[118] These may still exhibit increased T1 and T2 relaxation characteristics in our experience.

## Dermoid Tumors and Teratomas

Dermoid tumors are midline congenital neoplasms resulting from abnormal neural tube closure and possessing a squamous epithelial lining plus skin appendages. Sites of

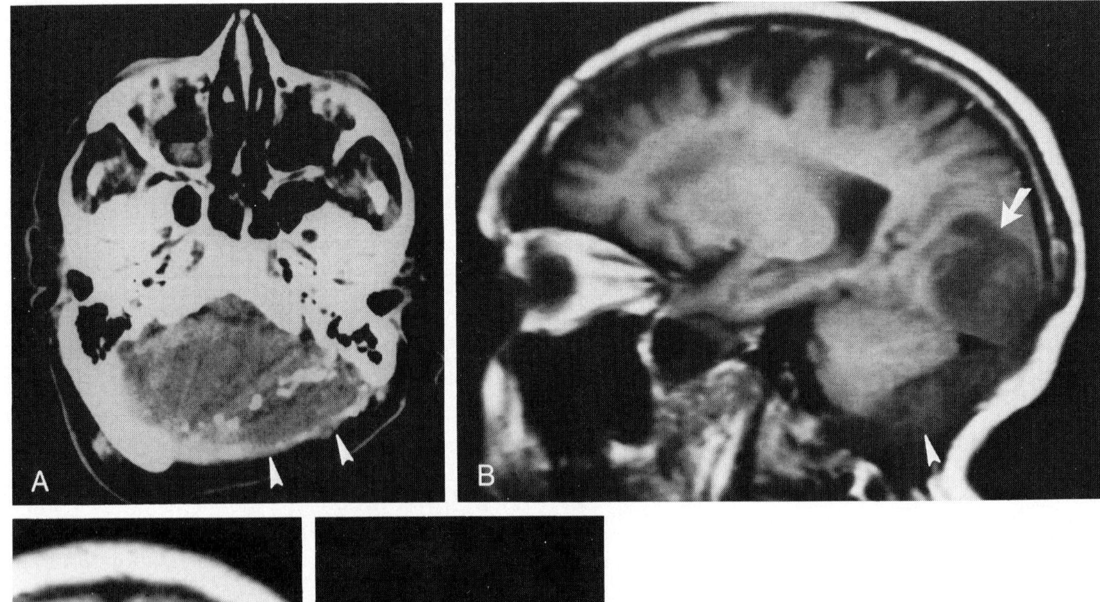


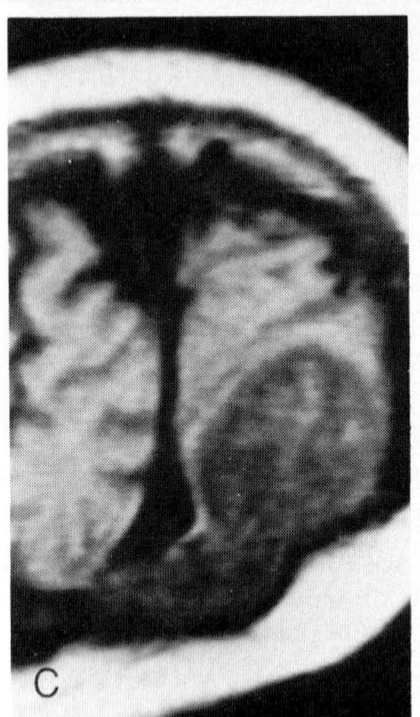


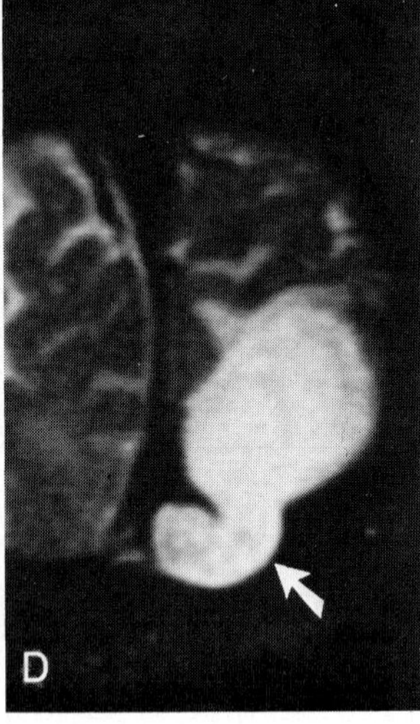


**Figure 8–31. Epidermoid, recurrent.** A 62-year-old man with calvarial lesion resected 29 years ago who presented with seizures (1.5 T). *A,* Axial CECT shows hypodensity in the prior surgical bed (arrowheads). *B,* Sagittal T1WI shows an inhomogeneous hypointense mass with infratentorial component seen on CT (arrowhead) and an invaginating supratentorial portion (arrow). *C* and *D,* Coronal multiecho N(H)WI and T2WI (TR 2000/TE 20/100 msec) depicts its extra-axial location (arrow).

involvement include suprasellar, subfrontal, and posterior fossa or peripineal regions. Posterior fossa lesions are frequently associated with sinus tracts or linear foci of T2 prolongation connecting lesion to the skin surface. Dermoids are the most frequent intracranial tumors to spontaneously rupture. These sharply marginated, rounded, low attenuation (−30 to −100 HU) lesions on CT more frequently calcify and have thicker walls than epidermoids. Dermoid tumors exhibit short T1 relaxation (Fig. 8–32), unlike cysts, epidermoidoma, and cystic neoplasms. Although signal intensity does not perfectly match subgaleal fat as in lipoma (Fig. 8–33), differentiation from a hemorrhagic lesion and detection of subarachnoid fat owing to rupture is greatly assisted by T1-weighted and chemical shift images. Dense or heavily calcified dermoid tumors still contain foci of bright signal on T1 images admixed with calcium-producing foci of signal dropout.

Teratomas contain ectodermal, mesodermal, and endodermal elements and are discussed with neoplasms of the pineal region, their most common site. Sellar and perisellar teratomas may occur. A solid component of intermediate signal intensity can be identified within, and larger bulky calcific foci of signal dropout are more frequent with teratoma than other congenital neoplasms.[19–21]

## Ganglioglioma

Ganglioglioma is an uncommon neoplasm of children and young adults, 30% occurring in those under 30 years of age.[122] Equal sex distribution or a slight male predominance

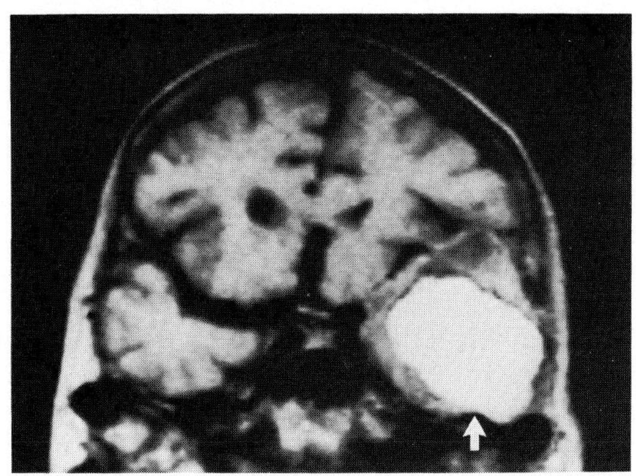

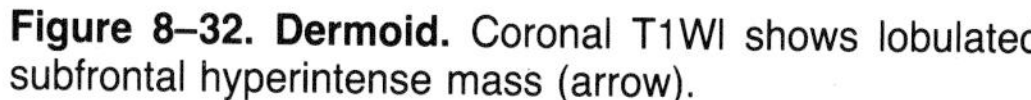

**Figure 8–32. Dermoid.** Coronal T1WI shows lobulated subfrontal hyperintense mass (arrow).

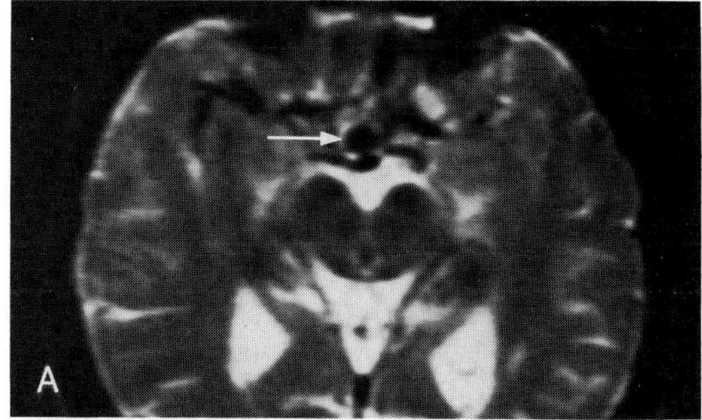


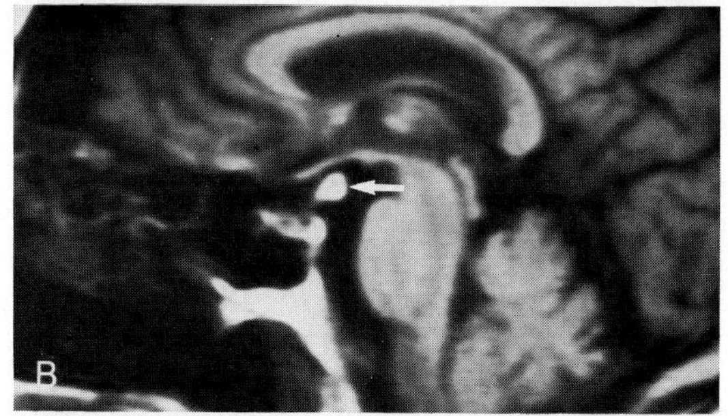


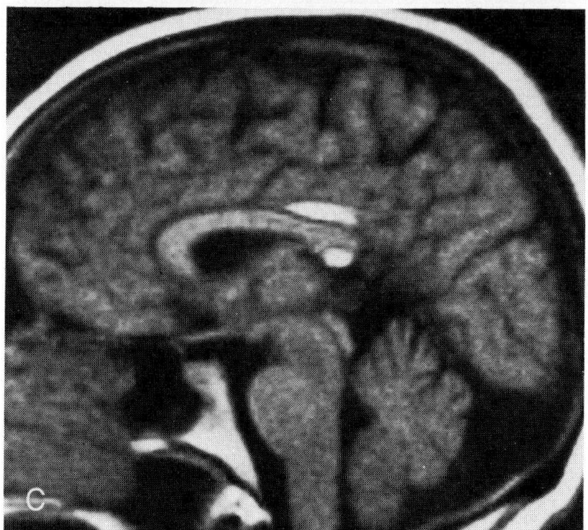


**Figure 8–33. Intracranial lipomas.** Two patients with nonspecific headaches and intracranial lipoma. *A,* Axial (1.5 T) T2WI (TR 2000/TE 100). *B,* Sagittal (1.5 T) T1WI (TR 600/TE 20). *C,* Sagittal (0.35 T) T1WI (TR 500/TE 16). Axial and sagittal images from the first patient (*A* and *B*) demonstrate hyperintense signal on T1WI (short arrow) and expected hypointense signal on T2WI (long arrow) relative to CSF with a lesion harboring fat. Sagittal section from the second patient *(C)* demonstrates another typical supratentorial location of lipoma, the corpus callosum. (Courtesy of J. Tobias, M.D., Radiology Dept., Mount Sinai Hospital, Miami Beach, Fla.)

has been noted.[123] Slow growth of this tumor often results in progressively frequent seizures. Malignant degeneration is unusual; it most often involves glial elements (glioblastoma) and less frequently, ganglion cells (neuroblastoma). If ganglion cells predominate heavily, ganglioneuroma is the histologic diagnosis.

The MR findings of ganglioglioma are not specific. Lesions are sharply marginated with mild mass effect and only mild-to-moderate high-signal edema. Markedly prolonged T2 relaxation and an intermediate signal nodule may occur in its cystic variant. Isodensity or hypodensity with moderate contrast enhancement is typical on CT. Optimal visualization with gadolinium-enhanced T1WI has been shown on MR.[124] Approximately 10% to 20% are calcified. A young patient with an insidious seizure history and signal abnormalities in the appropriate location (temporal lobe or anterior third ventricle) should suggest the correct diagnosis. Gangliogliomas do not typically yield bright signal on a T1WI, which assists in their differentiation from colloid cysts in the third ventricular region.

## Colloid Cyst

Colloid cyst is a developmental anomaly arising from the paraphysis, embryologic ependymal tissue thought to represent extraventricular choroid plexus. These lesions arise in the most anterosuperior third ventricle; typically, they occur in young persons over age ten years,[125] are 1 to 3 cm in size when symptomatic, and may produce intermittent hydrocephalus and headache.

The most anterosuperior third ventricular roof is its typical location. No third ventricular CSF signal should be seen anterior or superior to the lesion. Mild widening of the septum pellucidum, lateral ventricular dilation, and posterior third ventricular collapse is frequent.[126] Isodensity or hyperdensity on NCCT with a thin rimlike or a faint, diffuse central enhancement on CECT is typical. Rarely, hypodense lesions on CT can be seen.[127] This situation may arise when cuboidal epithelial ependymalike cells line the cyst and secrete a fluid of CSF composition. The result is a neuroepithelial cyst on MR with long T1 and T2 relaxation characteristics (cystic type).[128] More commonly, a ciliated epithelium secreting mucinous, not colloidal material, lines these lesions. Approximately 60% of colloid cysts are of this type and exhibit short T1 relaxation (Fig. 8–34) and variable shortening of T2 relaxation (paramagnetic type). This most typical MR appearance may be partially related to heavy protein or mucoid content. More than one half of cysts exhibiting bright signal on T1WI exhibit centrally shortened T2 relaxation with a circumferentially hyperintense T2WI capsule.[129] This central paramagnetic effect may be related to spectroscopically confirmed cyst contents such as magnesium, copper, or iron.[130] An atypical, hypodense colloid cyst on NCCT exhibited mild T1WI and marked T2WI signal hypointensity with a T1WI circumferentially hyperintense rim.[131]

The signal of many colloid cysts allows differentiation from most forniceal metastases (long or intermediate T1/T2 relaxation), glial tumors (long T1/T2 relaxation), hamartomas (isointense with cerebral cortex), and aneurysms (flow-related signal void). Only craniopharyngiomas or metastases from melanoma may exhibit similar T1 relaxation in this region. Melanoma metastases may exhibit shortened T1 and T2 but are differentiated by the presence of edema, multiplicity, and clinical history. Third ventricular craniopharyngiomas, a rare occurrence, are differentiated on the basis of their short T1 and long T2 relaxation. Correlation of the CT and MR appearances (hyperdense CT, short T1/T2 relaxation and hypodense CT, long T1/T2 relaxation) is inconsistent.[20] Previously, authors have recommended contrast ventriculography for evaluation of idiopathic lateral ventricular dilation and a normal CT.[132] We believe that this procedure is unnecessary and that MR and CEMR should supplant this examination.

## Lymphoma and Leukemia

Primary central nervous system lymphoma is more common than secondary involvement by systemic lymphoreticular disease. Primary lesions are probably neoplastic counterparts of normal lymphocytic transformation.[133] An increased incidence exists in allograft recipients,[134] patients with acquired immune deficiency syndrome (AIDS),[135] chemotherapy patients, and those with another existing primary malignancy.

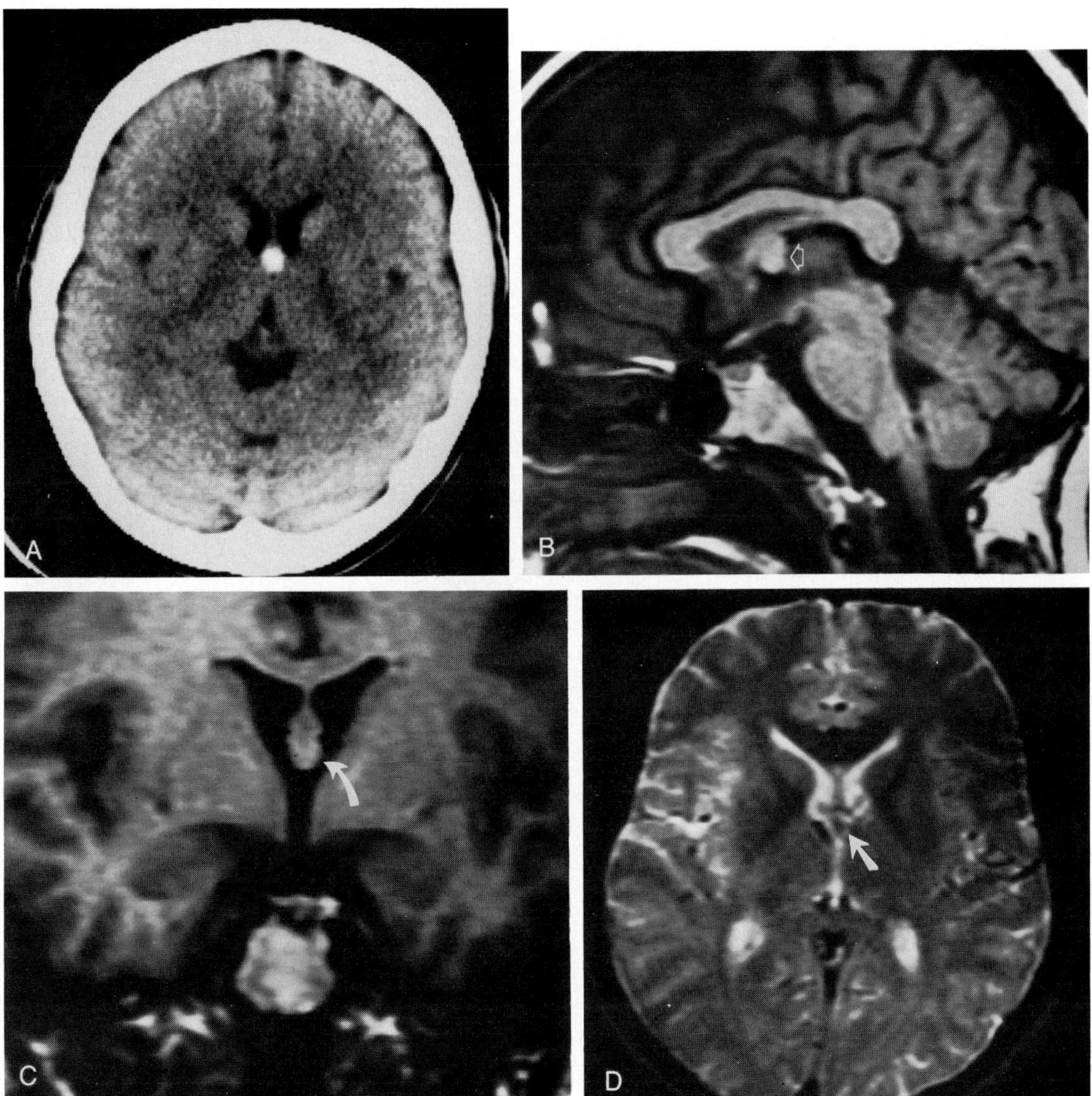


**Figure 8–34. Colloid cyst, paramagnetic type** (1.5 T). *A,* Axial NCCT. *B,* Sagittal T1WI. *C,* Coronal T1WI. *D,* Axial T2WI. CT shows a hyperdense, rounded mass. Hyperintense lesion on sagittal (open arrow) and coronal (curved arrow) T1WI is localized to the anterosuperior third ventricle. Hypointensity on T2WI (arrow) is compatible with paramagnetic effect.

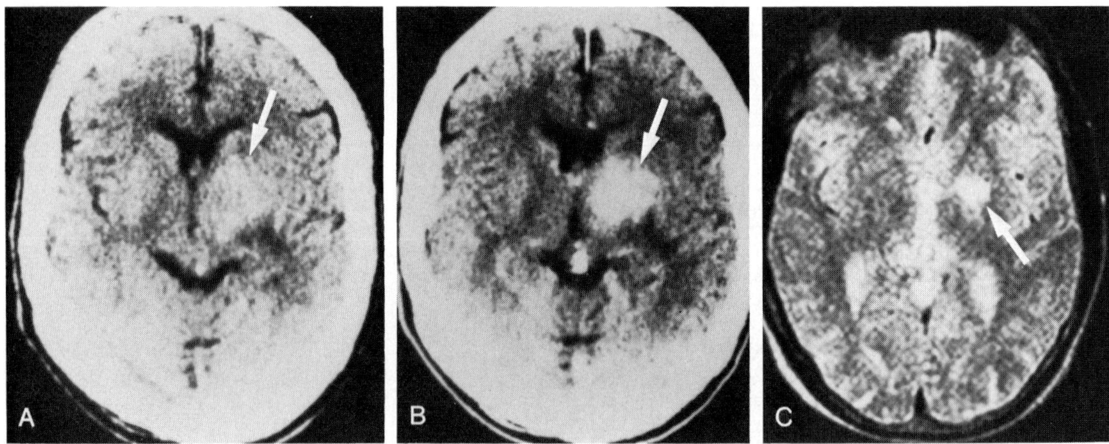

**Figure 8–35. Primary brain lymphoma.** *A–C,* Axial CT, CECT, and T2WI (0.35 T) MR. Enhancing leftward basal ganglia and thalamic mass enhances on CECT (arrow, to reader's right), and after two weeks on therapy, has diminished in size on noncontrast MR (arrowhead). (Courtesy of J. Tobias, M.D., Radiology Dept., Mt. Sinai Hospital, Miami Beach, Fla.)

Primary brain lymphoma typically involves the basal ganglia (50%), corpus callosum, periventricular white matter, cerebellar vermis, and septum pellucidum. Approximately 45% of lesions are multiple,[136] and 30% of patients demonstrate leptomeningeal involvement. Single lesions are usually large. Masses are often sharply marginated, round or oval, and isointense or hyperintense on T2WI (Figs. 8–35 and 8–36). Isointensity on multiple pulsing sequences is not rare, and periventricular high-signal edema may obscure lesions in this location. Focal areas of necrosis or hemorrhage are rare. For these reasons, we prefer NCCT and CECT in the initial evaluation of these lesions. Leptomeningeal, subarachnoid, and subependymal or ependymal tumor spread is difficult to detect on noncontrast MR but is detected more accurately with CEMR than CECT. CECT homogeneously enhancing, high-density, multiple, deep parenchymal lesions are characteristic with this modality. Nevertheless, MR is more accurate than CT in assessing lesion multiplicity, and the correct diagnosis may therefore be deduced following MR when only a single lesion of appropriate character is detected on CT. Furthermore, solitary, large, enhancing, high-attenuation lesions on CT may simulate meningioma or even glial neoplasms. The dural-based nature and short T2 of many meningiomas, or the disproportionate edema, mass effect, and poor margination of glioma assists in differentiation from lymphoma on MR. Transient spon-

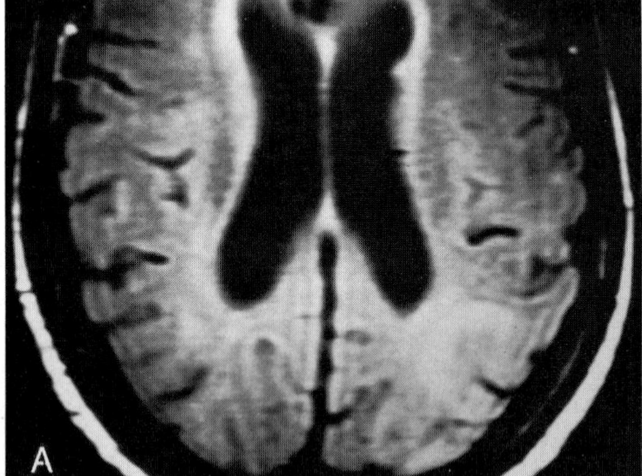

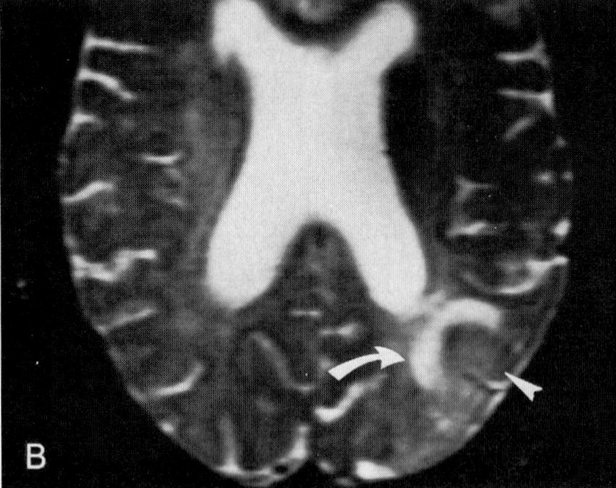

**Figure 8–36. Lymphoma.** *A* and *B,* A 59-year-old woman with spinal lymphoma presents with acute dysphagia and right-sided weakness (1.5 T). Axial multiecho N(H)WI and T2WI (TR 2000/TE 20/100 msec). Wedge-shaped signal hyperintensity (curved arrow) and paucity of mass effect suggest infarction. Cortical lesion (arrowhead) is inapparent.

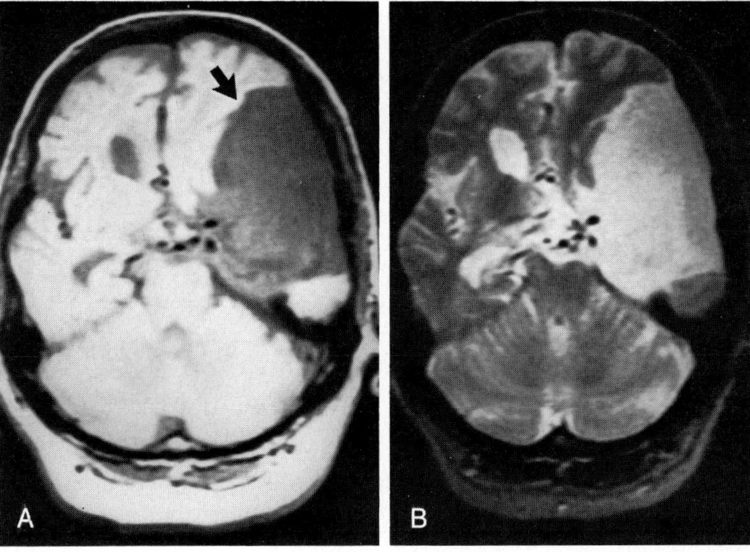

**Figure 8–37. Leptomeningeal arachnoid cyst.** A 52-year-old veterinarian with persistent left-sided headaches. *A,* Axial N(H)WI (TR 1800/TE 20). *B,* Axial T2WI (TR 1800/TE 100). An extra-axial mass (arrow) demonstrates signal intensity similar to CSF in the lateral ventricle and demonstrates a dural-based margin laterally. A remote history of head trauma was subsequently elicited after examination.

taneous regression of lymphoma has been reported,[137] and symptoms of reversible ischemia may occur owing to marked perivascular lymphoreticular invasion.

## Arachnoid Cyst

Arachnoid cysts account for 1% of intracranial masses and are congenital lesions arising from splitting of the arachnoid membrane. The middle cranial fossa, cerebral convexity, posterior fossa/retrocerebellar region, and suprasellar or quadrageminal cisterns are the most commonly affected sites. This surgically treatable mass lesion may produce obstructive hydrocephalus. Communication with the normal subarachnoid space is common.

The MR findings of arachnoid cyst are characteristic. A mass in the appropriate location exhibits homogeneous T1 and T2 prolongation, matches CSF in signal intensity (Figs. 8–37 and 8–38) on multiple pulsing sequences, and has sharp margins; edema is absent. A straight posterior margin may be present in middle fossa cysts with hypoplasia or mass effect on the temporal lobe and bulging of the temporal calvarium. Diagnostic features helpful in evaluation of suprasellar arachnoid cysts (see Fig. 10–19) include (1) oval or square appearance of the suprasellar cistern, (2) cisternal eccentricity, (3) splaying of cerebral peduncles, (4) carotid terminus separation, (5) trigeminal or crural cistern widening, (6) anterior displacement of the optic chiasm, (7) diamond-shaped mid-third ventricle, (8) asymmetric dilatation of the lateral ventricles with asymmetric expansion of one foramen of Monroe, (9) a pseudo third ventricle enlarged out of proportion to the remaining ventricles, (10) dilatation of the third ventricle with relative sparing of the suprapineal recesses, and (11) superolateral displacement of the forniceal columns.[138]

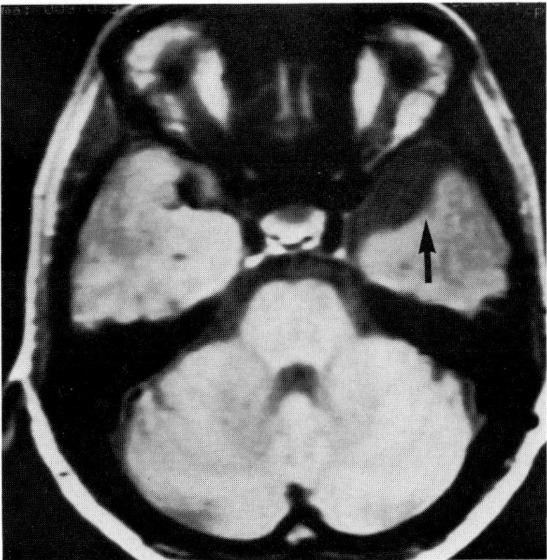

**Figure 8–38. Congenital arachnoid cyst.** A 42-year-old woman with frontal headaches. *A,* Axial T1WI (TR 500/TE 20) (arrow). Anterior to the left temporal tip (arrow) is a region of signal hypointensity matching the CSF signal in the fourth ventricle and the prepontine cistern. The signal is homogeneous and the location is typical.

The enlarged third ventricle of aqueductal stenosis may simulate suprasellar arachnoid cyst. These findings are particularly useful in confirming the diagnosis of aqueductal stenosis: (1) star-shaped, symmetric suprasellar cistern; (2) lack of basal cistern expansion; (3) marked suprapineal recess expansion; (4) inferoposterior displacement of the optic chiasm by the enlarged chiasmatic recess; (5) symmetric ventricular enlargement; and (6) lack of superolateral separation of the forniceal columns. Ependymal or nonependymal lined simple cysts may be differentiated by their location, intra-axial position, and less marked mass effect.

MR is the preferred modality in the evaluation of these lesions. Other cystic lesions on CT including dermoid tumors, teratoma, lipoma, and craniopharyngioma exhibit short T1 relaxation, unlike arachnoid cyst. The signal characteristics of craniopharyngioma and intracranial dermoid tumors (short T1/long T2) approximate that of sphenoid sinus mucocele.[139] Although most epidermoidomas exhibit long T1 and T2 relaxation, they in no way match CSF in signal intensity on various pulsing sequences as do arachnoid cysts. Cystic gliomas almost always exhibit high signal edema on T2WI. Parasitic cysts (echinococcal, cysticercosis), when suspected, are best evaluated on CT, since calcium detection is of great diagnostic value in these lesions.

The CT findings of arachnoid cyst include a smooth, homogeneous, low attenuation (− 20 to + 20 HU) mass, noncalcified and nonenhancing.

## References


1. Rosen BR, Pykett IL, Brady TJ, et al. NMR chemical shift imaging. In James TL, Margulis AR, eds. Biomedical magnetic resonance. San Francisco, Radiology Research and Education Foundation, 1984.
2. Bradley WG Jr. Pathophysiologic correlates of signal alterations. In Brant-Zawadski M, Norman D, eds. Magnetic Resonance Imaging of the Central Nervous System. New York, Raven Press, 1987:24.
3. Mills CM, Crooks LE, Kaufman L, et al. Cerebral abnormalities: use of calculated T1 and T2 magnetic resonance images for diagnosis. Radiology 150:87, 1984.
4. Englund E, Brun A, Larrson E-M, et al. Tumors of the central nervous system: proton and magnetic resonance relaxation times T1 and T2 and histopathologic correlates. Acta Radiol Diagn 27:653, 1986.
5. Pusey E, Kortman KE, Bradley WG, et al. MR of craniopharyngiomas: tumor delineation and characterization. AJNR 8:439, 1987.
6. Freeman MP, Kessler RM, Allen JH, et al. Craniopharyngioma: CT and MR imaging in nine cases. Comput Assist Tomogr 11:810, 1987.
7. Brant-Zawadski M, Kjos B, Newton TH, et al. Magnetic resonance imaging and characterization of normal and abnormal intracranial cerebrospinal (CSF) spaces. Neuroradiology 27:3, 1985.
8. Davis PC, Friedman NC, Fry SM, et al. Leptomeningeal metastasis: MR imaging. Radiology 163:449, 1987.
9. Olsen WL, Dillon WP, Kelly WM, et al. MR imaging of paragangliomas. AJNR 7:1039, 1986.
10. Sipponen JT, Sepponen RE, Sivula A. Nuclear magnetic resonance (NMR) imaging of intracerebral hemorrhage in the acute and resolving phases. Comput Assist Tomogr 7:954, 1983.
11. DeLaPaz RL, New PFJ, Buonanno FS, et al. NMR imaging of intracranial hemorrhage. Comput Assist Tomogr 8:599, 1984.
12. Scott M. Spontaneous intracerebral hematoma caused by cerebral neoplasms: report of eight verified cases. J Neurosurg 42:338, 1975.
13. Zimmerman HM. The pathology of primary brain tumors. Semin Roentgenol 19:129, 1984
14. Mandybur TI. Intracranial hemorrhage caused by metastatic tumors. Neurology 27:650, 1977.
15. Davis JM, Zimmerman RA, Bilaniuk LT. Metastases to the central nervous system. Radiol Clin North Am 20:417, 1982.
16. Atlas SW, Grossman RI, Gomori JM, et al. Hemorrhagic intracranial malignant neoplasms: spin-echo MR imaging. Radiology 164:71, 1987.
17. Sze G, Krol G, Olsen WL, et al. Hemorrhagic neoplasms: MR mimics of occult vascular malformations. AJNR 8:795, 1987.
18. Fullerton GD, Cameron IL, Ord VA. Frequency dependence of magnetic resonance spin-lattice relaxation of protons in biological materials. Radiology 151:135, 1984.
19. Bradley WG Jr. Pathophysiologic correlates of signal alterations. In Brant-Zawadski M, Norman D, eds. Magnetic Resonance Imaging of the Central Nervous System. New York, Raven Press, 1987:27.
20. Fishman RA. Brain edema. N Engl J Med 293:706, 1975.
21. Hilal SK, Ra JB, Silver AJ, et al. In vivo sodium imaging using a very short echo time: potential for selective imaging in intracellular sodium and extracellular space. Radiology 157(P):188, 1985.
22. Turski PA, Perman WH, Hald JF, et al. Clinical and experimental vasogenic edema: In vivo sodium MR imaging. Radiology 160:821, 1986.
23. Perman WH, Turski PA, Houston LW, et al. Methodology of in vivo human sodium MR imaging at 1.5 T. Radiology 160:811, 1986.
24. Spagnoli MV, Goldberg HI, Grossman RI, et al: Intracranial meningiomas: high-field MR imaging. Radiology 161:369, 1986.
25. Young IR, Khenia S, Thomas DGT, et al. Clinical susceptibility mapping of the brain. Comput Assist Tomogr 1:2, 1987.
26. Bradley WG, Crooks LE, Newton TH. Physical principles of NMR. In Newton TH, Potts DG, eds. Modern Neuroradiology, Vol 2: Advanced Imaging Techniques. San Francisco, Clavadel Press, 1983:15.
27. Wesbey GE, Moseley ME, Ehman RL. Translation

molecular self-diffusion in magnetic resonance imaging: effects and applications. In James TL, Margulis AR, eds. Biomedical Magnetic Resonance. San Francisco, Radiology Research and Education Foundation, 1984:63.
28. Waluch V, Bradley WG. NMR even-echo rephasing in slow laminar flow. J Comput Assist Tomogr 8:594, 1984.
29. Higgins CB, von Schulthess GK. Blood flow imaging with MR: Spin-phase phenomena. Radiology 157:687, 1985.
30. Roosen N, Gahlen D, Stork W, et al. Magnetic resonance imaging of colloid cysts of the third ventricle. Neuroradiology 29:10, 1987.
31. Atlas SW, Grossman RI, Gomori JM, et al. MR imaging of intracranial metastatic melanoma. J Comput Assist Tomogr 11:577, 1987.
32. Graif M, Bydder GM, Steiner RE, et al. Contrast-enhanced MR imaging of malignant brain tumors. AJNR 6:855, 1985.
33. Brasch RC, Weinmann HJ, Wesbey GE. Contrast-enhanced NMR imaging: animal studies using gadolinium-DTPA complex. AJR 142:625, 1984.
34. Strich G, Hagan PL, Gerber KH, et al. Tissue distribution and magnetic resonance spin-lattice relaxation effects of gadolinium-DTPA. Radiology 154:723, 1985.
35. Runge VM, Clanton JA, Lukehart CM, et al. Paramagnetic agents for contrast-enhanced NMR imaging: a review. AJR 141:1209, 1983.
36. Weinmann HJ, Brasch RC, Press WR, et al. Characteristics of gadolinium-DTPA complex: a potential NMR contrast agent. AJR 142:619, 1984.
37. Drago RS. Physical Methods in Chemistry. Philadelphia, WB Saunders, 1977.
38. Runge VM, Clanton JA, Herzer WA, et al. Intravascular contrast agents suitable for magnetic resonance imaging. Radiology 153:171, 1984.
39. Wehrli FW, Macfall JR, Glover GH, et al. The dependency of NMR image contrast on intrinsic and pulse sequence timing parameters. Magn Reson Imag 2:3, 1984.
40. Niendorf HP, Laniado M, Semmler W, et al: Dose administration of gadolinium-DTPA in MR imaging of intracranial tumors. AJNR 8:803, 1987.
41. Wolf GL, Joseph PM, Goldstein EJ. Optimal pulsing sequences for MR contrast agents. AJR 147:367, 1986.
42. Claussen C, Laniado M, Schorner W, et al. Gadolinium-DTPA in MR imaging of glioblastomas and intracranial metastases. AJNR 6:669, 1985.
43. Bradley WG, Waluch V, Yadley RA, et al. Comparison of CT and MR in 400 patients with suspected disease of the brain and cervical spinal cord. Radiology 152:695, 1984.
44. Bradley WG, Brant-Zawadski M, Brasch RC, et al. Initial clinical experience with Gd-DTPA in North America: MR contrast enhancement of brain tumors. Radiology 157(P):125, 1985.
45. Schaible TF, Goldstein HA, Haughton VM, et al. Diagnostic efficacy of gadolinium-DTPA/dimeglumine in MR imaging of intracranial tumors. Presented at the American Society of Neuroradiology 25th Annual Meeting, New York, May 10–15, 1987.
46. Brant-Zawadski M, Berry I, Osaki L, et al. Gd-DTPA in clinical MR of the brain: 1. Intraaxial lesions. AJR 147:1223, 1986.
47. Schorner W, Laniado M, Kornmesser W et al. Intracranial tumors: comparison of multi-echo and Gd-DTPA–enhanced images. Presented at the American Society of Neuroradiology 25th Annual Meeting, New York, May 10–15, 1987.
48. Berry I, Brant-Zawadski M, Osaki L, et al. Gd-DTPA in clinical MR of the brain. 2. Extraxial lesions and normal structures. AJR 147:1231, 1986.
49. Kilgore DP, Breger RK, Daniels DL, et al. Cranial tissues: normal MR appearance after intravenous injection of Gd-DTPA. Radiology 160:757, 1986.
50. Schorner W, Laniado M, Niendorf HP, et al. Time-dependent changes in image contrast in brain tumors after gadolinium-DTPA. AJNR 7:1013, 1987.
51. Bydder GM, Kingsley DPE, Brown J, et al. MR imaging of meningiomas including studies with and without gadolinium-DTPA. J Comput Assist Tomogr 9:690, 1985.
52. Koschorek F, Jensen H-P, Terwey B. Dynamic MR imaging: a further possibility for characterizing CNS lesions. AJNR 8:259, 1987.
53. Felix R, Schorner W, Laniado M, et al. Brain tumors: MR imaging with gadolinium-DTPA. Radiology 156:681, 1985.
54. Breger RK, Papke RA, Pojunas KW, et al. Benign extraxial tumors: contrast enhancement with Gd-DTPA. Radiology 163:427, 1987.
55. Khandji AG, Post KD, Hilal JA, et al. Study of pituitary microadenomas with gadolinium DTPA and ultra-thin section MRI. Presented at the American Society of Neuroradiology 25th Annual Meeting, New York, May 10–15, 1987.
56. Dwyer AJ, Frank JA, Doppman JL, et al. Pituitary adenomas in patients with Cushing's disease: initial experience with Gd-DTPA–enhanced MR imaging. Radiology 163:421, 1987.
57. Holland BA, Kucharcyzk W, Brant-Zawadski M, et al. MR imaging of calcified intracranial lesions. Radiology 157:353, 1985.
58. Atlas SW, Grossman RI, Hackney DB, et al. The utility of MR imaging with gradient-recalled signal acquisition in the steady state (GRASS) for the detection of calcified intracranial lesions. Presented at the American Society of Neuroradiology 25th Annual Meeting, New York, May 10–15, 1987.
59. Bradley WG, Waluch V. Blood flow: magnetic resonance imaging. Radiology 154:443, 1985.
60. Bradley WG, Waluch V, Lai K, et al. The appearance of rapidly flowing blood on magnetic resonance images. AJR 143:1167, 1984.
61. Mills CM, Zawadski MB, Crooks LE, et al. Nuclear magnetic resonance: principles of blood flow imaging. AJR 142:165, 1984.
62. Axel LA. Blood flow effects in magnetic resonance imaging. AJR 143:1157, 1984.
63. Zimmerman HM. Brain tumors: their incidence and classification in man and their experimental production. Ann NY Acad Sci 159:337, 1969.
64. Williams AL, Haughton VM. Cranial Computed Tomography: a Comprehensive Text. St. Louis, CV Mosby Co., 1985.
65. Gonzalez CF, Grossman CB, Masdeu JC. Head and Spine Imaging. New York, John Wiley & Sons, 1985.
66. Spagnoli MV, Grossman RI, Packer RJ, et al. Magnetic resonance imaging determination of gliomatosis cerebri. Neuroradiology 29:15, 1987.
67. Bydder GM, Pennock JM, Steiner RE, et al. The

NMR diagnosis of cerebral tumors. Magn Reson Imag Med 1:5, 1984.
68. Brant-Zawadski M, Badami JP, Mills CM, et al. Primary intracranial tumor imaging: a comparison of magnetic resonance and CT. Radiology 150:435, 1984.
69. Brant-Zawadski M, Norman D, Newton TH. Magnetic resonance of the brain: the optimal screening technique. Radiology 152:71, 1984.
70. Smith AS, Weinstein MA, Modic MT, et al. Magnetic resonance with marked T2-weighted images: improved demonstration of brain lesions, tumor, and edema. AJNR 6:691, 1985.
71. Aaron J, New PFJ, Strand R, et al. NMR imaging in temporal lobe epilepsy due to gliomas. J Comput Assist Tomogr 8:608, 1984.
72. Laster DW, Perry JK, Moody DM, et al. Chronic seizure disorders: contribution of MR imaging when CT is normal. AJNR 6:177, 1985.
73. Sostman HD, Spencer DD, Gore JC, et al. Preliminary observations on magnetic resonance imaging in refractory epilepsy. Magn Reson Imaging 2:301, 1984.
74. Schorner W, Meencke H-J, Felix R. Temporal lobe epilepsy: comparison of CT and MR imaging. AJNR 8:773, 1987.
75. McLachlan RS, Nicholson RL, Black S, et al. Nuclear magnetic resonance imaging: A new approach to the investigation of refractory temporal lobe epilepsy. Epilepsia 26:555, 1985.
76. Ormson MJ, Kispert DB, Sharbrough FW, et al. Cryptic structural lesions in refractory partial epilepsy: MR imaging and CT studies. Radiology 160:215, 1986.
77. Posin JP, Ortendahl DA, Hylton NM, et al. Variable magnetic resonance imaging parameters: effect on detection and characterization of lesions. Radiology 155:719, 1985.
78. Bradley WG Jr, Kortman KE, Burgoyne B, et al. Flowing cerebrospinal fluid in normal and hydrocephalic states: appearance on MR images. Radiology 159:611, 1986.
79. Ehman RL, McNamara MT, Brasch RC, et al. Influence of physiologic motion on the appearance of tissue in MR images. Radiology 159:777, 1986.
80. Kjos BO, Brant-Zadawski M, Kucharczyk, et al. Cystic intracranial lesions: magnetic resonance imaging. Radiology 155:363, 1985.
81. Feinberg DA, Mills CM, Postin JP, et al. Multiple spin-echo magnetic resonance imaging. Radiology 155:437, 1985.
82. Mills CM, Crooks LE, Kaufman L, et al. Cerebral abnormalities: use of calculated T1 and T2 magnetic resonance images for diagnosis. Radiology 150:87, 1984.
83. Kjos BO, Ehman RL, Brant-Zawadski M, et al: Reproducibility of relaxation times and spin density calculated from routine MR imaging sequences: clinical study of the CNS. AJR 144:1165, 1985.
84. Curnes JT, Laster DW, Ball MR, et al. MRI of radiation injury to the brain. AJR 147:119, 1986.
85. Shuman WP, Griffin BR, Haynor DR, et al. The utility of MR in planning the radiation therapy of oligodendroglioma. AJNR 8:93, 1987.
86. Mork SJ, Lindegaard KF, Halvorsen TB, et al. Oligodendroglioma: incidence and biological behavior in a defined population. J Neurosurg 63:881, 1985.
87. Swartz JD, Zimmerman RA, Bilaniuk LT. Computed tomography of intracranial ependymomas. Radiology 143:97, 1982.
88. Kelly WM, Brant-Zawadski M. Magnetic resonance imaging and computed tomography of supratentorial tumors. In Radiology: Diagnosis-Imaging-Intervention, Vol 3. Philadelphia, JB Lippincott Co. 1986:16.
89. Peterman SB, Steiner RE, Bydder GM. Magnetic resonance imaging of intracranial tumors in children and adolescents. AJNR 5:703, 1984.
90. Diebler C, Ponsot G. Hamartomas of the tuber cinereum. Neuroradiology 25:93, 1983.
91. Pomeranz SJ, Sheldon JJ, Tobias J, et al. MR of the visual pathways in patients with neurofibromatosis. AJNR 8:831, 1987.
92. Lee BCP, Deck MDF. Sellar and juxtasellar lesion detection with MR. Radiology 157:143, 1985.
93. Russell EJ, George AE, Kricheff II, et al. Atypical computed tomographic features of meningioma. Radiology 135:673, 1980.
94. Zimmerman RA, Bilaniuk LT, Grossman RI, et al. Cerebral NMR: diagnostic evaluation of brain tumors by partial saturation technique with resistive NMR. Neuroradiology 27:9, 1985.
95. Zimmerman RD, Fleming CC, Saint-Louis LA, et al: Magnetic resonance imaging of meningiomas. AJNR 6:149, 1985.
96. McGeachie RE, Gold LHA, Latchaw RE. Periventricular spread of tumor demonstrated by computed tomography. Radiology 125:407, 1977.
97. Gonzalez CF, Grossman CB, Masdeu JC. Head and Spine Imaging. New York, John Wiley & Sons, 1985:275.
98. Davis PC, Friedman NC, Fry SM, et al. Leptomeningeal metastasis: MR imaging. Radiology 163:449, 1987.
99. Rao KCVG, Williams JP: Intracranial tumors: metastatic. In Lee SH, Rao KCVG, eds. Clinical Computed Tomography. New York, McGraw-Hill Book Co, 1983.
100. Ginaldi S, Wallace S, Shalen P, et al: Cranial computed tomography of malignant melanoma. AJR 136:145, 1981.
101. Little JR, Dial JB, Belanger G, et al: Brain hemorrhage from intracranial tumor. Stroke 10:283, 1979.
102. Gildersleeve N Jr, Koo AH, McDonald CJ. Metastatic tumor presenting as intracerebral hemorrhage. Radiology 124:109, 1977.
103. Scott M. Spontaneous intracerebral hematoma caused by cerebral neoplasms. Report of eight verified cases. J Neurosurg 42:338, 1975.
104. Willia RA. Secondary tumors. In Minkler J, ed. Pathology of the Nervous System, Vol 2. New York, McGraw-Hill Book Co., 1971.
105. Pomeranz SJ, Sheldon JJ, Soila K, et al. Sensitivity of MRI in metastatic neoplasia. Magn Reson Imag 3:291, 1985.
106. Healy JF, Rosenkrantz H. Intraventricular metastases demonstrated by cranial computed tomography. Radiology 136:124, 1980.
107. Zimmerman RA, Bilaniuk LT. Age-related incidence of pineal calcification detected by computed tomography. Radiology 142:654, 1982.
108. Mamourian AC, Towfighi J. Pineal cysts: MR imaging. AJNR 7:1081, 1986.
109. Tapp E, Huxley M. The histologic appearance of the human pineal gland from puberty to old age. J Pathol 108:137, 1972.

110. Sevitt S, Schorstein J. A case of pineal cyst. Br Med J 2:490, 1947.
111. Lee DH, Norman D, Newton TH. MR imaging of pineal cysts. Comput Assist Tomogr 11:586, 1987.
112. Kobayashi T, Kageyama N, Kida Y, et al. Unilateral germinomas involving the basal ganglia and thalmus. J Neurosurg 55:55, 1981.
113. Kilgore DP, Strother CM, Starshak RJ, et al. Pineal germinoma: MR imaging. Radiology 158:435, 1985.
114. Kawakami Y, Kamada O, Tabuci K, et al. Primary intracranial choriocarcinoma. J Neurosurg 53:369, 1980.
115. Davidson HD, Ouchi T, Steiner RE. NMR imaging of congenital intracranial germinal layer neoplasms. Neuroradiology 27:301, 1985.
116. Latack JT, Kartash JM, Kemink JL, et al. Epidermoidomas of the cerebellopontine angle and temporal bone: CT and MR aspects. Radiology 157:361, 1985.
117. Weinstein MA, Masaryk TJ, Modic MT, et al. Magnetic resonance of fatty CNS tumors. Presented at the American Society of Neuroradiology 22nd Annual Meeting, Boston, June 2–7, 1984.
118. Braun IF, Naidich TP, Leeds NE, et al. Dense intracranial epidermoid tumors. Computed tomographic observations. Radiology 122:717, 1977.
119. Smoker WRK, Biller J, Moore SA, et al. Intradural spinal teratoma: case report and review of the literature. AJNR 7:905, 1986.
120. Monajati A, Spitzer RM, Wiley JL, et al. MR imaging of a spinal teratoma. J Comput Assist Tomogr 10:307, 1986.
121. Ganti SR, Hilal SK, Stein BM, et al. CT of pineal region tumors. AJNR 7:97, 1986.
122. Dorne HL, O'Gorman MA, Melanson D. Computed tomography of intracranial gangliogliomas. AJNR 7:281, 1986.
123. Rommel T, Hamer J. Development of ganglioglioma in computed tomography. Neuroradiology 24:237, 1983.
124. Claussen C, Laniado M, Kazner E, et al. Application of contrast agents in CT and MRI (NMR): their potential in imaging of brain tumors. Neuroradiology 27(2):164, 1985.
125. Okazaki H. Fundamentals of Neuropathology. Tokyo, Igaku-Shoin, 1983:201.
126. Ganti SR, Antunes JL, Louis KM, et al. Computed tomography in the diagnosis of colloid cysts of the third ventricle. Radiology 138:385, 1981.
127. Michels LD, Rutz D. Colloid cysts of the third ventricle. Arch Neurol 33:640, 1982.
128. Czervionke LF, Daniels DL, Meyer GA, et al: Neuroepithelial cysts of the lateral ventricles: MR appearance. AJNR 8:609, 1987.
129. Scotti G, Scialfa N, Colombo N, et al. MR in the diagnosis of colloid cysts of the third ventricle. AJNR 8:370, 1987.
130. Donaldson JO, Simon RH. Radiodense ions within a third ventricular colloid cyst. Arch Neurol 37:246, 1980.
131. Roosen N, Gahlen D, Stork W, et al. Magnetic resonance imaging of colloid cysts of the third ventricle. Neuroradiology 29:10, 1987.
132. Latchaw RE. Primary tumors of the brain: neuroectodermal tumors and sarcomas. In Latchaw RE. Computed Tomography of the Head, Neck and Spine. Chicago, Year Book Medical Publishers, 1985:223.
133. Lukes RJ, Parker JW, Taylor CR, et al. Immunologic approach to non-Hodgkin's lymphomas and related leukemias: analysis of the results of multiparameter studies in 425 cases. Semin Hematol 15:322, 1979.
134. Penn I. Development of cancer as a complication of clinical transplantation. Transplant Proc 9:1121, 1977.
135. Levy RM, Rosenbloom S, Perrett LV. Neuroradiologic findings in AIDS: a review of 200 cases. AJNR 7:833, 1986.
136. Enzmann DR, Krikorian J, Norman D, et al: Computed tomography in primary reticulum cell sarcoma of the brain. Radiology 130:165, 1979.
137. Weingarten KL, Zimmerman RD, Leeds NE. Spontaneous regression of intracerebral lymphoma. Radiology 149:721, 1983.
138. Gentry LR, Smoker WRK, Turski PA, et al: Suprasellar arachnoid cysts. 1. CT recognition. AJNR 7:79, 1986.
139. Sartor K, Karnaze MG, Winthrop JD, et al. MR imaging in infra-, para-, and retrosellar mass lesions. Neuroradiology 29:19, 1987.

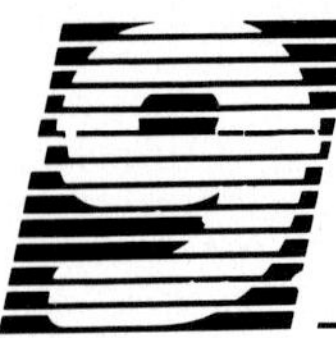

Stephen J. Pomeranz, M.D.

# POSTERIOR FOSSA, SKULL BASE, CRANIOCERVICAL JUNCTION

Magnetic resonance (MR) is the modality of choice when pathology in the brain stem, posterior fossa, or craniocervical junction is suspected and bony skeletal anatomy is not the primary concern (Table 9–1). Direct multiplanar imaging, superior contrast resolution and a lack of petrous bone or skull-base artifact lend credence to this philosophy. MR is now utilized as the initial and often sole modality in assessment of acoustic neuroma, of the cerebellopontine angle, and in selected skull-base lesions. Uncal, transtentorial, and tonsillar herniation are diagnoses easily made with axial or sagittal MR.

## INTRA-AXIAL LESIONS

### Metastases

The most common intra-axial posterior fossa lesions in the adult are metastatic. The cerebellum is most often affected, and 50 per cent of the lesions may be solitary. The MR appearance of metastatic disease in the posterior fossa differs little from metastases elsewhere and is described in detail in Chapter 8 of this text. T1 and T2 relaxation times, as expected, are prolonged in the majority of cases. Hemorrhagic lesions or those exhibiting paramagnetic effect may exhibit shortened relaxation times, as with melanoma. MR is particularly useful in the detection of brain stem metastases and in the detection of multiple pin-sized metastatic lesions or "tumorlets" (carcinomatous encephalitis) (Figs. 9–1 and 9–2).[1] We have detected these small lesions in the cerebellum or brain stem with breast and lung carcinoma and normal contrast-enhanced computed tomography (CECT) (Fig. 9–3). Although the majority of metastases (90 per cent) enhance on CECT, artifacts may make interpretation confusing. MR is more sensitive than CT in detecting the presence, extent, and number of metastatic lesions.[2,3] MR detection of these lesions may precede CECT by months. MR has become an invaluable tool for surgical and especially for radiation treatment-port planning.[4]

### Hemangioblastoma

Hemangioblastoma is the most common primary intra-axial tumor of the adult posterior fossa, constituting 10 per cent of posterior fossa malignancies. Ten per cent of hemangioblastomas are multiple, and at least 10 per cent of patients exhibit stigmata of von Hippel-Lindau syndrome.[5,6] An increased family incidence is probably present in 20 per cent of patients. At least 20 per cent of lesions are solid. The classic CECT descriptions of this lesion is that of a noncalcified, sharply marginated, peripherally enhancing cyst, the contents of which are iso- or slightly hyperdense compared with cerebrospinal fluid (CSF). An enhancing mural nodule is located on the wall closest to

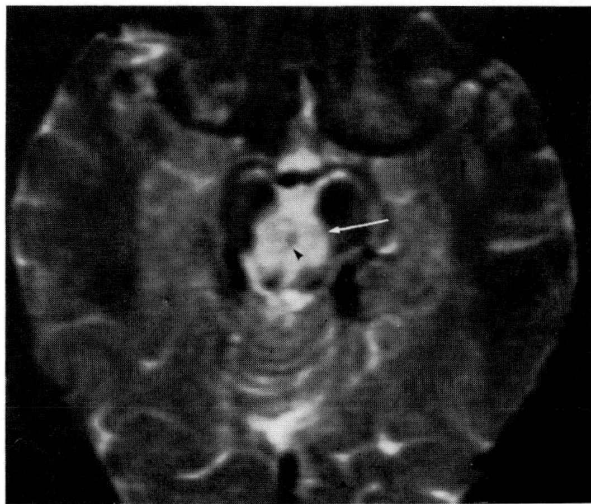

**Figure 9–1. Melanoma metastasis.** A 62-year-old woman with melanoma, third nerve palsy, and normal CECT (1.5 T). Axial T2WI (TR 2000/TE 100 msec). Bilateral midbrain hyperintense edema (arrow) with intermediate signal metastatic nodule (arrowhead) and punctate hyperintense necrosis within nodule are present.

the pial surface of the brain and is said to be more easily visualized with arteriography than CT.[7]

MR descriptions of hemangioblastomas are scant (Fig. 9–4).[8, 9] T1-weighted images (T1WI) demonstrate a hypointense signal of the cyst that is similar but slightly hyperintense relative to CSF. The mural nodule exhibits intermediate signal intensity that becomes relatively hyperintense as echo-time is lengthened. The cyst contents are hyperintense relative to brain or CSF on T2-weighted images (T2WI). Depending on the T2 parameters selected, the mural nodule may be "hidden" among the cyst contents or may be hypointense relative to the cyst when long echo times are selected. A surrounding thin region of moderate T2W signal hyperintensity corresponds pathologically to surrounding gliosis and edema. Serpiginous foci of flow-related signal void may be present from dilated feeding vessels with noncontrast MR. Solid hemangioblastomas have a nonspecific MR appearance (T1/T2 prolongation). Lesion location and clinical history may suggest the correct diagnosis. Only recently, vertebral angiography and digital subtraction vertebral angiography were suggested as means of searching for spinal lesions in patients with documented cerebellar hemangioblastoma.[10] Sagittal and axial T2W MR make this additional diagnostic step obsolete.

## Brain Stem Gliomas

Brain stem gliomas account for 25 per cent of neuroglial tumors in children and 3 per cent in adults. Approximately 80 per cent of these lesions occur in children.[11] Since contrast enhancement is minimal and calcification is infrequent, only indirect signs of

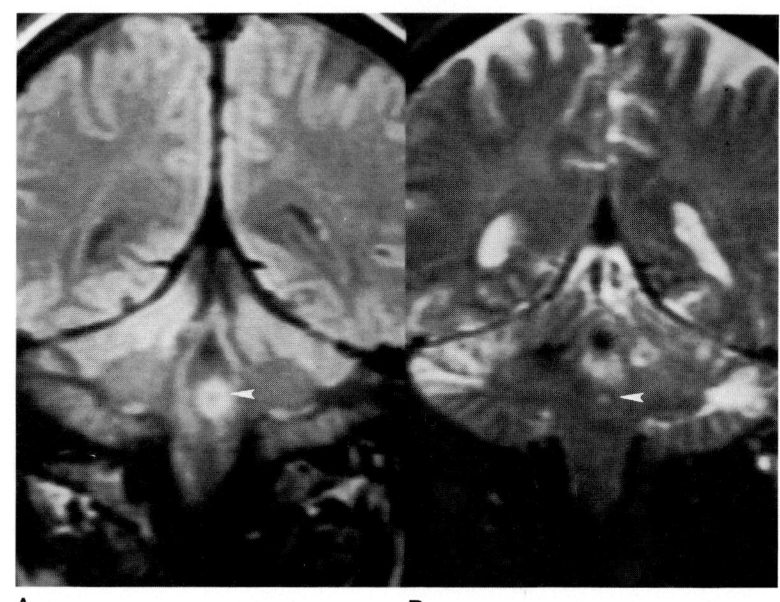


**Figure 9–2. Brain stem metastasis.** A 49-year-old woman with N(H)WI breast carcinoma, abducens palsy, and normal CECT (not shown) (1.5 T). *A* and *B,* Coronal multiecho N(H)WI and T2WI (TR 1800/TE 20/80 msec) show rounded hyperintense brain stem mass (arrowhead) with central hypointense necrosis on N(H)WI. The mass is inapparent on T2WI, and only punctate, central, hyperintense necrosis is visualized (arrowhead).

**Table 9–1.** MR FEATURES OF NEOPLASMS WITH A POSTERIOR FOSSA PREDILECTION

| Tumor/ Incidence | Location | Peak Age | Relaxation T1 | Relaxation T2 | Signal Uniformity | Ca⁺ | Enhancement Gd-DTPA | T2WI Edema | Other |
|---|---|---|---|---|---|---|---|---|---|
| ***Intra-axial*** | | | | | | | | | |
| Metastases (4+) | Cerebellum | 40–50 | + | + | Variable | Rare | 2–4+ ring | 1–4+ | Hypointense signal with T2WI colon, melanoma, prostate, osteogenic sarcoma; hyperintense T1WI with melanoma, choriocarcinoma |
| Hemangioblastoma (3+) | Cerebellar hemisphere | 30–40 | +++ | +++ | Yes | No | 4+ uniform | 0–1+ | Cyst with T1WI signal > CSF; mural nodule |
| Cerebellar (2+) astrocytoma | Cerebellar hemisphere | 5–20 | +++ | +++ | Yes | No | 1+ uniform | 1+ | Larger size (> 5 cm), younger age presentation than hemangioblastoma |
| Medulloblastoma (2+) | Superior vermis; 4th ventricular roof | 0–10 | + | +/= | Variable | 5% | 2+ uniform | 2+ | Punctate T2WI foci due to microcyst formation; low spin density common |
| Brain stem astrocytoma (2+) | Brain stem pons > medulla > midbrain | 5–15 | + | ++ | Variable | No | 0–1+ Mixed | 2–3+ | T2WI almost always hyperintense; invades cerebellar peduncle |
| Ependymoma (2+) | 4th ventricle, growth toward lateral recess | 10–20 | + | ++ | Mixed | 35% | 2+ mixed | 2+ | Frequent microcystic foci of T2WI hyperintensity; irregular margin |
| Choroid plexus papilloma (1+) | 4th ventricle | 0–20 | + | ++ | Variable | 7% | 3+ uniform | 0+ | Infratentorial lesions in older age group |

| | | | | | | | | | |
|---|---|---|---|---|---|---|---|---|---|
| ***Extra-axial*** | | | | | | | | | |
| Meningioma (4+) | Tentorium; petrous bone; CP angle | 40–70 | + | −/+/= | mixed | 40% | 4+ uniform | 1–3+ | Hypointense pseudocapsule; microcystic hyperintense T2 foci; low spin density; hemorrhage occasional; hypointense T1; hypo- or hyperintense adjacent bone |
| Neuroma (2+) | CP angle/eighth nerve complex > Meckel's cave > jugular foramen | 20–50 | + | +/= | uniform | rare | 3–4+ uniform | 0+ | Increased frequency T1, T2 isointensity with smaller lesions; cystic variant rare; round shape; wide cistern; 80% of CP angle tumors |
| Epidermoid (1+) | 4th ventricle, CP angle | 20–40 | ++ | +++ | mixed | 30% | 0+ | 0+ | Irregular margin; signal does not match normal CSF |
| Dermoid (1+) | Midline posterior | 20–40 | −− | ++ | variable | 50% | 0+ | 0+ | May rupture; may have T2WI hyperintense sinus tract |
| Lipoma (1+) | Quadrigeminal plate; CP angle | 20–40 | −− | − | uniform | 7% | 0+ | 0+ | Incidental finding; signal matches subgaleal fat |
| Paraganglioma (1+) | Jugular foramen, middle ear | 20–40 | + | + | mixed | rare | 0+ | 0+ | Invasion of jugular vein; petroclival fat signal; interrupted T2WI "speckled" appearance |
| Arachnoid cyst (1+) | Retrocerebellar; CP angle | 5–30 | +++ | +++ | uniform | no | 0+ | 0+ | Closely matches CSF signal |

1–4+: incidence 4+ most frequent, 1+ least frequent.
+: mild relaxation time (not signal) prolongation
++: moderate relaxation time prolongation
+++: marked relaxation time prolongation
0–4+: 4+ greatest, 0+ least edema or enhancement.
−: mild relaxation time shortening.
−−: moderate relaxation time shortening.
=: isointense appearance with brain on a given pulsing sequence.

T1 relaxation prolongation, hypointense; T1 relaxation shortening, hyperintense; T2 relaxation prolongation, hyperintense; T2 relaxation shortening, hypointense signal.

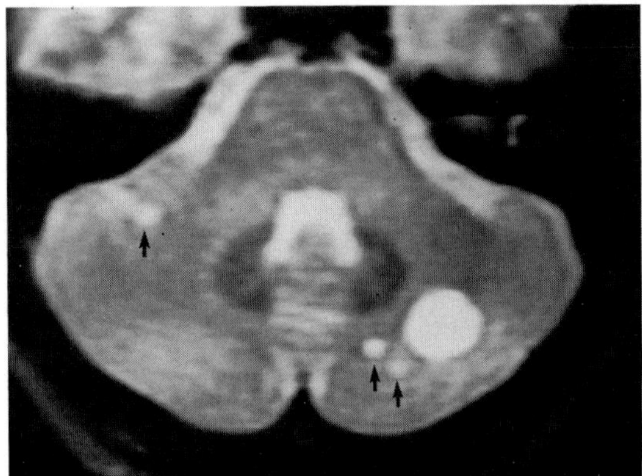

**Figure 9–3. Cerebellar metastases.** A 59-year-old woman with breast carcinoma and progressive ataxia (1.5 T). Axial T2WI (TR 1800/TE 100 msec) shows left (of patient) cerebellar hemispheric metastasis with smaller left- and right-sided satellite lesions (arrows) undetected on CECT (not shown).

fourth ventricular displacement or anterolateral bulging of the pontine belly may suggest the CT diagnosis.[12] Correlation of contrast enhancement and histologic grade is poor. Nonastrocytic brain stem tumors, ependymoma and ganglioglioma, do occur but are rare.

MR is the imaging procedure of choice for suspected brain stem disease and has supplanted CECT and water-soluble CT cisternography (WSCTC). As in CT, bulging contours of the posterior midbrain tectum, anterior pontine belly, or posterior medullary clava can be seen (Figs. 9–5, 9–6, 9–7). Likewise, the prepontine or perimesencephalic cisterns and fourth ventricles, respectively, may be effaced.[13, 14] A range of normal MR anteroposterior brain stem diameters in the sagittal orientation are as follows: midbrain tegmentum, 11 to 15 mm; pons, 24 to 29 mm; pontomedullary junction, 14 to 17 mm; and cervicomedullary junction, 8 to 11 mm.[15]

Most often, confluent but infiltrating foci of signal hyperintensity are present on T2WI images of patients with brain stem glial neoplasms (Fig. 9–6). Therefore, contour alterations of the brain stem are not the sole criteria for diagnosis. Isointense brain stem glioma with MR, even when heavily calcified, is rare, and the sensitivity of MR in depicting these lesions is excellent.[16] Extension of signal alterations into the ipsilateral middle cerebellar peduncle or upper cervical cord is common.[17] Signal inhomogeneity is frequent and is likely related to the high incidence of necrosis and cyst (33 per cent) formation appreciated histologically. Confluent cysts may be surgically aspirated with symptomatic improvement.

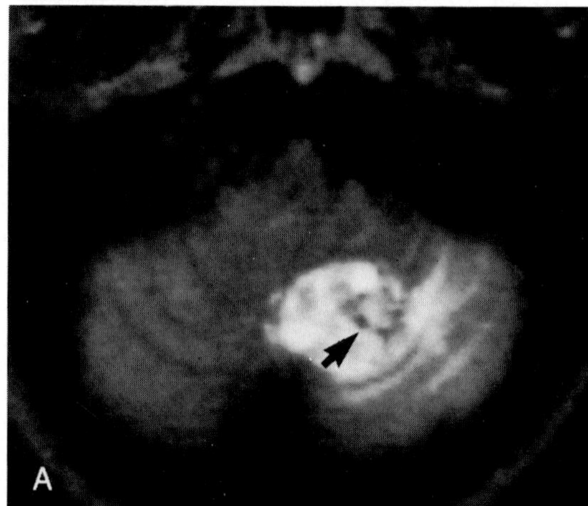


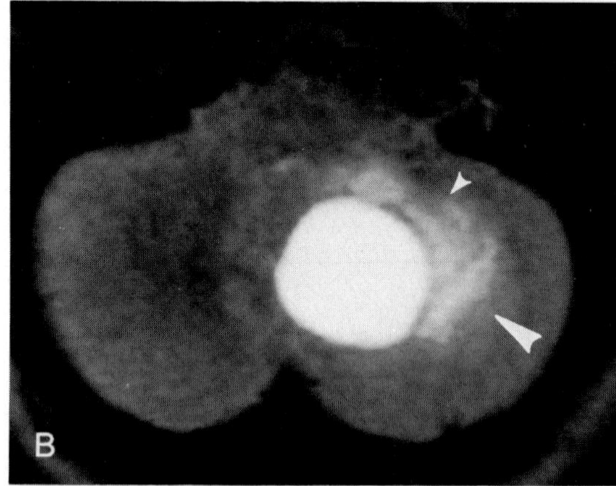


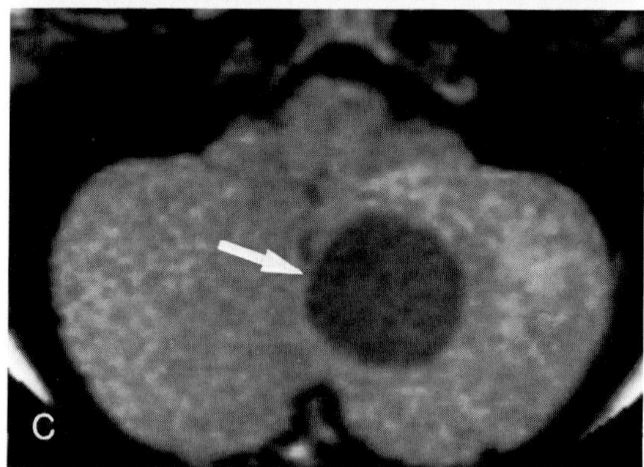


**Figure 9–4. Hemangioblastoma.** *A* and *B*, Axial 0.5T T2WI (TR 2000/TE 120 msec) show a rounded, well-circumscribed, hyperintense cerebellar mass with mild hyperintense edema (arrowheads). Intermediate signal tumor nodule is only apparent on T2WI in A (black arrowhead). *C*, Axial T1WI (TR 800/TE 20 msec) shows homogeneous, hypointense mass (arrow) compatible with cystic lesion character. Edema is inapparent on T1WI. (Courtesy of R. Lukin, M.D., Wellington Diagnostics, Cincinnati, Ohio.)

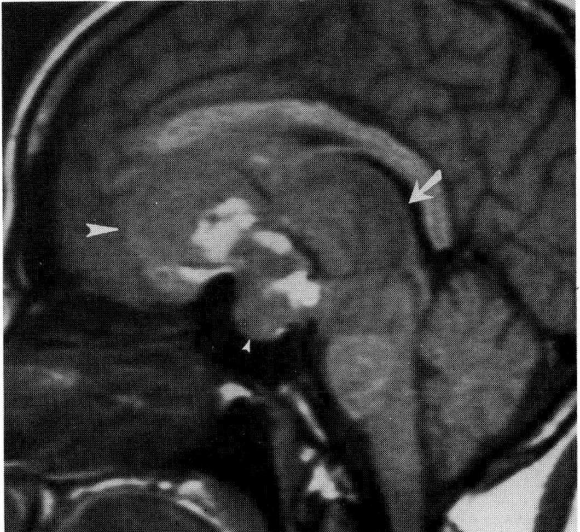

**Figure 9–5. Brain stem glioma.** Sagittal (1.5 T) T1WI (TR 700/TE 20 msec). A mass, of which the origin is difficult to define on axial sections, appears to expand the midbrain and thalmus (arrow), invades the pituitary fossa (small arrowhead), and extends into the anterior cranial fossa (arrowhead). Hyperintense hemorrhagic foci are present. (Courtesy of R. Lukin, M.D., Neuroradiology Dept., University Hospital, Cincinnati, Ohio.)

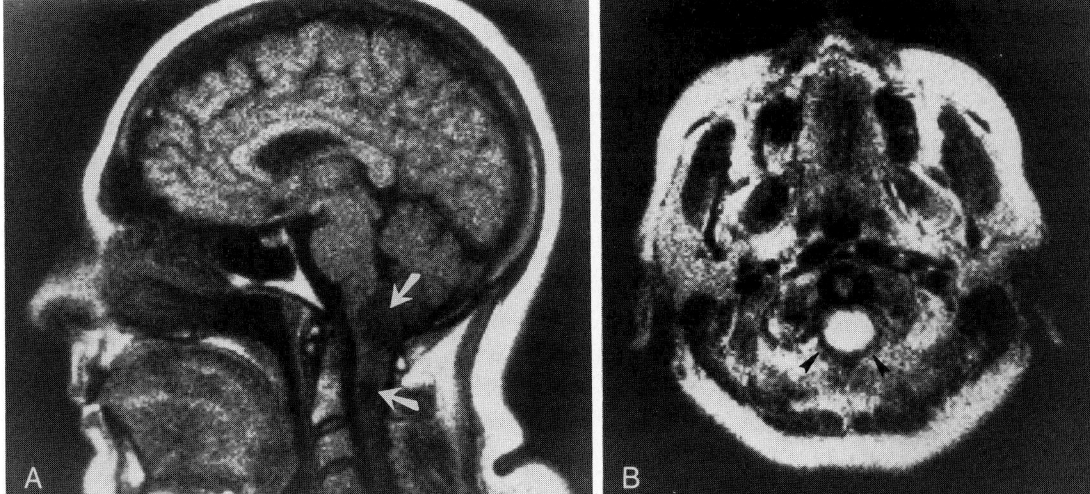


**Figure 9–6. Infiltrative brain stem glioma.** A 27-year-old woman with bulbar signs and myelopathy. *A,* Sagittal T1WI (0.35 T). *B,* Axial T2WI. Foci of signal hypointensity in the brain stem medullary clava and upper cervical cord (arrows) exhibit mass effect and produce cord enlargement at the level of the foramen magnum and marked signal hyperintensity, which is confluent (arrowheads) on T2WI.

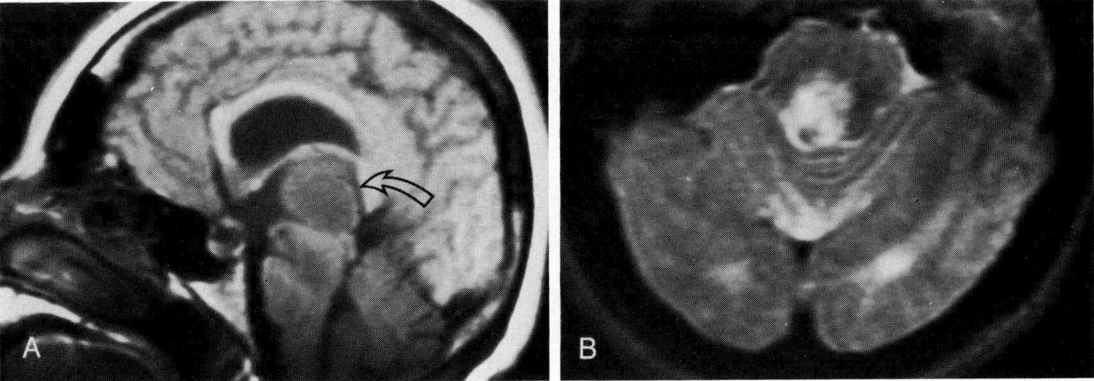


**Figure 9–7. Brain stem glioma.** A 36-year-old woman with seizures (1.5 T). *A,* Sagittal T1WI. *B,* Axial T2WI (TR 1800/TE 80). Mass on sagittal T1WI (arrow) could arise from pineal gland, midbrain, or posterior third ventricle. Axial T2WI shows intra-axial signal hyperintensity in the posterior brain stem mesencephalon, where the lesion has arisen. (Courtesy of R. Lukin, M.D., Neuroradiology Dept., University Hospital, Cincinnati, Ohio.)

Nodular extruding tumors, more focal and occasionally cystic, may occur in the tectal region.[18] The normal tectal collicullar anteroposterior diameter is approximately 5 mm (superior collicullus) and 6 mm (inferior colliculus) in the sagittal projection. Tumors in this region are easily distinguished from mesencephalic beaking or non-neoplastic tectal enlargement by their T2WI hyperintensity, T1WI hypointensity, or both.[19, 20] Tectal cystic neoplasms[21] exhibit rounded nodules or irregular foci of T2WI hyperintensity, and these should be sought out with thin sections (Fig. 9–7). High-resolution sagittal and axial T2WI MR should be the examination of choice to detect occult tectal pathology in patients with "idiopathic" obstructive hydrocephalus. However, care should be taken not to confuse phase-related flow artifacts or point artifacts for neoplasms when they project over the brain stem.[22] These artifacts can be eliminated by using flow-correction software.

## Cerebellar Astrocytoma

The most common posterior fossa neuroglial tumor is the cerebellar astrocytoma. It occurs most frequently in children (peak, 4 years) and involves the cerebellar hemispheres (75 per cent) more frequently than the vermis.[23] More than 50 per cent of cases appear cystic radiographically, and solid or microcystic variants occur in adults.[24] Moderate hydrocephalus may occur.

A benign form of this tumor consists of a focal, enhancing nodule of neoplastic tissue along a non-neoplastic gliotic cyst wall, whereas a more malignant form exhibits neoplastic tissue along the entire cyst wall.[25] Areas of necrosis or hemorrhage are not infrequent in the latter. Some series report a 20 per cent incidence of calcification.[26]

The more benign form of astrocytoma must be differentiated from hemangioblastoma, arachnoid cyst, ependymal- or nonependymal-lined cysts, and trapped fourth ventricle.[27] The latter demonstrates contiguity with the fourth ventricle, which is particularly well demonstrated by utilizing sagittal T1WI MR. Nodular foci of signal hyperintensity (tumor nodule) or perilesional hyperintense T2WI edema are not seen in trapped fourth ventricle or posterior fossa cysts. These findings are present in cerebellar astrocytoma (Fig. 9–8).[28] Heavily T2WI may produce a hyperintense cyst containing a hypointense nodule. These neoplastic cysts exhibit signal hyperintensity relative to CSF on T1WI. Non-neoplastic cysts (arachnoid or ependymal) are homogeneous in signal intensity, and this signal more closely approximates known CSF structures (Fig. 9–9). In addition, signal hypointensity on T1WI corresponds exactly to sites of signal hyperintensity on T2WI; that is, there is no edema. Differentiation of hemangioblastoma from the benign form of cystic astrocytoma is difficult with MR or CT, but lesion size less than 5 cm (90 per cent) and patient's age of more than 25 years

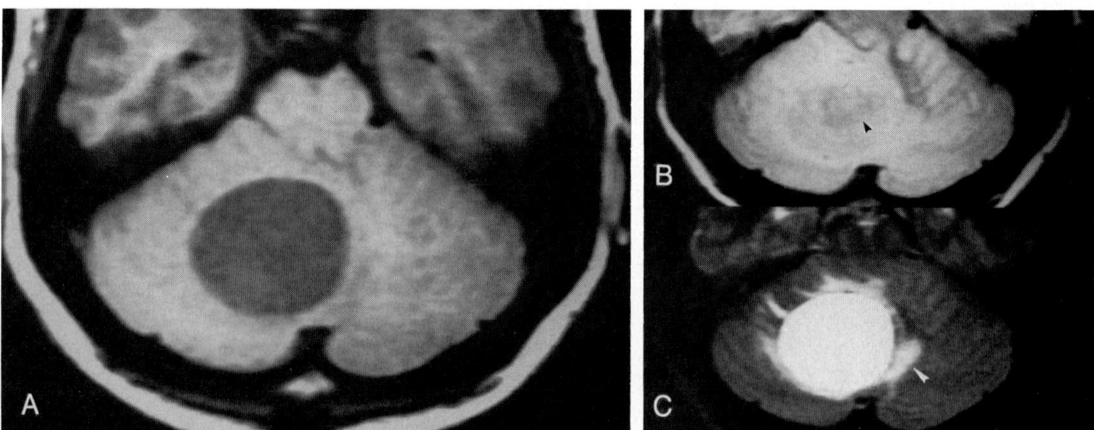


**Figure 9–8. Cystic astrocytoma.** A 28-year-old woman with progressive ataxia (1.5 T). *A*, Axial T1WI (TR 600/TE 20 msec). Hypointense mass exhibits homogeneous signal. *B* and *C*, Axial multiecho N(H)WI and T2WI (TR 1800/TE 20/100 msec). Signal inhomogeneity exists on N(H)WI (black arrowhead), making a benign cyst unlikely. Mild hyperintense T2WI edema (white arrowhead) is present.

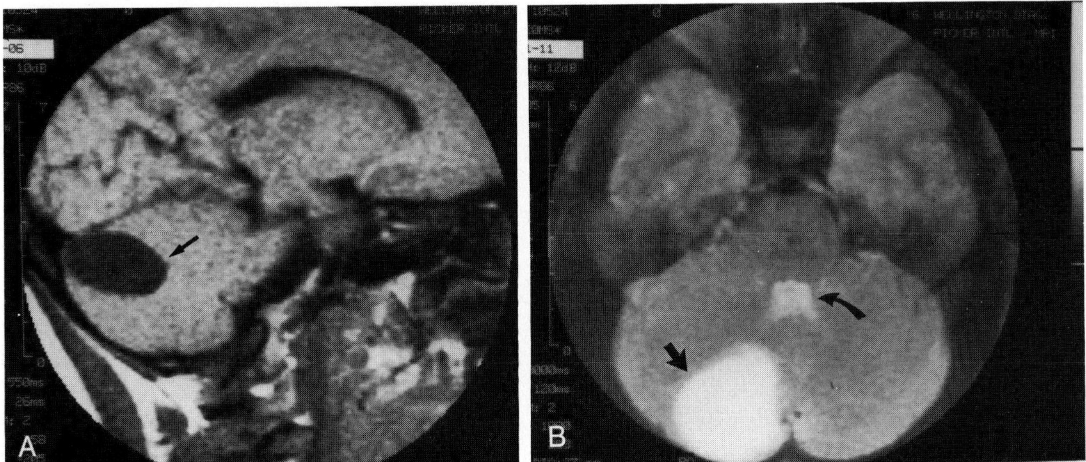

**Figure 9–9. Nonependymal-lined cyst.** A 37-year-old man with headaches (0.5 T). *A,* Sagittal T1WI (TR550/TE 26). *B,* Axial T2WI TR 3000/TE 120). A well-circumscribed mass in the right cerebellar hemisphere (arrow) has signal intensity identical to CSF. On axial T2WI, signal intensity is homogeneous (arrow) and matches the fourth ventricle (curved arrow). (Courtesy of A. Chambers, M.D., Neuroradiology Dept., University Hospital, Cincinnati, Ohio.)

(95 per cent) favor hemangioblastoma. Cystic astrocytomas tend towards slight eccentricity, large size (> 6 cm), and a higher incidence of hydrocephalus. Calcification is unusual and occurs only in more solid lesions.

The more malignant form of astrocytoma appears as a poorly defined region of midhemispheric signal hyperintensity, difficult to differentiate from medulloblastoma, ependymoma, and solitary metastasis. Extension into the brain stem or spinal cord is not uncommon. Medulloblastoma in adults is often dural based, and T2WI signal hyperintensity appears minimal. Ependymomas exhibit poorly defined inhomogeneous foci of T2WI hyperintensity. A periventricular or ventricular location with signal extension toward the foramina of Lushka or cerebellopontine angle cistern favors ependymoma. An intraventricular location is most easily appreciated in the sagittal projection.

## Medulloblastoma

Medulloblastoma originates from primitive neuroectodermal cells in the fourth ventricular roof and after astrocytoma is the second most frequent primary tumor of the posterior fossa in children. At least 50 per cent of these tumors occur in the first decade; boys are more frequently affected, and one third of lesions occur between 15 and 35 years. Small age peaks are seen at 1, 7 to 8, and 13 years of age. The classic CT description is that of a midline (85 per cent), well-marginated, hyperdense, homogeneously enhancing mass (4 to 5 cm) with cystic areas, infrequent calcification (2 per cent to 10 per cent) and obstructive hydrocephalus (75 per cent).[29, 30] A propensity for subarachnoid, ventricular, and ependymal seeding (30 per cent) or spinal drop metastases exists.[31] The fourth ventricle may be filled by tumor. A suprasellar or spinal mass may be a presenting manifestation. Nodular drop metastases are detectable with MR but sheet-like tumor spread may go unrecognized without Gd-DTPA MR or CECT.

The atypical medulloblastoma occurs in an older age group and is a hyperdense and moderately enhancing dural-based mass along the lateral cerebellar hemisphere, cerebellar tonsil, or cerebellopontine angle.[32] Desmoplasia and fibrosis in these atypical lesions has prompted a histologic diagnosis of cerebellar sarcoma.

Because the CT findings of medulloblastoma are so characteristic and the diagnosis of intracranial subarachnoid tumor spread is difficult with noncontrast MR, we believe multiplanar MR serves only as an aid in treatment planning. The tumor epicenter, in the fourth ventricular roof, is easily recognized in the sagittal projection. We have observed that the T2WI signal intensity of medulloblastoma is less than for other brain neoplasms and may be related to lesion density. Low spin density is particularly prominent in the adult form, or hemispheric medulloblastoma (Fig. 9–10). Thus less contrast between lesion and normal brain is produced. Punctate foci of T2WI signal hyperintensity occur (10 per cent) owing to cyst formation. Gd-DTPA enhancement may be homogeneous or inhomogeneous and results in T1WI hyperintensity.

A supratentorial lesion that may be histologically mislabeled as medulloblastoma is primary neuroblastoma. Unlike medulloblastoma, this lesion has yielded marked T2WI signal hyperintensity and exhibits a hemorrhagic tendency.

## Ependymoma

Ependymoma is the second most common neuroglial tumor (6 per cent) and often occurs in the posterior fossa of children and young adults. For this reason, MR diagnosis will be discussed in greater detail in Chapter 7. Infratentorial ependymomas are far less common than medulloblastoma and astrocytoma. Two peak ages, 5 and 34 years, are seen.[33] The typical CT appearance is that of a fourth ventricular heterogeneous mass, frequently calcified (50 per cent), enhancing (80 per cent), and with occasional cyst formation. Aggressive (ependymomoblastoma) and benign (subependymoma) variants occur. Supratentorial ependymomas occur in 40 per cent, but when occurring in children they are more frequently aggressive, with cystic components.

A mass exhibiting the expected T1 and T2 prolongation is appreciated in its true intraventricular position with sagittal MR. Ventricular expansion with extension toward the foramen of Lushka or cerebellopontine angle (60 per cent) and tonguelike projection into the vallecula cerebelli or cisterna magna is recognized with multiplanar MR. Direct extension into the cerebellum or brain stem occurs in 35 per cent of cases. A hyperintense (T2) or hypointense (T1) circumferential rim of fourth ventricular fluid is frequently appreciated. Subarachnoid tumor spread, common with ependymoma, is difficult to appreciate with MR, but nodular hyperintense T2WI drop metastases are easily detectable. Punctate T2WI hyperintense foci owing to cyst formation are smaller than those of cystic astrocytoma.

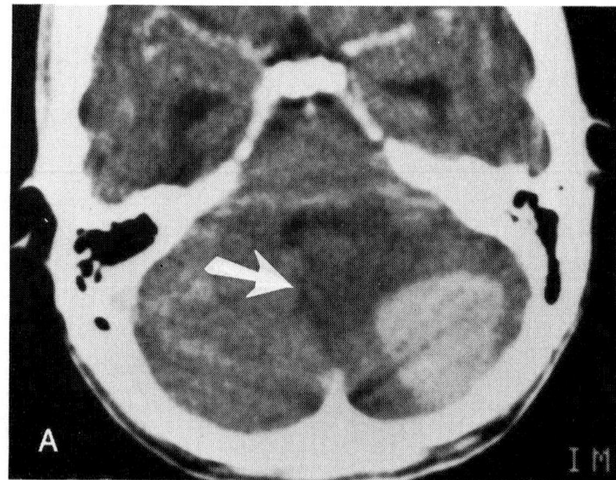


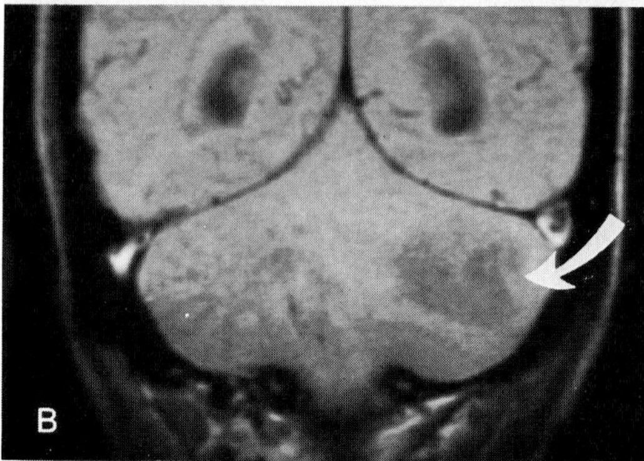


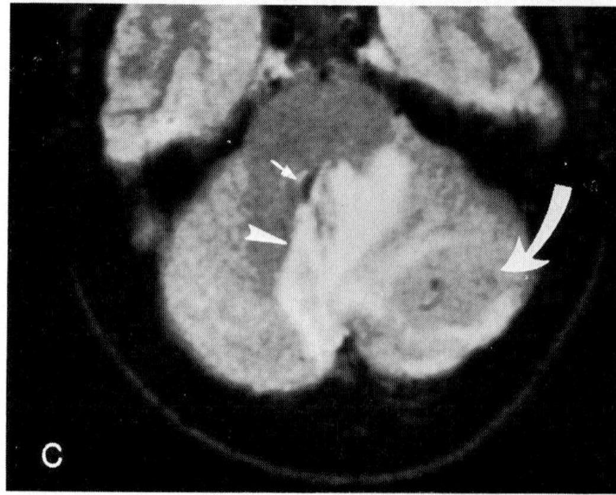


**Figure 9–10. Primary cerebellar sarcoma (hemispheric medulloblastoma.** *A, B,* and *C,* Axial CECT, coronal (1.5 T) N(H)WI (TR 1800/TE 25), and axial T2WI (TR 1800/TE 100), respectively. CT shows enhancing, juxtadural, hyperdense left (of patient) cerebellar mass and hypodense edema (arrow). Mass is hypointense on N(H)WI and isointense on T2WI (curved arrows), compatible with its fibrous, dense nature. Hyperintense edema (arrowhead) and fourth ventricular displacement (small arrow) are identified on T2WI, along with signal inhomogeneity in the lesion not seen on CT. The intra-axial nature of the lesion is better appreciated with MR than CT since edema circumscribes the dural margin. (Courtesy of D. Chakeres, M.D., Department of Radiology, Ohio State University Hospital, Columbus, Ohio.)

Features that favor ependymoma over medulloblastoma include expansion rather than compression of the fourth ventricle, marked inhomogeneous T2 signal hyperintensity, growth laterally and inferiorly into basal cisterns, smaller size, patchy inhomogeneous Gd-DTPA enhancement and an epicenter on sagittal MR closer to the foramen magnum than to the superior cerebellar vermis.

### Choroid Plexus Papillomas

Posterior fossa choroid plexus papillomas are tumors of adults. Their supratentorial counterparts are more common in children. The left atrial trigone of the lateral ventricle is the classic location in the pediatric population and afflicts patients in the first decade of life. Choroid plexus carcinoma can occur in an older group but peaks at 3 years of age. Posterior fossa papillomas affect the midline fourth ventricle or its lateral recess. Cerebellopontine angle extension is common. Relaxation times are prolonged, as expected; however, the lesion is difficult to distinguish from ependymoma with MR signal alone. Homogeneous, intense Gd-DTPA enhancement (producing T1WI signal hyperintensity) and a fourth ventricular location in the adult age group suggests papilloma. Differentiation of hyperintense T2WI choroid plexus tumors from intraventricular arteriovenous malformation or aneurysm (flow-void signal [FVS]) is obvious with MR.

## CEREBELLOPONTINE ANGLE AND EXTRA-AXIAL LESIONS OF THE POSTERIOR FOSSA

### Acoustic Neuroma

The cerebellopontine angle (CPA) is a favored site for extra-axial posterior fossa masses. Acoustic neuroma is the most common neoplasm of this region (85 per cent) and accounts for 8 per cent of all intracranial neoplasms. Schwann cells that envelope the eighth cranial nerve, particularly its peripheral superior vestibular branch (60 per cent), proliferate and may produce neurosensory hearing loss, tinnitus, or both. Large neuromas (> 3 cm) may produce fifth and seventh nerve symptoms, brain stem compression, or even hydrocephalus. The peak incidence usually occurs between 40 and 60 years of age. Bilateral neuromas, particularly in children, may occur in neurofibromatosis and in a familial form not associated with neurofibromatosis.

Typical CT findings of acoustic neuroma include a homogeneously enhancing, rounded or oval noncalcified mass centered on the internal auditory meatus and producing cisternal widening and canal enlargement (90 per cent). The criteria for canal enlargement (discrepancy of 2 mm in width and 3 mm in length) and crista falciformis displacement (2 mm) have been detailed elsewhere.[34, 35] Lesions less than 0.5 cm in size and completely intracanalicular previously required gas cisternography CT (GCCT) or WSCTC.[36]

The four components of the seventh and eighth nerve complex are visualized with multiplanar MR (Fig. 9–11). Individual nerves are identified on coronal and axial projections with T1WI but are often obscured with T2WI. The seventh (anterior) and superior vestibular nerve (posterior) are superiorly oriented with the cochlear (anterior) and inferior vestibular nerve (posterior) beneath. All course in an anteroinferolateral to posterosuperomedial orientation. These four components are simultaneously visualized in the sagittal projection. The cochlea is positioned inferoanteriorly with respect to nerves and vestibule. Its apex points anterolaterally. When the cochlea is asymmetrically imaged in the coronal plane a pedunculated intracanalicular pseudolesion is simulated. The vestibule and semicircular canals lie posterosuperior to the cochlea.

The facial nerve enters the anterosuperior internal auditory canal and exits anterolaterally as the geniculate ganglion above the cochlea (Fig. 9–11). It then reverses direction (the genu) and courses directly posteriorly along the medial middle ear as the tympanic or horizontal portion of the facial nerve underneath the lateral semicircular canal. It turns inferiorly toward the stylomastoid foramen as the mastoid segment. Occasionally, the greater superficial petrosal nerve extending anteriorly from the facial nerve geniculate ganglion is demonstrated.[37, 38]

We believe that high-resolution multiplanar MR is the examination of choice for

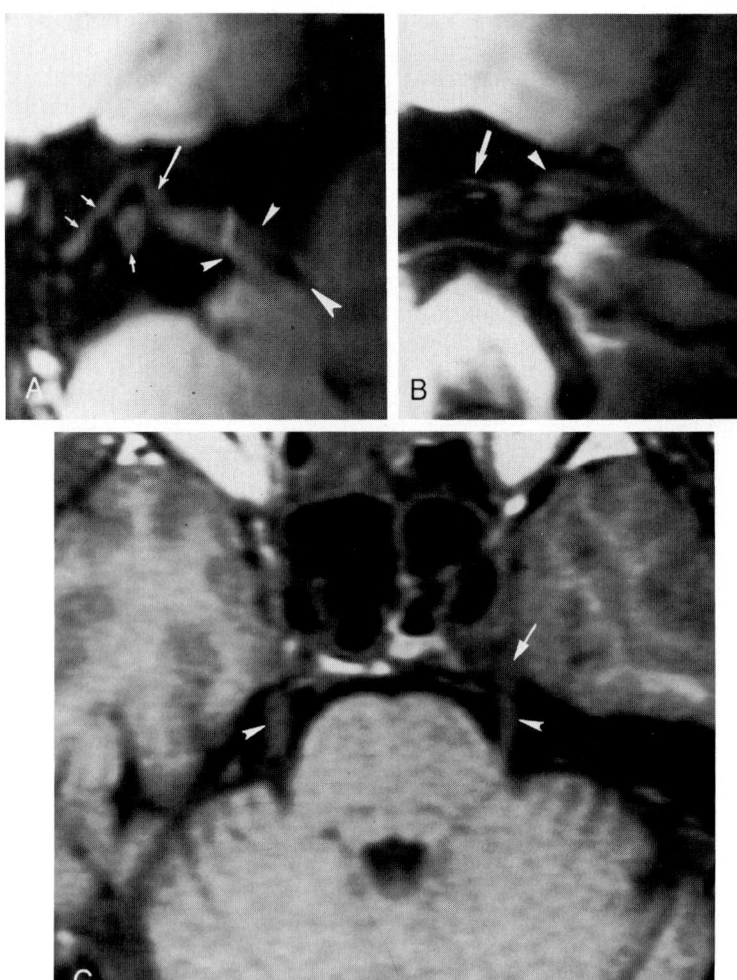


**Figure 9–11.** *A* and *B,* Axial and coronal (1.5 T) T1WI (TR 600/TE 20 msec) 3-mm sections; 3-in surface coil; 12-cm FOV of normal seventh and eighth nerve complex. *A,* Anterior and posterior portions of eighth nerve complex (arrowheads) are separated by normal cleft (large arrowhead). Vestibule (arrow), cochlea (long arrow), and facial nerve (paired arrows). *B,* Superior (arrowhead) and inferior portions of complex are separated by normal cleft. Arrow shows lateral semicircular canal. *C,* Axial 3-mm T1WI shows fifth nerves (arrowheads) and their entrance into Meckel's cave (arrow).

acoustic neuroma evaluation. The reasons are as follows: (1) improved spatial resolution utilizing small FOV head coil or surface coil imaging; (2) innate superior tissue contrast without intravenous contrast enhancement; (3) direct multiplanar thin (≤ 3-mm) sections; (4) absence of petrous bone artifact; (5) exclusion of false positives owing to vascular loop; and (6) detectability of intracanalicular lesions without GCCT or WSCTC. Since isolated intracanalicular lesions may occur in 8 per cent (only 5 per cent are totally extracanalicular), GCCT or WSCTC have been recommended for these small lesions (< 1 cm). False positives with these examinations owing to very small canals or meatal arachnoiditis are reduced with MR.[39] In view of the anteroinferior eighth nerve course, we have found that high-resolution multiplanar nonorthogonal MR is equal to or more sensitive than GCCT and WSCTC for acoustic neuroma detection.[40] We initially examine the eighth nerve complex and CPA in a standard whole-volume head coil, utilizing T1WI coronal and axial series. The coronal sections are centered around the posterior one third of the dens, which is visualized on a sagittal scout sequence. Three-millimeter gapless sections are used. Depending on the quality of the signal demonstrated on a scout image, patient cooperation, and lesion size, a choice exists with regard to field-of-view (FOV) and matrix size. When small lesions are suspected, high-resolution 3-mm sections may be obtained with 20 FOV, 128 × 256 matrix and six excitations at 1.5 tesla (T). This sequence may be employed in one or both imaging planes. However, if one high-resolution scanning plane demonstrates normal anatomy, the second scanning plane may be obtained with 128 × 256 matrix and four or two excitations. For problem cases or to assess the intracanalicular extent of small lesions, flow-compensated T2WI and CEMR using T1-weighted axial or coronal images are routinely implemented. Fast scan (GRASS), oblique images, or small FOV (8 to 16 cm), high-resolution surface coil MR may be employed. An optimal multiplanar sequence utilizes repetition times of 800 msec and echo times of 20 msec at 1.5 T.[41] False-negative MR examinations have been reported when 5-mm sections were obtained and when CSF pulsations produced pseudosignal alterations.[42] False-positive readings may result from trapped intracanalicular CSF or partial volume averaging of adjacent petroclival fat. Thin sections, multiprojection oblique MR, small FOV, cardiac gating, and flow-correction software may help resolve some of these disparities. Contrast-enhanced MR (CEMR) markedly improves diagnostic specificity.

Most neuromas exhibit some T2WI signal increase, assisting in differentiation from meningioma.[43,44] However, smaller neuromas or intracanalicular lesions may not exhibit increased T2 relaxation (Fig. 9–12). Intracanalicular neuromas are identified by contour alterations and signal slightly greater than CSF on T1WI (Fig. 9–13). They occasionally exhibit a central linear hypointense signal that bisects the lesion. Neuromas, unlike meningiomas, are more rounded than sessile in configuration, exhibit acute angles between lesion and petrous bone, are centered in or over the porus acousticus, rarely extend to the middle fossa, and less often exhibit T2WI signal hypointensity owing to low spin density or calcification (Fig. 9–14).[45] Sensorineural hearing loss, common with neuroma, is rare with meningioma and is unusual with epidermoid. The signal alteration of epidermoid is inhomogeneous. T1WI hypointensity and T2WI hyperintensity is more marked in epidermoidoma than in meningioma or neuromas. Vascular lesions of the CPA such as aneurysm or vertebrobasilar dolichoectasia are easily differentiated from other lesions by their characteristic flow-void signal (FVS).

Atypical signal characteristics of eighth nerve neuromas may occur on MR. We have encountered large eighth nerve neuromas with marked T1 and T2 relaxation prolongation that were pathologically cystic (Fig. 9–15). These were indistinguishable from epidermoidoma. Large, noncystic cerebellopontine angle neuromas may exhibit pronounced T1WI hypointensity and T2WI hyperintensity, particularly at low field strengths (0.15 T).[46]

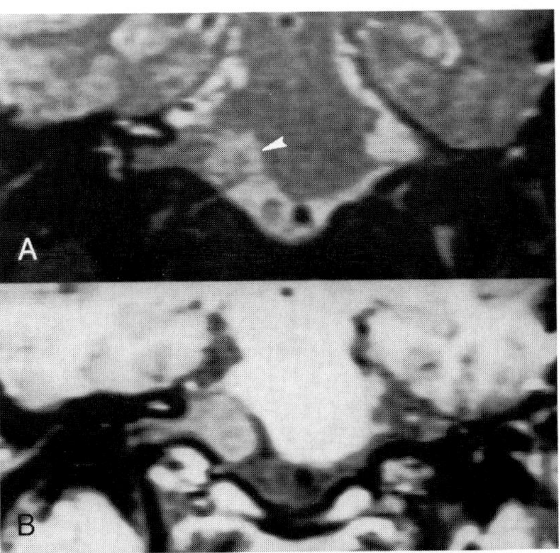


**Figure 9–12. Acoustic neuroma.** *A* and *B*, A 23-year-old woman with neurofibromatosis, bilateral deafness, and prior left-sided neuroma (1.5 T). Coronal T2WI (TR 1800/TE 80) and T1WI (TR 600/TE 20 msec). Rightward (on patient) is a cerebellopontine angle mass isointense on T2WI with subtle focus of hyperintensity (arrowhead). The lesion is hypointense and more obvious on T1WI.

The issue of contrast administration in MR eighth nerve evaluation is unresolved. Although CECT may actually double or triple the sensitivity of neuroma detection over NCCT, T1WI Gd-DTPA, while more sensitive than CECT and NCMR, is not often necessary (Fig. 9–13).[47] It may prove helpful in distinguishing neuroma from other lesions and in assessing postoperative neuroma recurrence and nontumoral nerve enlargement or in the rare instance of trapped intracanalicular fluid.[48,49] Gd-DTPA enhancement of meningioma, as expected, is more homogeneous, immediate, and persistent when compared with neuroma.

In summary, we use MR and often CEMR as the examination of choice for acoustic neuroma evaluation. Size, shape, location, and lesion contour are more helpful than signal in improving diagnostic specificity. We, like others, believe that MR is more helpful in characterization of neuromas, cholesterol granulomas, or cysts of the pet-

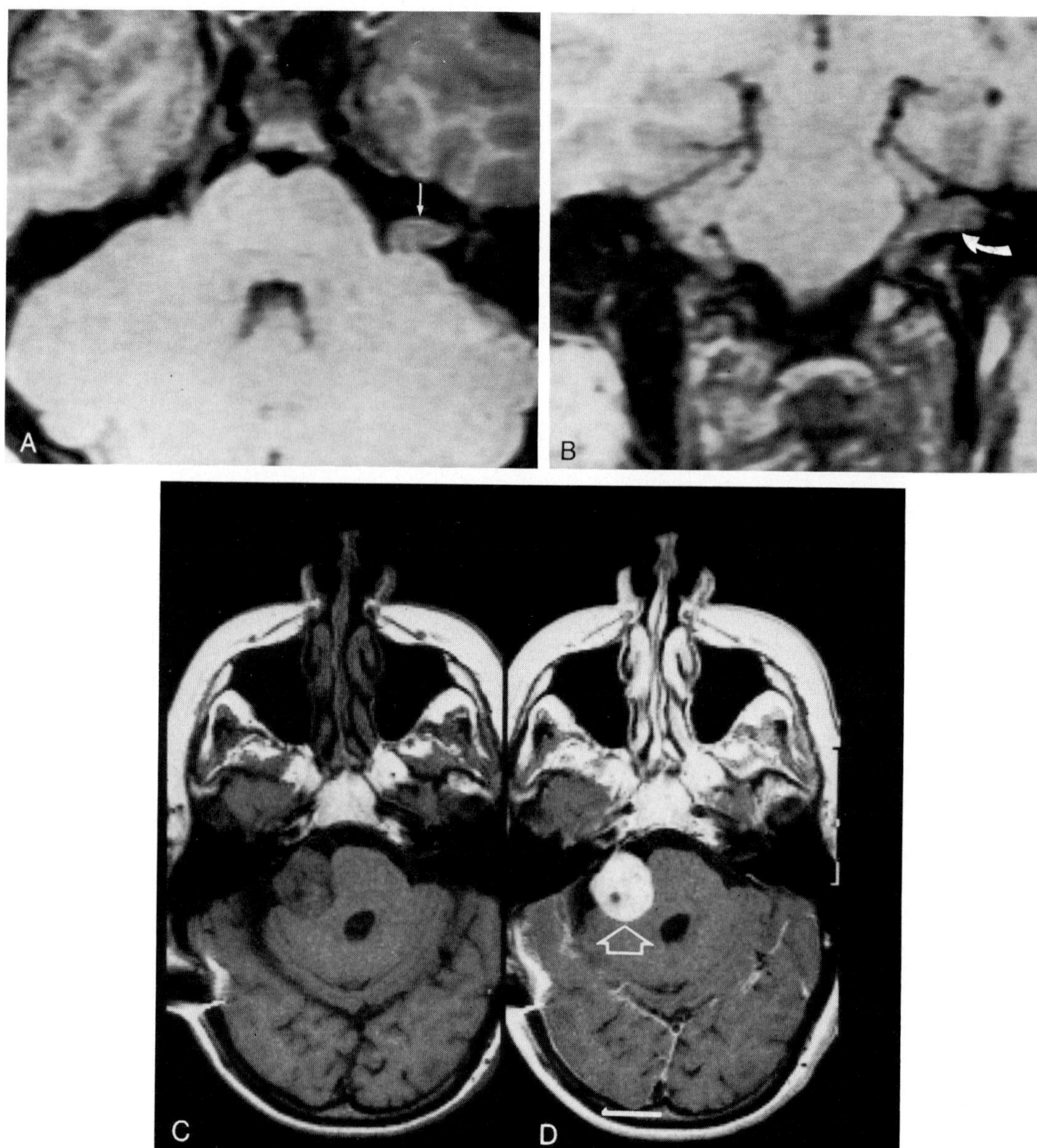

**Figure 9–13. Intracanalicular (*A* and *B*) and enhancing CP-angle (*C* and *D*) acoustic neuromas.** A 32-year-old male with tinnitus (1.5 T) (*A* and *B*). *A,* Axial T1WI (TR 700/TE 20 msec). *B,* Coronal T1WI. *C* and *D,* Axial T1WI pre- and post–Gd-DTPA (0.1 mmol/kg IV) 1.0 T. Intracanalicular (*A* and *B*) mass (arrow) is isointense with gray matter and encompasses superior and inferior vestibular nerves (curved arrow). Neuroma in another patient at 1.0 T (*C* and *D*) is hypointense on T1WI and markedly enhances on postcontrast T1WI (open arrow). (*C* and *D,* courtesy of V. Runge, M.D., Radiology Department, New England Medical Center, Tufts University, Boston, Mass.)

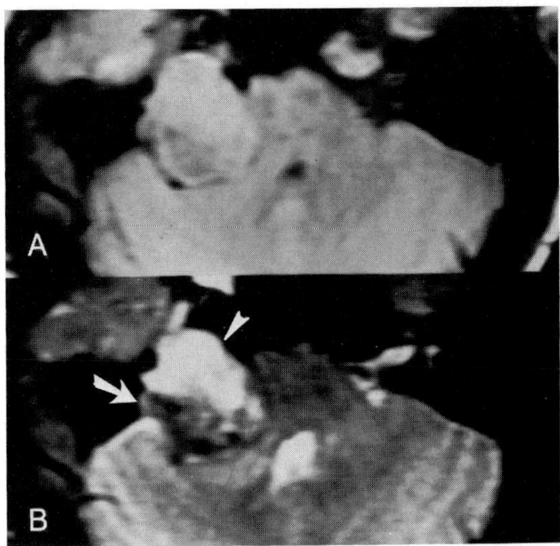


**Figure 9–14. Calcified acoustic neuroma.** *A* and *B*, A 21-year-old female with a hearing loss since infancy. Axial multiecho N(H)WI and T2WI (TR 2000/TE 20/80 msec) show right-sided cerebellopontine angle mass, hyperintense anteriorly (arrowhead), and hypointense posteriorly (arrow) owing to proven calcification.

rous bone; epidermoidomas; vascular lesions; and exophytic glial neoplasms. On the other hand, CT is more revealing in the diagnosis of tympanomastoiditis, middle ear disease, secondary cholesteatoma, and meningioma.[50]

## Meningioma

The posterior fossa or foramen magnum is the site of 10 per cent to 12 per cent of all meningiomas, and the majority of these arise in the CPA. Still, the incidence of CPA neuroma is three to four times that of meningioma. However, meningioma is the most common benign extra-axial lesion of the foramen magnum, and 2 per cent to 4 per cent of all meningiomas occur here. The clivus, tentorium cerebelli, jugular tubercle, and cerebellar hemispheric dura are other common posterior fossa locations.

The MR findings of posterior fossa meningioma differ little from the supratentorial compartment (Figs. 9–16 and 9–17). T2WI signal is less hyperintense relative to gray matter when compared with neural tumors. Hypointense pseudocapsule formation is observed on MR in a significant percentage (65 per cent) of meningiomas. Signal inhomogeneity or microcyst cyst formation (20 per cent) is common, but frank cyst formation (confluent foci of T2WI hyperintensity) is rare (2 per cent). Our series of meningiomas showed that perilesional intra-axial T2WI hyperintense edema occurred in 75 per cent of cases and was sometimes profound. A helpful finding in differentiating meningioma from neuroma is a lack of intracanalicular signal alteration or lack of intracanalicular contour abnormality produced by meningioma with direct coronal MR (Fig. 9–16). As with CT, rounded masses with a broad base ("global meningiomas"), obtuse margins, and eccentric lesion orientation relative to the porus acusticus support a diagnosis of meningioma. Multiplanar MR greatly assists in demonstration of a flat dural lesion margin (Fig. 9–18; see also Fig. 9–16). Marked punctate or confluent foci of T2WI hypointensity usually indicate calcification (25 per cent), a finding that is unusual with neuroma (5 per cent). Alteration of adjacent skeletal signal intensity (hypointense T1WI may occur when meningioma induces bone sclerosis or reactive hyperemic flow phenomena in bone (hypointense T1WI, hyperintense T2WI).[51, 52] It is well known that hyperostosis in the temporal bone owing to meningioma occurs less commonly than with meningiomas located elsewhere.[53]

Meningiomas along the skull base may assume a flattened contour (meningioma en plaque). Gd-DTPA contrast MR imaging parallels conventional iodinated contrast agents with homogeneous, early, prolonged, and

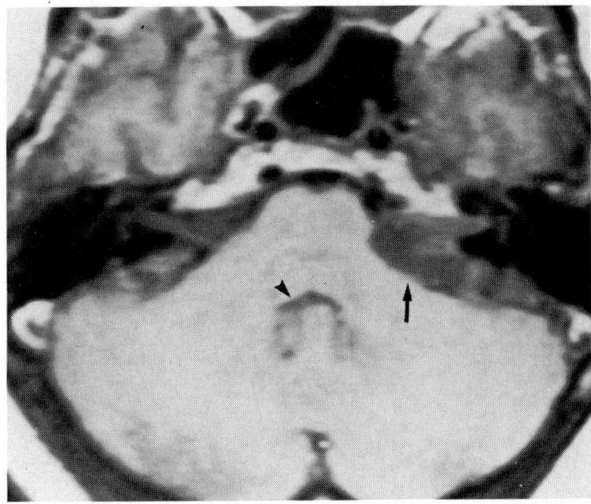

**Figure 9–15. Cystic acoustic neuroma.** Axial (1.5 T) T1WI (TR 700/TE 20 msec). Rounded mass at cerebellopontine angle (arrow) with similar signal to adjacent fourth ventricle (arrowhead). (Courtesy of S. Weinberg, M.D., Medi-Center North, Cincinnati, Ohio.)

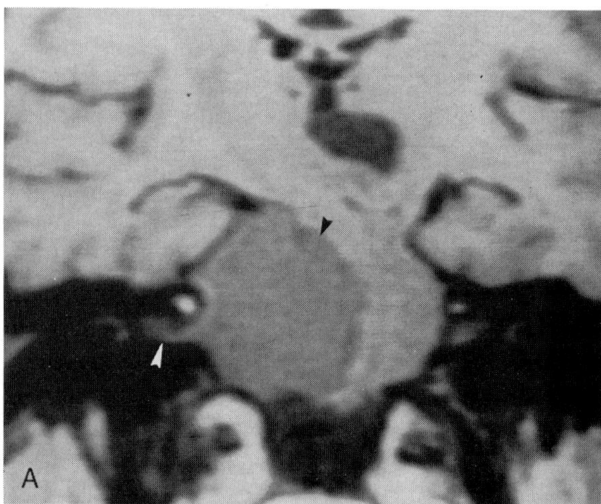


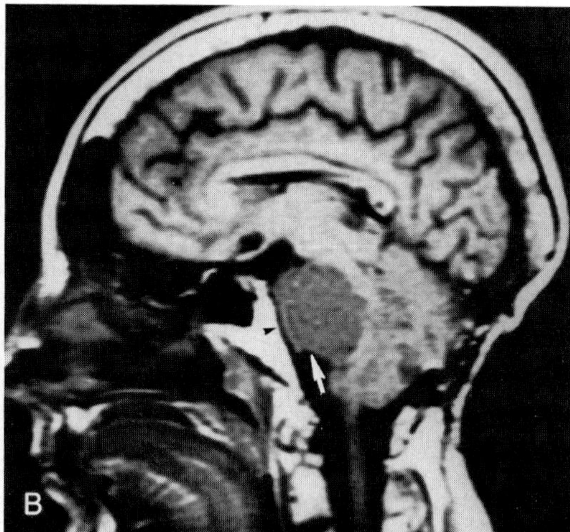


**Figure 9–16. Clival/CP angle meningioma.** *A,* Coronal (1.5 T) T1WI (TR 600/TE 20). Extra-axial hypointense mass (black arrowhead) at right cerebellopontine (CP) angle spares intracanalicular neural anatomy (white arrowhead). Differentiation of meningioma and neuroma is difficult. *B,* Sagittal T1WI shows hypointense extra-axial mass (arrow) with broad, clival-based margin (arrowhead) apparent only in this projection. (Courtesy of R. Lukin, M.D., Neuroradiology Department, University Hospital, Cincinnati, Ohio.)

pronounced enhancement. Gd-DTPA–enhanced MR may improve detection of these en plaque lesions. Enhancement is appreciated on T1WI as progressive lesion hyperintensity.

### Epidermoidomas

Epidermoidomas constitute 0.5 per cent of intracranial neoplasms and are less common CPA lesions than neuroma or meningioma. Inclusion of squamous epithelium at the time of neural groove closure may produce either an intra- or an extradural location. Frequently, patients are middle aged and exhibit a paucity of neurologic deficits for the size of the lesion. Posterior fossa epidermoids are most often found in the CPA, fourth ventricular region, petrous apex, and occipital calvarium. A predilection for the geniculate ganglion has been reported but is not widely appreciated.[54] Tympanomastoid congenital epidermoidomas do occur but are more often acquired.

The MR findings of congenital epidermoidomas are characteristic. T1WI hypointensity and T2WI inhomogeneous signal hyperintensity is the rule (Fig. 9–19). Cases of

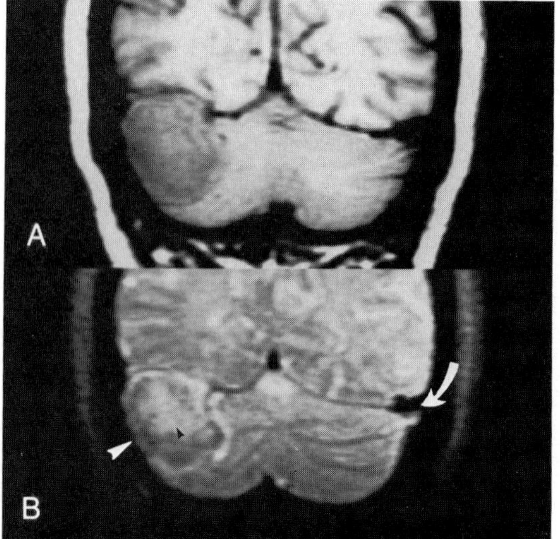


**Figure 9–17. Tentorial meningioma.** *A* and *B,* White coronal (1.5 T) T1WI (TR 600/TE 20) and T2WI (TR 1800/TE 100) show rightward extra-axial mass (white arrowhead), hypointense on T1WI and isointense on T2WI. Central foci of hyperintensity (black arrowhead) exist on T2WI. The patient's right transverse sinus appeared invaded and the left, patent (curved arrow); however, only marked sinus compression and occlusion was found at surgery.

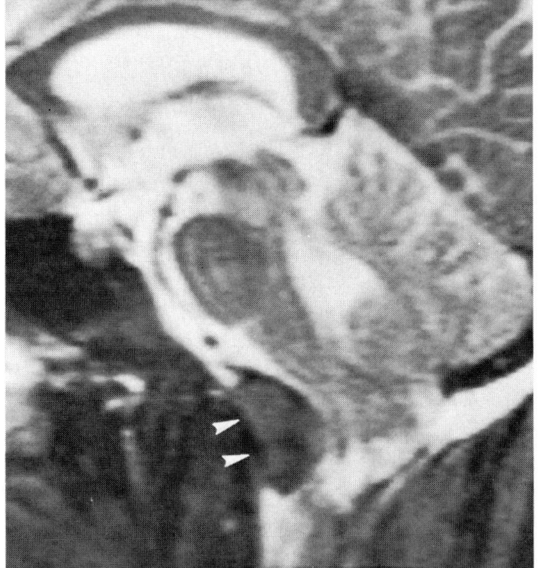

**Figure 9–18. Foramen magnum meningioma.** Sagittal (0.5 T) T2WI (TR 1700/TE 80 msec) shows a dural-based mass with a flat margin (arrowheads) displacing the brain stem. The signal is hypointense to gray matter on T2WI. (Courtesy J. Mantil, M.D., Department of Radiology, Kettering Medical Center and Wright State Medical School, Kettering, Ohio.)

T1WI hyperintense epidermoidomas rarely occur (< 3 per cent), and several of these reported cases are pathologically unproved.[55] Some may correspond to the hyperdense epidermoidoma on CT.[56] Acquired cholesteatomas may appear hyperintense on T1WI.[57] The signal characteristics of most congenital epidermoidomas may be related to the manner in which lipid cholesterin moieties are arranged with regard to large macromolecular complexes, unlike normal adipose tissue. Intercalation of these moieties about the bound hydrogen of adjacent water may account for the unexpected "waterlike" signal characteristics of congenital epidermoidomas.

Epidermoids must be differentiated from other lower attenuation CT lesions. Besides their T1 and T2 relaxation characteristics, sharp but scalloped or serpiginous margins, eccentric anatomic location, absence of T2WI hyperintense edema, and signal inhomogeneity assist in their identification. Minimal peripheral Gd-DTPA contrast enhancement approximates that seen with CECT. Hypointense calcific foci, common in meningioma, are rare in neuroma and infrequent in epidermoidomas. Differentiation

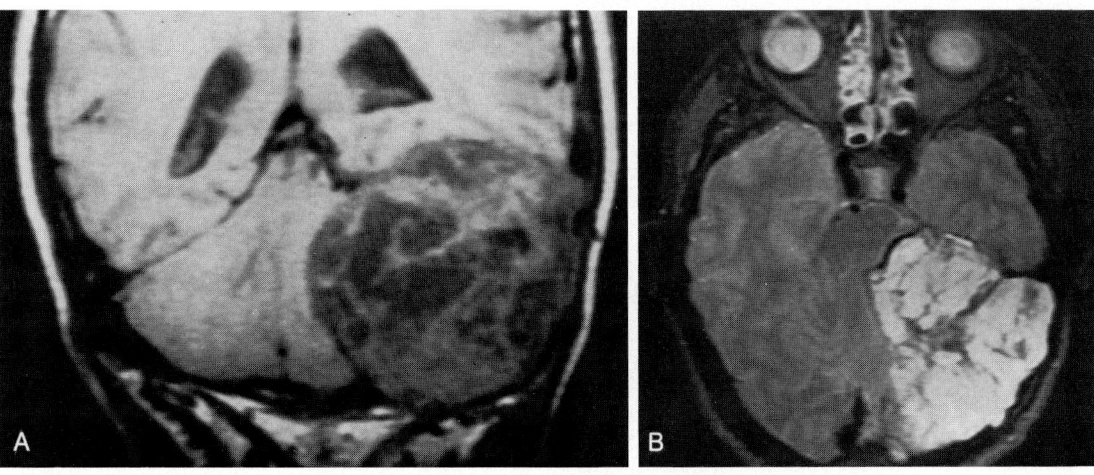


**Figure 9–19. Epidermoidomas.** *A* and *B*, Coronal (1.5 T) T1WI (TR 600/TE 20) and axial T2WI (TR 2000/TE 100 msec) show a leftward (of patient) posterior fossa extra-axial mass exhibiting T1 and T2 prolongation and signal inhomogeneity. (Courtesy of T. Seward, M.D., Medi-Center North, Cincinnati, Ohio.)

from cystic acoustic neuroma may be impossible with MR or CT; however, sensorineural hearing loss and signal homogeneity heavily favor neuroma.

### Other Tumors or Tumorlike Lesions

MR adds specificity to the differential diagnosis of cerebellopontine angle pathology. The signal characteristics of aneurysm or vascular ectasia are discussed in Chapter 11 of this text but are easily recognized by the lamellated appearance of flow-signal void, intermediate intensity vascular wall, or variable intensity crescent-shaped thrombus. Lipomas produce a pathognomonic MR appearance of T1WI hyperintensity and T2WI hypointensity that approximates the signal of subgaleal fat (Fig. 9–20).[58] The quadrageminal plate and CPA are the most frequent posterior fossa locations of lipoma. The frequency of detection in the quadrageminal plate and anterior third ventricular regions is higher on MR than CT.[59] Unlike the supratentorial compartment, where 50 per cent of lesions are symptomatic, most posterior fossa lipomas are asymptomatic. Cerebellar vermian agenesis is rarely associated with posterior fossa lipomas.

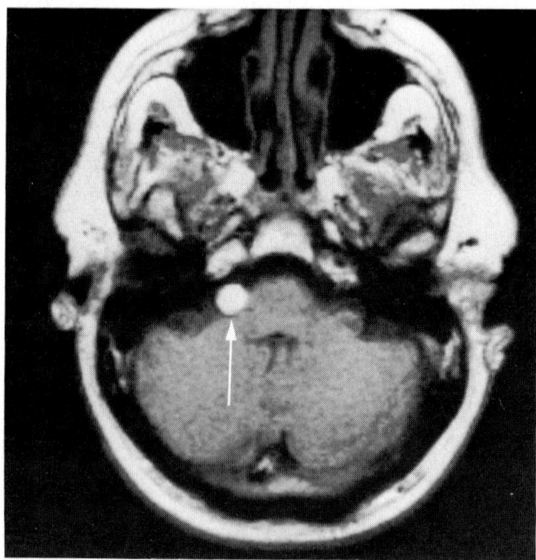

**Figure 9–20. CP-angle lipoma.** Axial T1WI (0.5 T) (TR 800/TE 25 msec) shows a rounded, hyperintense, cerebellopontine (CP) angle mass with signal similar to subgaleal and petroclival fat/marrow. (Courtesy of A. Chambers, M.D., Wellington Diagnostic Center, Cincinnati, Ohio.)

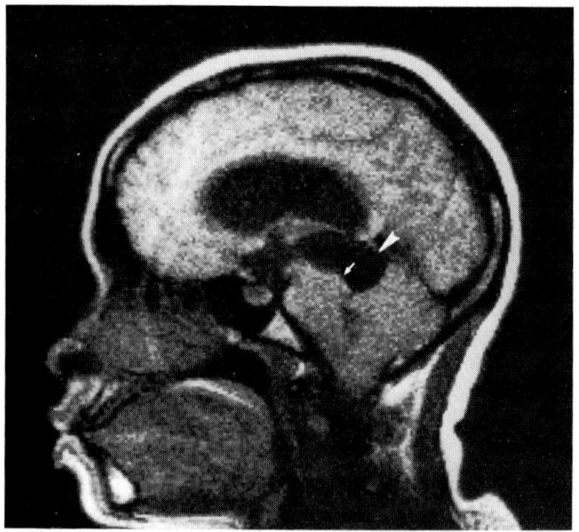

**Figure 9–21. Arachnoid cyst.** Sagittal (0.35 T) T1WI (TR 300/TE 35 msec). A cyst in the quadrigeminal cistern with signal matching the adjacent CSF. Tectal plate (arrow) is displaced anteriorly. Pineal recesses of the third ventricle are not identified as in aqueductal stenosis. The posterior cyst margins (arrowhead) of the mass are smooth and rounded. (Courtesy of J. Sheldon, M.D., Radiology Dept., Mount Sinai Hospital, Miami Beach, Fla.)

The majority of arachnoid cysts lie in the supratentorial space. Most infratentorial cysts are developmental. When involving the posterior fossa, the CPA is the second most common site and arachnoid cysts are found almost exclusively in adults.[60] A midline or lateral retrocerebellar location is the most common infratentorial site and affects young adults or adolescents. Quadrageminal plate cistern and juxtaclival arachnoid cysts are least common and occur in childhood or infancy.[61]

Arachnoid cysts are smooth rounded masses with T1WI and T2WI relaxation prolongation that nearly match CSF in signal intensity. T1 and T2 relaxation times are more prolonged than with epidermoidomas, and signal is quite homogeneous. The subarachnoid/prepontine cisternal location of juxtaclival cysts is easily demonstrated with sagittal T1WI. MR is also ideally suited for evaluating quadrageminal plate cysts (Fig. 9–21). Their true intra-arachnoidal location is confirmed by observing anterior collicular or tectal displacement on sagittal MR. In addition, herniation of cyst contents above the tentorial notch (25 per cent) and subsequent downward compression of the tentorium is easily appreciated.[62] Unlike arachnoid cysts, aqueductal stenosis with diverticular-like third ventricular enlargement displaces the tectal plate posteriorly in the sagittal plane. The intra-axial nature of ependymal cyst, a lesion confused with extra-axial arachnoid cyst, is easily recognized with multiplanar axial and sagittal MR.

Retrocerebellar arachnoid pouch (Fig. 9–22) is an entity that likely is identical to mega–cisterna magna and may be misconstrued as arachnoid cyst. A hypointense eccentric line courses through the CSF in this region and exhibits signal intensity compatible with eccentric dural venous sinus complex. The cerebellum may appear displaced or hypoplastic but not compressed.

Posterior fossa dermoid tumors are rare, frequently midline in location, may exhibit a linear T2WI hyperintense sinus tract, thickened, rounded walls, and hypointense calcific foci. Hyperintense T1WI signal is common with dermoid tumors and is not unexpected since their CT attenuation approximates fat.

A lesion confused initially with epidermoidoma and recognized with increased frequency on MR is cholesterol granuloma or cyst (Fig. 9–23). This lesion may involve the petrous apex, middle ear, or mastoid, listed in order of frequency. A petrous apex location, smooth margins, T1WI signal hyperintensity, absent neurologic symptomatology, and bilateral tendency allow differentiation from other abnormalities in this region. These lesions are likely of postinflammatory origin. Another inflammatory lesion, acquired tympanomastoid cholesteatoma, may exhibit T1WI signal hyperintensity.[63] These acquired inflammatory lesions are best evaluated with CT.

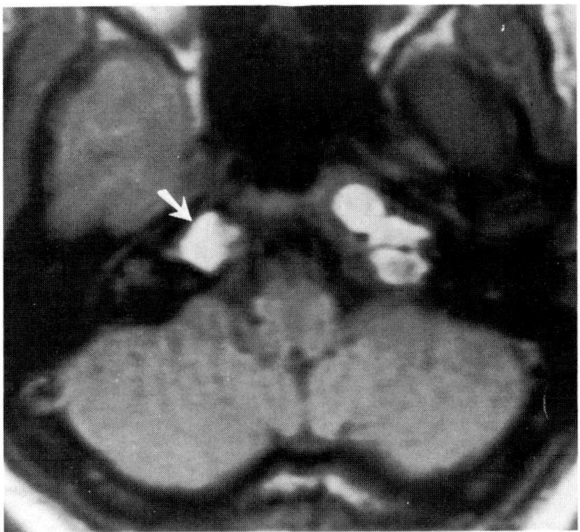

**Figure 9–23. Cholesterol cysts of the petrous apex.** Axial (1.5 T) T1WI (TR 600/TE 20 msec) shows bilateral, multifocal, hyperintense petrous signal (arrow) in a 27-year-old woman. The signal is hyperintense on T2WI (not shown), allowing differentiation from normal petroclival fat or lipoma. (Courtesy of S. Weinberg, M.D., Medi-Center North Diagnostics, Cincinnati, Ohio.)

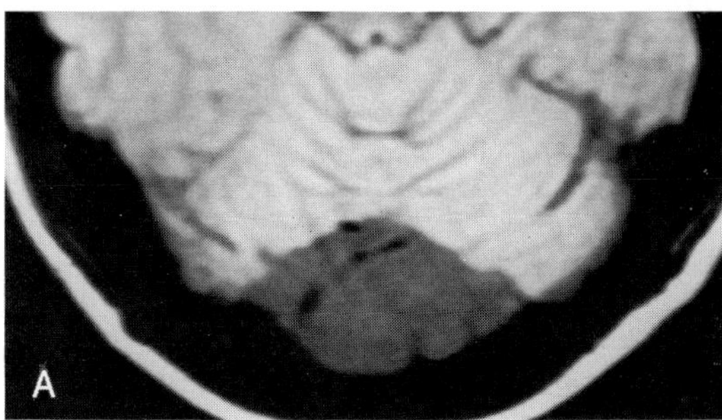


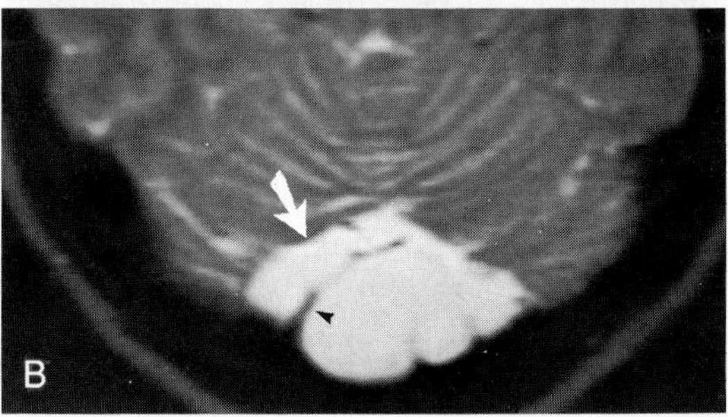


**Figure 9–22. Retrocerebellar arachnoid cyst.** *A* and *B*, A 27-year-old woman with persistent occipital headaches (1.5 T). *A* and *B*, Axial multiecho N(H)WI and T2WI (TR 1800/TE 20/80 msec). A posterior, homogeneous CSF signal (arrow) displaces the dural venous anatomy toward the patient's right (arrowhead).

## TEMPORAL BONE AND SKULL BASE

CT provides excellent bone detail in evaluating the normal and abnormal bone of the skull base and also the cranial nerves (Figs. 9–24 and 9–25). It is the favored modality in evaluating middle and external ear and bony skull base trauma. Nevertheless, MR remains a useful adjunctive tool.[64, 65] Bone undershoot or overshoot artifact may obscure detail in this region. MR can depict disease that has invaded vital vascular anatomy or neural foramina but, if it has not produced expansion of vessel or bone destruction, is barely detectable with NCCT. MR is far superior to CT in detecting soft tissue, extra-axial, and temporal lobe complications of skull base trauma.

Brain anatomy is reviewed in Chapter 5, but selected MR anatomic features are illus-

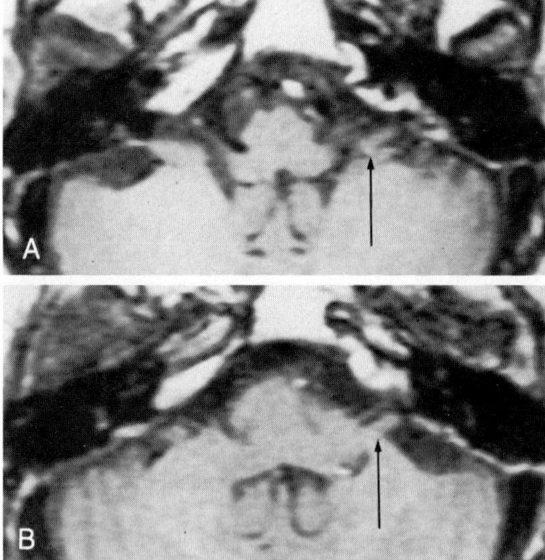


**Figure 9–24. Nerve complex (arrow).** *A* and *B*, Axial 3-mm T1W images at the level of the medulla demonstrate the patient's normal left IX, X, and XI.

trated in this chapter. The jugular bulb contains an anteromedial pars vascularis housing cranial nerve IX, a posterolateral pars nervosa containing cranial nerves X and XI, and a variable third compartment that includes the inferior petrosal sinus. On sagittal sections, these nerves have an oblique course from superoposterior to anteroinferior. Identification of individual nerves is possible with MR and virtually excludes tumor.[66] The right jugular bulb is often larger than the left, and any increased flow state may enlarge the pars vascularis. Flow phenomena are common in this region and may simulate jugular venous or lateral/sigmoid sinus thrombosis. This is particularly true on partial saturation sequences using relatively long TR (> 800) and short TE.

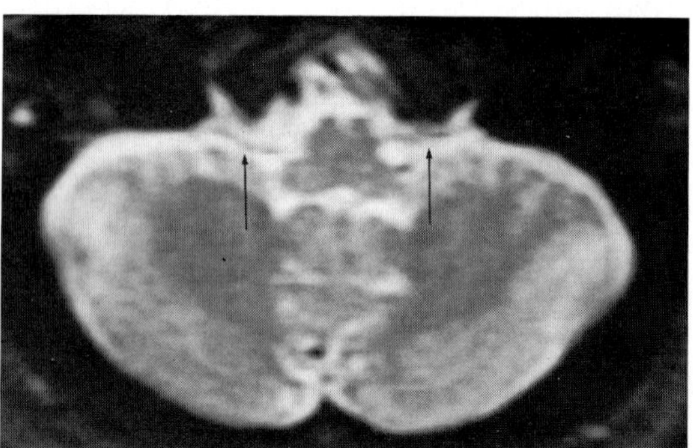

**Figure 9–25. Axial (1.5 T) T2WI (TR 1800/TE 20).** The twelfth nerves (arrows) are demonstrated at the level of the caudal medulla.

Our protocol for examining the skull base includes coronal and axial 5-mm gapless T1WI (TR 600 to 1000/TE 20 msec). If a specific disease site is suspected on clinical grounds, then 3-mm sections are substituted. These sections are selected from a sagittal or coronal one excitation scout. Most often, a 20-cm FOV is employed. Either two or four excitations (nex) are used, depending on time constraints and patient cooperation. Only if an abnormality is detected will other sequences be employed for further lesion characterization. Spin-echo 5-mm sections in the plane that best demonstrates the pathology are utilized (TR 1600 to 2000/TE 20/80 msec; 2 nex; 24 FOV; 128 × 256 matrix). When confusing flow phenomena in the jugular bulb, vein, or dural venous sinus occur, fast-scan imaging can be a quick and useful problem-solving technique (5-mm gapless sections; 5° to 11° flip angle; TR 20 to 40 msec; TE 12 msec; 24 cm FOV; 128 × 256 matrix; 4–6 nex).

## Glomus Tumor and Chemodectoma

Glomus tumors are neoplasms that arise from proliferation of cells arising along the jugulotympanic ganglia. Therefore these lesions may arise along the tympanic branch (Jacobson's nerve) of the glossopharyngeal nerve, forming a glomus tympanicum tumor (20 per cent to 30 per cent); along the auricular branch (Arnold's nerve) of the vagus nerve, forming a glomus vagale tumor (10 per cent); and paraganglia adjacent and inferior to the jugular foramen, a glomus jugulare tumor (50 per cent). In the head and neck, paraganglial cells are found most often at the carotid bifurcation (carotid body tumor). Middle-aged females are most often affected; 10 per cent of patients have multiple lesions, and 8 per cent harbor other neoplasms. Glomus tumor is the most common primary middle ear tumor and the second most common temporal bone neoplasm.

CECT is the preferred method of evaluating the middle ear. However, MR is sensitive in detection of jugular foramen mass or abnormality. Glomus tumors appear as serpiginous foci of intermediate T1WI signal intensity and mild to marked T2WI signal hyperintensity. A characteristic appearance

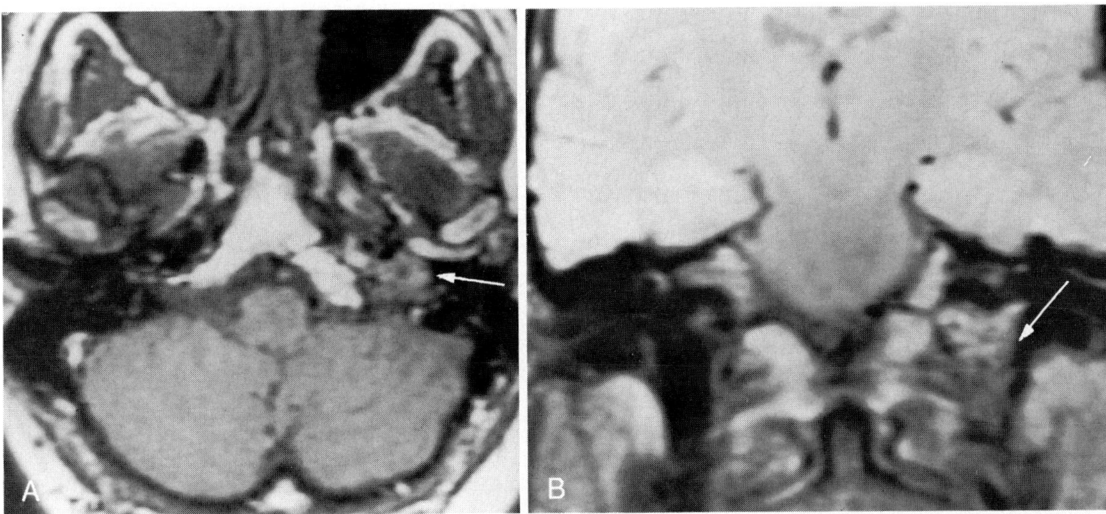


**Figure 9–26. Glomus jugulare.** *A* and *B,* Axial N(H)WI (TR 1800/TE 20) and coronal T1WI (TR 600/TE 20 msec) in a man with pulsatile tinnitus. A mass in the jugular bulb invading the jugular vein (arrow) has a "speckled" signal, or hypointense punctate foci, within.

of larger paragangliomas has been suggested. It consists of a "salt-and-pepper" appearance that includes punctate foci of signal void owing to lesion hypervascularity amongst the hyperintense T2WI signal of solid tumor (Fig. 9–26).[67] Although CT more easily demonstrates adjacent bone destruction, interruption of petroclival and jugular tubercular hyperintense T1WI marrow signal is easily demonstrable with MR. Coronal images optimally demonstrate jugular venous and bulb occlusion and coronal T1-weighted CEMR readily shows cranio-caudad tumor extent. Since dense calcification can go undetected with MR, isointense or hypointense lesions in this region suggest a diagnosis of jugular tubercle meningioma (Fig. 9–27). Neuromas in this region are more rounded in configuration but are otherwise difficult to differentiate from glomus tumor.

## Chordoma

Intracranial chordomas most commonly arise in the third to fourth decades of life from notochordal remnants in the spheno-occipital synchondrosis, or clival region. MR is extremely well suited to diagnose and stage these neoplasms. T1WI will depict destruction or replacement of the hyperintense T1WI clival marrow signal by intermediate signal intensity. Similar findings can be seen in the dorsum sella, posterior clinoids, and sellar floor. The hypointense linear signal of cortical bone is often interrupted in this region. Vascular encasement is well illustrated with MR.

Signal homogeneity and relaxation characteristics roughly approximate tumor density and calcification. Often, a "frondlike or cauliflower-like" appearance is simulated in the sagittal projection (Fig. 9–28). T1WI hypointensity and T2WI hyperintensity is often present (80 per cent); however, intermediate and inhomogeneous T2WI signal characteristics occur with heavily calcified lesions. Neoplasm is easily contrasted with

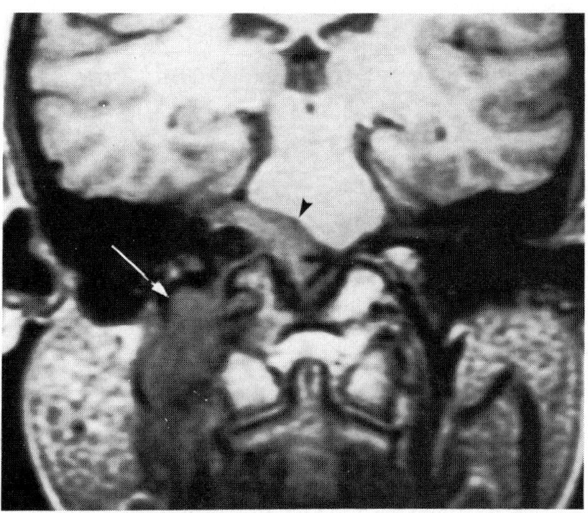

**Figure 9–27. Jugular tubercle meningioma.** A 24-year-old woman with otalgia and IX, X, and XI cranial nerve palsies. Coronal (1.5 T) T1WI (TR 700/TE 20 msec). Hypointense mass (arrowhead) above the jugular tubercle invades the jugular bulb and vein (arrow).

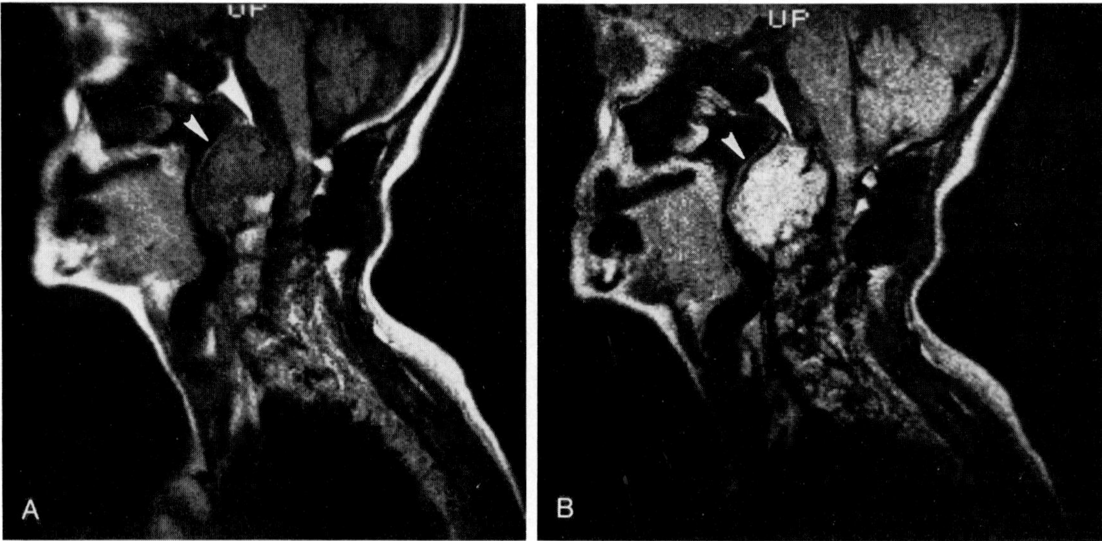


**Figure 9–28. Chordoma.** *A* and *B,* A 36-year-old woman with dysphagia (0.35 T). T1WI (TR 400/TE 35 msec) and N(H)WI (TR 1500/TE 35 msec). T1WI shows a hypointense mass replacing marrow signal of C2 (arrowhead) and the clival tip. A hyperintense mass on N(H)WI encroaches on brain stem and nasopharynx. (Courtesy of K. Soila, M.D., Radiology Dept., Mount Sinai Hospital, Miami Beach, Fla.)

brain stem on T2WI, and sagittal T1WI provide accurate nasopharyngeal and airway assessment. Therefore examination with sagittal T1 and T2WI and axial T1WI is recommended.

Typical CT findings include an isodense or hyperdense calcified (30 per cent to 50 per cent) mass with variable contrast enhancement. Bone destruction may involve the clivus, sella, petrous bone, orbit, middle fossa, jugular tubercle, atlas, and foramen magnum in decreasing order of frequency.

## Trigeminal and Other Neuromas

Trigeminal neuromas are the second most common intracranial neuroma, occurring in the third to fourth decade and arising from the gasserian ganglion in 50 per cent of cases. Similarly, 50 per cent arise as extradural middle fossa masses, but of these 25 per cent arise from the trigeminal nerve root ganglion and appear in the intradural CPA. The remaining 25 per cent involve both the middle and posterior fossae. Gasserian gan-

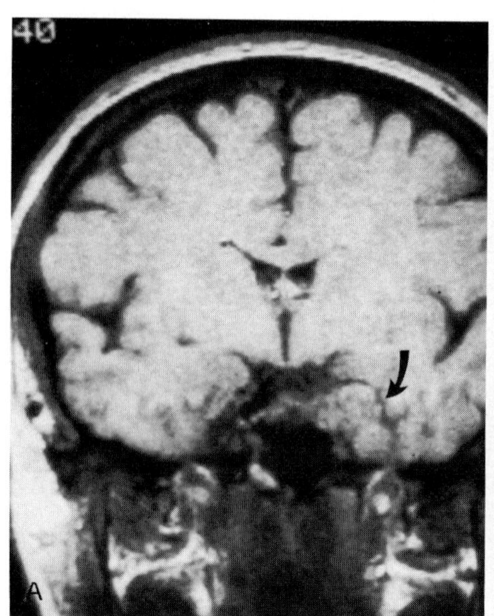


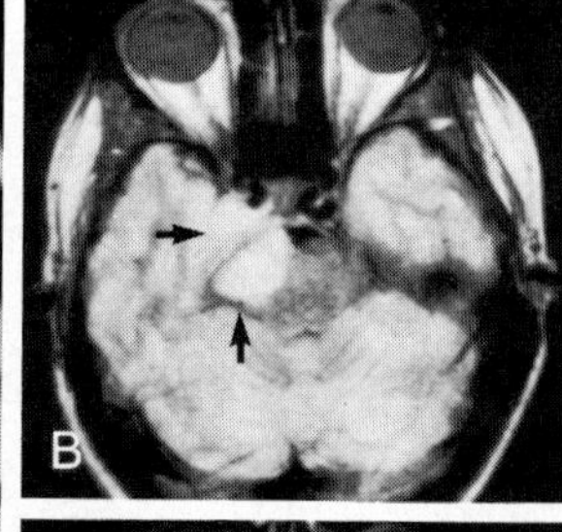


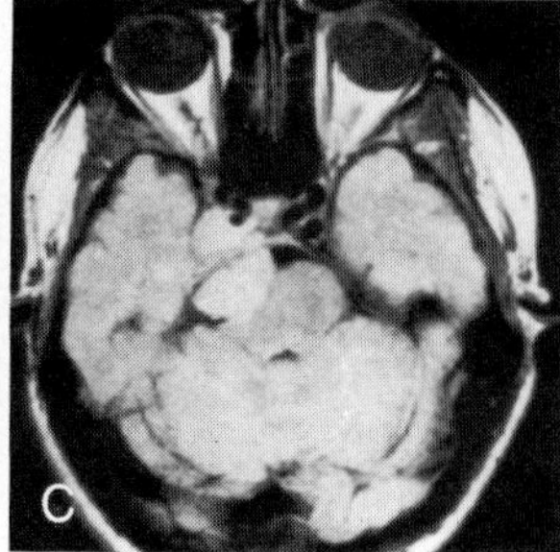


**Figure 9–29. Trigeminal neuromas.** *A,* Coronal (1.5 T) T1WI. *B,* Axial N(H)WI. *C,* Axial T1WI. The coronal image shows a normal hypointense CSF signal in the cistern of Meckel's cave on the patient's right but an intermediate signal mass (curved arrow) on the left. Axial images (*B* and *C*) in a patient with the same diagnosis as in *A* show a dumbell-shaped mass (arrows) with a ventral component in the middle fossa (Meckel's cave) and a dorsal component in the posterior fossa. (Courtesy of Neuroradiology Dept., New York University Hospital, New York, N.Y.)

glion or Meckel's cave lesions are manifested clinically with ipsilateral facial hypesthesia, corneal anesthesia or hypesthesia, and headache. Posterior fossa lesions may present with hearing loss, facial nerve palsy, or ataxia.[68] Females are more often affected.

The signal alterations of trigeminal neuroma approximate acoustic neuroma (Fig. 9–29). Location and symptomatology provide the key to diagnosis. Location anterior to the CPA, near to or interrupting the hyperintense petrous tip signal, or extension into Meckel's cave and the middle fossa on axial and coronal images are supportive findings. T2WI signal hyperintensity favor trigeminal neuroma over meningioma, the primary differential diagnostic consideration. Marked Gd-DTPA enhancement favors the latter. Epidermoids are easily distinguished by their marked T1 and T2 relaxation prolongation. Temporal lobe gliomas may resemble trigeminal neuroma on CT, but their intra-axial nature is definitive with coronal MR.

Seventh nerve neuromas occur in the descending intrapetrous facial canal or in the geniculate ganglion.[69,70] Because of the diminutive canal size, lesions in the descending segment are more apt to cause facial paralysis. Lesions in the porus acusticus present with sensorineural hearing loss, whereas neuromas located near the tympanic cavity result in conductive hearing loss. Neuromas account for 5 per cent of patients with persistent Bell's palsy (80 per cent are idiopathic).[71,72] Neoplastic causes of Bell's palsy are slowly progressive, unlike more common causes such as idiopathic, trauma, herpes zoster, and otitis media, which have acute onset. Most geniculate ganglion lesions present in the middle fossa. Fifth and seventh nerve neuromas are easily distinguished from intrapetrous carotid aneurysms by their lack of flow-void signal.[73] CPA facial neuromas may be indistinguishable from acoustic neuroma but, on sagittal, small FOV, surface coil images, the anterosuperior branch of the four-nerve complex is affected. Neuromas of the ninth, tenth (Fig. 9–30), and eleventh nerves may be indistinguishable from glomus tumors on MR; however, large glomus tumors exhibit a "speckled" pattern owing to hypervascular flow-void signal alteration. Patients with neurofibromatosis and suspected neoplasm of the skull base or foramen magnum are best assessed with MR.[74]

### Other Lesions

MR is an adjunctive tool to CT in detection of both large and small skull base lesions (Fig. 9–31). Some may have characteristic signal or location allowing specific diagnoses. Nasopharyngeal carcinomas may involve the skull base (Fig. 9–32) via the for-

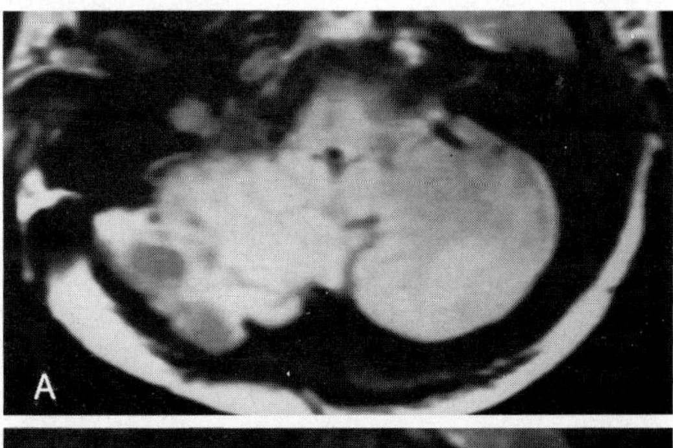


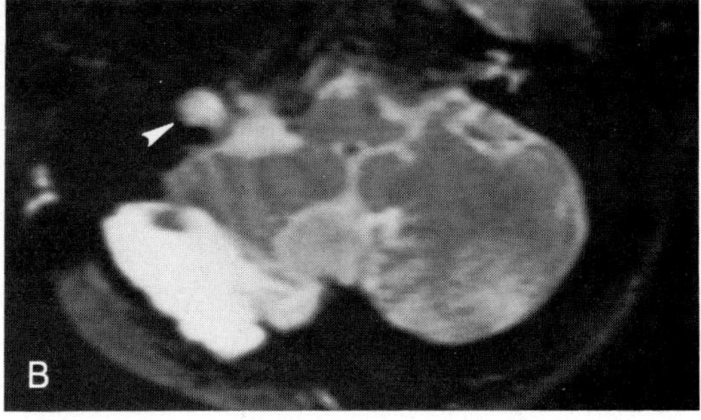


**Figure 9–30. Vagus nerve neuroma.** A 27-year-old woman with dysphagia and prior meningioma resection (1.5 T). *A,* Axial multiecho N(H)WI, and *B,* T2WI (TR 2000/TE 20/100 msec). A rounded mass with prolonged T2 relaxation lies in the patient's right jugular foramen (arrowhead). Rightward (to reader's left), a retrocerebellar subdural collection is also present from prior surgery.

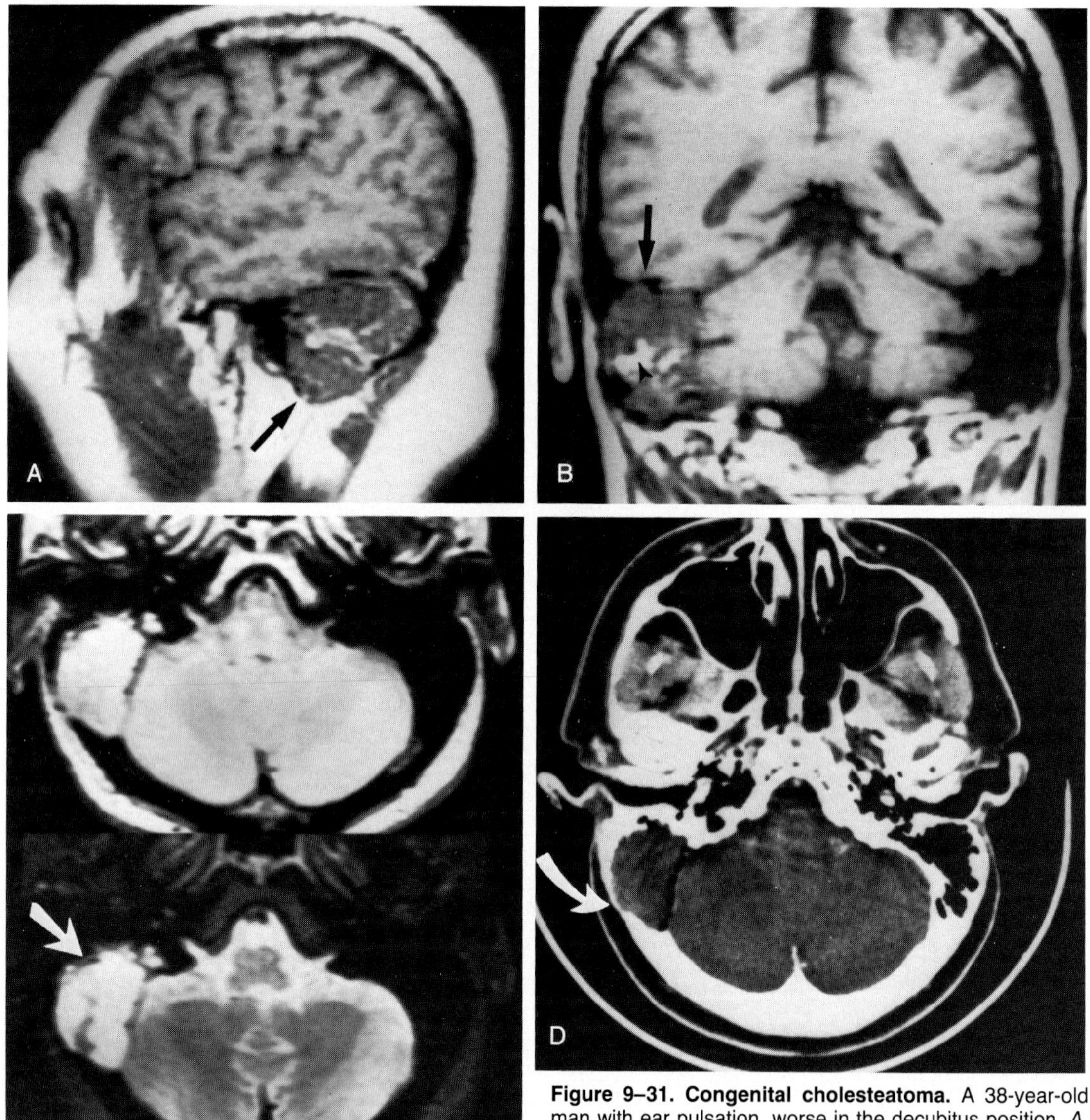


**Figure 9–31. Congenital cholesteatoma.** A 38-year-old man with ear pulsation, worse in the decubitus position. *A,* Sagittal T1WI (TR 600/TE 20). *B,* Coronal T1WI (TR 600/TE 20). *C,* Axial N(H)WI and T2WI. *D,* Axial CECT. Intermediate attenuation mass (curved arrow, *D*) replaces the entire mastoid region but spares the middle ear on CECT. *B,* note that within the mass (black arrow), a focus of signal hyperintensity is present (arrowhead), representing pathologic components of cholesterin and keratin. *C,* The axial T2WI demonstrates an inhomogeneous signal hyperintensity (arrow), not unexpected for this lesion.

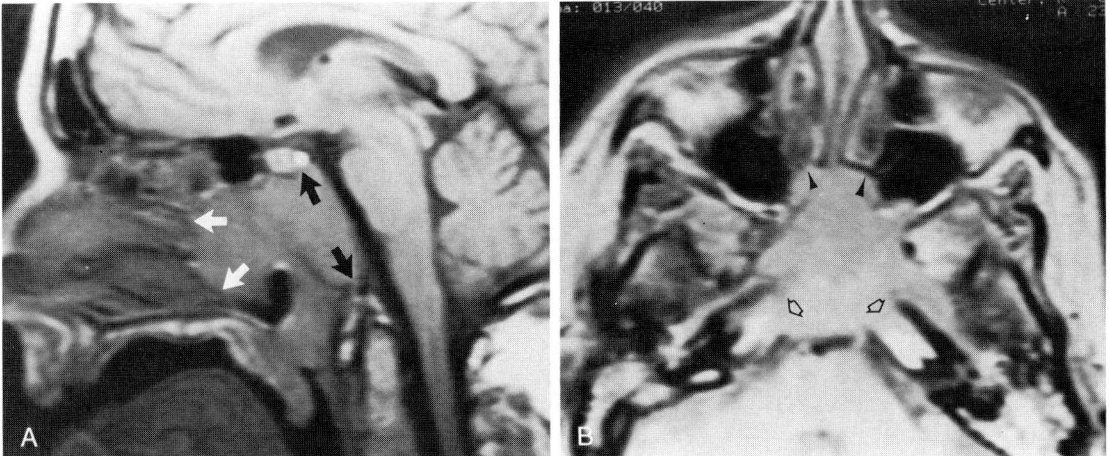

**Figure 9–32. Nasopharyngeal carcinoma with nasal and skull base invasion.** A 36-year-old Chinese woman with dysphagia. *A,* Sagittal T1WI (TR 900/TE 20). *B,* Axial N(H)WI (TR 2300/TE 20). Sagittal T1WI shows cephalad and caudad extension along the mucosal and submucosal planes of the nasopharynx and invasion of the clivus and sellar floor (black arrows). Extension into the nasal cavity and ethmoid region is present (white arrows). On N(H)WI, the pharyngobasilar fascia is transgressed with invasion of the clivus and petrous bone (open arrows) and with nasal cavity extension (black arrowheads).

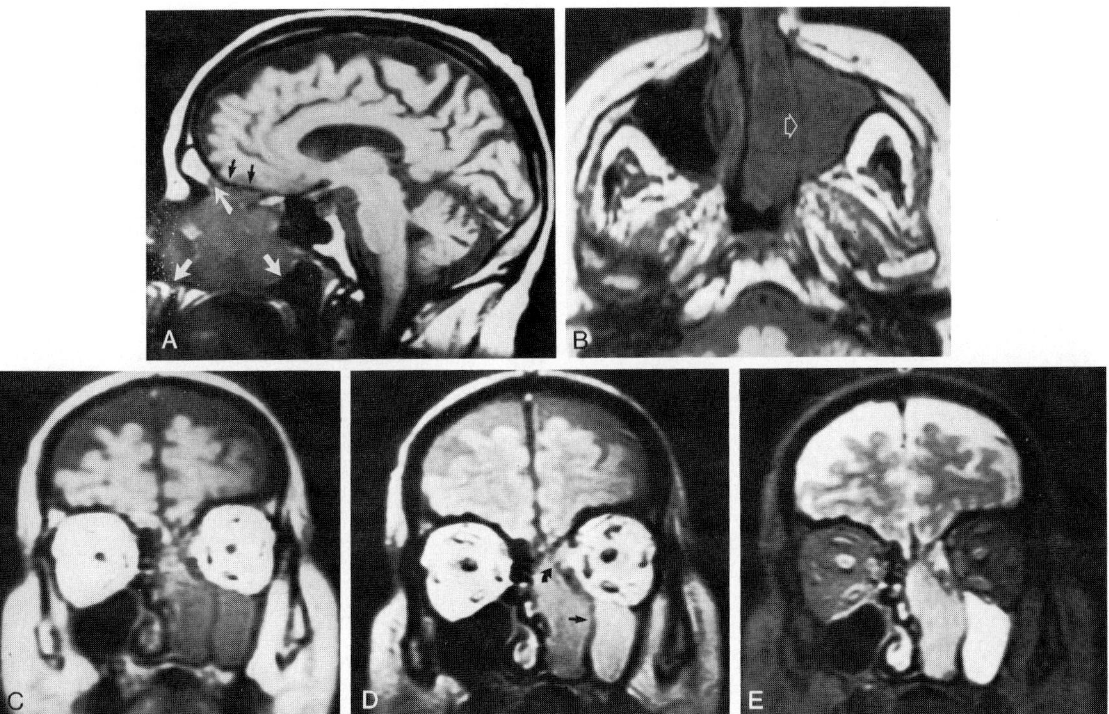

**Figure 9–33. Esthesioneuroblastoma.** A 62-year-old man with anosmia, nasal congestion, and nasal discharge (1.5 T). *A,* Sagittal T1WI. *B,* Axial T1WI. *C,* Coronal T1WI. *D* and *E,* Coronal N(H)WI and T2WI. A mass (arrows) of intermediate signal intensity has invaded the nasal fossa and has interrupted the hyperintense signal in the crista galli region (upper white arrow). The hypointense signals of dura, CSF, and cortical bone are preserved (black arrows) and the hyperintense signal in the frontal sinus is due to sinus obstruction on the sagittal T1WI. In *B,* the medial maxillary sinus wall is intact (open arrow). Coronal T1WI and CT (not shown) suggest that the mass has invaded the maxillary sinus; however, N(H)WI and T2WI confirm that mass has different signal intensity from the obstructed sinuses and has not transgressed the maxillary (black arrow) or ethmoid (curved arrow) sinus walls.

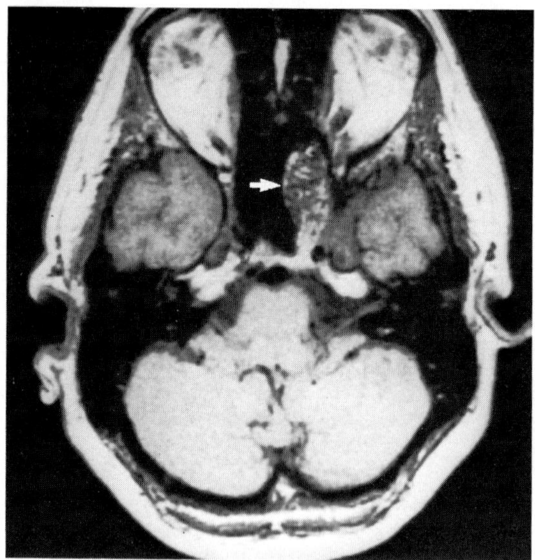

**Figure 9–34. Fibrous dysplasia.** Axial (1.5 T) T1WI (TR 800/TE 20 msec). Mass extending from patient's leftward sphenoid bone (arrow) exhibits "gyriform" internal signal. (Courtesy of L. Eynon, M.D., Radiology Dept., Mercy Hospital, Fairfield, Ohio.)

amen lacerum and often extend into or arise near the fossa of Rosenmüller. The nasopharyngeal epicenter on sagittal T1WI permits differentiation from other skull base lesions such as chordomas. Similarly, the typical crista galli location and involvement by esthesioneuroblastomas (Fig. 9–33) is easily appreciated on sagittal MR. When these patients present with cranial nerve deficits, subtle or marked T2WI signal hyperintensity in foramina, in the cavernous sinus region, or in the skull base itself may be present. When such deficits are present, examination with 3-mm, contiguous, 20-cm FOV coronal T1WI is carried out over the region of interest. If anatomical asymmetry is demonstrated, then T2WI coronal sections may be performed.

We have encountered numerous cases of fibrous dyplasia (Fig. 9–34) and Paget's disease of the skull base on MR. CT or conventional radiography are superior methods of diagnosis; however, the MR appearance should be recognized. Fibrous dysplasia results in replacement of normal cancellous bone with fibrous tissue. It exhibits intermediate signal intensity on multiple pulsing sequences but contains serpiginous or gyri-

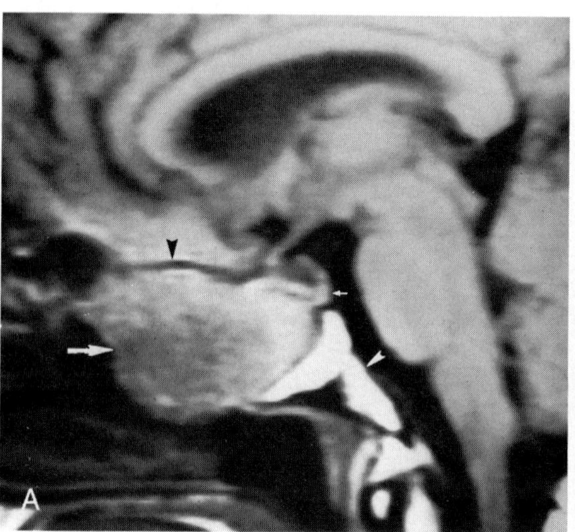


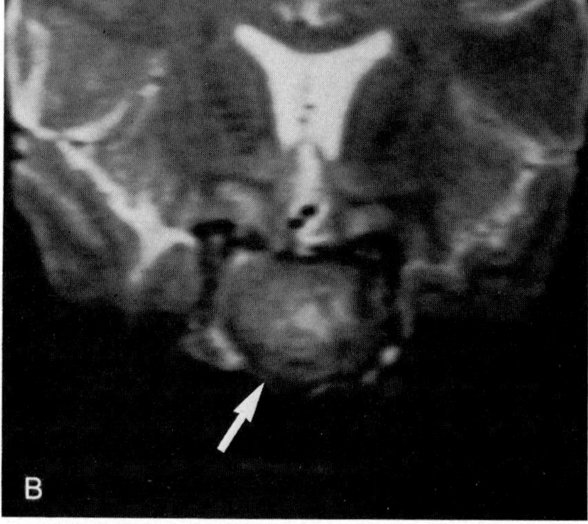


**Figure 9–35. Sphenoid sinus meningioma.** *A,* Sagittal (1.5 T) T1WI (TR 600/TE 20), and *B,* coronal T2WI (TR 1800/TE 100 msec). Mass in sphenoid sinus (arrow) has remodeled the clivus (white arrowhead), uplifted the sellar floor (small arrow), and thickened the anterior cranial fossa floor (black arrowhead). T2WI isointensity is compatible with a fibrous, dense nature. T2 signal hyperintensity is present within the lesion.

form signal inhomogeneity that allows differentiation from skull base meningioma in some cases (Fig. 9–35). Paget's disease produces enlargement and increase in the signal of normally hypointense outer and inner cortical tables. Encroachment and occasional obliteration of the normal hyperintense intradiploic signal may occur.

## References


1. Olsen WL, Winkler ML, Ross DA. Carcinomatous encephalitis: CT and MR findings. AJNR 8:553, 1987.
2. Brant-Zawadski M, Badami JP, Mills CM, et al. Primary intracranial tumor imaging: a comparison of magnetic resonance and CT. Radiology 150:435, 1984.
3. Randell CP, Collins AG, Young IR, et al. Nuclear magnetic resonance imaging of posterior fossa tumors. AJR 41:489, 1983.
4. Pomeranz SJ, Soila K, Tobias JA, Sheldon JJ, et al. Sensitivity of MRI in metastatic neoplasia: a case report. Magn Reson Imag 3:291, 1985.
5. Seeger JF, Burke DP, Knake JE, et al. Computed tomographic and angiographic evaluation of hemangioblastomas. Radiology 138:65, 1981.
6. Fill WL, Lameill JM, Polk NO, et al. The radiologic manifestations of von Hippel-Lindau disease. Radiology 133:289, 1979.
7. Ganti SR, Silver AJ, Hilal SK, et al. Computed tomography of cerebellar hemangioblastomas. Comput Tomogr 6:912, 1982.
8. Brant-Zawadski M, Davis PL, Crooks PL, et al. NMR demonstration of cerebral abnormalities: comparison with CT. AJR 140:847, 1983.
9. Rebner M, Gebarski SS. Magnetic resonance imaging of spinal-cord hemangioblastoma. AJNR 6:287, 1985.
10. Di Chiro G, Rieth KG, Oldfield EH, et al. Digital subtraction angiography and dynamic computed tomography in the evaluation of arteriovenous malformations and hemangioblastomas of the spinal cord. J Comput Assist Tomogr 6:655, 1982.
11. Bilaniuk LT, Zimmerman RA, Littman P, et al. Computed tomography of brainstem gliomas in children. Radiology 34:89, 1980.
12. Leeds NE, Elkin CM, Zimmerman RD. Gliomas of the brain. Semin Roentgen 19:27, 1984.
13. Peterman SB, Steiner RE, Bydder GM, et al. Nuclear magnetic resonance imaging (NMR), (MRI), of brain stem tumors. Neuroradiology 27:202, 1985.
14. Bradac GB, Schorner W, Bender A, et al. MRI (NMR) in the diagnosis of brain-stem tumors. Neuroradiology 27:208, 1985.
15. Koehler PR, Haughton VM, Daniels DL, et al. MR measurement of normal and pathologic brainstem diameters. AJNR 6:425, 1985.
16. Hueftle MG, Han JS, Kaufman B, et al. MR imaging of brain stem gliomas. J Comput Assist Tomogr 9:263, 1985.
17. Lee BCP, Deck MDF, Kneeland JB, et al. MR imaging of the craniocervical junction. AJNR 6:863, 1985.
18. Okazaki H. Fundamentals of Neuropathology. Tokyo, Igaku-Shoin, 1983:193.
19. Sherman JL, Citrin CM, Barkovich AJ, et al. MR imaging of the mesencephalic tectum: normal and pathologic variations. AJNR 8:59, 1987.
20. Zimmerman RA, Bilaniuk LT, Packer R, et al. Resistive NMR of brain stem gliomas. Neuroradiology 27:21, 1985.
21. Kjos BO, Brant-Zawadski M, Kucharczyk W, et al. Cystic intracranial lesions: magnetic resonance imaging. Radiology 155:363, 1985.
22. Bellon EM, Haake EM, Coleman PE, et al. MR artifacts: a review. AJR 147:1271, 1986.
23. Naidich TP, Lin JP, Leeds NE, et al. Primary tumors and other masses of the cerebellum and fourth ventricle: differential diagnosis by computed tomography. Neuroradiology 14:153, 1977.
24. Weisberg LA. Computed tomographic findings in cerebellar astrocytoma. Comput Radiol 6:137, 1982.
25. Zimmerman RA, Bilaniuk LA, Bruno L, et al. Computed tomographic findings in cerebellar astrocytoma. Comput Radiol 6:137, 1982.
26. Segall HD, Zee CS, Naidich TP, et al. Computed tomography in neoplasms of the posterior fossa in children. Radiol Clin North Am 20:237, 1982.
27. Lee BCP, Kneeland JB, Deck MDF, et al. Posterior fossa lesions: magnetic resonance imaging. Radiology 153:137, 1984.
28. Zimmerman RA, Bilaniuk LT, Goldberg HI, et al. Cerebral NMR imaging: early results with a 0.12 T resistive system. AJR 141:1187, 1983.
29. Schott LH, Naidich TP, Gan J. Common pediatric brain tumors: typical computed tomographic appearances. J Comput Assist Tomogr 7:3, 1981.
30. Davis KR, Richardson EP. High attenuation lesions of the posterior fossa. J Comput Assist Tomogr 4:704, 1980.
31. North C, Segall HD, Stanley P, et al. Early CT detection of intracranial seeding from medulloblastoma. AJNR 6:11, 1985.
32. Zee CS, Segall HD, Miller C, et al. Less common CT features of medulloblastoma. Radiology 144:97, 1982.
33. Swartz JD, Zimmerman RA, Bilaniuk L. Computed tomography of intracranial ependymomas. Radiology 143:97, 1982.
34. Levine HL, Kleefield J, Rao KCVG. The base of the skull. *In* Lee SH, Rao KCVG, eds. Cranial Computed Tomography. New York, McGraw-Hill Co. 1983:446.
35. Wu E, Tang Y, Zhang Y, et al. CT in diagnosis of acoustic neuromas. AJNR 7:645, 1986.
36. Pinto RS, Kricheff II, Bergeron RT, et al. Small acoustic neuromas: detection by high resolution gas CT cisternography. AJR 139:129, 1982.
37. Daniels DL, Schenck JF, Foster T, et al. Surface-coil magnetic resonance imaging of the internal auditory canal. AJNR 6:487, 1985.
38. Daniels DL, Herfkins R, Koehler RR, et al. Magnetic resonance imaging of the internal auditory canal. Radiology 151:105, 1984.
39. Solti-Bohmann LG, Magaram DL, Lo WWM, et al. Gas-CT cisternography for detection of small acoustic nerve tumors. Radiology 150:403, 1984.
40. New PFJ, Bachow TB, Wismer GL, et al. MR imaging and small acoustic neuromas at 0.6 T: prospective study. AJR 144:1021, 1985.
41. Enzmann DR, O'Donohue J. Optimizing MR imaging for detecting small tumors in the cerebellopontine and internal auditory canal. AJNR 8:99, 1987.

42. Barkovich AJ, Wippold FJ, Brammer RE. False-negative MR imaging of an acoustic neuroma. AJNR 7:363, 1986.
43. Bydder GM, Steiner RE, Young IR, et al. Clinical NMR imaging of the brain: 140 cases. AJR 139:215, 1982.
44. Mawhinney RR, Buckley JH, Worthington BS. Magnetic resonance imaging of the cerebello-pontine angle. Br J Radiol 59:961, 1986.
45. Curati WL, Graif M, Kingsley DPE, et al. MRI in acoustic neuroma: a review of 35 patients. Neuroradiology 28:208, 1986.
46. Kingsley DPE, Brooks GB, Leung AWL, et al. Acoustic neuromas: evaluation by magnetic resonance imaging. AJNR 6:1, 1985.
47. Daniels DL, Millen SJ, Meyer GA, et al. MR detection of tumor in the internal auditory canal. AJNR 8:249, 1987.
48. Curati WL, Graif M, Kingsley DPE, et al. Acoustic neuromas: Gd-DTPA in MR imaging. Radiology 158:447, 1986.
49. Valvanis A, Dabir K, Hamdi R, et al. Current state of the radiologic diagnosis of acoustic neuroma. Neuroradiology 23:7, 1982.
50. Gentry LR, Jacoby CG, Turski PA, et al. Cerebellopontine angle-petromastoid mass lesions: comparative study of diagnosis with MR imaging and CT. Radiology 162:513, 1987.
51. Zimmerman RD, Fleming CC, Saint-Louis LA, et al. Magnetic resonance imaging of meningiomas. AJNR 6:149, 1985.
52. Spagnoli MV, Goldberg HI, Grossman RI, et al. Intracranial meningiomas: high-field MR imaging. Radiology 161:369, 1986.
53. Valvanis A, Schubiger O, Hayek J, et al. CT of meningiomas of the posterior surface of the petrous bone. Neuroradiology 22:11, 1981.
54. Fisch V, Ruttner J. Pathology of intratemporal tumors involving the facial nerve. *In* Fisch V, ed. Facial Nerve Surgery. Amstelveen, The Netherlands, Kugler, 1977:448.
55. Houston LW, Hinke ML. Neuroradiology case of the day. AJR 146:637, 1986.
56. Braun IF, Naidich TP, Leeds NE, et al. Dense intracranial epidermoid tumors. Computed tomographic observations. Radiology 122:717, 1977.
57. Latack JT, Kartush JM, Kemink JL, et al. Epidermoidomas of the cerebellopontine angle and temporal bone: CT and MR aspects. Radiology 157:361, 1985.
58. Kean DM, Smith MA, Douglas RHB, et al. Two examples of CNS lipomas demonstrated by CT and low-field (0.08 T) MR imaging. J Comput Assist Tomogr 9:494, 1985.
59. Zimmerman RA, Bilaniuk LT, Dolinskas C. Cranial computed tomography of epidermoid and congenital fatty tumors of maldevelopment origin. Comput Tomogr 3:40, 1979.
60. Little JL, Gomez MR, McCarty CS. Infratentorial arachnoid cysts. J Neurosurg 39:380–387, 1973.
61. Menezes AH, Bell WE, Perret GE. Arachnoid cysts in children. Arch Neurol 37:168, 1980.
62. Choi SK, Meyey GA, Kovnar EH, et al. Arachnoid cyst of the quadrageminal plate cistern: report of two cases. AJNR 7:725, 1986.
63. Koenig H, Lenz M, Sauter R. Temporal bone region: high-resolution MR imaging using surface coils. Radiology 159:191, 1986.
64. Han JS, Huss RG, Benson JE, et al. MR imaging of the skull base. J Comput Assist Tomogr 8:944, 1984.
65. Paling MR, Black WC, Lavine PA, et al. Tumor invasion of the anterior skull base: a comparison of MR and CT studies. J Comput Assist Tomogr 11:824, 1987.
66. Daniels DL, Schenck JF, Foster T, et al. Magnetic resonance imaging of the jugular foramen. AJNR 6:699, 1985.
67. Olsen WL, Dillon WP, Kelly WM, et al. MR imaging of paragangliomas. AJNR 7:1039, 1986.
68. Goldberg R, Byrd S, Winter J, et al. Varied appearance of trigeminal neuromas on CT. AJR 134:57, 1980.
69. Horn KL, Crumley RL, Schindler RA. Facial neurilemmomas. Laryngoscope 91:1326, 1981.
70. Latack JT, Gabrielsen TO, Knake JE, et al. Facial nerve neuromas: radiologic evaluation. Radiology 149:731, 1983.
71. Neely JG, Alford BR. Facial nerve neuromas. Arch Otolaryngol 100:298, 1974.
72. Jackson CG, Glasscosk ME 3rd, Hughes G, et al. Facial paralysis of neoplastic origin: diagnosis and management. Laryngoscope 90:1581, 1980.
73. Kelly WM, Harsh GR IV. CT of Petrous carotid aneurysms. AJNR 6:830, 1985.
74. Mayer JS, Kulkarni MV, Yeakley JW. Craniocervical manifestations of neurofibromatosis: MR versus CT studies. J Comput Assist Tomogr 11:839, 1987.

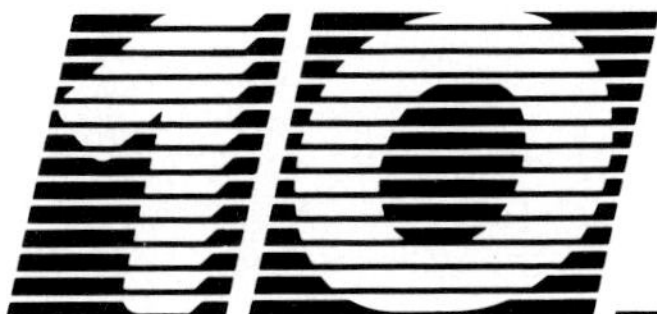

Jerome J. Sheldon, M.D.

# MRI OF THE SELLA

Magnetic resonance imaging (MRI) has shown increasing promise as the primary imaging procedure in the evaluation of the pituitary and perisellar region.[1–6] Reports to date have indicated that MRI is competitive with computed tomography (CT) imaging in its ability to detect lesions in this area.[4,5] In addition, because of its ability to directly image in orthogonal projections (i.e., axial, sagittal, and coronal), it provides unique anatomic information as to the relationship of pathology to the surrounding normal juxtasellar anatomy.[2,5] MRI in certain instances may suggest the etiology of the lesion.[5] It can identify hydrolyzed cholesterol in craniopharyngiomas,[4] differentiate the spinal fluid in an empty sella from the fluid in cystic pituitary lesions,[1,7] and identify flowing blood in aneurysms.[3,4,8–10] MRI does not use ionizing radiation nor does it require the injection of intravenous contrast. Because MRI is becoming more readily available and because of the advantages listed, it is superceding CT as the imaging procedure of choice in the evaluation of the sellar region.

## IMAGING PROTOCOL

MR imaging of the sella and the perisellar region necessitates optimum patient positioning and examination parameters to optimize the resolution and contrast of the images. The patient is positioned on the gantry table with the head placed inside the 30-cm diameter head coil with the canthomeatal plane perpendicular to the gantry table and to the Z axis of the magnet. A spin-echo pulse sequence is utilized to obtain sagittal and coronal images through the sella.[11]

A T1-weighted (T1W) sequence is the preferred screening sequence, as it provides maximum contrast between the spinal fluid (CSF) of the suprasellar cistern and the pituitary gland and adjacent hypothalamic structures.[12] A T2-weighted (T2W) sequence does not give as sharp an interface between the CSF and the surrounding anatomy and is obtained to screen for abnormalities in signal intensity within the pituitary gland and in the perisellar region. The operator-determined variables of TR (time of repetition) and TE (time of echo), will determine the degree of T1 and T2 weighting.[8] The optimal TR and TE to maximize the degree of T1 and T2 weighting with an acceptable imaging time and signal-to-noise ratio (SNR) are dependent on magnet field strength and the device.[12,13] The latter is a reflection of the individual manufacturer's engineering and computer programming parameters. The optimal imaging parameters are therefore individualized to each MR device, and the parameters indicated in this chapter should be considered as guidelines. The basic principle is that the optimal T1W and T2W sequence for the particular MR imager should be used.

Our image data are acquired using a 512 × 256 matrix. The 512 axis is frequency encoded, whereas the 256 axis is phase encoded. This provides for a pixel size of 0.5 mm × 1 mm with the phase-encoded axis determining the imaging time, which is within an acceptable range. Good quality, thin section slices of 5-mm thickness or less can be obtained on modern MR imagers. Thin sections are necessary for sella evaluation to avoid volume averaging.

The images shown in this chapter were obtained on four different MR imaging systems. Three were superconducting systems manufactured by the Siemens Corporation. These include 0.5 tesla (T), 1.0 T, and 2.0 T magnets operating at 0.35 T, 0.5 T, and 0.5 T, respectively. The 0.35 T system was a prototype system and is no longer in operation. The fourth system was manufactured by Fonar Corporation and is a permanent magnet operating at 0.3 T at another institution. The imaging protocols utilized on the 0.35 T and the Fonar system are not presented here but are indicated in the legends of the appropriate figures.

The sella region is screened with seven multislice, 5-mm thick, sagittal T1W images obtained with a slice gap of 2 mm. The gap is to avoid cross excitation between slices, which would reduce the signal-to-noise ratio. This sagittal projection yields excellent detail as to pituitary size, the pituitary stalk, the suprasellar cistern, the optic chiasm, the tuber cinereum, the mamillary bodies, and the third ventricle (Fig. 10–1*A* and *B*). The images are reviewed, and if no abnormality is evident, the "microadenoma" sequence is used (see Table 10–1). This consists of seven multislice 3-mm T1W coronal images obtained with a 2-mm gap. The thin, 3-mm slice maximizes the resolution at the expense of a decreased SNR. The gap is interlaced with a second set of 3-mm T1W images. Hence there is a 0.5-mm overlap between adjacent images (Fig. 10–5*A–D*). This is followed by a dual-echo, T2W, 5-mm coronal sequence yielding seven contiguous images at each echo. The T2W images are obtained with a single acquisition to keep the image time within a reasonable time frame. Consequently, they tend to have a lower signal-to-noise ratio than the T1W images and 5-mm thick images are utilized in an attempt to counter this problem. The coronal images provide for maximum assessment of pituitary symmetry and cavernous sinus anatomy.[14]

The macroadenoma protocol (Table 10–2) is used when after review of the 5-mm thickness sagittal T1W images, the pituitary is noted to be enlarged or a perisellar mass is demonstrated. The problem here is not one of high resolution necessary for detection, as the lesion is already detected. The problem is to define the relationship of the lesion to surrounding anatomy and if possible to

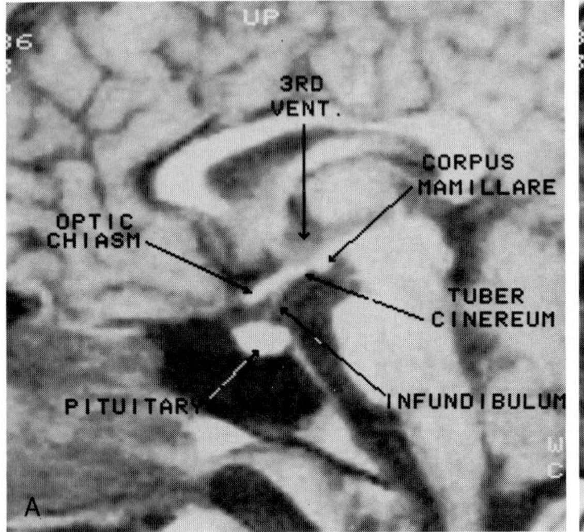


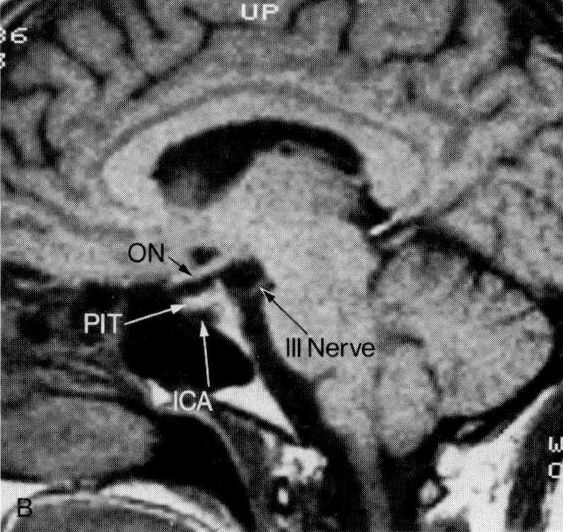


**Figure 10–1. Normal anatomy.** *A,* A 5-mm T1WI (TR 500/TE 16 msec) midline sagittal projection. The contrast between the CSF-filled suprasellar cistern and the adjacent pituitary and CNS structures is maximized with this sequence. Note that the signal intensity of the pituitary is the same as that of the pons. This is the first sequence obtained in all sella evaluations. If no masses are seen, further evaluation defaults to the microadenoma protocol. If a mass is demonstrated, the workup defaults to the macroadenoma-juxtasellar protocol. *B,* A 3-mm T1WI sagittal projection, 4 mm off the midline (TR 500/TE 35 msec). The projection is lateral to the midpoint of the optic chiasm, and the optic nerve (ON) is the horizontal structure in the suprasellar cistern above the pituitary (PIT). The tubular lucency in the posterior, inferior part of the pituitary, is averaging with the flow void of the posterior portion of the cavernous segment of the internal carotid artery (ICA). Note the third nerve extending toward the cavernous sinus.

**Table 10–1.** MICROADENOMA PROTOCOL

| Projection | Weighting | Thickness (mm) | Slice Gap (mm) | TR (sec) | TE (msec) | No. of Acquisitions | No. of Slices | Total Time (min) |
|---|---|---|---|---|---|---|---|---|
| Sagittal | T1W | 5 | 2 | 0.5 | 16 | 4 | 7 | 8.53 |
| Coronal* | T1W | 3 | 2 | 0.5 | 35 | 4 | 5 | 8.53 |
| Coronal | T2W | 5 | 2 | 2.0 | 35/80† | 1 | 7‡ | 8.53 |

*This is repeated to fill in the gaps so that there is a 0.5 mm overlap between slices.
†This is a dual-echo sequence.
‡There are 7 slices at each echo.

characterize its morphology and to predict the histology. Five-millimeter thickness images have a better SNR than 3-mm thickness images, and 5-mm is the slice thickness utilized. The original screening T1W sagittal images are followed by T1W coronal images and then by T2W sagittal (Fig. 10–2*A* and *B*) and coronal (see Fig. 10–6) images. These images are 5 mm thick with a 2-mm gap between the slices. The gap is interlaced if necessary. Axial T1W images (Table 10–2) could be obtained (see Fig. 10–7*A*–*C*) to better relate suprasellar pathology to structures in the suprasellar cistern.

After the images obtained with the protocols as outlined in Tables 10–1 and 10–2 are

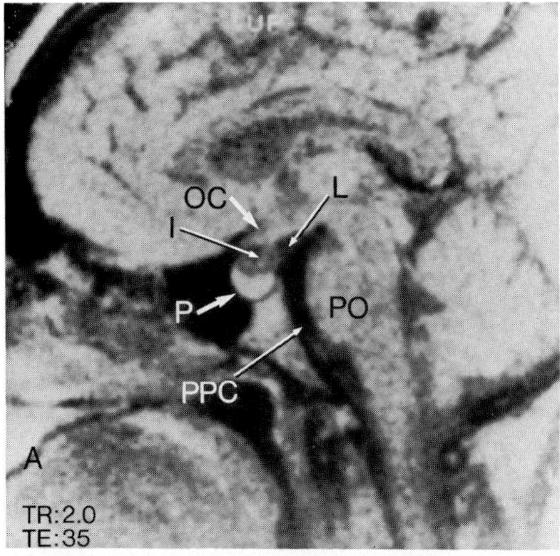


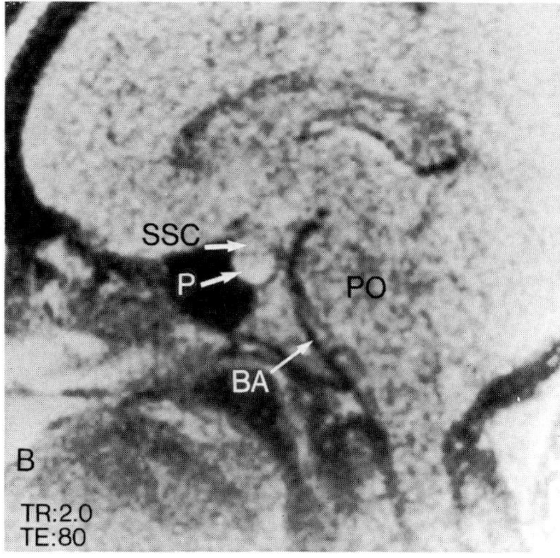


**Figure 10–2. Normal anatomy.** *A,* A 5-mm N(H)WI midline sagittal projection (TR 2000/TE 35 msec). The pituitary (P) has a slightly greater signal intensity than the pons (PO), indicating a longer T2 relaxation. The CSF above the pituitary has an intermediate signal equal to that of the third ventricle (not labeled). This intermediate signal decreases the contrast between the suprasellar CSF and infundibulum (I) and optic chiasm (OC). The CSF in the prepontine cistern (PPC) has hypointense signal, secondary to CSF pulsations from the basilar artery as well as the basilar artery flow void. It is speculated that the sharp interface (L) between the suprasellar and prepontine cistern is probably due to the damping of the CSF-transmitted basilar artery pulsations by the membrane of Liliequist. *B,* A 5-mm T2WI, midline sagittal projection (TR 2000/TE 80 msec). The signal from the pituitary (P) is now significantly brighter than the pons (PO), emphasizing the longer T2 relaxation. The CSF has now turned gray and is isointense with the structures of the suprasellar cistern (SSC). There is no contrast between the CSF and the optic chiasm and infundibulum; consequently, they are not visualized. The basilar artery (BA) flow void is well seen.

**Table 10–2.** MACROADENOMA OR JUXTASELLAR MASS PROTOCOL

| Projection | Weighting | Thickness (mm) | Slice Gap (mm) | TR (sec) | TE (msec) | No. of Acquisitions | No. of Slices | Total Time (min) |
|---|---|---|---|---|---|---|---|---|
| Sagittal | T1W | 5 | 2 | 0.5 | 16 | 4 | 7 | 8.53 |
| Sagittal | T2W | 5 | 2 | 2.0 | 35/80* | 1 | 7 | 8.53 |
| Coronal | T1W | 5 | 2 | 0.5 | 16 | 4 | 7 | 8.53 |
| Coronal | T2W | 5 | 2 | 2.0 | 35/80* | 1 | 7 | 8.53 |
| Axial† | T1W | 5 or 3 | 2 | 0.5 | 16 or 35 | 4 | 5 | 8.53 |

*Dual-echo sequence

†Not routinely obtained. Good visualization of the intracranial portion of the optic nerves. The thickness will be either 5 mm or 3 mm; our system is programmed to give a 35-msec echo as the shortest echo.

reviewed, further lesion characterization may be desired (Table 10–3). An inversion recovery (IR) sequence may sometimes be useful specifically to emphasize the T1 relaxation if a meningioma is suspected.[11] Our MR imager allows a maximum of four multislice IR images to be obtained with a full slice-thickness slice gap. A more heavily weighted T2 sequence may be desired, and this can be obtained with an eight-pulse image train to maximize the T2 contrast (Fig. 10–3*A–H*). A calculated T2 map image can be retrospectively calculated from these data (Fig. 10–4).

The above special sequences are obtained in the sagittal or coronal projection, whichever best shows the pathology as determined from the original images.

The basic imaging examination for sella evaluation, either for a microadenoma or a macroadenoma, takes approximately 34 to 35 minutes of sequencing time. If special sequences are obtained, the examination time will increase according to the time and number of additional sequences.

## NORMAL ANATOMY

**The Pituitary Gland.** The pituitary gland is located within the bony confines of the sella turcica and projects as an oblong or elliptical structure in both the sagittal (Fig. 10–1*A*) and coronal projections (Fig. 10–5*A* and *B*). It has the same signal intensity as hemispheric white matter on T1W coronal images and as the pons on T1W sagittal images.[15] The gland has a relatively homogeneous bright signal except for its posterior inferior portion. In the majority of sagittal images there is a crescent-shaped region of high signal intensity in this region that has been attributed either to fat in the pituitary fossa outside of the gland, to a paramagnetic substance, or to fat in the pituicytes of the posterior lobe.[16–18] A hypointense area just anterior to the posterior lobe is thought to be due to a chemical shift artifact.[19]

The signal intensity of the pituitary gland (with the possible exception of the posterior lobe)[18] relative to the pons and white matter of the cerebral hemispheres progressively

**Table 10–3.** SPECIAL SEQUENCES

**Inversion Recovery for Suspected Meningioma**

| *Projection* | *Weighting* | *Thickness (mm)* | *Slice Gap (mm)* | *TR (sec)* | *T1 (msec)* | *No. of Acquisitions* | *No. of Slices* | *Total Time (min)* |
|---|---|---|---|---|---|---|---|---|
| Sagittal or coronal | T1W | 5 | 5 | 2.1 | 400 | 1 | 4 | 8.96 |

**Spin-Echo Pulse Train for Lesion Characterization**

| *Projection* | *Weighting* | *Thickness (mm)* | *Slice Gap (mm)* | *TR (sec)* | *TE (msec)* | *No. of Acquisitions* | *No. of Slices* | *Total Time (min)* |
|---|---|---|---|---|---|---|---|---|
| Sagittal or coronal | T2W | 5 | — | 2.0 | 30/. . . /240* | 4 | 1† | 17.06 |

*This is an 8-echo pulse train at multiples of 30 msec.

†There is one slice at each echo.

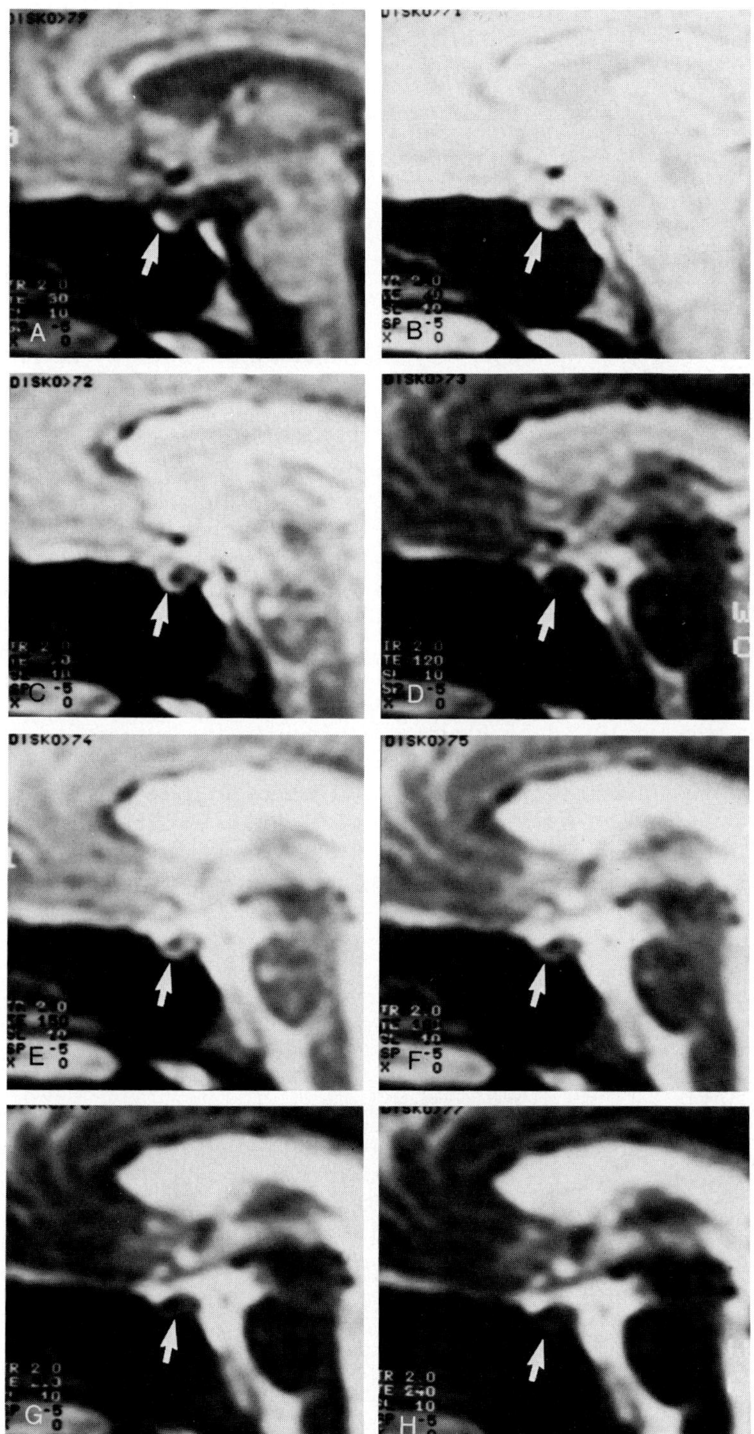


**Figure 10–3. A 10-mm, sagittal midline pulse train.** (TR 2100 msec with an 8-echo pulse train/TE 30, 60, 90, 120, 150, 180, 210, 240 msec is progressively demonstrated from *A* to *H*.) The pituitary (arrow) is brighter than the pons on the early echoes but becomes progressively isointense as the echo gets longer and the images become more T2W.

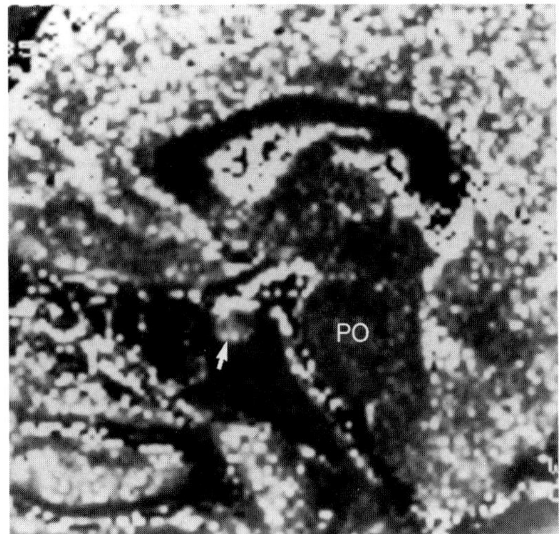


**Figure 10–4. Calculated sagittal T2 map image.** The eight images of the echo train (see Fig. 10–3) are used to calculate a pixel-by-pixel T2 map. The pituitary (arrow) is brighter than the pons (PO), indicating longer T2 values.

increases as the images become more T2W (Fig. 10–6; see also Fig. 10–2*A* and *B*). This increase is pronounced on the early echoes of the pulse train (see Fig. 10–3*A*–*C*). On delayed echoes (see Fig. 10–3*D*–*H*), the signal from the pituitary becomes increasingly isointense with the pons. The T2 calculated map image shows the pituitary to have a slightly greater signal than the adjacent pons (see Fig. 10–4), indicating a slightly prolonged T2 relaxation relative to white matter.

The size of the gland is variable. It has a maximum vertical height of 8 mm except in young or pregnant females in whom the height can be as high as 10 mm.[16, 20–22] The superior portion of the gland is either flat or upwardly concave. An upwardly convex configuration may be present in pregnant females or females of childbearing age.[21]

**The Infundibulum.** The pituitary infundibulum is sharply visualized on the T1W images and has a maximum thickness of 1.5 mm.[17] On sagittal images, it projects behind the optic chiasm and anterior to the tuber cinereum and corpus mamillare (see Fig. 10–1*A*). It is visualized from the gland to the hypothalamus.[23] On the coronal projection, it is a midline vertical structure, projecting upward from the gland (see Fig. 10–5C).

**The Optic Tracts.** The optic nerves extend posteriorly from the globe, enter the cranial cavity via the optic canal, form the optic chiasm in the suprasellar cistern, and become the optic tracts, which extend around the midbrain to synapse in the lateral geniculate bodies of the thalamus. MRI, with its

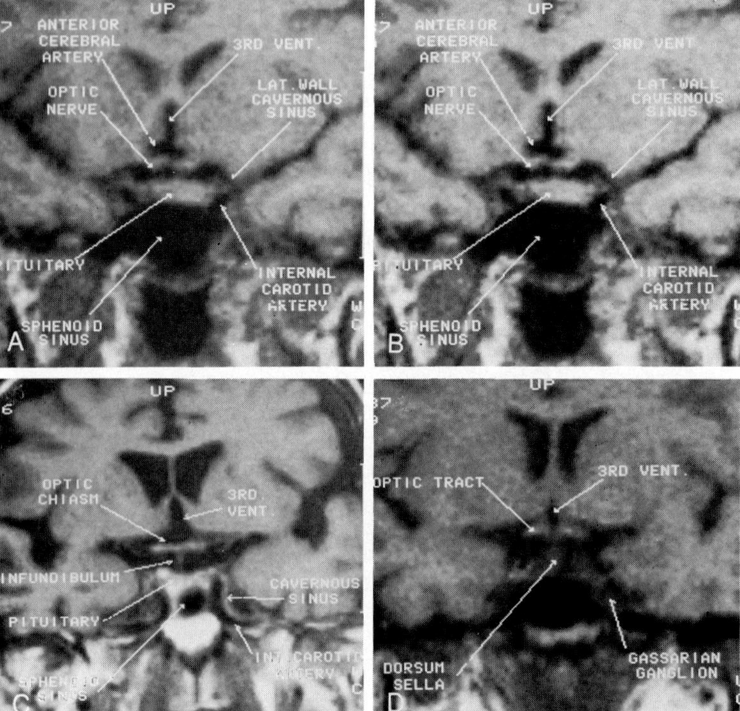


**Figure 10–5. A 3-mm coronal T1WI progressing from the anterior *(A)* to posterior *(D)*.** *A* through *D*, The coronal projection gives the maximum transverse and craniocaudad information. It is the best projection to evaluate the cavernous sinus. The intensity of the pituitary is similar to the white matter of the adjacent temporal lobe.

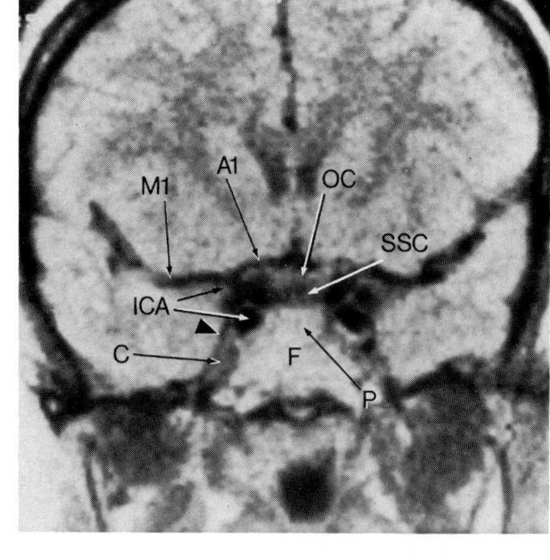


**Figure 10–6. A 5-mm coronal N(H)WI (TR 2000/TE 35 msec).** The cavernous sinus (C) is well demonstrated with this sequence. Note the hypointense signal from its fibrous dural wall (arrowhead).

The CSF in the suprasellar cistern (SSC) has an intermediate gray signal that outlines the flow void in the cerebral vasculature (A1 = horizontal segment of the anterior cerebral artery, M1 = horizontal segment of the middle cerebral artery, ICA = internal cerebral artery [upper arrow = supraclinoid segment; lower arrow = cavernous segment]). The optic chiasm (OC) is demonstrated, but there is a lack of contrast between it and the gray signal of the CSF in the suprasellar cistern. F = fatty marrow in the nonaerated bodies of the sphenoid and the clivus.

orthogonal projections and high contrast on T1W images, is ideal for visualizing the optic pathways. The midline sagittal projection and coronal images exhibit the optic chiasm, its size, and its relationship to the regional anatomy to maximum advantage.[24] The optic chiasm projects on the sagittal projection as a homogeneous signal anterior to the infundibulum. It has a tilted course from a slightly anterior, inferior position to a posterior, superior position as it is formed by the optic nerves anterolaterally (Fig. 10–7*A*; see also Fig. 10–1*B*), and it extends as the optic tract posterosuperiorly (Fig. 10–7*B* and *C*). On the coronal projection, it projects as a horizontal density above the pituitary, separated by the CSF in the suprasellar cistern (see Fig. 10–5*C*). On the more anterior coronal images, the optic nerves are lateral to the chiasm (see Fig. 10–5*A* and *B*), and on the more posterior images, the optic tracts extend laterally toward and around the midbrain (see Fig. 10–5*D*) on their way to the lateral geniculate bodies. Axial views are optimal for examining the optic nerves (especially the intracanalicular and intracranial segments) and the retrochiasmatic extension of the optic tracts around the midbrain (Fig. 10–7*A*–*C*).[24, 25] On all projections, the anatomy is best demonstrated on T1W images.[24, 25]

**The Cavernous Sinus.** The cavernous sinus is best visualized on coronal and axial projections (see Figs. 10–5*A*–*D* and 10–6); it forms the lateral boundary of the pituitary

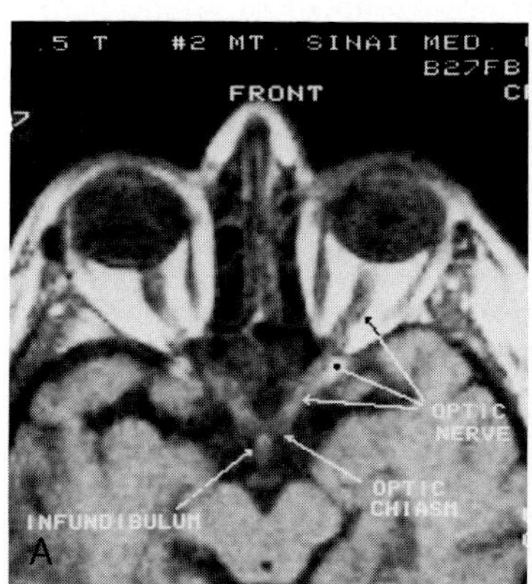


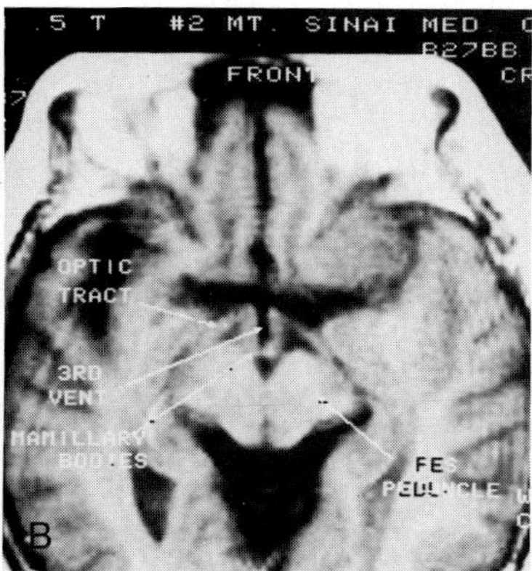


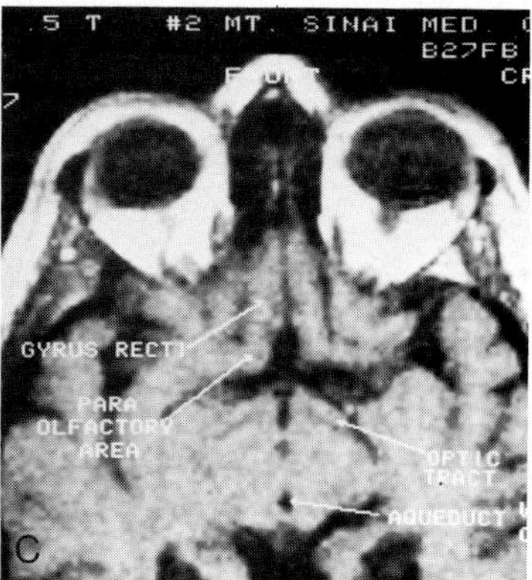


**Figure 10–7. The optic tracts as they extend around the midbrain on their way to the lateral geniculate bodies.** *A*, A 3-mm axial T1WI through the optic nerves and chiasm (TR 500/TE 35 msec). This projection demonstrates the intracranial portion of the optic nerves to best advantage. *B*, A 5-mm axial T1WI through the upper part of the suprasellar cistern (TR 500/TE 16 msec). The optic tract and mamillary bodies are well demonstrated. *C*, A 3-mm axial T1WI through the most craniad portion of the suprasellar cistern (TR 500/TE 35 msec).

fossa. Its medial wall is usually not visualized, whereas its thicker lateral wall is generally seen (see Fig. 10–5*B*). The cavernous segment of the internal carotid artery is consistently demonstrated as a flow void within the sinus. The third, fourth, ophthalmic ($V_1$), and maxillary ($V_2$) divisions of the fifth cranial nerve make up the neural components of the cavernous sinus and have been demonstrated with MR imaging.[14] In our experience, their visibility within the sinus has not been consistent. However, the cisternal portion of the third cranial nerve as it extends from the intracrural cistern is routinely visualized on parasagittal images (see Fig. 10–1*A*), and the gasserian ganglion within Meckel's cave as a rule is also demonstrated (see Fig. 10–5*D*). The venous portion of the sinus has a stippled appearance that has a signal intensity equal to or slightly less intense than the pituitary on a T1W image and less intense than the pituitary on T2W images (see Figs. 10–5 and 10–6). Even-echo rephasing, yielding a bright signal, may be present on the second echo of a dual-echo sequence, emphasizing the slow flow of blood within the sinus.[9] The lateral wall of the sinus is either straight or is slightly concave laterally.

**The Bony Sella.** The normal bony sella and the air-filled sphenoid sinus have a relative lack of mobile protons and project as a signal void. They are not imaged to advantage on MR. The fatty marrow of the nonaerated portion of the sella gives a bright signal on all imaging sequences (see Fig. 10–6). A pathologic process that replaces the fatty marrow, the air in the sphenoid sinus, or the bone of the sella and body of the sphenoid can be identified and generally will appear as a dark gray lesion on the T1W and will have a bright signal on the T2W images.

## PATHOLOGY

### Pituitary Adenoma

Pituitary adenomas arise from the anterior lobe of the pituitary.[26] They may be functioning or nonfunctioning. The functioning tumors cause recognized overproduction syndromes. The particular syndrome depends on the type of trophic hormone produced, as the following examples illustrate: growth hormone produces acromegaly (25% of functioning adenomas may be associated with eosinophilic tumors); adrenocorticotropic hormone (ACTH)-secreting adenoma produces adrenal hyperplasia, causing Cushing's syndrome (5% of functioning adenomas, usually associated with basophilic tumors); prolactin-secreting adenomas (35% of functioning tumors); thyroid-stimulating hormone (TSH)-secreting adenomas (< 1% of functioning tumors); or mixed secreters (adenomas producing two or more trophic hormones, 10% of functioning tumors).[26] A functioning adenoma causes symptoms because of its production of a trophic hormone, and the patient will more likely seek medical attention when the tumor is small. With modern laboratory techniques allowing for more precise endocrinologic data, the incidence of adenomas that do not secrete some type of active hormone is about 25% of pituitary adenomas.[26] The nonfunctioning adenomas (principally adenomas of the chromophobe type) silently grow large before becoming clinically evident. Symptoms are then due to the mass effect of the tumor on surrounding structures. More than half of these patients have pituitary insufficiency owing to pressure on the normal gland, or they have a bitemporal visual field defect as a result of encroachment on the optic chiasm.[27]

Pituitary adenomas can be subclassified as to size. A microadenoma is less than 10 mm in diameter, whereas macroadenomas are larger.[28] Functioning tumors, because they cause symptoms early, are most often microadenomas.[26] However, not all microadenomas secrete hormones. Incidental microadenomas have been found in 8.5% to 27% of autopsies of patients who had no pituitary symptoms during life.[29–31]

The MR imaging problem reflects the clinical presentation. The hormone-secreting tumors are microadenomas mostly confined to the gland. The nonsecreting lesions are macroadenomas with a good probability of extrapituitary extension into the juxtasellar territory.[26, 27]

#### *Microadenomas*

The tumor is usually confined to the gland and is identified as a well-circumscribed region of low signal intensity on T1W images at least 3 mm or more in diameter.[12, 32] This indicates a long T1 relaxation time relative to that of the pituitary and is direct evidence of the lesion (Figs. 10–8 to 10–11). The T2 relaxation time is variable, and on T2W images, the signal from the lesion may be greater than, equal to, or less than that of the gland, respectively reflecting a T2 relaxation time that is faster than, equal to, or longer than that of the pituitary (Figs. 10–8 and 10–9).[32] The variable MR appearance of microadenomas may be related to the secretory activity of the hormone-producing cells or to the effects of bromocriptine therapy.[32, 33] In the latter instance, about one third of the patients will show a change in the MR signal when compared with the pretreatment examination.[33] The T1 relaxation time may become shorter, and the T2 relaxation time may also change, becoming either shorter or longer (Fig. 10–11C).[33] The cause of the change is not well understood. Histologically, there is an increase in the number of secretory granules and lysosomes. The lesion may become reduced in size secondary to reduction in the cytoplasmic volume, loss of ribosomes, decreased num-

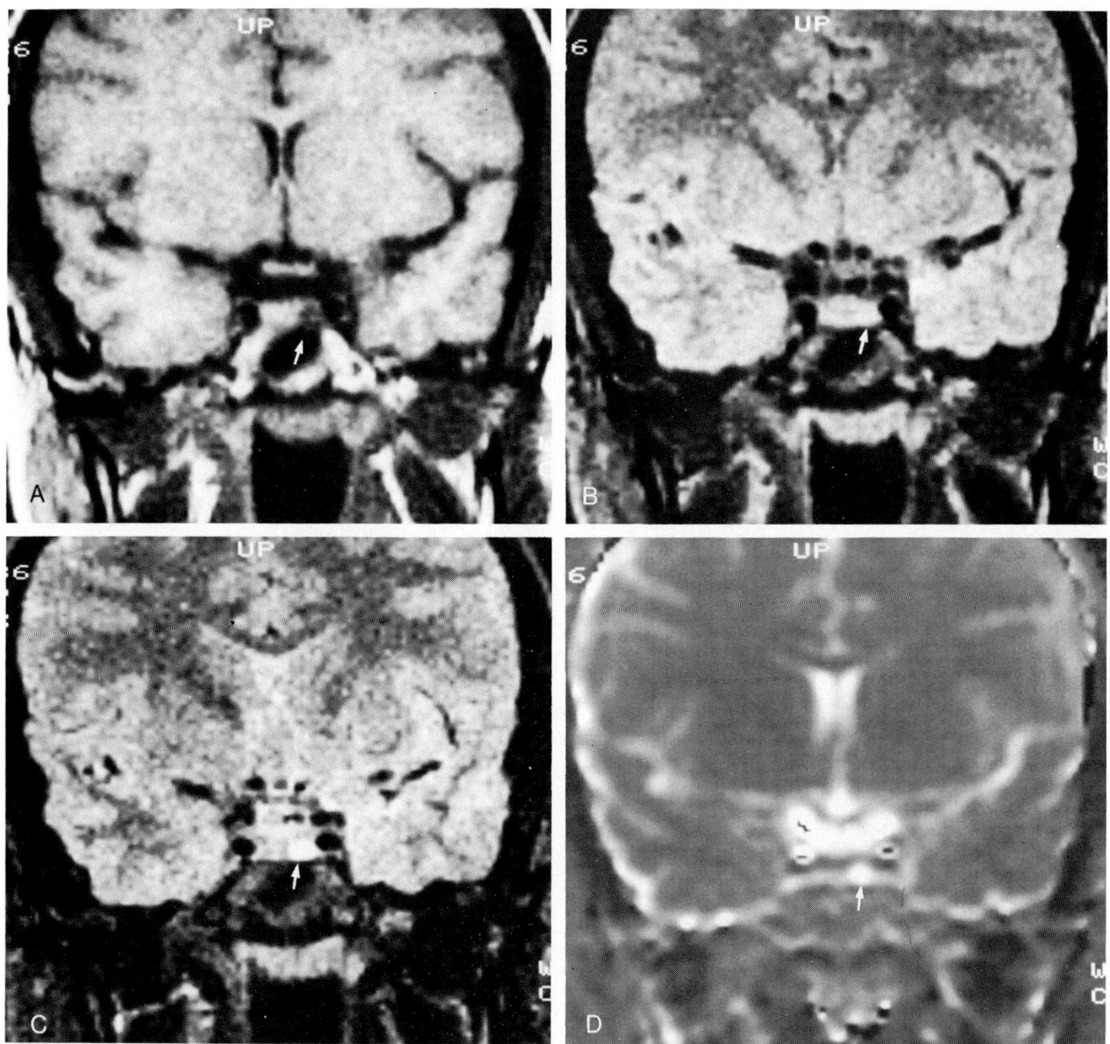


**Figure 10–8. Prolactinoma.** A 17-year-old woman with amenorrhea, galactorrhea, and a prolactin level of 240 ngm % (15 ngm % is maximum normal). *A,* A 3-mm coronal T1WI (TR 500/TE 35 msec) reveals an area of decreased signal intensity (arrow) in the left side of a gland that is normal in size and shape. *B,* A 3-mm coronal, multi-echo T2WI (TR 2500/TE 35 msec) demonstrating increased signal (arrow) in the lesion. *C,* A 3-mm coronal, second-echo T2WI (TR 2500/TE 80 msec) demonstrating the lesion (arrow) to be brighter than the adjacent pituitary. *D,* A T2 map image reveals the lesion (arrow) to have a T2 relaxation longer than the pituitary gland as evidenced by the bright signal.

*Illustration continued on following page*

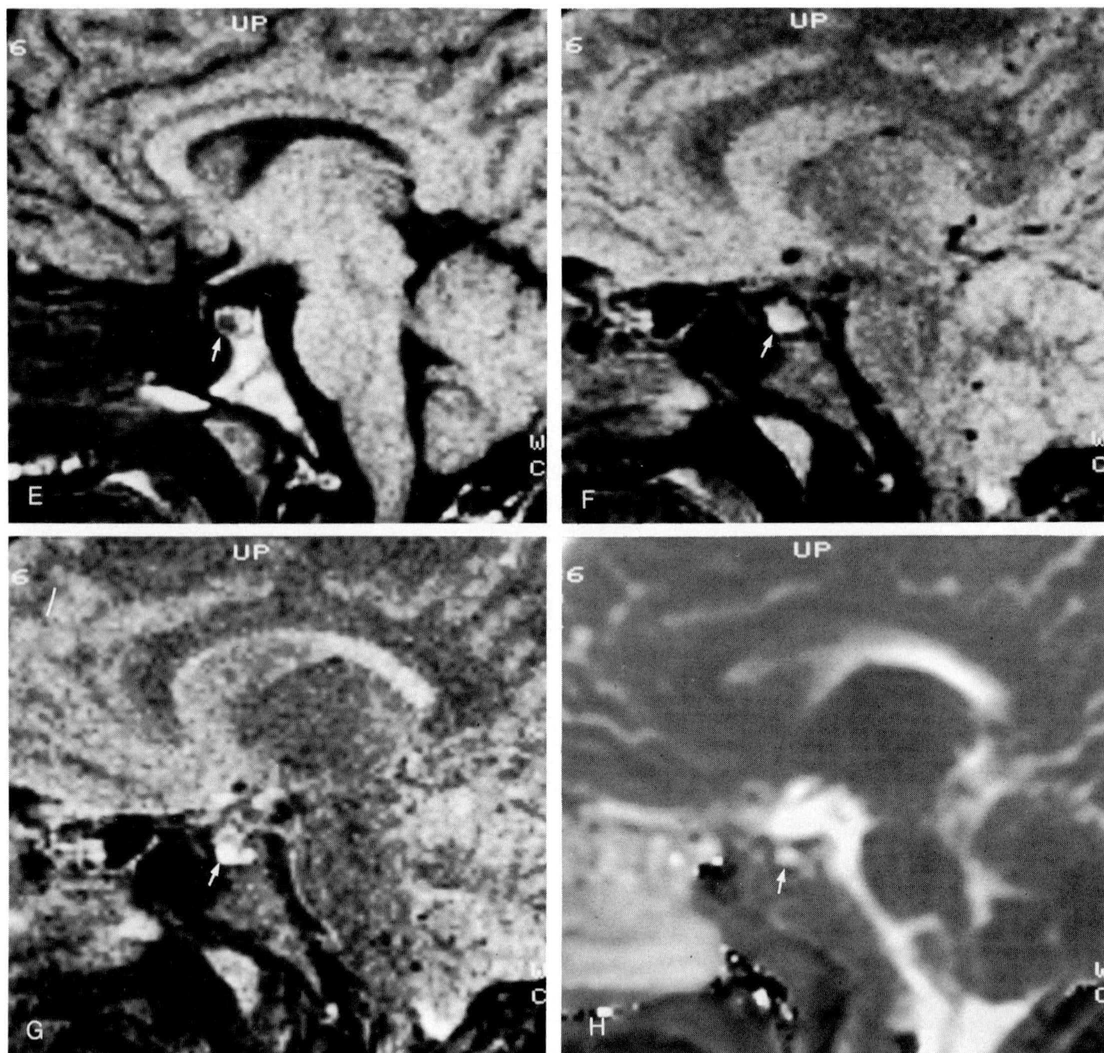


**Figure 10–8** *Continued E,* A 3-mm sagittal T1WI (TR 500/TE 35 msec) reveals an area of decreased signal intensity (arrow) in the anterior portion of the gland in the topography of the anterior lobe. *F,* A 3-mm sagittal T2WI (TR 2500/TE 35 msec) demonstrates increased signal (arrow) in the lesion. *G,* A 3-mm sagittal T2WI (TR 2500/TE 80 msec) demonstrating the lesion (arrow) to be brighter than the adjacent anterior lobe and slightly brighter than the hyperintense signal from the posterior lobe. *H,* A T2 map image reveals the lesion (arrow) to have a T2 relaxation longer than the anterior lobe, slightly longer than the posterior lobe, and not as long as the CSF, as indicated by the relative brightness of the signals from these various anatomic regions.

ber of Golgi complexes, and clumping of nuclear protein.[33] Hemorrhage or infarction is rare.

Although the only MRI abnormality allowing for identification of the tumor may be the abnormal signal intensity (Fig. 10–8), an associated mass effect occurs as the lesion gets larger. A midline shift of the infundibulum (Fig. 10–10), asymmetric, unilateral upward convexity of the superior gland surface (Figs. 10–10 and 10–11), and eccentric erosion of the sella floor (Figs. 10–9*B* and 10–11) are indirect evidence of a mass.[12] This indirect evidence may be the only indication of an abnormality, as the adenoma may be isointense with the rest of the gland. Reports have indicated a sensitivity of detection of 55% to 91%.[12, 32] This will probably continue to improve as higher resolution and thinner slices become available. We currently utilize MR as the primary imaging modality for microadenoma evaluation and are reserving CT for those instances in which MRI is normal.

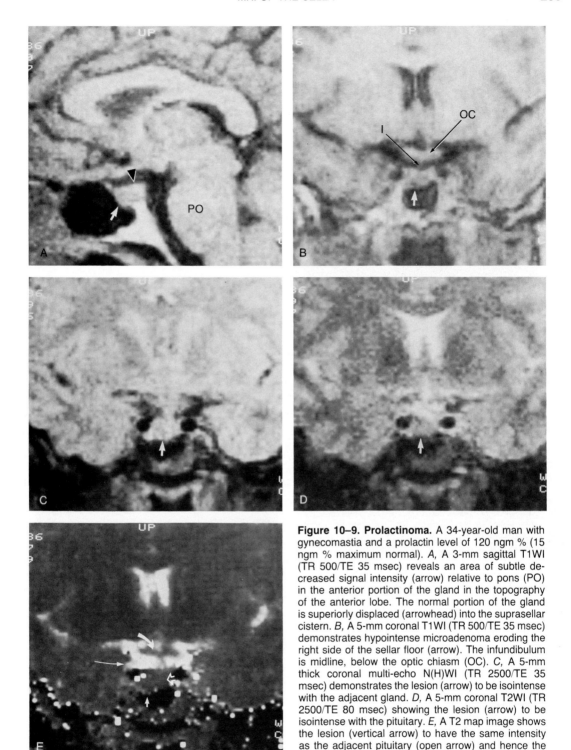

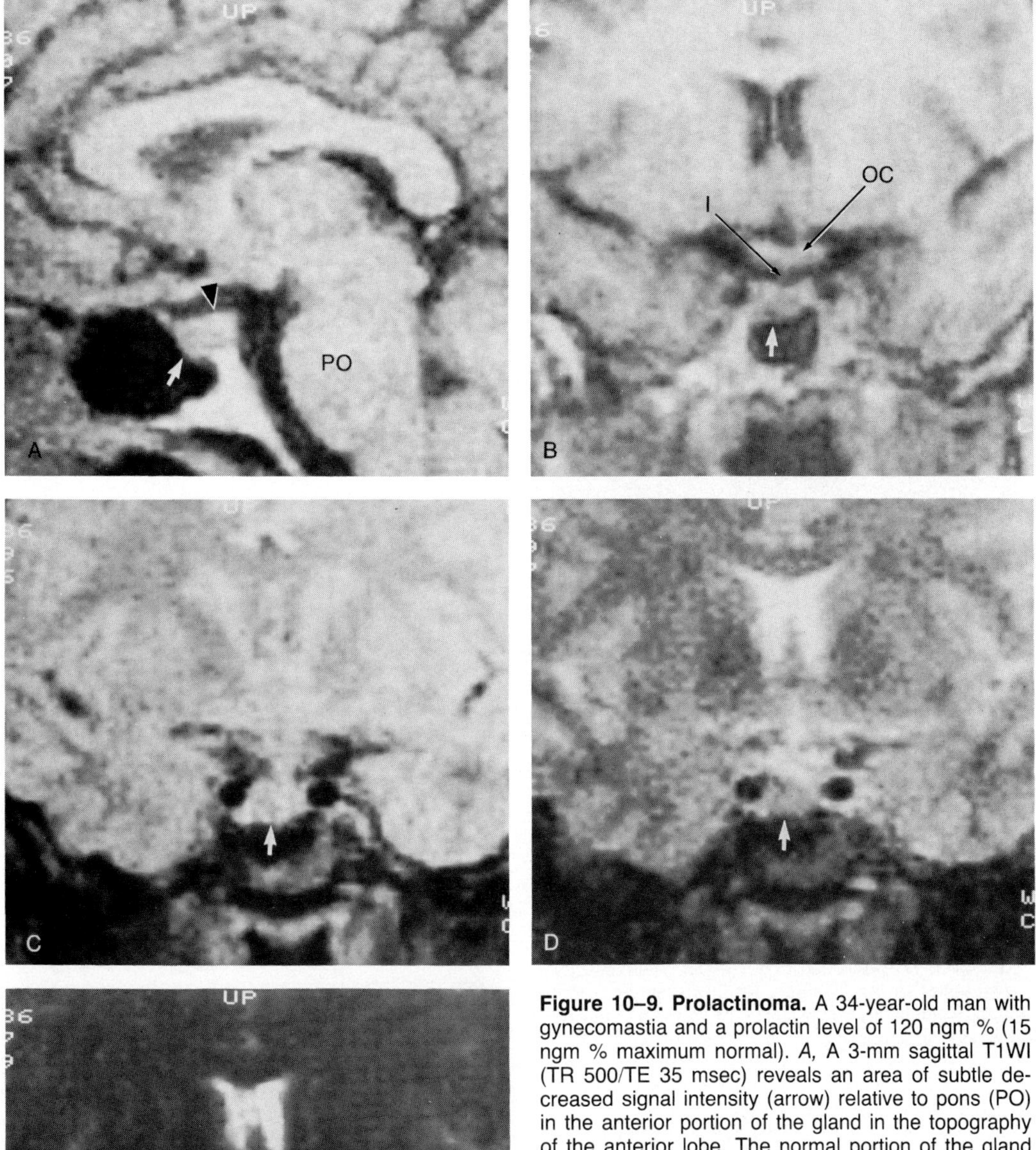


**Figure 10–9. Prolactinoma.** A 34-year-old man with gynecomastia and a prolactin level of 120 ngm % (15 ngm % maximum normal). *A,* A 3-mm sagittal T1WI (TR 500/TE 35 msec) reveals an area of subtle decreased signal intensity (arrow) relative to pons (PO) in the anterior portion of the gland in the topography of the anterior lobe. The normal portion of the gland is superiorly displaced (arrowhead) into the suprasellar cistern. *B,* A 5-mm coronal T1WI (TR 500/TE 35 msec) demonstrates hypointense microadenoma eroding the right side of the sellar floor (arrow). The infundibulum is midline, below the optic chiasm (OC). *C,* A 5-mm thick coronal multi-echo N(H)WI (TR 2500/TE 35 msec) demonstrates the lesion (arrow) to be isointense with the adjacent gland. *D,* A 5-mm coronal T2WI (TR 2500/TE 80 msec) showing the lesion (arrow) to be isointense with the pituitary. *E,* A T2 map image shows the lesion (vertical arrow) to have the same intensity as the adjacent pituitary (open arrow) and hence the same T2 relaxation. CSF in the suprasellar cistern (horizontal arrow) is bright owing to its long T2 relaxation, whereas the optic chiasm (curved arrow) is isointense with the lesion.

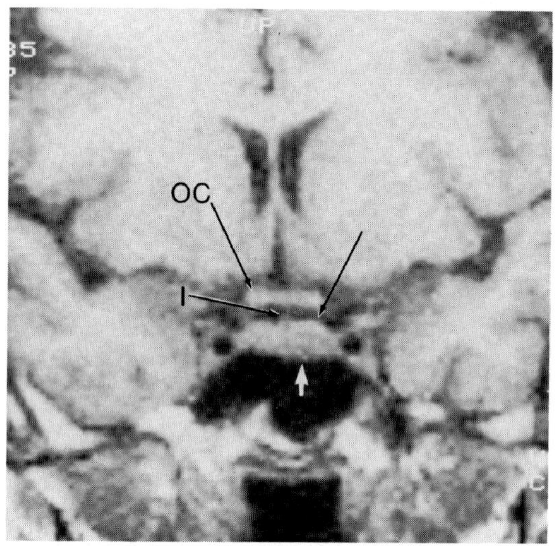


**Figure 10–10. Prolactinoma on bromocriptine therapy.** A 34-year-old woman with a history of high prolactin levels who had had bromocriptine therapy for the past two years and then had near-normal prolactin levels (0.35 T). A 5-mm coronal T1WI (TR 300/TE 30 msec) reveals a hypointense lesion (vertical arrow) replacing the left side of the gland, which bulges convexly upward (upper slanted arrow). The infundibulum (I) is displaced slightly to the left. The optic chiasm (OC) is outlined by the CSF in the suprasellar cistern.

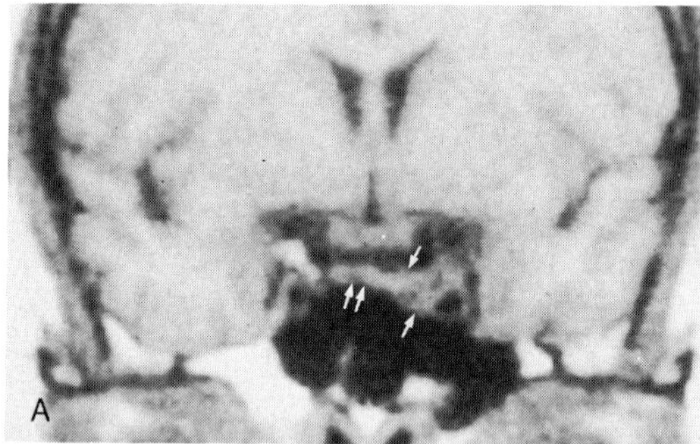


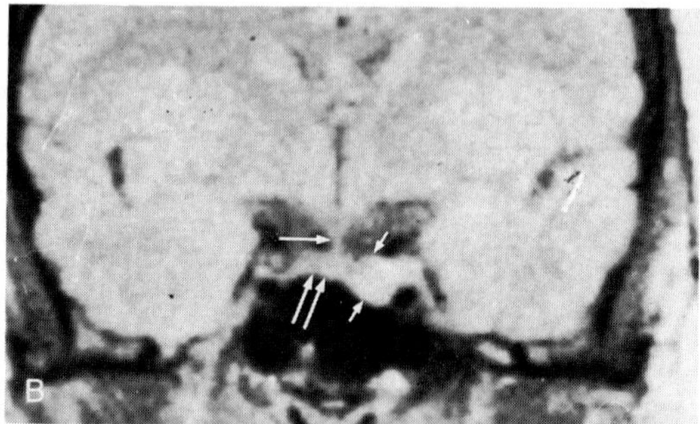


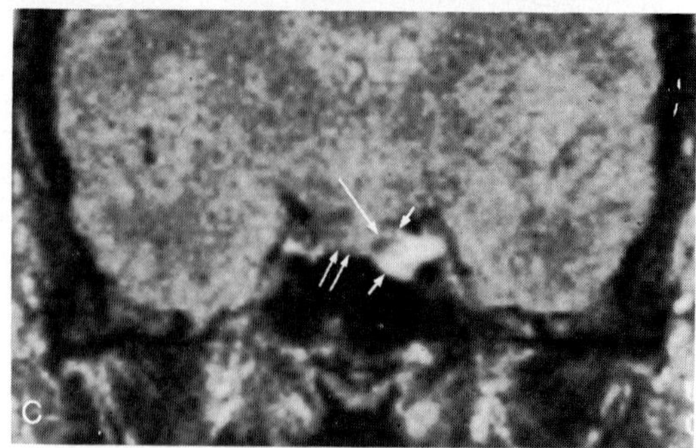


**Figure 10–11. Prolactinoma.** A 23-year-old woman experiencing amenorrhea and galactorrhea for the preceding nine months and who had been on bromocriptine therapy. The prolactin levels were still elevated (0.35 T). *A,* A 3-mm coronal T1WI (TR 300/TE 30 msec) reveals a hypointense lesion on the patient's left (lower single arrow) eroding the sella floor and producing an upward convexity to the gland (upper single arrow). The normal pituitary gland (double arrow) is identified. *B,* A 3-mm coronal first-echo N(H)WI (TR 1500/TE 35 msec) shows the lesion (lower single arrow) to have a slightly greater intensity than the adjacent pituitary (double arrows) producing a superior convexity (upper single arrow) to the left side of the gland (on reader's right). The infundibulum (horizontal arrow) is now demonstrated and is midline. *C,* A 3-mm coronal second-echo T2WI (TR 1500/TE 70 msec) reveals pronounced increased signal in the lesion, which indicates a prolonged T2 relaxation and the eccentric erosion of the sella floor (lower single arrow). Just below the upward convexity of the gland (upper single arrow) there is a crescent-shaped region of hypointensity (long arrow) indicating a faster T2 relaxation. The normal gland and sella floor (double arrows) are demonstrated to the right.

### Macroadenomas

These lesions are usually nonfunctioning and have become quite large, extending beyond the confines of the sella when first discovered. The lesions may be solid (Fig. 10–12), or they may be necrotic and may appear cystic (Fig. 10–13). Both the solid and the cystic lesions will have prolongation of the T1 relaxation times, leading to a signal intensity that is decreased when compared with adjacent white matter.[12, 15, 18] The T2W images differentiate the cystic from the solid lesion. The T2 relaxation of the solid adenoma is only slightly prolonged when compared with the adjacent pons (Fig. 10–12*J*), whereas it is markedly prolonged in the cystic lesion (Fig. 10–13*I*).

MRI, because of its orthogonal projections, can precisely demonstrate the relationship of the pituitary mass to the surrounding anatomy.[12] The inferior extension of the mass enlarging the sella into the sphenoid sinus or undermining the tuberculum or both is best visualized on the sagittal projection (Figs. 10–12*B* and 13*A*; see also Fig. 10–15*B*). It is difficult to determine if the tumor has remodeled the sella floor or has broken through into the sphenoid sinus. The absent signal of the cortical bone making up the sella floor blends with the absent signal of the air in the sinus. Symmetrical enlargement (e.g., ballooning) speaks for remodeling, whereas focal lobulation suggests local erosion and invasion of the sinus.[12, 18]

Lateral extension of the tumor brings it into contact with the thin medial wall of the cavernous sinus. This wall is usually not visualized, and it cannot therefore be determined if the adenoma is displacing the wall laterally via contiguity or is invading it.[12, 34] The cavernous segment of the internal carotid artery projects as a flow void in the cavernous sinus. Its relationship to the lesion and the sella is shown to best advantage on the coronal projection, obviating the necessity for neuroangiography.[18] Lateral displacement of this segment of the carotid artery with a normal, speckled signal in the sinus and a normal, straight or slightly concave lateral sinus wall suggests collison and displacement (Fig. 10–14; see also Fig. 10–12*C*) but not invasion. The findings of cavernous sinus invasion are loss of the normal speckled signal from the sinus, encasement of the internal carotid artery, T1 and T2 relaxation and consequent T1W and T2W signal intensity equal to that of the tumor, and a lateral convexity of the lateral cavernous sinus wall (Fig. 10–15).[12, 34] The signal intensity of the tumor within the cavernous sinus is greater than that of cavernous sinus blood.[14]

Superior extension of the tumor may occur through the diaphragm sella. Lateral notching of the tumor by the fibrous diaphragm sella may occur (Fig. 10–15*A*).[35] In the suprasellar cistern, the adenoma may come into contact with the optic chiasm (Fig. 10–12*B*). The chiasm may be superiorly displaced and may be draped over the tumor. Effacement of the third ventricle may also occur (Fig. 10–15*A* and *B*). The tumor may grow sufficiently large and may extend high enough to obstruct the foramen of Monro. It may grow anteriorly over the tuberculum and under the frontal lobes, or it may spill over the dorsum sella and impinge on the brain stem.[26]

The differential diagnosis of pituitary masses of all sizes includes colloid cysts (Rathke's cleft cyst) of the pars intermedia, metastatic disease (from breast and lung), and in the case of microadenomas, pituitary infarcts.[26, 27, 30, 36]

## Postsurgical Evaluation

The surgical treatment of pituitary adenomas can be divided into transcranial and transsphenoidal procedures.[26] The transcranial approach may be paramedian subfrontal (along the medial floor of the anterior fossa), pterional (along the sphenoid wing), or subtemporal (across the floor of the middle fossa). In right-handed patients, the approach is from the right side. The first two approaches are ideal in patients with a postfixed chiasm where the tumor can be removed anteriorly between the two optic nerves. In the paramedian subfrontal approach, the tuberculum sella may be drilled off to get better exposure. The tumor is removed, leaving adherent capsule behind, and the surgically emptied sella is packed with temporalis muscle to prevent retraction of the optic chiasm and nerves into the sella. The subtemporal approach is ideal for the prefixed chiasm, for extension of the mass behind the dorsum sella, or for primary suprasellar masses.

*Text continued on page 292*

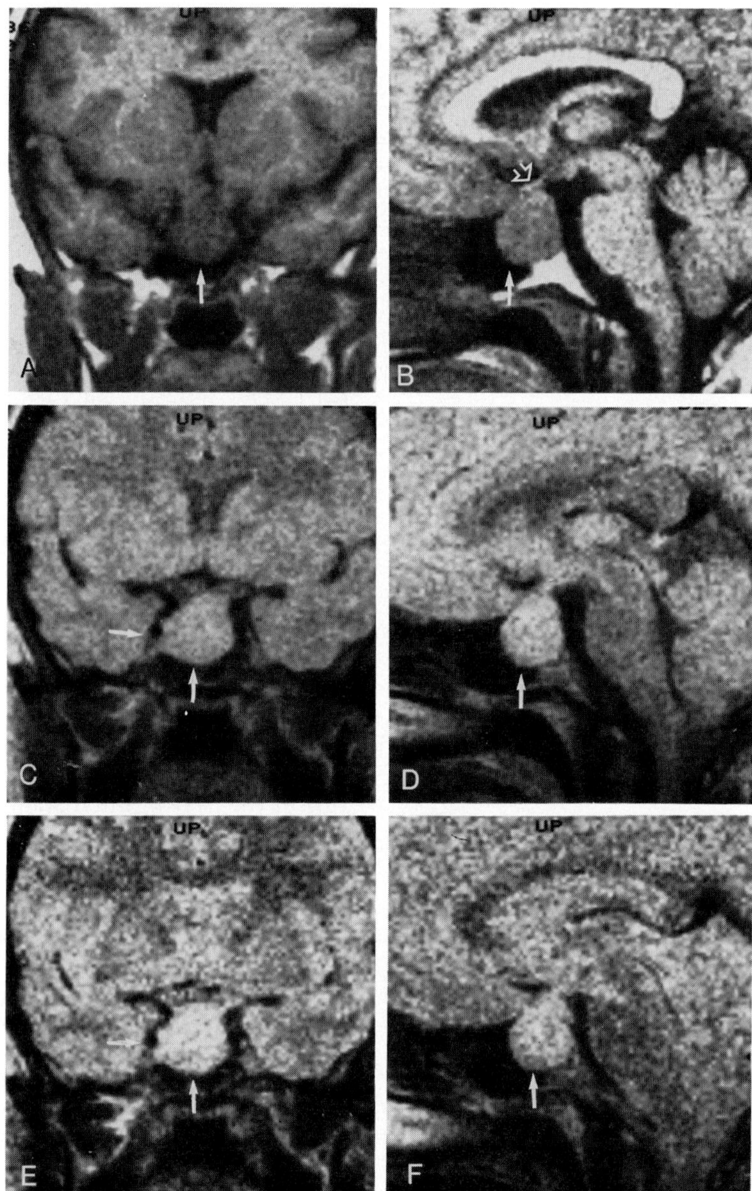


**Figure 10–12. Chromophobe adenoma (solid).** A middle-aged woman with headache and early bitemporal field defect (0.35 T). *A,* A 5-mm coronal T1WI (TR 500/TE 30 msec) demonstrating a solid pituitary mass (arrow) with an intensity less than that of white matter. *B,* A 5-mm sagittal T1WI. The adenoma has a signal intensity less than that of the pons (TR 500/TE 30 msec). It has remodeled the sella floor (vertical arrow) and eroded the dorsum. There is suprasellar extension and collision with the optic chiasm (open arrow). *C,* A 5-mm coronal first-echo N(H)WI (TR 1500/TE 35 msec) demonstrating a slightly increased signal intensity in the tumor (vertical arrow) relative to white matter. There is lateral displacement of the cavernous sinus on the patient's right (reader's left) as evidenced by the lateral displacement of the cavernous segment of the internal carotid artery (horizontal arrow). Note the normal speckled appearance of the cavernous sinus, which is less intense than the tumor.

*D,* A 5-mm sagittal first-echo N(H)WI (TR 1500/TE 35 msec). The signal in the adenoma (arrow) is brighter than the pons. *E,* A 5-mm coronal second-echo, T2WI (TR 1500/TE 70 msec). The tumor (arrow) is now much brighter than the cerebral white matter, indicating a prolonged T2 relaxation time. The flow void in the internal carotid (horizontal arrow) is now better contrasted against the bright signal of the tumor and is laterally displaced. The appearance of the venous blood in the cavernous sinus is still less intense than that of the tumor. *F,* A 5-mm sagittal second-echo, T2WI (TR 1500/TE 70 msec). The signal in the adenoma (arrow) has become even brighter relative to the pons.

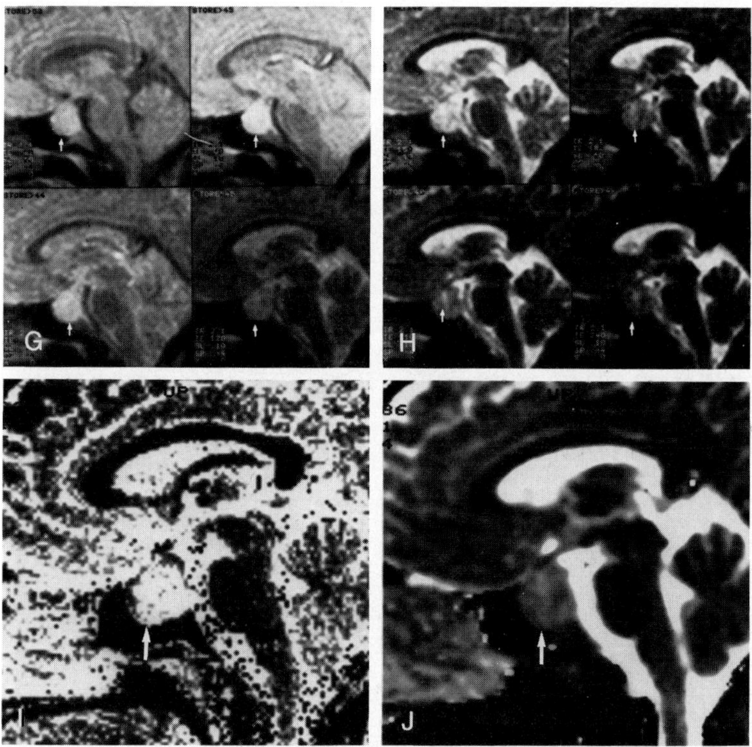

**Figure 10–12** *Continued G* and *H,* Eight 10-mm sagittal images (TR 2100/TE 30, 60, 90, 120, 150, 180, 210, and 240 msec) from an 8-image pulse train, characterizing the signal and reflecting the T2 relaxation of the adenoma. Note that the signal in the early echos is at first brighter than the pons but then decreases on the latter part of the pulse train (vertical arrows).

*I,* A T1 map image calculated from the sagittal T1WI (TR 500/TE 30 msec) and the first sagittal N(H)WI of the pulse train *G* (TR 2100/TE 30 msec). The tumor is much brighter than the pons, indicating that the T1 relaxation time is much greater than the pons. (Note: On a T1 map image the pixels are assigned calculated T1 values, and the gray scale reflects these values. Hence the longer the T1 relaxation time, the greater the pixel value, and the brighter the signal. A bright signal therefore means a long T1 relaxation.) *J,* A T2 map image calculated from the 8 images of the pulse train. The tumor is slightly brighter than the pons (vertical arrow), indicating a T2 relaxation time only slightly prolonged relative to the pons. The tumor is not as bright as CSF, which has the longest T2 relaxation time on this image.

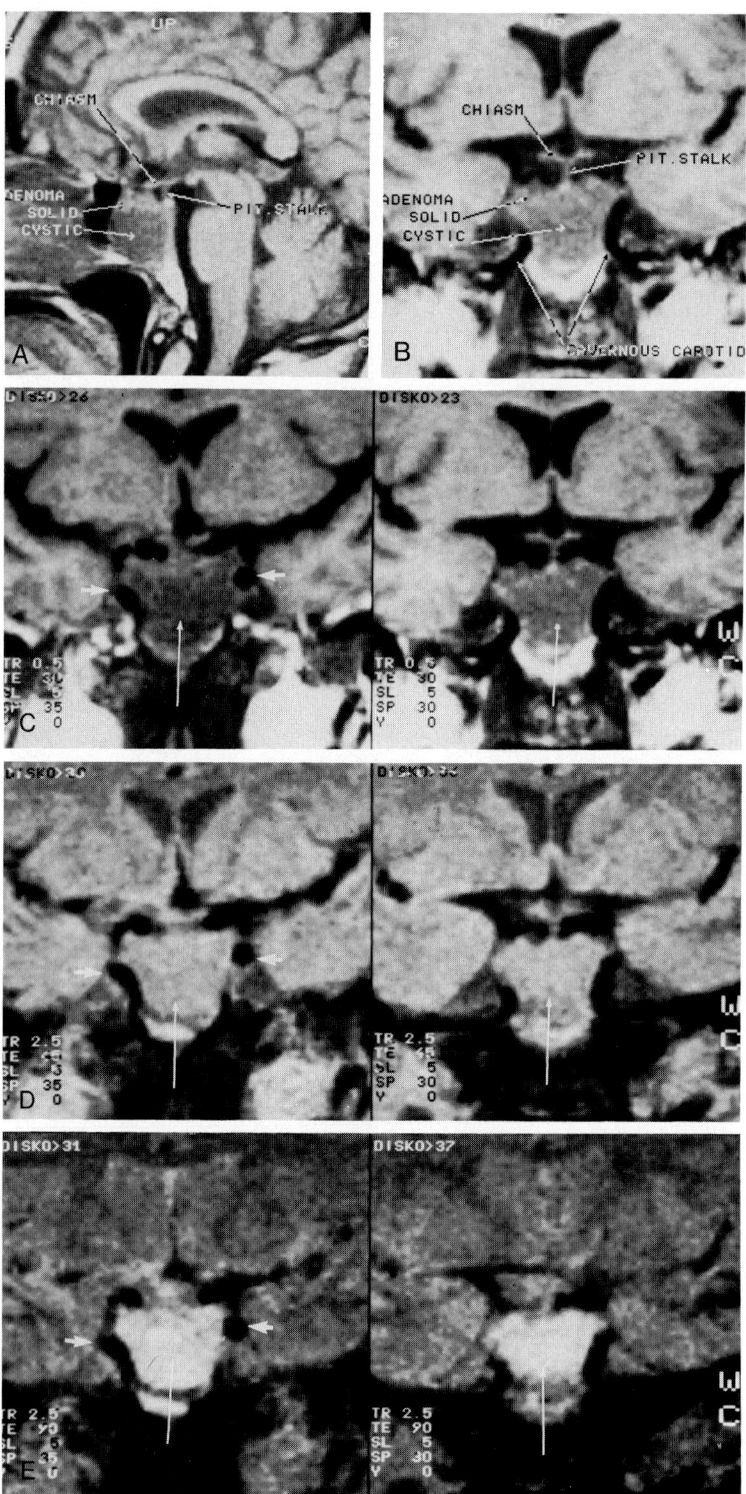


**Figure 10–13** *See legend on opposite page*

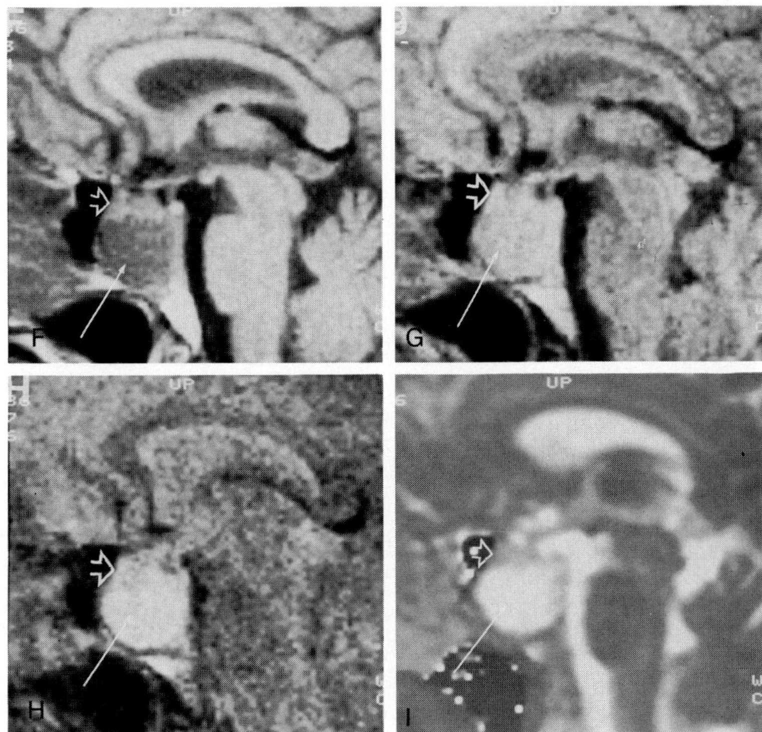


**Figure 10–13. Chromophobe adenoma (cystic).** A 57-year-old woman with headache and evidence of hypofunction of the pituitary. *A,* A 5-mm sagittal T1WI (TR 500/TE 30 msec) demonstrating the cystic component of the tumor within the ballooned sella. This component has a signal less intense than the adjacent pons. The solid component of the lesion and probably also some normal pituitary are superiorly displaced up to but not quite in contact with the optic chiasm. The infundibulum is posteriorly displaced. *B,* A 5-mm coronal T1WI (TR 500/TE 30 msec) demonstrating the decreased signal in the cystic component of the tumor relative to cerebral white matter. The infundibulum is midline below the optic chiasm. The posterior portion of the cavernous segment of the internal carotid arteries is in normal position.

*C,* A 5-mm coronal T1WI (TR 500/TE 30 msec). The image to the reader's left is at the level of the anterior portion of the carotid siphon whereas the image on the right is at the level of the posterior portion. The signal from the lesion (vertical arrows) is decreased relative to white matter. The anterior portion of each carotid siphon is laterally displaced (horizontal arrows) indicating lateral displacement of the cavernous sinuses. The venous blood within the sinus has a normal signal that is slightly greater than the tumor on this imaging sequence. In the anterior image there is focal upward extension of the tumor toward the right side of the optic chiasm (not labeled). The infundibulum (not labeled) is midline on the more posterior image. *D,* A 5-mm coronal first-echo N(H)WI (TR 2500/TE 45 msec) at the same anatomic locations as those in image *C*. The signal from the lesion (vertical arrow) is now slightly brighter than cerebral white matter. The CSF is becoming slightly gray.

*E,* A 5-mm coronal second-echo T2WI (TR 2500/TE 90 msec) at the same anatomic locations as those in *C* and *D*. The lesion now has the brightest signal on the image (vertical arrow), brighter than the CSF. This brightness differentiates cystic from solid lesions. In the latter, the CSF still has a brighter signal. The flow void in the laterally displaced carotid siphons (horizontal arrows) is better contrasted by the relatively increased signal from the venous blood in the cavernous sinus. The signal from the sinus is still less intense than the tumor, indicating patency. *F,* A 5-mm sagittal T1WI (TR 500/TE 30 msec). The cystic intrasellar portion of the tumor (lower arrow) is hypointense relative to the pons. The solid superior portion (open arrow) is only slightly less intense than the pons. This indicates the diverse T1 relaxation times in the different tumor regions.

*G,* A 5-mm sagittal first-echo N(H)WI (TR 2500/TE 45 msec). The signal from the cystic component of the lesion (lower arrow) is now almost isointense with the solid portion (open arrow). Both areas are hyperintense relative to the pons. *H,* A 5-mm sagittal second-echo T2WI (TR 2500/TE 90 msec). The signal from the solid portion of the lesion (open arrow) has decreased, so that it is now less intense than the signal from the cystic component (solid arrow). The signal from the latter is brighter than the signal from the CSF, confirming the cystic nature of the lesion.

*I,* A T2 map image calculated from an 8-echo pulse train (not shown). The intrasellar portion of the adenoma (solid arrow) is as bright as spinal fluid, indicating relatively equal T2 relaxation times and confirming the cystic nature of the lesion. The solid portion of the tumor (open arrow) is not as bright as CSF and is slightly brighter than the pons (compare with the solid tumor in Fig. 10–12*J*), which indicates a T2 relaxation intermediate between the cyst and the pons.

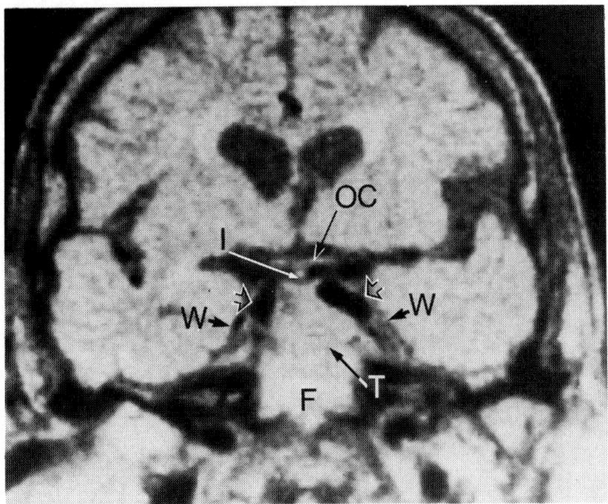


**Figure 10–14. A chromophobe adenoma with lateral displacement of the cavernous sinuses.** A 5-mm coronal first-echo T2WI (TR 1500/TE: 35 msec, 0.35 T). The signal intensity of the lesion (T) is slightly brighter than cerebral white matter. The cavernous segments of the internal carotid arteries (open arrows) are laterally displaced. The lateral wall of each cavernous sinus (W) has a normal straight-to-convex lateral configuration. The venous blood within the sinus has a normal speckled appearance and is less intense than the mass. (I = infundibulum; OC = optic chiasm; F = fat in the body of the sphenoid).

The transsphenoidal procedures may originate from the sublabial transseptal region, the transantral region, or the transethmoidal region. Regardless of the approach, an opening is made in the anterior wall of the sphenoid sinus and then through the sinus, and the sella is entered through its anterior wall below the tuberculum. A small tumor confined to the sella can easily be removed. A lesion with direct suprasellar extension can also be delivered through this opening. After tumor removal, the sella and sphenoid sinus are packed with Gelfoam, Surgicel, muscle, or fat and may accumulate various amounts of fluid.[26]

The MR appearance of the postsurgical pituitary depends upon the operative approach. A craniotomy defect is seen in the transcranial approaches, with evidence of postsurgical encephalomalacia of the gyrus rectus, the orbitofrontal gyri, or the temporal lobe, depending upon whether a paramedian subfrontal, a pterion, or a subtemporal technique was used. This defect appears as a region of long T1 and T2 relaxation on T1W and T2W images.[37] In the transsphenoidal approach, the resulting bony defect in the anterior wall of the sella is not usually demonstrated on the MR examination. Fat or muscle packing and fluid accumulations in the sphenoid sinus are well demonstrated. The fat, because of its rapid T1 relaxation, appears as a bright signal on T1W images, whereas the signal from muscle is intermediate because of its longer T1 relaxation time. These signals appear in the sphenoid sinus, the sella, or both, depending upon the surgical approach (Fig. 10–16). With time, fat eventually loses its bright signal.[18]

It is important to image the sella soon after surgery to establish a baseline for future follow-up. Any soft tissue outside the confines of the sella is either recurrent or residual tumor. The appearance of the intrasellar contents is variable, depending upon the surgical approach and the type of packing used at surgery. Tumor recurrence cannot be detected unless there is a postoperative baseline for comparison. Inasmuch as there should be postoperative retraction of sellar contents, any increase in size compared with a baseline study should be considered tumor recurrence.

## The Empty Sella

An empty sella is usually an incidental finding,[26, 38] and its recognition is important so that it can be differentiated from cystic pituitary lesions or suprasellar subarachnoid cysts. This distinction can be a vexing problem (Figs. 10–17 and 10–18), especially if CT is the primary imaging modality. There are two types of empty sella. The primary type is thought to be due to a large opening in the diaphragm sella and downward pulsation of arachnoid filled with CSF into the sella.[38–40] The pituitary gland is atrophic and is displaced posteriorly and inferiorly against the dorsum.[7, 38–41] The infundibulum crossing the CSF-filled sella and suprasellar cistern is always present (Fig. 10–17). This is an important differential point, because the infundibulum either is not demonstrated or is not in a normal position in patients with a cystic pituitary lesion (Fig. 10–18) or a subarachnoid cyst (Fig. 10–19).[18, 42] The fluid within the sella is contiguous with fluid of the suprasellar cistern, and on all imaging sequences, it has the same signal intensity as the CSF elsewhere.[5]

The empty sella is more frequently seen in women than in men, usually in the fourth or fifth decade, and may be associated with

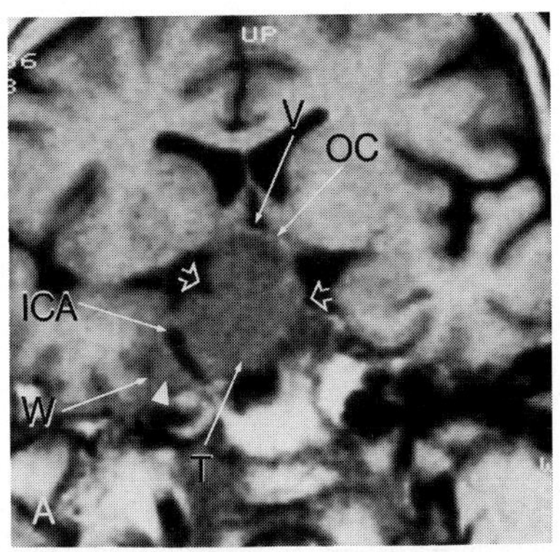


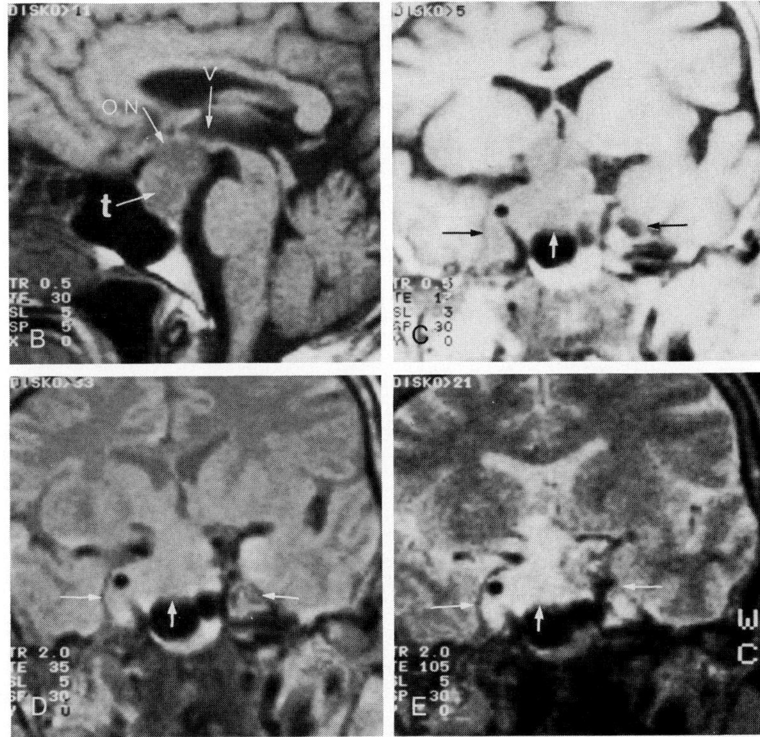


**Figure 10–15. Chromophobe adenoma with invasion of the right cavernous sinus.** *A,* A 5-mm coronal T1WI (TR 500/TE 17 msec). The signal intensity of the tumor (T) is the same as that of the right cavernous sinus (arrowhead). The lateral wall of the right (reader's left) cavernous sinus (W) is convex lateral as compared with the straight-to-concave lateral configuration of the patient's left cavernous sinus wall (not labeled). The cavernous segment of the internal carotid artery (ICA) is laterally displaced. The tumor extends upward and is notched laterally by the diaphragm sella (open arrows). The optic chiasm (OC) is superiorly displaced and is draped over the lesion. The inferior recess of the third ventricle (V) is effaced by the tumor and the superiorly displaced chiasm. *B,* A 5-mm sagittal T1WI (TR 500/TE 30 msec). The tumor (t) is slightly less intense than the pons and extends superiorly displacing the optic chiasm and optic nerve (ON) anteriorly and superiorly. The inferior portion of the third ventricle is effaced. *C,* A 5-mm coronal T1WI (TR 500/TE 17 msec) demonstrating the tumor (vertical arrow) to have the same signal intensity as the venous blood in the right cavernous sinus (horizontal arrow). *D,* A 5-mm coronal first-echo N(H)WI (TR 2000/TE 35 msec). The tumor (vertical arrow) is slightly brighter than the cerebral white matter but is equal in intensity to the venous blood within the right cavernous sinus (right horizontal arrow). The blood within the left cavernous sinus (left horizontal arrow) is less intense than the tumor and has a normal speckled appearance.

*E,* A 5-mm coronal second-echo T2WI (TR 2000/TE 80 msec). The tumor (vertical arrow) is almost as bright as CSF and much brighter than cerebral white matter. The signal in the right cavernous sinus (right horizontal arrow) has paralleled the tumor, indicating sinus invasion. The tumor is lateral to the laterally displaced siphon (flow void in the sinus, not labeled) thus encasing the artery. A normal left cavernous sinus (left horizontal arrow) is present.

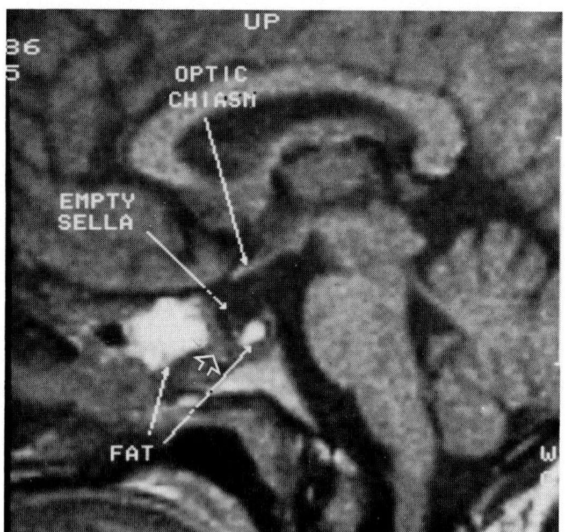


**Figure 10–16. Postsurgical sella one year after a transsphenoidal hypophysectomy for pituitary macroadenoma.** A 3-mm sagittal T1WI (TR 500/TE 35 msec) demonstrating the bright signal from fat in the pituitary fossa and the sphenoid sinus. The intermediate signal from muscle (open arrow) is also present in the sphenoid sinus. There is a postsurgical empty sella with the optic chiasm in normal position.

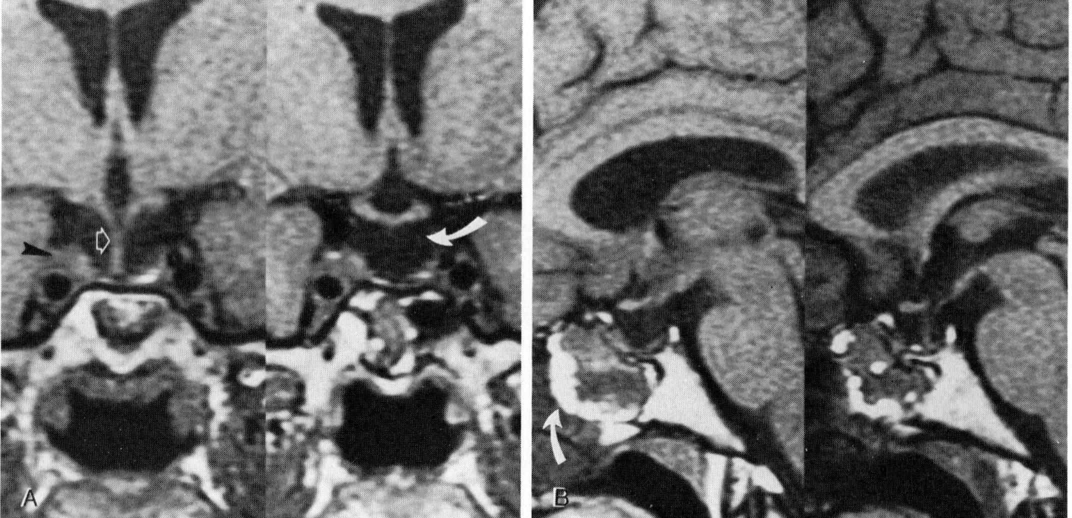


**Figure 10–17. Secondary empty sella.** A patient two years post transsphenoidal hypophysectomy for macroadenoma, currently asymptomatic (1.5 T). *A,* Coronal T1WI-multiformat. *B,* Sagittal T1WI-multiformat.

Coronal image shows CSF signal in the pituitary fossa (curved arrow) with the pituitary stalk (open arrow) in its midline position. Residual neoplasm is identified in the right cavernous sinus (arrowhead). Muscle and fat plug (postoperative) are identified on sagittal T1WI (curved arrow). The pituitary stalk is also seen in the sagittal plane. (Courtesy of S. J. Pomeranz, M.D., The Christ Hospital, Cincinnati, Ohio.)

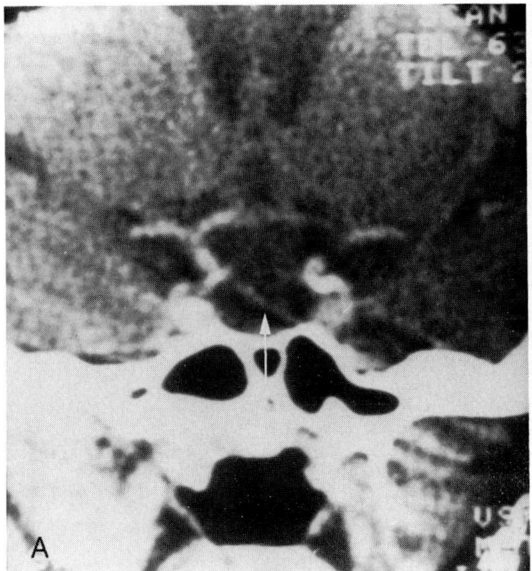


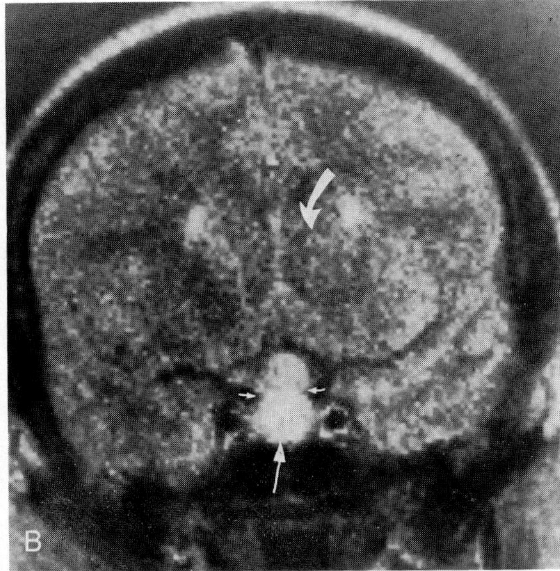


**Figure 10–18. Cystic pituitary adenoma mimicking an empty sella on the CT.** A 60-year-old woman with headache (0.35 T). *A,* Coronal CT with contrast demonstrates fluid hypodensity within the sella (vertical arrow). *B,* A 5-mm coronal second-echo T2WI (TR 1500/TE 80 msec) demonstrates increased signal within the well-marginated lesion (vertical arrow) that extends out of the sella into the suprasellar cistern. The lesion is notched (horizontal arrows) by the diaphragm sella and has a greater signal than the CSF within the ventricle (curved arrow), indicating that this is not an empty sella but the proteinaceous debris of a cystic pituitary adenoma. (Reprinted with permission from Wallace C, Sheldon JJ. MR imaging of the sella and juxtasellar regions. In MRI Update Series, Vol. 2, Book 9, Challenges 17 and 18.)

obesity and hypertension.[26, 38, 39, 41] In a minority of patients there may be mild evidence of endocrine, mainly pituitary, hypofunction.[38] However, most patients are asymptomatic, and the entity is discovered because of a slight enlargement of the sella seen on skull radiographs taken for trauma or on CT evaluation for headaches. The secondary empty sella is due to successful treatment of pituitary lesions (Fig. 10–16). The significance of the latter is that the optic chiasm may be retracted into the sella by adhesions and can result in recurrent visual disturbances.[26]

## Arachnoid Cyst

These lesions are commonly located in the sylvian fissure, the cisterna magna, or the suprasellar cistern. A developmental origin is speculated. The wall of the cyst is composed of a cleaved arachnoid membrane lined by ependymal or meningothelial cells. The cyst is filled with clear fluid,[43] it may be confined to the suprasellar cistern, may be within the sella, or may be both intra- and suprasellar. A cyst may act as a mass and may cause clinical symptoms associated with a compressive lesion.[44]

The appearance on MRI is that of a well-circumscribed lesion having the same signal intensity as CSF on all imaging sequences.[45] The wall is too thin to be detected. Unlike an empty sella, there may be displacement of surrounding structures, and the infundibulum either is not visualized or is displaced (Fig. 10–19).[44] The differential diagnostic features of suprasellar arachnoid cyst are discussed in greater detail in Chapter 8 of this text.

## Craniopharyngioma

Craniopharyngiomas account for 3% to 5% of all intracranial tumors.[43, 46] There is a biphasic incidence peaking in the first two decades and the fifth decade of life.[27, 36, 47, 48] The lesion most often is located in the suprasellar cistern (Fig. 10–20); less frequently, it is confined to the sella, and sometimes it occurs in both locations (Figs. 10–21 and 10–22).[43] Rare instances of a third ventricular location have been described.[43]

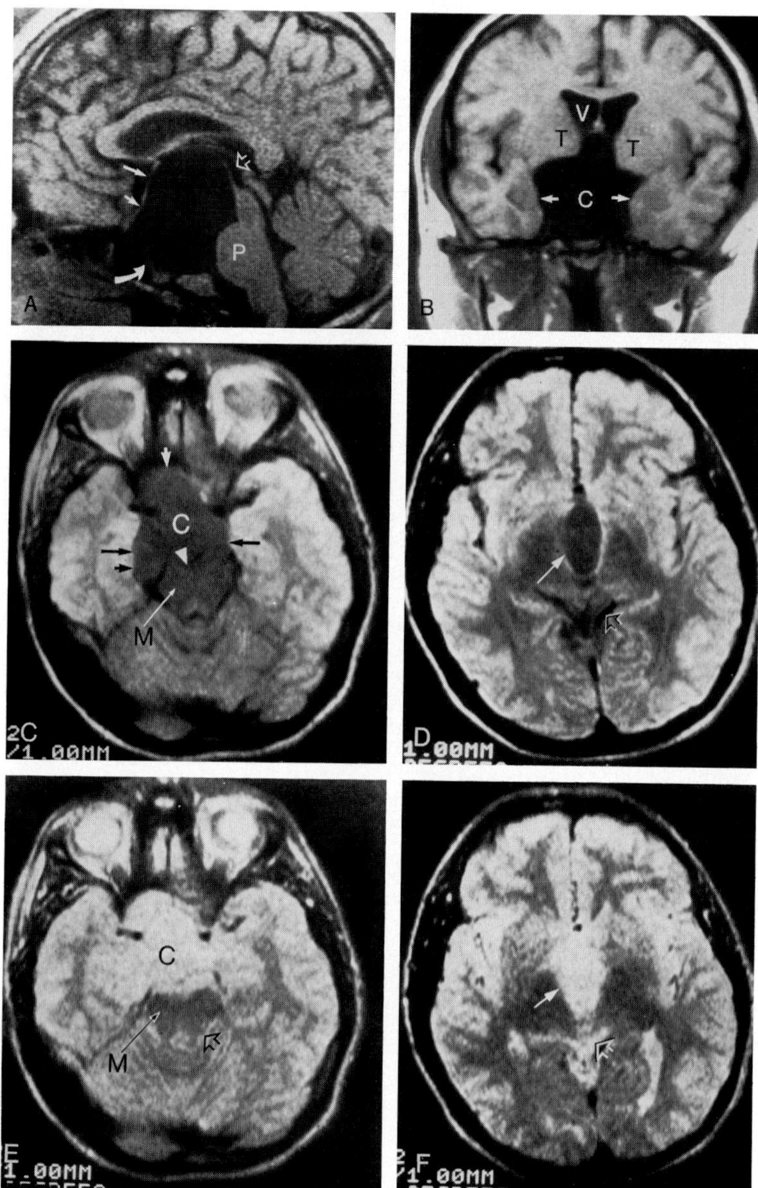


**Figure 10–19. Arachnoid cyst.** A 23-year-old man with clinical evidence of a sella mass (0.3 T). *A,* Sagittal T1WI (TR 722/TE 28 msec). A mass expands the sella and erodes the dorsum (curved arrow). It has markedly elevated the third ventricle (open arrow). The pituitary and the infundibulum have been displaced and cannot be identified. The intracranial portion of the optic nerve (lower anterior arrow) and the chiasm (upper anterior arrow) are elevated and anteriorly displaced. P = pons. *B,* Coronal T1WI (TR 499/TE 28 msec). The cyst (C) has spread the medial aspect of the temporal lobes laterally (arrows) and has insinuated itself between the thalami (T). The cyst has the same signal intensity as does the CSF in the ventricle (V). *C,* Axial first-echo N(H)WI (TR 2039/TE 28 msec). The cyst (C) is in the suprasellar cistern and has extended into the intracrural cistern (arrowhead) anterior to the midbrain (M). It has extended to the right around the midbrain (posterior horizontal arrow) and anteriorly over the tuberculum and roof of the right optic canal (anterior white arrow). It has spread the medial aspect of the temporal lobes (horizontal arrows).

*D,* Axial first-echo N(H)WI (TR 2039/TE 28 msec). The cyst (solid arrow) has insinuated between the thalami and has the same signal intensity as the CSF in the quadrigeminal cistern (open arrow). *E,* Axial second-echo T2WI (TR 2039/TE 84 msec). The cyst (C) anterior to the midbrain (M) is almost isointense with gray matter and has the same signal as CSF in the quadrigeminal cistern (open arrow). *F,* Axial second-echo T2WI (TR 2039/TE 84 msec). The cyst (solid arrow) is isointense with the CSF in the quadrigeminal cistern (open arrow). (Courtesy of Dr. Martin Stern, Radiologist, Department of Radiology, Holmes Regional Medical Center, Melbourne, Fla.)

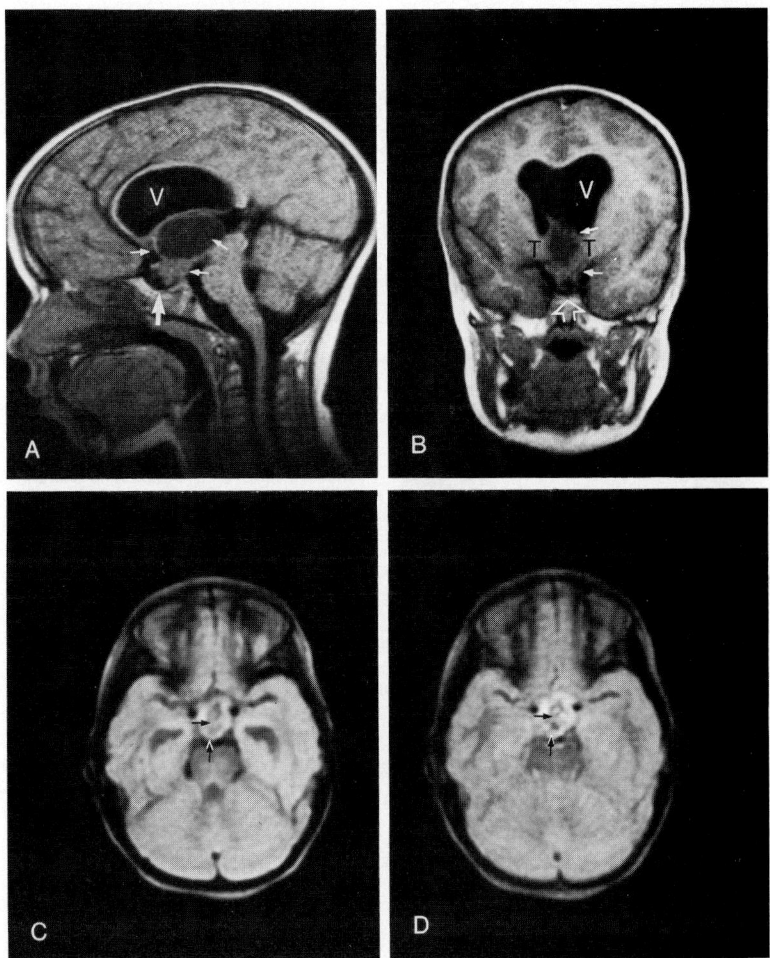


**Figure 10–20. Craniopharyngioma with solid and fluid-filled cystic compartment.** A 10-year-old girl with headache and bitemporal visual field defect (0.3 T). *A,* A 2-mm sagittal T1WI (TR 499/TE 14 msec). The sella is eroded (vertical arrow). The suprasellar mass has a solid (lower horizontal arrow) and a cystic (upper horizontal arrow) component. The solid component is slightly hypointense relative to the pons, whereas the cystic component is slightly hyperintense relative to CSF in the dilated lateral ventricle (V). The optic chiasm (anterior horizontal arrow) is anteriorly displaced. *B,* A 2-mm coronal T1WI (TR 499/TE 14 msec). The solid component of the lesion (lower horizontal arrow) is above the eroded sellar floor (open arrow). The cystic component is between the thalami (T) obstructing the foramen of Monro and dilating the lateral ventricles (V). *C,* A 2-mm axial first-echo N(H)WI (TR 2039/TE 42 msec). The thick wall of the cystic component of the lesion (vertical arrow) is hyperintense and more apparent. The signal from its fluid-detritus center (horizontal arrow) is not isointense with CSF. *D,* A 2-mm axial second-echo T2WI (TR 2039/TE 84 msec). The signal from the cyst wall (vertical arrow) with fluid and detritus contents (horizontal arrow) is more hyperintense, indicating the prolonged T2 relaxation time. (Courtesy of Dr. Nolan Altman, Neuroradiologist, Department of Radiology, Miami Children's Hospital, Coral Gables, Fla.)

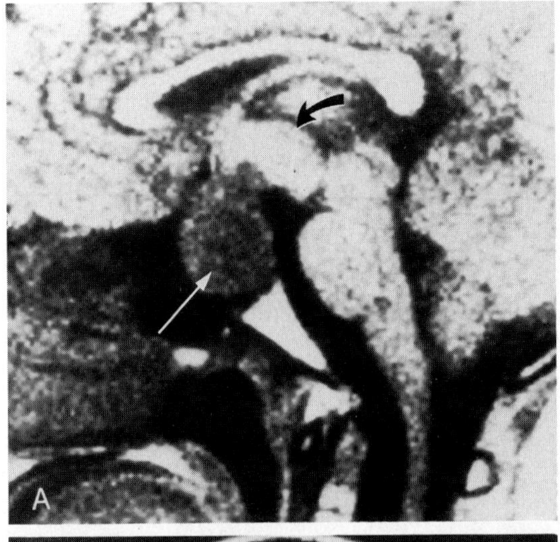


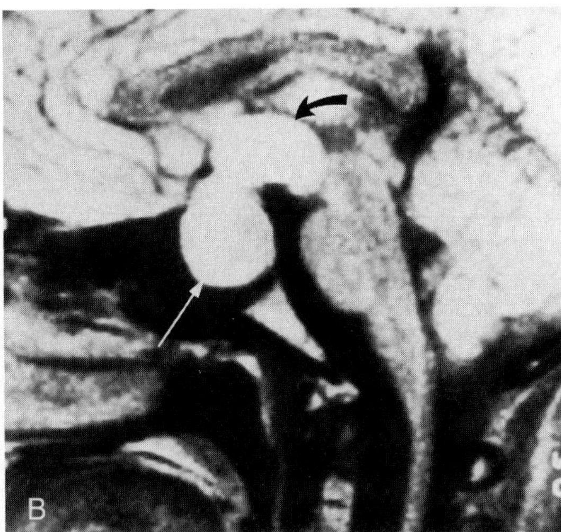


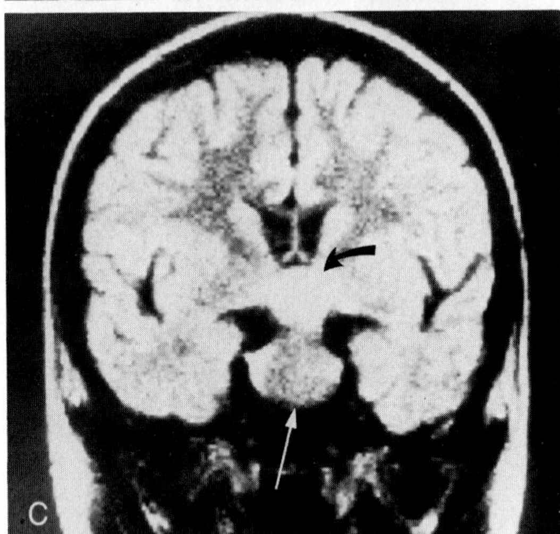


**Figure 10–21. Craniopharyngioma with fluid and fatty component.** A middle-aged woman with headache and bitemporal visual field defect (0.35 T). *A,* A 5-mm sagittal T1WI (TR 300/TE 30 msec). The hypointense signal relative to the pons from the fluid-filled portion of the lesion is within the eroded sella (lower arrow). The cystic mass has extended upward toward the foramen of Monro and has a bright signal indicating fat (hydrolyzed cholesterol; curved arrow). *B,* A 5-mm sagittal second-echo T2WI (TR 1500/TE 70 msec). The signal from the fluid-detritus portion of the cyst has become brighter, so that it is almost isointense with the bright signal from the fat compartment (curved arrow).

*C,* A 5-mm coronal first-echo N(H)WI (TR 1500/TE 35 msec). The signal from the fluid-detritus portion of the cyst (lower arrow) is brighter than on the T1W image but has not yet become as bright as the fatty compartment (curved arrow). The varying signal intensities with the different imaging sequences allow for discrimination of the lesion's different compartments. The bright signal on the T2W (brighter than spinal fluid) indicates that the lesion is not solid but cystic.

It has been speculated that the tumor arises from remnants of Rathke's pouch.[43, 46] Grossly, the lesion may be solid, cystic, or mixed, with both solid and cystic components. The cysts contain an oily straw- to brown-colored fluid with cholesterol crystals.[43, 46] Histologically, columnar and squamous epithelial cells, cholesterol crystals, keratin, fluid, necrotic debris, and areas of calcification are found.[43] The calcifications can be detected on skull radiographs in 81% of children and 40% of adults.[49] In 85% of the tumors, calcification is demonstrated on CT (Figs. 10–22 and 10–23).[46] The tumor produces symptoms by causing pressure on surrounding structures, especially the pituitary and the optic chiasm. It may extend superiorly and obstruct the foramen of Monro (Fig. 10–20), causing symptoms of increased intracranial pressure.[36]

The MRI appearance is variable and depends upon the gross and histologic components of the neoplasm. Fluid has long T1 and T2 relaxation times, and a decreased signal on T1W images (T1WI) and an increased signal on T2WI (Fig. 10–20). When hydrolyzed, cholesterol has a rapid T1 relaxation time and appears as a bright signal on T1WI.[5, 45] The extent of signal hyperintensity may vary greatly in all tumors derived from Rathke's remnants (compare Figs. 10–21 through 10–24). If the cyst contains fluid, there may be separation and layering between the cholesterol and the fluid (Fig. 10–21*A*). Keratin, fibrous tissue, and calcium have few mobile protons, and these areas

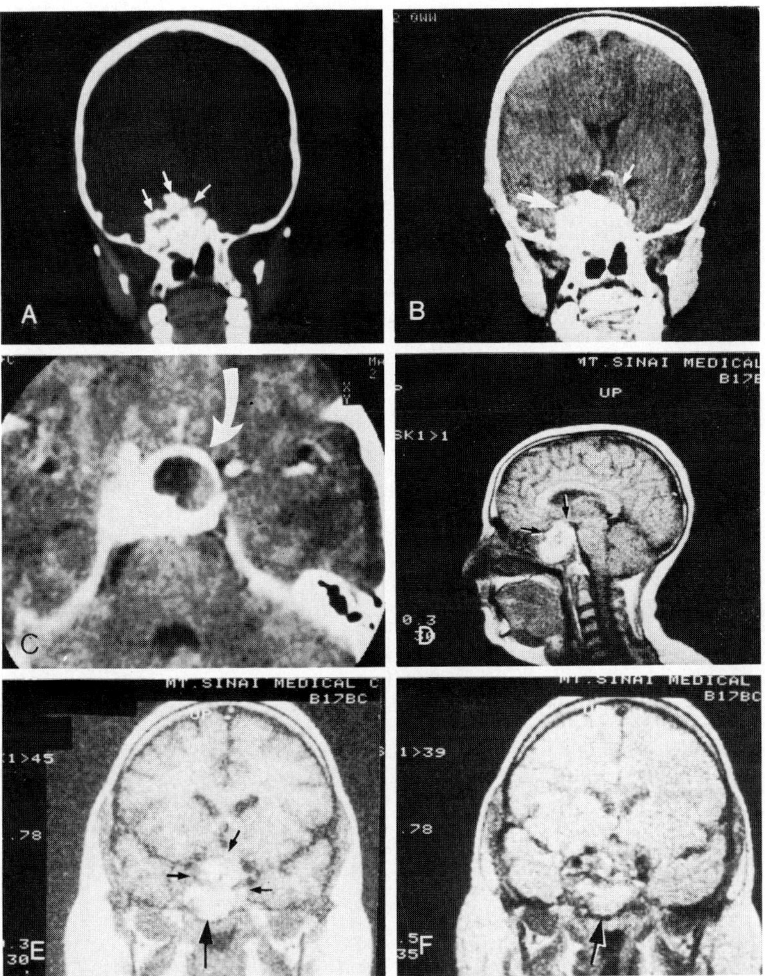


**Figure 10–22. Craniopharyngioma (calcified).** A 34-year-old man with a temporal field defect in his right eye (0.35 T). *A,* Coronal CT shows a calcified sellar mass (arrows). *B,* Coronal contrast CT reveals rim enhancement (upper arrow) of the cystic portion of the lesion above the calcification (large horizontal arrow). *C,* Axial contrast CT shows the ring-enhancing cyst (curved arrow) in the suprasellar cistern. *D,* Sagittal T1WI (TR 300/TE 30 msec). The lesion (horizontal arrow) extends out of the sella into the suprasellar cistern, elevating the optic chiasm (upper vertical arrow). The signal is bright, indicating a fast T1 relaxation secondary to hydrolyzed cholesterol and fatty components. The signal from the soft tissue components of the lesion overwhelms the signal dropout from the calcium except in the center, which appears darker.

*E,* Coronal T1WI (TR 300/TE 30 msec). The lesion (lower vertical arrow) has a bright signal and extends out of the sella to elevate the optic chiasm (upper vertical arrow). It is notched on each side by the diaphragm sella (horizontal arrows). *F,* Coronal first-echo N(H)WI (TR 1500/TE 35 msec). The mild degree of T2W has given the lesion (lower vertical arrow) a mottled appearance which indicates variable T2 relaxation times. This is a reflection of the multiple detritus and fatty components of the cyst. (Reprinted with permission from Wallace C, Sheldon JJ. MR imaging of the sella and juxtasellar regions. In MRI Update Series, Vol. 2, Book 9, Challenges 17 and 18.)

may appear as regions of signal dropout on all imaging sequences, or they may appear as regions with different degrees of decreased signal intensities owing to signal averaging from mobile protons in the surrounding matrix.[45] The same variable signal intensity on T1 and T2WI can be seen in intrasellar epithelial, colloid, or pituitary cysts (Fig. 10–24) as alluded to above. They have been previously referred to as Rathke's cleft cysts or intrasellar craniopharyngiomas, since they are derived from the Rathke's pouch of ectodermal cells lying in the roof of the primitive oral cavity. These cells eventually form the anterior hypophysis, intermediate lobe, and pars tuberalis. Rathke's cysts with a single epithelial lining occur in 20% of glands sectioned pathologically. These lesions (single-layered epithelium) are differentiated from craniopharyngiomas (multilayered, complex epithelial lining) by histology and lack of aggressiveness clinically. Symptoms are rare but can be attributed to local mass effect when lesions are large. Cysts contain serous or mucous fluid and variable amounts of debris, thus accounting for their varied MR signal as either "waterlike" (hypointense T1; hyperintense T2) or "fatlike" (hyperintense T1; hypointense T2). Noncontrast CT may reveal increased or decreased attenuation. These so-called tumors typically do not calcify. Recurrence of these lesions following surgical extirpation may occur in 15%.

The diagnosis of a craniopharyngioma on MRI would depend upon the demonstration of a sellar or suprasellar cystic lesion containing areas of bright signal on the T1WI representing hydrolyzed cholesterol and areas of signal dropout on all imaging sequences suggesting calcification or keratinization. Blood within a pituitary adenoma may also yield a bright signal on a T1W image. However, the abrupt clinical onset and the pituitary location of the lesion distinguish the latter from a craniopharyngioma. Comparison with CT will also differentiate blood from fat. At high field, the

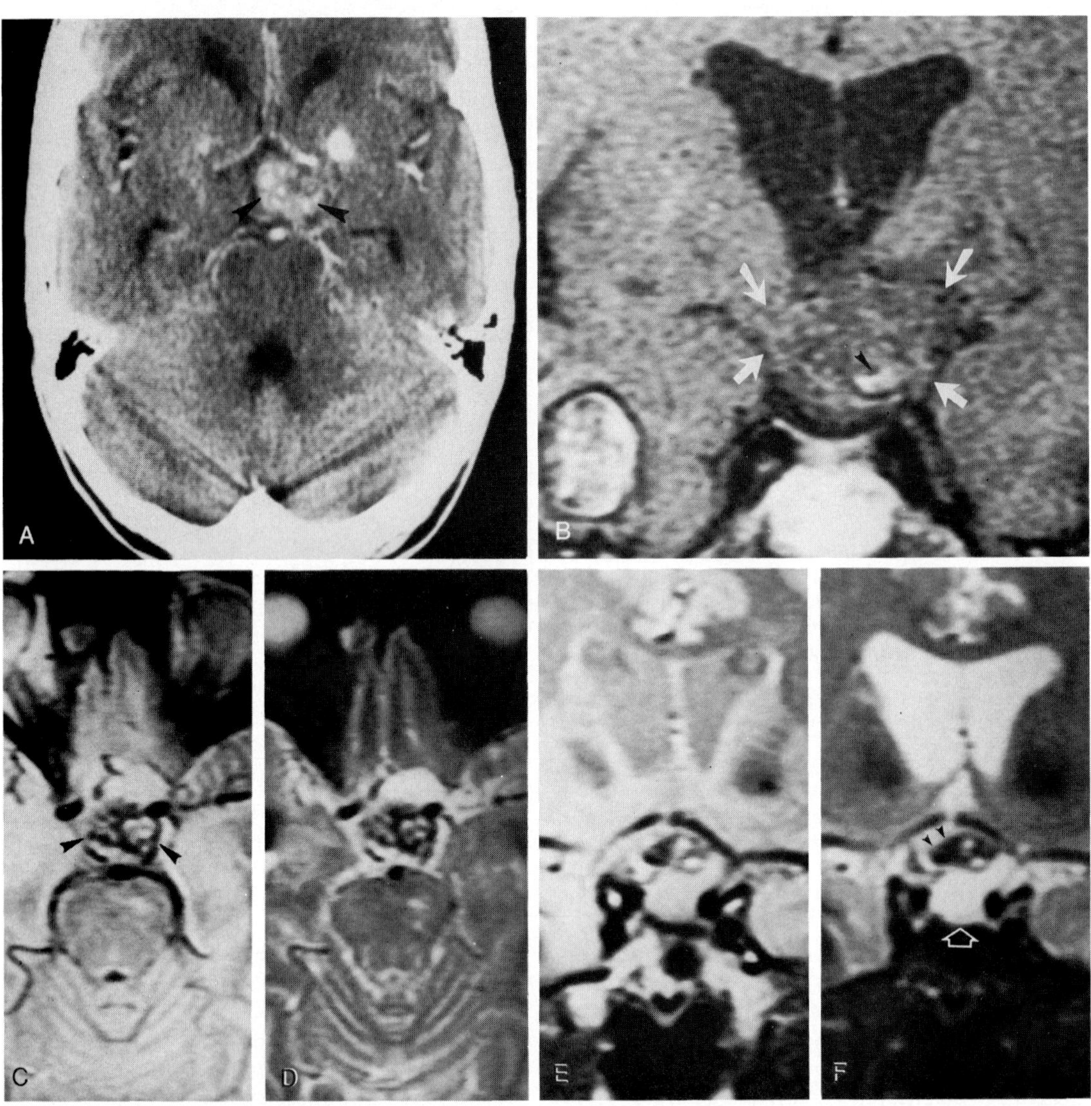


**Figure 10–23. Solid craniopharyngioma (calcified).** A 32-year-old man with blurred vision and chronic headaches. *A,* Axial CECT. *B,* Coronal T1WI. *C* and *D,* Axial multiecho N(H)WI & T2WI. *E* and *F,* Coronal multiecho N(H)WI & T2WI. Calcified suprasellar mass (arrowheads) on CT has solid isointense signal on coronal T1WI (white arrows), and only punctate hyperintense signal corresponding to fat (arrowhead [*B*]). Intrasellar or solid component of this lesion is hyperintense on T2WI (open arrow) and calcification is hypointense on T2WI (arrowheads [*D* and *F*]). Note the paucity of hyperintense fat signal on T1WI in this patient.

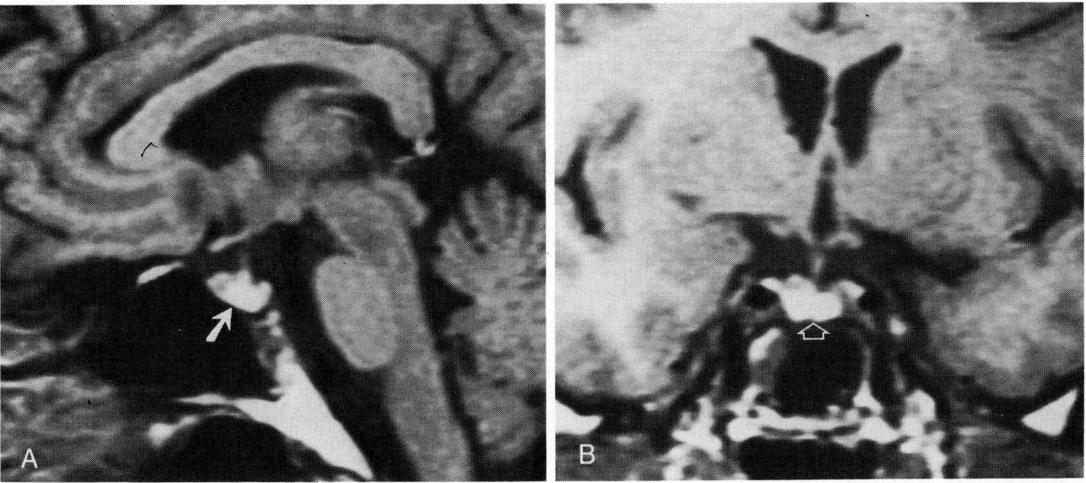


**Figure 10–24. Rathke's cyst (intrasellar craniopharyngioma).** A 22-year-old woman with headache (1.5 T). *A* and *B*, Sagittal and coronal T1WI. Intrasellar focus of signal hyperintensity (white and open arrows) on T1WI corresponds to fat or hydrolyzed cholesterol or both within this lesion. Subacute or chronic hemorrhagic loci could also produce a similar signal.

presence of chemical shift artifact would support a fat-containing rather than a hemorrhagic lesion; however, one must keep in mind that hemorrhagic elements may exist in craniopharyngiomas.

## Meningiomas

Meningiomas constitute about 15% of intracranial neoplasms.[27, 47] Approximately 10% to 20% will occur in the perisellar region.[47, 50] These may arise from the diaphragm sella (Fig. 10–25), the tuberculum sella, the planum sphenoidale area, the anterior clinoid and adjacent medial third of the lessor sphenoid wing, the walls of the cavernous sinus (Fig. 10–26), or the dorsum sella and adjacent anterolateral tentorial incisura.[27, 36] A purely intrasellar origin may occur.[46] There are no anatomic boundaries separating the listed perisellar regions. Meningiomas arising there have a tendency to spread along meningeal surfaces and to involve more than one territory.[27] They are more frequently seen in females than males, with a numerical peak in the third through the fifth decades of life.[27, 51] Symptoms are related to pressure on adjacent structures, including the optic nerve (causing monocular blindness), the optic chiasm, and the third through sixth cranial nerves.[26, 36]

Grossly, the meningiomas that arise in the perisellar region tend to spread in sheetlike fashion (en plaque) along a dural surface, the globoid mass associated with its growth occurring later. A simplified microscopic classification would include the meningothelial (syncytial) type, composed of nests of large cells thought to be of arachnoid origin; and the fibroblastic type, consisting of interlacing strands of fibrous collagen tissue and reticulin fibers containing scattered nests of elongated cells; and a transitional type that embodies features of both the meningothelial and fibroblastic forms.[43, 51, 52] Psammomatous calcifications can occur in any of the types described.[43] Sarcomatous transformation may also occur. Still another type is angioblastic meningioma, which may consist of two histologic subdivisions: hemangiopericytomas and hemangioblastomas.[43]

CT is more sensitive than MRI in imaging meningiomas.[46] The classic findings of hyperostotic bone changes, blistering, and calcifications that have been described on routine skull films are exquisitely demonstrated on CT.[46, 50, 53] These changes, along with an isodense to hyperdense mass on plain CT coupled with homogenous enhancement after intravenous contrast injection, strongly suggest a diagnosis of meningioma.[36, 46, 50] MRI, because of its multiplanar orthogonal projections, does show the relationship of the lesion to the surrounding anatomy to better advantage. This is especially true re-

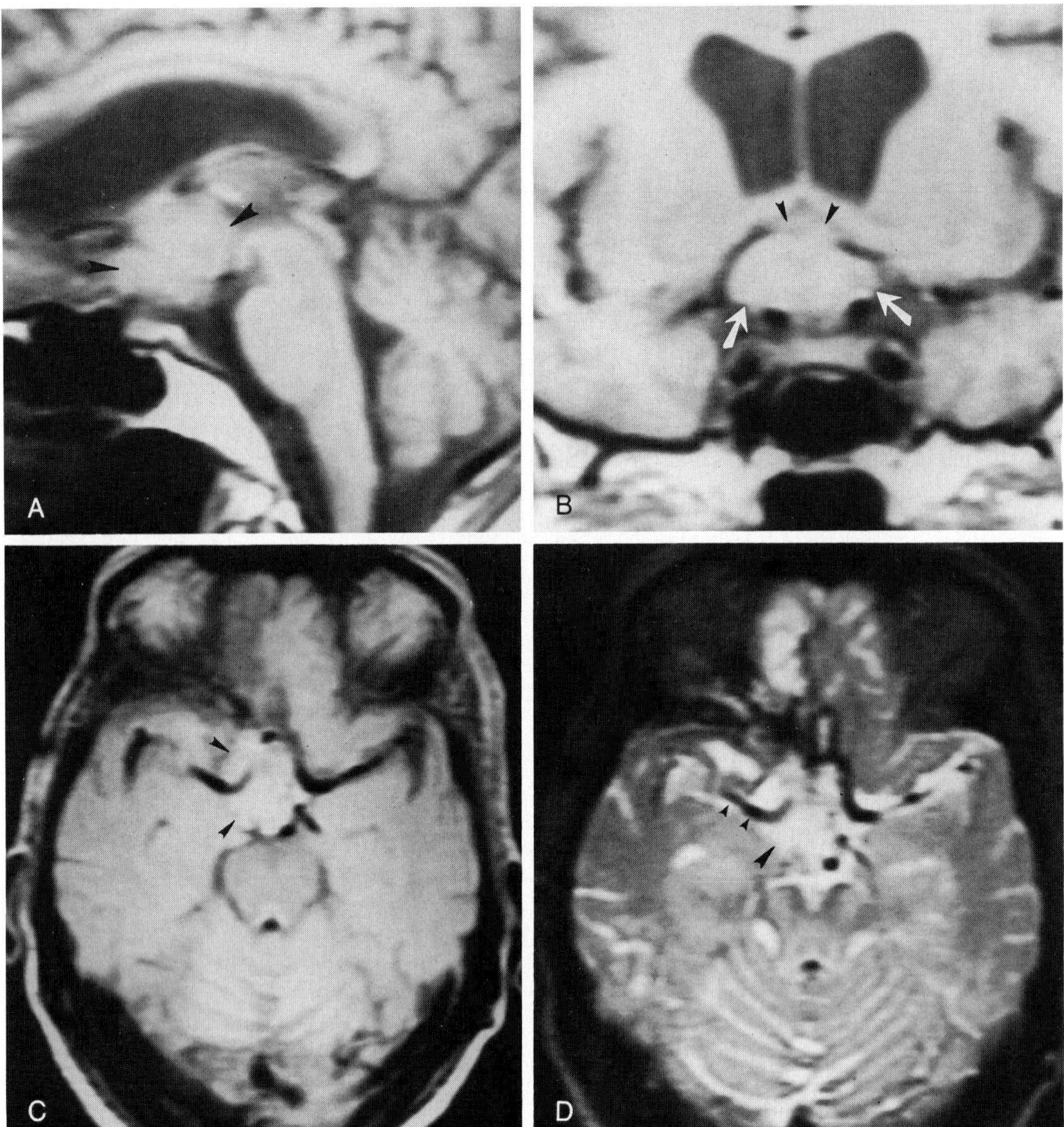


**Figure 10–25. Suprasellar meningioma.** A 42-year-old woman with progressive visual loss (1.5 T). *A,* Sagittal T1WI. *B,* Coronal T1WI. *C,* Axial N(H)WI. *D,* Axial T2WI. Suprasellar mass is isointense with white matter on T1WI (arrowheads [*A*]), and mass (white arrows [*B*]) effaces the chiasm (arrowheads [*B*]) superiorly on coronal T1WI. Mass encases right middle cerebral artery (small arrowheads [*D*]), is isointense (arrowheads) on axial N(H)WI, and is hyperintense on T2WI (large arrowhead [*D*]). (Courtesy of S. J. Pomeranz, M.D., The Christ Hospital, Cincinnati, Ohio.)

garding compression of the optic chiasm and the optic nerve and encasement of the carotid artery (Figs. 10–25*D* and 10–26*F*).[5]

While MRI currently is not as sensitive as CT in the detection of meningiomas, contrast-enhanced MR (CEMR) may change this.[46] This is probably because the T1 and T2 relaxation times from the tumor are approximately the same as adjacent cerebral gray matter and yield a signal similar to cerebral cortex (Fig. 10–26).[54] It is speculated that this circumstance is due to volume averaging of the mobile protons of the hydrogen-rich cytoplasmic cellular matrix with a lack of such protons in the fibrous stroma. If present, this circumstance is accentuated by psammomatous calcification within the neoplasm.[55] Vasogenic cerebral edema with a bright signal on T2WI may be the only sign of the mass (Fig. 10–26*C*–*E*).[3, 54] Occasionally, the lesion may show a bright signal on the T2WI, probably owing to a more cellular

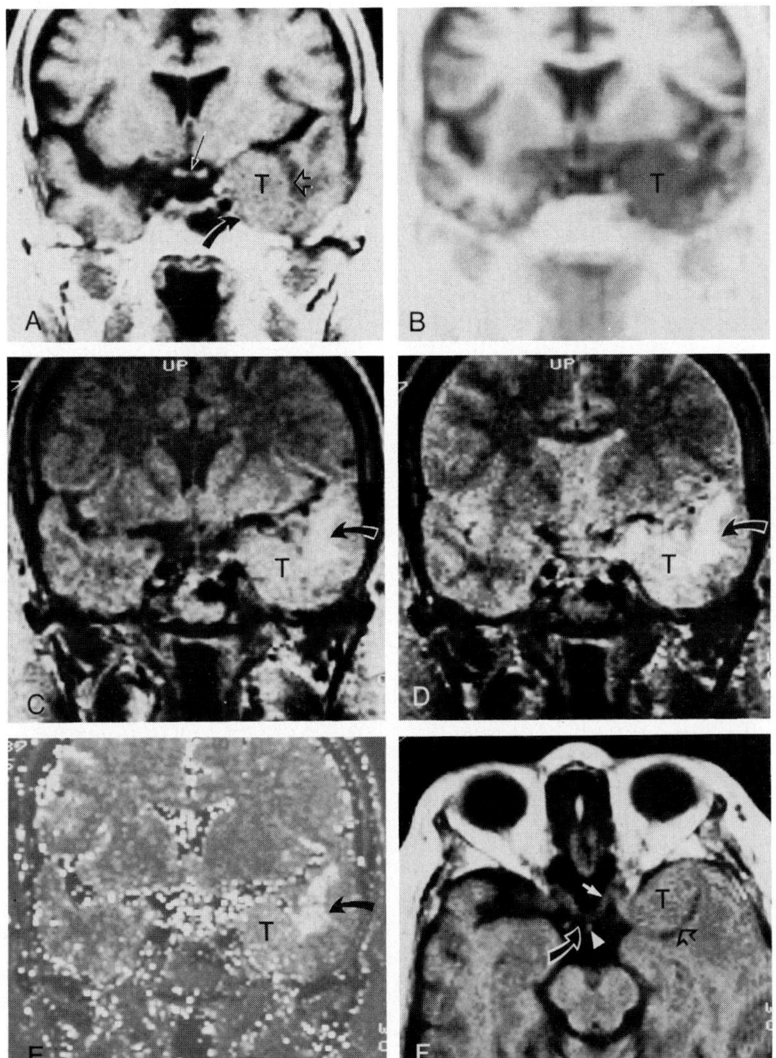


**Figure 10–26. Meningioma (lateral wall of left cavernous sinus).** A 48-year-old woman with headache and left third-nerve palsy. *A,* A 5-mm coronal T1WI (TR 500/TE 16 msec). The tumor (T) is isointense with adjacent gray matter and displaces the left temporal lobe laterally. It is marginated by a dark rim (open arrow). The lateral wall of the cavernous sinus (curved arrow), which is giving rise to the lesion, retains its identity and remains hypointense. *B,* A 5-mm coronal IR T1WI (TR 2100/TI 400/TE 35 msec). The subtle differences in T1 relaxation time between the gray matter and the lesion are more apparent on this imaging sequence. The signal from the tumor (T) has become relatively more hypointense.

*C,* A 5-mm coronal first-echo N(H)WI (TR 2000/TE 35 msec). The tumor (T) is almost isointense with adjacent gray matter. Hyperintense edema (curved arrow) is present in the temporal white matter. *D,* A 5-mm coronal second-echo T2WI (TR 2000/TE 35 msec). The tumor (T) is still almost isointense with adjacent gray matter. The hyperintense signal from the edema (curved arrow) in the temporal white matter is even brighter on this sequence. *E,* A calculated T2 map image. The signal from the tumor (T) is isointense with that of the adjacent brain, indicating equivalent T2 relaxation times. Edema (curved arrow) has a bright signal compatible with its long T2 relaxation time. *F,* A 5-mm axial T1WI (TR 500/TE 16 msec). The tumor (T) is displacing the intracranial portion of the left optic nerve (anterior arrow). (Curved arrow = optic chiasm; arrowhead = infundibulum).

lesion (e.g., meningothelial meningioma) containing more water and therefore more mobile protons.

Consequently, detection is usually not due to a recognizable signal difference but rather to the recognition of the mass effect of the tumor displacing adjacent brain (Fig. 10–26*A* and *F*) or causing cerebral edema (Fig. 10–26*C* and *D*) or both.[54] Although the mass effect is illustrated on T1W spin-echo images, it is better visualized with an inversion recovery sequence (Fig. 10–26*B*).[3, 56] This latter sequence may show the lesion to have a slightly decreased signal relative to adjacent gray matter owing to its greater sensitivity to subtle differences in T1 relation times.[3] It also contrasts the gray-white matter interface of the brain to better advantage. Consequently, it will have greater sensitivity to an extra-axial mass that displaces the brain and produces white-matter buckling.[3, 57]

Not infrequently, a dark rim surrounding the meningioma is demonstrated (Fig. 10–26). It is thought that this may be due to a venous or vascular tumor capsule, a fibrous tumor capsule, or compressed adjacent leptomeninges and brain.[58]

Currently, if a perisellar meningioma is suspected, a plain and contrast high resolution CT is most sensitive for detection. It is suggested that this procedure be followed by MRI to relate the mass to perisellar anatomy.[3, 5, 46, 56]

## Aneurysms

Perisellar aneurysms arise either from the supraclinoid or the cavernous segment of the internal carotid artery (Figs. 10–27 and 10–28). They may be asymptomatic or may cause symptoms either because they have bled or because of their mass effects on adjacent structures.[59] Morphologically, they are saccular outpouchings with a lumen 3 mm or more in diameter, usually arising from the junction of a branching or originating vessel. The etiology is unknown but is thought to be either congenital or atherosclerotic.[36, 59]

The lesions may be demonstrated on plain CT as isodense or slightly hyperdense masses in the perisellar region that homogeneously enhance on CT after intravenous contrast infusion (Fig. 10–27*A* and *B*). They may be indistinguishable from pituitary adenomas or other solid perisellar masses (e.g., meningiomas).[10, 46] The imaging problem confronting MRI is to make the distinction between a solid lesion and an aneurysm, thus guiding further treatment strategies. If the lesion is an aneurysm, the ultimate evaluation for definitive treatment is neuroangiography.

The MR appearance of an aneurysm depends upon the velocity of the blood flowing through it, the degree of turbulence, the presence of a thrombus, and the presence of hemosiderin deposits if the lesion has bled in the past.[60] High-velocity blood flow through the aneurysm appears as a signal void on all imaging sequences (Figs. 10–27, 10–28, 11–22, 11–23, 11–25, and 11–26).[5, 10, 46, 61] A thrombus may show a high signal intensity on T1W and T2W images secondary to methemoglobin deposition.[60] Turbulent slow flow may be seen as an absolute increase in signal intensity on the second echo of a multiecho sequence owing to even-echo rephasing.[10] Hemosiderin facilitates T2 relaxation, so that it appears hypointense on T2W spin-echo sequences, usually surrounding the aneurysm or outlining the basilar cisterns.[60] This phenomenon of T2-dependent dephasing and signal loss is field dependent and more apparent at high field. The MRI appearance depends upon the biodynamics of the blood within the aneurysm and degree to which the above processes are present. A common appearance is a high-velocity flow void and a bright signal on the second echo in regions of even-echo rephasing.[10]

## Chiasmal Gliomas

Chiasmal gliomas most often occur in children between the ages of 2 and 9 years.[36] Seventy-five percent of the patients are under 10 years of age.[62] The average age is 5 years; the oldest recorded patient was aged 79 years.[63] Approximately 30% of patients have associated neurofibromatosis, and 16% of those with neurofibromatosis have a glioma of the optic nerve or optic chiasm or both.[62]

The extent of the tumor is variable. It may be confined to the optic chiasm, may extend to the adjacent hypothalamus, involve one or more optic nerves, the optic tract, or both (Figs. 10–29, 10–30, and 10–31, respec-

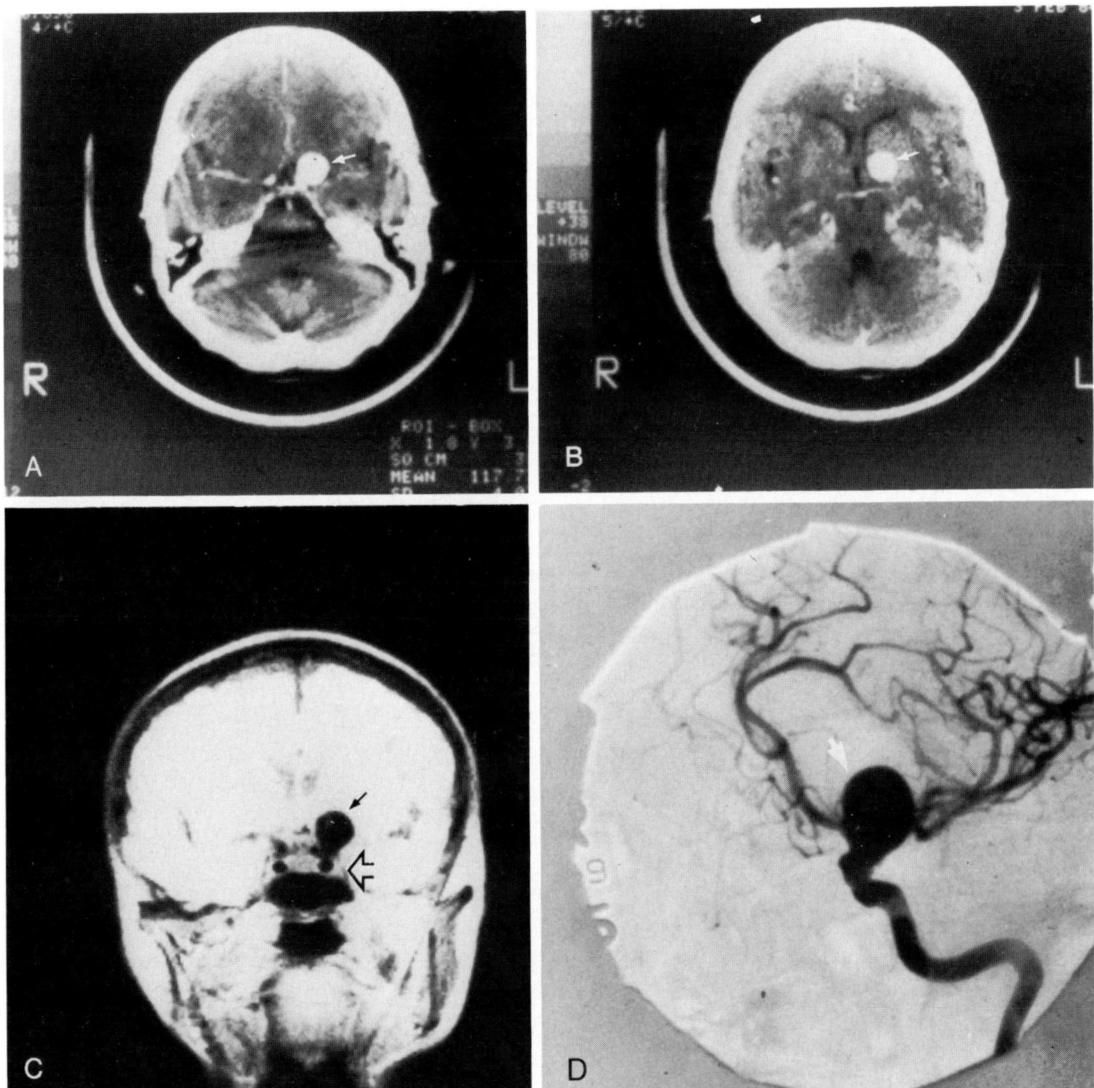


**Figure 10–27. Aneurysm (supraclinoid left internal carotid artery).** A 57-year-old woman with headaches and left third-nerve palsy (0.35 T). *A,* The contrast CT shows a well-circumscribed, homogeneously enhancing mass (arrow) in the left side of the suprasellar cistern (to reader's right). On plain CT (not shown), the mass was isodense. *B,* The enhancing mass (arrow) indents the thalmus.

*C,* A 5-mm coronal T1WI (TR 300/TE 30 msec) shows the absent signal compatible with high-velocity flow void within the lesion (arrow). The lesion arises from the supraclinoid segment of the left internal carotid artery just above the patient's left cavernous sinus (open arrow). *D,* A selective left internal carotid arteriogram in the contralateral oblique projection demonstrates the aneurysm (arrow). (*A–C* reprinted with permission from Wallace C, Sheldon JJ. MR imaging of the sella and juxtasellar regions. In MRI Update Series, Vol. 2, Book 9, Challenges 17 and 18. *D,* courtesy of Dr. Robert Quencer, Professor of Radiology, University of Miami School of Medicine.)

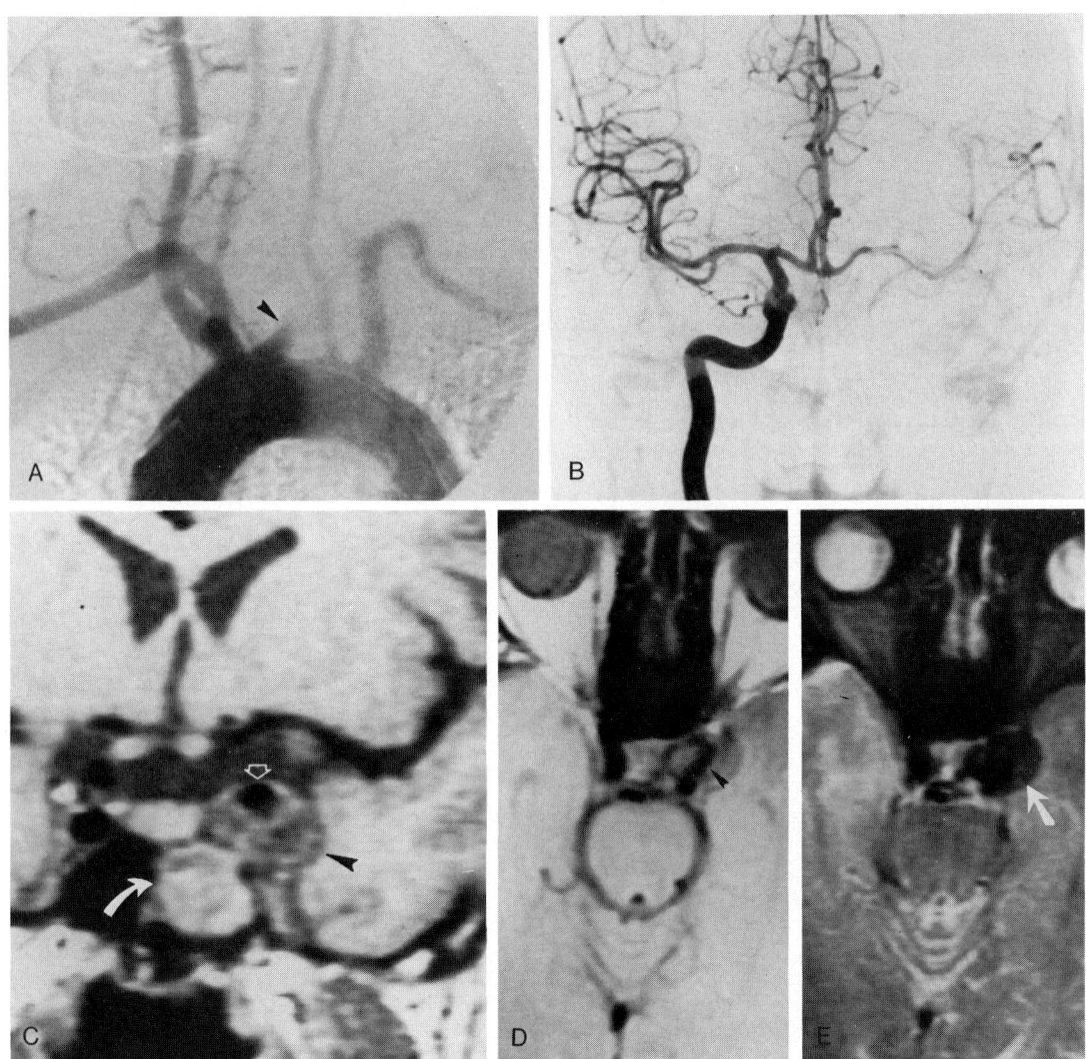


**Figure 10–28. Carotid artery aneurysm with thrombus proved.** A 72-year-old man with right-sided hemiparesis (1.5 T). *A,* Digital angiography–aortic arch. *B,* Right internal carotid angiogram—AP Caldwell. *C,* Coronal T1WI. *D* and *E,* Axial multiecho N(H)WI and T2WI.

Left common carotid artery is occluded (arrowhead) and no filling of the parasellar left internal carotid artery (LICA) is apparent from the right carotid injection. Coronal T1WI shows a dumbbell-shaped parasellar mass containing flow void of LICA (open arrow), acute thrombus (arrowhead), and chronic thrombus (curved arrow). Axial images show carotid flow void (arrowhead) and hypointense signal of acute clot (arrow) at high-field strength. (Courtesy of S. J. Pomeranz, M.D., The Christ Hospital, Cincinnati, Ohio.)

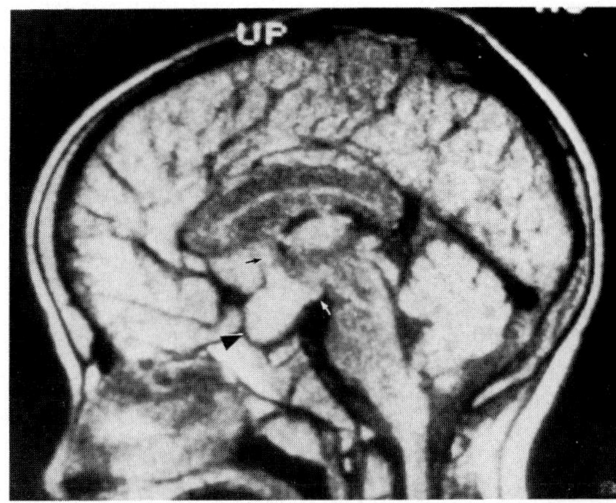


**Figure 10–29. Optic chiasm glioma with hypothalamic extension.** A 9-year-old boy with bilateral progressive visual loss (0.35 T). Sagittal N(H)WI (TR 1500/TE 35 msec) demonstrates a mass (arrowhead) with increased signal arising from the optic chiasm. It has extended into the lamina terminalis (upper anterior arrow) and the tuber cinereum (upper posterior arrow) of the hypothalamus. (Reprinted with permission from Wallace C, Sheldon JJ. MR imaging of the sella and juxtasellar regions. In MRI Update Series, Vol. 2, Book 9, Challenges 17 and 18.)

tively).[64] Morphologically, the lesion may be solid or may have cystic components.[46]

The clinical presentation depends on the location of the glioma. If confined to the optic chiasm, visual loss is the most common presenting complaint. The visual field may show dense scotomas. If the hypothalamus has been invaded, there may be diabetes insipidus, obesity, dwarfism, and precocious puberty. Extension to the optic nerve may be manifested as proptosis and monocular loss of vision.[62]

MRI is more sensitive than CT in demonstrating the relationship of the lesion to surrounding anatomy and extra-chiasmal extension.[4, 5, 24, 25] T1W images in the sagittal projection are most sensitive in evaluating the chiasm. The coronal projection demonstrates lateral extent.[4, 5, 24, 25] Axial and coronal projections are better suited to evaluate the optic nerves and optic tracts (Figs. 10–30 and 10–31), respectively.[24, 25] Enlargement of the optic chiasm is the most common MRI finding (Fig. 10–30*A*).[24] The signal intensity is variable. The tumor may be isointense or hypointense (Fig. 10–30) on T1W images and isointense or hyperintense on T2W images (Fig. 10–31). The changes in signal intensity have been ascribed to cystic changes in the glioma.[4]

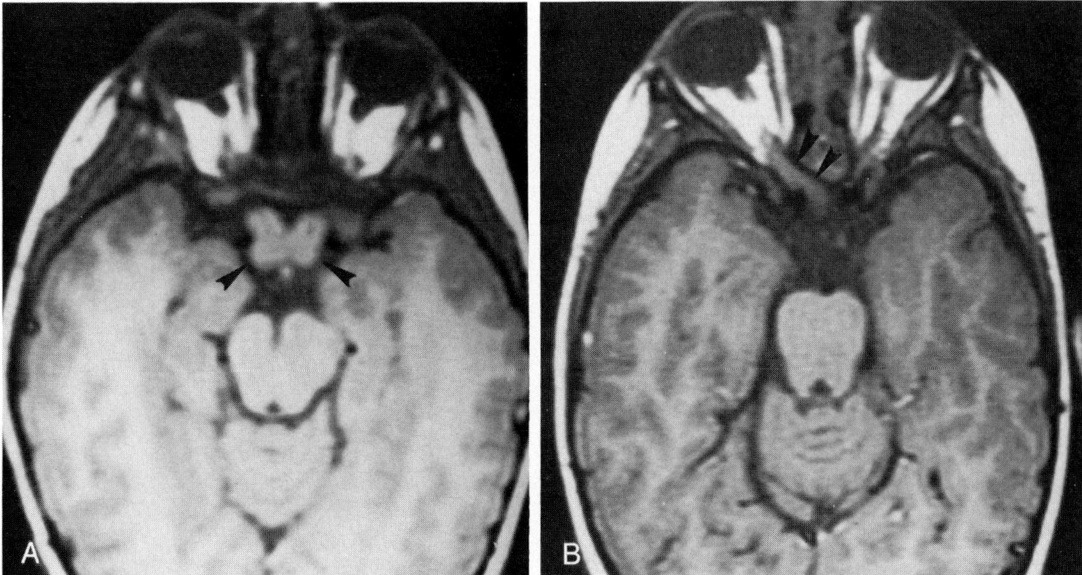


**Figure 10–30. Chiasmatic and intracanalicular nerve optic gliomas.** Visual symptoms in two patients with neurofibromatosis, eight and ten years old, respectively (1.5 T). *A,* Axial T1WI. *B,* Axial T1WI. A mass symmetrically enlarges the optic chiasm (arrowheads) in patient *A.* In patient *B,* a mass involves the right intracanalicular optic nerve (arrowheads). (Courtesy of William Ball, M.D., Department of Radiology, Children's Hospital Medical Center, Cincinnati, Ohio.)

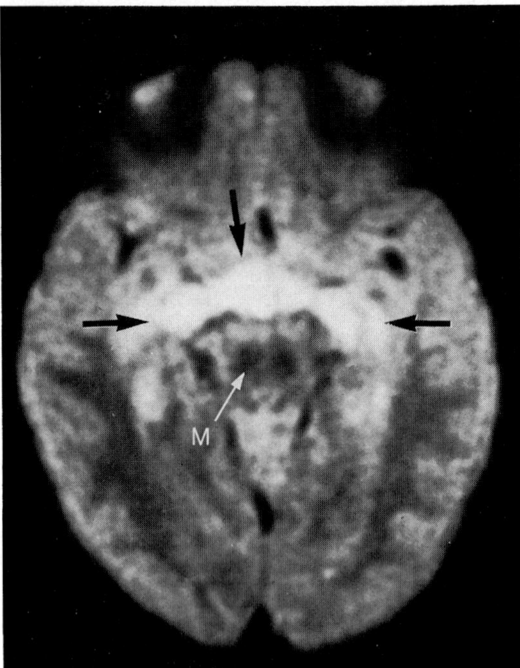


**Figure 10–31. Optic chiasm glioma with extension into both optic tracts.** Early childhood patient with neurofibromatosis (0.3 T). Axial T2WI (TR 2039/TE 84 msec) demonstrates increased signal in the glioma of the optic chiasm (vertical arrow) extending into both optic tracts (horizontal arrows). (M = midbrain). (Courtesy of Nolan Altman, M.D., Department of Radiology, Miami Children's Hospital, Coral Gables, Fla.)

## Hamartoma

This is a rare benign lesion arising from the hypothalamic region in the topography of the tuber cinereum. It is not a true neoplasm and is probably developmental in origin.[27] The tumor usually is discovered in early childhood and is more common in males than females. The lesion causes precocious puberty. Seizures, mental changes, behavioral disorders, and diabetes insipidus may be present.[65, 66, 67] The mass is usually 1 to 2 cm in diameter and projects into the interpeduncular cistern (Fig. 10–32). It may displace and deform the floor of the third ventricle.[65]

The appearance on MRI is that of a mass arising from the tuber cinereum and projecting above and slightly behind the dorsum sella into the intracrural cistern. It is isointense with brain on T1W and isointense or slightly hyperintense on T2W (not shown) imaging sequences (Fig. 10–32). The etiology of the lesion can be suggested by the clinical history, the typical site of origin, its relatively noninvasive appearance, and the relatively isointense signal on all imaging sequences.[54]

## Chordoma

These are well-circumscribed malignant tumors that arise most commonly in the sacrococcygeal region (50%) and the clivus (35%) in the topography of the spheno-occipital synchondrosis.[68] It is the most common primary tumor of the clivus and arises from notochordal remnants.[69] The lesion is soft in consistency and grayish white. It is surrounded by a pseudocapsule except in the region of bone destruction.[68] Microscopically, there are areas of cystic degeneration and hemorrhage.[27] Nodular flecks of calcification are present in 33% to 50% of lesions.[50] There is osteolysis of the bone at the site of origin; the lesion can extend anteriorly into the sphenoid sinus and nasopharynx as well as posterosuperiorly into the basilar cistern. Even though these tumors arise near the midline, they tend to grow eccentrically.[69]

Chordomas of the clivus arise in the fourth to fifth decades of life. The tumors are slow growing and the overall five-year survival for chordomas from all locations is 50% to 60%.[68]

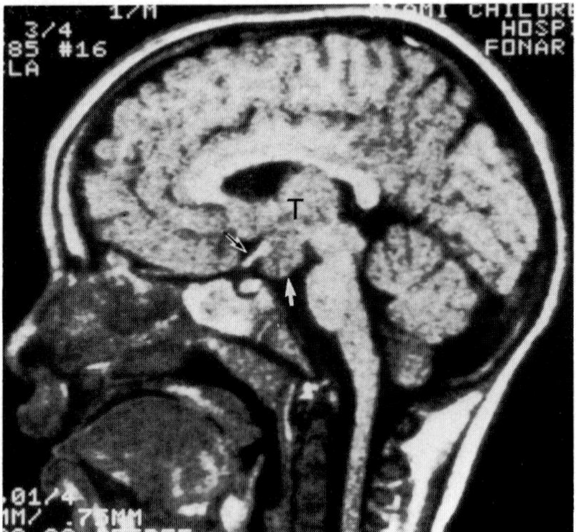


**Figure 10–32. Hamartoma of the tuber cinereum.** A 2-year-old boy with precocious puberty (0.3 T). A sagittal T1WI (TR 499/TE 14 msec). A 2-cm isointense (relative to the thalamus, T) mass (posterior arrow) arising from the tuber cinereum just posterior to the optic chiasm (anterior arrow). (Courtesy of Nolan Altman, M.D. Department of Radiology, Miami Children's Hospital, Coral Gables, Fla.)

CT is useful to demonstrate the extent of bone destruction and the presence of calcification. MRI with its sagittal projection and its excellent soft tissue contrast resolution is useful to demonstrate the cephalocaudal extent of the tumor and its relationship to the brain stem, thalmus, and third ventricle (Fig. 10–33). The prolonged T1 and T2 relaxation times, resulting in decreased signal on T1W images and increased signal on T2W images, along with the bone destruction, help to distinguish this tumor from clival meningiomas.[45]

## Cavernous Sinus Lesions

Perisellar lesions may also arise in a parasellar or infrasellar location. The cavernous sinus is in the immediate parasellar location,

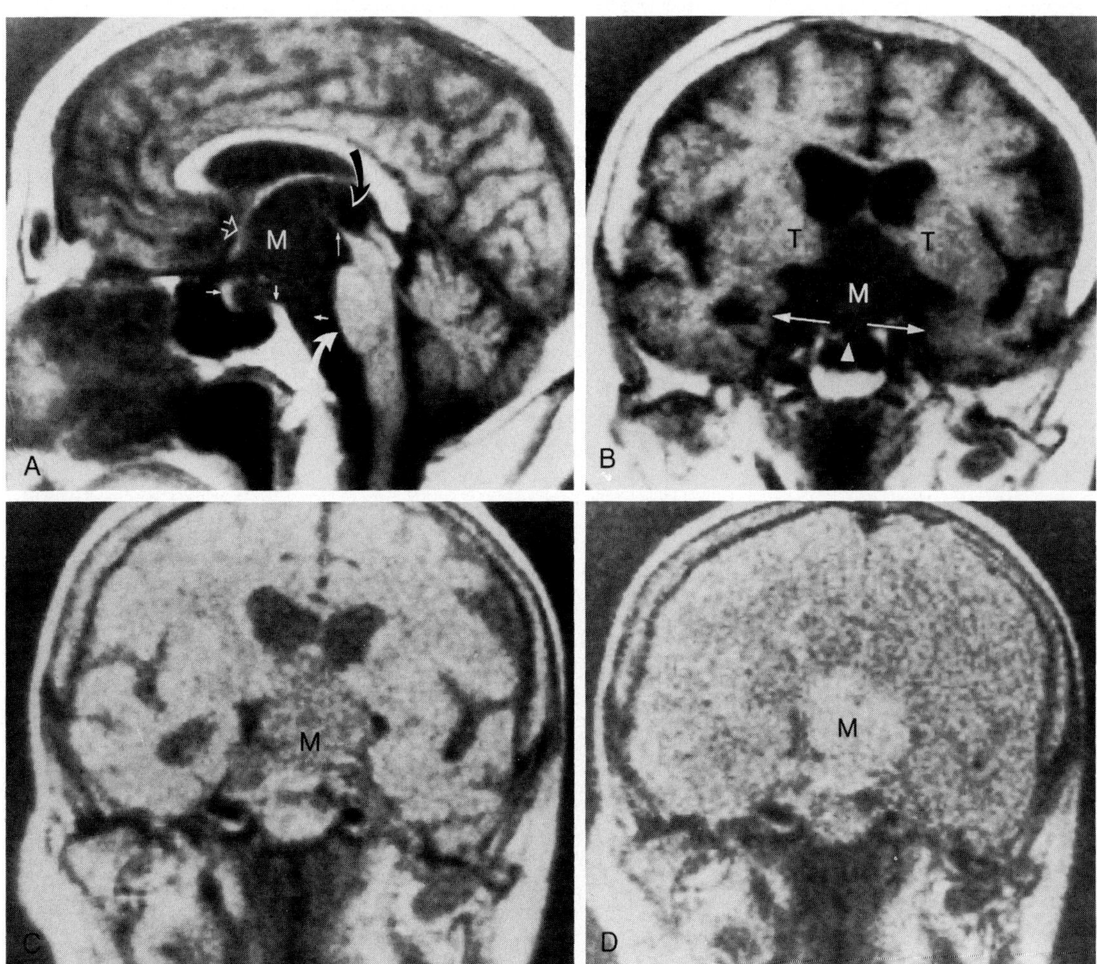


**Figure 10–33. Chordoma of the clivus.** A 60-year-old woman who has had head trauma, but is asymptomatic (0.35 T). *A,* Sagittal T1WI (TR 300/TE 30 msec). The mass (M) is hypointense but slightly brighter than CSF. It has eroded the dorsum (lower vertical arrow) and has extended down the upper portion of the clivus (posterior horizontal arrow). The brain stem is displaced posteriorly (lower curved arrow). The pituitary (anterior horizontal arrow) is displaced against the anterior wall of the sella. The optic chiasm (open arrow) is anterosuperiorly displaced. The tuber cinereum (upper vertical arrow) and the third ventricle (upper curved arrow) are superiorly displaced.

*B,* Coronal T1WI (TR 300/TE 30 msec). The mass (M) is above the sellar floor (arrowhead) and has spread the thalami (T) and the temporal lobes (horizontal arrows). *C,* Coronal first-echo N(H)WI (TR 1500/TE 35 msec) demonstrates increased signal in the mass (M) with an increase in the TR in keeping with a prolonged T1 relaxation time. The signal from the ventricles is darker than that of the lesion, in keeping with the longer T1 relaxation time of the CSF. *D,* Coronal second-echo T2WI (TR 1500/TE 70 msec). The signal from the mass (M) is even brighter in keeping with the long T2 relaxation. It is brighter than spinal fluid, which is almost isointense with the brain on this sequence. (Reprinted with permission from Wallace C, Sheldon JJ. MR imaging of the sella and juxtasellar regions. In MRI Update Series, Vol. 2, Book 9, Challenges 17 and 18.)

and mass lesions may be involved.[46] A rare lesion is the trigeminal neuroma. Pathologically, this is usually a schwannoma. Fifty percent arise from the gasserian ganglion located within Meckel's cave. Extension into the cavernous sinus or an origination from the cavernous portion of the trigeminal nerve (ophthmalic division) may occur. Symptoms may include tic douloureux, corneal anesthesia or hyposthesia, and headache (Fig. 10–34).[69] More infrequently, the cavernous segment of the third, fourth, or sixth cranial nerve may give rise to the neuroma.[46] When it is small, MR demonstrates the lesion within the cavernous sinus, along with the nonspecific signs that indicate a cavernous sinus mass, including asymmetry of the cavernous sinuses, enlargement of the side with the lesion, straight or lateral convexity to the lateral wall of the sinus, and loss of the normal signal of venous sinus blood (Fig. 10–34).[70] The lesion itself may have long T1 and T2 relaxation times and may appear as a hypointense signal on T1W images and a bright signal on T2W images (Fig. 10–34*A* and *B*). Metastasis to the body of the sphenoid may extend into the cavernous sinus (Fig. 10–35). CT clearly demonstrates the bony destruction (Fig. 10–35*A*), whereas MRI demonstrates the relationship of the soft tissue mass to the cavernous sinus and the perisellar anatomy (Fig. 10–35*B* and *C*). Meningiomas may arise directly from within the sinus or may invade the sinus after arising from its external dural wall. MRI will show encasement of the cavernous or supraclinoid segment of the internal carotid artery. A pituitary adenoma may also invade the sinus and encase the carotid artery (Fig. 10–15).[34] An aneurysm of the cavernous segment of the internal carotid artery may also present as a cavernous sinus mass with third, fourth, or sixth cranial nerve palsy. In addition to the nonspecific imaging signs of a cavernous sinus space–occupying lesion, the aneurysm will have a high-velocity flow void on MRI that is specific for a vascular lesion.

## Miscellaneous Lesions

Malignant neoplasms may arise within the sphenoid sinus or the nasopharynx. These may extend superiorly and destroy the bony body of the sphenoid; they may even extend laterally to invade the cavernous sinus (Fig. 9–32). Suprasellar intracranial extension

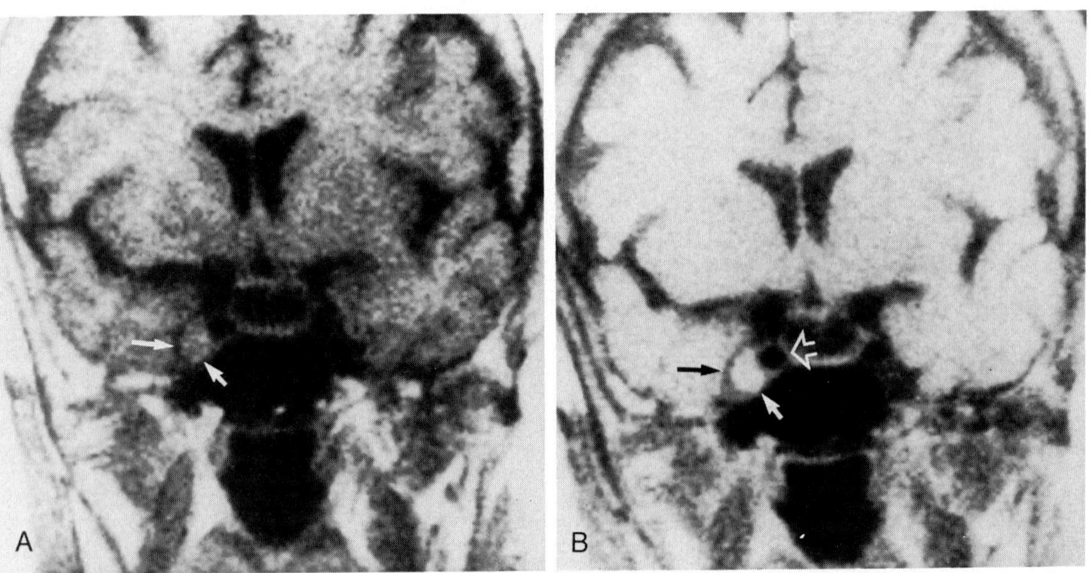


**Figure 10–34. Neurofibroma of the ophthalmic division of the trigeminal nerve.** A 76-year-old woman with corneal anesthesia and right third nerve palsy (0.35 T). *A,* A 5-mm coronal T1WI (TR 300/TE 30 msec). A mass (lower arrow) in the patient's right cavernous sinus (to reader's left) having a signal isointense with the adjacent temporal lobe. The mass is bulging the lateral wall (horizontal arrow) of the sinus convexly and laterally. *B,* A 5-mm coronal N(H)WI (TR 1500/TE 35 msec). The signal from the mass (lower arrow) is now brighter relative to brain, reflecting its longer T2 relaxation time. The lesion is just lateral to the high-flow signal void of the cavernous segment of the internal carotid artery (open arrow). Horizontal arrow = lateral wall of the cavernous sinus.

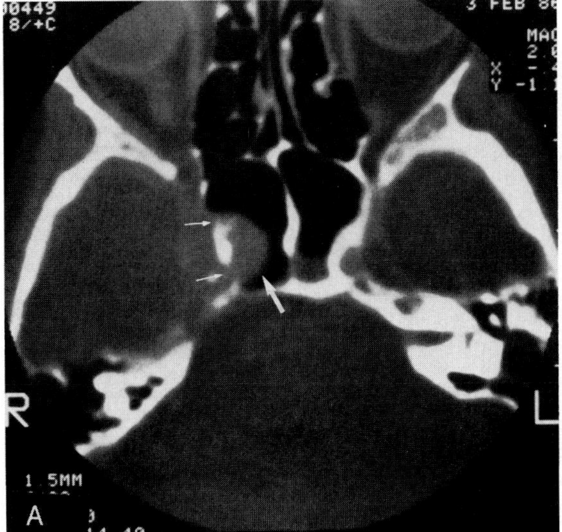


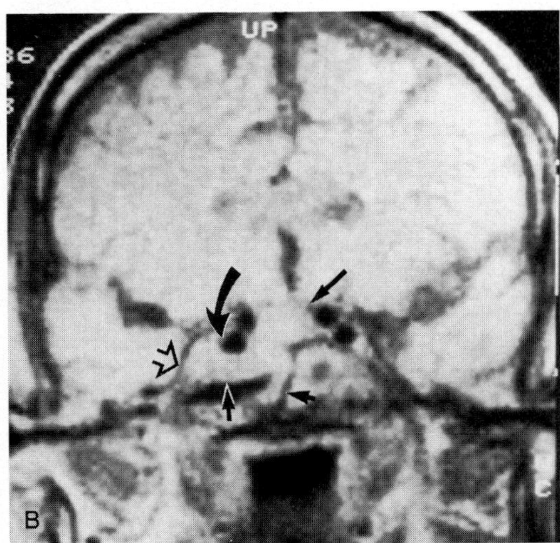


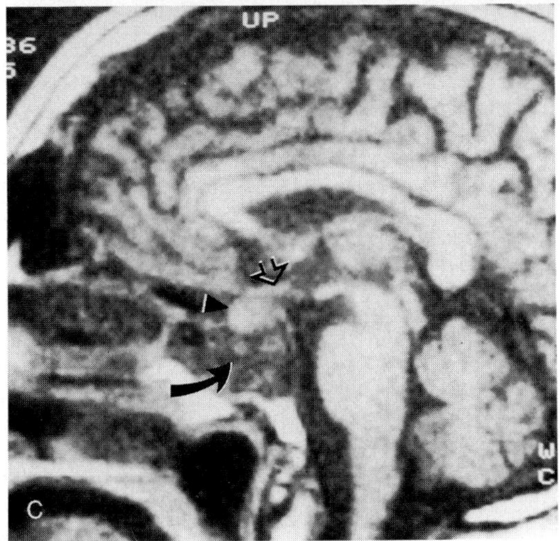


**Figure 10–35. Metastatic renal cell carcinoma to the body of the sphenoid with extension into the sphenoid sinus and cavernous sinus.** A 62-year-old man with right third nerve palsy and with a history of right nephrectomy 12 years earlier for renal cell carcinoma (0.35 T). *A,* A CECT-bone window setting demonstrates a mass (angled arrow) in the patient's right sphenoid sinus with bone destruction of the lateral wall (horizontal arrows). *B,* Coronal N(H)WI (TR 1500/TE 35 msec). The mass (lower vertical arrow) has invaded the cavernous sinus, pushing the lateral wall laterally (open arrow). The lesion has encased the internal carotid artery (curved arrow). The pituitary (upper, angled arrow) is elevated and displaced laterally by the intrasellar extension of the mass. The bony septa (horizontal arrow) forms the medial boundary of the mass. *C,* Coronal T1WI (TR 300/TE 30 msec) demonstrates the mass (curved arrow) within the body of the sphenoid. There are mottled high-signal areas most likely persistent fatty sphenoid marrow. The pituitary (arrowhead) is elevated and has impinged upon the optic chiasm (open arrow).

may also occur.[46, 71] MRI is as sensitive as CT for demonstrating bony destruction;[72] however, CT has better spatial resolution and will show the bony destruction in more detail.[71] MRI is more sensitive than CT in defining the margins of the lesion and their relationship to the normal perisellar anatomy.[72]

The last lesion to be addressed in this section is suprasellar germinoma (Fig. 10–36), or ectopic pinealoma.[73, 74] Peak incidence is in the second and third decades and, unlike its counterpart in the pineal region, it is more common in females. Coexistence of a mass in the pineal region is suggestive of the diagnosis. Because of the proclivity of germinomas to seed the CSF, it was initially thought that all suprasellar germinomas were actually metastatic implants of a pineal primary. However, isolated germinomas of the suprasellar region do occur. In fact, primary germinomas have been reported in the basal ganglia and thalamus.[75] On MR a suprasellar or hypothalamic mass is seen with or without a pineal region lesion. However, no signal characteristics provide further diagnostic specificity. Intermediate signal on N(H)WI and increased signal on T2WI have been seen in our cases, and marked enhancement with CEMR is expected as occurs on contrast-enhanced CT.

In summary, thin-section MRI has become the primary imaging modality for evaluation of pituitary, sella, and perisellar lesions. Because of the high contrast resolution and multiplanar projections, MRI is sensitive in

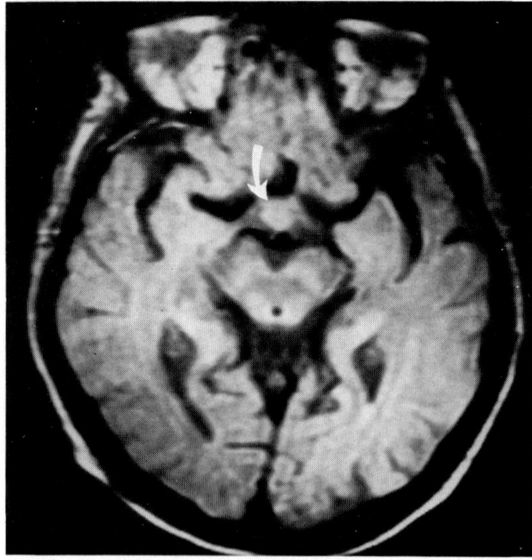

**Figure 10–36. Suprasellar germinoma (ectopic pinealoma).** A 21-year-old man with headache (1.5 T). Axial N(H)WI. A mass (arrow) in the suprasellar cistern is round, isointense with adjacent brain, and hyperintense on T2WI (not shown). The pineal gland was normal.

its ability to detect lesions, define their margins, and determine their relationship to surrounding perisellar anatomy. It is sensitive in demonstrating the relationship of the lesion to blood vessels, which appear as flow signal void on all imaging sequences. MRI can also detect bone destruction, probably with the same sensitivity as CT. However, CT has better spatial resolution and shows the bone destruction with better detail. In addition, meningiomas are brightly enhanced on CT after intravenous contrast injection and may more readily be detected than on noncontrast MRI, where they tend to be isointense with the surrounding anatomy.

Imaging of the sella and perisellar region is a complementary process involving both of these modalities. It is suggested that high-resolution MRI be used as the primary imaging modality and that the role of CT be to evaluate bone destruction. Contrast-enhanced CT is reserved for the evaluation of selected perisellar processes such as meningiomas or until CEMR is available.

## References


1. Glaser B, Sheinfeld M, Benmar J, et al. Magnetic resonance imaging of the pituitary gland. Clin Radiol 37:9, 1986.
2. Hawkes RC, Holland GN, Moore WS, et al. The application of NMR to the evaluation of pituitary and juxtasellar tumors. AJNR 4:221, 1983.
3. Huk WJ, Fahlbusch R. Nuclear magnetic imaging of the region of the sella turcica. Neurosurg Rev 8:141, 1985.
4. Karnaze MG, Sartor K, Winthrop JD, et al. Suprasellar lesions: evaluation with MR imaging. Radiology 161:77, 1986.
5. Lee BCP, Deck MDF. Sellar and juxtasellar detection with MR. Radiology 157:143, 1985.
6. Oot R, New PF, Buonano FS, et al. MR imaging of pituitary adenomas using a prototype resistive magnet: preliminary assessment. AJNR 5:131, 1984.
7. Petrykowski WV, Reinwein H, Ostertag C, et al. Asymptomatic primary empty sella in a 14-year-old girl. Comparison of computer tomography and nuclear magnetic resonance imaging. Hormone Res 22:58, 1985.
8. Wehrli FW, MacFall JR, Newton TH. Parameters determining the appearance of NMR images. In Newton TH, Potts DG, eds. Advanced Imaging Techniques. San Anselmo, Calif., Clavadel Press, 1983:81.
9. Bradley WG. Magnetic resonance appearance of flowing blood and cerebrospinal fluid. In Brandt-Zawadski M, Norman D, eds. Magnetic Resonance Imaging of the Central Nervous System. New York, Raven Press, 1987:83.
10. Alverez O, Hyman O. Even-echo MR rephasing in the diagnosis of giant intracranial aneurysm. J Comput Assist Tomogr 10:699, 1986.
11. Bradley WG, Newton TH, Crooks LE. Physical principles of nuclear magnetic resonance. In Newton TH, Potts DG, eds. Advanced Imaging Techniques. San Anselmo, Calif., Clavadel Press, 1983:15.
12. Kucharczyk W, Davis DO, Kelly WM, et al. Pituitary adenomas: high-resolution MR imaging at 1.5 T. Radiology 161:761, 1986.
13. Bilaniuk LT, Zimmerman RA, Wehrli FW, et al. Magnetic resonance imaging of pituitary lesions using 1.0 to 1.5 T field strength. Radiology 153:415, 1984.
14. Daniels DL, Pech P, Mark L, et al. Magnetic resonance imaging of the cavernous sinus. AJR 144:1009, 1985.
15. Kaufman B. Magnetic resonance imaging of the pituitary gland. Radiol Clin North Am 22:795, 1984.
16. Mark L, Pech P, Daniels D, et al. The pituitary fossa: a correlative anatomic and MR study. Radiology 153:453, 1984.
17. Nishimura K, Fujisaw I, Togashi K, et al. Posterior lobe of the pituitary: identification by lack of chemical shift artifact in MR imaging. J Comput Assist Tomogr 10:899, 1986.
18. Kucharczyk W. The pituitary gland and sella turcica. In Brandt-Zawadski M, Norman D, eds. Magnetic Resonance Imaging of the Central Nervous System. New York, Raven Press, 1987:187.
19. Haughton VM, Prost R. Pituitary fossa: chemical shift effect in MR imaging. Radiology 158:461, 1986.
20. Wiener SN, Rzeszotarski MS, Droeg RT, et al. Measurement of pituitary gland height with MR imaging. AJNR 6:717, 1985.
21. Swartz JD, Russell KB, Basile BA, et al. High-resolution computed tomography of the intrasellar contents: normal, near-normal and abnormal. Radiographics 3:229, 1983.

22. Swartz JD, Russell KB, Basile BA, et al. High-resolution computed tomographic appearance of the intrasellar contents in woman of childbearing age. Radiology 147:115, 1983.
23. Gomori JM, Grossman RI, Goldberg HI, et al. Wall of infundibular recess: a CT and MR study. J Comput Assist Tomogr 9:705, 1985.
24. Albert A, Lee BCP, Saint-Louis L, et al. MRI of the optic chiasm and optic pathways. AJNR 7:255, 1985.
25. Daniels DL, Herfkins R, Gager WE, et al. Magnetic resonance imaging of the optic nerves and chiasm. Radiology 152:79, 1984.
26. Landolt AM, Wilson CB. Tumors of the sella and parasellar area in adults. In Youmans JR, ed. Neurologic Surgery: A Comprehensive Reference Guide to the Diagnosis and Management of Neurosurgical Problems, Vol. 5. Philadelphia, W. B. Saunders Co., 1982:3107.
27. Wilson B, Moossy J, Boldrey EB. Pathology of intracranial tumors. In Newton TH, Potts DG, eds. Radiology of the Skull and Brain. Anatomy And Pathology, Vol. 3. St Louis, C. V. Mosby Co., 1977:3016.
28. Hardy J. Transsphenoidal surgery of the normal and pathological pituitary. Clin Neurosurg 16:185, 1969.
29. Burrow GN, Wortzman G, Rewcastle NB, et al. Microadenomas of the pituitary and abnormal sellar tomograms in an unselected autopsy series. N Engl J Med 304:156, 1981.
30. Chambers EF, Turski PA, LaMasters D, et al. Regions of low density in the contrast-enhanced pituitary gland: normal and pathologic process. Radiology 144:109, 1982.
31. Parent AD, Bebin J, Smith RR. Incidental pituitary adenomas. J Neurosurg 54:228, 1981.
32. Pojunas KW, Daniels DL, Williams AL, et al. MR imaging of prolactin-secreting microadenomas. AJNR 7:209, 1986.
33. Weissbuch SS. Explanation and implications of MR signal changes within pituitary adenomas after bromocriptine therapy. AJNR 7:214, 1985.
34. Ahmadi J, North MC, Segall HD, et al. Cavernous sinus invasion by pituitary adenomas. AJR 146:257, 1986.
35. Daniels DL, Pojunas KW, Kilgore DP, et al. MRI of the diaphragm sellae. AJNR 7:765, 1985.
36. Sheldon JJ, Leborgne MJ. Computed tomography in the evaluation of the sella and juxtasella region. In Smith JL, ed. Neuro-Ophthmology Focus 1980. New York, Masson Publishing, USA. 1980:261.
37. Bradley WG Jr. Pathophysiologic correlates of signal alterations. In Brandt-Zawadski M, Norman D, eds. Magnetic Resonance Imaging of the Central Nervous System. New York, Raven Press, 1987:23.
38. Lachtow RE, Ropolloo HM. Radiographic evaluation of the normal pituitary gland. In Taveras JM, Ferucci JT, eds. Radiology Diagnosis-Imaging-Intervention Vol. 3. Philadelphia, J. B. Lippincott Co., 1986.
39. Neelon FA, Goree JA, Lebovitz HE. The primary empty sella: clinical and radiographic characteristics and endocrine function. Medicine 32:73, 1973.
40. Kaufman B. The "empty" sella turcica—a manifestation of the intrasellar subarachnoid space. Radiology 90:931, 1968.
41. Shore RN, DeCherney AH, Stein KM, et al. The empty sella syndrome. Virilization in a 59-year-old woman. JAMA 227:69, 1974.
42. Haughton VM, Rosenbaum AE, Williams AL, et al. Recognizing the empty sella by CT: the infundibulum sign. AJNR 1:527, 1980.
43. Burger PC, Vogel SF. The region of the sella turcica. In Burger PC, Vogel SF, eds. Surgical Pathology of the Nervous System and Its Coverings. New York, John Wiley & Sons, 1976:407.
44. Kaufman B. Pituitary gland and other intrasellar abnormalities. In Taveras JM, Ferucci JT, eds. Radiology Diagnosis-Imaging-Intervention Vol. 3. Philadelphia, J. B. Lippincott Co., 1986.
45. Wallace C, Sheldon JJ. MR imaging of the sellar and juxtasellar regions. In Viamonte M Jr, Baum S, Evan RG, et al., eds. MRI Update Series, Challenges 17 and 18. Vol. 2, Book 9. Princeton, Continuing Professional Education Center, 1987:1.
46. Kaufman B. Perisellar lesions. In Taveras JM, Ferucci JT, eds. Radiology Diagnosis-Imaging-Intervention Vol. 3. Philadelphia, J. B. Lippincott Co., 1986.
47. Zimerman HM. The ten most common types of brain tumor. Semin Roentgenol 6:48, 1971.
48. Fitz CR, Weitzman C, Harwood-Nash DC, et al. Computed tomography in craniopharyngiomas. Radiology 127:687, 1978.
49. Hoff JT, Potuson RH Jr. Craniopharingiomas in children and adults. J Neurosurg 36:299, 1972.
50. Levine HL, Kleefield J, Krishna CVGR. The base of the skull. In Lee HS, Rao GK, eds. Cranial Computed Tomography. New York, McGraw-Hill Book Co., 1983:371.
51. Lee HS, Rao GK. Primary tumors in adults. In Lee HS, Rao GK, eds. Cranial Computed Tomography. New York, McGraw-Hill Book Co., 1983:241.
52. Minckler J. Nervous system. In Anderson WAD, ed. Pathology. St. Louis, CV Mosby Co., 1961:1286.
53. Pribram HW, du Boulay PG. Sella tursica. In Newton TH, Potts DG, eds. Radiology of the Skull and Brain. The Skull. Vol. 1/Book 1. St Louis, C. V. Mosby Co., 1971:357.
54. Brandt-Zawadzki M, Kelly W. Brain tumors. In Brandt-Zawadzki M, Norman D, eds. Magnetic Resonance Imaging of the Central Nervous System. New York, Raven Press, 1987:151.
55. Brandt-Zawadzki M, Norman TH, et al. Magnetic resonance of the brain: the optimal screening technique. Radiology 152:71, 1984.
56. Mawhinney RR, Buckley JH, Holland IM, et al. The value of magnetic resonance imaging in the diagnosis of intracranial meningiomas. Clin Radiol 37:429, 1986.
57. George AE, Russell EJ, Kricheff II. White matter buckling: CT sign of extra-axial intracranial mass. AJR 135:1031, 1980.
58. Zimmerman RD, Fleming CA, St. Louis LA, et al. Magnetic resonance imaging of meningiomas. AJNR 6:149, 1984.
59. Allcock JM. Aneurysms. In Newton TH, Potts DG, eds. Radiology of the Skull and Brain. Angiography. Vol. 2/Book 4. St. Louis, C. V. Mosby Co., 1974:2435.
60. Norman D. Vascular disease: hemorrhage. In Brandt-Zawadzki M, Norman D, eds. Magnetic Resonance Imaging of the Central Nervous System. New York, Raven Press, 1987:209.
61. Bradley WG Jr, Waluch V. Blood flow: magnetic resonance imaging. Radiology 154:443, 1985.
62. Lloyd LA. Gliomas of the optic nerve and chiasm in childhood. In Smith JL, ed. Neuro-Ophthalmology

Update. New York, Masson Publishing, USA, 1977:185.
63. Condon JR, Rose FC. Optic nerve glioma. Br J Ophthalmol 51:703, 1967.
64. Harward-Nash DC. Optic gliomas and pediatric neuroradiology. Radiol Clin North Am 10:83, 1972.
65. Newton TH, Hoyt WF, Glaser JS. Abnormal third ventricle. In Newton TH, Potts DG, eds. Radiology of the Skull and Brain. Ventricles and Cisterns, Vol. 4. St Louis, C. V. Mosby Co., 1978:3440.
66. Lin SR, Bryson MM, Gobien RP, et al. Radiologic findings of hamartomas of the tuber cinereum and hypothalmus. Radiology 127:697, 1978.
67. Mori K, Handa H, Takeuchi J. Hypothalamic hamartoma. J Comput Assist Tomogr 5:519, 1981.
68. Smith J. Chordoma. In Taveras JM, Ferucci JT, eds. Radiology Diagnosis-Imaging-Intervention, Vol. 5. Philadelphia, J. B. Lippincott Co., 1986.
69. McGinnis BD, Davis KR. Radiology of extra-axial posterior fossa tumors. In Taveras JM, Ferucci JT, eds. Radiology Diagnosis-Imaging-Intervention, Vol. 3. Philadelphia, J. B. Lippincott Co., 1986.
70. Kline LB, Acker JD, Post MJD, et al. The cavernous sinus: a computed tomographic study. AJNR 2:299, 1981.
71. Han JS, Huss RG, Benson JE, et al. MR imaging of the skull base. J Comput Assist Tomogr 8:944, 1984.
72. Sartor K, Karnaze JD, Winthrop M, et al. MR imaging in infra-, para-, and retrosellar mass lesions. Neuroradiology 29:19, 1987.
73. Swishchuk LE, Bryan RN. Double midline intracranial atypical teratomas. AJR 122:517, 1974.
74. Zimmerman RA, Bilaniuk LT, Wood JH, et al. Computed tomography of pineal, parapineal, and histologically related tumors. Radiology 137:699, 1980.
75. Kobayashi T, Kageyama N, Kida Y, et al. Unilateral germinomas involving the basal ganglia and thalamus. J Neurosurg 55:55, 1981.

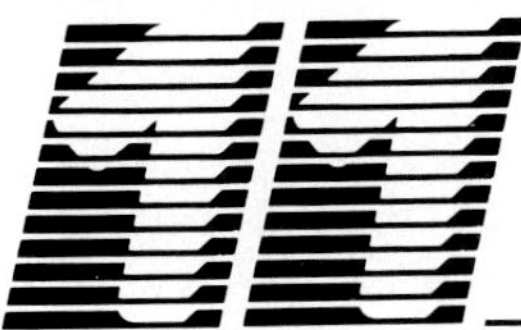

Jeffrey A. Tobias, M.D.

# MRI OF INTRACRANIAL VASCULAR DISEASE WITH EMPHASIS AT LOW AND INTERMEDIATE FIELD STRENGTHS (IMAGES AT 0.35-1.0 T)

Magnetic resonance imaging (MRI) is well suited to the detection and evaluation of vascular diseases of the brain. Its superb contrast sensitivity enables it to detect subtle areas of abnormal signal associated with ischemia. The use of multiple imaging projections can better confirm and localize abnormalities, especially around the cerebral convexities and skull base. The ability of magnetic resonance (MR) to routinely visualize a lesion in two anatomic projections also reduces the problems of partial volume averaging of brain and bone.

Intracerebral hemorrhage is uniquely studied by MRI. The degradation of hemoglobin results in paramagnetic breakdown products that have characteristic MR appearances. Other variables that may influence the MR imaging of blood include the age of the hemorrhage, the pulse sequences utilized (i.e., spin echo, gradient echo), and the magnetic field strength of the MR unit.

MRI permits direct visualization of cerebral vessels and other vascular abnormalities without the use of intravenous contrast agents. The presence or absence of complex MR phenomena, including signal flow void, second-echo rephasing, and flow-related enhancement, yields important diagnostic information regarding blood flow and thrombosis.

## MRI OF INTRACRANIAL HEMORRHAGE AND HEMATOMA (< 0.5 T)

The MR appearance of intracranial hemorrhage is complex and controversial. Multiple factors, including field strength, the age of the hemorrhage, and the pulse sequences used, must be considered in the analysis of the MR image. The presence of various hemoglobin breakdown products (e.g., deoxyhemoglobin and methemoglobin) and the local environment of surrounding brain tissue are important variables. Cerebral edema, macrophage activity, and the integrity of the blood-brain barrier (BBB) also influence the evolving MR appearance of intracerebral hemorrhage.

There has been extensive research on MRI of blood.[1–5] The T1 and T2 relaxation values of blood are directly related to blood pH and inversely related to osmolality and hemoglobin concentration.[6–8] The concentration of both hemoglobin and methemoglobin tends to increase over time as methemoglobin is being formed and the blood clot progressively organizes and dehydrates.[9] The breakdown of hemoglobin (ferrous state) by oxidative denaturation results in methemoglobin (ferric state), which is paramagnetic and shortens the T1 relaxation time of the hematoma.[10] The brain tissue that surrounds a focal collection of extravasated blood becomes acidic in pH owing to the catabolic state of metabolism. The hematoma also acts as an inflammatory focus that causes vasogenic edema within the adjacent brain tissue.

### Acute Intracerebral Hemorrhage

Gomori and co-workers have described in detail the evolution of intracranial hemorrhage (ICH) in clinical high field MR.[11,12] In the acute stage (less than seven days old), the T1-weighted images (TR < 600 msec) reveal the hematoma to be either isointense or slightly hypointense to gray matter (Fig. 11–1*A*). The center of the blood clot has a marked hypointensity on the T2-weighted images (T2WI) at 1.5 tesla (T) (TR > 1500 msec). This hypointensity is present but less obvious in acute hematomas imaged at low field strengths (Fig. 11–1*B*). The central hypointensity has been linked to the formation of intracellular deoxyhemoglobin within intact, extravasated red blood cells (RBCs). The $Fe^{2+}$ deoxyhemoglobin has four unpaired electrons, is paramagnetic, and has been shown to preferentially shorten the T2 relaxation values of protons.[11] The phenomenon of preferential T2 proton relaxation enhancement (PRE) seen with acute intracerebral hemorrhage theoretically increases with the square of the magnetic field. It also increases with the concentration of intracellular deoxyhemoglobin and intracellular methemoglobin.[11] The effect disappears after lysis of the red blood cell.[13] Other investigators suggest that the measured relaxation times of hemoglobin and its breakdown products (deoxyhemoglobin, oxyhemoglobin, methemoglobin, and ferritin) do not adequately account for the extremely low signal seen

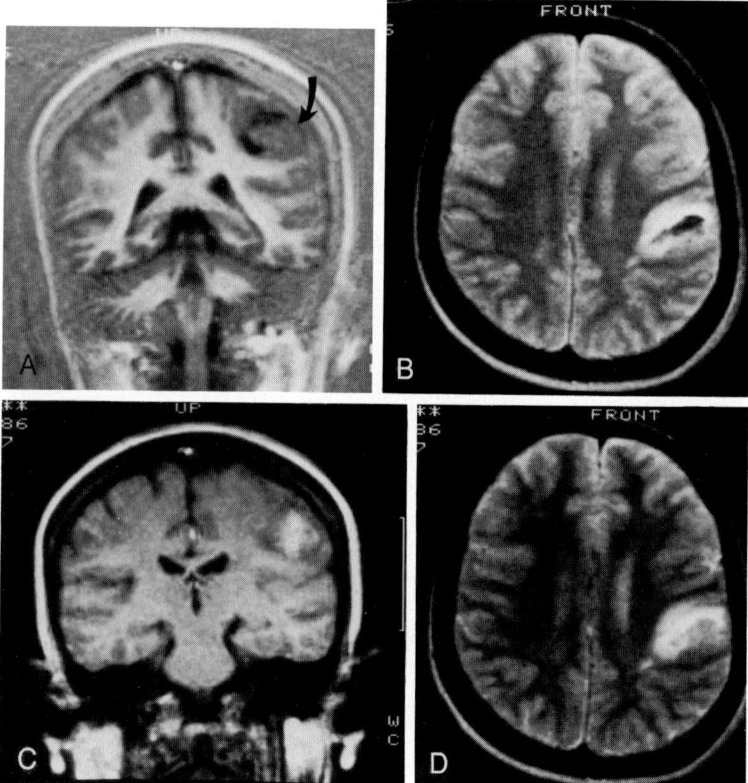


**Figure 11–1. Acute-subacute cortical hemorrhagic infarction.** A 35-year-old woman with a one-day history of dysphasia. CT on admission (not shown) revealed a left parietal hemorrhagic cortical infarct with edema (0.5 T).

*A*, Coronal T1WI (IR TI 400/TR 2100/TE 35). *B*, Axial T2WI (SE TR 2000/TE 80). *C*, Coronal T1WI (SE TR 500/TE 16). *D*, Axial T2WI (SE TR 2000/TE 80).

Initial MR (day of admission). There are no hyperintense areas demonstrated within the isointense acute hemorrhage (curved black arrow in *A*) on the T1WI. The surrounding edema is hypointense. The cortical hemorrhage is moderately hypointense to adjacent cortex on the T2WI *(B)* owing to deoxyhemoglobin formation. The surrounding hyperintense signal is due to edema. On a followup MR (three days later), the subacute hemorrhage has become hyperintense to cortex on T1WI as methemoglobin is formed *(C)*. The blood is now isointense to cortex on the T2WI, with continued hyperintense edema surrounding it.

on T2WI at high field strengths.[14] Many investigators have emphasized the contribution of blood clot retraction, with its associated increase in hematocrit, toward this low signal on spin-echo T2WI.

Although the preferential T2 proton relaxation effect is more noticeable at higher field strengths when utilizing conventional spin-echo sequences, it has also been observed at lower field strengths (0.5 T and 0.6 T).[15] The use of specially modified partial saturation (PS) pulse sequences with gradient echoes has permitted even more rapid detection of magnetic susceptibility effects associated with acute hemorrhage on intermediate field images.[15] Gradient echo sequences appear to be much more sensitive than conventional spin-echo (SE) sequences in detecting magnetic susceptibility phenomena, attributed to the paramagnetic properties of deoxyhemoglobin (acute hematomas) and hemosiderin (nonacute hematomas). The spin-echo pulse sequences tend to minimize the effects of magnetic field inhomogeneity and are thus less sensitive than the gradient-echo sequences in demonstrating them.[16]

Using these sequences, it will therefore be possible for a lower field strength MR to detect acute hemorrhage as well as a high field unit using the spin-echo T2WI.[16] This can be done because the gradient-echo sequences are sensitive to minor inhomogeneities in the local magnetic fields caused by the paramagnetic agents associated with hemorrhage. The subtle variations in the local magnetic fields in and around the hematoma affect the diffusion of protons through the region and diminish the spin-echo signal intensity on strongly T2-weighted images.

Approximately 24 to 48 hours after hematoma formation, cerebral edema develops in the adjacent brain. It is visible as an area of either isointensity or slight hypointensity on T1WI (Fig. 11–1*A*), and high intensity on T2WI (Fig. 11–1*B*). This vasogenic edema is noted at all field strengths and is often visualized on CT studies as hypodensity in the white matter surrounding the hematoma. The edema resolves slowly within the following weeks.

The appearance of hyperacute and early acute intracranial hemorrhage is not yet widely documented. Early reports suggest high signal intensity on T2WI. Zimmerman and co-workers reported that hematomas studied between 12 and 24 hours posthemorrhage appeared mildly hyperintense on short TR/short TE scans and markedly hyperintense on long TR (with intermediate and long TE) spin-echo sequences.[17] An intracerebral hematoma that developed during an MR examination was heterogeneous in appearance with slightly high signal on saturation recovery images. The hyperacute hemorrhage appeared as moderately low intensity on inversion recovery and as high signal on spin-echo T2WI.[18]

## Subacute and Chronic Intracranial Hematoma

After approximately one week (three to nine days), the periphery of the hematoma (located within the ring of edema) will develop a high signal intensity on the T1WI, which is followed by a similar high signal rim on the T2WI (Figs. 11–2 and 11–3).[19] This hyperintensity progresses to fill in the subacute hematoma from the periphery to the center over the course of several weeks. The high-intensity appearance of the hematoma may persist for over one year. The appearance of the high-intensity ring on the T1WI is largely due to the paramagnetic effect of intracellular methemoglobin, which shortens the T1 relaxation values of the hematoma. It has been observed regularly on low, intermediate, and high magnetic fields. There is also evidence that the high spin density of intracranial subacute hemorrhage may contribute significantly to its hyperintense appearance on T1WI.[20]

The high signal intensity of the subacute hematoma on T2WI occurs after lysis of the RBC with release of intracellular methemoglobin and deoxyhemoglobin into the extracellular space. The homogeneous distribution of these substances removes the local magnetic gradients that caused the shortening of T2 relaxation times. This allows the intrinsic prolonged T2 relaxation times and high proton density of dilute blood to show as high signal on the T2WI. Prior to RBC lysis, intracellular methemoglobin and deoxyhemoglobin cause preferential shortening of T2 proton relaxation. The high signal intensity of evolving hematomas is routinely seen on T1WI before its appearance on the T2WI. This suggests that intracellular methemoglobin (causing short T1 relaxation) is

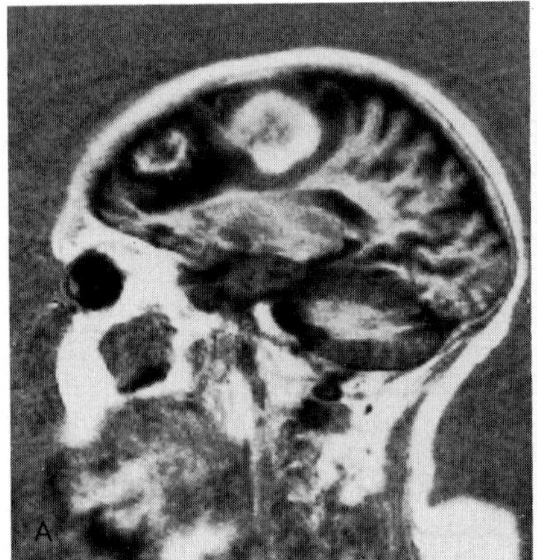


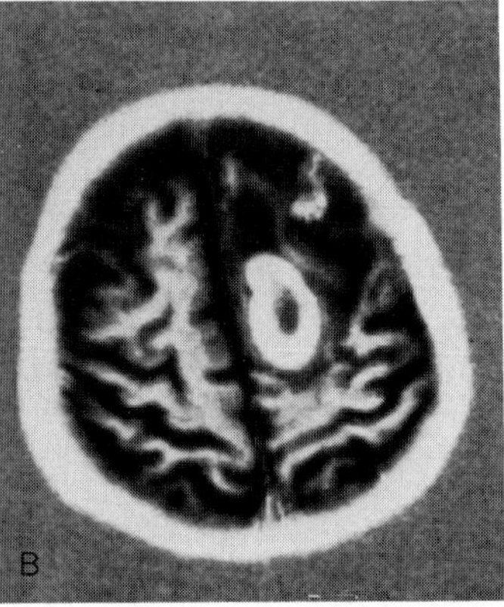


**Figure 11–2. Multiple subacute left frontoparietal hematomas.** Severe head trauma occurred four days before the MR study (0.35 T). *A,* Sagittal T1WI (IR TI 400/TR 2100/TE 35). *B,* Axial T1WI (IR TI 400/TR 2100/TE 35). The typical ring of high signal on T1WI is present in the periphery of these subacute hematomas.

formed prior to the lysis of the RBC, which releases extracellular methemoglobin and prolongs the T2 relaxation within the hematoma.

At approximately one week, a ring of markedly low signal appears in the cerebral parenchyma, immediately adjacent to the hematoma, on the T2WI (Fig. 11–4). This ring is isointense or slightly hypointense on the T1WI and was noted to appear after the hematoma periphery had become hyperintense on both T1 and T2WI. It may persist indefinitely. The appearance of this low signal area on T2WI suggests the presence of a

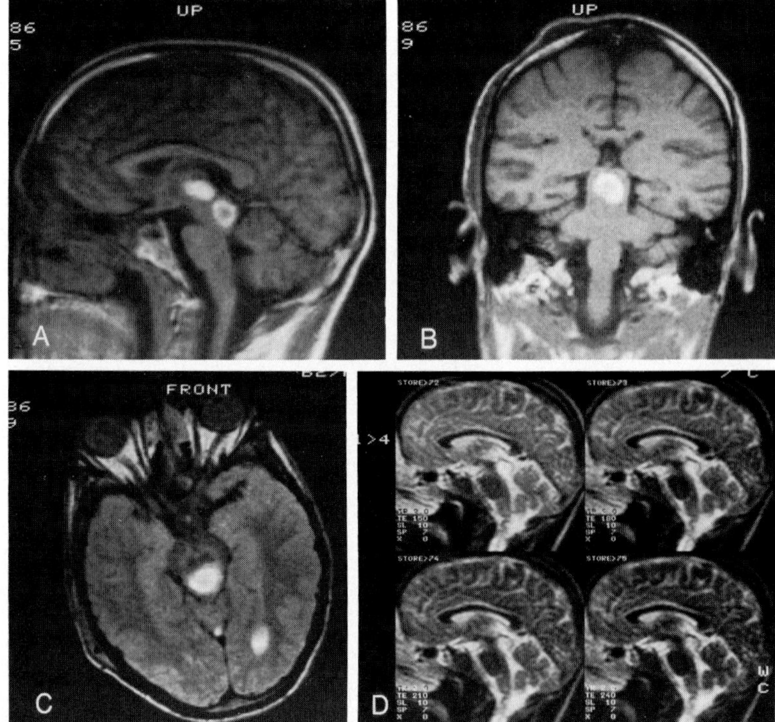


**Figure 11–3. Brain stem hemorrhages.** Spontaneous brain stem hemorrhages in a 35-year-old man (0.5 T). *A,* Sagittal T1WI (SE TR 500/TE 16). *B,* Coronal T1WI (SE TR 500/TE 16). *C,* Axial N(H)WI (SE TR 2000/TE 35). *D,* Sagittal T2WI (SE TR 2000/TE 150, 280, 210, 240).

One week posthemorrhage, two subacute hematomas are seen in the dorsal midbrain on the T1WI. A rim of high signal surrounds the more recent hematoma. The older, cephalad hematoma has filled in completely. The hematomas have high signals on the T2WI, with progressively longer TEs ("echo train") owing to long T2 relaxations. The lesions become less conspicuous as their signals approach that of surrounding CSF in the quadrigeminal ciŝtern.

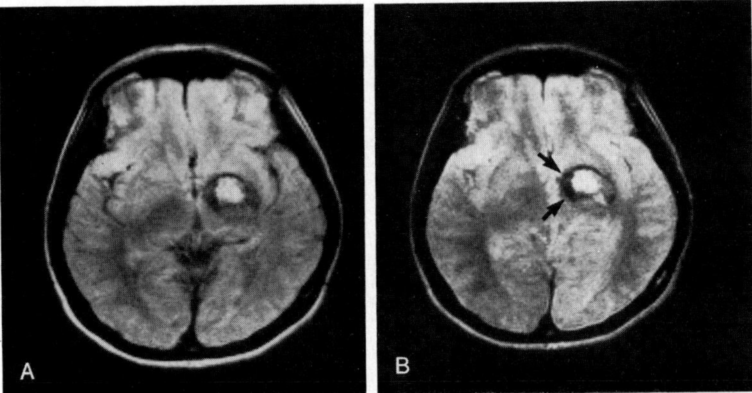


**Figure 11–4. Chronic thalamic hematoma with hemosiderin ring.** Spontaneous hematoma in left thalamus occurred one year before the MR study. CT (not shown) at time of MRI revealed a slightly hyperdense area without significant mass effect or enhancement (0.5 T).

*A,* Axial N(H)WI (TR 2000/TE 35). A thin rim of mildly decreased signal (hemosiderin) surrounds the centrally located hyperintense region of chronic hematoma. *B,* Axial T2WI (TR 2000/TE 80). The hemosiderin rim (arrows) becomes broader and more hypointense. The central hematoma remains hyperintense on all sequences. There is no surrounding high signal due to edema as would be seen with a more recent hemorrhage.

preferential T2 proton relaxation effect from a paramagnetic agent. It is thought that this agent is hemosiderin within the macrophages that are in the capsular rim surrounding and resorbing the hematoma. Other studies, however, have shown this low signal ring to be present, even in acute hematomas, when gradient echo sequences are used instead of conventional spin echoes.[16] This observation suggests that the hypointense rings around the hematomas, on T2WI, are not always due to hemosiderin deposition. They may be due in part to subtle differences in local magnetic fields between the hematomas and normal brain (i.e., magnetic susceptibility effects).[16] Similar rims of low signal have been consistently seen surrounding abscesses and occasionally around metastatic foci.[17]

In the chronic stage (longer than one month), the hematoma appears bright on all sequences (Fig. 11–4). The rim of brain directly adjacent to the hematoma is isointense on T1WI and hypointense on the T2WI (owing to the hemosiderin capsule). The vasogenic edema in the adjacent white matter has usually resolved by this time.

In the presence of an atypical-appearing hematoma, the possibility of hemorrhage within an underlying neoplasm should always be considered (Figs. 11–5 and 11–6). A markedly heterogenous signal intensity, delayed appearance of expected signal intensity changes within the evolving hematoma, or evidence of associated nonhemorrhagic tumor tissue may be clues to the correct diagnosis.[21] Persistent or prominent white matter edema and the absence of a well-formed hemosiderin ring have also been described in association with hemorrhagic neoplasms.[21] In many cases, only one or two of these characteristics may be present, and it should be remembered that none of them are pathognomonic for hemorrhagic neoplasm (Fig. 11–7). Likewise, an intracranial hemorrhage with a homogeneous appearance and peripheral rim of hypointensity is not necessarily nonmalignant in origin. Further characterization of the hemorrhagic lesion may sometimes be aided by correlation with a contrast-enhanced CT or possibly by MR with paramagnetic contrast to evaluate the integrity of the blood-brain barrier.

## CEREBRAL ISCHEMIA AND INFARCTION (< 0.5 T)

MRI is unsurpassed in the detection of cerebral ischemia. It is especially advantageous in the examination of the brain stem and posterior fossa, in which CT is limited by beam-hardening artifacts arising from adjacent bone. The superior contrast sensitivity of MRI permits earlier detection of ischemic changes than on CT (especially within the first 48 hours).[22–24] Experimental models have shown that MR can detect ischemia within 30 minutes to two hours of the insult, possibly while it is still reversible (i.e., be-

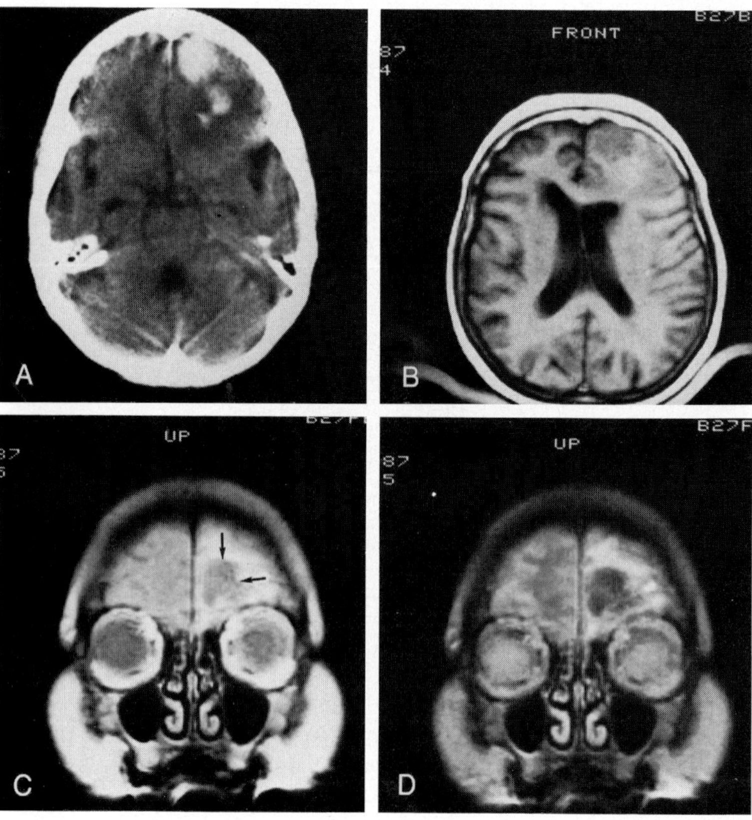


**Figure 11–5. Acute hemorrhagic metastasis from lung carcinoma.** MR study performed one day following CT (0.5 T).

*A,* On axial CT (noncontrast), there is hemorrhage within a metastatic lesion in the patient's left frontal lobe, with surrounding edema and mass effect. Study obtained on the day of admission. *B,* Axial T1WI (SE TR 300/TE 17). The acute left frontal hemorrhage has not yet formed the hyperintense elements associated with methemoglobin. There is mass effect effacing the adjacent cortical sulci. *C,* Coronal N(H)WI (TR 2000/TE 35). The area of acute hemorrhage (arrows) appears mildly hypointense to cortical sulci. There is a hyperintense rim of surrounding edema. *D,* Coronal T2WI (TR 2000/TE 80). The acute hemorrhage becomes hypointense on this sequence due to its short T2 values. High-signal edema is again seen in the periphery.

fore infarction).[23] Shifts of intracellular and extracellular water result in changes in cerebral water content. These regions are seen as foci of bright signal on T2WI. It is for this reason that T2WI are the most sensitive images for the detection of cerebral infarcts (Figs. 11–8 and 11–9).[25] The ischemic lesions are usually less apparent on T1, where they appear hypointense, owing to prolongation of T1 relaxation (Fig. 11–10). The ischemic abnormalities on T1 sequences have been found within six hours of the onset of symptoms.[26] Unfortunately, abnormal areas of long T1 and T2 values may be seen in many conditions that cause cerebral edema (e.g., neoplasms, trauma, and infections) as well as in demyelinating processes and gliosis. They are not specific for either ischemia or cerebral infarction.

The evaluation of cerebrovascular disease requires a screening study of the brain with T2WI. Routine imaging in the axial and coronal projection is often helpful in confirming and localizing lesions. Any regions of abnormal increased T2 signal can then be evaluated in the appropriate imaging plane for high signal on T1WI. The presence of high-signal regions (short T1 areas) may indicate the presence of methemoglobin within subacute or chronic hemorrhage. The possibility of high signal on T1WI owing to atypical intracranial marrow deposition (e.g., ossified falx cerebri) or within intracranial lesions with fat content (dermoids, lipoma) should also be considered.

### Hemorrhagic Cortical Infarction

The appearance of hemorrhagic cortical infarction (HCI) has been described on high-field MRI by Hect-Leavitt et al.[27] In the acute stage, areas of cortical hemorrhage have mildly decreased signal intensity on T2WI (Fig. 11–1). This is felt to be related to the presence of deoxyhemoglobin within the hemorrhage. As with intracerebral hematomas, this phenomenon is more apparent at higher magnetic field strengths. A surrounding subcortical area of high signal is due to cerebral edema, which will not be present in the chronic stages.

Hemorrhagic infarcts may appear acutely

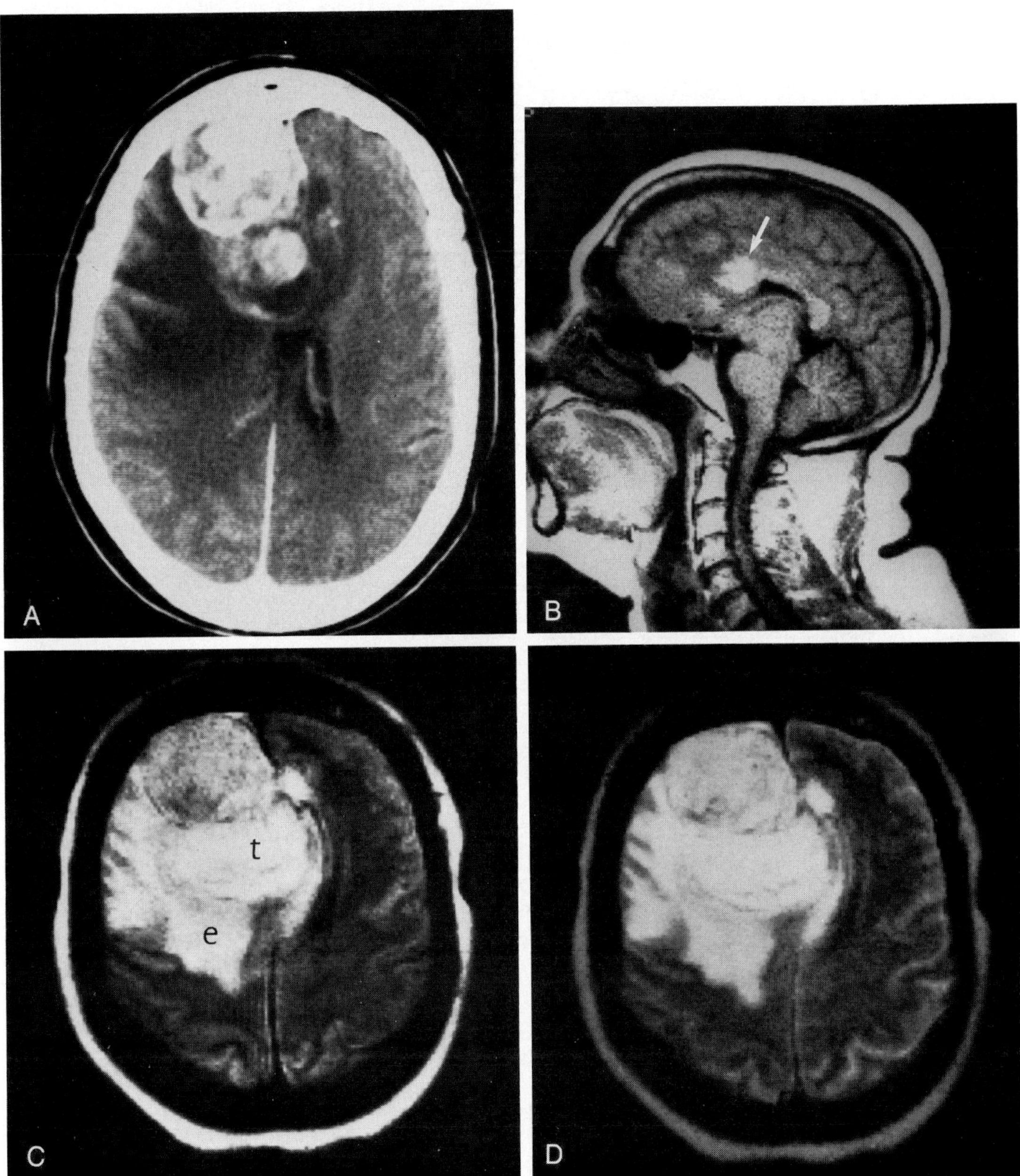


**Figure 11–6. Glioblastoma multiforme with subacute hemorrhage.** (0.5 T). *A,* CT (with contrast). Inhomogeneous ring-enhancing right frontal lobe mass crossing the midline with marked mass effect and surrounding edema. Hyperdense areas were present in the noncontrast study (not shown). *B,* Sagittal T1WI (SE TR 300/TE 17). The posterior aspect of the glioma has high signal owing to subacute hemorrhage (arrow). The invasion of the genu of the corpus callosum is well demonstrated. *C,* Axial N(H)WI (TR 2000/TE 35). The edema (e) and hyperintense elements of the tumor (t) posteriorly are not well differentiated on this sequence because they both have similar signals. *D,* Axial T2WI (TR 2000/TE 80). The glioma has higher signal intensity (longer T2 relaxation) posteriorly owing to the cystic, necrotic, and hemorrhagic components.

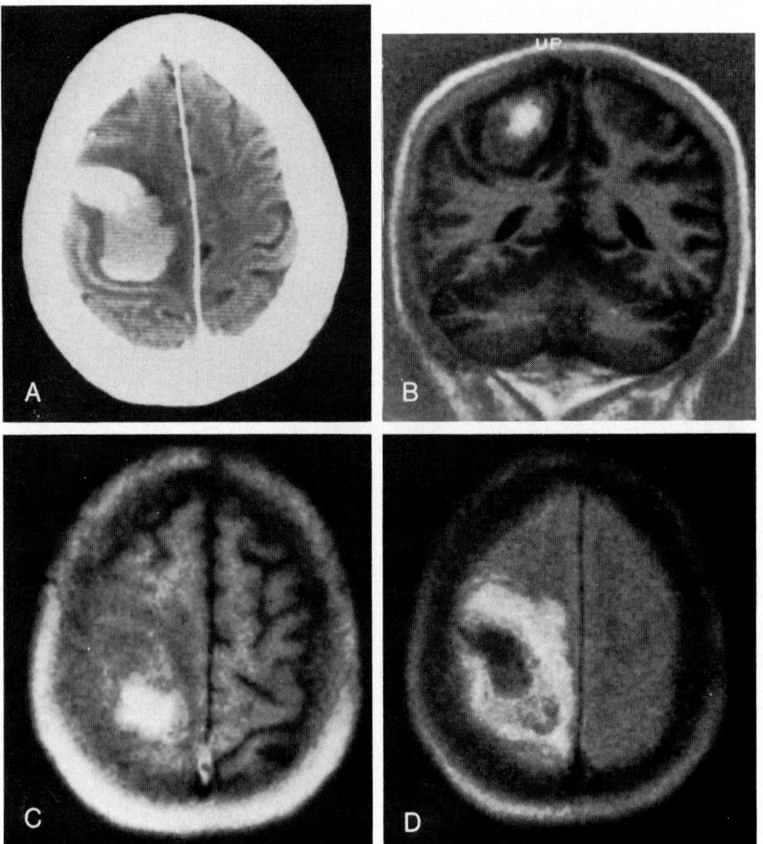


**Figure 11–7. Atypical intracerebral hemorrhage (amyloid angiopathy).** An elderly woman with a history of breast carcinoma presents in the emergency department with an acute neurologic deficit. The intracerebral hematoma was surgically evacuated (0.35 T).

*A,* CT (noncontrast). There is a right parietal convexity hematoma surrounded by edema. The hematoma is not homogeneous. The posterior area appears less dense (less recent) than the anterior portion. *B,* Coronal T1WI (IR TI 400/TR 2000/TE 35). The central portion of the hematoma has become hyperintense. Typically, the peripheral portion of a hematoma should become bright first with the high signal filling towards the center in time. The appearance suggested the possibility of a central hemorrhage within a neoplastic mass. *C,* Axial T1WI (SE TR 500/TE 16). The hematoma does not have a well-defined hyperintense rim. The anterior portion is not yet hyperintense because it is a more recent area of hemorrhage. *D,* Axial T2WI (TR 2000/TE 80). The hypointense anterior portion of the hematoma is due to acute hemorrhage with subacute hemorrhage present posteriorly. A multifocal hemorrhage with old and new areas of bleeding is suggestive of a neoplasm but is not an unusual feature of amyloid angiopathy.

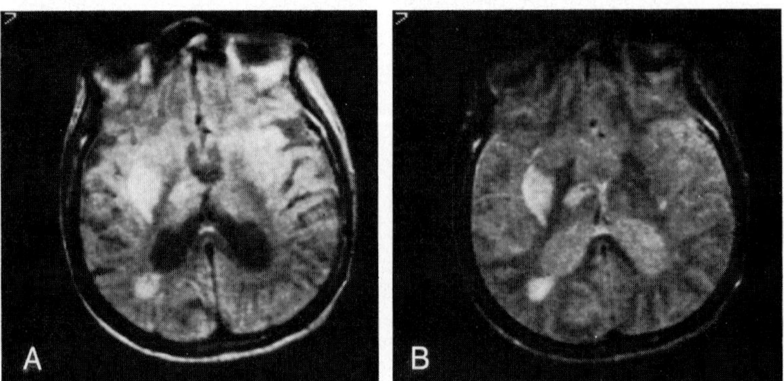


**Figure 11–8. Multiple nonhemorrhagic cerebral infarctions.** An elderly man with multiple cerebrovascular accidents according to the history and a CT (0.5 T).

*A,* Axial N(H)WI (TR 2000/TE 35). *B,* Axial T2WI (TR 2000/TE 80). There are multiple areas of abnormal increased signal due to cerebral infarctions. These lesions become brighter and more conspicuous on the T2WI *(B)*. The largest is located in the right basal ganglia. Smaller ischemic lesions are also present in the right periatrial region and the thalamus. There were no hyperintense areas to suggest associated subacute hemorrhage on T1WI (not shown).

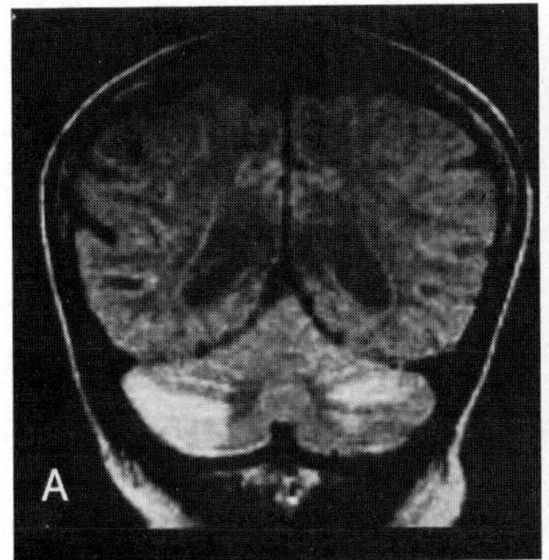


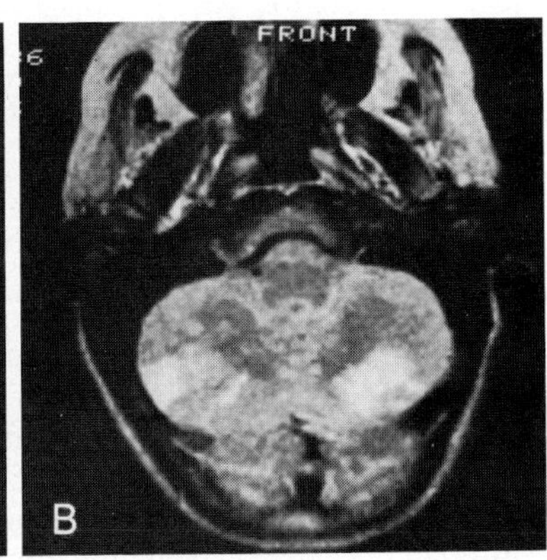


**Figure 11–9. Acute nonhemorrhagic cerebellar infarctions.** A 70-year-old hypertensive woman with a sudden onset of ataxia. CT study on admission was negative for cerebral infarction (0.5 T). *A,* Coronal N(H)WI (TR 2000/TE 35). *B,* Axial T2WI (TR 2000/TE 80). The bilateral hyperintense areas are due to acute cerebellar infarcts that are without mass effect.

isointense to normal cortex on the T1WI. During the subacute stage, the T1WI will begin exhibiting high signal followed by high signal on the T2WI. In the chronic stage, on the T2WI the cortical hemorrhage may exhibit low intensity that may persist indefinitely owing to the presence of hemosiderin. There may be associated cortical atrophy around an old infarct that lacks mass effect and is surrounded by CSF intensity signal. The T1WI shows the old cortical hemorrhage as isointense with normal cortex or, more commonly, as an area of hypointense CSF signal at porencephalic sites.

Cortical hemorrhagic infarcts have reportedly demonstrated relatively less hypointensity than similar-appearing parenchymal hematomas on T2WI.[27] A possible explanation for this observation is the relatively higher local $PO_2$ in cortical infarcts owing to luxury perfusion and revascularization. This circumstance would result in a smaller percentage of deoxyhemoglobin within the extravasated red cells. With less paramagnetic deoxyhemoglobin, there would be less associated preferential T2 proton relaxation enhancement (PRE) present and less hypointensity within a HCI on T2WI. The T2 relaxation effects of hemosiderin are not related to local $PO_2$ but are proportional to the strength of the magnetic field.[28]

Hemorrhage within cerebral infarcts, including watershed infarcts, embolic events, vasculitis, and reperfusion of thrombotic infarcts, is more often seen in clinical settings.[29] Hemorrhagic cortical infarcts may also be associated with hypertension, anticoagulation, and compression of the posterior cerebral arteries owing to uncal herniation.[27]

The high sensitivity of MR has permitted the unparalleled detection of ischemic white matter lesions in the aging brain.[30] Pathologic correlation has shown that many of these areas correspond to clinically silent white matter infarcts, ischemic demyelination, and isomorphic gliosis in otherwise normal brains from elderly patients. Initial clinical experience has not shown a strong correlation between the MR appearance of periventricular lesions and the presence or absence of dementia.[31] Therefore the pres-

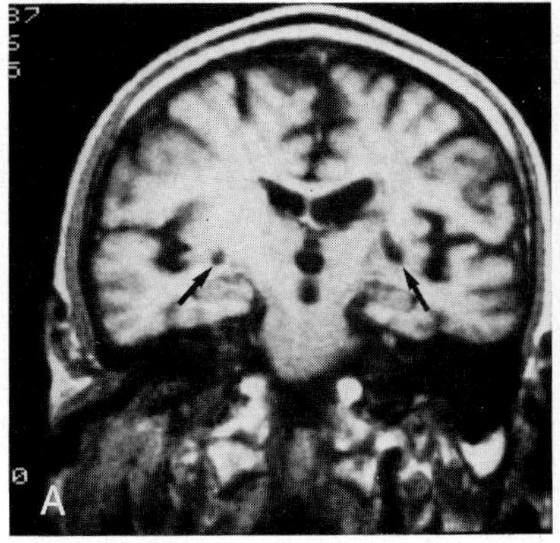


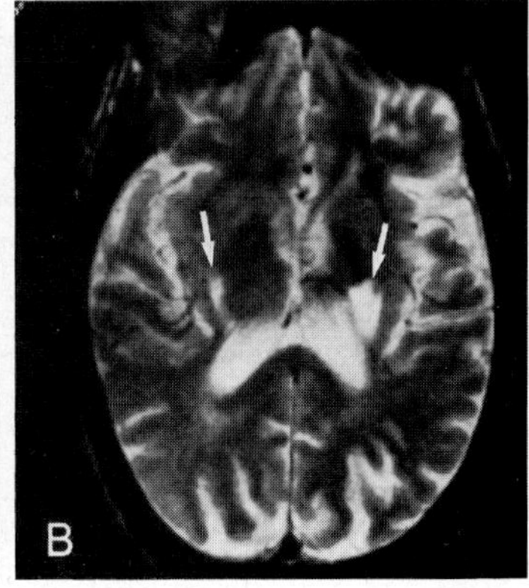


**Figure 11–10. Chronic bilateral infarcts.** (1.0 T). *A,* Coronal T1WI (SE TR 500/TE 17). The chronic infarcts are hypointense (arrows) owing to their long T1 relaxation values. The left (to reader's right) body of the lateral ventricle is dilated as a result of ipsilateral central atrophy. *B,* Axial T2WI (TR 2500/TE 80). Both infarcts exhibit very long T2 values with high intensities that rival that of the adjacent CSF. These are probably areas of porencephaly or microcyst formation.

ence of severe periventricular white matter lesions in the aged is not pathognomonic for dementia, symptomatic infarction, or demyelination.[32]

## Pathophysiology of Cerebral Ischemia

The ability of MR to detect an ischemic lesion in the brain is largely related to changes in water content with the development of cerebral edema. The first changes are related to cytotoxic edema, which is followed later by vasogenic edema.[33] Cytotoxic edema is due to a series of biochemical breakdowns leading to an inability to produce adequate ATP. There is loss of cell membrane integrity, disruption of the cell's sodium pump with influx of extracellular sodium, and loss of intracellular potassium, leading to osmotic gradients that permit extracellular water to move intracellularly. The formation of excess lactate and free fatty acid also leads to increased intracellular water content in the first 30 minutes following the ischemic insult. These shifts of water within the cell are detectable by MRI as areas of long T1 and T2. These abnormalities may be seen even in the absence of increased net tissue protons and prior to the breakdown in blood-brain barrier.[34] In most clinical instances, when there is preservation of collateral blood flow to the infarct, cytotoxic edema is followed by vasogenic edema. Vasogenic edema results from the loss of vascular autoregulation, with hydrostatic and osmotic gradients leading to a net movement of fluid from the vascular space into the extracellular and then the intracellular space. When endothelial damage occurs (usually 12 to 24 hours after the ischemia) there is breakdown of the blood-brain barrier

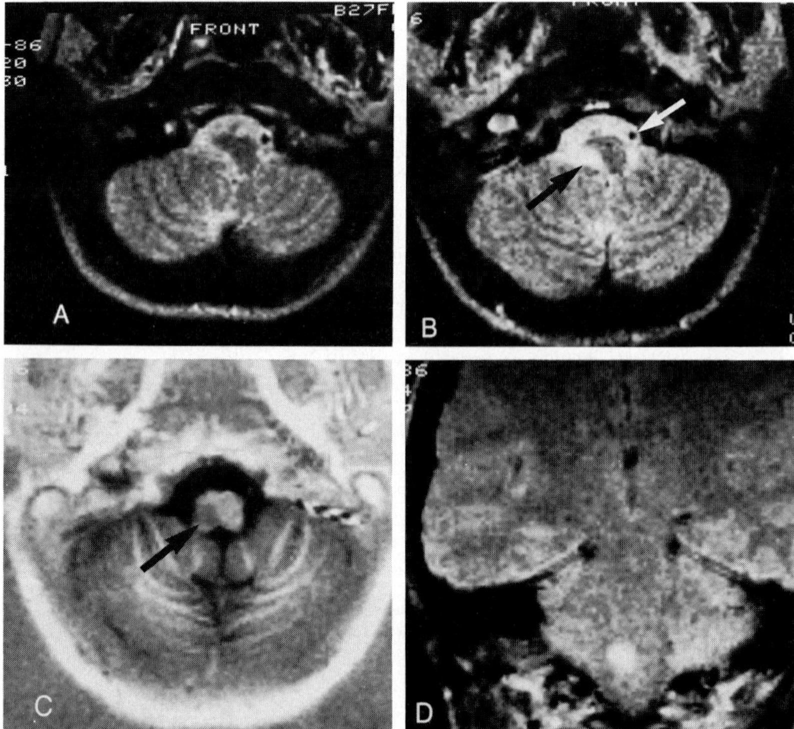


**Figure 11–11. Acute lateral medullary nonhemorrhagic infarct.** A 27-year-old woman with acute onset of neurologic deficit typical of a Wallenberg's syndrome. CT of the posterior fossa on the day of admission was negative (0.5 T).

*A*, Axial T2WI (TR 2000/TE 90) obtained 24 hours after the onset of the patient's symptoms. *B*, Axial T2WI (TR 2000/TE 80), repeated at 72 hours. *C*, Axial T1WI (IR TI 400/TR 2100/TE 35) at 72 hours. *D*, Coronal N(H)WI (TR 2000/TE 35) at 72 hours.

*A*, Initial MR study: the right lateral border of the medulla is poorly defined, but the infarct is not yet well visualized on T2WI. Follow-up MR at 72 hours: The infarct is now well visualized as a discrete, hyperintense region in the right lateral aspect of the medulla (black arrow in *B*) on both the N(H)WI and T2WI. The infarct is hypointense on the T1WI (arrow in *C*). Note that normal signal void is demonstrated within the patent left vertebral artery (white arrow in *B*). Flow void within the right vertebral artery was never visualized.

with additional leakage of fluid, proteins, and other macromolecules into the extravascular space. All of these factors lead to shifts or increases in cerebral water content that are readily detected by magnetic resonance imaging.

### Factors Affecting Detection of Ischemic Lesions

Difficulty in visualizing an infarct may be due either to its small size, the inappropriate timing of the MR study, or both. Several of the factors that affect lesion detectability may be influenced by the imaging parameters selected. The proper choice of imaging factors is especially critical on low field strength units.

Small infarcts may sometimes be highly symptomatic, yet difficult to detect. The high signal associated with an acute infarct on T2WI is due to the development of cytotoxic and, later, vasogenic edema that increase in intensity over time. An acute lesion may not be visualized if there has been insufficient time for that edema to develop. An infarct that is not detected in the first 24 hours is sometimes readily apparent when the MR is repeated at 48 to 72 hours (Fig. 11–11).

Attempts to visualize small brain stem lesions with high-resolution techniques (thin-section images and 256 × 256 matrix) are not always advantageous and may actually make it more difficult to detect certain infarcts. This is especially true in low field strength MR systems (0.35 T) in which there are marginal signal-to-noise ratio (SNR) characteristics. Work by Bradley and colleagues has shown that the detection of small, low-contrast lesions may be improved at 0.35 T by emphasizing maximum signal/noise through the use of 128 × 128 instead of 256 × 256 matrices and by in-

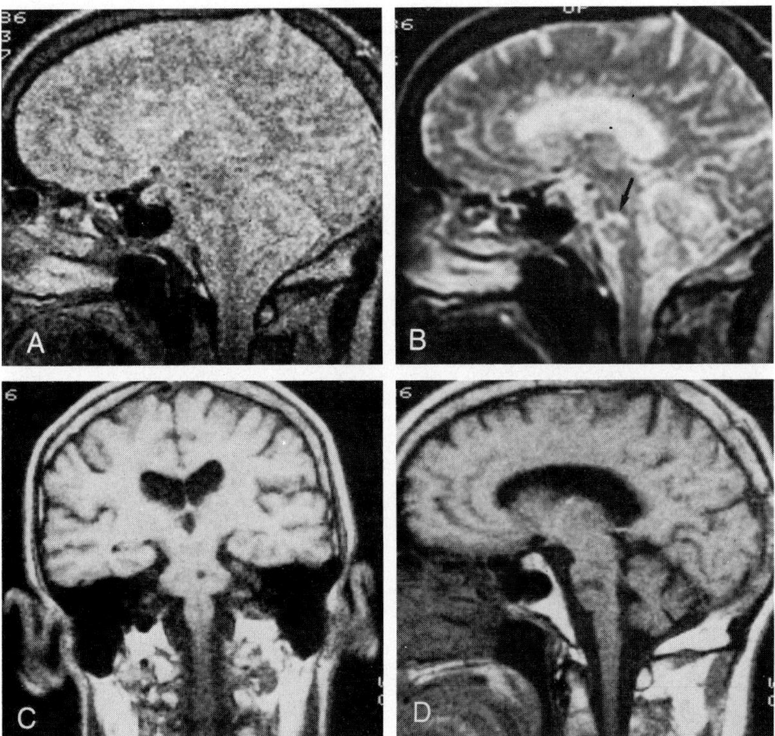


**Figure 11–12. Importance of imaging parameters at low field strength: brain stem infarct.** (0.35 T). *A,* Sagittal T2WI (TR 1500/TE 70), 5-mm thickness, 256 × 256 matrix. *B,* Sagittal T2WI (TR 1500/TE 105), 10-mm thickness, 128 × 256 matrix. *C,* Coronal T1WI (SE TR 300/TE 16), 5-mm thickness, 256 × 256. *D,* Sagittal T1WI (SE TR 300/TE 16), 5-mm thickness, 256 × 256.

The standard thin-section T2WI (5-mm and $256^2$ matrix) images are too noisy on this low-field image *(A)* to confidently distinguish the brain stem infarct from background noise. The lesion is more conspicuous (arrow in *B*), even with thicker slices (10-mm), because the selected imaging parameters have improved the overall contrast-to-noise ratio of the image. The coronal *(C)* and sagittal *(D)* T1WIs confirm the presence of this lesion.

creasing the number of acquisitions.[35] High spatial resolution techniques result in fewer resonating protons within smaller voxel volumes. The relative decrease in signal reduces the scan's signal/noise. The net result may be a decrease in the resolving power of the scan and a greater likelihood that a small infarct will be missed. Although the thin sections and $256^2$ matrix provide better spatial resolution, they may not adequately separate an abnormality from the surrounding background noise. On occasion, the use of 10-mm echo train sequences (progressively longer TE images, with 128 matrix size) may sometimes succeed in detecting small lesions not seen with 5-mm thin images (Fig. 11–12).

In high field strength MR units (1.5 T), there is much better overall signal-to-noise ratio than on a low field strength unit. Therefore thin image sections and large matrix sizes can be obtained without a significant degradation in resolving power. Small infarctions within the medulla as well as ipsilateral vertebral occlusions have been reported on high field strength MRI (Fig. 11–13).[36]

## The Use of Gadolinium-DTPA in Infarcts

Gadolinium-diethylenetriaminepenta-acetic acid (Gd-DTPA) is a rare earth metal chelate whose use in cerebral ischemia is being investigated in clinical and experimental settings. Various other compounds such as Gd-DOTA and nonionic Gd-DO3A are also being developed. The paramagnetic agent strongly enhances proton relaxation and causes shortening of T1 values within ischemic areas in which it accumulates. It does not change the T2 values of infarcts significantly.

The role of intravenous paramagnetic agents in MR imaging is still unclear. Early clinical investigation, however, has suggested certain trends.[37, 38] Subacute infarcts that were poorly seen on T1WI were better

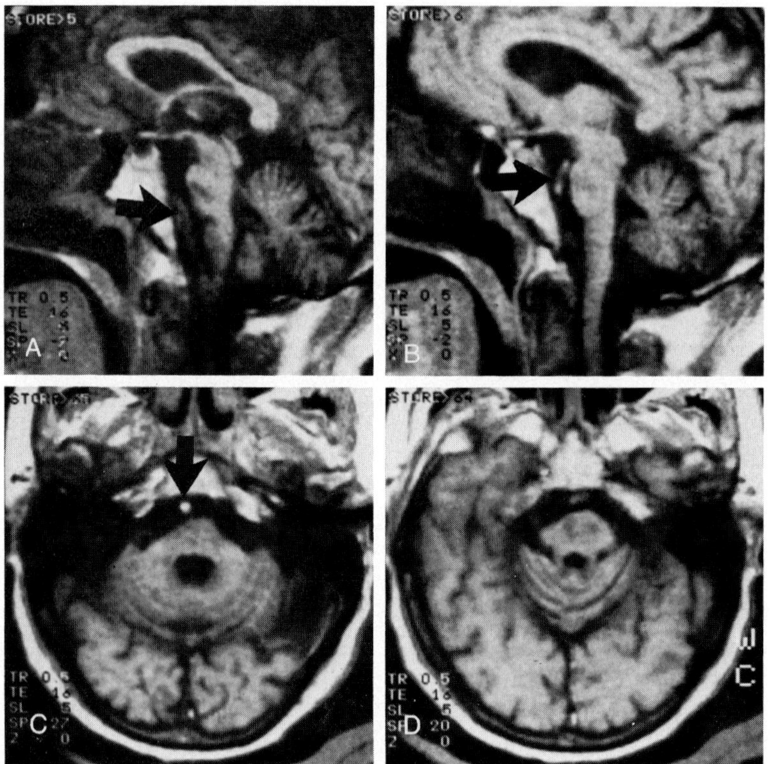


**Figure 11–13. Brain stem infarction with basilar artery thrombosis.** (0.5 T). *A*, Sagittal T1WI (SE TR 500/TE 16). *B*, Sagittal T1WI (SE TR 500/TE 16). *C*, Axial T1WI (SE TR 500/TE 16). *D*, Axial T1WI (SE TR 500/TE 16). There is a persistent signal arising from the basilar artery within the prepontine cistern on all T1WI owing to intraluminal thrombus (arrows). An associated hypointense pontine infarct is also present.

visualized, matching the contrast-enhanced appearance of the CT scans. Enhancement in human subjects was not seen until several days after the infarct occurred, although experimental studies have shown enhancement within 16 to 24 hours of ischemic change.[36] In many cases, the degree of enhancement on MRI was greater than that seen on CT. Enhancement in asymptomatic and periventricular lesions and chronic asymptomatic lacunar infarcts was not seen.[38] The Gd-DTPA enhancement was maximal in the subacute and late infarcts.

The appearance of enhancement is related to the leakage of Gd-DTPA through a damaged blood-brain barrier in vessels leading to the infarct during the phase of vasogenic edema. If there is no collateral circulation to the infarct (only cytotoxic edema) or collapse of the capillary bed from edema within the infarct, then Gd-DPTA cannot reach the site and extravasate. In these cases, which are probably uncommon, there is no T1 enhancement within the infarct. However, the T2WI still shows the shifts in water content (edema) as a bright signal within the infarct. Gadolinium does not appear to visualize flow in the capillary space as well as iodinated contrast does in CT. Therefore Gd-DTPA may not reveal perfusion abnormalities such as luxury perfusion, only areas of breakdown in blood-brain barrier.[37]

While T2W images are sometimes more sensitive than Gd-DTPA–enhanced T1WI, they are still nonspecific. Gd-DTPA–enhanced T1WI offer the possibility of adding specificity, similar to that of contrast-enhanced CT, in characterizing areas of abnormal T2 signal. The presence of Gd-DTPA enhancement signifies a lesion with breakdown in the BBB, and the pattern of enhancement may help differentiate a clinically insignificant ischemic lesion from neoplastic lesions. MR is probably more sensitive than CT in demonstrating subacute breakdown of the BBB and may possibly have prognostic value in the evaluation of ischemic lesions and their future potential for hemorrhage.

### Limitations of MRI in Ischemic Disease

Among the current limitations of MR imaging is its inability to easily determine acute from chronic infarcts. Both acute and nonacute bland infarcts may demonstrate areas of long T1 and T2 values, and a given lesion may be difficult to date by MRI. A chronic infarction can sometimes be identified by the presence of associated cortical atrophy and the well-defined appearance of the altered region of increased T2 signal. The precise etiology of MR lesions in patients with clinically reversible symptoms (transient ischemic attacks) is not yet resolved. They may represent areas of silent infarction or, possibly, pathologically reversible ischemia.

MR's high sensitivity but lack of specificity may lead to difficulty in separating clinically significant from insignificant abnormalities. The high sensitivity of MR results in the detection of asymptomatic white matter and lacunar infarcts in up to 30% of the population over 65 years of age.[30] Although these lesions may be clinically unimportant, they may appear radiographically similar to lesions related to demyelination or even neoplastic disease. Thus MRI findings must always be interpreted in conjunction with the patient's age and the clinical setting. If MRI is used as a screening modality in the elderly, care must be taken not to dismiss an important lesion (e.g., metastasis) that could be superimposed on the ischemic white lesions that are commonly seen in the aging brain. This could result in a false-negative study for a clinical significant abnormality. The use of Gd-DTPA (or contrast-enhanced CT) in the evaluation of these patients may be helpful in characterizing abnormal areas.

Occasionally, MR may have difficulty in determining if an atypical abnormality is an infarction or a neoplasm. This problem may occur when the infarct is large, has mass effect, or shows prominent contrast enhancement (often in the subacute stage) (Figs. 11–14 and 11–15). Considerable care should be taken if an attempt is made to characterize the lesion by MR appearance alone. Infarcts would not typically cross vascular boundaries, have disproportionate amounts of associated edema, or invade the corpus callosum. The use of coronal images is often helpful in better defining the borders and location of the lesion. When clinically feasible, a follow-up MR or CT should be performed approximately four to six weeks later. The resolution or improvement of mass effect and signal abnormality (or contrast

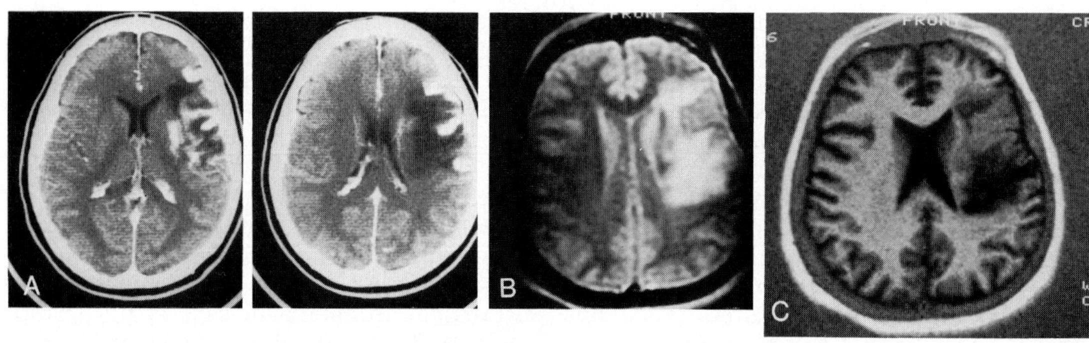

**Figure 11–14. Subacute infarct with CT enhancement.** A 50-year-old South American woman with acute onset of right hemiplegia two weeks before admission. Arteriography at the time symptoms began revealed a high-grade stenosis at the bifurcation of the left common carotid artery (0.5 T).

*A,* CT (with contrast) obtained two weeks post-CVA reveals a subacute infarct in the distribution of the patient's left middle cerebral artery, with gyral enhancement. *B,* Axial T2WI (TR 2000/TE 60). *C,* Axial T1WI (IR TI 400/TR 2100/TE 35). The MR appearance of this infarct on *(B)* could be confused with a neoplasm surrounded by edema. Note, however, that the lesion has no mass effect, is confined to a single vascular boundary (the middle cerebral artery), and has well-defined, sharp margins.

enhancement) is a reliable means of distinguishing infarct from tumor.

The inability of MR to easily and reliably detect acute hemorrhage is an important limitation in imaging patients with acute cerebrovascular accidents. The presence of hemorrhage within a cerebral infarction may be of paramount clinical importance to the management of stroke patients, and the MR appearance of acute hemorrhage is highly variable on current spin-echo sequences. CT remains the modality of choice for the workup of acute supratentorial stroke patients because of its lower cost, rapidity, and ability to easily detect acute hemorrhage.

MRI may also fail to detect cortical infarcts that show contrast enhancement on CT.[39] The high signal of these lesions on T2WI is often indistinguishable from that of the CSF in adjacent cortical sulci. The use of Gd-DTPA will probably improve the detection of those cortical lesions that are associated with breakdown in the blood-brain barrier. Cortical infarcts that enhance on CT owing to luxury perfusion however may still be difficult to detect on enhanced MR because the current paramagnetic agents (Gd-DTPA) do not effectively visualize the arterial or capillary vascular bed.[37, 40] Conversely, cortically based infarcts in the temporal lobes, brain vertex, and occipital poles may be more easily seen on MR owing to absence of beam-hardening artifacts. Therefore, when strong clinical suspicion of infarct is present but CT is normal, MR may still be indicated.

Many of the current limitations in MR imaging of cerebrovascular disease may be resolved by technical innovations in the near future. The use of new intravascular paramagnetic contrast agents and the development of special pulse sequences (e.g., gradient echo) promise to improve both the sensitivity and specificity of MRI. The use of fast-imaging techniques should also significantly decrease examination times and more readily permit identification of the acute intracerebral hemorrhage.

## MRI OF VASCULAR MALFORMATIONS

Vascular malformations of the brain have been histologically classified into four categories: (1) arteriovenous malformation (AVM), (2) capillary telangiectasis, (3) cavernous malformation, and (4) venous malformation.[41] They may present with intracerebral or subarachnoid hemorrhage, seizures, headaches, or focal neurologic symptoms. In many cases they are incidental findings. Their CT appearance can mimic calcified, low-grade gliomas. MR offers unique advantages in visualizing vascular malformations. It is able to visualize flow within feeding and draining vessels without intravascular contrast. MR has unparalleled sensitivity in detecting the presence of subacute or chronic hemorrhage that may strongly suggest the correct diagnosis. There are no

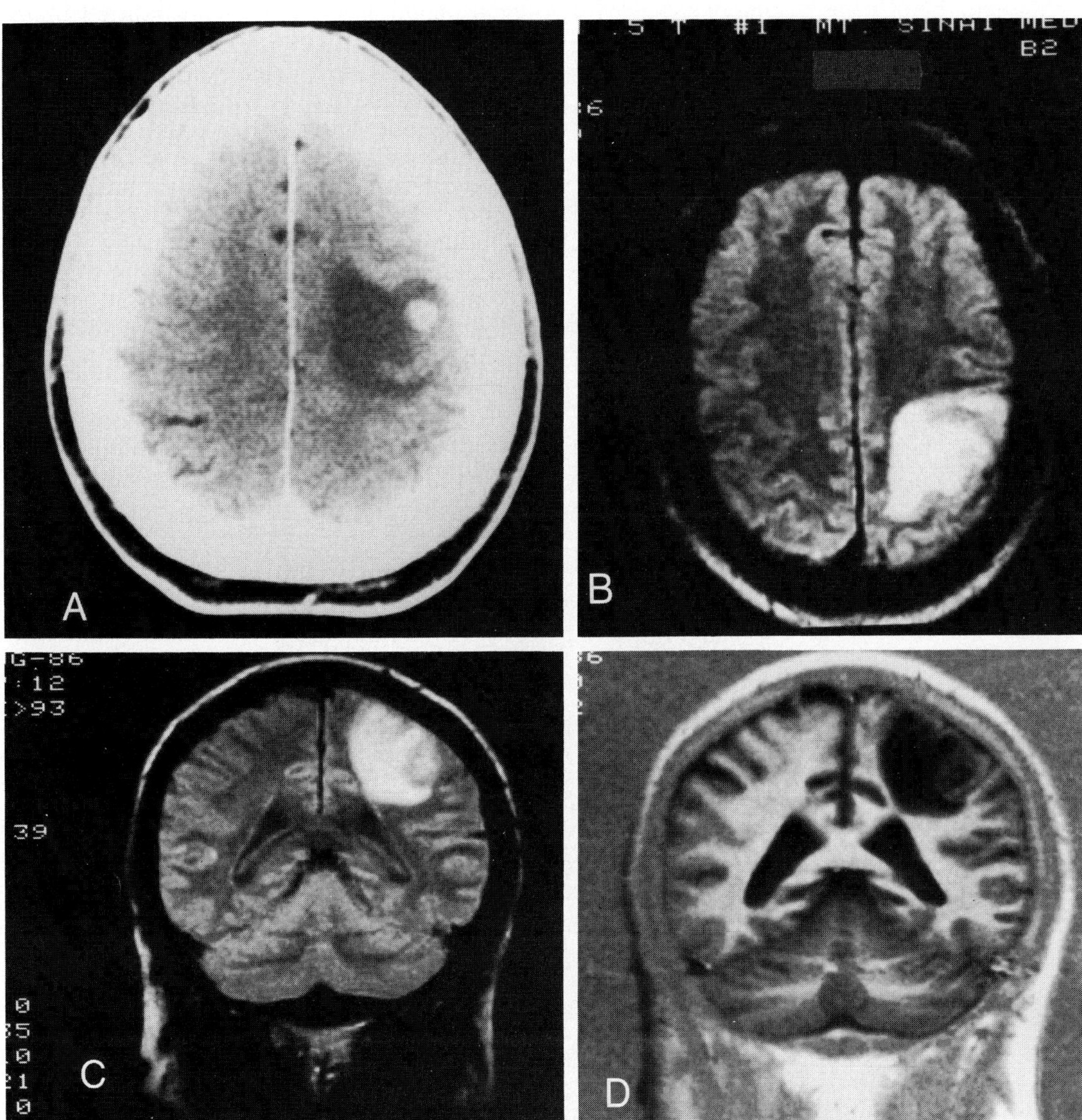


**Figure 11–15. Atypical infarct that mimics a metastatic lesion.** An elderly man with acute left cerebral hemisphere dysfunction compatible with a cerebrovascular accident. History of hypernephroma 20 years before present illness (0.5 T).

*A,* CT (with contrast) demonstrates an enhancing left parietal lesion with surrounding edema suggestive of metastasis. *B,* Axial N(H)WI (TR 2000/TE 35). *C,* Coronal N(H)WI (TR 2000/TE 35). *D,* Coronal T1WI (IR TI 400/TR 2100/TE 35). The MR study, especially the coronal images, reveals no associated mass effect on the adjacent ventricle. This lack of mass effect is unusual for a metastasis. The borders of the lesion are sharply defined and end abruptly at the confines of the left middle cerebral artery. These features favored an infarction and prompted conservative management. Follow-up double-dose CT (not shown) and MRI six weeks later showed complete resolution of all abnormalities.

streak artifacts arising from bone to obscure lesions of the posterior fossa. The multiplanar capability of MR also gives excellent anatomic information for planning surgical or radiation therapy.

Angiographically apparent intracerebral AVMs can be routinely demonstrated by MR.[42] The larger feeding and draining vessels can be visualized as a cluster of serpiginous regions of signal void (Figs. 11–16 and 11–17). The draining venous structures can sometimes be identified by their larger size and anatomic relationship to the deep venous system. Areas of venous or slow flow often display increased signal intensity on the second echo of the double-echo T2WI owing to even-echo rephasing. Rapid blood flow within the arterial components of the AVM often have no signal on either T1WI or T2WI. The presence of increased signal intensity on both the T1WI and T2WI is evidence of methemoglobin formation owing to subacute or chronic hemorrhage. An associated rim of low signal around the AVM (best seen on intermediate and high-field MR) may occur on the T2WI. This hypointense rim represents either chronic hemosiderin deposition or a magnetic susceptibility phenomenon from subtle differences in the local magnetic fields between normal brain and hematoma. The brain parenchyma adjacent to this low signal rim may exhibit a high signal on the T2WI. This may be due to vasogenic edema, ischemia, or gliosis. There is generally little mass effect associated with these lesions unless there has been hemorrhage. CT studies performed with and without contrast media are highly sensitive in detecting these angiographically evident AVMs. The contrast study shows intense homogenous or vermiform contrast enhancement within the tortuous dilated feeding vessels (Fig. 11–17).[44]

Unruptured AVMs may be difficult to detect on the noncontrast CT if the feeding vessels are only slightly hyperdense. The

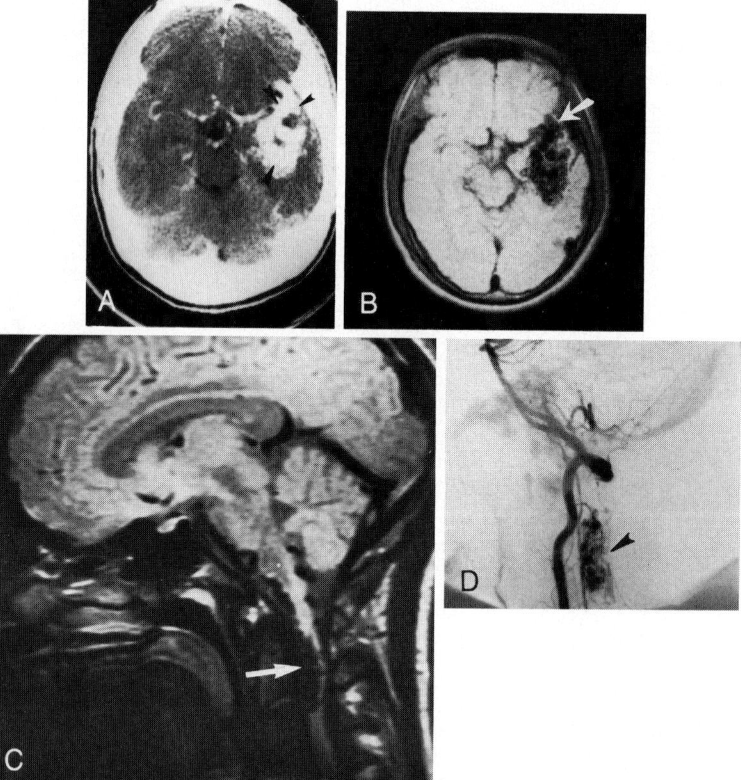


**Figure 11–16. Left temporal arteriovenous malformation (AVM).** (0.35 T). **Spinal AVM.** (1.5 T). *A,* CT (with contrast). *B,* Axial N(H)WI (TR 2000/TE 35). *C,* Sagittal N(H)WI (TR 2000/TE 20). *D,* Vertebral angiogram, lateral view. The large vermiform enhancing vessels of the AVM on *A* and *D* (arrowheads) are seen as tubular areas of signal void on the corresponding MR images *B* and *C* owing to rapid blood flow (arrows). (*C* and *D,* courtesy of Radiology Department, Schumpert Medical Center, Shreveport, La.)

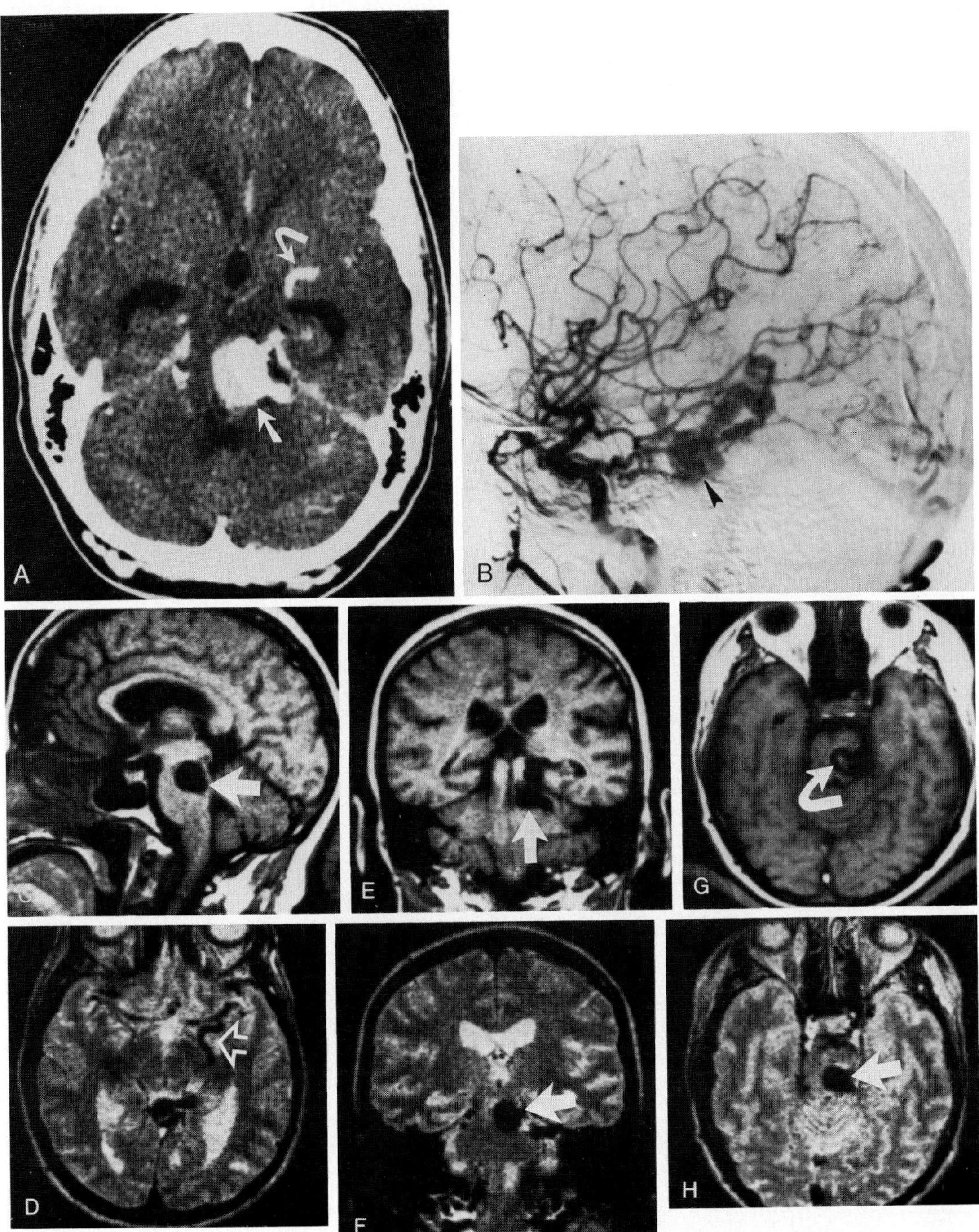


**Figure 11–17. Tentorial AVM with varix.** (0.5 T). *A,* CT (with contrast). *B,* Left carotid arteriogram (lateral, arterial phase). *C,* Sagittal T1WI (SE TR 500/TE 16). *D,* Axial T2WI (TR 2000/TE 80). *E,* Coronal T1WI. *F,* Coronal T2WI. *G,* Axial T1WI. *H,* Axial T2WI.

Feeding vessel on CT (curved arrow), varix on CT (arrow) and angiogram (arrowhead) are apparent. The rounded signal void of the varix is present at the level of the brain stem on multiple images (straight arrows). A feeding vessel supplying the vascular malformation is noted (open arrow). A small amount of intraluminal signal is present on T1WI *(G)* owing to entry-slice phenomenon (curved arrow).

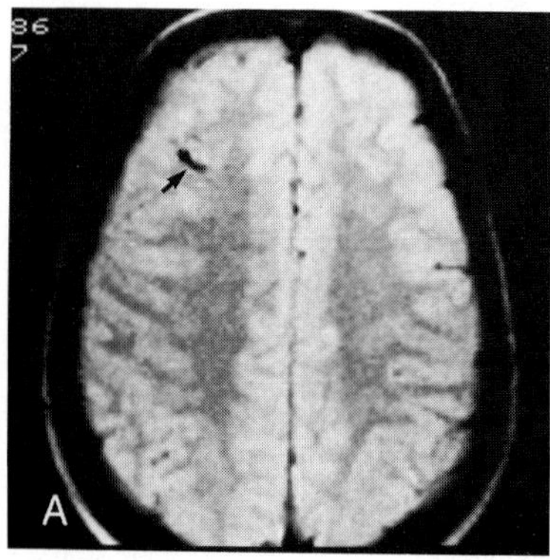


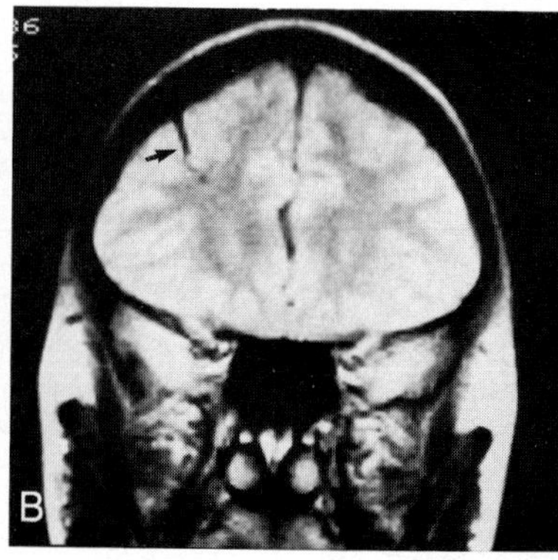


**Figure 11–18. Venous angioma.** A 24-year-old woman with headache (0.5 T). *A,* Axial N(H)WI (TR 2000/TE 35). *B,* Coronal N(H)WI (TR 2000/TE 35). A CT with contrast (not shown) revealed a curvilinear enhancing structure in the right frontal lobe without surrounding mass effect or edema. The presence of signal void (arrow) on the N(H)WI shows this structure to represent a vessel. Angiography revealed a draining vein with a typical venous angioma.

presence of calcium or an adjacent region of cerebral injury from previous hemorrhage may be a clue to their presence. Both calcification and hemorrhage within an AVM may result in a hyperdense appearance on noncontrast CT. Old areas of hemorrhage within an AVM cannot be specifically characterized by CT. These resolving hematomas may have ring enhancement and may be confused with neoplasms. MR can be helpful in showing the presence of the old hemorrhage because of its bright signal on both T1WI and T2WI associated with hypointense T2 hemosiderin effects.

Venous malformations are seen as curvilinear structures of little or no signal intensity on T1-weighted and proton density sequences (Fig. 11–18). These veins may show increased signal on the second echo of the double-echo T2WI owing to slow blood flow

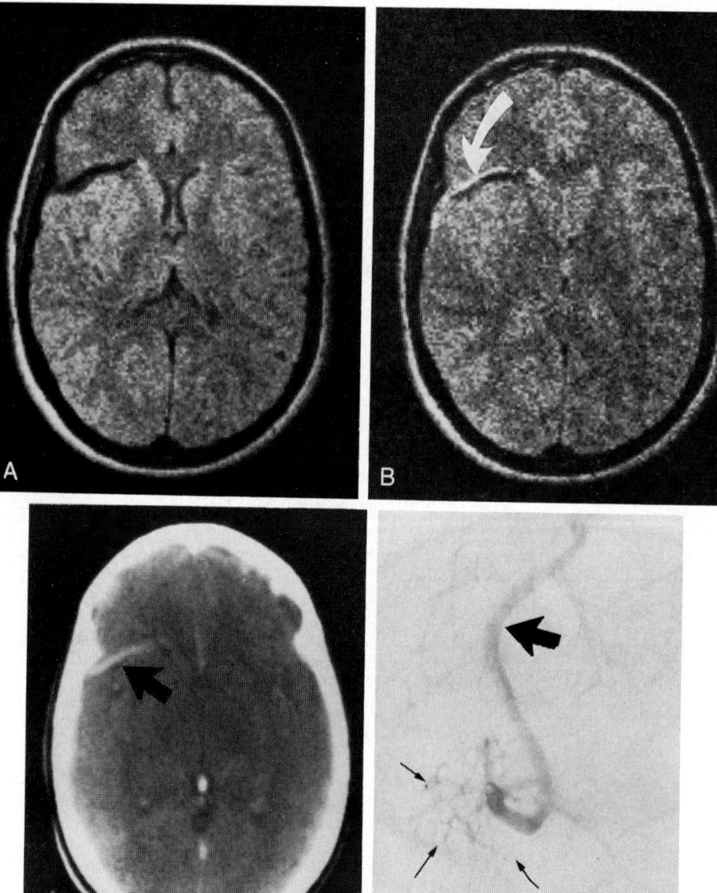


**Figure 11–19. Venous Angioma.** (0.35 T). *A,* Axial N(H)WI (TR 1500/TE 35). *B,* Axial T2WI (TR 1500/TE 70). *C,* CT (with contrast) reveals a curvilinear area of enhancement. *D,* Right carotid arteriogram (lateral, venous phase) shows the venous angioma (small arrows) and its draining cortical vein (large arrow).

*A* and *B,* Curvilinear signal void is seen within the draining vein of the venous angioma. Note the increased signal resulting from slow flow (second-echo rephasing) projects outside the vessel lumen on the T2WI (curved arrow, *B*). This phenomenon is due to the oblique plane of flow through the image. (Courtesy of The Department of Radiology, Mercy Hospital, Miami, Fla.)

and second-echo rephasing (Fig. 11–19*B*).[45] Most reports have found the T2-weighted spin-echo images to be most helpful in visualizing venous malformations.[46, 47] They may be supratentorial or infratentorial in location.

Angiographically, venous angiomas appear as multiple, small, dilated medullary veins that empty into a single, large draining vein (Fig. 11–19*D*).[48] They may drain into either a superficial cortical vein or a dural sinus and deep venous system. It is the draining transcerebral vein that can be seen by MRI. The blood pool within the body of the angioma may also be visualized as an area of increased signal on the T2WI.[47] There are no associated arterial abnormalities. Hemorrhage has been reported within venous angiomas (especially the infratentorial ones) but is more commonly seen with true arteriovenous malformations (Fig. 11–20). The clinical presentation of these lesions is variable. Headaches and seizures are most typical, but these lesions may be incidental findings in patients examined for other reasons. Both axial and coronal imaging planes may be necessary to demonstrate the long axis of the draining vein. If the vessel is imaged only in cross section, it may blend with the CSF in the cortical sulci and be undetected on the MR study. Superficially located supratentorial angiomas and cerebral varices may be especially difficult to detect for this reason. Similar problems have been reported in the detection of periventricular angiomata.[47] The use of short TR/short TE spin-echo and gradient-echo sequences may be helpful in demonstrating signal from intravascular flow within these lesions. Cerebral varices are simply dilated cerebral veins located either within the brain parenchyma or the leptomeninges. They probably result from a congenital weakness in the wall of the vessel. They have a smooth saclike appearance with an associated large superficial or deep draining vein. These are rare lesions, but there have been isolated reports of their association with venous angiomas.[49] The brain parenchyma adjacent to a venous angioma may appear normal or may show mixed signal abnormalities thought to represent focal ischemia, gliosis, or calcification.[47] Angiomatous malformations of the choroid plexus have also been described and

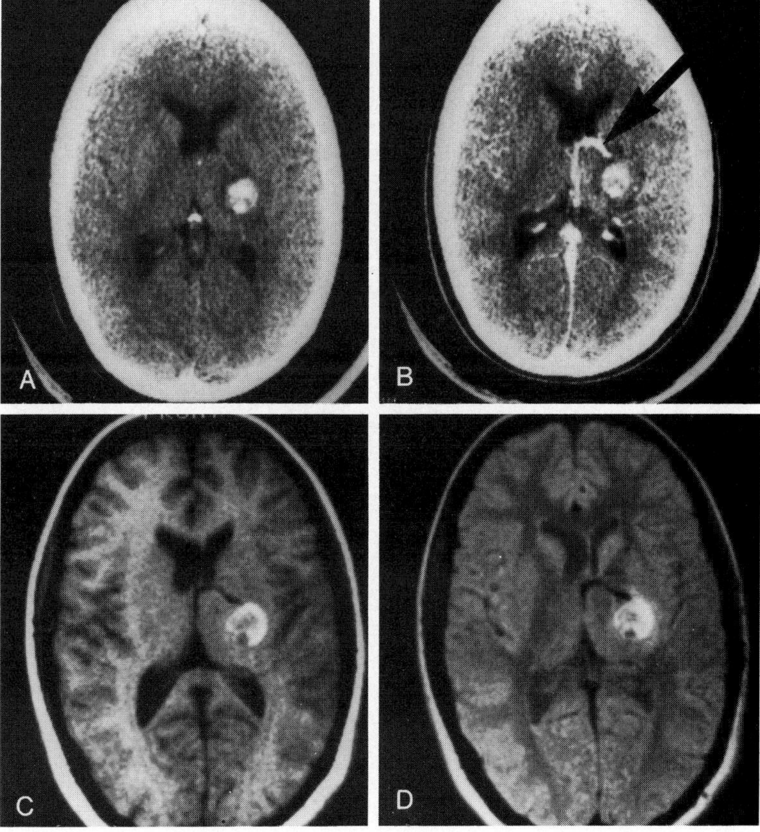


**Figure 11–20. Hemorrhagic vascular malformation.** A 26-year-old woman with acute onset of a mild left cerebral hemisphere deficit (0.35 T). *A,* CT (noncontrast). *B,* CT (with contrast). *C,* T1WI (SE TR 300/TE 30). *D,* N(H)WI (TR 1500/TE 35).

The noncontrast CT demonstrates a deep left basal ganglionic hematoma. The contrast CT shows a single aberrant draining vessel that arises from the hemorrhage and is directed toward the patient's left foramen of Monro and internal cerebral vein (arrow). The bright signal seen on the T1WI confirms the presence of subacute hemorrhage, and flow void within the draining vein is also apparent. There is no surrounding edema on the N(H)WI or T2WI because the hematoma is not acute. Cerebral angiography confirmed the presence of an enlarged draining vein with no evidence of neovascularity or arteriovenous shunting.

are likely more common than previously thought in patients with Sturge-Weber syndrome.[50] The CT scans show calcification, enlargement, and increased enhancement of the choroid plexus on the same side as the patient's facial and leptomeningeal angiomas. On MRI these lesions have bright signal on T2WI, probably owing to slow flow of venous blood or increased fluid content.[51]

MRI is useful in the evaluation of angiographically occult (cryptic) arteriovenous malformations (Fig. 11–21). These lesions display no abnormal vascularity or blush on conventional angiography. Occult AVMs are a diverse histologic group that encompasses cavernous angiomas, capillary telangiectasias, and thrombosed AVMs.[41] The distinction between small neoplasms containing calcium and occult AVMs may be difficult by CT evaluation alone.

Occult AVMs are typically small (2 to 3 cm), circumscribed, hyperdense regions that can appear mottled or homogenous on the noncontrast CT. Less commonly, they appear hypodense or isodense on the unenhanced CT. There is often subtle contrast enhancement, but surrounding edema is unusual, unless there has been recent hematoma formation. As with other vascular malformations that have bled, a ring-enhancing pattern associated with a resolving hematoma can be seen. Mild mass effect is found in approximately one third to one half. Multiple lesions are not unusual.[52] They are most commonly seen in the brain stem periventricular white matter and subcortical region. They may be clinically manifested by seizures, headache, or hemorrhage. When these lesions occur within the brain stem, they may cause severe debilitating symptoms that mimic brain stem gliomas. Vascular malformations in the brain stem are often telangiectasias or cavernous lesions that are rarely demonstrated on angiography. The MR demonstration of chronic hemorrhage within the lesion is helpful, although not totally specific, in supporting the diagnosis of AVM.[43, 53]

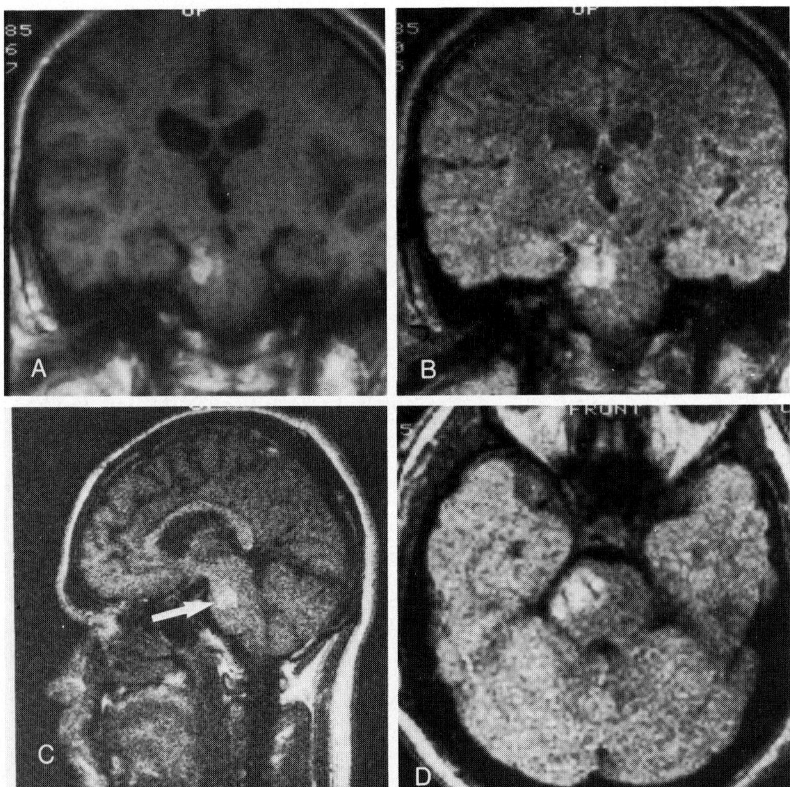


**Figure 11–21. Occult brain stem AVM with subacute hemorrhage.** A 30-year-old man with a previous history of subarachnoid hemorrhage due to right frontal lobe AVM (0.35 T). *A,* Coronal T1WI (SE TR 300/TE 30). *B,* N(H)WI (TR 1500/TE 35). *C,* Sagittal T1WI (SE TR 300/TE 30). *D,* N(H)WI (TR 1500/TE 35). The T1WI shows high signal (arrow) in the right upper pons and right cerebral peduncle secondary to a subacute hemorrhage. There is no associated mass effect or evidence of associated edema on the N(H)WI. The patient remained clinically stable over a two-year period.

The sensitivity of MRI in the detection of occult AVMs is still under clinical investigation. The presence of calcification within an AVM is generally not well appreciated on MR and is better detected by CT. MR fast scan facilitates detection of parenchymal calcification. If the only CT manifestation of the AVM is a calcific lesion without hemorrhage or mass effect, it may be missed on MRI. In summary, CT appears to be more sensitive in the detection of small calcified malformations, and MRI is more sensitive in detecting the subacute and chronic hemorrhagic foci commonly associated with these occult lesions. The ability of MR to detect dural-based AVMs is not yet known. Early experience suggests that both CT and MR may have difficulty in detecting these lesions.[42, 44, 53, 54] High-field (1.5 T) MR detected more of these vascular lesions than either low-field (0.5 T and less) MR or CT (with and without contrast).[43] Occult AVMs on MR appear as circumscribed lesions with peripheral low signal and heterogeneous mixture of centrally increased and decreased signal. Areas of methemoglobin appear bright on both T1WI and T2WI. High-field MR is especially sensitive to the presence of hemosiderin within macrophages that surround the periphery of chronic hemorrhage around occult AVMs. The hemosiderin ring appears as an area of low signal intensity on T1-weighted images and becomes broader and more hypointense on the T2-weighted sequences.

It is important and often difficult with MR to distinguish between calcium and flow void within a lesion. The hypointensity seen within an AVM may be due to flow-related signal void, dense calcification, hemosiderin deposition, or a combination of these. The presence of vascular flow may be confirmed by demonstrating flow-related enhancement or second-echo rephasing on spin-echo sequences. The use of short TR (100 msec), single-slice, spin-echo sequences or gradient-echo images will show bright signal arising from flow within vascular lesions. Calculated T2 images can also emphasize this effect.[16, 42] Calcium is usually seen centrally within the AVM and often has mild, constant hypointensity on all sequences. The low-signal ring of hemosiderin is present in the periphery of the AVM and usually has smooth margins. The heterogeneous appearance of the hemorrhage within an occult AVM is suggestive of recurrent bleeding episodes.[43] These areas of hemorrhage are in different stages of evolution and therefore have differing T1 and T2 values. Hematomas from hypertension, trauma, and surgery more often lie within a single cavity and evolve in the typical fashion described earlier in this chapter.

The presence of hemorrhage within a lesion with surrounding areas of hemosiderin deposition is helpful in suggesting occult AVM in the proper clinical setting. The diagnosis is not completely specific since small primary and metastatic neoplasms may, on occasion, also have areas of hemorrhage.[53, 54] In one study, almost one third of cerebral neoplasms showed a partial or complete rim of alteration in local magnetic field.[55] This was thought to be related to the presence of paramagnetic breakdown products of blood (deoxyhemoglobin, methemoglobin, free ferric iron, and hemosiderin). Therefore neither hemosiderin deposition nor central foci of hemorrhage may be totally specific for occult AVMs. The absence of hemorrhage within the lesion, especially if there is mass effect, should suggest the possibility of an alternate diagnosis, especially a neoplasm.[42, 53]

## ANEURYSMS AND SUBARACHNOID HEMORRHAGE (< 05 T)

Intracranial aneurysms can often be seen by MRI because of its ability to directly visualize areas of rapid blood flow. An aneurysm characteristically appears as a well-defined circular or elliptical region of signal void contiguous with the parent cerebral vessel (Figs. 11–22 and 11–23). The presence of thrombus or turbulent flow within the aneurysm may be associated with signal arising within its lumen (Fig. 11–24).

The detection of intracerebral aneurysms is dependent on several technical and anatomic factors. The visualization of small lesions demands both high spatial resolution and images with adequate signal-to-noise characteristics. This is best accomplished by thin-section (5-mm or thinner) images at high field strengths in multiple projections, using both T1- and T2-weighted spin-echo pulse sequences. The T1WI yields satisfactory anatomic detail and reveals evidence of

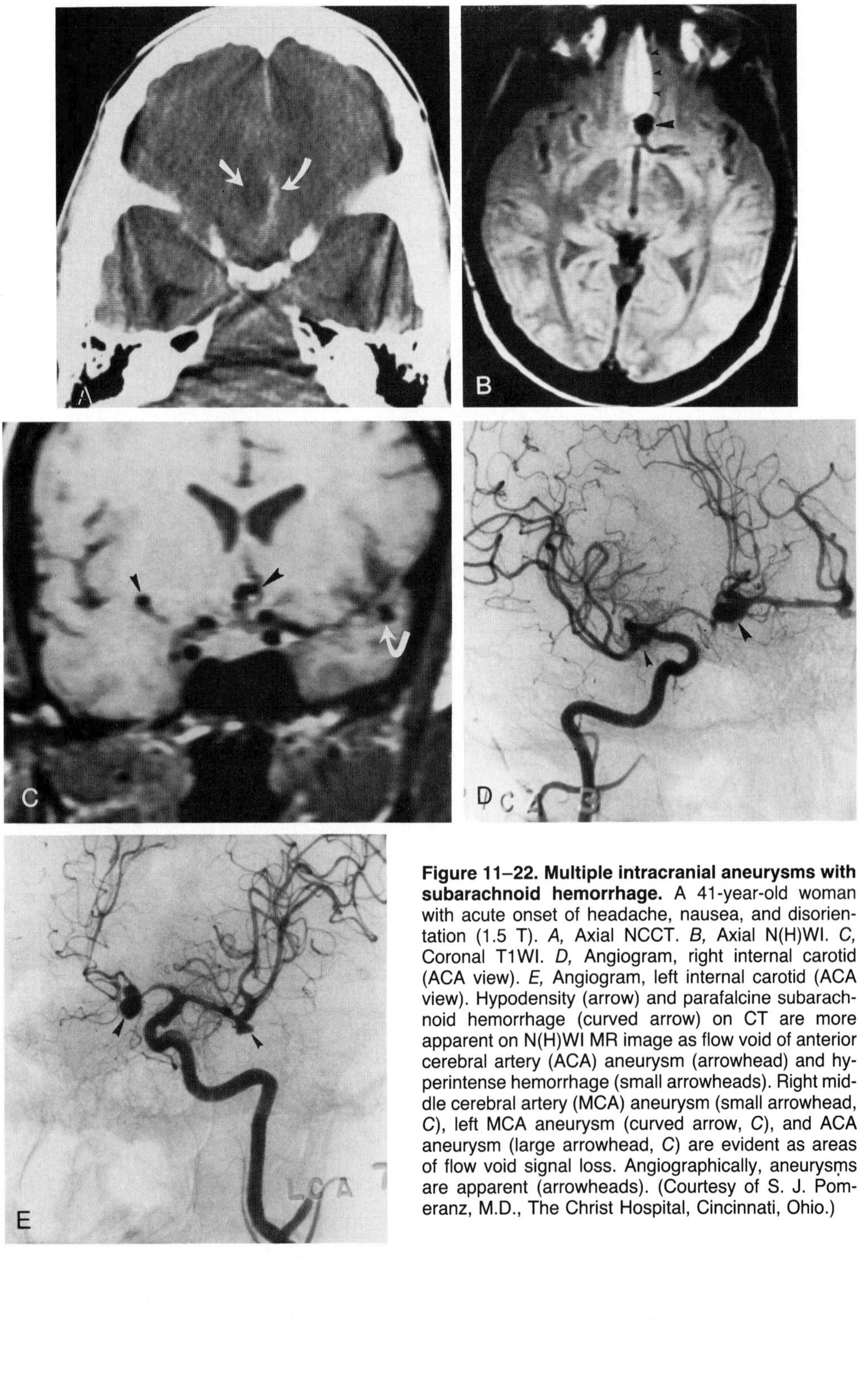

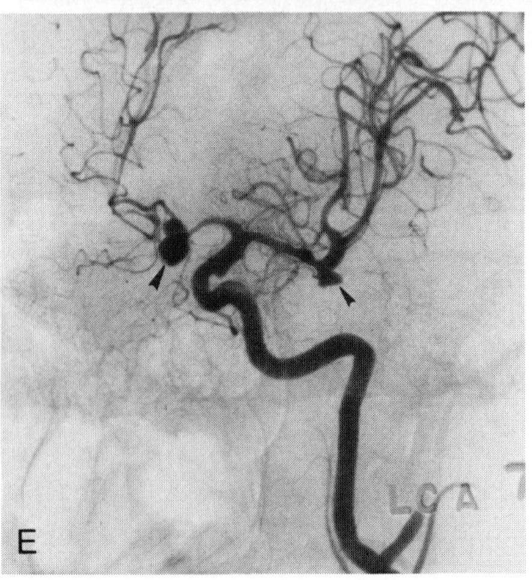

**Figure 11–22. Multiple intracranial aneurysms with subarachnoid hemorrhage.** A 41-year-old woman with acute onset of headache, nausea, and disorientation (1.5 T). *A,* Axial NCCT. *B,* Axial N(H)WI. *C,* Coronal T1WI. *D,* Angiogram, right internal carotid (ACA view). *E,* Angiogram, left internal carotid (ACA view). Hypodensity (arrow) and parafalcine subarachnoid hemorrhage (curved arrow) on CT are more apparent on N(H)WI MR image as flow void of anterior cerebral artery (ACA) aneurysm (arrowhead) and hyperintense hemorrhage (small arrowheads). Right middle cerebral artery (MCA) aneurysm (small arrowhead, *C*), left MCA aneurysm (curved arrow, *C*), and ACA aneurysm (large arrowhead, *C*) are evident as areas of flow void signal loss. Angiographically, aneurysms are apparent (arrowheads). (Courtesy of S. J. Pomeranz, M.D., The Christ Hospital, Cincinnati, Ohio.)

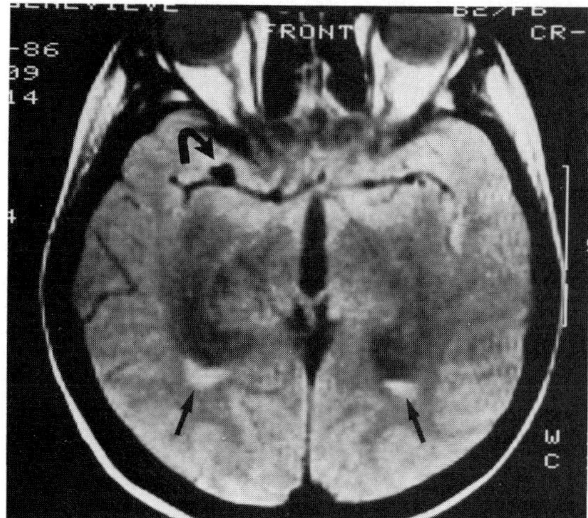

**Figure 11–23. Middle cerebral aneurysm with intraventricular hemorrhage (0.5 T).** The patient experienced sudden onset of severe headache, followed by coma. CT on admission (not shown) demonstrated marked subarachnoid and intraventricular hemorrhage. Axial N(H)WI (TR 2000/TE 35) reveals a lobulated region of signal void contiguous with the distal right middle cerebral artery (curved arrow). This aneurysm was confirmed by arteriography and surgery. High signal, due to intraventricular hemorrhage, is seen lying dependently within the atria (straight arrows).

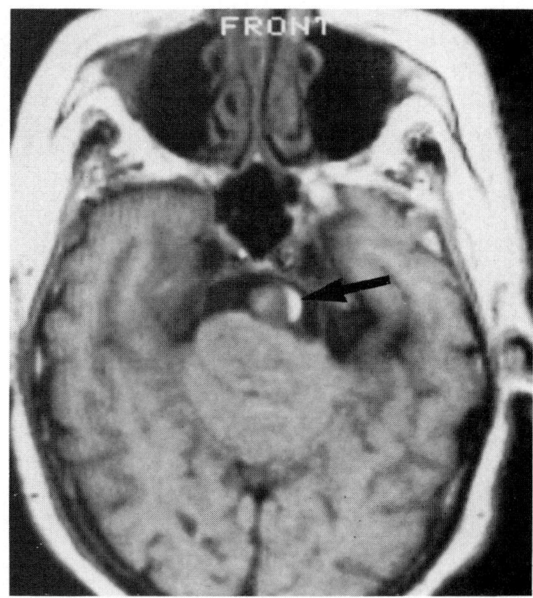


**Figure 11–24. Mural thrombus within the basilar artery.** Axial T1WI (SE TR 500/TE 16). An eccentric region of high signal (arrow) is seen within a subacute or chronic thrombus lying in the dilated basilar artery of this elderly man.

intraluminal thrombus or perianeurysmal hemorrhage. As in other areas, subacute or chronic hemorrhage will be hyperintense on T1WI owing to methemoglobin. The T2WI will show any areas of perianeurysmal ischemia or hemorrhage as hyperintense. In the acute stage (less than five days), intracerebral hematomas may appear hypointense on high-field units owing to the presence of deoxyhemoglobin (short T2 values). The T2WI may also make the aneurysm more detectable by increasing the contrast between the hypointense signal void and the adjacent structures of the brain.

The proper imaging projection is an important factor in detecting intracerebral aneurysms. Unfortunately, the optimum imaging plane is not always known in advance of the MR study. Intracavernous carotid artery aneurysms may be difficult to visualize on sagittal images owing to partial volume averaging with the aerated sphenoid sinus. The signal void of the aneurysm may be indistinguishable from the air within the sphenoid sinus (Fig. 11–25). The use of coronal projections in such cases will highlight the low-signal aneurysm surrounded by high signal within the cavernous sinus on T2WI (Fig. 11–26). The coronal projec-

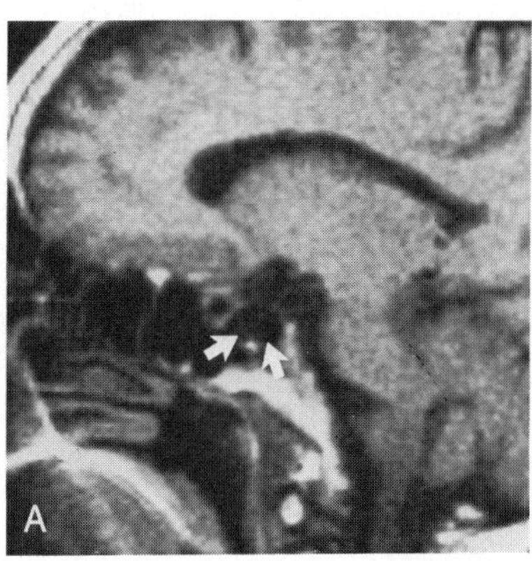


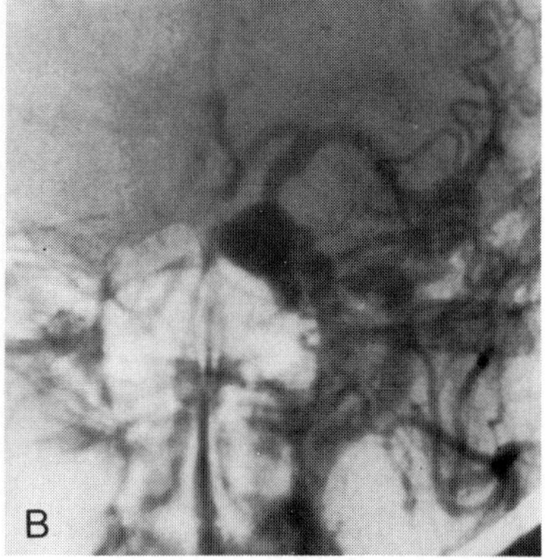


**Figure 11–25. Imaging techniques and intracranial aneurysms.** An incidental intracavernous carotid artery aneurysm in a 59-year-old woman (0.35 T). *A,* Left parasagittal T1WI (SE TR 300/TE 30, 10 mm). *B,* Left common carotid arteriogram (AP projection). There is a large left intracavernous carotid artery aneurysm seen on the arteriogram in *B* (to reader's right). The signal void of the aneurysm on the parasagittal MR (arrows in *A*) is indistinguishable from the adjacent air-filled sphenoid sinus in this projection see Figure 11–26*A*.

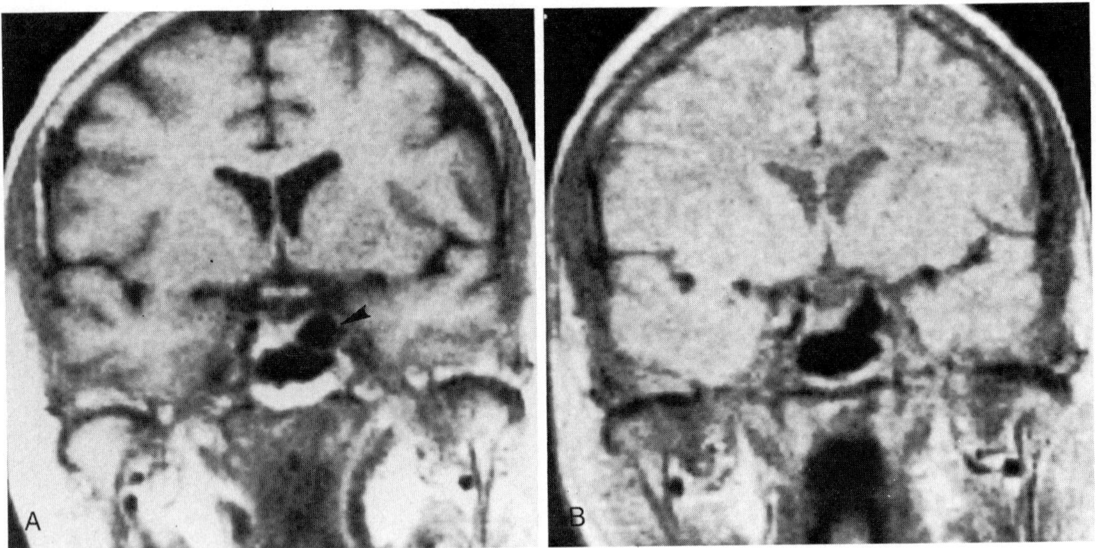


**Figure 11–26. Intracavernous aneurysm.** The same patient as in Figure 11–25 (0.35 T). *A,* Coronal T1WI (SE TR 300/TE 30). *B,* Coronal N(H)WI (TR 1500/TE 30). The left intracavernous aneurysm is easily appreciated on the coronal projections as a focal rounded area of persistent signal void (arrowhead).

tion also permits comparison within the normal intracavernous carotid artery on the other contralateral side. Areas of vessel tortuosity or redundancy can mimic aneurysms because of inadequate MR resolution of fine anatomic detail (Fig. 11–27). The superior spatial resolution of conventional or intra-arterial angiography is required in questionable cases and prior to surgical intervention for definitive diagnosis. Future advances in surface coil technology, thin-section imaging, and three-dimensional image acquisition may resolve these MR limitations.

The presence of thrombus, flow-related signal increase, or both within an aneurysm may result in a variable amount of intraluminal signal. The lack of signal void within such an aneurysm may make its appearance atypical or heterogenous. Such lesions, especially giant aneurysms (> 2 cm), may mimic extra-axial neoplastic lesions in the prepontine or cerebellopontine cistern. T1WI can show the extra-axial origin and the high signal of subacute or old thrombus within the lumen of the "mass" (Fig. 11–28). The thrombus within an aneurysm may

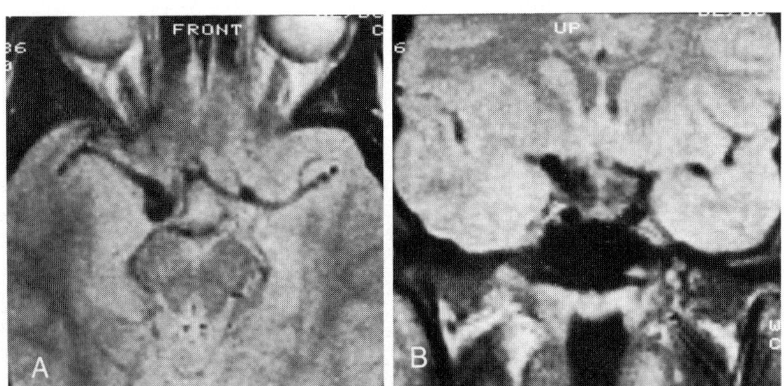


**Figure 11–27. Tortuous vessel mimics aneurysm.** A 23-year-old woman with headache and a strong family history of subarachnoid hemorrhage. A contrast CT revealed an enhancing suprasellar density suggestive of an aneurysm (0.5 T). *A,* Axial T2WI (TR 2000/TE 70). *B,* Coronal N(H)WI (TR 2000/TE 35). The axial and coronal images reveal a prominent rounded area of signal void in the right suprasellar region. This finding persisted on all projections and sequences, and an aneurysm could not be excluded. An arteriogram revealed only a highly tortuous, redundant supraclinoid carotid and right middle cerebral artery.

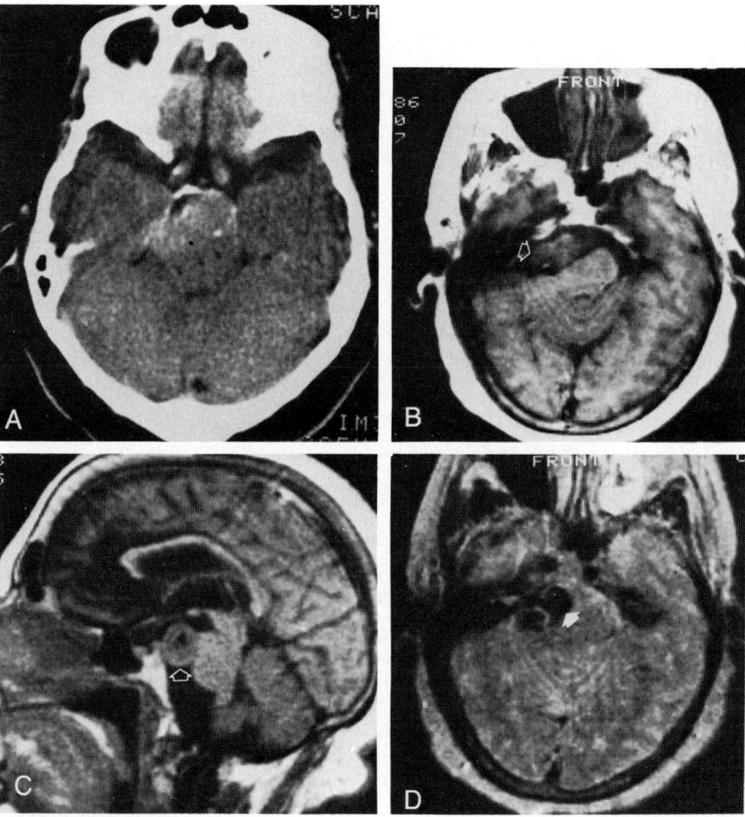


**Figure 11–28. Fusiform basilar artery aneurysm.** An elderly man with vertebrobasilar insufficiency (0.5 T). *A,* CT (noncontrast). There is a hyperdense tubular structure with peripheral calcification adjacent to the pons and the right CP angle cistern. *B,* Axial T1WI (SE TR 300/TE 30). *C,* Sagittal T1WI (SE TR 500/TE 16). *D,* Axial T2WI (TR 2000/TE 80).

The basilar artery aneurysm demonstrates heterogeneous signal intensity on the MR study. The extra-axial origin (clear arrow) of the lesion and extrinsic compression of the brain stem are well demonstrated. The presence of turbulent flow, slice entry phenomenon (arrow), and mural thrombi of differing ages are responsible for the variable appearance of these aneurysms. (Courtesy of L. Ripstein, M.D., Coral Gables Hospital, Miami, Fla.)

have a laminated appearance from both methemoglobin and hemosiderin deposition.[56] MR will show the presence of signal void within the residual lumen if there is rapid flow. A characteristic rim of low signal has also been described in the periphery of many ruptured aneurysms on both T1WI and T2WI. Mechanisms for this finding include high–blood flow signal void, calcium, and hemosiderin within hemosiderin-laden macrophages. In one report of a giant vertebral aneurysm, this area pathologically correlated with a nonhemosiderin-containing mural thrombus (RBCs) adherent to a hemosiderin-laden fibrous capsule.[57] Intact red blood cells with high deoxyhemoglobin concentration within hematomas may also result in low signal intensities on T2WI. In selected cases, correlation with CT may make the diagnosis obvious by showing peripheral calcium around the aneurysm or typical pattern of contrast enhancement.

Vein of Galen aneurysms are due to arteriovenous malformations and usually are manifested by cyanotic congestive heart failure in neonates. Rarely, they may even occur in adults, who may have various symptoms, including seizures, enlarged scalp veins, subarachnoid hemorrhage, chronic headaches, or syncope.[58, 59] Hydrocephalus may occur but is more common in neonates and young children. The MR appearance of this anomaly shows a typical large, rounded or ovoid area of signal void in the region of the vein of Galen on T1WI. There may be areas of high signal within the aneurysm owing to flow effects, especially on the heavily T2WI.[60]

The detection of acute subarachnoid hemorrhage by conventional spin-echo or inversion recovery techniques is currently very limited on MR. In vitro studies by Chakeres and associates have shown that MR relaxation times are theoretically more sensitive to subtle differences in normal and dilute CSF hemorrhages than CT Hounsfield units.[61] Occasionally acute clot within the subarachnoid space may be appreciated by a subtle focally abnormal increase in intensity within the CSF on T1WI. This may be related to the fortuitous early formation of methemoglobin. In the usual clinical setting, however, CT is more sensitive than MR in detecting acute subarachnoid hemorrhage.[62] Various factors such as partial volume averaging with the slitlike subarachnoid space, CSF pulsatile flow, isointensity of bloody CSF with cerebral cortex and clot oxygenation may all influence and limit detection of acute subarachnoid blood. Therefore patients suspected of having acute subarachnoid hemorrhage are currently studied first by CT. Computed tomography is however also limited in sensitivity, and false-negative findings can occur. An acute bleed into the subarachnoid space appears hyperdense on CT if there is concentrated hemorrhage (> 70% blood).[61] An extensive but dilute CSF hemorrhage (< 40% blood, 60% CSF) appears to be essentially isodense with CSF or brain and may go undetected.[61] Patients who are anemic (hematocrit < 20%) can also have false-negative CTs for subarachnoid hemorrhage, because acute hemorrhage in these patients is of low density.[63] The characteristic high Hounsfield values of blood (primarily hemoglobin and protein) are directly related to the hematocrit.[64] Therefore a lumbar puncture may still be indicated, even with negative CT and MR studies, if there is strong clinical suggestion of acute subarachnoid hemorrhage.

In the subacute stage of subarachnoid hemorrhage (approximately one week post ictus), MR imaging becomes more useful. Clot formation within the subarachnoid space may appear hyperintense on the T1WI owing, in part, to the formation of methemoglobin.[65] Therefore the detectability of subarachnnoid blood increases on MR in the subacute stage. At the same time, the detectability of blood on CT is decreasing as the blood becomes more isodense with CSF. Subacute intraventricular hemorrhage may also be seen as an area of high-signal layering dependently within the ventricular system (Fig. 11–23). Chronic or remote subarachnoid hemorrhage may appear as gyriform cortical foci of signal hypointensity on the brain surface with T2WI, so-called superficial siderosis.

## MRI OF INTRACRANIAL TRAUMA (< 0.5 T)

CT has long been a diagnostic cornerstone in the evaluation of intracranial trauma. It provides an accurate, rapid, noninvasive means of determining which patients require emergency evacuation of intracerebral and extra-axial hematomas. Early experience with MR in trauma patients has suggested that it may add important diagnostic and prognostic information. This is especially true in the subacute and chronic trauma patients with profound neurologic deficits and only a minimally abnormal CT study.

MR has been found to be equal or superior to CT in the detection of most extracerebral and intracerebral post-traumatic abnormalities.[66–69] The contrast resolution of MR, its ability to provide multiplanar imaging, and the absence of bone artifacts all contribute to its high sensitivity. In the acute setting (first few days), CT however remains the modality of choice because of its greater speed and the ability to easily monitor unstable patients in the CT suite.

Acute extra-axial or intracerebral hemorrhage appears markedly hypointense on T2-weighted SE images (on high-field MR) and moderately hypointense on the T1-weighted sequences (Fig. 11–29).[11, 66] Acute intraventricular hematoma appears markedly hy-

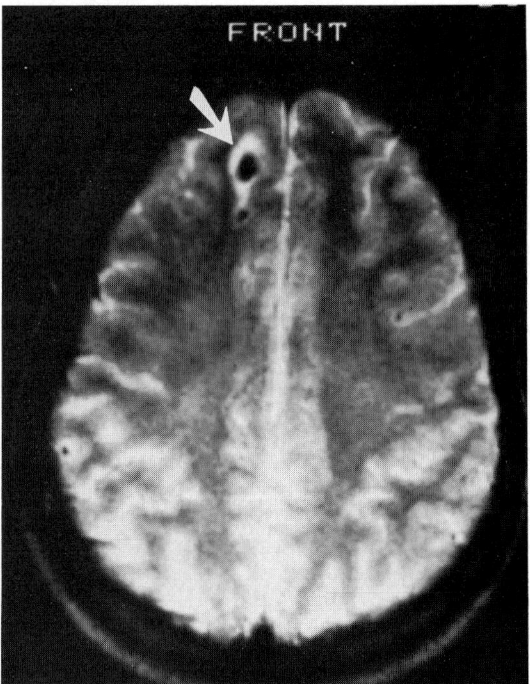


**Figure 11–29. Acute post-traumatic hemorrhagic contusion.** A 21-year-old woman with head trauma one day before the MR study (1.0 T). The CT on admission (not shown) revealed a hemorrhagic contusion in the right superior frontal gyrus, with surrounding edema. Axial T2WI (TR 2500/TE 90). The hemorrhagic contusion exhibits markedly hypointense signal (arrow), owing to the paramagnetic effects of deoxyhemoglobin. There is a thin rim of hyperintense edema in the adjacent brain (arrow).

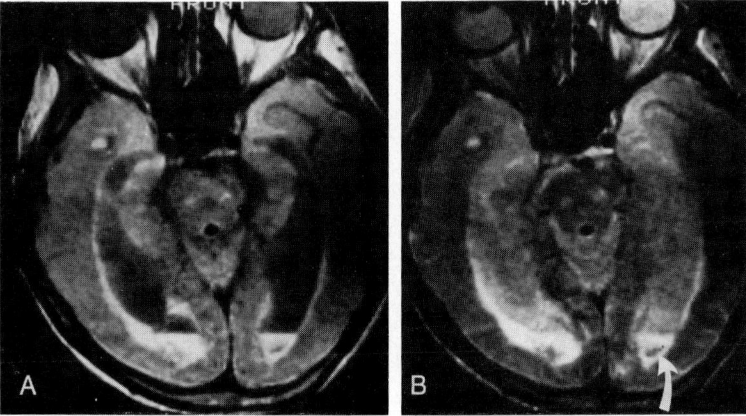

**Figure 11–30. Acute post-traumatic intraventricular hemorrhage.** (0.5 T). The MR study was obtained two days after an automobile accident. The patient had hydrocephalus and intraventricular hemorrhage on the CT examination. *A,* Axial N(H)WI (TR 2000/TE 40). *B,* Axial T2WI (TR 2000/TE 80).

There are enlarged ventricles with a prominent aqueductal flow void. The high signal, which is layering dependently within the ventricles, corresponded to the intraventricular hemorrhage seen on CT. A rounded area of decreased signal is seen within the high signal and is better seen on the T2WI (curved arrow in *B*). This presumably represents an area of acute clot formation with short T2 values.

pointense to CSF on T2WI and slightly hyperintense to CSF on the T1WI obtained on high-field MR (Fig. 11–30).[66] The evolving appearance of intracerebral hemorrhage and the possibility of visualizing acute hemorrhage on low-field MR units with gradient-echo sequences is discussed in the section on intracerebral hematoma.

MR is superior to CT in the evaluation of the subacute trauma patient (approximately, days 5 to 30). The high signal of subacute hemorrhage on T1WI permits the detection of the 10% to 25% of subdural hematomas that are isodense with adjacent cerebral cortex on CT.[69] Areas of hemorrhagic contusion are also easily seen owing to their high signal on T1WI (Fig. 11–31). The multiplanar capability of MR permits easy identification of hematomas located within the interhemispheric fissure or in subfrontal or infratem-

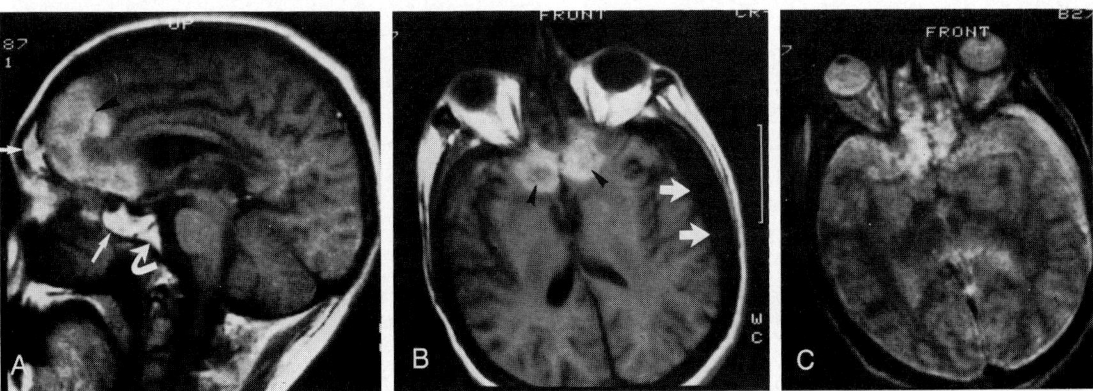

**Figure 11–31. Subacute hemorrhagic contusion and subdural hygroma.** The patient fell from a ladder and suffered head trauma ten days before the MR study (0.5 T). *A,* Sagittal T1WI (SE TR 300/TE 17). *B,* Axial T1WI (SE TR 500/TE 16). *C,* Axial T2WI (TR 2000/TE 80).

There is high signal on the T1WI throughout the frontal lobes (arrowheads) on *A* and *B* owing to subacute hemorrhagic contusion. High signal is also seen arising from blood that fills the frontal and sphenoid sinuses (straight arrows in *A*). The intensity of the subacute hemorrhage within the sphenoid sinus is similar to the hyperintense signal of normal clival fat (curved arrow in *A*). Care must be taken not to overlook this finding. Further evaluation with T2WI should resolve any questions.

The axial T1WI shows effacement of the left temporal lobe (arrows in *B*) by a hypointense subdural hygroma. The low signal of the extra-axial collection is indistinguishable from the hypointense temporal bone on the T1WI. A subdural hematoma, if subacute or chronic in age, would have high signal on the T1WI (see Fig. 11–32). The subdural hygroma is directly visualized on the T2WI as a hyperintense lenticular region between the temporal lobe and inner table.

poral regions. The ability to choose different pulse sequences allows the differentiation between subdural hygroma and chronic subdural hematoma. Both collections appear hypodense on CT and hyperintense on MR T2WI. Only the chronic subdural hematoma exhibits bright signal on T1WI owing to the presence of methemoglobin (Fig. 11–32). Trauma patients should be routinely scanned in at least two projections with T2WI to exclude extra-axial collections. Any abnormal areas of increased or decreased signal intensity can then be further characterized by T1WI. Care should be taken not to confuse the chemical shift artifacts on high-field MR, which result in high signal adjacent to the inner table of the calvarium, with extra-axial fluid collections. These high signal artifacts are present along the frequency encoding axis and are more evident with higher field strengths (1.5 T) and low bandwidth sequences.

MR is also better able to visualize white matter shear injuries, which are often the result of high-speed motor vehicle accidents. The rapid acceleration of one cerebral hemisphere relative to the other can disrupt white matter tracts, predominantly in the region of the corpus callosum. These patients may be rendered comatose, although their CT shows only mild cerebral edema or small focal hemorrhages.[70] MR is also superior to CT in the detection of brain stem and hippocampal infarcts, edematous contusions, and hemorrhagic contusions. Both MR and CT can show areas of atrophy and porencephaly in the chronic patient (imaged one month to several years after the trauma), but MR is superior in its ability to anatomically depict the abnormalities. MR can also detect areas of chronic hemorrhage, which appear hyperintense on T1WI and have a hypointense rim on T2WI owing to hemosiderin deposition within macrophages. Incidental findings such as associated transverse sinus thrombosis and post-traumatic osteomyelitis of the skull have also been reported on follow-up MR studies of trauma patients.[66, 68]

In conclusion, the nonhemorrhagic sequelae of trauma are better visualized by MR than CT, including infarction, edematous contusion, and white matter shear injuries.[66] MR is superior in demonstrating extra-axial hematomas in the subacute patient, in whom hemorrhage is more likely to be isodense on CT. Computed tomography is still the modality of choice for the emergency patient who needs rapid diagnosis for a decision between medical and surgical treatment. In patients with depressed fractures or penetrating injuries, there also is better visualization of small bone fragments on CT.[68]

## MR OF VENOUS SINUS THROMBOSIS (< 0.5 T)

Several studies have suggested that MR is the imaging modality of choice for the study of venous sinus thrombosis.[71–73] Occlusive disease of the cerebral venous system may be associated with steroids (especially oral contraceptives), pregnancy, dehydration, mastoiditis, hematologic disorders, neoplasms, and idiopathic cases.[44] It may be manifested by nonspecific symptoms (emesis, headache, confusion) from increased intracranial pressure or catastrophic neurologic deficits. The clinical diagnosis is often unsuspected. Definitive diagnosis by digital subtraction or conventional arteriography

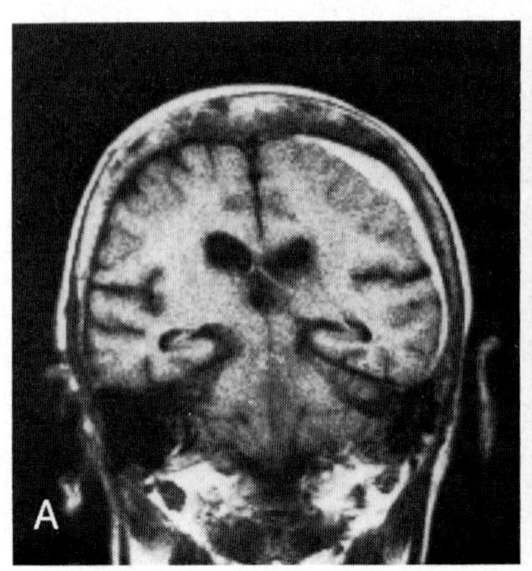


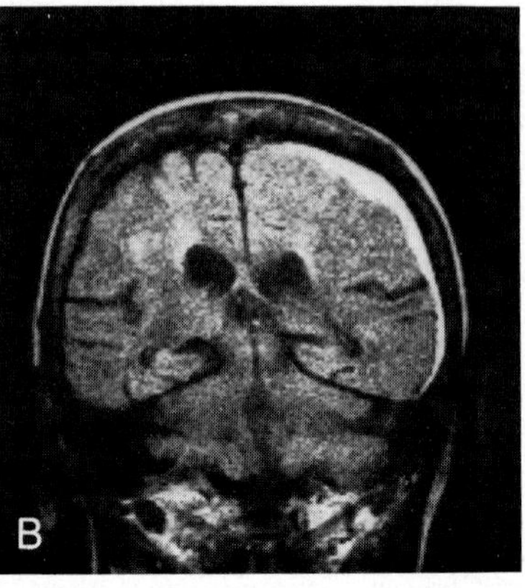


**Figure 11–32. Subacute subdural hematoma.** (0.35 T). *A*, Coronal T1WI (SE TR 300/TE 35). *B*, Coronal N(H)WI (TR 1500/TE 35). The patient's left temporal-parietal hemorrhagic subdural collection exhibits high signal on both T1WI and T2WI. Note the displacement and effacement of the adjacent cortical sulci. A subdural hygroma would be hypointense on the T1WI (see Fig. 11–31*B*).

involves invasive procedures and strong clinical suggestion. Evaluation by CT requires intravenous contrast and wide window settings to detect an intraluminal clot within the dural sinuses.[73] MR has the advantage of directly and noninvasively visualizing the presence or absence of intravascular flow. This information is especially useful when evaluating tumor invasion of adjacent venous dural sinuses (Fig. 11–33). Associated complications, like venous infarction, are also well visualized on MR (Fig. 11–34C).

The major dural sinuses normally show a lack of signal on both long and short TR, first-echo sequences, except for flow-related enhancement on the entrance slices (Fig. 11–35).[74] The absence of signal from flowing blood within a vessel may be related to either time-of-flight phenomena or first-echo dephasing phenomena. Time-of-flight phenomena are related to protons that flow perpendicularly through the plane of imaging. If the protons are moving rapidly enough, they will enter and leave the imaging plane before a spin echo can be detected. This results in high-velocity signal loss.[74, 75] Loss of signal on the first-echo image can also be related to dephasing phenomena.[76] Spin-phase changes occur when flowing protons in blood move under the influence of a magnetic gradient. This effect is most easily appreciated in vessels that are coursing within the imaging plane since these vessels are free of time-of-flight effects. In the presence of turbulence, which may be associated with blood flow, the protons within each voxel exhibit a nonuniform, or nearly random, velocity of protons within each voxel. The spins of these protons point in different directions on the first echo. This spread of phases leads to a loss of coherence and results in signal of lower intensity.[76] These vessels however show increased intraluminal signal on the second and fourth echoes if there is slow laminar flow (even-echo rephasing).

The presence of a thrombus within a venous sinus results in intraluminal signal. It is the absence of flow void, which persists on all imaging sequences and in all imaging planes, that is the most characteristic feature of venous thrombosis. Macchi and colleagues described the high-field MR appearance of acute cerebral venous thrombosis as isointense on T1WI and hypointense on

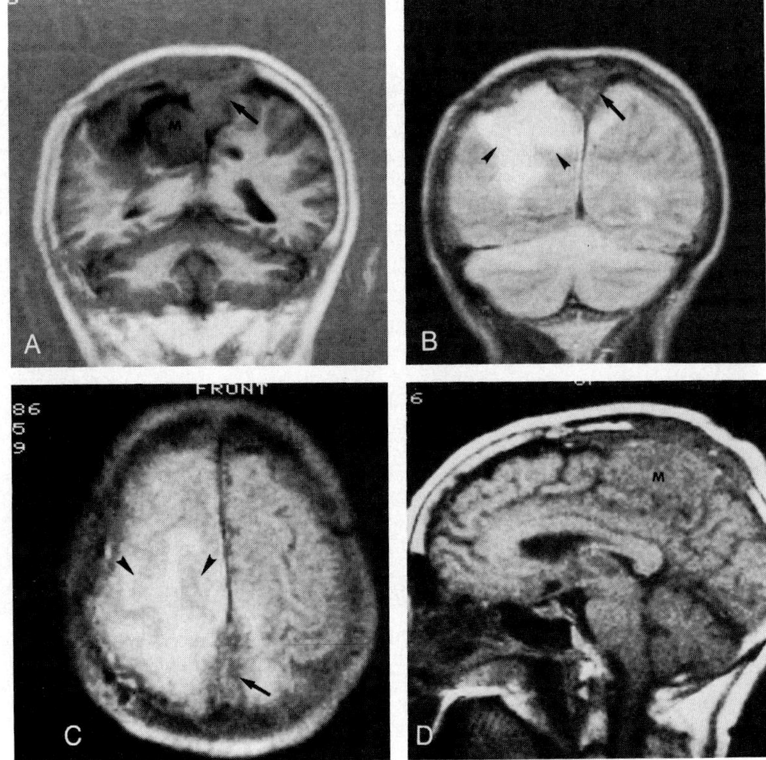


**Figure 11–33. Parafalcine meningioma with sagittal sinus invasion.** An 80-year-old woman with recurrent meningioma and intractable seizures (0.5T). *A,* Coronal T1WI (IR TI 400/TR 2100/TE 35). *B,* Coronal T2WI (TR 2000/TE 80). *C,* Axial N(H)WI (TR 1500/TE 35). *D,* Sagittal T1WI (SE TR 300/TE 30).

The coronal images reveal a right parafalcine mass (M) that has extended into the superior sagittal sinus (SSS). The normal signal void in the SSS has been replaced by abnormal signal owing to tumor invasion (arrows *A, B,* and *C*). Tumor extension and postsurgical changes are present in the right parietal bone in *D.* The high signal (arrowheads) surrounding the meningioma on T2WI may be secondary to cerebral edema, ischemia, or venous infarction related to occlusion of the sagittal sinus.

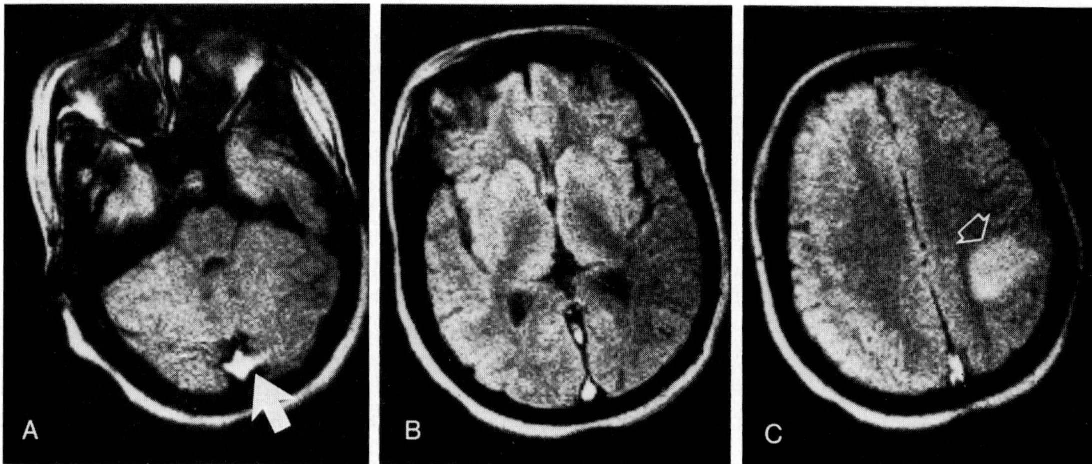

**Figure 11–34. Sagittal sinus thrombosis with venous infarction.** A patient with coagulopathy and history of renal vein thrombosis who presents with left cerebral hemisphere dysfunction (0.35 T). Axial N(H)WI (TR 2000/TE 35). High signal due to thrombus is present within the superior sagittal sinus replacing the normal signal void (arrow). The thrombus is hyperintense to adjacent cortex. A venous infarction is visible within the left centrum semiovale (open arrow) on *C*.

T2WI.[71] They described an orderly pattern of thrombus evolution over time, similar to that described in high-field MR of intracerebral hematomas.[11] In the intermediate stage, high signal intensity was eventually seen within the thrombus, initially on T1WI (as methemoglobin was formed) and then on the T2WI. These changes in MR signal did not correlate with either thrombus extension or clinical deterioration. Late changes (after approximately two weeks) may include the resumption of flow void within the vessel as the thrombus is recanalized. The signal on T2WI at high field with acute thrombosis may pass through an isointense phase as it matures from acute (hypointense) to chronic (hyperintense) phases.

Chronic cavernous sinus thrombosis re-

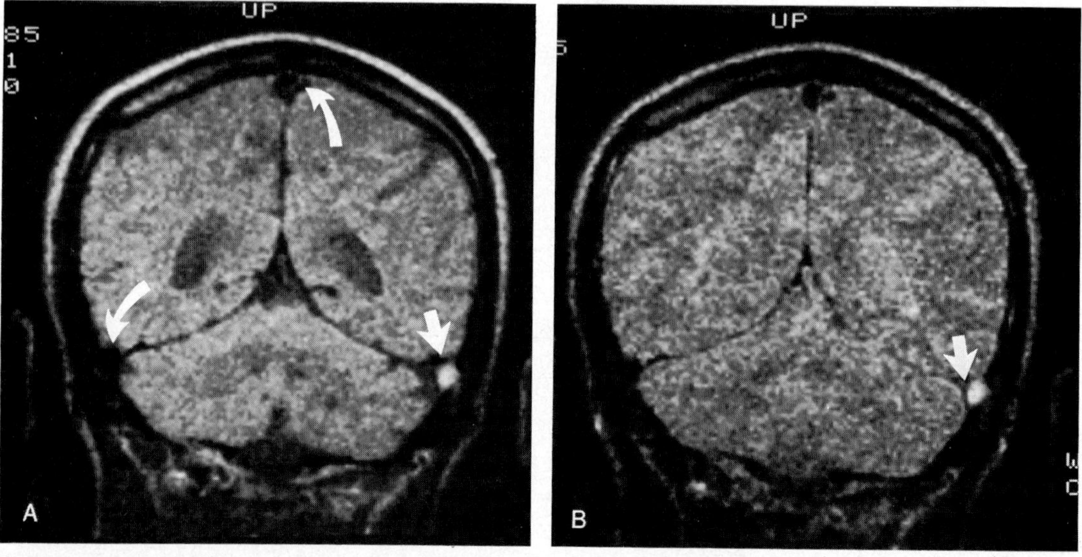


**Figure 11–35. Thrombosis of the transverse sinus.** An elderly man with metastatic involvement of the left petrous bone and extension into the adjacent transverse sinus. Angiography confirmed thrombosis of the right transverse sinus (0.35 T). *A*, Coronal N(H)WI (TR 1500/TE 35). *B*, Coronal T2WI (TR 1500/TE 70). A focus of high signal is seen arising from the thrombus in the left transverse sinus (straight arrows on *A* and *B*). Note the flow void phenomena within the normal superior sagittal sinus and right transverse sinus (curved arrows in *A*). The high signal was reproducible in axial projections as well.

sults in a high signal intensity on both T1- and T2WI on high-field MR.[77] The high signal in the anterior portion of the cavernous sinus may extend into the thrombosed posterior portion of the ipsilateral superior ophthalmic vein.

The description of dural sinus thrombosis at 0.35 T has shown high signal intensity from the thrombus on all imaging sequences (Figs. 11–34 and 11–35).[73, 78] Sequential MR studies at this field strength failed to show any significant change in signal pattern of the thrombus over a three-week period. This was true of both experimentally induced and clinical thrombi.[78] It has been suggested that low- or intermediate-field MR may have an advantage over high-field MR in the detection of acute venous thrombosis.[73, 78] An acute thrombus, which appears hypointense to brain on high-field T2WI, may be confused with vessel patency and go unrecognized. The relatively bright appearance of the thrombus at 0.35 T may appear more conspicuous.

A single thrombus may often show multiple stages of evolution (early, intermediate, and late) in a single patient. This corresponds with the spectrum of histologic changes seen within an organizing thrombus and is true at all field strengths. It may therefore be difficult to determine the age of a thrombus on the basis of a single MR study.[78] Sequential studies, however, should be useful in following the resolution and recanalization of venous sinus thrombosis.

### Differentiation of Flow from Thrombus-Phase Display Imaging

Intraluminal signal related to flow phenomena may present a difficult diagnostic problem. Its appearance may closely mimic partial or complete vascular occlusion by tumor or thrombus. The persistence of the signal on both T1WI and T2WI in multiple imaging projections is usually indicative of a thrombus (or tumor invasion). An increased signal on second-echo compared with first-echo images, owing to even-echo rephasing, is seen with slowly moving blood.[74] Even-echo rephasing has also been reported in areas of turbulent flow.[75] Increased signal from flow-related enhancement is most prominent on short TR sequences, especially in the first few contiguous entrance sections of the imaged volume. In some cases, however, differentiation between thrombus and flow-related signal may not be possible without special, phase-sensitive, reconstructed images.[78] The flow sensitivity of these images is determined not by the intensity of the NMR signal but by its phase, another intrinsic property of the signal. Protons within flowing blood, which pass through a magnetic gradient, experience a different phase-shift than do stationary protons.[76] This information is contained but not directly displayed in the usual MR image. One technique for flow imaging by phase display was developed by Wedeen and co-workers and is commonly referred to the "zebra-stripe" method.[79–81] The same data acquisition is used to generate two sets of images. One set consists of the conventional anatomic images. A second set of reconstructed, phase-sensitive images contains information about blood flow. These zebra-stripe images show areas of constant phase with a series of black and white bands superimposed on the conventional images. Areas without flow have continuous stripes, whereas areas with flow result in displacement of the stripes. The amount of displacement is related to the velocity and direction of the flow. Hence, the zebra-stripe images give both qualitative and quantitative information about flow. Any offset of the zebra stripes is a highly specific indication of flow. This MR technique is especially useful in demonstrating the presence of flow around small lesions partially occluding the vessel lumen. Phase-shift imaging may be helpful in differentiating luminal patency from obstruction by thrombus or tumor. Major advances in MR angiography may permit the direct noninvasive visualization of vessel patency or thrombosis in the near future.

## MRI OF VASCULITIS

A large number of poorly understood inflammatory and immunologic disorders may directly or secondarily involve the cerebral blood vessels. The causes of vasculitis include but are not limited to the following: infectious agents (*Mycobacterium*, fungus, yeast, bacteria, spirochete, *Leptospira*, *Rickettsia*, or virus), drug-induced (amphetamines, birth control pills, heroin), necrotizing arteritis (periarteritis nodosa, systemic lupus erythematosus, Wegener's granulomatosis, Behçet's disease, rheumatoid, temporal arteritis, hypersensitivity, allergic arteritis), granulomatous disease (sarcoidosis), and radiation-induced arteritis.[82, 83] Blood vessels of all sizes may be affected, often in a segmental fashion. Typical histologic findings include infiltration of the vessel wall by mononuclear cells or neutrophils, with variable amounts of thrombosis, extravasated RBCs, and fibrinoid necrosis. The classic angiographic features of vasculitis include vessel irregularity, "beaded" appearance, multiple aneurysms, segmental stenosis, and thrombosis.[84] The CT findings of vasculitis are nonspecific. The study may be normal and may show diffuse atrophy or focal areas of low attenuation, either with or without contrast enhancement.[44] The hypodense areas are likely related to underlying vascular compromise resulting in cerebral edema, infarction, or both. The contrast enhancement is related to a breakdown in blood-brain barrier from ischemia or abnormal vessel permeability.[44] Enhancement may also be due to collateral flow in leptomeningeal vessels.

The MR diagnosis of vasculitis is also nonspecific. It may, however, be suspected in patients with multiple foci of increased signal in the corticomedullary junction of the coronal radiata (vascular watershed zones). The presence of hemorrhagic foci (hemorrhagic infarcts), especially in the basal ganglia, with these periventricular lesions may suggest the proper diagnosis.[85] It is possible that the microangiopathy often seen pathologically with the vasculitides may predispose these younger patients to ischemic deep white matter lesions.

Patients with systemic lupus erythematosus (SLE) have been found to have more cerebral abnormalities visualized by MR than CT.[86, 87] This is not surprising in view of the known sensitivity of MR in detecting cerebral abnormalities related to edema, ischemia, and gliosis. This disease most commonly manifests itself as a small vessel angiitis but may rarely involve or occlude major cerebral arteries. The CT studies in patients with SLE have generally shown either diffuse atrophy, infarctions, or no abnormality.[88] The presence of atrophy may be related to microinfarction or may be partially induced by steroid therapy or both. Early experience with MR has shown signal abnormalities predominantly in the deep white matter. These have appeared as either large focal lesions or multiple small punctate areas of high signal on T2-weighted images within the white matter. Although these lesions usually represent white matter infarctions, reversible high-signal abnormalities, predominantly in the cortical gray matter, have also been described on sequential MR studies in some of these patients.[86] It is uncertain whether these lesions are due to cerebral edema, transient ischemia, or some other vascular phenomena. The prospective identification and significance of potentially reversible ischemic lesions requires further investigation.

## MR OF NEUROVASCULAR ARTERIAL DISSECTION

Dissections of the extracranial carotid or vertebral arteries have been recognized with increasing frequency in the recent medical literature.[89, 90] They may occur spontaneously or following minor trauma to the artery. Hemorrhage into the subintimal, medial, or, rarely, into the subadventitial layer of the carotid compromises the true lumen and may thrombose the vessel. The intramural hematoma may be circumferential or may involve a segment of the vessel wall. The incidence of dissection among patients presenting with strokes varies between 2.5% and 4%.[89, 90] The clinical features that suggest the diagnosis of carotid dissection consist of unilateral headache or neck pain and unilateral, incomplete Horner's syndrome (oculosympathetic paresis) with a transient ischemic attack or stroke. Patients with vertebral dissection may present with posterior neck cramping, bulbar signs, or Wallenberg's syndrome. The patient may exhibit mild transient neurologic deficits or a major cerebral infarction, resulting in death. Extracranial carotid dissections are most commonly seen in middle-aged adults (mean age approximately 40 to 45 years). Men are affected slightly more often than women.

The diagnosis of arterial dissection has previously required a compatible clinical presentation with typical angiographic features. One series reported that in only 17% of arterial dissections was there a suggestive clinical presentation and that therefore the diagnosis was uncertain before angiography.[89] The characteristic features of carotid dissection include a long, gradually tapered narrowing or occlusion of the internal carotid artery, beginning 2 to 5 cm beyond the carotid bifurcation and extending to the skull base.[89–92] Pseudoaneurysms may also be seen. Occlusions of the intracerebral arteries owing to emboli may be seen in patients presenting with large infarcts. These angiographic features, while suggestive, are not completely specific. Visualization of a double lumen (false lumen), commonly seen in aortic dissection, is rarely observed. Intracranial extension of the dissection, often associated with subarachnoid hemorrhage, may occur. There may also be evidence of associated fibromuscular dysplasia.

MR has the potential of diagnosing extracranial arterial dissection noninvasively (Fig. 11–36). The intramural hematomas appear as crescentic or circumferential hyperintense masses on both T1WI and T2WI obtained in the subacute or early chronic stage of the clot evolution (after approximately seven days).[93] Since only subacute or early chronic blood clot exhibits these characteristics, the MR appearance is quite specific for dissection. Fat surrounding the carotid artery or vertebral arteries in the cervical soft tissues also exhibits high signal on the T1WI. The mural hyperintensity is

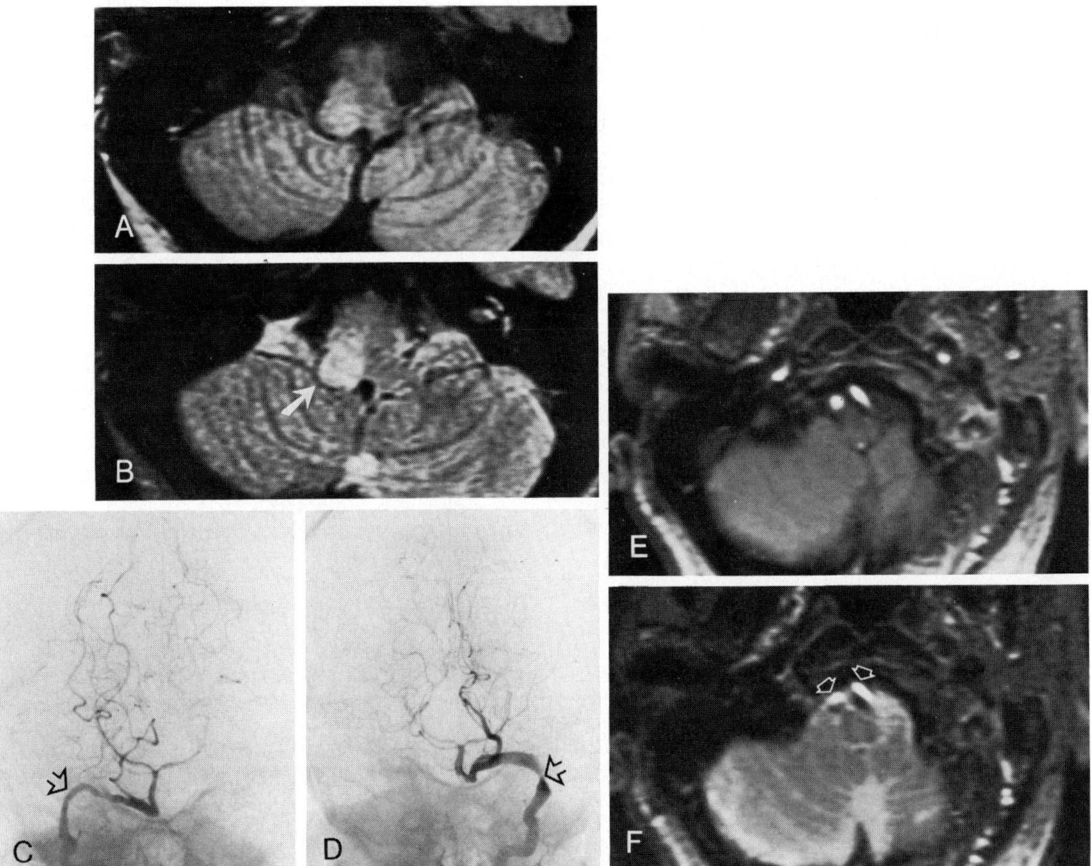


**Figure 11–36. Bilateral vertebral artery dissection with Wallenberg's syndrome and medullary infarction.** A 31-year-old woman, three months post partum, with a nine-week history of persistent neck pain and subtle bulbar signs (1.5 T). *A,* Axial N(H)WI. *B,* Axial T2WI. *C,* Right vertebral angiogram, Towne's view. *D,* Left vertebral angiogram, Towne's view. *E,* Axial N(H)WI, cervicomedullary junction. *F,* Axial T2WI, cervicomedullary junction.

The axial T2WI demonstrates right posterolateral signal hyperintensity involving the medulla (arrow) and compatible with clinical Wallenberg's syndrome. Vertebral angiography demonstrates segmental areas of narrowing (open arrows) before entrance into the foramen magnum. More caudal axial images (*E* and *F*) demonstrate bilateral intravascular signal hyperintensity (open arrows). On T2WI *(E)*, notice that hyperintense signal does not fill the entire lumen. (Courtesy of S. J. Pomeranz, M.D., The Christ Hospital, Cincinnati, Ohio.)

however separated from the surrounding interstitial fat by the hypointense rim of the adventitia.[93] The intensity of cervical fat also decreases on the T2WI, whereas the dissecting hematoma appears hyperintense. The internal carotid or vertebral artery lumen and wall are best examined by thin (5-mm or less) axial images through the upper cervical region. Sagittal images of the neck are more difficult to interpret owing to tortuosity of the carotid or vertebral arteries and partial volume problems with surrounding soft tissues and fat. The presence of signal void within those vessels assures their continued patency. Fast-scan MR may be of assistance in confirming vessel patency. This information may have potentially important prognostic and management implications. Patients with a good clinical outcome often have early reopening of their occluding dissections on heparin. Patients with poor outcomes usually have persistent carotid or vertebral occlusion owing to intraluminal thrombus formation, distal embolization, and large cerebral infarctions.[89] It is possible that MR may permit accurate, noninvasive assessment of carotid or vertebral dissections so that appropriate therapy can be initiated and followed without angiography. Sequential MR studies have been able to document resolution or recanalization of the mural thrombus in carotid dissection over a period of seven weeks.[93] The appearance and sensitivity of MR in detecting acute dissection (first seven days) requires further study.

## References


1. Swenson SJ, Keller PL, Berquist TH, et al. Magnetic resonance imaging of hemorrhage. AJR 145:921, 1985.
2. Friedmann GB, Sandu HS. NMR in blood. Magn Reson Rev 6:247, 1981.
3. Sandhu HS, Friedmann GB. Proton spin-spin relaxation time and hemoglobin content. J Clin Eng 4:357, 1979.
4. Sipponen JT, Sipponen RE, Sivula A. Nuclear magnetic resonance (NMR) imaging of intracerebral hemorrhage in the acute and resolving phases. J Comput Assist Tomogr 7:954, 1983.
5. Cohen MD, McGuire W, Cory DA, et al. MR appearance of blood and blood products: an in vitro study. AJR 146:1293, 1986.
6. Chuang AH, Waterman MR, Yamaoka K, et al. Effect of pH, carbamylation and other hemoglobins on deoxyhemoglobin S aggregation inside intact erythrocytes as detected by proton relaxation rate measurements. Arch Biochem Biophys 167:145, 1975.
7. Zipp A, James TL, Kuntz ID. Water proton magnetic resonance studies of normal and sickle erythrocytes: temperature and volume dependence. Biochem Biophys Acta 428:291, 1976.
8. Singer JR, Crooks LE. Some magnetic studies of normal and leukemic blood. J Clin Eng 3:237, 1978.
9. Norman D, Price D, Boyd, Fishman R, et al. Quantitative aspects of computed tomography of the blood and cerebrospinal fluid. Radiology 123:335, 1977.
10. Davidson N, Gold R. The nuclear magnetic relaxation time of water protons in ferrihemoglobin solutions. Biochem Biophys Acta 26:370, 1957.
11. Gomori JM, Grossman RI, Goldberg HI, et al. Intracranial hematomas: imaging by high-field MR. Radiology 157:87, 1985.
12. Hect-Leavitt C, Gomori JM, Grossman RI. High-field MRI of hemorrhagic cortical infarction. AJNR 7:581, 1986.
13. Gomori JM, Grossman RI, Yu C, et al. Physical and chemical mechanisms underlying hematoma evolution. Paper Presented at The Annual Meeting of the Radiological Society of North America, Chicago, November 30–December 5, 1986.
14. Round M, Nolte E, Mims M, et al. Relaxation times of hemoglobin and its degradation products. Presented at The Annual Meeting of the Radiological Society of North America, Chicago, 1986.
15. Zimmerman RD, Deck MDF. Intracranial hematoma: imaging by high-field MR. Letter. Radiology 159:565, 1986.
16. Edelman RR, Johnson K, Buxton R, et al. MR of hemorrhage: a new approach. AJNR 7:751, 1986.
17. Zimmerman RD, Heier LA, Snow RB, et al. Acute intracranial hemorrhage: intensity changes on sequential MR scans at 0.5 T. AJR 150:651, 1988.
18. Nose T, Enomoto T, Hyodo A, et al. Intracerebral hematoma developing during MR examination. J Comput Assist Tomogr 11:184, 1987.
19. Dooms GC, Uske A, Brant-Zawadzki M, et al. Spin-echo MR imaging of intracranial hemorrhage. Neuroradiology 28:132, 1986.
20. Hackney DB, Atlas SW, Grossman RI, et al. Subacute intracranial hemorrhage: contribution of spin density to appearance on spin-echo MR images. Radiology 165:199, 1987.
21. Atlas SW, Grossman RI, Gomori JM, et al. Hemorrhagic intracranial malignant neoplasms: spin-echo MR imaging. Radiology 164:71, 1987.
22. Heiss WD, Herholz K, Bocher-Schwarz HG, et al. PET, CT, and MR imaging in cerebrovascular disease. J Comput Assist Tomogr 10:906, 1986.
23. Brant-Zawadzki M, Pereira B, Weinstein P, et al. MR imaging of acute experimental ischemia in cats. AJNR 7:7, 1986.
24. Buonanno FS, Pykett IL, Brady TJ, et al. Proton NMR imaging in experimental ischemic infarction. Stroke 14:178, 1983.
25. Bryan RN, Willcott RM, Schneiders NJ. Nuclear magnetic resonance evaluation of stroke. Radiology 149:189, 1983.
26. Sipponen JT. Visualization of brain infarction with nuclear magnetic resonance imaging. Neuroradiology 26:387, 1984.
27. Hect-Leavitt C, Gomori JM, Grossman RI, et al. High-field MRI of hemorrhagic cortical infarction. AJNR 7:581, 1986.
28. Gomori JM, Grossman RI, et al. Intracranial hematomas: imaging by high-field MR. Radiology 157:87, 1985.

29. Fisher CM, Adams RD. Observations on brain embolism with special reference to the mechanism of hemorrhagic infarction. J Neuropathol Exp Neurol 10:92, 1951.
30. Bradley WG, Waluch V, Brant-Zawadzki M, et al. Patchy, periventricular white matter lesions in the elderly: common observation during NMR imaging. Noninvas Med Imag 1:35, 1984.
31. George AE, de Leon MJ, Gentes CI, et al. Leukoencephalopathy in normal and pathologic aging. 2. MRI of brain lucencies. AJNR 7:567, 1986.
32. Brant-Zawadzki M, Fein G, Van Dyke C, et al. Magnetic resonance imaging of the aging brain: patchy white matter lesions and dementia. AJNR 675, 1985.
33. Fishman RA. Brain edema. N Engl J Med 293:706, 1975.
34. Bederson JB, Bartkowski HM, Moon K, et al. Nuclear magnetic resonance imaging and spectroscopy in experimental brain edema in a rat. J Neurosurg 64:795, 1986.
35. Bradley WG, Kortman KE, Crues JV. CNS high resolution MRI: effect of increasing spatial resolution on resolving power. Radiology 156:93, 1985.
36. Fox AJ, Bogousslavksy J, Carey LS, et al. Magnetic resonance imaging of small medullary infarctions. AJNR 7:229, 1986.
37. McNamara MT, Brant-Zawadzki M, Berry I. Acute experimental cerebral ischemia: MR enhancement using Gd-DTPA. Radiology 158:701, 1986.
38. Virapongse C, Mancuso A, Quisling R. Human brain infarcts: Gd-DTPA–enhanced MR imaging. Radiology 161:785, 1986.
39. Weinstein MA, LaValley A, Rosenbloom SA, et al. Limitations of MRI for the detection of gray matter lesions. Presented at the Annual Meeting of the American Society of Neuroradiology, San Diego, January 18–23, 1986.
40. Brant-Zawadzki M, Weinstein P, Bartkowski H, et al. MR imaging and spectroscopy in clinical and experimental cerebral ischemia: a review. AJNR 8:39, 1987.
41. Russell DS, Rubinstein LJ. Pathology of Tumors of the Nervous System, 4th ed. Baltimore, Williams & Wilkins, 1977:129.
42. Kucharczyk W, Lemme-Plaghos L, Uske A, et al. Intracranial vascular malformations: MR and CT imaging. Radiology 156:383, 1985.
43. Gomori JM, Grossman RI, Goldberg HI. Occult cerebral vascular malformations: high field imaging. Radiology 158:707, 1986.
44. Williams AL, Haughton VM. Cranial Computed Tomography. A Comprehensive Text. St Louis, C. V. Mosby Co., 1985.
45. Lee BCP, Herzberg L, Zimmerman RD, et al. MR imaging of cerebral vascular malformations. AJNR 6:863, 1985.
46. Cammarata C, Han JS, Haaga JR, et al. Cerebral venous angiomas imaged by MR. Radiology 155:639, 1985.
47. Augustyn GT, Scott JA, Olson E, et al. Cerebral venous angiomas: MR imaging. Radiology 155:639, 1985.
48. Olson E, Gilmor RL, Richmond B. Cerebral venous angiomas. Radiology 151:97, 1984.
49. Dross P, Raji MR, Dastur KJ. Cerebral varix associated with a venous angioma. AJNR 8:373, 1987.
50. Wohlwill FJ, Yakovlev PI. Histopathology of meningofacial angiomatosis (Sturge-Weber disease): report of four cases. J Neuropathol Exp Neurol 16:341, 1957.
51. Stimac GK, Solomon MA, Newton TH. CT and MR of angiomatous malformations of the choroid plexus in patients with Sturge-Weber disease. AJNR 7:623, 1986.
52. Patel SC, Sanders WP, Fuentes J, et al. Angiographically occult vascular malformations of the brain: MR imaging at 1.5 T. Presented at the Annual Meeting of the Radiological Society of North America, Chicago, November 30–December 5, 1986.
53. Lemme-Plaghos L, Kucharczyk W, Brant-Zawadzki M, et al. MRI of angiographically occult vascular malformations. AJR 146:1223, 1986.
54. New PFJ, Ojemann RG, Davis KR. MR and CT of occult vascular malformations of the brain. AJNR 7:771, 1986.
55. Young IR, Khenia S, Thomas DGT, et al. Clinical magnetic susceptibility mapping of the brain. J Comput Assist Tomogr 11:2, 1987.
56. Atlas SW, Grossman RI, Hackney DB, et al. High-field MR imaging of giant intracranial aneurysms: radiologic-pathologic correlation. Presented at the Annual Meeting of the Radiological Society of North America, Chicago, November 30–December 5, 1986.
57. Hahn FJ, Ong E, McComb R, et al. Peripheral signal void ring in giant vertebral aneurysm: MR and pathology findings. J Comput Assist Tomogr 10:1036, 1986.
58. Black KL, Farhat SM. Giant arteriovenous malformation of the vein of Galen in an adult. Surg Neurol 22:382, 1984.
59. Anderson SC, Murtagh FR, Schnitzlein HN. Vein of Galen aneurysm in a 38-year-old white female. Rev Interam Radiol 11:169, 1986.
60. Roosen N, Schirmer M, Lins E. MRI of an aneurysm of the vein of Galen. AJNR 7:733, 1986.
61. Chakeres DW, Bryan RN. Acute subarachnoid hemorrhage: in vitro comparison of magnetic resonance and computed tomography. AJNR 7:223, 1986.
62. DeLaPaz RL, New PFJ, Buonanno FS, et al. NMR imaging of intracranial hemorrhage. J Comput Assist Tomogr 8:599, 1984.
63. New PFJ, Aronow S. Attenuation measurement of whole blood and blood fractions in computed tomography. Radiology 121:635, 1976.
64. Norman D, Price D, Boyd D, et al. Quantitative aspects of computed tomography of the blood and cerebrospinal fluid. Radiology 123:335, 1977.
65. Bradley WG, Schmidt PG. Effect of methemoglobin formation on the MR appearance of subarachnoid hemorrhage. Radiology 156:99, 1985.
66. Zimmerman RA, Bilaniuk LT, Hackney DB, et al. Head injury: Early results of comparing CT and high-field MR. AJR 147:1215, 1986.
67. Gandy SE, Snow RB, Zimmerman RD, et al. Cranial nuclear magnetic resonance imaging in head trauma. Ann Neurol 16:254, 1984.
68. Han JS, Kaufman B, Alfidi RJ, et al. Head trauma evaluated by magnetic resonance and computed tomography: a comparison. Radiology 150:71, 1984.
69. Moon KL, Brant-Zawadzki M, Pitts LH, et al. Nuclear magnetic resonance imaging of CT-isodense subdural hematomas. AJNR 5:319, 1984.
70. Zimmerman RA, Bilaniuk LT, Gennarelli T. Computed tomography of shearing injuries of the cerebral white matter. Radiology 127:393, 1978.

71. Macchi PJ, Grossman RI, Gomori JM, et al. High field MR imaging of cerebral venous thrombosis. J Comput Assist Tomogr 10:10, 1986.
72. Savino PJ, Grossman RI, Schatz NJ, et al. High-field magnetic resonance imaging in the diagnosis of cavernous sinus thrombosis. Arch Neurol 43:1081, 1986.
73. McMurdo SK, Brant-Zawadzki M, Bradley WG, et al. Dural sinus thrombosis: study using intermediate field strength MR imaging. Radiology 161:83, 1986.
74. Bradley WG, Waluch V. Blood flow: magnetic resonance imaging. Radiology 154:443, 1985.
75. Bradley WG, Waluch V, Lai KS, et al. The appearance of rapidly flowing blood on magnetic resonance images. AJR 143:1167, 1984.
76. von Schulthess GK, Higgins CB. Blood flow imaging with MR: spin-phase phenomena. Radiology 157:687, 1985.
77. Savino PJ, Grossman RI, Schatz NJ, et al. High field magnetic resonance imaging in the diagnosis of cavernous sinus thrombosis. Arch Neurol 43:1081, 1986.
78. Erdman WA, Weinreb JC, Cohen JM, et al. Venous thrombosis: clinical and experimental MR imaging. Radiology 161:233, 1986.
79. Wedeen VJ. Flow MRI holds promise in vascular diagnosis. Diagn Imag 8:84, 1986.
80. Wedeen VJ, Rosen BR, Chesler D, et al. MR velocity imaging by phase display. J Comput Assist Tomogr 9:530, 1985.
81. White EM, Edelman RR, Wedeen VJ. Intravascular signal in MR imaging: use of phase display for differentiation of blood-flow signal from intraluminal disease. Radiology 161:245, 1986.
82. Ferris EJ, Levin HL. Cerebral arteritis. Radiology 109:327, 1973.
83. Gabrielsen TO, Knake JE, Gebarski SS. Inflammatory and immunologic arterial lesions. In Radiology: Diagnosis-Imaging-Intervention, Vol. 3. Philadelphia, J. B. Lippincott, 1986.
84. Ferris EJ: Arteritis. In Newton TH, Potts DG, eds. Radiology of the Skull and Brain. Angiography. St. Louis, C. V. Mosby, 1974.
85. Brant-Zawadzki M, Norman D, eds. Magnetic Resonance Imaging of the Central Nervous System. New York, Raven Press, 1987.
86. Aisen AM, Gabrielsen TO, McCune WJ. MR imaging of systemic lupus erythematosus involving the brain. AJR 144:1027, 1985.
87. Vermess M, Bernstein RM, Bydder GM, et al. Nuclear magnetic resonance (NMR) imaging of the brain in systemic lupus erythematosus. J Comput Assist Tomogr 7:461, 1983.
88. Bilaniuk LT, Patel S, Zimmerman RA. Computed tomography of systemic lupus erythematosus. Radiology 124:119, 1977.
89. Bogousslavsky J, Despland P, Regli F. Spontaneous carotid dissection with acute stroke. Arch Neurol 44:137, 1987.
90. Hart RG, Easton JD. Dissections of cervical and cerebral arteries. Neurol Clin 1:155, 1983.
91. Fisher CM, Ojemann RG, Roberson GH. Spontaneous dissection of cervico-cerebral arteries. Can J Neurol Sci 5:9, 1978.
92. Ojemann RG, Fisher CM, Rich JC. Spontaneous dissecting aneurysm of the cervical internal carotid artery. Stroke 3:434, 1972.
93. Goldberg HI, Grossman RI, Gomori JM. Cervical internal carotid artery dissecting hemorrhage: diagnosis using MR. Radiology 158:157, 1986.

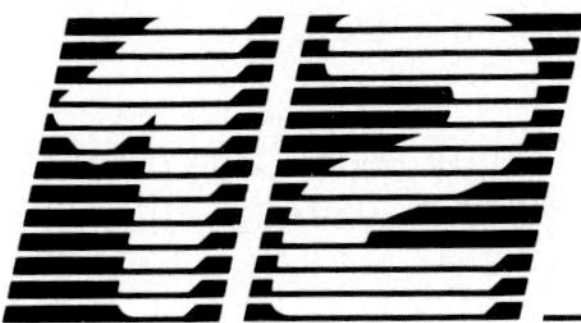

James J. Masters, M.D.

# ISCHEMIA, HYDROCEPHALUS, ATROPHY, AND NEURODEGENERATIVE DISORDERS: MRI EXPERIENCE AT HIGH FIELD STRENGTH (1.5 T)

Approximately 500,000 new strokes will be sustained in America this year, most occurring in individuals more than 55 years of age. Of the 1.5 million citizens in this country who have survived stroke, two in five are so afflicted they require specialized services.[1,2] Stroke may be defined as a sudden focal neurologic deficit (exclusive of seizure, the cause of which is vascular). Stroke is the expressed clinical manifestation of cerebrovascular disease and may be caused by one or more of the following: intraparenchymal hemorrhage or subarachnoid hemorrhage (15%), and ischemia that may or may not progress to infarction.[3]

Major etiologies of brain infarction are known. These emcompass arterial occlusion by thrombosis or embolism, inadequate cerebral circulatory support, and arterial spasm (often secondary to a subarachnoid hemorrhage). Vasculitis, anoxia, moyamoya disease, venous thrombosis, and small penetrating artery disease (lacunes) are other known causes of infarction.

The pathophysiologic response of brain cells to the interruption of cerebral blood flow is characterized by a rapidly moving chain of events. These events have been well reviewed and summarized.[4,5] Research, primarily in mammals, has elucidated several fundamental principles in understanding recovery, partial recovery, or nonrecovery from cerebral ischemia. Hossmann and coworkers showed in animal brains that after one hour of total ischemia at least partial neuronal activity could still occur.[6,7] Later research has shown that depth and duration of ischemia are two basic determinants of outcome; in other words, local cerebral blood flow defines *thresholds* for reversible paralysis and infarction.[8]

A corollary to the concept of thresholds in cerebral ischemia is the ischemic *penumbra*.[9] This descriptive term usually refers to a peripheral zone of nonfunctional but still viable tissue that is capable of complete recovery. This zone surrounds a central locus of brain infarction. However, the term *penumbra* may also be applied in global ischemic states. Another definition is this: a volume of tissue that has not deteriorated enough to make recovery impossible.

Edema is a sequel of cerebral ischemia. Brain edema can be defined as an increase in brain tissue volume secondary to an increase in its fluid content. Two main types of cerebral edema were initially classified, cytotoxic and vasogenic.[10] To *cytotoxic* edema and *vasogenic* edema a third general category, *interstitial* edema, has been added.[11] In the cytotoxic form, all brain cells in the gray and white matter may undergo swelling. The swollen neurons, glia, and endothelial cells serve to decrease the extracellular fluid volume, but capillary permeability remains normal. Conversely, vasogenic edema, the most common type, chiefly affects white matter. Its pathogenesis is characterized by increased permeability of brain capillary endothelial cells. Once the blood-brain barrier has been broken, increased extracellular fluid volume may result. The third type of edema, interstitial edema, is best exemplified in obstructive hydrocephalus in which transependymal movement of CSF across ventricular walls causes an increase in the sodium and water content of the periventricular white matter. This may be reversible with neurosurgical shunting.

Water content is increased in ischemic and infarcted brain tissue. The increase is maximal at two days.[12] However, certain ischemic flow and time thresholds must be violated before edema begins to form.[13] Cerebral ischemic edema is of more than one type. Vasogenic (extracellular) edema occurs first, followed by cytotoxic (intracellular) edema.[14] Changes in brain water caused by edema-producing brain lesions can be detected by magnetic resonance imaging (MRI).[15] There is also evidence that brain edema can be analyzed as to type with MRI.[16] Optimal pulsing sequences determine the conspicuity of brain edema.[17]

Certain facts regarding the clinical usefulness of MR in stroke have been established. Evidence exists that MR can characterize acute, subacute, and chronic intracerebral hematomas as well as similar states of hemorrhagic infarction.[18–20] Subarachnoid hemorrhage has been studied with MR both in vitro and in vivo. Unfortunately, acute subarachnoid hemorrhage less than one week old is difficult to detect with MR and is

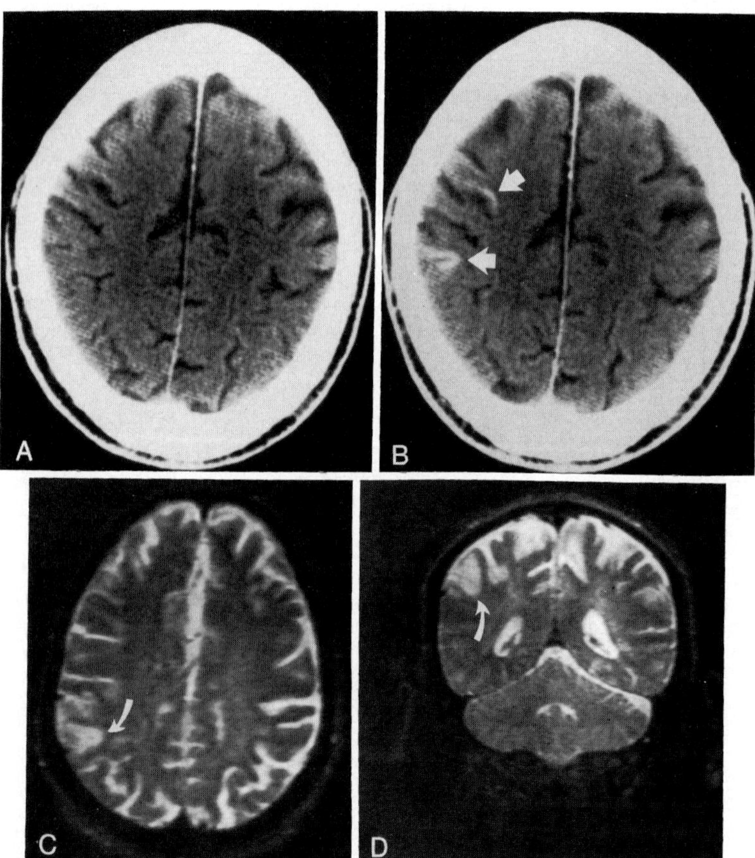


**Figure 12–1. Cortical infarction, poorly seen on MR.** A 70-year-old man with left hemiparesis, whose previous CT (not shown) was interpreted as normal. *A,* CT. *B,* CECT. *C,* Axial T2WI. *D,* Coronal T2WI. Computed tomography *(A* and *B*), performed one week later, shows right parietal cortical enhancement (arrows), a subacute cortical infarct. T2WI MR shows subtle cortical signal increase (curved arrows), easily misconstrued as a prominent cortical sulcus.

nearly isointense with normal brain.[21, 22] Conversely, computed tomography (CT) can identify subarachnoid blood within the first few hours after ictus.[23, 24] Clearly, this capability gives CT the early imaging advantage for this diagnosis.

Given the 20% to 30% false-negative rate for CT in detecting brain ischemic infarcts within the first 24 hours, a more sensitive diagnostic tool such as MR is welcome.[25, 26] In experimental animals, MR imaging has detected cerebral infarction as early as 30 minutes post ictus.[27] Abundant evidence in humans indicates that MR is generally more sensitive than CT in demonstrating infarcts and their extent, both above and, especially, below the tentorium.[28–37] However, diagnostic difficulties have been reported in the MR diagnosis of small purely cortical gray matter infarcts (Fig. 12–1).[38] Scattered white matter foci of signal hyperintensity may occur in the following clinical syndromes: (1) ischemic disease, (2) hypertension, (3) Binswanger's disease, (4) normal aging, and (5) demyelination.

Sodium, the second most favorable nuclei for MR imaging, is also being evaluated in animals and humans in CNS disease in general and ischemia in particular.[39–42] Very large differences in sodium concentrations exist among both normal and diseased tissues. The differences are greater than those resulting from hydrogen proton concentrations. In clinical images, these differences mean increased contrast in areas of cerebral infarction and the potential for earlier or more complete lesion detection or both.[39] However, sodium MR imaging is hindered by low signal-to-noise levels, high operating fields, and increased imaging time.[39–41]

Early results indicate low specificity with MR for findings of infarction, as many lesions do not correlate with the clinical history or examination.[32, 35, 37] However, while there is still a relative paucity of specific data on infarction, hints of MR's ability to diagnose reversible ischemia in humans prior to actual infarction have appeared in the literature, but this awaits adequate proof.[43–45]

Although neither CT nor proton MR is the perfect imaging method for acute stroke, we believe that, on balance, CT should remain the initial supratentorial screening examination at present. If CT does not provide an answer to the clinical problem, then MRI should follow.

# ISCHEMIA AND INFARCTION

## Ischemic Infarct

Despite the presence of several different etiologies for ischemic strokes, their MR appearance is rather uniform and is demonstrable on machines of all field strengths (Table 12–1). Post ictus, the earliest reported onset of signal changes seems to vary from 30 minutes to 6 hours.[27, 46–49] In general, the signal changes are due to postinfarction edema, which causes T1 (hypointense signal) and T2 (hyperintense signal) prolongation.[46–48, 50, 51] These changes increase for at least the first 24 hours.[46, 48] Of the two parameters, T1 and T2, prolonged T2 (hyperintense signal) seems to be the more sensitive marker of infarction.[30] This conclusion is bolstered by some T1-weighted images (T1WI) in which the infarct is not seen as an area of hypointensity. This phenomenon can be explained by the presence of several opposing processes in edematous tissue. Increased water in the tissue, that is, edema, increases the number of protons available to resonate and also serves to lengthen their coherent resonance following radiowave stimulation. Therefore, T2 relaxation is lengthened. Alone, these circumstances produce increased signal. Countering this is the signal-lowering tendency of incomplete magnetization in edematous tissue on short TR (T1-weighted) sequences. The net result, at times, is a lack of contrast between normal brain and the infarct.[52] Therefore long TR/long TE, spin-echo (SE) T2-weighted images are optimal for early detection.[52, 53] Occasionally, in spin-echo imaging, creating an echo train or calculated images will clarify an uncertain distinction between tumor or hemorrhagic infarct and a recent, simple ischemic infarct.[54] Either of these two tech-

**Table 12–1.** CAUSES OF BRAIN INFARCTION

| |
|---|
| Arterial occlusive disease |
| Atherosclerotic occlusion |
| Embolism |
| Hemodynamic ischemia |
| Arteriolosclerosis (lacunar disease) |
| Vasculitis |
| Moya moya disease |
| Anoxic ischemia |
| Venous thrombosis |

*Source:* Goldberg H, Lee SH. Stroke in Cranial Computed Tomography, 2nd ed. New York, McGraw-Hill Book Co., 1987, p. 645, with permission.

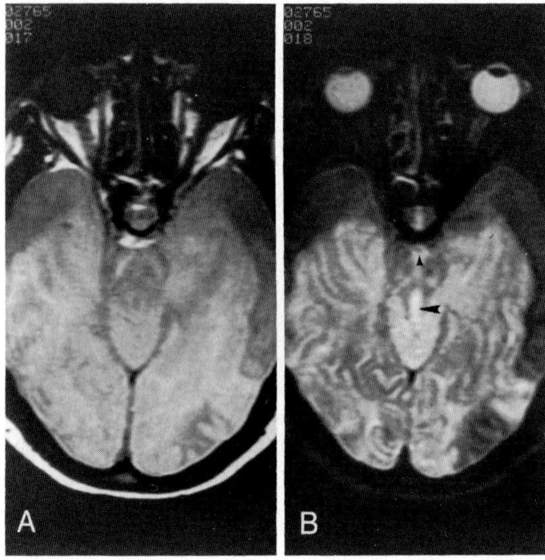

**Figure 12–2. Basilar artery occlusion; posterior circulation infarction; clinical "locked-in" syndrome.** An 80-year-old man with suspected hypertension made hypointensive by clinicians in the emergency room. A clinical "locked-in" syndrome ensued (1.5 T). *A,* Axial N(H)WI (TR 1800/TE 20). *B,* T2WI (TR 1800/TE 100). Diffuse hyperintense edema and cerebral swelling appear in the distribution of the posterior circulation. Brain swelling has eliminated aqueductal flow void (arrowhead). Normal basilar artery flow-void signal is eliminated (small arrowhead).

niques may increase contrast between the bed of edema and the tumor or hemorrhage lying within it. Other MR features of infarction should be familiar from CT. Multiplanar MR allows one to identify that a signal abnormality lies in a vascular territory, allowing distinction from neoplasm. Serial scans are also useful. Infarcts evolve and change in the near-term whereas tumors do not, assuming the patient is not on steroids. Infarct mass effect is related to the expansile property of edematous tissue and is maximal at two to four days, subsiding thereafter.[25] Unless the infarct is large, mass effect is usually subtle. Ventricular compression and sulcal effacement are readily detected. Loss of gray-white matter contrast occurs in both new and old infarction.[51] Infarct contour becomes more sharply marginated with time. In addition, the diagnosis of vessel occlusion can be made with MR by noting persistent increased or isointense signal

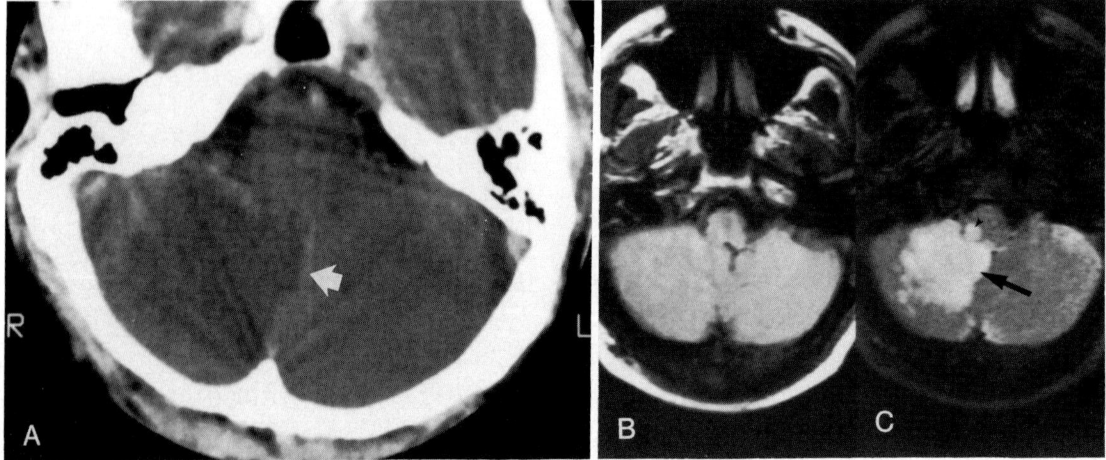

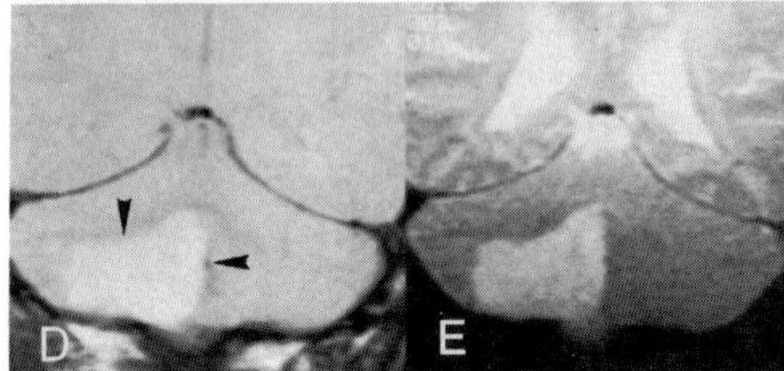

**Figure 12–3. PICA infarct (36 hours).** A 58-year-old man with acute onset of ataxia (1.5 T). *A,* Axial CECT. *B* and *C,* Axial multiecho N(H)WI and T2WI. *D* and *E,* Coronal multiecho N(H)WI and T2WI. Hypodensity in the right cerebellar hemisphere produces mild mass effect (white arrow): An axial MR reveals hyperintense signal on T2WI (arrow) and unsuspected restiform body involvement (arrowhead). A coronal MR shows typical vascular distribution of a posterior inferior cerebellar artery (PICA) infarct and a wedge shape (arrowheads). More acute infarcts may not appear on N(H)WI.

within the appropriate vessel (Fig. 12–2). The signal in an acute or early subacute vascular occlusion often decreases between the first and second echoes of a spin-echo pulse sequence, particularly at high field strengths.[55]

Infarct dating by MR without intravenous contrast has proven to be an imprecise and difficult exercise. Acute and subacute infarction (Figs. 12–2 to 12–8) may be difficult to differentiate by MR alone unless paramagnetic contrast agents are given. Both acute and subacute infarcts may produce signal hyperintensity on T2WI at 1.5 tesla (T). However, hypointensity is more pronounced on T1WI with subacute infarcts and may be undetectable acutely on T1WI or N(H)WI. A chronic infarct consisting of either gliosis or porencephaly (Figs. 12–9 to 12–12) can be confidently diagnosed. Marked homogeneous T1 and T2 prolongation, similar to CSF, is often accompanied by neighboring areas of "negative" mass effect indicating adjoining brain shrinkage. Focal, prominent mass effect suggests cystic neoplasm (Fig. 12–13). Localized sulcal enlargement with secondary widening of the neighboring subarachnoid space and regional ventricular enlargement toward the lesion are examples of negative mass effect.

The computed tomographic findings of infarction may be summarized as follows:

*Acute infarction* (zero to five days): De-

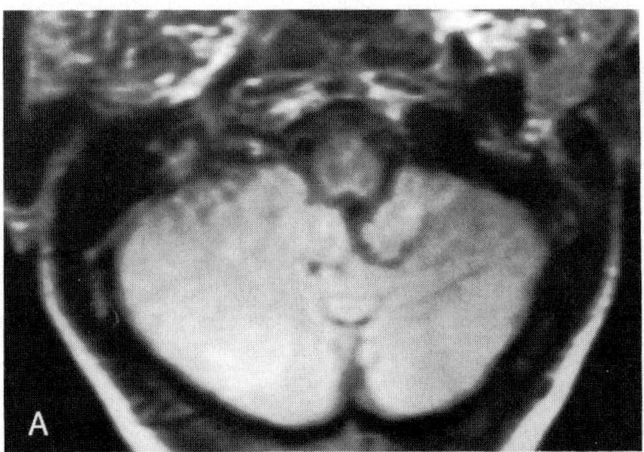


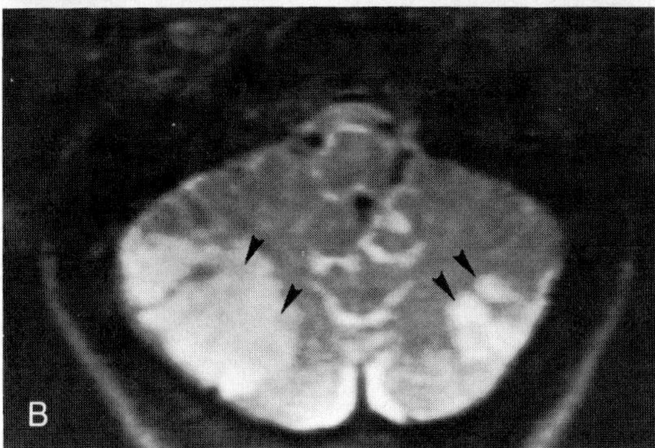


**Figure 12–4. Acute bilateral PICA infarcts (42 hours).** An 84-year-old woman with ataxic gait (1.5 T). *A* and *B*, Axial multiecho N(H)WI and T2WI. Bilateral cerebellar lesion hyperintensity on T2WI (arrowheads) is virtually inapparent on N(H)WI.

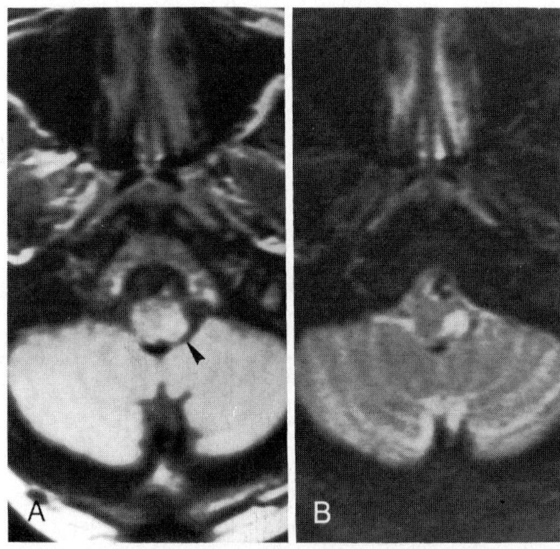


**Figure 12–5. Acute restiform body infarct.** A 59-year-old man with acute onset of diplopia, slurred speech, and left hemiparesis (1.5 T). *A*, Axial N(H)WI (TR 2300/TE 20). *B*, Axial T2WI (TR 2300/TE 100). A rounded focus of increased signal is present in the patient's left restiform body; it is barely visible on N(H)WI (arrowhead) but is easily seen on T2WI. No mass effect is present.

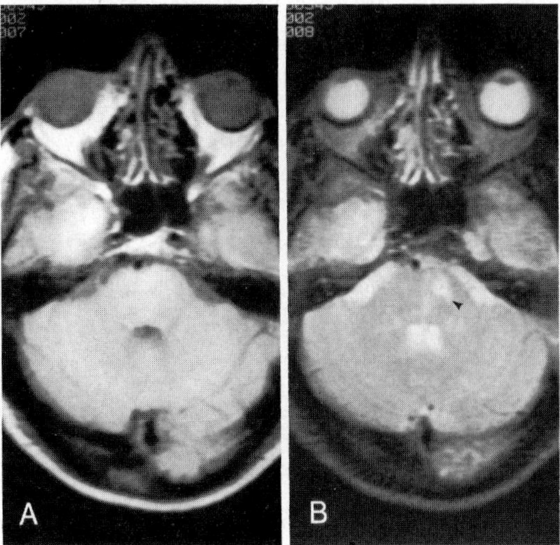


**Figure 12–6. Acute pontine infarct (24 hours).** A 66-year-old man with a two-day history of bulbar signs and a normal CECT (not shown) (1.5 T). *A* and *B*, Axial multiecho N(H)WI and T2WI (TR 1800/TE 20/80). Hyperintensity is appreciated only on T2WI (arrowhead); it is "hidden" on N(H)WI, not unusual with acute (< 72-hour) infarcts.

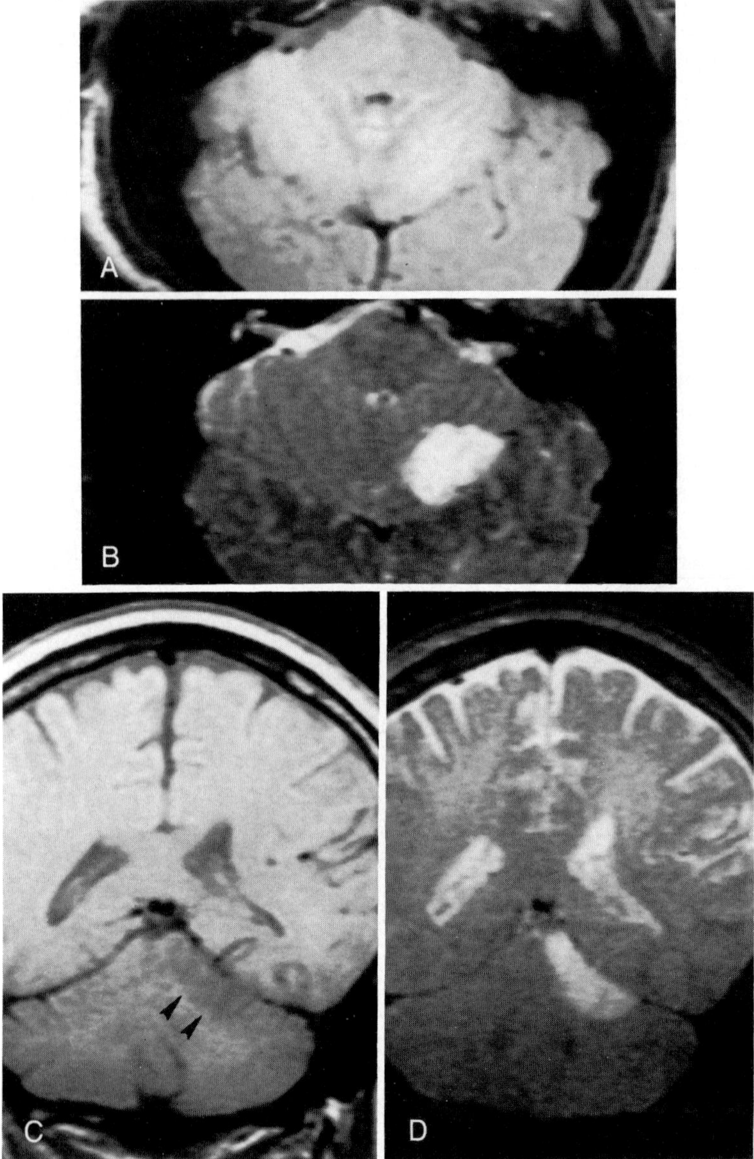


**Figure 12–7. Acute superior cerebellar artery infarction.** A 54-year-old man with dizziness and ataxia (1.5 T). *A* and *B,* Axial multiecho N(H)WI and T2WI. *C* and *D,* Coronal multiecho N(H)WI and T2WI. The axial images demonstrate a focal signal increase in the left superior cerebellar hemisphere, exhibiting little mass effect on T2WI. Paucity of mass effect supports the diagnosis of ischemia/infarction. Direct coronal MR confirms the wedge shape, peripheral location, and vascular territory of the signal alteration (arrowheads).

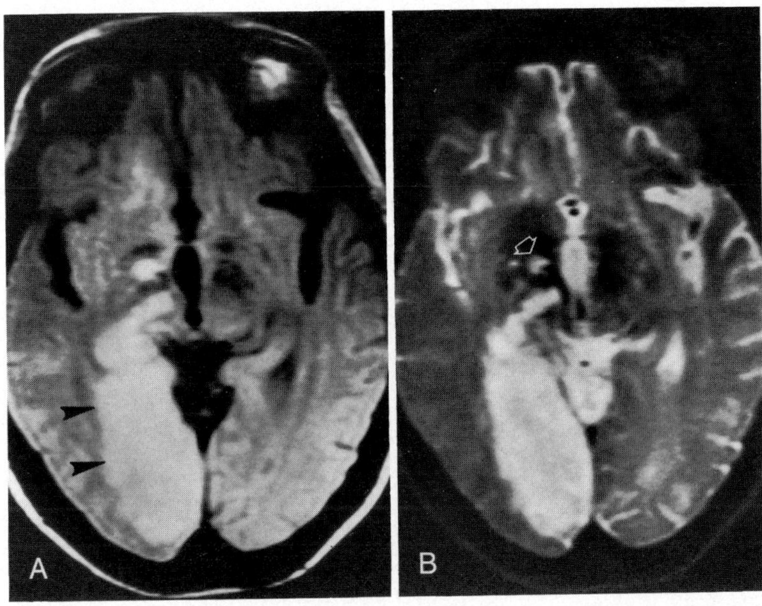

**Figure 12–8. Nonhemorrhagic posterior cerebral artery infarction (48 hours).** A 62-year-old woman with 48-hour-old visual symptoms (1.5 T). *A* and *B,* Axial multiecho N(H)WI and T2WI (TR 1800/TE 20/80. Hyperintense signal in the right occipital lobe (arrowheads) follows a vascular distribution. Hyperintense thalamic signal (open arrows) corresponds to thalamogeniculate vascular territory.

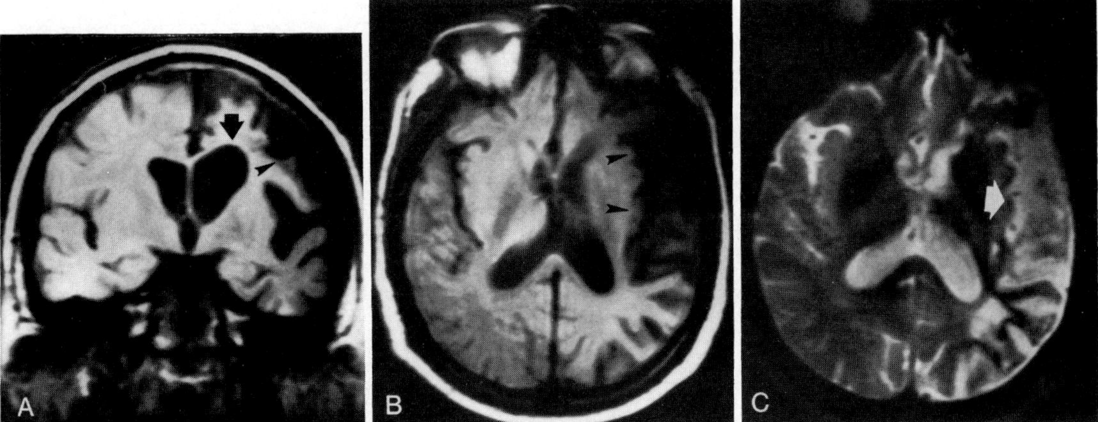

**Figure 12–9. Remote left middle cerebral infarction.** A 59-year-old man. Atrophy and encephalomalacia produces CSF-like signal hypointensity on T1WI (arrowheads) and hyperintensity on T2WI (white arrow) in the middle cerebral artery distribution. "Ex vacuo" enlargement of the left ventricle is present (black arrow).

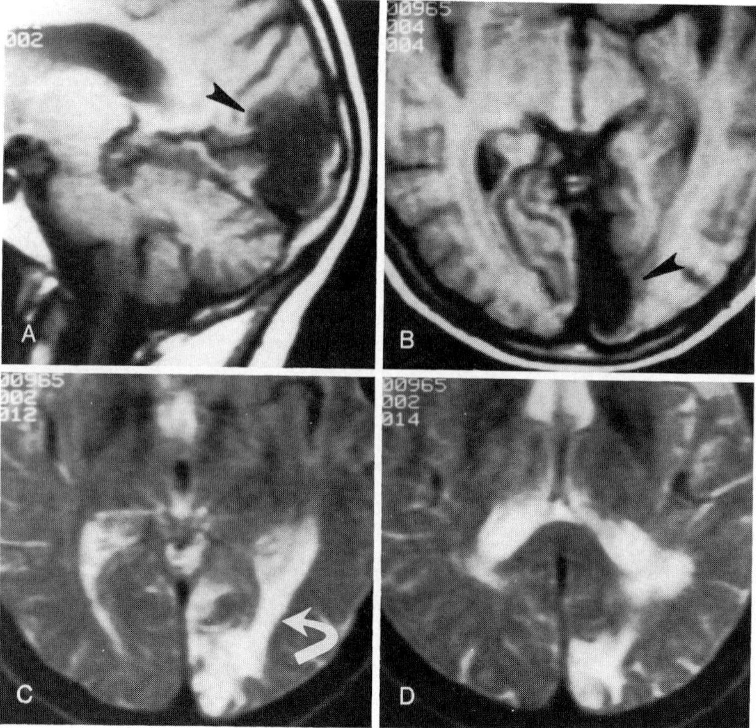


**Figure 12–10. Chronic (five months) posterior cerebral artery infarct.** A 74-year-old woman with a known five-month-old ischemic effect (1.5 T). *A,* Sagittal T1WI. *B,* Axial T1WI. *C* and *D,* Axial T2WI. Left (of patient) occipital hypointense signal (arrowheads) matches the signal of CSF on T1WI and has resulted in compensatory ventricular occipital horn enlargement (curved arrow).

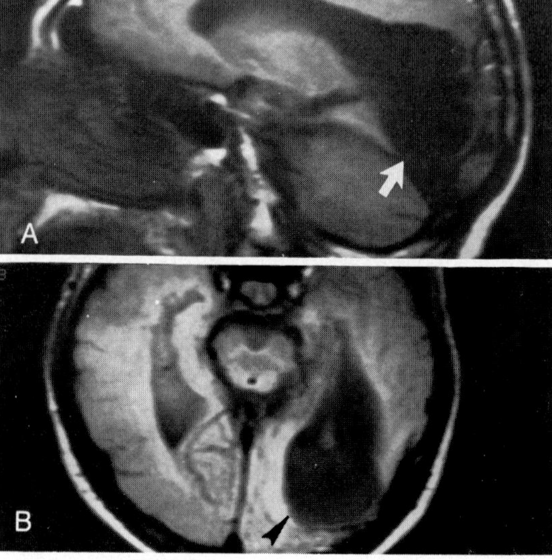


**Figure 12–11. Porencephaly, remote (three years) occipital infarct.** A 68-year-old man who has had a prior ischemic event (1.5 T). *A,* Sagittal T1W1. *B,* Axial N(H)WI. A focal, old, left occipital infarct has resulted in porencephaly with ipsilateral enlargement and communication with the ventricular occipital horn on T1WI (arrow) and N(H)WI (arrowhead).

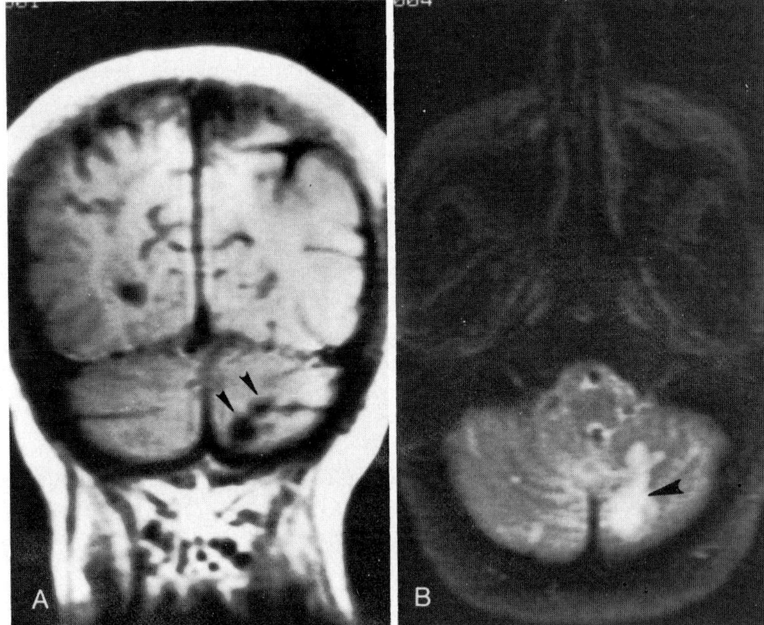


**Figure 12–12. Remote PICA infarct.** A 68-year-old woman with known posterior inferior cerebellar (PICA) infarct two years previously. Focal hypointensity similar to CSF in signal (arrowheads) on T1WI and hyperintense on T2WI (arrowhead) is compatible with porencephaly secondary to remote infarct.

creased attenuation appears within 12 hours in 66% of instances and in 80% by 24 hours; mass effect (maximal at two to four days) may be seen.

*Subacute infarction* (7 to 30 days): As edema resolves, the infarct may become isodense to normal brain (fogging effect) on noncontrast CT; nonhomogeneous contrast enhancement occurs in 70% of cases.

*Chronic infarction* (more than 1 month): Lesion density evolves to less than normal brain (gliosis) or to CSF attenuation (porencephaly); focal atrophic changes in brain and neighboring CSF-filled structures yield negative mass effect; generally, no contrast enhancement is seen, except for rare cases in which enhancement may occur for weeks or months post ictus.

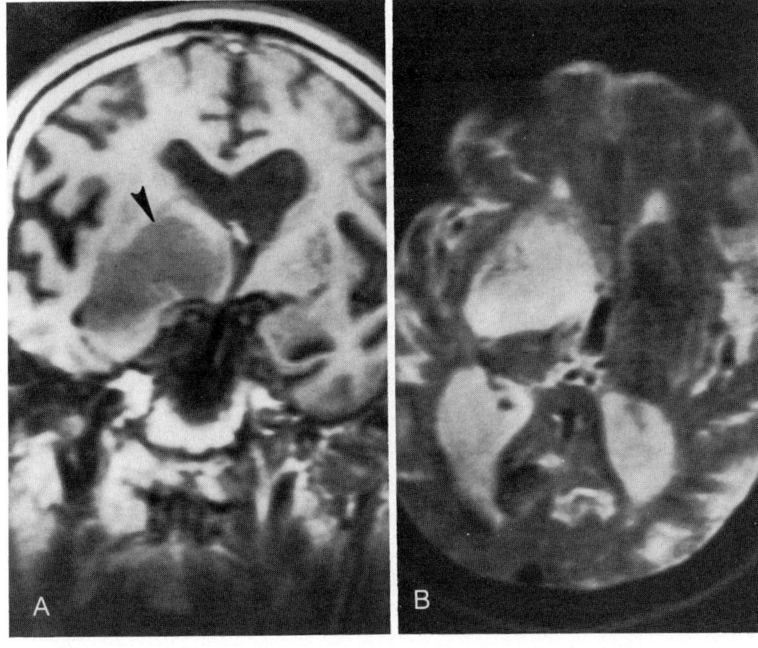


**Figure 12–13. Colon carcinoma metastasis.** An 84-year-old man with altered mental status (1.5 T). *A,* Coronal T1WI (TR 600/TE 20). *B,* Axial T2WI (TR 1800/TE 100). A hypointense region (arrowhead) on T1WI exhibits a signal that differs from that of the CSF. The hyperintense signal on T2WI exhibits moderate mass effect and does not follow a vascular territory. It should not be misconstrued as a subacute infarct.

### Hemorrhagic Infarction at 1.5 T

The great majority of hemorrhagic brain infarctions are due to cerebral embolism followed by high-pressure arterial reperfusion of the ischemic brain through damaged capillaries.[56] Most cerebral emboli come from atheroma of major neck arteries and cardiac valvular or ischemic problems.[2] But hemorrhagic infarction can also be associated with hypertension and anticoagulation.[57, 58] Ordinarily, the hemorrhage involves the gray matter of the cortex or basal ganglia.[59] Evidence exists that both intermediate- and high-field MR units can detect and categorize hemorrhage into acute, subacute, and chronic phases (Figs. 12–14 to 12–18) provided proper pulse sequences are used.[18, 20] In addition, MRI can distinguish a hemorrhagic cortical infarct from both a purely ischemic infarct and from an intraparenchymal hematoma.[19]

Chronologic MR staging of hemorrhagic infarction is possible. Acutely, isointense signal with normal gray matter and cortex appears on T1WI. White matter edema may produce acute T1 signal hypointensity. T2WI shows serpiginous or gyriform cortical hypointensity (at higher field strengths) interdigitating with high-intensity subcortical white matter edema (Fig. 12–14). Subacutely, progressive gyriform T1WI hyperintensity (Figs. 12–15 and 12–16) occurs as cortical T2WI hypointensity begins to become less apparent. Subcortical hyperintense white matter edema again is present at this stage on T2WI. Chronically, hyperintense signal (Figs. 12–17 and 12–18) may be present along with focal atrophy on T1WI; T2WI yield increased signal intensity.[19] However, hypointense infarct residua on T2WI may result from parenchymal hemosiderin. These temporal changes are related to the evolution of red blood cell degradation products.[18, 19]

### Transient Ischemic Attack

A transient ischemic attack (TIA) is presently defined as a short incident of focal neurologic disturbance resolving completely within 24 hours, in a patient with vascular disease. At least 10% of strokes are preceded by a TIA. Those TIAs that recur within 24 hours, within a few days, or last more than one hour are more likely to be harbingers of stroke. The current belief is that 95% of TIAs are caused by small emboli, and that the remaining 5% result from hemodynamic factors or spasm.[60]

Although complete remission of signs and symptoms is part of the definition of a TIA, this should not imply that no structural ischemic damage ever results from an attack. Post-TIA infarcts have been found.[61–63] Some sources have raised the question whether TIAs, reversible ischemic neurologic deficits

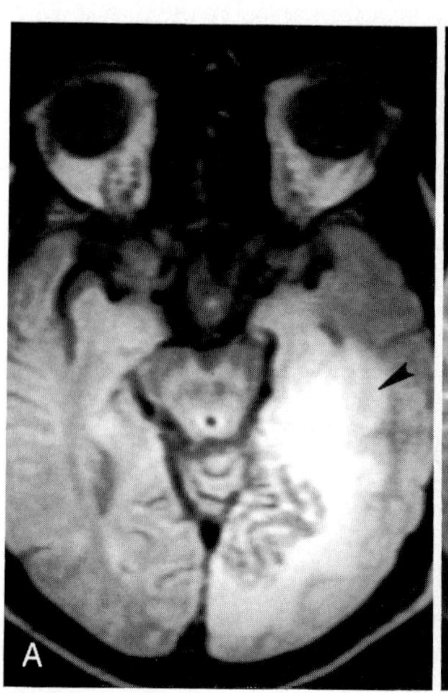


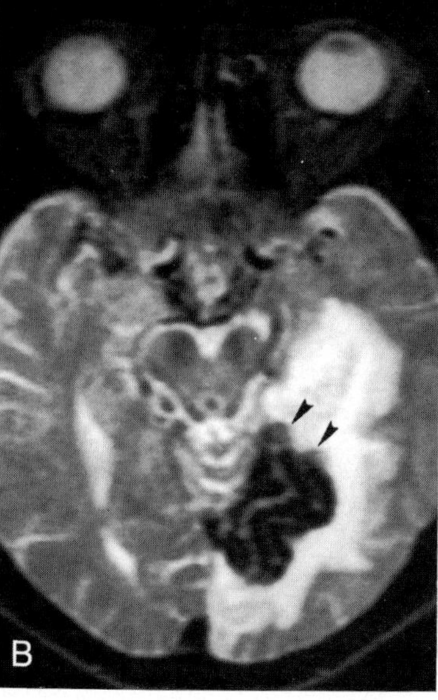


**Figure 12–14. Hemorrhagic posterior cerebral artery infarction (48 hours).** A 72-year-old man with acute onset of ataxia 48 hours earlier (1.5 T). *A* and *B,* Axial multiecho N(H)WI and T2WI (TR 1800/TE 20/80). Left parieto-occipital infarct edema (arrowhead) and preferential T2-relaxation shortening effect due to intracellular deoxyhemoglobin and methemoglobin (arrowheads).

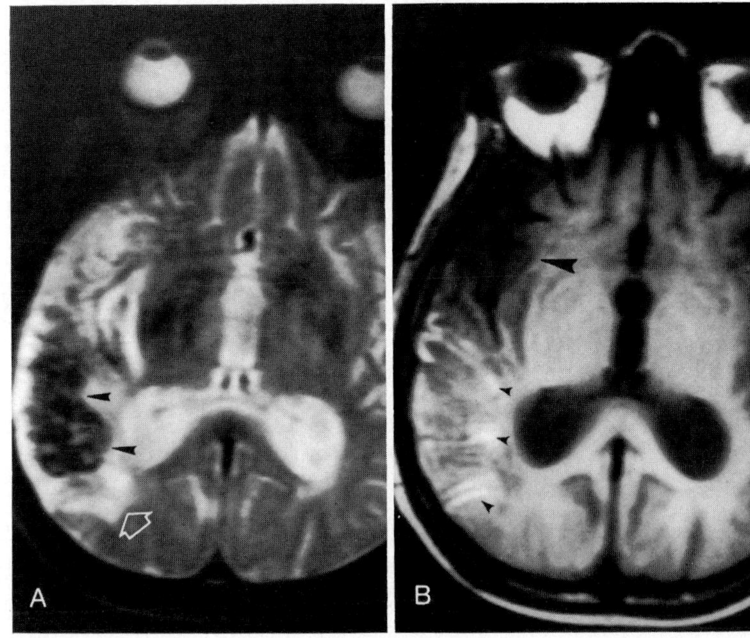


**Figure 12–15. Chronic nonhemorrhagic infarct; superimposed early subacute hemorrhagic infarct.** A 79-year-old man with a history of right middle cerebral artery infarct, treated with anticoagulants, two months earlier (1.5 T). *A,* Axial T2WI (TR 1800/TE 20). *B,* Axial T1WI (TR 600/TE 20). The older infarct appears as a CSF-like hypointense signal on T1WI (large arrowhead) and is hyperintense on T2WI. Subacute hemorrhagic infarction (three days) exhibits hyperintense edema (open arrow), T2 preferential shortening due to intracellular deoxyhemoglobin and methemoglobin (arrowhead), and a hyperintense proton-electron dipole-dipole effect on T1WI (small arrowheads) due to extracellular methemoglobin.

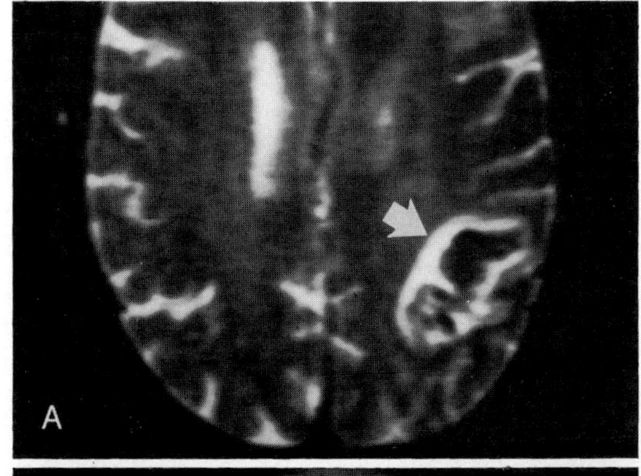


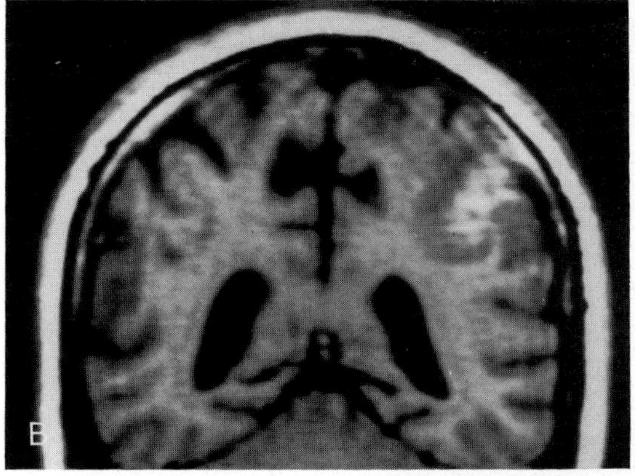


**Figure 12–16. Subacute (six days) hemorrhagic infarction.** A 74-year-old man with right hemiparesis and a normal CT six days previously (not shown) who was placed on heparin (1.5 T). *A,* Axial T2WI (TR 2300/TE 100). *B,* Coronal T1WI (TR 600/TE 20). T2W1 shows hyperintense parietal infarct edema (arrow) and preferential T2-relaxation shortening caused by intracellular deoxyhemoglobin and methemoglobin of acute/early subacute hemorrhage. T1WI shows hyperintensity of methemoglobin (extracellular) in subacute hemorrhagic phenomena.

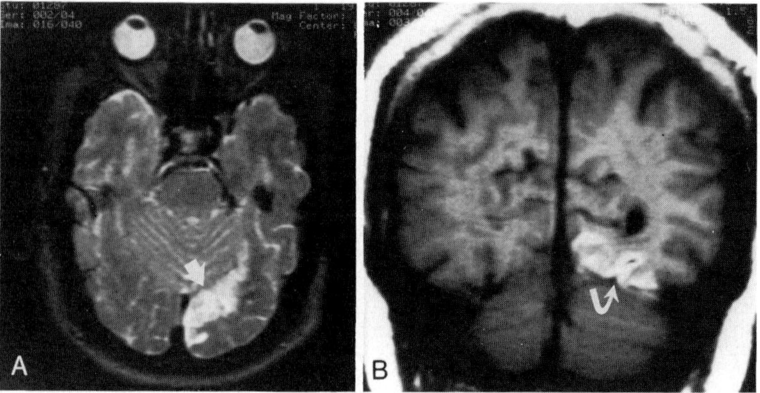


**Figure 12–17. Chronic hemorrhagic occipital infarct (three weeks).** A 51-year-old man (1.5 T). *A,* Axial T2WI. *B,* Coronal T1WI. Serpiginous gyriform signal hyperintensity without mass effect involves the left parahippocampal and occipital cortex (arrow) on T2WI. Signal hyperintensity on T1WI (curved arrow) and T2WI identifies process as hemorrhagic and chronic.

(RINDs), and strokes with minimal residua should even be considered different groups since the structural ischemic lesions identified show no differences in size and location.[64] We agree with one authority who has called for redefinition of the classification of ischemic episodes once a large MRI imaging data base has been collected.[65] For now, early MRI data show focal parenchymal changes in approximately three fourths of TIA patients, while CT is positive in about one third. Focal areas of increased signal intensity on T2WI constitute the findings, with some, but not all, seen less conspicuously on T1WI. Correlation with the clinical findings is confusing as a high frequency of similar changes in the contralateral nonsymptomatic vascular territory is often present as well.[32]

### Watershed Infarction

Boundary or border zones exist between neighboring vascular territories in the brain. Examples include the anterior and middle cerebral arteries, the middle and posterior cerebral arteries, and the superior and infe-

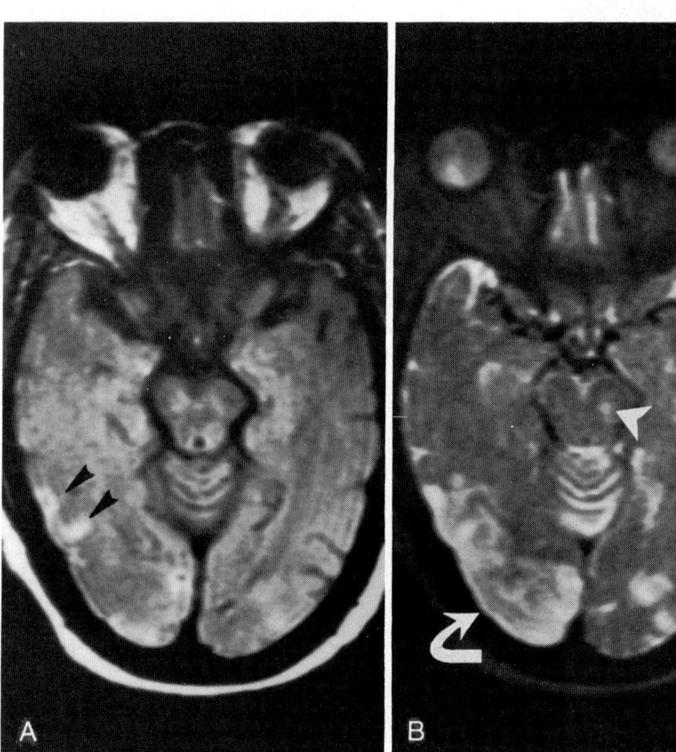


**Figure 12–18. Chronic hemorrhagic infarct; left cerebral peduncle infarct.** An 84-year-old woman with left-sided weakness (1.5 T). *A,* T1WI (TR 600/TE 20). *B,* T2WI (TR 1800/TE 100). Gyriform signal hyperintensity appears in the patient's right parieto-occipital cortex on T2WI (curved arrow). Hyperintense foci (arrowheads) on T1WI identify the process as hemorrhagic. Hyperintensity on both T1WI and T2WI identify the hemorrhage as chronic. There is also a left cerebral peduncle infarct (arrowhead).

rior cerebellar arteries. Small end-branches of these arteries anastomose with one another, serving as potential sources of collateral blood supply if needed. These zones are usually predictable and bilaterally symmetric. Cerebral blood flow may be harmfully diminished in these "watershed" zones owing to occlusion of large arteries, to systemic hypotension, or to decreased cardiac output.[66] The parieto-occipital cortex is the most vulnerable of the boundary zones. Depending on the chronology and severity of the perfusion pressure reduction, the patient may sustain a TIA or complete infarction.[67]

The ischemic signal change may be localized to the proximal white matter, the peripheral cortical gray matter (Fig. 12–19), or both.[2, 68] MR findings in the evolution of purely ischemic and hemorrhagic infarctions have already been described in this chapter.

## DISEASES STRONGLY RELATED TO HYPERTENSION

### Lacunar Disease

Lacunes are small infarcts, deep within the brain, ranging in size from 3 mm to 20 mm. They may or may not be symptomatic, depending on size and location. The most frequent sites of lacunes in declining order are as follows: putamen, caudate, thalamus, pons, internal capsule, and convexity white matter. In 90% of patients, these small cavities are associated with chronically elevated systemic blood pressure.[69] Whatever the method of stenosis or occlusion, the arteries involved are the small penetrating twigs of larger vessels such as the lenticulostriate branches of the anterior and middle cerebral arteries.[70]

Often conical in shape because of the small vascular territories involved, lacunes are seen on axial MR images as distinct foci of T2 prolongation yielding hyperintense signal and in their more chronic phase as areas of low signal on T1WI (Fig. 12–20). Lacunes are part of the differential diagnosis for small white matter lesions seen on MR as foci of T2 prolongation. When acute or subacute (Fig. 12–21), they appear hyperintense on balanced or proton density weighted images (N[H]WI) and T2WI, making distinction from many causes of punctate signal alteration on MR difficult. Lacunar infarcts less than 24 hours old may produce signal alteration on T2WI, but not N(H)WI or T1WI. Other processes producing such signal changes include multiple sclerosis (Fig. 12–22), chronic hypertension, carcinomatous encephalitis of metastatic disease, normal aging changes (Fig. 12–23), Binswanger's disease (Fig. 12–24), and infection. Two recent additions to the differential diagnostic list include Sjögren's syndrome and migraine headache.[71, 72] These UBOs (unknown bright objects), or foci of T2WI hyperintensity, are indistinguishable on MR

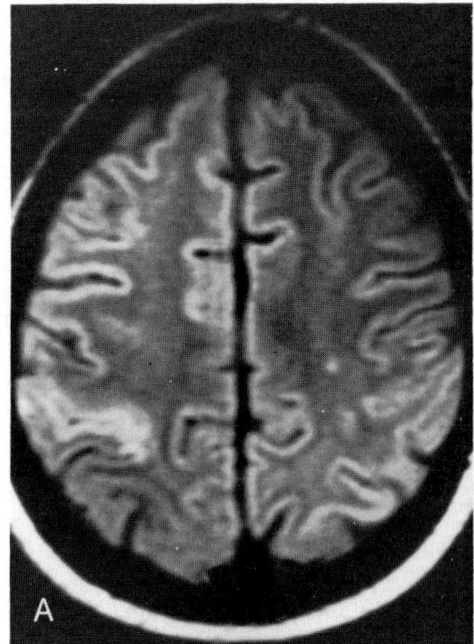


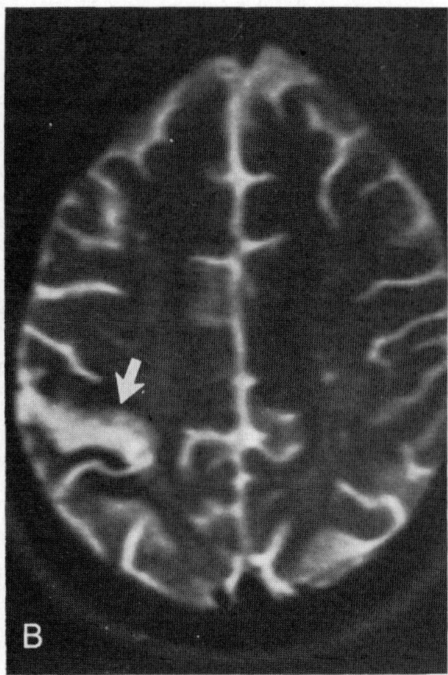


**Figure 12–19. Watershed zone, parietal cortical infarct.** A 39-year-old woman with sudden left sensorimotor deficit dating to a generalized seizure and global anoxia (1.5 T). *A* and *B*, Axial multiecho N(H)WI and T2WI (TR 1800/TE 20/80). A localized gyral signal hyperintensity on N(H)WI and T2WI (arrow) identifies the lesion as a cortical infarct. The lesion was inapparent on T1WI (not shown).

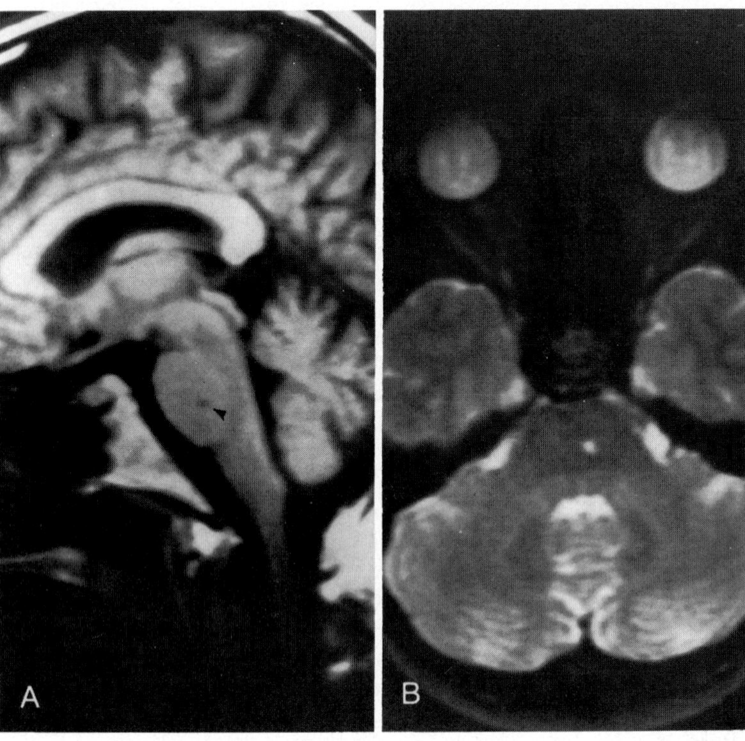


**Figure 12–20. Chronic pontine lacunar infarction.** A 40-year-old woman with known systemic lupus erythematosus (1.5 T). *A,* Sagittal T1WI. *B,* Axial T2WI. A focal, punctate, hypointense signal on T1WI (arrowhead) and hyperintensity on T2WI in the patient's leftward pons.

and usually cannot be differentiated from one another based on MR appearance alone.[32, 38, 73] Although these UBOs are seen in the asymptomatic elderly population, they have been pathologically correlated with microinfarction.

### Binswanger's Disease (Subcortical Arteriosclerotic Encephalopathy—SAE)

More common than previously suspected, this condition is generally thought to be a variant of hypertensive arteriosclerotic vasculopathy affecting mainly the long, penetrating medullary arteries of deep cerebral white matter. Pathologically, focal and diffuse loss of myelin, axonal loss, and fibrosis within the walls of small arteries may be identified. Hydrocephalus ex vacuo, lacunes, and cortical infarcts are often associated with SAE.[74] This disease, which often begins in the sixth decade of life, has highly variable clinical symptomatology. One third of patients have no neurologic deficits, whereas others may present with stroke, gait disturbance, or slowly progressive dementia.[75] There is no specific treatment.

Three MR grades of severity have been described, all of which cause T1 and T2 prolongation. In the mildest degree, discrete small focal lesions are present in anterior, posterior, or mid periventricular locations (Fig. 12–24). Intermediate involvement yields focal or partially confluent hyperintense lesions best seen on T2WI. The severest form shows confluent lesions of white matter circumferentially about the ventricles (Fig. 12–25).[75]

When the lesions are punctate, the UBO differential diagnosis pertains. When confluent periventricular signals are present, the span of diagnostic possibilities includes demyelinating diseases and transependymal absorption of CSF. In the latter, enlarged temporal horns and other criteria for obstructive hydrocephalus should be present. Furthermore, transependymal CSF reabsorption signal zones are said to be centered anteriorly to the frontal horns, to have sharp transition to normal white matter along their outer margins, and often to extend fully through the corpus callosum. SAE, in contradistinction, usually is centered anterolaterally to the frontal horns, has poorly defined margins, and rarely extends into the corpus callosum.[74]

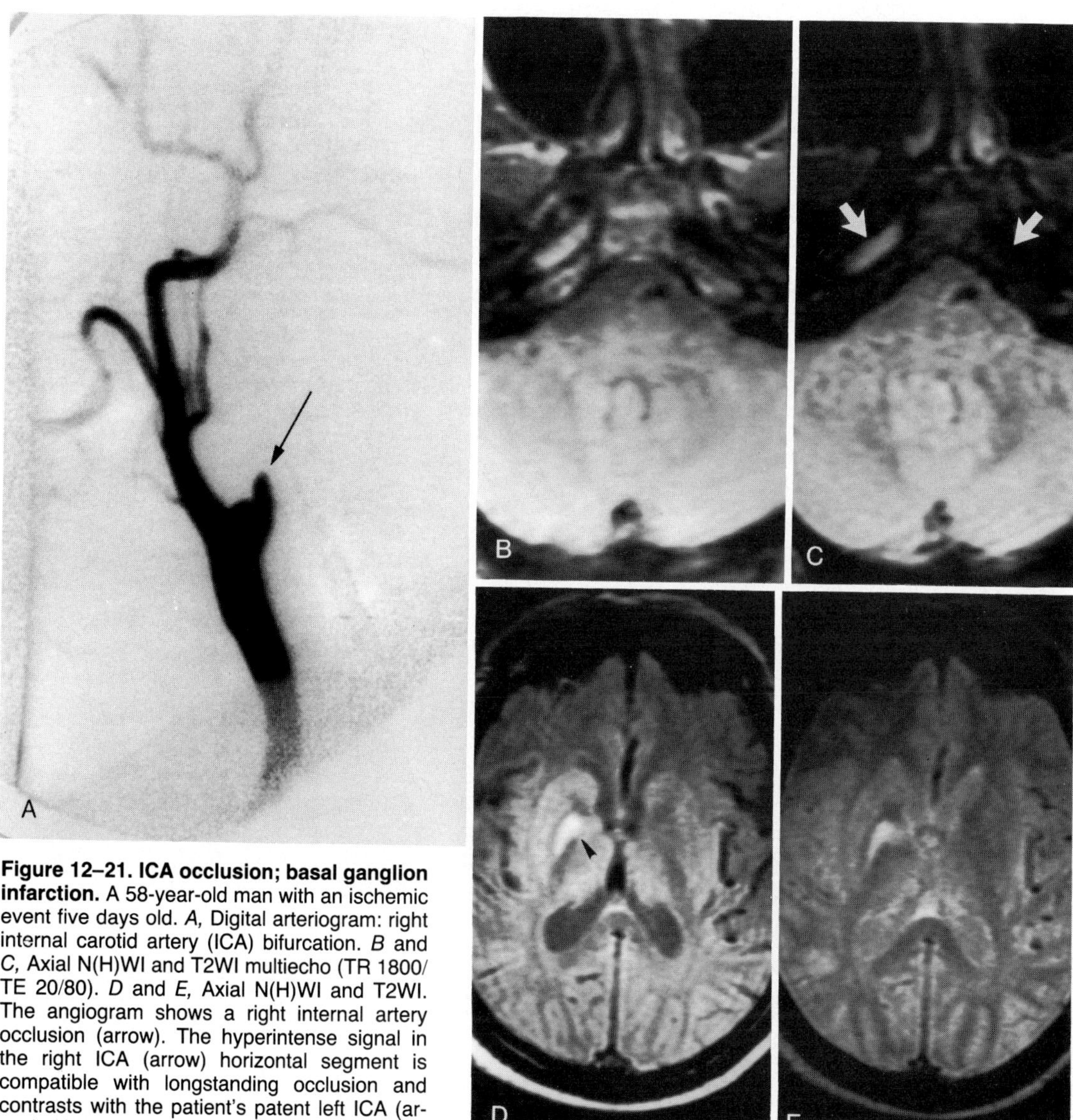


**Figure 12–21. ICA occlusion; basal ganglion infarction.** A 58-year-old man with an ischemic event five days old. *A,* Digital arteriogram: right internal carotid artery (ICA) bifurcation. *B* and *C,* Axial N(H)WI and T2WI multiecho (TR 1800/TE 20/80). *D* and *E,* Axial N(H)WI and T2WI. The angiogram shows a right internal artery occlusion (arrow). The hyperintense signal in the right ICA (arrow) horizontal segment is compatible with longstanding occlusion and contrasts with the patient's patent left ICA (arrow). Hyperintensity in the globus pallidus on N(H)WI (arrowhead) and T2WI is compatible with subacute infarction.

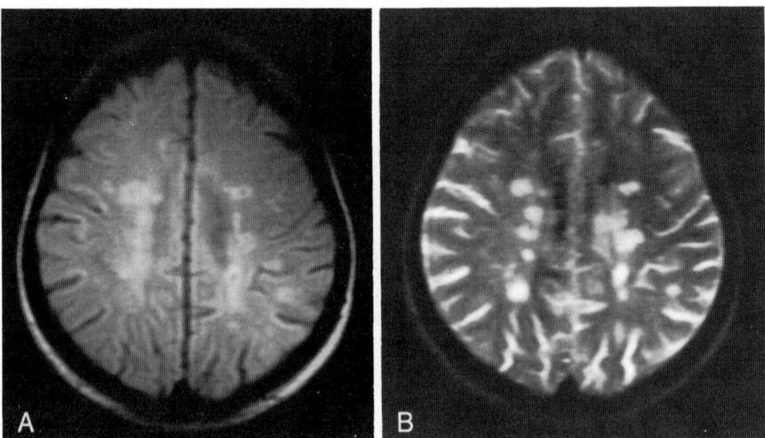

**Figure 12–22. Multiple sclerosis.** A 51-year-old woman (1.5 T). *A,* Axial N(H)WI. *B,* Axial T2WI. Multiple punctate foci of signal hyperintensity affecting the centrum semiovale bilaterally. Differential diagnosis of these unidentified bright objects (UBOs) might include demyelination, ischemic disease, hypertensive encephalopathy, Binswanger's disease, neurodegenerative disorders, and even microinfarction associated with aging. A diagnosis of MS would only be made in the presence of a positive clinical test: visual or auditory evoked response, classic history and physical exam, or positive CSF oligoclonal bands.

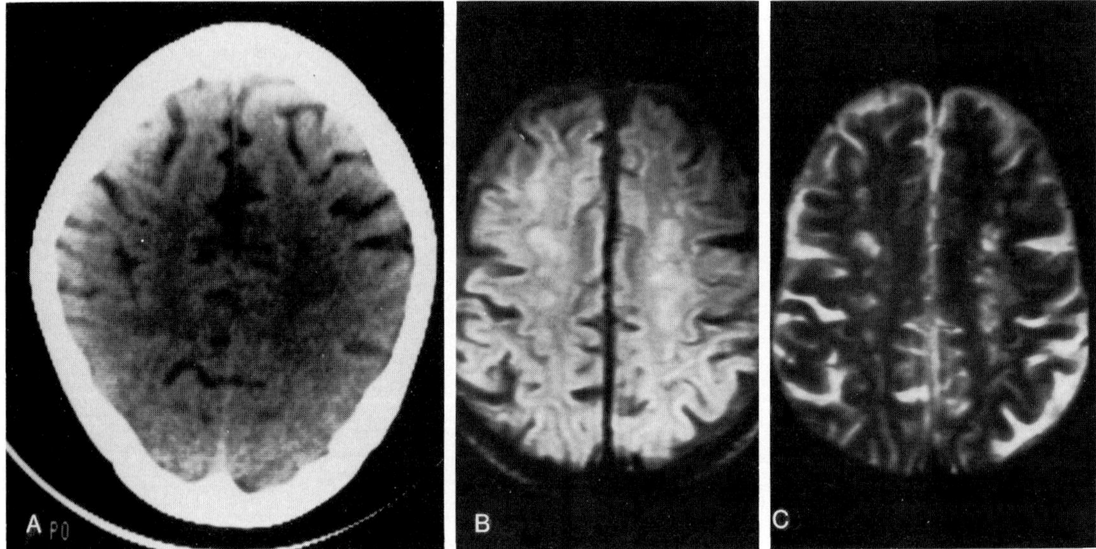

**Figure 12–23. Normal aged brain.** A 69-year-old male evaluated for metastases. *A,* Axial, noncontrast CT. *B* and *C,* Axial, multiecho N(H)WI and T2WI. Multifocal signal hyperintensity is present in the centrum semiovale bilaterally. The differential diagnosis of these unidentified bright objects (UBOs) includes normal aging, demyelination, ischemic disease, hypertension, and inflammatory disease.

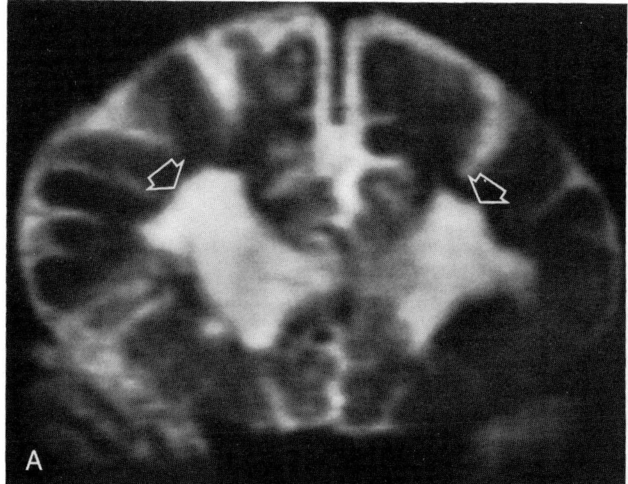


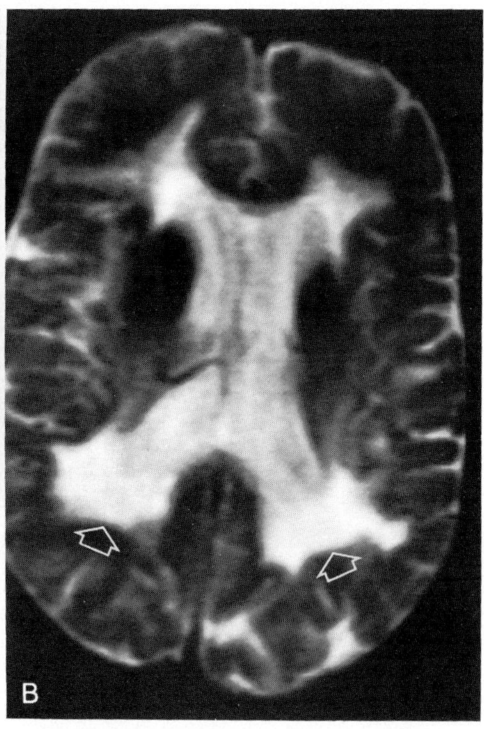


**Figure 12–24. Binswanger's disease (subcortical arteriosclerotic encephalopathy).** A 56-year-old male (1.5 T). *A,* Coronal T2WI. *B,* Axial T2WI. Periventricular signal hyperintensity (open arrows), polar in distribution, is not specific and can even be seen in the aged brain on T2WI (see text).

### Hypertensive Encephalopathy

Uncommonly seen today, owing to more widespread, effective clinical blood pressure control, this is a condition that is manifested by severe headaches, fits, emesis, focal neurologic signs, or coma. Normally, small arteries within the brain are able to reflexively vary their caliber so as to maintain constant blood flow over reasonable blood pressure ranges. This is called autoregulation. However, this physiologic mechanism may fail with resultant increase in cerebral blood flow if the blood pressure is increased 40% to 60% above normal. Vasodilatation, increased cerebral blood flow, blood-brain barrier abnormalities, and cerebral edema follow.[76, 77] Petechial hemorrhages and microinfarcts also occur in those portions of the CNS involved, which include in decreasing order of severity the brain stem, basal ganglia (Fig. 12–26), cerebral white matter, cerebral cortex, and spinal cord.[78]

MR descriptions of this state are still lacking, but CT has shown bilateral cerebral edema resolving.[79] Our experience has revealed poorly marginated signal hyperintensity on T2WI in the centrum semiovale bilaterally.

### Multi-Infarct Dementia (MID)

Approximately 15% of dementias diagnosed in patients over the age of 65 years are caused by multiple infarctions, and another 15% is caused by the mixed involvement of MID and Alzheimer's disease. Dementia usually occurs when the combined volume of cerebral tissue destroyed by stroke exceeds 50 ml. The infarcts generally are bilateral, multiple, and of varying ages. Cortex, basal ganglia, and white matter can be involved. Usually, geographic predominance of one of these three regions is present.[80] Mental deterioration from cerebrovascular disease results from the infarction of brain tissue.[81]

Be aware that no novel findings have been described for CT or MR in MID. One may see ventriculomegaly and multiple infarcts of varying ages. Foci of T2WI signal hyperintensity that are inapparent, hyperintense, or hypointense on T1 or N(H)WI images (Fig. 12–27) are present. Yet MID remains a clinical diagnosis. But MRI and CT are useful in that they confirm a vascular etiology for the clinical deterioration. The advantage of MR is its superiority in diagnosing small but debilitating posterior fossa lesions. A recent

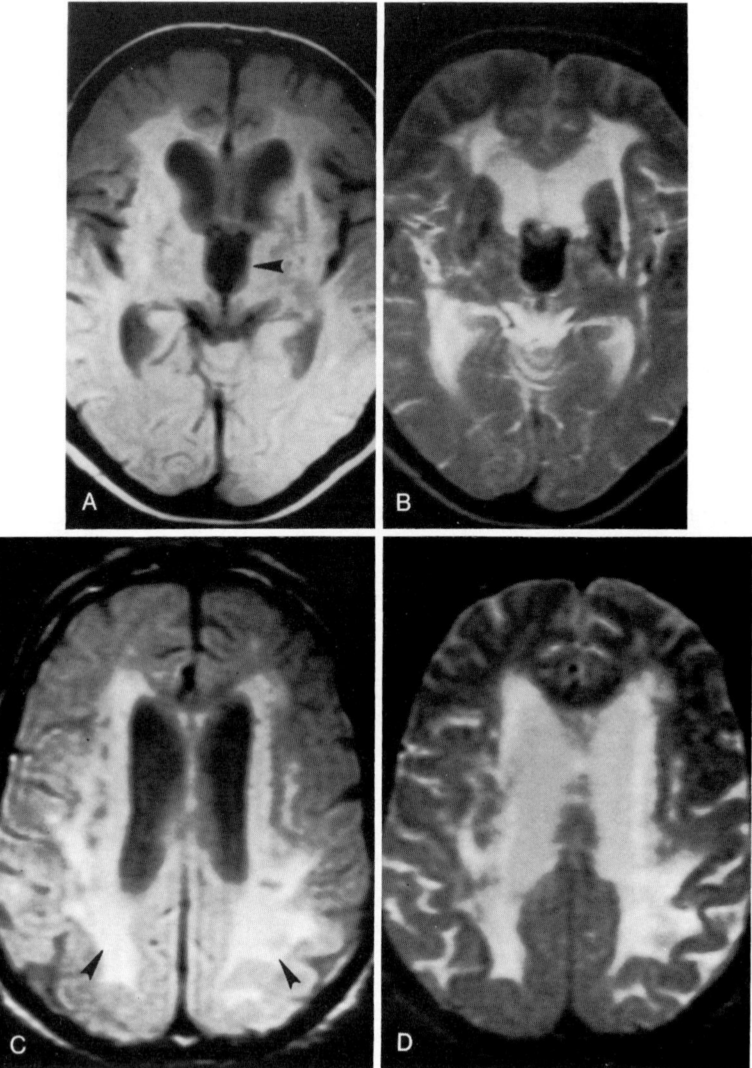


**Figure 12–25. Binswanger's disease (subcortical arteriosclerotic encephalopathy), severe.** A 62-year-old man with progressive memory loss and altered behavior (1.5 T). *A* and *B,* Axial multiecho N(H)WI and T2WI, third ventricular level. *C* and *D,* Axial N(H)WI and T2WI, centrum semiovale level. Diffuse periventricular hyperintensity, or "cloaking," involves the anterior, mid, and posterior white matter (paired arrowheads). Ventricular enlargement due to atrophy is present, and persistent flow-void signal is noted in the third ventricle (arrowhead) on N(H)WI and T2WI (*A* and *B*) image.

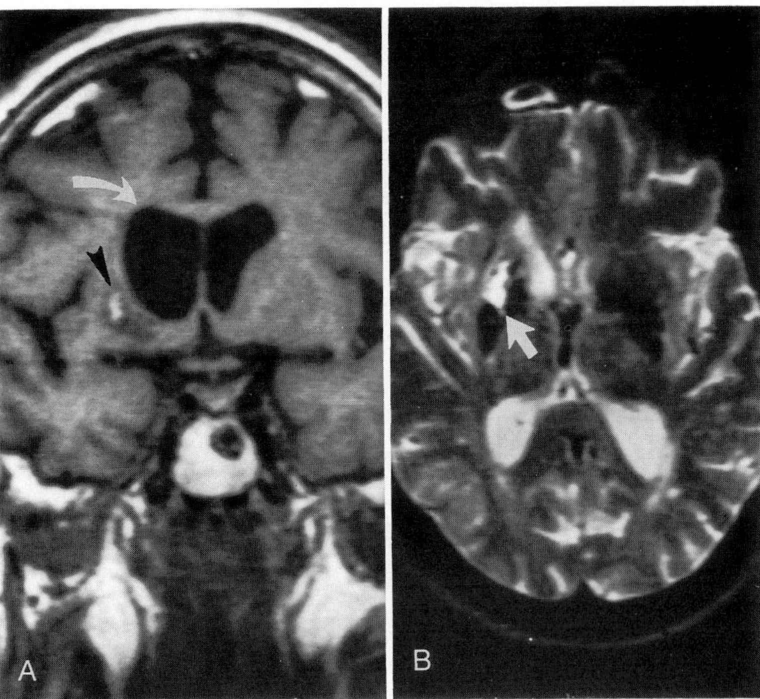


**Figure 12–26. Chronic putamenal hypertensive hemorrhage (eight months).** A 64-year-old man with aortic stenosis, hypertension, carotid stenosis, and vertebrobasilar insufficiency (1.5 T). *A,* Coronal T1WI. *B,* Axial T2WI. Rightward putamenal signal hyperintensity on T1WI (arrowhead) and T2WI (arrow) represents chronic hemorrhage. Ex vacuo enlargement ("negative mass effect") of the ipsilateral ventricle (curved arrow) identifies the process as chronic.

review emphasizes that although MID is relatively uncommon, its early recognition is important because of its association with the treatable conditions of thromboembolism and hypertension.[82]

## OTHER VASCULAR DISEASES

### Moyamoya Disease

Occurring primarily in children and young adults, this cerebrovascular disorder is of unknown etiology and has no specific treatment. The disease predominantly strikes the Japanese, but people of other races may be afflicted as well.[83, 84] Clinically, the initial manifestations in children relate to cerebral ischemic symptomatology, whereas in adults, intracranial bleeding often marks the presentation. Focal, progressive narrowing or occlusion of the supraclinoid segment of the internal carotid artery and proximal portions of the anterior and middle cerebral arteries is present. The basilar artery tip may occasionally be involved. Failure to identify the normal flow-void signal of these vessels is an important MR clue. Extensive arterial collaterals, leptomeningeal, transdural, parenchymal, or a combination of these, develop. The latter are chiefly numerous fine vessels in the basal ganglia that appear like a cloud on angiography, thus the name *moya moya*, meaning "puff of smoke" in Japanese.

It is now known that these arterial features may be seen in young patients in a variety of conditions such as tuberculous meningitis, sickle cell disease, neurofibromatosis, post irradiation, and cerebral embolism.[2] T1WI have shown the multiple pinpoint areas of signal void that correspond to hypertrophied coiled perforating arteries in the thalami and basal ganglia at the base of the brain (Fig. 12–28).[85, 86]

### Arteritis (1.5 T)

A great variety of conditions are capable of causing cerebral vasculitis (Table 12–2). It is useful to think of the arteritic process as primary or secondary. Arteries may be primarily affected by a disease or secondarily affected by way of extension from a neighboring brain or meningeal lesion.[67] Any portion of the cerebral arterial tree and any size vessel may be involved, with some but not all diseases favoring one or more segments.[87]

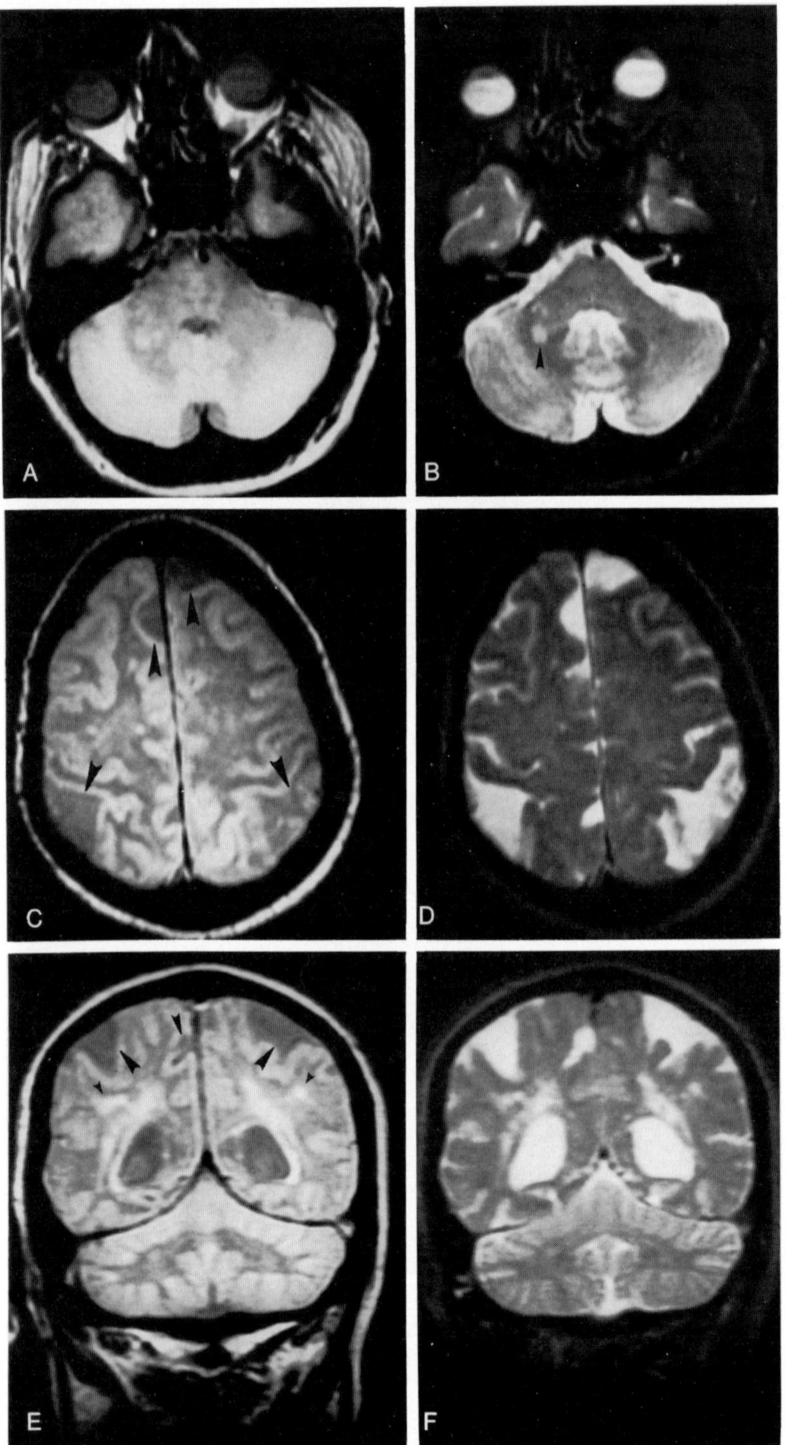


**Figure 12–27. Multi-infarct dementia.** A 58-year-old woman with progressive dementia (1.5 T). *A* and *B,* Axial multiecho N(H)WI and T2WI (TR 1800/TE 20/80), pons level. *C* and *D,* Axial multiecho N(H)WI and T2WI, corona radiata level. *E* and *F,* Coronal multiecho N(H)WI and T2WI. Multiple foci of signal hyperintensity, infratentorial (arrowhead *B*) and supratentorial (arrowheads *C–F*), represent infarcts of varying ages. Older infarcts have resulted in focal cortical atrophy (large arrowheads *C–F*) and give specificity to more recent periventricular foci of ischemia (small and intermediate arrowheads).

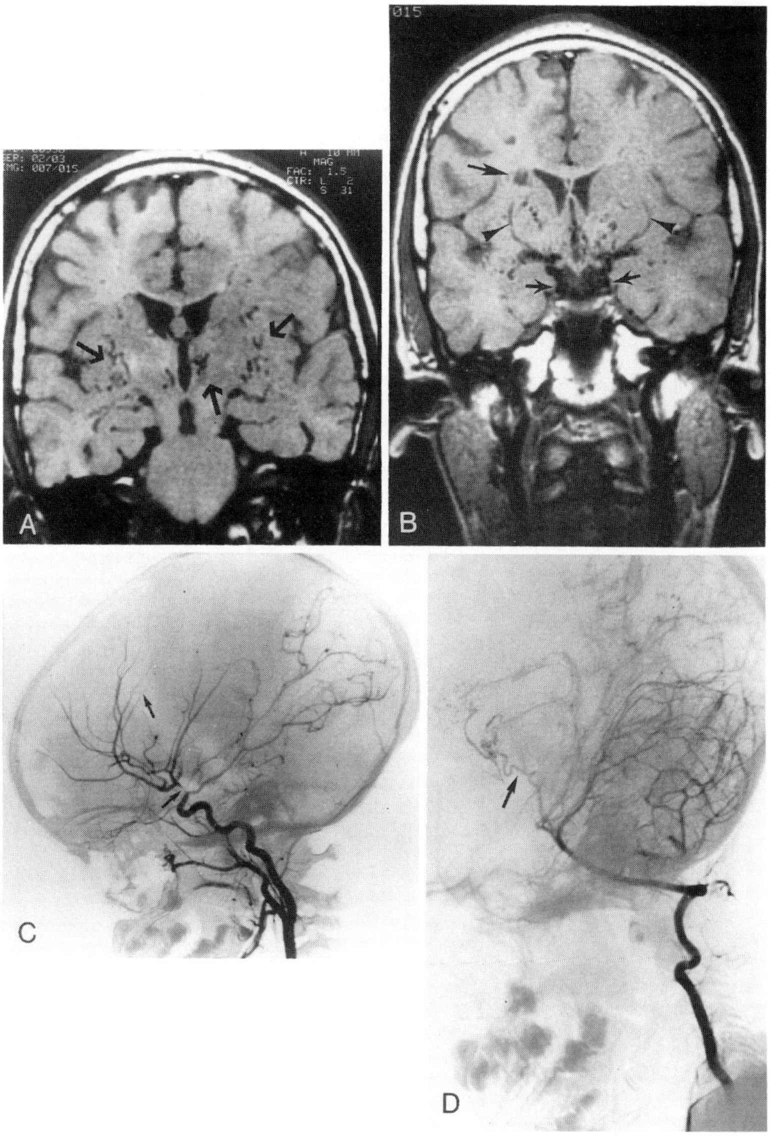

**Figure 12–28. Moyamoya disease.** A 4-year-old black girl with left arm and leg weakness (1.5 T). *A,* Coronal T1WI (TR 800/TE 25). *B,* Coronal T1WI. *C* and *D,* Lateral common and vertebral subtraction angiograms. Multiple foci of flow-void signal are due to collateral moyamoya vessels in the basal ganglia and thalamus (arrows) in *A.* In *B,* a right frontal infarct is present (solid long arrow). Lenticulostriate arteries are identified (arrowheads). *C,* carotid angiogram shows supraclinoid segment narrowing and branch vessel narrowing (arrows). Serpiginous collaterals from the posterior circulation (arrow) are identified in *D.* (From Brooks BS, et al. AJNR 8:178, © Williams & Wilkins, 1987, with permission.)

Infiltration of the vascular wall by mononuclear cells or neutrophils, with variable degrees of thrombosis, extravasated red blood cells, and fibrinoid necrosis are noted histologically. Vessel irregularity, "beaded" appearance, aneurysm formation, segmental stenosis, and thrombosis are typical angiographic features.[88] The CT findings of vasculitis are nonspecific and may show diffuse atrophy, focal low attenuation with or without contrast enhancement, or may be normal. CT changes may reflect cerebral edema, infarction, or both. The MR diagnosis of vasculitis is nonspecific. Multiple foci of signal hyperintensity in the corticomedullary junction of the corona radiata (vascular watershed zone) are suggestive of the diagnosis when associated with hemorrhagic infarcts in the basal ganglia.[89]

Cerebral MR findings for systemic lupus erythematosus (SLE) have been described and are more easily detected with MR (Fig. 12–29) than CT.[90, 91] SLE is characteristically a small vessel arteritis, but may involve major cerebral arteries. CT findings include diffuse atrophy, infarction, or normal examination.[92] Atrophy may reflect prior microinfarction or may be a result of previous steroid therapy. Three patterns have been noted on MR: the first pattern reflects large

**Table 12–2.** CLASSIFICATION OF CEREBRAL ANGIITIS

| |
|---|
| **Arteriopathy and Arteritis Caused by Degeneration** |
| Arteriolosclerosis: hyalin, hyperplastic and arteriolonecrosis |
| Arteriosclerosis: atheromatosis and atherothrombosis |
| Calcifying sclerosis of the tunica media (Monckeberg) |
| **Necrosing Arteritis** |
| Arteritis with obliteration of the supra-aortic trunks (Takayasu) |
| Temporal arteritis |
| **Infectious Viral or Bacterial Arteritis** |
| Viral meningoencephalitis |
| Purulent meningitis |
| Tuberculous meningitis |
| Syphilitic meningitis |
| **Arteritis Caused by Collagen Disease** |
| Polyarteritis nodosa |
| Arteritis of lupus erythematosus |
| Arteritis of hypersensitivity |
| Arteritis of rheumatoid arthritis |
| Granulomatous allergic arteritis |
| Granulomatous arteritis of Wegener |
| **Miscellaneous** |
| Thromboangiitis obliterans (Buerger) |
| Thrombotic microangiopathy (Moschowitz) |
| Neoplastic angiitis |
| Arteritis caused by irradiation |
| Arteritis caused by chemical agents |
| Mycotic arteritis |
| Sarcoidosis of Boeck |

From Sole-Llenas J, Pons-Tortella E. Neuroradiology 15:1, 1978, with permission.

confluent areas of T2 signal hyperintensity in cerebral white matter, suggesting prior infarction; second, single or multiple punctate foci of T2 prolongation may be present; and third, transient foci of T2WI signal hyperintensity in the gray matter, often resolved within two to three weeks.[43] We have identified three cases of connective tissue disease in which subtle intra-axial and multiple occult posterior fossa subdural hematomas were detected on MR. No other risk factors predisposing toward hemorrhage were present.

## Global Anoxic/Hypoxic-Ischemic Encephalopathy (1.5 T)

A diverse spectrum of events may cause global anoxic/hypoxic-ischemic encephalopathy. In general terms, these events can be categorized as cardiocirculatory problems, tracheopulmonary causes, inhalation of toxic substances, or deficiencies in the normal gaseous components of inspired air. Some specific examples include asystole, shock of all types, suffocation, Guillain-Barré syndrome, carbon monoxide inhalation, anesthesia accidents, and confined space entrapment.[93]

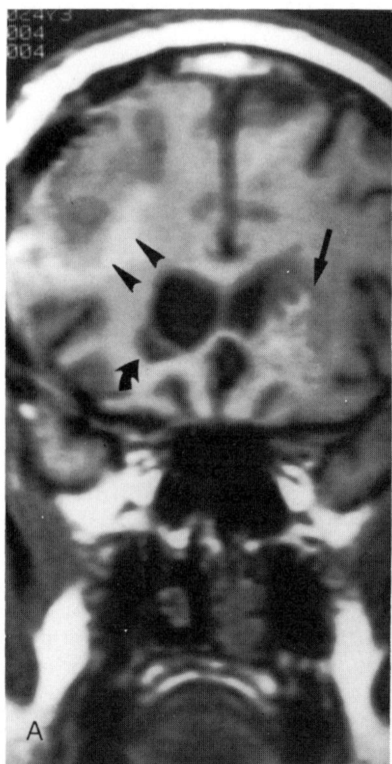


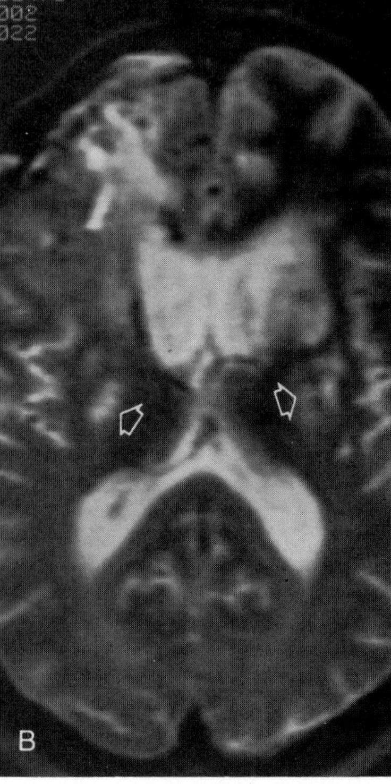


**Figure 12–29. Lupus cerebritis and vasculitis.** A 26-year-old woman with systemic lupus erythematosus. *A,* Coronal T1WI (TR 600/TE 20). *B,* Axial T2WI (TR 1800/TE 100). Multiple infarctions and hemorrhages of varying ages are visible: (1) Remote infarct producing focal encephalomalacia (curved arrow), (2) a two-week-old left basal ganglia hemorrhage (arrow), (3) multiple unidentified bright objects (UBOs, open arrows), (4) remote hematoma (arrowheads), excised and thought to represent arteriovenous malformation but found pathologically to be vasculitis.

Minor degrees of hypoxia/anoxia produce only transient clinical symptoms, but with prolonged hypoxia or anoxia, those who do not die immediately present with coma. Still others initially regain consciousness and improve, some days later falling victim to the delayed onset of neurologic deterioration.[94, 95]

Pathologic changes resulting in the brain from global hypoxic/anoxic ischemia vary considerably in relation to ischemia. Major factors in the injury equation are magnitude, duration, totality, and the differing vulnerability of different types of neuronal tissues to deoxygenation.[96] Especially vulnerable to global hypoxic/anoxic ischemia are portions of the neocortex, striatum, hippocampus, cerebellar cortex, and brain stem.[2] Be aware that no injury pattern is specific for any one cause of global hypoxic/anoxic ischemia. Indeed, in any one case, gray matter changes, white matter changes, or a combination of the two may predominate.[97–103]

This neuropathologic polymorphism should be reflected in the MR as well as the CT scan. History and bilateral symmetry of findings in susceptible tissues are valuable hints to explain the foci of T2 prolongation seen on MR.[104] Reversible or irreversible T2WI signal hyperintensity in the globus pallidus, occipital poles, or periaqueductal gray (Fig. 12–30) watershed vascular territories are not uncommon. Diffuse edema can be present. Later, atrophic changes occur as with any chronic ischemic process.

## Cerebral Venous and Dural Sinus Thrombosis (1.5 T)

The venous drainage system of the brain is composed of three main components: the superficial veins of the cortex; the deep veins; and the dural sinuses. One or more of these subsystems may become involved by the process of thrombosis. Since cerebral sinovenous occlusion may be lethal, early detection and treatment are a necessity.

The clinical manifestations of this dangerous condition are rather characteristic. The development of a severe headache is followed by increasing obtundation and a rise in intracranial pressure as the CSF drainage is impaired. Papilledema and sixth nerve palsy are soon followed by fits and transient postictal hemiparesis.[60]

Sinovenous thrombosis may have primary (aseptic) or secondary (septic) origins. Primary thrombosis may be seen complicating heart disease, dehydration, malnutrition,

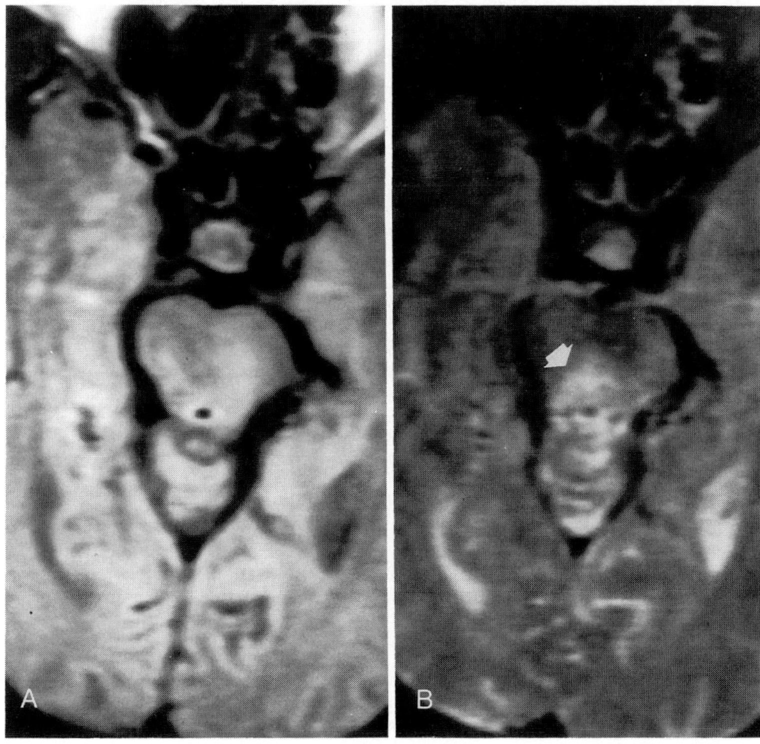


**Figure 12–30. Carbon monoxide poisoning.** A 57-year-old man in a coma following accidental carbon monoxide exposure (1.5 T). *A* and *B,* Axial multiecho N(H)WI and T2WI. Periaqueductal signal hyperintensity (arrow) on T2WI was resolved seven weeks later on follow-up MR (not shown).

pregnancy, the puerperium, the postoperative state, neoplasia, use of birth control pills, trauma, and a host of hematologic disorders such as polycythemia, sickle cell anemia, leukemia, cryofibrinogenemia, and disseminated intravascular coagulation.[2, 105] The superior sagittal sinus is commonly involved initially, with subsequent extension into adjoining venous structures.[2] Secondary occlusion is usually due to a pyogenic process in the paranasal sinuses, middle ear, mastoid air cells, subdural space, or facial tissues.[2]

The MR findings for cerebral venous thrombosis (Fig. 12–31) have been described (Table 12–3) for both intermediate- and high-field MR units (and are demonstrated at low field elsewhere in this text [Fig. 11–34]).[106–109] Initially, absence of a normal flow void in the dural sinus is detected and secondary collateral venous channels may be observed. Early thrombosis on high-field MR appears isointense to brain on T1WI and hypointense on T2WI. At low field strengths ($< 0.35$ T), acute thrombus may appear isointense or mildly hyperintense on T2WI. In the early subacute phase (48 to 72 hours), thrombus converts centripetally (seen best in large channels) to hyperintensity on T1WI. Signal increase on T2WI is slower and may go through a phase of isointensity from two to six days at high field. After 10 to 14 days, hyperintensity on both T1- and T2WI may be present. After two weeks, vascular recanalization may produce central hypointensity owing to reappearance of the flow-void signal.[107] By careful attention to location, one should be able to differentiate the expected MR signal evolution of a known venous thrombus from new thrombus formation.

**Table 12–3.** INTRAVASCULAR THROMBI AT LOW-FIELD (LF) AND HIGH-FIELD (HF) MR

| | T1 | T2 (HF) | T2 (LF) | Miscellaneous |
|---|---|---|---|---|
| Acute | = | – | =/+ | |
| Subacute | =/+ | =/+ | + | A hyperintense rim may exist on T1WI |
| Chronic | + | + + | + + | A hypointense rim and center may exist on T2WI (see text) |

Equal sign (=), intermediate signal intensity.
En dash (–), hypointense signal.
Plus (+), hyperintense signal.
Equal/plus (=/+), intermediate or hyperintense signal.
Plus plus (+ +), marked signal intensity.

Although focal thrombus usually does not interfere with venous drainage in the brain, more extensive thrombosis, encompassing a dural sinus and some of its venous feeders, can do so, and this may lead to complicating *venous infarction* (Fig. 12–32).[2] Often hemorrhagic, and not infrequently multiple, venous infarcts do not always confine themselves to one arterial territory. In addition, a venous infarct often exhibits more mass effect than a comparably sized arterial infarct and tends to possess rounded irregular edges, instead of the sharper geometric margin of an arterial infarct.[67] The signal characteristics of a venous infarct are the same as those of an ischemic or hemorrhagic infarction. Dural venous sinus thrombosis must be differentiated from slice entry phenomena, second-echo rephasing, and other flow effects peculiar to MR imaging.[110–112] Clot within a dural sinus is signal generating on all echoes of all pulse sequences in all planes, whereas flow phenomena are not.[106] Bear in mind that hypointensity, a field-dependent, preferential T2 susceptibility effect, may occur on T2WI at 1.5 T and may be misconstrued for vessel patency. Nevertheless, MR has become the modality of choice in making this diagnosis.

The CT findings of dural sinus thrombosis include the following: small ventricles, hemorrhagic infarction, visualization of a high-attenuation thrombosed vein ("cord sign"), negative defect in a contrast-enhanced posterior superior sagittal sinus ("delta sign"), and a normal scan.

## HYDROCEPHALUS

Hydrocephalus refers to an increase in ventricular size. This includes an increase in CSF volume within the cranial cavity and a present or past increase in intraventricular pressure. Most commonly, it is the result of a degree of *obstruction* that may be located anywhere along the intracranial CSF flow pathways. Rarely, it may be caused by *increased CSF production* (choroid plexus papilloma).

The obstructive form of hydrocephalus may be subdivided into two main varieties. In *noncommunicating* (intraventricular) hydrocephalus, the obstruction is located between the CSF-forming choroid plexus of the lateral ventricles and the exit foramina of the fourth ventricle. If the obstruction is

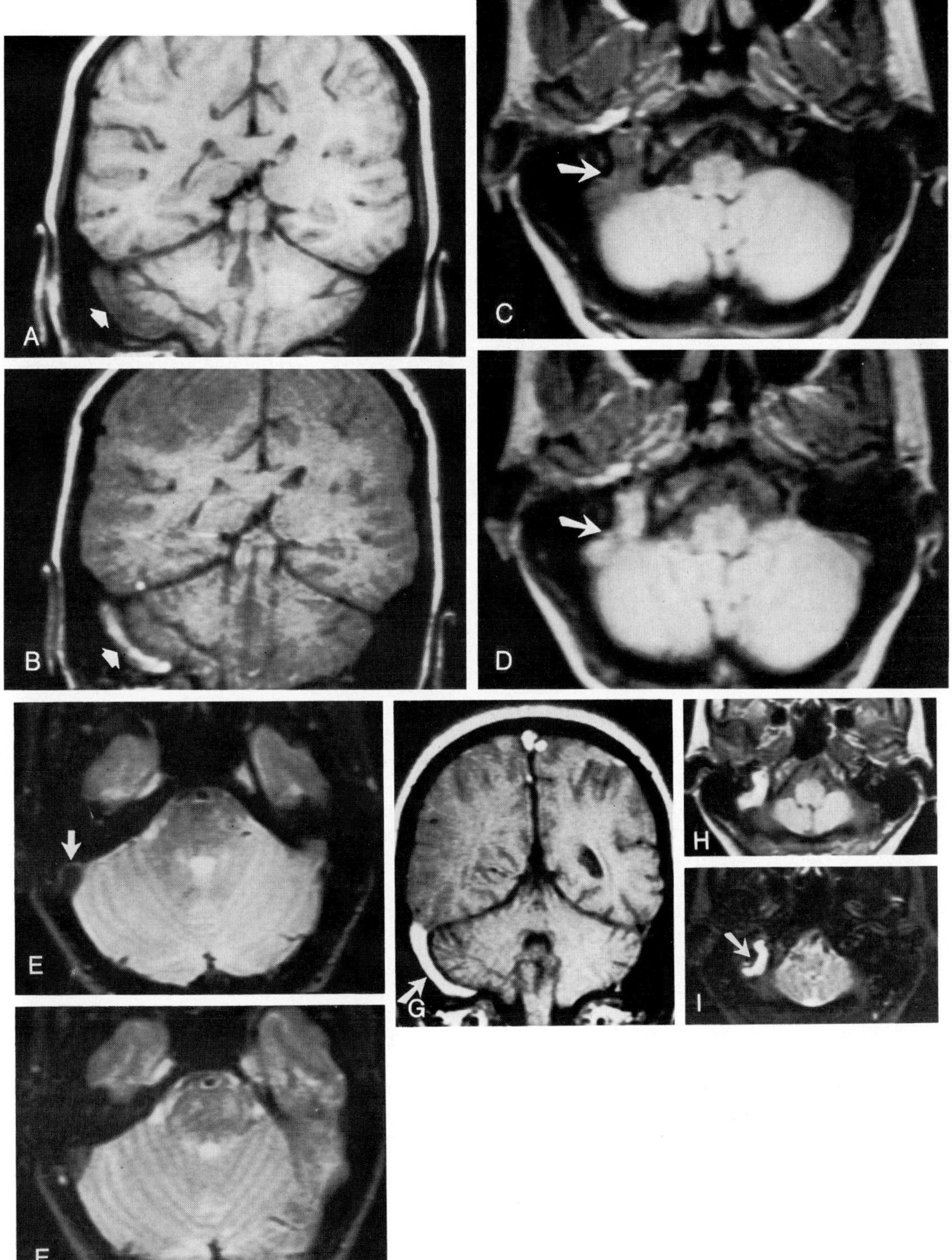


**Figure 12–31. A 20-year-old woman with multifocal dural sinus thrombosis.** Paired images are presented at 36 hours and 6 days post ictus *(A–F)* and at 14 days *(G–I)*. *A* and *B*, Coronal T1WI (TR 600/TE 20 msec). At 36 hours *(A)*, lateral sinus thrombosis is hypointense (arrowhead) and at 6 days *(B)* exhibits progressive hyperintensity. *C* and *D*, Axial N(H)WI (TR 1800/TE 20 msec). Jugular venous sinus clot (arrows) is hypointense at 36 hours *(A)* but is isointense with cerebellum at six days *(B)* and could be overlooked.

*E* and *F*, Axial T2WI (TR 1800/TE 100 msec). Thrombus in the lateral sinus *(E)* is hypointense acutely (arrow) and hypointense or isointense at six days *(F)* owing to T2* relaxation shortening, a field-dependent susceptibility effect accentuated at 1.5 tesla. T2WI signal hypointensity could be misconstrued as vessel patency. *G*, Coronal T1WI at 14 days. Signal in the right lateral sinus (arrow) and superior sagittal sinus is hyperintense. *H* and *I*, Axial multiecho N(H)WI and T2WI at 14 days. Signal hyperintensity is present in the jugular bulb (arrow) at this chronic stage.

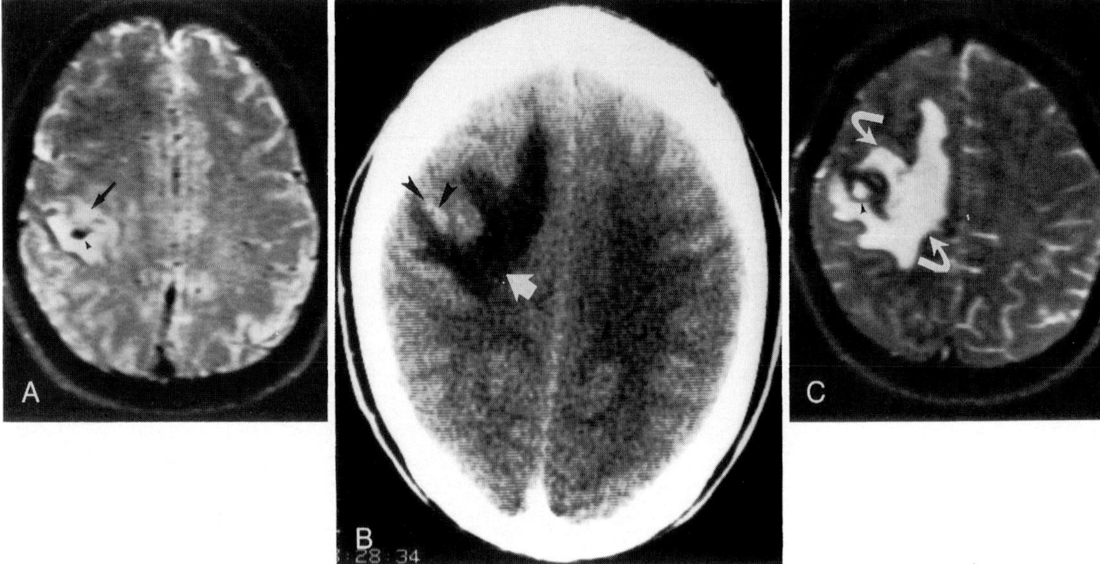


**Figure 12–32. Venous infarction, hemorrhage.** A 20-year-old woman with acute left arm hemiparesis and normal CT (not shown) (1.5 T). *A,* Axial T2WI (day 2). *B,* CECT (day 6). *C,* Axial T2WI (day 14) same level as CECT. In *A,* hyperintense edema (arrow) and hypointense early subacute hemorrhagic focus (arrowhead) are apparent. Susceptibility effect of intracellular deoxyhemoglobin and methemoglobin produces preferential T2 relaxation enhancement/shortening. CECT shows vasogenic hypodense edema (arrow) and hyperdense hemorrhagic focus (arrowheads). In *C,* edema (curved arrows) is more extensive and chronic hemorrhagic focus is hyperintense (arrowhead).

between the foramina of Luschka/Magendie and the CSF-absorbing arachnoid villi, then *communicating* (extraventricular) hydrocephalus is present (Table 12–4). Neurosurgical shunting of the CSF is usually required for relief in obstructive hydrocephalus owing in part but not exclusively to the law of Laplace. Applying this principle is helpful in understanding that once the hydrocephalus has been established, progressively less transmural pressure is required to continue the process.[113] An exception is *arrested* hydrocephalus. In this state, the intraventricular pressure has returned to a low enough value to remove the stimulus for further ventricular enlargement, and a new steady state is attained with continued large ventricles. Clinically, obstructive hydrocephalus may develop rapidly or slowly, depending on the nature and location of the offending lesion. With rapid development, signs and symptoms of acute elevation of intracranial pressure may be recognized, whereas with slow expansion of the system, the clinical course may be insidious.

**Table 12–4.** ETIOLOGIES OF COMMUNICATING HYDROCEPHALUS

| |
|---|
| Meningitis |
| Subarachnoid hemorrhage |
| Posterior fossa extra-axial masses |
| Subdural hematoma |
| Normal-pressure hydrocephalus |
| Venous pathway occlusion |
| Congenital abnormalities of extraventricular pathways |
| Neoplastic meningeal involvement |
| Increased CSF protein |

Compensatory enlargement of the intracranial CSF spaces, including the ventricles, may occur with increased CSF volume under normal pressure. This condition is produced by shrinkage of the brain from aging or disease and is referred to as *brain atrophy.* An older term, *hydrocephalus ex vacuo,* is now used less commonly. CSF shunt surgery in this condition is contraindicated, as it is of no value.

Both MR and CT portray the enlarged ventricular system in a similar fashion.[51] They both show ventricular size and location as well as the sulcal width and breadth of basilar cisterns. But to this MR is able to add valuable dynamic information (Fig. 12–33) about CSF movement (flow).[114–116]

Direct sagittal and coronal images may add valuable differential diagnostic information not seen on CT. The following MR findings are suggestive of CSF pathway obstruction (Figs. 12–34 to 12–37) rather than ventricular enlargement owing to atrophy: (1) dila-

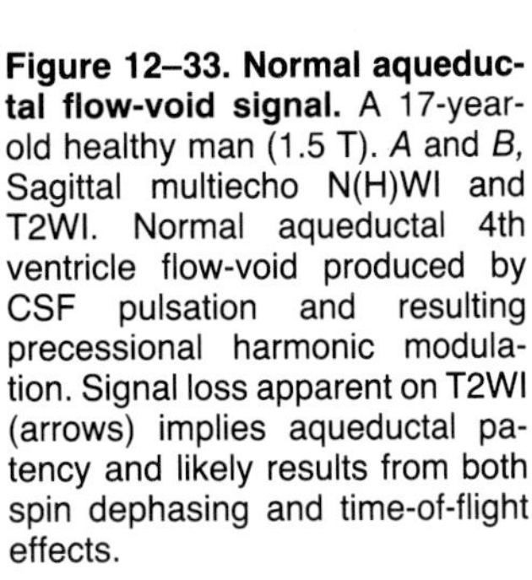

**Figure 12–33. Normal aqueductal flow-void signal.** A 17-year-old healthy man (1.5 T). *A* and *B,* Sagittal multiecho N(H)WI and T2WI. Normal aqueductal 4th ventricle flow-void produced by CSF pulsation and resulting precessional harmonic modulation. Signal loss apparent on T2WI (arrows) implies aqueductal patency and likely results from both spin dephasing and time-of-flight effects.

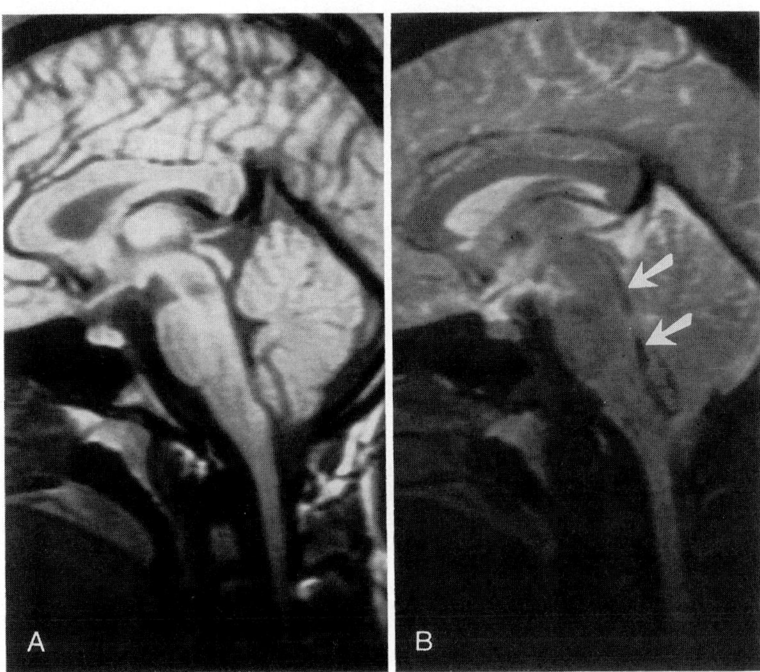


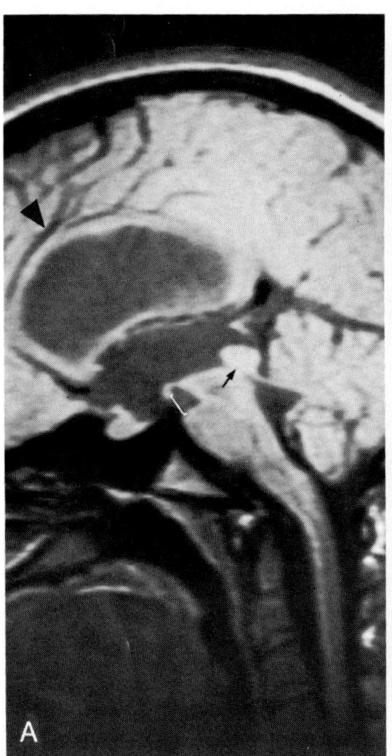


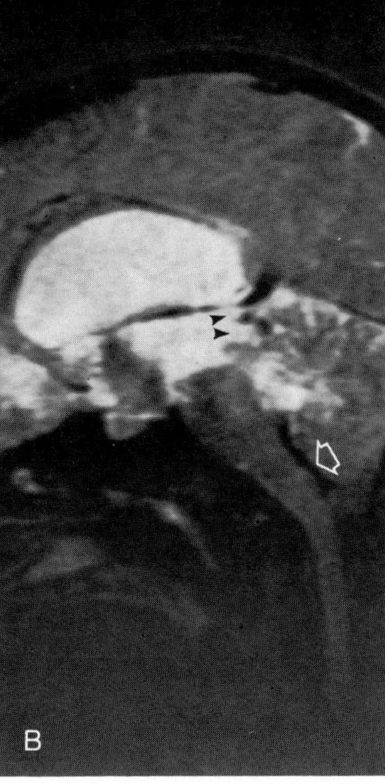


**Figure 12–34. Tectal glioma with aqueductal stenosis.** A 21-year-old woman with headache following a motor vehicle accident (1.5 T). *A,* Sagittal N(H)WI (TR 1800/TE 20). *B,* T2WI (TR 1800/TE 100). A tectal mass (arrow) produces aqueductal stenosis. The normal flow-void signal is seen below (open arrow), but not at or above the level of obstruction; the corpus callosum is bowed superiorly (large arrowhead). The mamillopontine distance (white line) is decreased (see text), and the supra- and infrapineal recesses (arrowheads) of the third ventricle are enlarged. All are signs compatible with obstructive hydrocephalus.

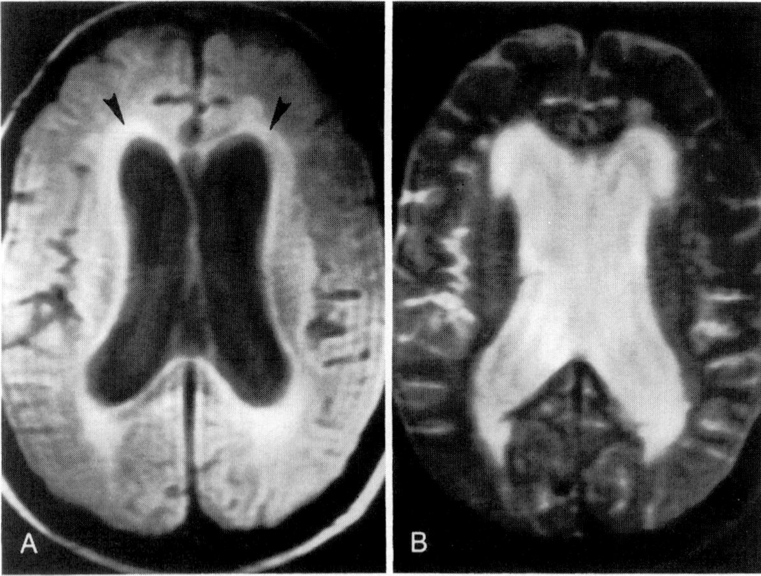

**Figure 12–35. Obstructive hydrocephalus with transependymal CSF migration.** A 75-year-old woman with breast carcinoma (1.5 T). *A* and *B*, Axial multiecho N(H)WI and T2WI. Ventricular dilation with smooth periventricular signal hyperintensity more prominent anteriorly (arrowheads) and posteriorly.

tion of the anterior third ventricle, (2) inferior bowing and displacement of the hypothalamus in the sagittal projection with reduction in the mamillopontine distance (< 1 cm), (3) depression of the posterior fornix with increase in the superior-inferior dimensions of the lateral ventricles, (4) uniform thinning (< 6 mm) and elevation rather than depression of the corpus callosum, (5) loss of intraventricular flow-void signal owing to CSF movement, and (6) periventricular signal hyperintensity on N(H)WI and T2WI.[117]

Furthermore, posterior fossa and skull base CT artifacts caused by the petrous bones are eliminated with MR, making the aqueduct of Sylvius and temporal lobes routinely well seen. In our judgment, MR matches and goes beyond the information provided by CT and is indicated as the initial examination

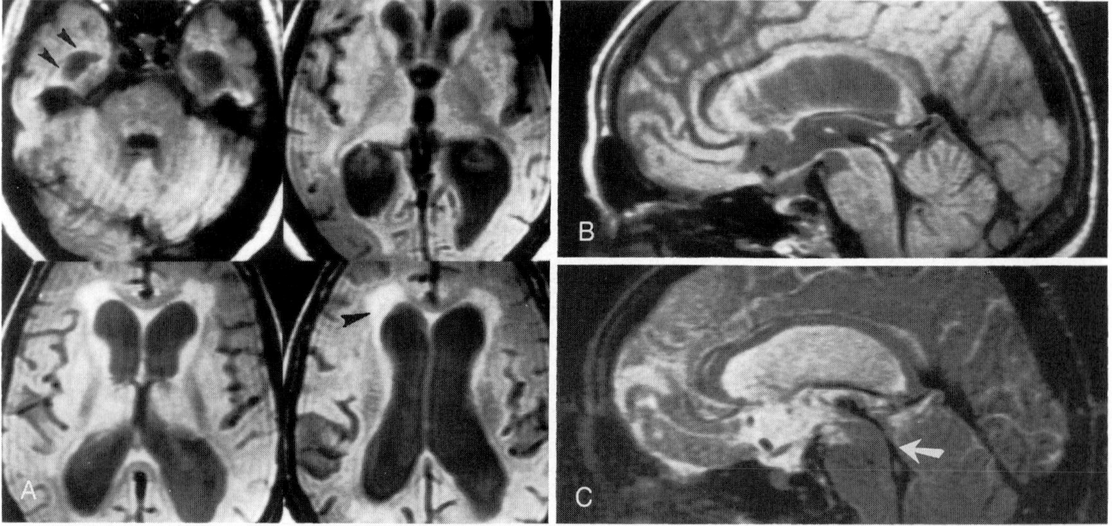

**Figure 12–36. Normal-pressure hydrocephalus.** An 86-year-old woman with progressive dementia over a one-year period (1.5 T). *A,* Axial N(H)WI (multiformat). *B,* Sagittal N(H)WI (TR 1800/TE 20). *C,* Sagittal T2WI (TR 1800/TE 80). Axial images demonstrate ventricular dilation, periventricular hyperintensity (arrowhead), and temporal horn enlargement (arrowheads). Aqueductal flow void is present on sagittal T2WI (arrow).

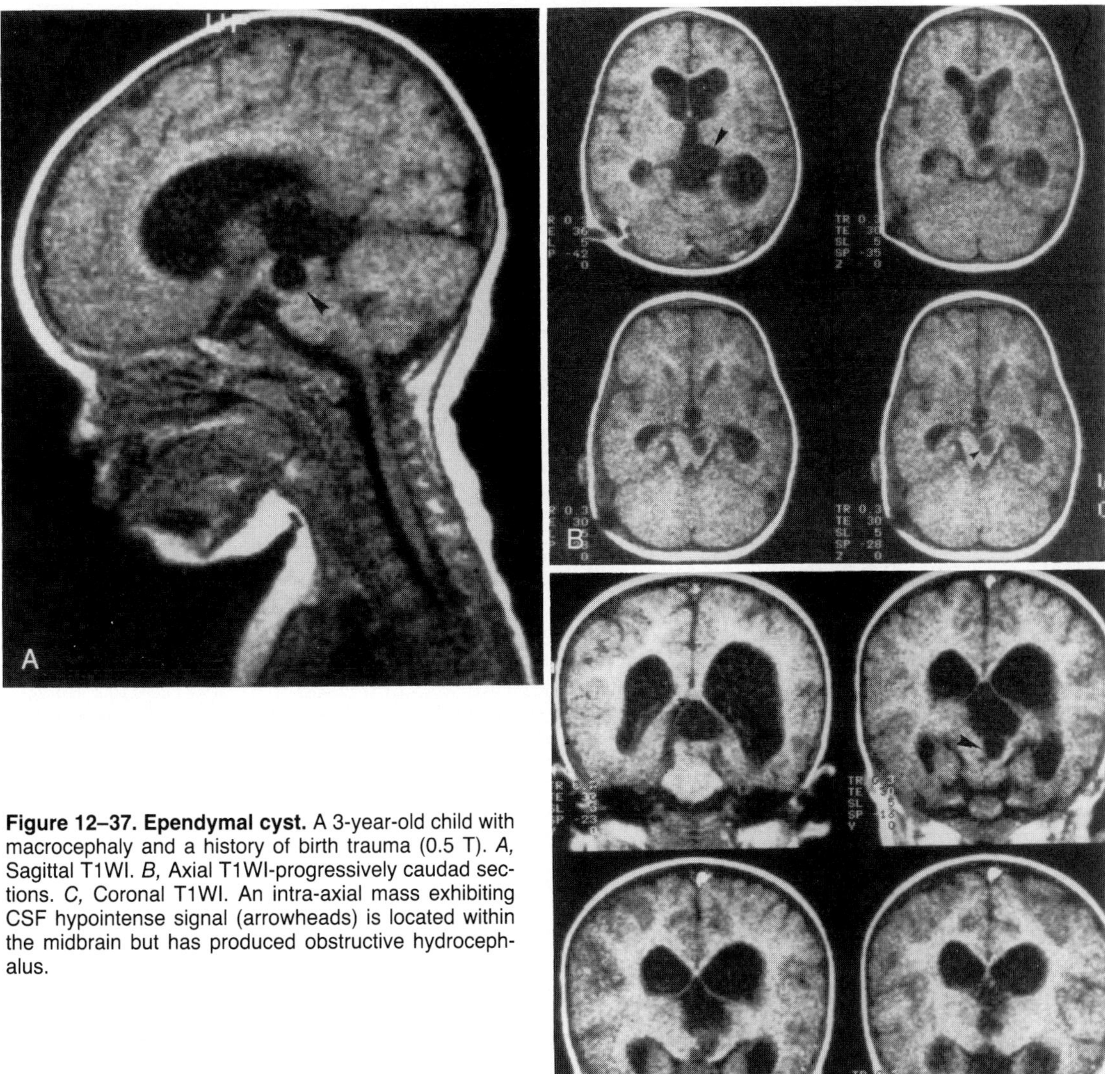

**Figure 12–37. Ependymal cyst.** A 3-year-old child with macrocephaly and a history of birth trauma (0.5 T). *A,* Sagittal T1WI. *B,* Axial T1WI-progressively caudad sections. *C,* Coronal T1WI. An intra-axial mass exhibiting CSF hypointense signal (arrowheads) is located within the midbrain but has produced obstructive hydrocephalus.

for suspected hydrocephalus. We further recommend its use for follow-up and post-shunting evaluation of patients.

## Obstructive Hydrocephalus

Of fundamental importance is the separation of obstructive hydrocephalus from the enlarged ventricles of cerebral atrophy. Differentiation is based on determination of which ventricles are dilated and the shape of these dilated components. In general, the ventricular system proximal to the point of blockage enlarges in obstructive hydrocephalus; however, this alone often does not differentiate obstruction from atrophy. Two key observations need emphasis. Prominent temporal horns (Fig. 12–36) are a valuable sign of nonatrophic (obstructive) ventricular enlargement. Symmetrical enlargement of the temporal horns in obstructive hydrocephalus was initially found by Sjaastad and co-workers on pneumoencephalograms and confirmed by others on CT.[118–120] Of added value is the fact that the dilated temporal horn tips appear early and exhibit a linear relation to the degree of obstruction.[119, 120] Temporal horns are more easily assessed with angled axial MR sections parallel to the canthomeatal line or with direct coronal images. A second highly useful sign of obstructive hydrocephalus is "ballooning" (like Mickey Mouse ears) of the frontal horns of the lateral ventricles in contradistinction to brain atrophy, in which the frontal horns may be enlarged but retain their more curved, sausagelike configuration.

The differential diagnosis of obstructive hydrocephalus and brain atrophy is usually readily accomplished by careful inspection of the images. However, in difficult cases one may resort to ventricular measurements and ratios.[119–121]

With use of spin-echo T2WI, periventricular hyperintensity (PVH) has been identified, regardless of diagnosis, in approximately 90% of a large series of consecutive patients. Five patterns have been described.[122] If mild, PVH may be a normal finding. However, when moderate, PVH is always abnormal and is an indicator of either demyelinating disease or transependymal absorption of CSF (interstitial edema) in hydrocephalic patients (Fig. 12–35). Unfortunately, pattern overlap between the two conditions occurs. But it has been noted that in severe hydrocephalus, the peripheral margins of the PVH are irregular but unpointed and do not extend to the corticomedullary junction. In demyelinating diseases, extension of the PVH to the corticomedullary junction is more frequent, along with sharp angulation to the PVH margins.[122] Although MR is more sensitive than CT for diagnosing periventricular edema, disappointing evidence exists indicating that PVH cannot be used as a predictor for shunting success in hydrocephalus.[122]

CSF is constantly in motion along its bulk-flow pathways. This flow is intermittent and primarily reflects cardiac pulsations, it is believed.[123] Disregarding other variables, the signal intensity of the CSF can vary, depending upon its state of motion.[114] Rapidly flowing CSF exhibits decreased signal when flowing through narrowed portions of the ventricular system. This is most easily observed at the aqueduct of Sylvius (Fig. 12–33) but may also be seen at the foramina of Monro, at the fourth ventricle outlet foramina, and in the posterior third ventricle. This phenomenon has been termed the CSF flow-void sign (CFVS).[114] Signal loss in CFVS occurs owing to spin-dephasing and time-of-flight effects.[116] The CFVS appears more conspicuous on thinner section T2WI and can be observed in any imaging plane.

Determining the presence or absence of the CFVS may have diagnostic significance. When observed, it indicates that the ventricular pathway in which it is located is at least partially patent. In noncommunicating hydrocephalus, CFVS absence connotes the possible presence of an obstructive lesion, but this sign's absence is not specific for lesion level.[115] For example, a lesion blocking the foramen of Monro could cause the loss of CFVS in the aqueduct of Sylvius. Alternatively, absence of the aqueductal CFVS (Fig. 12–34) could indicate aqueductal obstruction. Absence of the CFVS is most useful when placed within the framework of other scan observations such as presence or absence of large ventricles or a detectable mass.

### Noncommunicating Hydrocephalus

Part or all of one ventricle may be "trapped" and therefore enlarged by an intraventricular lesion with continued CSF production behind the point of obstruction. MR shows the enlarged ventricle or segment of ventricle and often characterizes the mass (see Chap. 8). Similarly, CT will show the mass and sequential ventricular enlargement. Some lesions have characteristic locations, and systematic ventricular analysis assists in lesion localization. An example is the colloid cyst. Intraventricular colloid cysts involve one or both foramina of Monro and lie in the anterosuperior third ventricle. Intermittent lateral ventricular obstruction and normal-to-small third and fourth ventricles may result. Aqueductal stenosis is a specific subtype of obstructive hydrocephalus. Non-neoplastic causes include congenital stenosis or atresia and postinflammatory gliosis. Neoplastic causes include pineal tumors, mesencephalic gliomas (Fig. 12–34), posterior third ventricular ependymoma, medulloblastoma, vermian tumors, or tentorial meningioma. MR identifies the offending mass or may show the primary intra-aqueductal stenosis or web directly on sagittal images.[124] As on CT, the lateral and third ventricles show dilatation, whereas the size of the fourth ventricle remains normal or small.[125] In addition, the normal CSF aqueductal flow void may be absent on thin-section T2WI.

In our experience, cisternal disease is difficult to detect on MR. If present in Magendie/Luschka foraminal blockage, differentiation from communicating hydrocephalus is necessary, as the gross scan appearance may be similar. To date, there is a lack of reported MR experience in this differential diagnostic dilemma, but perhaps observation of the CSF flow-void sign from at least one fourth ventricular exit foramen will prove to be of value. If necessary, differentiation can be made by radionuclide cisternography or ventriculography with iodinated contrast.

In a trapped fourth ventricle, both the aqueduct of Sylvius and the fourth ventricular exits are blocked, yielding supratentorial hydrocephalus and enlargement of the fourth ventricle. Usually, this is due to antecedent meningitis or subarachnoid hemorrhage.[126] The diagnosis is made when the fourth ventricle remains dilated after successful shunting of supratentorial ventricular chambers.

### Communicating Hydrocephalus

The causes of communicating hydrocephalus are numerous and varied (Table 12–4).[127] CSF flow is blocked in an extraventricular location distal to the fourth ventricular foramina. A specific disease process may eliminate the subarachnoid spaces. Alternatively, the organs of CSF absorption, the arachnoid villi, may be impaired. The cause of the communicating hydrocephalus may or may not be seen on the MR scan. The examination will show expanded lateral, third, and usually fourth ventricles. Bizarre signal intensity patterns in lateral ventricles owing to intraventricular CSF flow phenomena are common. Sulci may exhibit progressive elimination as the ventricles swell. The temporal horns typically enlarge, as communicating hydrocephalus is an obstructive process with the block located external to the ventricles. CT findings mirror the MR pattern of ventricular enlargement.

### Normal-Pressure Hydrocephalus

This syndrome, a subset of communicating hydrocephalus, was initially described in 1965 and consists of hydrocephalus along with the clinical triad of dementia, gait disturbance, and urinary incontinence in older patients.[128, 129] Although the intraventricular pressure is usually normal, it may not be so at all times. Prolonged monitoring has shown transient elevations in intraventricular pressure.[130, 131] There may or may not be a possible antecedent cause for the communicating hydrocephalus. Many but not all patients show complete or partial improvement when shunted.[132]

The search for reliable diagnostic and prognostic tests has proved frustrating.[133] Typically, the pattern of ventricular enlargement and sulcal nonenlargement is that of communicating hydrocephalus. But some patients with the clinical symptom triad and excellent shunt response have had a normal scan or one suggesting atrophy.[134] Thus there is no novel appearance pathognomonic for NPH. Recent preliminary MR work suggests that the CFVS is much more likely to be present in NPH (Fig. 12–36) than in normal individuals, in atrophy, or in other forms of communicating hydrocephalus.[116] The CT pattern of ventriculomegaly is identical to that seen on MRI.

### Hydrocephalus Caused by Increased CSF Production

Choroid plexus papilloma, the MR characteristics of which are described in Chapter 8, can cause a nonobstructive hydrocephalus. The pathophysiology is most likely increased CSF production with concomitant local CSF pressure increase.[135] The ventricle containing the neoplasm increases in size. In adults, the fourth ventricle is most often affected, but the tumor may also occur in the third ventricle, the trigone, or the body of the lateral ventricle.[136, 137] MR and CT will show the enlarged ventricle(s) and the mass.

## ATROPHY, NEURODEGENERATIVE DISEASES, AND MOVEMENT DISORDERS

A potpourri of selected neurodegenerative and atrophic states, both focal and diffuse, are discussed in this section (Tables 12–5 and 12–6). MR imaging represents a significant step forward in the evaluation of many of these disorders because of its unique ability to provide information about brain iron, subtle differences in water content in both white and gray matter, and posterior fossa pathoanatomy undistorted by petrous bone CT artifacts. However, in a few conditions MR has not, to date, added to knowledge beyond that provided by CT. When pertinent, this is addressed in the discussion of these entities.

MR affords us the ability to map the distribution of macromolecular complexes such as $Fe^{3+}$ utilizing heavy T2WI. This T2* effect results from local magnetic field inhomogeneity that increases spin dephasing and results in signal loss, a susceptibility effect.[138] This signal loss varies according to the macromolecular complex concentration and the square of the field strength. The characteristic distribution of iron varies with age.

**Table 12–5.** MR DEMENTIA

| Disease | MR Findings |
|---|---|
| Alzheimer's and Parkinson's | Atrophy: ↑ sulci, ↑ temporal horns, ↑ III, ↑ mesencephalic cisterns<br>T2: ↑ SI (↓ on T1) medial temporal, ↓ SI parietal gyri (↑ iron), +/− ↑ SI subcortical (WM/BG) |
| Pick's | Atrophy: frontotemporal dominant; spares posterosuperior temporal gyrus, caudate (↑ frontal horns) |
| Wernicke-Korsakoff | Atrophy: generalized sulci, superior vermian, mamillary bodies<br>T2: increased signal periaqueductal gray and medial thalamus |
| Vascular | Atrophy: ventricles, sulci<br>T2: confluent ↑ SI cerebral WM (infarction, pallor, gliosis); ↑ SI in BG, thalamus, pons (infarction); +/− ↑ SI owing to residual slitlike iron (hypertensive hemorrhage) |
| Hydrocephalic (NPH) | Preferential ventricular enlargement, rounded temporal and frontal horns; periventricular increased signal; +/− exaggerated aqueductal and ventricular flow void; +/− anterosuperior bowing of the CC and mamillopontine distance (< 1 cm) on sagittal MR if secondary to chronic obstruction |

*Source:* Modified from Drayer BP. Imaging of the aging brain. Part II. Pathologic considerations. Radiology 166:801, 1988.

↑ = increase; ↓ = decrease; SI = signal intensity; +/− = present or absent; III = third ventricle; WM = white matter; BG = basal ganglia.

**Table 12–6.** MR PARKINSONIAN/PSEUDOPARKINSONIAN SYNDROMES

| Disease | MR Abnormality/Localization |
|---|---|
| Parkinson's | Atrophy<br>T2: +/− ↓ SI putamen/SN compacta, +/− ↑ SI subcortical |
| Parkinson-plus syndromes | |
| Striatonigral degeneration | Atrophy |
| Shy-Drager syndrome | T2: ↓ SI putamen/SN compacta (most profound in multisystem atrophy); +/− ↑ SI subcortical (WM/BG) |
| Olivopontocerebellar atrophy | Severe pons, medulla, inferior cerebellar atrophy |
| Progressive supranuclear palsy | Atrophy: tectal<br>T2: ↑ periaqueductal SI due to gliosis; ↓ SI in putamen or superior colliculus due to ↑ iron |
| Hallervorden-Spatz disease | Atrophy<br>T2: severe ↓ ↓ SI in globus pallidus, red nucleus, and SN reticulata |
| Hypothyroidism | Atrophy<br>T2: severe ↓ ↓ SI in normal anatomic locales |

*Source:* Modified from Drayer BP. Imaging of the aging brain. Part II. Pathologic conditions. Radiology 166:797, 1988.

↑ = increase; ↓ = decrease; +/− = present or absent; SI = signal intensity; SN = substantia nigra; WM = white matter; BG = basal ganglia.

Although none is present at birth, a rapid accumulation of iron ensues between 8 and 25 years of age. Subsequently, progressive accumulation is noted in the globus pallidus, putamen, and substantia nigra with advancing age.[139, 140] Lesser amounts of iron accumulate in the red nucleus, dentate nucleus, nigrostriatal tract, caudate nucleus, and fifth layer of cortical gray matter.[141]

## MR Findings in Atrophy and Neurodegeneration

### *Focal Atrophy*

After a localized insult to the brain, focal atrophy may ultimately result. Possible etiologies include brain abscess, intracerebral hematoma, ischemic infarction, trauma, surgical amputation of tissue, and an arteriovenous malformation (pulsatile pressure effects) (see Figs. 12–9 to 12–11). After weeks or months, focal parenchymal brain loss,

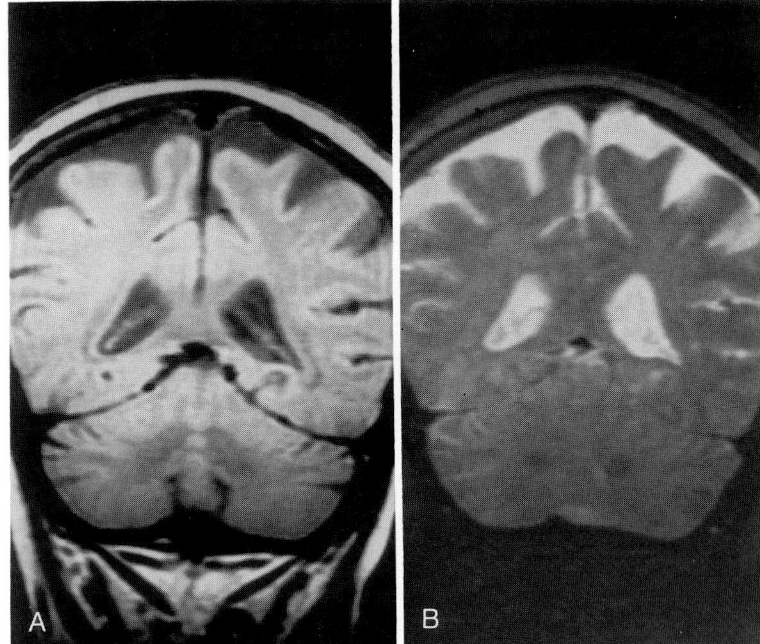


**Figure 12–38. "Peripheral" cerebral supratentorial atrophy.** A 71-year-old woman with suspected clinical infarct. *A,* Coronal N(H)WI (TR 2000/TE 20). *B,* Coronal T2WI (TR 2000/TE 100). Diffuse cortical atrophy is present with normal ventricular size. No infarct was found.

subarachnoid channel dilatation in the affected area, focal enlargement of a neighboring segment of the ventricular system, and T1 or T2 prolongation or both can be observed (Figs. 12–38 and 12–39). Signal intensities vary according to the pathologic process involved (e.g., hemorrhage, ischemia, and so forth). Note that most of the aforementioned signs are really those of negative mass effect as opposed to the positive mass effect seen in most neoplastic processes (see Fig. 12–13). This is a key differential diagnostic point. Identifying the location of the atrophic zone in the brain may provide a specific hint as to its etiology. For example, a hypertensive hemorrhage occurs in the basal ganglia. Nevertheless, clinical history is often important in discerning the specific nature of the original insult.

*Cerebral hemiatrophy* is a form of focal brain atrophy. Clinically characterized by hemiplegia and seizures, with or without mental retardation, the Dyke-Davidoff-Masson syndrome may be caused by a variety of prenatal and postnatal conditions.[142, 143] Infarction, hemorrhage, and infection have all been implicated. MR demonstrates atrophy, including most or all of the hemicerebrum (Fig. 12–40). Ventricles shift toward the involved side, and ipsilateral hydrocephalus ex vacuo is present. Ipsilateral sulci are widened or, less commonly, not seen. Relatively larger areas of focal signal abnormality may or may not be present, depending on

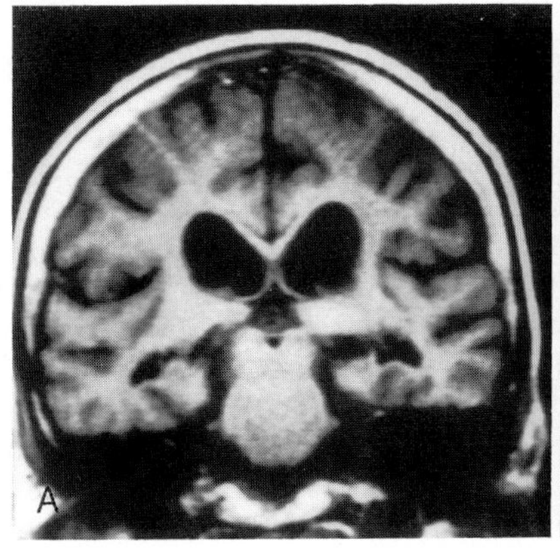


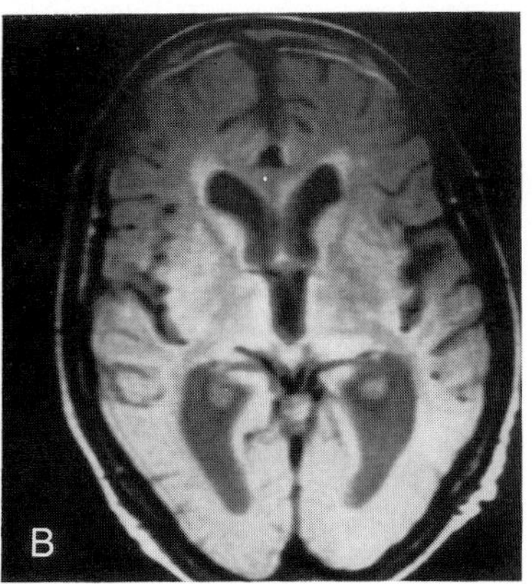


**Figure 12–39. Central atrophy.** A 69-year-old woman with known lymphoma who had received prior CNS irradiation and steroid administration (1.5 T). *A,* Coronal T1WI. *B,* Axial N(H)WI. Normal sulcal/cortical contour for age with prominent ventricles is apparent. Parenchymal signal was normal.

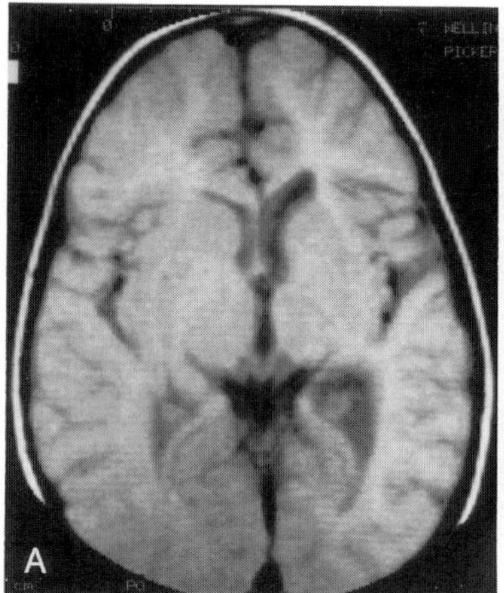


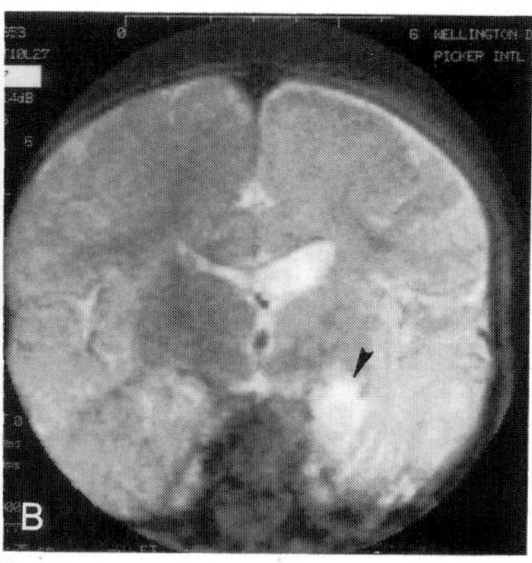


**Figure 12–40. Dyke-Davidoff-Masson syndrome; mesial temporal sclerosis.** A 17-year-old patient with chronic partial complex temporal lobe seizures (0.5 T). *A,* Axial T1W. *B,* Coronal T2WI. Left ventricular/sulcal prominence compatible with cerebral hemiatrophy. Left parahippocampal gliosis (mesial temporal sclerosis) is present (arrowhead). (Courtesy of Wellington Diagnostics; Cincinnati, Ohio.)

the nature of the prior insult. Focal T2 intra-axial signal hyperintensity should not be present unless a chronic seizure disorder exists. In this instance, T2WI signal hyperintensity may be seen in the hippocampal formation (mesial temporal sclerosis).

Differential diagnosis of cerebral hemiatrophy includes the Sturge-Weber syndrome, which exhibits the flow-void signal of a cortical angioma along with the characteristic port-wine nevus on the ipsilateral side of the face. Recognition of a tumor ipsilateral to the atrophy indicates the rare association of a brain neoplasm (usually a germinoma) and ipsilateral cerebral hemiatrophy in a young male.[144] We have also observed white matter signal increase (demyelination) on the affected side on T2WI in several cases.

## MR Findings in Diffuse Atrophy

### *Alzheimer's Disease*

Afflicting those in middle or later life, this progressive dementia is neuropathologically characterized by senile plaques, Hirano bodies, granulovacuolar degeneration, and neurofibrillary tangles. To date, no novel MR findings with pathologic correlations have been described. MR and CT generally show diffuse, atrophic brain changes (Fig. 12–41) most commonly but not in every case in the frontal, parietal, and temporal regions. Some have reported exaggerated periventricular hyperintensity in Alzheimer's patients compared with normal controls, although the value of this finding, when related to diagnostic specificity, is limited.[145] Be aware that normal scans can be obtained in some of these demented patients, but more commonly one sees the abnormal but nonspecific findings of symmetrical ventricular atrophic enlargement and prominent cortical sulci.[146] Unfortunately, the normal aging process can produce identical changes.[147] Thus the imaging diagnosis of Alzheimer's disease remains one of exclusion.

### *Pick's Disease*

Slightly more common in females, this progressive dementing disorder has an age peak around 60 years and is considerably less common than Alzheimer's disease, with which it can be clinically confused. Heredofamilial factors are known in some cases.[148] Because the atrophy usually shows frontotemporal accentuation (Fig. 12–42), it has been called lobar atrophy. Other strange features of the disease include the fact that the anterior third of the superior temporal gyrus is involved, and its posterior portion is spared; in two thirds of cases, the hemispheric shrinkage is asymmetric, with left-sided predominance.[149] Extension of the atrophy to the parietal lobes is occasionally seen. White matter as well as the cortex are typically affected; deep gray matter is less commonly involved. The corresponding portions of the ventricular system are dilated on a hydrocephalus ex vacuo basis. Sylvian fissures and cisterns are expanded as well. Neuronal intracytoplasmic argentophilic Pick's bodies are characteristic microscopically.

Although no unique signal characteristics have been described in this disease, MR, like CT, reflects the aforementioned gross anatomic changes and therefore suggests the diagnosis. Hyperintense T2 foci may or may

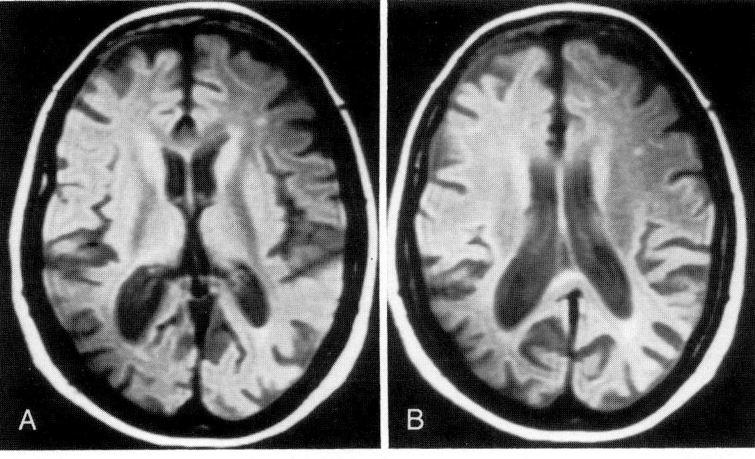


**Figure 12–41. Alzheimer's disease.** A 52-year-old woman with progressive dementia (1.5 T). *A* and *B,* Axial N(H)WI (TR 1800/TE 20). Gyral and sulcal prominence in the posterior parieto-occipital cortex has resulted in mild posterior ventricular enlargement. Punctate foci of signal increase in the left forceps minor and centrum semiovale are not specific.

not be present and are nonspecific. Differential diagnosis may prove difficult, because the imaging findings are quite similar to advanced Alzheimer's disease and can resemble Huntington's disease.

### *Huntington's Disease*

It is now known that the gene responsible for this neurodegenerative disorder with autosomal dominant inheritance that predominantly afflicts males can be traced to a locus on the short arm of chromosome 4.[150] A specific set of cholinergic and GABA-nergic neurons in the neostriatum are lost. Usually manifesting in the third to fifth decades, symptoms result from premature neuronal cell death, most prominent in the basal ganglia. Emotional disturbances, chorea, and dementia are the clinical hallmarks. Although the disease may involve the basal ganglia, cerebral cortex, thalami, and spinal cord, the earliest and most severe changes are seen in the caudate nucleus and putamen (striatum).[151]

MR and CT studies reveal characteristic progressive expansion of the frontal ventricular horns (Fig. 12–43) secondary to predominating caudate atrophy.[152–154] In addition, MR demonstrates hypointense signal in the caudate, putamen, and neostriatum.[155] Later, nonspecific cortical atrophy occurs,

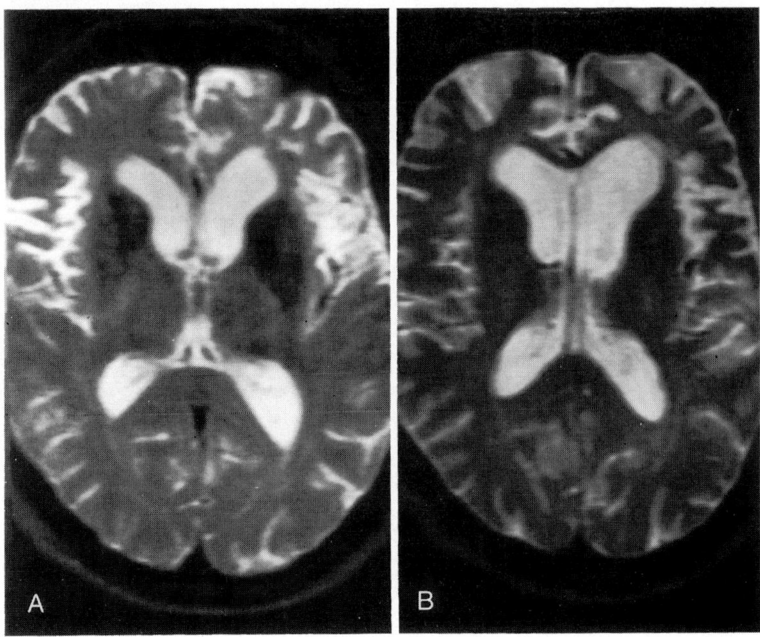


**Figure 12–42. Pick's disease.** A 61-year-old man with progressively agitated behavior, emotional lability, and dementia (1.5 T). *A* and *B,* Axial T2WI. Rostral-frontal cortical atrophy and ventricular prominence. No intra-axial signal alterations were present.

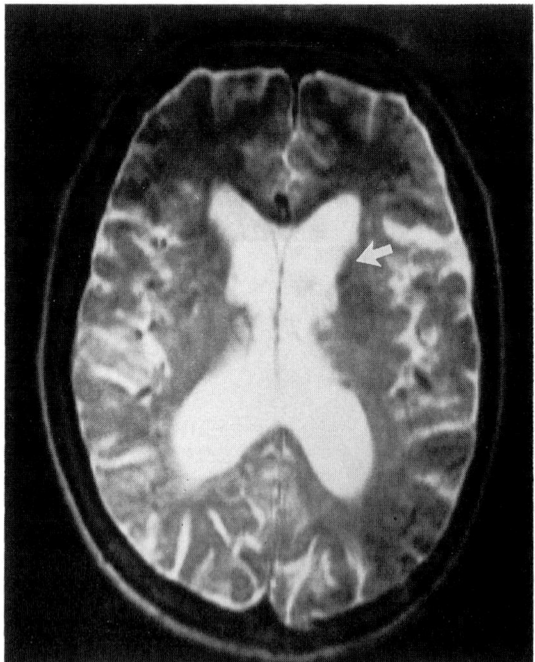

**Figure 12–43. Huntington's chorea.** Axial T2WI (1.5 T). Severe atrophy of the caudate nucleus and putamen (arrow) is associated with biventricular enlargement in this patient. (Courtesy of B. Drayer, M.D., Barrow Neurological Institute, Phoenix, Ariz.)

beginning frontally and progressing posteriorly. A similar pathologic entity, chorea-acanthocytosis, exhibits MR changes identical to those in Huntington's disease, which suggests a common pathoanatomic etiology for the chorea syndrome.

## MR Findings in Movement Disorders and Neurodegeneration

### *Wilson's Disease*

Hepatolenticular degeneration, or Wilson's disease, is an autosomal recessive problem usually diagnosed biochemically. Low blood ceruloplasmin levels permit abnormal deposits of copper in the brain and liver. Symptoms are frequently manifested in the late teens. Early diagnosis and therapy of this rare disease can prevent severe neurologic consequences, which may include dementia and dystonia.

Key pathologic changes include loss of neurons, gliosis, and cavitation in the brain. As the name of this affliction implies, the lentiform nucleus, especially the putamenal division, is most commonly involved. Not uncommonly, the caudate nuclei, thalami, midbrain, and dentate nuclei demonstrate changes as well. Less frequent alterations are exhibited by the white matter and the cerebral and cerebellar cortices.

MR findings at low field strengths have been described and consist of focal prolongation of T1 and T2 in the involved areas. At high field (1.5 T), the potential for preferential T2 paramagnetic shortening exists (Fig. 12–44). Gray matter lesions show characteristic bilateral symmetry, whereas white matter involvement, if present, is typically asymmetric and is most frequent in the frontal lobes. Diffuse atrophy may occur. MR seems to be generally more sensitive than CT in this disease; however, MR and the

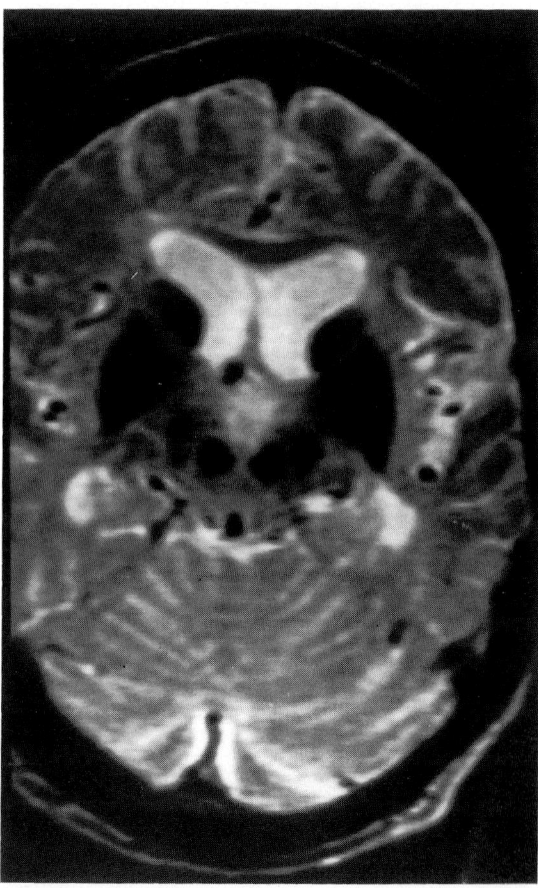

**Figure 12–44. Wilson's disease.** A 52-year-old man with tremor and abnormal serum ceruloplasmin (1.5 T). Axial T2WI. Susceptibility or paramagnetic effect is apparent in the lateral aspect of the lentiform nucleus (putamen), the red nucleus, and in the caudate nucleus, both exhibiting marked T2 signal hypointensity. Normally, hypointensity in the putamen and caudate nucleus is mild and less hypointense than the medially positioned globus pallidus in this age group.

clinical findings do not always correlate well.[156,157] On CT decreased attenuation in the basal ganglia without enhancement and with variable atrophy may be present. The CT scan may be normal.

## Parkinsonian Syndromes

### *Parkinson's Disease*

The major clinical features of this disorder are widely recognized and include the following tetrad: rigidity, postural instability, resting tremor, and bradykinesia. Slowly progressive, this neuroatrophic process appearing in later life involves primarily the lentiform nuclei, substantia nigra, and caudate nuclei. Dementia may ultimately ensue.

Although CT has been largely unrewarding in the study of this disease, MR mapping of brain iron may ultimately offer new insights. In normal adult individuals, spin-echo T2WIs at 1.5 T have shown dominant decreased signal intensity (shortened T2) at specific brain sites such as the cerebellar dentate nucleus, red nucleus, reticular substantia nigra, and globus pallidus. These sites of decreased signal correlate with accentuated deposition of ferric iron.[158] In Parkinson's disease, at high field strengths on T2WI, increased signal hypointensity was first reported in the putamen and lateral zone of the substantia nigra (pars compacta). These findings were manifest as focal signal hypointensity on T2WI that were not appreciated on T1WI.[159] However, we and others have observed restoration of signal in the dorsal lateral substantia nigra that may coincide with iron depletion, local cell death, edema, and increased cellular metabolic activity. This has proved to be an inconsistent finding and therefore is not a reliable marker for this disease.

Secondary parkinsonian syndromes may exhibit signal alterations that can be seen in normal aging, Parkinson-plus syndromes (see following), Huntington's chorea, motor neuron disease, and multiple sclerosis.[160] By the eighth decade in normal patients, putamenal iron approaches that of the globus pallidus. In Parkinson-plus syndromes, the MR findings in the putamen and substantia nigra compacta may be difficult to differentiate from other entities. Huntington's chorea patients should demonstrate excess iron in the caudate and putamen in addition to other non–iron-related findings. Motor neuron disease can produce excess putamenal iron detectable on MR. Finally, multiple sclerosis with its characteristic white matter signal abnormalities can also exhibit excess iron, detectable by MR, in the putamen and thalamus.[158,159]

### *Parkinson-Plus Syndromes*

**Progressive Supranuclear Palsy.** Usually occurring in the sixth decade, this is the most common Parkinson-plus syndrome. Postural instability, pseudobulbar palsy, and supranuclear ophthalmoplegia are clinical features. Dementia follows eventually. A high preponderance of males is afflicted, and no familial cases are known. Microscopically, symmetrical severe gliosis and neuronal loss which is worse in the globus pallidus, subthalamic nucleus, red nucleus, substantia nigra, tectum, periaqueductal gray matter, and dentate nucleus can be observed.[161] High-field MR in six patients has identified focal midbrain atrophy with tectal accentuation and secondary enlargement of the cerebral aqueduct, posterior third ventricle, and quadrigeminal plate cistern (Fig. 12–45). MR findings may precede the clinical syndrome manifestations. In half the patients, T2WI showed periaqueductal increased signal. This may reflect an earlier stage of the disease, before development of atrophy.[155] Conversely, one report emphasized decreased signal intensity on T2WI, felt to represent excess iron accumulation, in the superior colliculi and especially in the putamen.[162]

**Multisystem Atrophies.** This term refers to a set of four syndromes previously thought to be separate ailments. Shy-Drager syndrome, olivopontocerebellar atrophy (OPC), striatonigral degeneration, and parkinsonism-amyotrophy syndrome are now considered to be variants of the same entity, multisystem atrophy.[163] First afflicted in their thirties or forties, these patients usually perish within a decade. Antiparkinsonian drugs are of little help.

**Shy-Drager Syndrome.** Affecting males and females in equal numbers, this progressive syndrome usually presents in one of two neurologic forms: (1) autonomic dysfunction (particularly orthostatic hypotension) with Parkinson-like symptoms and (2) autonomic dysfunction with ataxia. Patho-

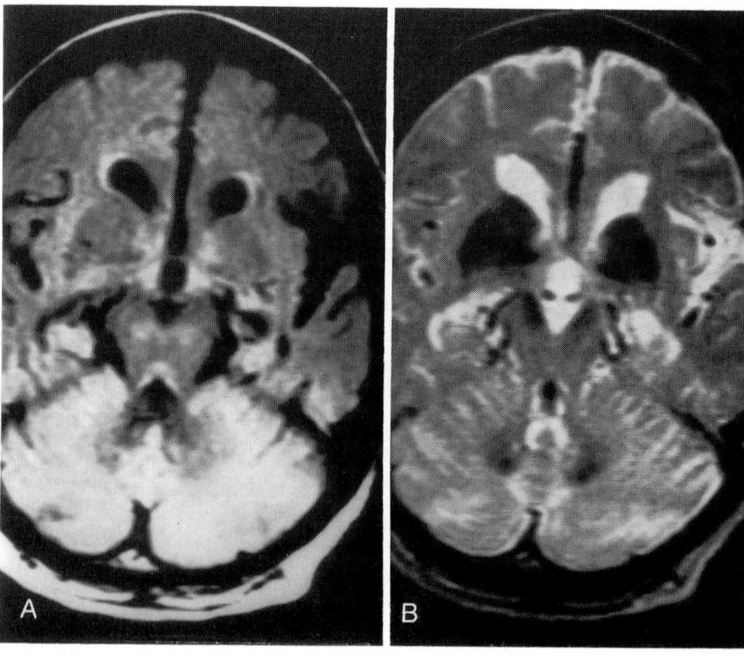


**Figure 12–45. Supranuclear palsy, progressive.** A 49-year-old man with parkinsonian syndrome, ophthalmoplegia, and dementia refractory to therapy (1.5 T). *A,* Axial N(H)WI (TR 1800/TE 20). *B,* Axial T2WI (TR 1800/TE 100). Midbrain atrophy with tectal "pointing" or atrophy is present in conjunction with excessive T2WI signal hypointensity in the lateral aspect of the lentiform nucleus (the putamen).

logically, involvement of the intermediolateral horn cells, striatum, substantia nigra, and cerebellum is common. MRI shows putamenal atrophy (T1WI) and decreased signal (T2WI) in this part of the brain.[164] Atrophic changes similar to olivopontocerebellar atrophy or striatonigral degeneration may also occur.[155] Some consider Shy-Drager and olivopontocerebellar atrophy as overlap syndromes. However, increased globus pallidus signal on T2WI may occur in Shy-Drager, but has not been reported in OPC.

**Olivopontocerebellar Atrophy.** The medullary olive, pons, and cerebellum show degenerative changes along with the substantia nigra and striatum. Intermediolateral horn cells are not involved vis-à-vis Shy-Drager.[165] MRI, like CT, will reveal pontine, brachium pontis, and cerebellar atrophy. These findings are most conspicuous on sagittal T1WI MR (Fig. 12–46). Hemispheric cerebellar atrophy should be equal to or more severe than that of the vermis.[166] Clinically, the manifestations are dysarthria, gait

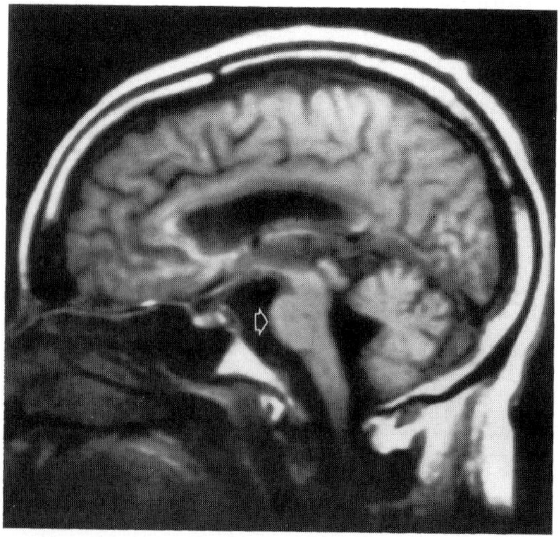

**Figure 12–46. Pontocerebellar atrophy, heredofamilial.** A 47-year-old man with ataxia, tremor, and refractory parkinsonian symptoms (1.5 T). Sagittal T1WI (TR 600/TE 20) shows pontine atrophy (open arrow) and cerebellar vermian atrophy.

abnormalities, and symptoms of Parkinson's disease.

**STRIATONIGRAL DEGENERATION.** In this part of the multisystem atrophy spectrum, parkinsonian symptoms precede rigidity and restlessness. Tremor and cerebellar symptoms are absent. Atrophy of the caudate may occur.[155]

**PARKINSON-AMYOTROPHY SYNDROME.** This disorder involves the nigrostriatum and anterior horn cells. MR findings have not been addressed, as only a few cases have been described.

## Dystonias

Dystonias comprise a subgroup of movement disorders that may be primary (dystonia musculorum deformans and spasmodic torticollis) or secondary—Meige's syndrome. Signal alterations on MR in primary dystonic disease have not been observed. Patients with secondary, delayed-onset, or sudden dystonia may demonstrate signal hyperintensity in the caudate nucleus, putamen, or globus pallidus. Mixed or predominantly hypointense signal may be seen in a similar distribution, and the MR findings therefore are extremely heterogeneous. Yet secondary dystonic disorders such as Wilson's disease or Hallervorden-Spatz syndrome may have more consistent findings. Leigh's disease, a defect in pyruvate metabolism, is a third dystonic disorder with more consistent signal alterations on MR. For these reasons, these entities are discussed as separate disorders. Other secondary dystonias, including those related to infection or inflammations, may produce hyperintense signal and atrophy in the putamen on T2WI. Infarct-induced dystonia produces putamenal signal alteration that may be hemorrhagic or nonhemorrhagic. Therefore signal hyperintensity or hypointensity may exist on T2WI. The pathophysiologic MR changes of neonatal asphyxia and subsequent dystonic disease have yet to be fully elucidated.

### *Cytoplasmically Inherited Striatal Degeneration*

Best labeled as a familial striatal degeneration, this most uncommon disorder is likely transmitted by mitochondrial (cytoplasmic) inheritance. Most patients are under 20 years of age. Dystonia, the predominant clinical feature, may be associated with Leber's neuroretinal degeneration, short stature, muscle atrophy and weakness, and intellectual deficits.[167] However, each patient does not exhibit every feature.[167]

The MR and CT findings of this condition have been described. On MRI, symmetric, sharply marginated putamenal T1 and T2 prolongations have been observed (Fig. 12–47). Similar signal changes were seen in the right caudate nucleus head. MR may show lesions CT does not. The absence of cerebral, cerebellar, and brain stem atrophy serves to distinguish this illness from other striatal disorders.[168] CT usually reveals symmetric low attenuation in the substantia nigra and caudate nuclei, indicating atrophy.[168]

### *Leigh's Disease (Cortical Subacute Necrotizing Encephalomyelopathy*

This is a form of dystonia producing signal hyperintensity in the putamen and associated more subtle signal hyperintensity in the midbrain and cerebral cortex. The latter signal alterations separate this disease from other dystonias.[169] Periaqueductal signal alterations in the midbrain correlate with foci of gliosis and vacuolation.[170]

### *Hallervorden-Spatz Disease*

This is a hereditary movement disorder that may present in childhood (more common) or in adulthood. Treatment is unrewarding. Histologically, pigmentation and iron deposition are noted in the globus pallidus and the reticular zone of the substantia nigra. In combination with the pigment changes, spheroids lend some specificity to the diagnosis when tissue is available. Demyelination is usually present as well as variable involvement of the cerebral cortex, Purkinje cells of the cerebellum, striatum, and spinal cord.[171]

MR at 1.5 T reveals decreased signal in the globus pallidus (Fig. 12–48) on T2WI. Superimposed small islands of increased signal are present within these pallidal zones of T2 shortening. Focal atrophy may not be present.[155] Bilateral caudate atrophy has been seen on CT, making differentiation from Huntington's disease difficult.[172] Perhaps the presence or absence of atrophy is a measure of the stage of the disease.

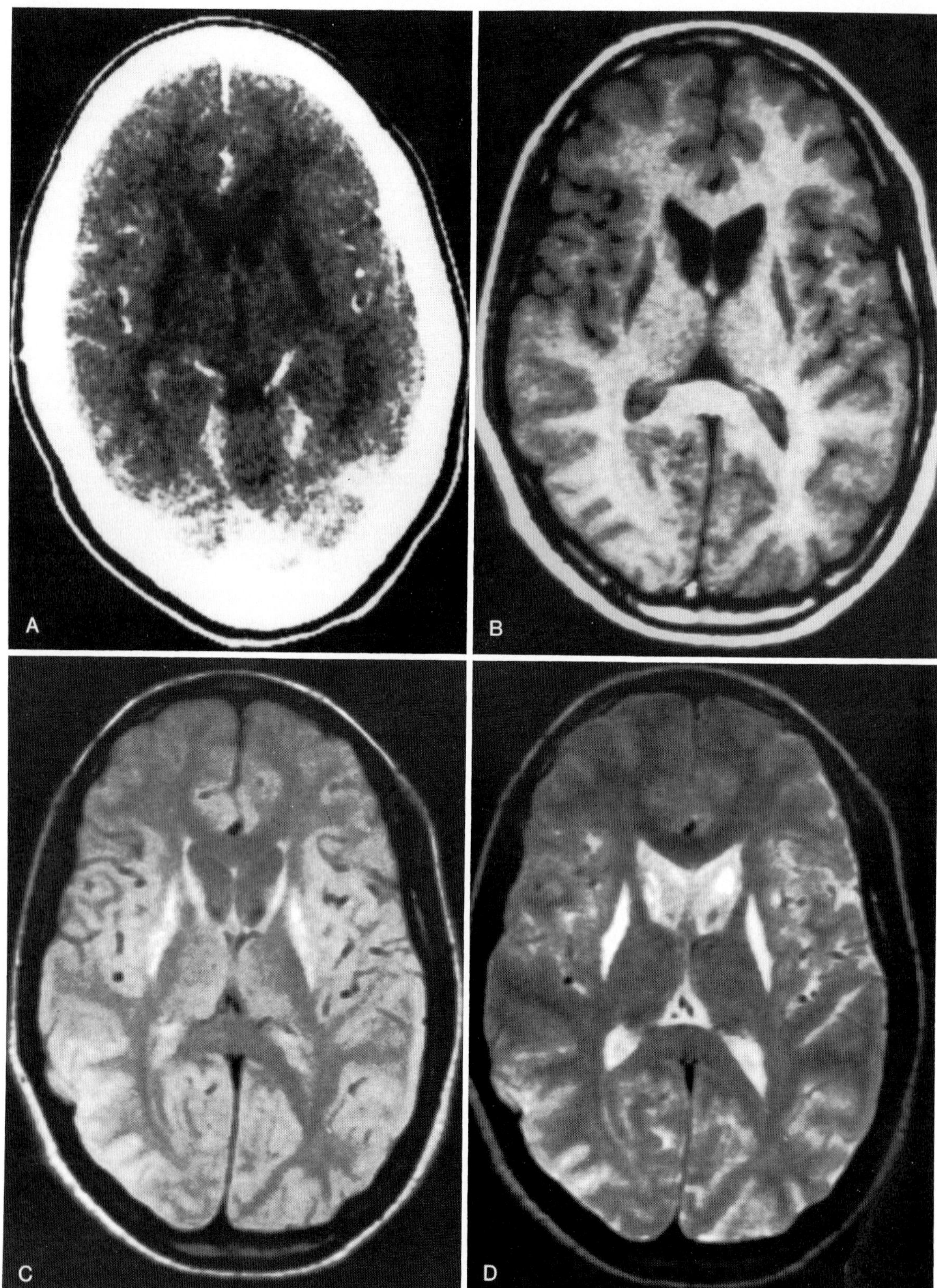


**Figure 12–47. Cytoplasmically inherited striatal degeneration.** An 18-year-old patient with rigidity, dystonia, and mental retardation (1.5 T). *A,* CECT. *B,* Axial T1WI (TR 400/TE 25). *C* and *D,* Axial N(H)WI and T2WI (TR 2000/TE 40/80). The CT shows low density in the putamen. Hypointensity on T1WI and hyperintensity on T2WI are apparent in the putamen and caudate nuclei. Putamenal signal alteration can also be seen in Wilson's disease and Leigh's disease. (From Seidenwurm D, et al. MR and CT in cytoplasmically inherited striatal degeneration. AJNR 7:629, © by American Society of Neuroradiology, 1986, with permission.)

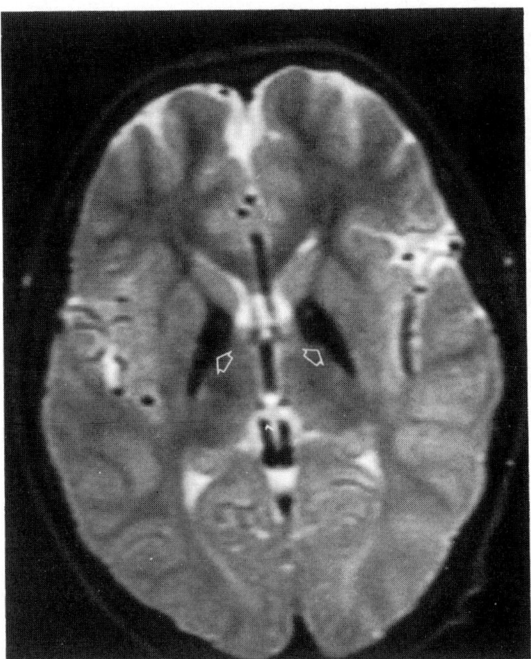

**Figure 12–48. Hallervorden-Spatz disease (HSD).** A 2-year-old child with dystonic movement. T2* relaxation shortening (open arrows), a field strength dependent paramagnetic effect, is due to premature iron deposition in the globus pallidus. Normal statistical iron accumulation in this location occurs between 8 and 25 years and should not appear in this age group. Focal globus pallidus central hyperintensity may be related to pathologic demyelination, neuronal loss, gliosis, and axonal swelling, which occur in this disease.

## Miscellaneous Atrophies, Neurodegenerations, and Movement Disorders

### *Hemiballismus*

This movement disorder is often categorized with the choreoathetoid movement disorders. It consists of spontaneous and abrupt flailing of an extremity. MR findings may demonstrate signal hyperintensity in the subthalamic nucleus contralateral to the clinical side of disease. MR evidence of subthalamic nuclear hemorrhage may also be present.

### *Marchiafava-Bignami Disease*

Most uncommon, Marchiafava-Bignami disease (see Fig. 15–23 in Chap. 15) is usually diagnosed in abusive drinkers of red wine or other alcoholic beverages but may be seen in nonalcoholic individuals, too. Pathogenesis is unknown. The clinical features are protean, so that the diagnosis may be missed before death. Necrosis of the central layer of the corpus callosum is the key pathologic marker. This may involve part of or the entire length of the corpus callosum. However, lesion extension to the lateral margins of the corpus callosum is the rule.[171]

MR spin-echo T2WIs accurately reflect the pathology with increased signal in the middle layer of the corpus callosum. Coronal or sagittal images often show this to best advantage. Small periventricular and subcortical white matter foci of increased signal may also be noted.[173] T1 images have shown decreased signal in the corpus callosum, at least in the chronic stage.[174, 175] Acutely, CT demonstrates decreased attenuation in the corpus callosum. In the subacute phase, enhancement is present. Finally, in the chronic stage atrophy of the corpus callosum and particularly the frontal cortex may be observed.[176]

### *Central Pontine Myelinolysis (CPM)*

This is another rare disorder seen primarily in alcoholics but also known to afflict adults and juveniles with liver disease, burns, cancer, sepsis, anorexia, malnutrition, Wilson's disease, Addison's disease, and marked electrolyte imbalances (especially hyponatremia). Rapid correction of chronic hyponatremia appears to be important in the pathogenesis of this demyelinating disease.[177–179] For this reason, the term *osmotic demyelination syndrome* has come into vogue. Spasticity or flaccid paraparesis or quadriparesis, mutism, dysarthria, and impaired swallowing are often observed. Some patients survive and recover.

MR findings are heterogeneous; however, symmetric, focal myelin destruction in the central pons, exhibiting T1 and T2 prolongation, may be seen (Fig. 12–49).[173, 180] The symmetry, paucity of mass effect, and lesion location in the right clinical setting allow proper diagnosis. Another appearance produces diffuse, symmetric, pontine T1 and T2 prolongation with sparing of the descending corticospinal tracts bilaterally and a peripheral rim of pontine tissue.[181] Extrapontine myelinolysis may occur and may involve the thalamus; putamen; midbrain; internal, external, and extreme capsule; claustrum; lateral geniculate bodies; corpus

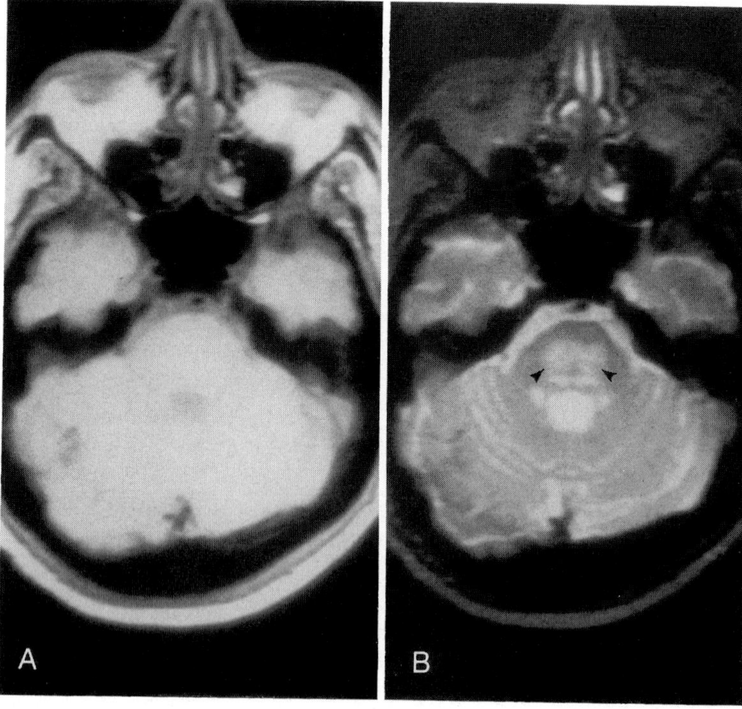


**Figure 12–49. Central pontine myelinolysis.** A 65-year-old alcoholic man found unconscious with serum sodium of 106 mg. *A* and *B*, Axial multiecho N(H)WI and T2WI (TR 1800/TE 20/80). Only on T2WI is bilateral symmetric central pontine hyperintensity (arrowheads) appreciated. The ventrolateral pons is spared.

callosum; gray-white matter junction; cerebral cortex; and spinomedullary-corticospinal tracts.[182] Yet another MR appearance involves bilateral, small, paramidline pontine foci, sparing the locations previously described in the pons and assuming a trident-shape of T1 hypointensity and T2WI hyperintensity.[183] Sparing of the pontine tegmentum and peripheral ventral pontine tissue characterizes this disease as demyelinating; however, symmetry and location allow differentiation from multiple sclerosis. When CT is abnormal, the disease is usually advanced. Frequently, CT is normal; MR findings may revert to normal over weeks or years.

### Behçet's Disease

Suspected to be a vasculitis, this disorder usually presents with recurrent oral and genital ulcers along with relapsing iridocyclitis or uveitis. There is no reliable therapy, and the clinical course is unpredictable and highly variable. Central nervous system involvement occurs in 10 to 25% of patients.[184] This involvement may antedate systemic expressions of the disease.[185] Any portion of the CNS may be involved, but a preference for the basal ganglia and brain stem exists. The neuropathology is nonspecific and consists of multifocal necrotizing lesions with an accompanying florid inflammatory cellular reaction.

MR may show normal T1WI and increased signal on T2WI in the upper brain stem with spin-echo pulsing. Inversion recovery has revealed a low signal focus.[186] Our cases have demonstrated decreased signal on T1WI and increased signal on T2WI in the cerebral peduncles and thalami, bilaterally (see Fig. 14–13).

### Cerebellar Atrophy

Several processes are known to be able to cause isolated cerebellar atrophy. These include the following: radiation; alcohol abuse; diphenylhydantoin toxicity; late cortical cerebellar atrophy; Hodgkin's disease; lung, breast, ovary, or other carcinomas.[187–193]

Both MR and CT can document cerebellar atrophy with enlargement of the superior vermian and cerebellopontine cisterns, the cerebellar sulci, and the fourth ventricle.[190, 194] The sagittal view is especially useful for assessing vermian atrophy (see Fig. 12–46). Usually, the clinical history lends more specificity to the diagnosis of the atrophy than the imaging findings.

Differential diagnosis encompasses chronic subdural hematomas of the posterior fossa or olivopontocerebellar atrophy. In the former, the sulci and fourth ventricle are not enlarged, even though the cerebellum appears shrunken. As the name implies, olivopontocerebellar atrophy demonstrates brain stem as well as cerebellar atrophy.

### *Reversible States Mimicking Atrophy*

True atrophy implies a static or progressive condition that does not improve or is irreversible.[195] Evidence exists that in the cerebrum, apparent atrophy in some instances may be partially or completely reversible when it results from steroid administration, adrenocorticotropic hormone therapy, Cushing's syndrome, anorexia nervosa, or alcoholism.[195–203] The reversibility of the atrophic appearance is not completely understood, but it appears to be associated with an improved nutritional state or removal of the offending drug or both. The amount of brain water may also play a role.[204] CT and MRI can show the changes of widened sulci and fissures, enlarged ventricles, and diminution of brain mass. Caution is therefore advised in the appropriate clinical setting when making the diagnosis of true cerebral atrophy based on only one CT or MRI scan.

## References


1. Wolf P, Kannel W. Controllable risk factors for stroke: preventive implications of trends in stroke mortality. In Meyer JS, Shaw T, eds. Diagnosis and Management of Stroke and TIAs. Reading, Mass., Addison-Wesley, 1982:25.
2. Brierley JB, Graham DI. Hypoxia and vascular disorders of the central nervous system. In Adams JH, Corsellis JAN, Duchen LW, eds. Greenfield's Neuropathology, 4th ed. New York, John Wesley & Sons, 1984:125.
3. Adams RD, Victor M. Principles of Neurology. New York, McGraw-Hill, 1977:496.
4. Raichle ME. The pathophysiology of brain ischemia. Ann Neurol 13:2, 1982.
5. Siesjo BK. Cell damage in the brain: a speculative synthesis. J Cereb Blood Flow Metabol 1:155, 1981.
6. Hossmann KA, Sato K. Recovery of neuronal function after prolonged cerebral ischemia. Science 168:375, 1970.
7. Hossmann KA, Kleihues P. Reversibility of ischemic brain damage. Arch Neurol 29:375, 1973.
8. Jones TH, Morawetz RB, Crowell RM, et al. Thresholds of focal cerebral ischemia in awake monkeys. J Neurosurg 54:773, 1981.
9. Astrup J, Siesjo BK, Symon L. Thresholds in cerebral ischemia—the ischemic penumbra. Stroke 12:723, 1981.
10. Klatzo I. Neuropathological aspects of brain edema. J Neuropath Exp Neurol 26:1, 1967.
11. Fishman RA. Brain edema. N Engl J Med 293:706, 1975.
12. O'Brien MD, Waltz AG, Jordan MM. Ischemic cerebral edema. Arch Neurol 30:456, 1974.
13. Bell BA, Symon L, Branston NM. CBF and time thresholds for the formation of ischemic cerebral edema, and effect of reperfusion in baboons. J Neurosurg 62:31, 1985.
14. O'Brien MD. Ischemic cerebral edema, a review. Stroke 10:623, 1979.
15. Go KG, Edzes HT. Water in brain edema. Arch Neurol 32:462, 1975.
16. Naruse S, Horikawa Y, Tanaka C, et al. Proton nuclear magnetic resonance studies on brain edema. J Neurosurg 56:747, 1982.
17. Brant-Zawadzki M, Davis PL, Crooks LE, et al. NMR demonstration of cerebral abnormalities: comparison with CT. AJR 140:847, 1983.
18. Gomori JM, Grossman RI, Goldberg HI, et al. Intracranial hematomas: imaging by high-field MR. Radiology 157:87, 1985.
19. Hecht-Leavitt C, Gomori JM, Grossman RI, et al. High-field MRI of hemorrhagic cortical infarction. AJNR 7:581, 1986.
20. Edelman RR, Johnson K, Buxton R, et al. MR of hemorrhage: a new approach. AJNR 7:751, 1986.
21. Bradley WG Jr, Schmidt PG. Effect of methemoglobin formation on the MR appearance of subarachnoid hemorrhage. Radiology 156:99, 1985.
22. Chakeres DW, Bryan RN. Acute subarachnoid hemorrhage: in vitro comparison of magnetic resonance and computed tomography. AJNR 7:223, 1986.
23. Scotti G, Ethier R, Melancon D, et al. Computed tomography in the evaluation of intracranial aneurysms and subarachnoid hemorrhage. Radiology 123:85, 1977.
24. Modesti LB, Binet EF. Value of computed tomography in the diagnosis and management of subarachnoid hemorrhage. Neurosurgery 3:151, 1978.
25. Inoue Y, Takemoto K, Miyamoto T, et al. Sequential computed tomography scans in acute cerebral infarction. Radiology 135:655, 1980.
26. Wall S, Brant-Zawadzki M, Jeffrey RB, et al. High-frequency CT findings within 24 hours after cerebral infarction. AJNR 2:553, 1981.
27. Brant-Zawadzki M, Pereira B, Weinstein P, et al. MR imaging of acute experimental ischemia in cats. AJNR 7:7, 1986.
28. Fox AJ, Bogousslavsky J, Carey LS, et al. Magnetic resonance imaging of small medullary infarctions. AJNR 7:229, 1986.
29. Sipponen JT. Visualization of brain infarction with nuclear magnetic resonance imaging. Neuroradiology 26:387, 1984.
30. Bryan RN, Willcott MR, Schneiders NJ, et al. Nuclear magnetic resonance evaluation of stroke. Radiology 149:189, 1983.
31. Ross MA, Biller J, Adams HP, et al. Magnetic resonance imaging in Wallenberg's lateral medullary syndrome. Stroke 17:542, 1986.

32. Awad I, Modic M, Little JR, et al. Focal parenchymal lesions in transient ischemic attacks: correlation of computed tomography and magnetic resonance imaging. Stroke 17:399, 1986.
33. Buonanno FS, Kistler JP, DeWitt LD, et al. Proton ($^1$H) nuclear magnetic resonance (NMR) imaging in stroke syndromes. Neurol Clin 1:243, 1983.
34. Kistler JP, Buonanno FS, DeWitt LD, et al. Vertebral-basilar posterior cerebral territory stroke—delineation by proton nuclear magnetic resonance imaging. Stroke 15:417, 1984.
35. Salgado ED, Furlan AJ, Modic MT, et al. Proton magnetic resonance imaging in cerebrovascular disease. Ann Neurol 18:122, 1985.
36. Simmons Z, Biller J, Adams HP Jr, et al. Cerebellar infarction: comparison of computed tomography and magnetic resonance imaging. Ann Neurol 19:291, 1986.
37. Biller J, Adams HP Jr, Dunn V, et al. Dichotomy between clinical findings and MR abnormalities in pontine infarction. J Comput Assist Tomogr 10:379, 1986.
38. Weinstein MA, Modic MT. Diagnosing non-neoplastic intracranial abnormalities. Arch Clin Imag 1:94, 1985.
39. Hilal SK, Maudsley AA, Ra JB, et al. In vivo NMR imaging of sodium 23 in the human head. J Comput Assist Tomogr 9:1, 1985.
40. Hilal SK, Maudsley AA, Simon HE, et al. In vivo NMR imaging of tissue sodium in the intact cat before and after acute cerebral stroke. AJNR 4:245, 1983.
41. Feinberg DA, Crooks LA, Kaufman L, et al. Magnetic resonance imaging performance: a comparison of sodium and hydrogen. Radiology 156:133, 1985.
42. Perman WH, Turski PA, Houston LW, et al. Methodology of in vivo human sodium MR imaging at 1.5 T. Radiology 160:811, 1986.
43. Aisen AM, Gabrielsen TO, McCune WJ. MR imaging of systemic lupus erythematosus involving the brain. AJR 144:1027, 1985.
44. Sipponen JT, Kaste M, Sepponen RE, et al. Nuclear magnetic resonance imaging in reversible cerebral ischema. (Letter.) Lancet 1:294, 1983.
45. Mauskop A, Wolintz AH, Valderrama R. Cerebral infarction and subdural hematoma. J Clin Neuro-ophthalmol 4:251, 1984.
46. Mano I, Levy RM, Crooks LE, et al. Proton nuclear magnetic resonance imaging of acute experimental cerebral ischemia. Invest Radiol 17:345, 1983.
47. Buonanno FS, Pykett IL, Brady TJ, et al. Proton NMR imaging in experimental cerebral ischemic infarction. Stroke 14:178, 1983.
48. Levy RM, Mano I, Brito A, et al. NMR imaging of acute experimental cerebral ischemia: time course and pharmacologic manipulations. AJNR 4:238, 1983.
49. Sipponen J, Kaste M, Ketonen L, et al. Serial nuclear magnetic resonance (NMR) imaging in patients with cerebral infarction. J Comput Assist Tomogr 7:585, 1983.
50. Mills CM, Crooks LE, Kaufman L, et al. Cerebral abnormalities: use of calculated T1 and T2 magnetic resonance images for diagnosis. Radiology 150:87, 1984.
51. Bydder GM, Steiner RE, Young IR, et al. Clinical NMR imaging of the brain: 140 cases. AJNR 3:459, 1982.
52. Brant-Zawadzki M, Solomon M, Newton TH, et al. Basic principles of magnetic resonance imaging in cerebral ischemia and initial clinical experience. Neuroradiology 27:517, 1985.
53. Brant-Zawadzki M, Norman D, Newton TH, et al. Magnetic resonance of the brain: the optimal screening technique. Radiology 152:71, 1984.
54. Feinberg DA, Mills CA, Posin JP, et al. Multiple spin-echo magnetic resonance imaging. Radiology 155:437, 1985.
55. Mills CM, Brant-Zawadzki M, Crooks LE, et al. Nuclear magnetic resonance: principles of blood flow imaging. AJR 142:165, 1984.
56. Fisher CM, Adams RD. Observations on brain embolism with special reference to the mechanism of hemorrhagic infarction. J Neuropathol Exp Neurol 10:92, 1951.
57. Faris AA, Hardin CA, Poser CM. Pathogenesis of hemorrhagic infarction of the brain. Arch Neurol 9:468, 1963.
58. Wood MW, Wakim KG, Sayre GP, et al. Relationship between anticoagluants and hemorrhagic cerebral infarction in experimental animals. Arch Neurol Psychiatr 79:390, 1958.
59. Davis KR, Ackerman RH, Kistler JP, et al. Computed tomography of cerebral infarction: hemorrhagic, contrast enhancement, and time of appearance. Comput Tomogr 1:71, 1977.
60. Marshall J, Thomas DJ. Vascular disease. In Asbury AK, McKhann GM, McDonald WI, eds. Diseases of the nervous system. Philadelphia, W. B. Saunders, 1986:1101.
61. Waxman SG, Toole JF. Temporal profile resembling TIA in the setting of cerebral infarction. Stroke 14:433, 1983.
62. Araki G, Mihara H, Shizuka M, et al. CT and arteriographic comparison of patients with transient ischemic attacks—correlation with small infarction of basal ganglia. Stroke 14:276, 1983.
63. Bogousslavsky J, Regli F. Cerebral infarction with transient signs (CITS): Do TIAs correspond to small deep infarcts in internal carotid artery occlusion? Stroke 15:536, 1984.
64. Calandre L, Gomara S, Bermejo F, et al. Clinical-CT correlations in TIA, RIND, and strokes with minimum residuum. Stroke 15:663, 1984.
65. Kricheff I. Arteriosclerotic ischemic cerebrovascular disease. Radiology 162:101, 1987.
66. Romanul FCA, Abramowicz A. Changes in brain and pial vessels in arterial border zones. Arch Neurol 11:40, 1964.
67. Goldberg HI. Stroke. In Lee SH, Rao KCVG, eds. Cranial Computed Tomography. New York, McGraw-Hill, 1983:583.
68. Einsiedel-Lechtape H, Kleihues P. Pathology of cerebral vascular insufficiency. In Newton TH, Potts DG, eds. Radiology of the Skull and Brain. Anatomy and Pathology. Vol. 1. St. Louis, C. V. Mosby, 1977:3173.
69. Fisher CM. Lacunar strokes and infarcts: a review. Neurology 32:871, 1982.
70. Fisher CM. Lacunes: small, deep cerebral infarcts. Neurology 15:774, 1965.
71. Kuhn MJ, Davis KR, Shoukimas GM, et al. Magnetic resonance imaging of migraine: comparison with CT. Presented at 25th Annual Meeting of the American Society of Neuroradiology, New York, May 10–15, 1987.

72. Kumar AJ, Rosenbaum AE, Wang H, et al. Magnetic resonance imaging in Sjögren's syndrome. Presented at 25th Annual Meeting of American Society of Neuroradiology, New York, May 10–15, 1987.
73. Brant-Zawadzki M, Fein G, VanDyke C, et al. MR imaging of the aging brain: patchy white-matter lesions and dementia. AJNR 6:675, 1985.
74. Lotz PR, Ballinger WE Jr, Quisling RG. Subcortical arteriosclerotic encephalopathy: CT spectrum and pathologic correlation. AJNR 7:817, 1986.
75. Kinkel WR, Jacobs L, Polachini I, et al. Subcortical arteriosclerotic encephalopathy (Binswanger's disease). Arch Neurol 42:951, 1985.
76. Strandgaard S. Autoregulation of cerebral circulation in hypertension. Acta Neurol Scand (Suppl 66) 57:11, 1978.
77. Mackenzie ET, Strandgaard S, Graham DI, et al. Effects of acutely induced hypertension in cats on pial arteriolar caliber, local cerebral blood flow, and the blood-brain barrier. Circ Res 39:33, 1976.
78. Chester EM, Agamanolis DP, Banker BQ, et al. Hypertensive encephalopathy: a clinicalpathologic study of 20 cases. Neurology 28:928, 1978.
79. Rail DL, Perkin GD. Computerized tomographic appearance of hypertensive encephalopathy. Arch Neurol 37:310, 1980.
80. Perl D, Pendlebury WW. Neuropathology of dementia. Neurol Clin 4:355, 1986.
81. Hachinski VC, Lassen NA, Marshall J. Multi-infarct dementia: a cause of mental deterioration in the elderly. Lancet 2:207, 1974.
82. Fields WS. Multi-infarct dementia. Neurol Clin 4:405, 1986.
83. Kudo T. Spontaneous occlusion of the circle of Willis. Neurology 18:485, 1968.
84. Taveras JM. Multiple progressive intracranial arterial occlusions: a syndrome of children and young adults. AJR 106:235, 1969.
85. Brooks BS, El Gammal T, Adams RJ, et al. MR imaging of moya moya in neurofibromatosis. AJNR 8:178, 1987.
86. Fujisawa I, Asato R, Nishimura K, et al. Moya moya disease: MR imaging. Radiology 1987:164, 103.
87. Sole-Llenas J, Pons-Tortella E. Cerebral angiitis. Neuroradiology 15:1, 1978.
88. Ferris EJ. Arteritis. In Newton TH, Potts DG, eds. Radiology of the Skull and Brain: Angiography. Vol. 2. St. Louis, C. V. Mosby Co., 1974:2583.
89. Brant-Zawadzki M, Norman D, eds. Magnetic Resonance Imaging of the Central Nervous System. New York, Raven Press, 1987:225.
90. Aisen AM, Gabrielson TO, McCune WJ. MR imaging of systemic lupus erythematosus involving the brain. AJR 144:1027, 1985.
91. Vermess M, Bernstein RM, Bydder GM, et al. Nuclear magnetic resonance (NMR) imaging of the brain in systemic lupus erythematosus. J Comput Assist Tomogr 7:461, 1983.
92. Bilaniuk LT, Patel S, Zimmerman RA. Computed tomography of systemic lupus erythematosus. Radiology 124:119, 1977.
93. Myers RE. A unitary theory of causation of anoxic and hypoxic brain pathology. In Fahn S, et al., eds. Advances in Neurology. Vol. 26. New York, Raven Press, 1979:195.
94. Plum F, Posner JB, Hain RF. Delayed neurological deterioration after anoxia. Arch Intern Med 110:56, 1962.
95. Adams RD, Victor M. Principles of Neurology. New York, McGraw-Hill, 1977:732.
96. Plum F, Pulsinelli WA. Cerebral metabolism and hypoxic-ischemic brain injury. In Asbury AK, McKhann GM, McDonald WI, eds. Diseases of the Nervous System. Philadelphia, W. B. Saunders, 1986:1086.
97. Brucher JM. Neuropathological problems posed by carbon monoxide poisoning and anoxia. Progr Brain Res 24:75, 1967.
98. Ginsberg MD. Delayed neurological deterioration following hypoxia. In Fahn S, et al., eds. Advances in Neurology. Vol. 26. New York, Raven Press, 1979:21.
99. Ginsberg MD, Hedley-Whyte ET, Richardson EP Jr. Hypoxic-ischemic leukoencephalopathy in man. Arch Neurol 33:5, 1976.
100. Yagnik P, Gonzalez C. White matter involvement in anoxic encephalopathy in adults. J Comput Assist Tomogr 4:788, 1980.
101. Kjos BO, Brant-Zawadzki M, Young RG. Early CT findings of global central nervous system hypoperfusion. AJR 141:1227, 1983.
102. Miura T, Mitomo M, Kawai R, et al. CT of the brain in acute carbon monoxide intoxication: characteristic features and prognosis. AJNR 6:739, 1985.
103. Kim KS, Weinberg PE, Suh JH, et al. Acute carbon monoxide poisoning: computed tomography of the brain. AJNR 1:399, 1980.
104. Davis PL. The magnetic resonance imaging appearances of basal ganglia lesions in carbon monoxide poisoning. Magn Reson Imag 4:489, 1986.
105. Buonanno FS, Moody DM, Ball MR, et al. Computed cranial tomographic findings in cerebral sinovenous occlusion. J Comput Assist Tomogr 2:281, 1978.
106. McMurdo SK Jr, Brant-Zawadzki M, Bradley WG, et al. Dural sinus thrombosis: study using intermediate field strength MR imaging. Radiology 161:83, 1986.
107. Macchi PJ, Grossman RI, Gomori JM, et al. High-field MR imaging of cerebral venous thrombosis. J Comput Assist Tomogr 10:10, 1986.
108. Bauer WM, Einhaupl K, Heywang SH, et al. MR of venous sinus thrombosis: a case report. AJNR 8:713, 1987.
109. McArdle CB, Mirfakhraee M, Amparo EG, et al. MR imaging of transverse/sigmoid dural sinus and jugular vein thrombosis. J Comput Assist Tomogr 11:831, 1987.
110. Bradley WG Jr, Waluch V. Blood flow: magnetic resonance imaging. Radiology 154:443, 1985.
111. Waluch V, Bradley WG. NMR even-echo rephasing in slow laminar flow. J Comput Assist Tomogr 8:594, 1984.
112. Axel L. Blood flow effects in magnetic resonance imaging. AJR 143:1157, 1984.
113. Early CB, Fink LH. Some fundamental applications of the law of LaPlace in neurosurgery. Surg Neurol 6:185, 1976.
114. Sherman JL, Citrin CM. Magnetic resonance demonstration of normal CSF flow. AJNR 7:3, 1986.
115. Sherman JL, Citrin CM, Bowen BJ, et al. MR demonstration of altered cerebrospinal fluid flow by obstructive lesions. AJNR 7:571, 1986.

116. Bradley WG, Kortman KE, Burgoyne B. Flowing cerebrospinal fluid in normal and hydrocephalic states: appearance on MR images. Radiology 159:611, 1986.
117. El Gammal T, Allen MB, Brooks BS, et al. MR evaluation of hydrocephalus. AJNR 8:591, 1987.
118. Sjaastad O, Skalpe IO, Engeset A. The width of the temporal horn in the differential diagnosis between pressure hydrocephalus and hydrocephalus ex vacuo. Neurology 19:1087, 1969.
119. LeMay M, Hochberg FH. Ventricular differences between hydrostatic hydrocephalus and hydrocephalus ex vacuo by computed tomography. Neuroradiology 17:191, 1979.
120. Heinz ER, Ward A, Drayer BP, et al. Distinction between obstructive and atrophic dilatation of ventricles in children. J Comput Assist Tomogr 4:320, 1980.
121. Hahn FJ, Rim K. Frontal ventricular dimensions on normal computed tomography. AJR 126:593, 1976.
122. Zimmerman RD, Fleming CA, Lee BCP, et al. Periventricular hyperintensity as seen by magnetic resonance: prevalence and significance. AJNR 7:13, 1986.
123. duBoulay GH. Pulsatile movements in the CSF pathways. Br J Radiol 39:255, 1966.
124. Novetsky GJ, Berlin L. Aqueductal stenosis: demonstration by MR imaging. J Comput Assist Tomogr 8:1170, 1984.
125. Naidich TP, Epstein F, Lin JP, et al. Evaluation of pediatric hydrocephalus by computed tomography. Radiology 119:337, 1976.
126. Zimmerman RA, Bilaniuk LT, Gallo E. Computed tomography of the trapped fourth ventricle. AJR 130:503, 1978.
127. Hughes CP, Gado M. Pathology of hydrocephalus and brain atrophy. In Newton TH, Potts DG, eds. Radiology of the Skull and Brain. Anatomy and Pathology. Vol. 3. St. Louis, C. V. Mosby, 1977: 3197.
128. Adams RD, Fisher CM, Hakim S, et al. Symptomatic occult hydrocephalus with a "normal" cerebrospinal fluid pressure. N Engl J Med 273:117, 1965.
129. Hakim S, Adams RD. The special clinical problem of symptomatic hydrocephalus with normal cerebrospinal fluid pressure observations on cerebrospinal fluid hydrodynamics. J Neurol Sci 2:307, 1965.
130. Gunasekera L, Richardson AE. Computerized axial tomography in idiopathic hydrocephalus. Brain 100:749, 1977.
131. Symon L, Hinzpeter T. The enigma of normal-pressure hydrocephalus. Clin Neurosurg 24:285, 1977.
132. Black PM. Idiopathic normal pressure hydrocephalus. J Neurosurg 52:371, 1980.
133. Huckman MS. Normal pressure hydrocephalus: evaluation of diagnostic and prognostic tests. AJNR 2:385, 1981.
134. TerBrugge KG, Rao KCVG. Hydrocephalus and atrophy. In Lee SH, Rao KCVG, eds. Cranial Computed Tomography. New York, McGraw-Hill, 1983:171.
135. Haughton VM. Hydrocephalus and atrophy. In Williams AL, Haughton VM, eds. Cranial Computed Tomography. St. Louis, C. V. Mosby, 1985:240.
136. Kendall B, Reider-Grosswasser I, Valentine A. Diagnosis of masses presenting within the ventricles on computed tomography. Neuroradiology 25:11, 1983.
137. Morrisson G, Sobel DF, Kelley WM, et al. Intraventricular mass lesions. Radiology 153:435, 1984.
138. Koenig SH, Brown RD, Peters TJ, et al. Relaxometry of ferritin solutions and the influence of the Fe(III) core ions. Magn Reson Med 3:755, 1986.
139. Hock A, Demmer U, Schicha K. Trace elements concentration in human brain: copper, zinc, iron, and magnesium. Clin Chim Acta 21:55, 1968.
140. Ule G, Volke A, Berlet H. Trace elements in human brain. Neurology 206:117, 1974.
141. Hallgren B, Sourander P. The effect of age on the non-haemin iron in the human brain. J Neurochem 3:41, 1958.
142. Zilkha A. CT of cerebral hemiatrophy. AJNR 1:255, 1980.
143. Jacoby CG, Go RT, Hahn FJ. Computed tomography of cerebral hemiatrophy. AJR 129:5, 1977.
144. Maehara T, Machida T, Tsuchiya K, et al. Brain tumors with ipsilateral cerebral hemiatrophy. AJNR 4:478, 1983.
145. Fazekas F, Chawluk JB, Alavi A, et al. MR signal abnormalities at 1.5 T in Alzeimer's dementia and normal aging. AJNR 8:421, 1987.
146. McGeer PL. Brain imaging in Alzheimer's disease. Br Med Bull 42:24, 1986.
147. Takeda S, Matsuzawa T. Brain atrophy during aging. J Am Geriatr Soc 32:520, 1984.
148. Groen JJ, Hekster REM. Computed tomography in Pick's disease: findings in a family affected in three consecutive generations. J Comput Assist Tomogr 6:907, 1982.
149. Tomlinson BE, Corsellis JAN. Aging and the dementias. In Adams JH, Corsellis JAN, Duchen LW, eds. Greenfield's Neuropathology, 4th ed. New York, John Wiley & Sons, 1984:951.
150. Gusella JF, Wexler NS, Conneally PM, et al. A polymorphic DNA marker genetically linked to Huntington's disease. Nature 306:234, 1983.
151. Martin JB, Gusella JF. Huntington's disease. Pathogenesis and management. N Engl J Med 315:1267, 1986.
152. Simmons JT, Pastakia B, Chase TN, et al. Magnetic resonance imaging in Huntington's disease. AJNR 7:25, 1986.
153. Terrence CF, Delaney JF, Alberts MC. Computed tomography for Huntington's disease. Neuroradiology 13:173, 1977.
154. Stober T, Wussow W, Schimrigk K. Bicaudate diameter—the most specific and simple CT parameter in the diagnosis of Huntington's disease. Neuroradiology 26:25, 1984.
155. Rutlege JN, Hilal SK, Silver AJ, et al. Study of movement disorders and brain ion by MR. AJNR 8:397, 1987.
156. Lawler GA, Pennock JM, Steiner RE, et al. Nuclear magnetic resonance (NMR) imaging in Wilson disease. J Comput Assist Tomogr 7:1, 1983.
157. Aisen AM, Martel W, Gabrielsen TO, et al. Wilson disease of the brain: MR imaging. Radiology 157:137, 1985.
158. Drayer B, Burger P, Darwin R, et al. Magnetic resonance imaging of brain ion. AJNR 7:373, 1986.

159. Drayer B: Degenerative brain disorders and brain ion. In Brant-Zawadzki M, Norman D, eds. Magnetic Resonance Imaging of the Central Nervous System. New York, Raven Press, 1987:123.
160. Drayer B, Burger P, Hurwitz B, et al. Reduced signal intensity on MR images of thalamus and putamen in multiple sclerosis: increased iron content? AJNR 8:413, 1987.
161. Oppenheimer RD. Diseases of the basal ganglia, cerebellum, and motor neurons. In Adams JH, Corsellis JAN, Duchen LW, eds. Greenfield's Neuropathology, 4th ed. New York, John Wiley & Sons, 1984:699.
162. Drayer BP, Olanow W, Burger P, et al. Parkinson plus syndrome: diagnosis using high-field MR imaging of brain ion. Radiology 159:493, 1986.
163. Bannister R, Oppenheimer D. Parkinsonism, system degenerations and autonomic failure. In Marsden CD, Fahn S, eds. Movement Disorders. London, Butterworth Scientific, 1982:174.
164. Pastakia B, Polinsky R, Di Chiro G, et al. Multiple system atrophy (Shy-Drager syndrome): MR imaging. Radiology 159:499, 1986.
165. Fahn S. Parkinson's disease and other basal ganglion disorders. In Asbury AK, McKhann GM, McDonald WI, eds. Diseases of the Nervous System. Philadelphia, W. B. Saunders, 1986:1217.
166. Savoiardo M, Bracchi M, Passerini A, et al. Computed tomography of olivopontocerebellar degeneration. AJNR 4:509, 1983.
167. Novotny EJ Jr, Singh G, Wallace DC, et al. Leber's disease and dystonia: a mitochondrial disease. Neurology 36:1053, 1986.
168. Seidenwurm D, Novotny E Jr, Marshall W, et al. MR and CT in cytoplasmically inherited striatal degeneration. AJNR 7:629, 1986.
169. Rutledge JN, Hilal SK, Silver AJ, et al. Study of movement disorders and brain iron by MR. AJNR 8:397, 1987.
170. Pincott EJ Jr, Wilson J, et al. Cortical subacute necrotizing encephalomyelopathy. Neuropediatrics 15:150, 1984.
171. Duchen LW, Jacobs JM. Nutritional deficiencies and metabolic disorders. In Adams JH, Corsellis JAN, Duchen LW, eds. Greenfield's Neuropathology, 4th ed. New York, John Wiley & Sons, 1984:573.
172. Dooling EC, Richardson EP Jr, Davis KR. Computed tomography in Hallervorden-Spatz disease. Neurology 30:1128, 1980.
173. Holland BA. Diseases of white matter. In Brant-Zawadzki M, Norman D, eds. Magnetic Resonance Imaging of the Central Nervous System. New York, Raven Press, 1987:259.
174. Clavier E, Thiebot J, Hannequin D, et al. Marchiafava-Bignami disease. Neuroradiology 28:376, 1986.
175. Kawamura M, Shiota J, Yagishita T, et al. Marchiafava-Bignami disease: computed tomographic scan and magnetic resonance imaging. Ann Neurol 18:103, 1985.
176. Raneurel G, Gardeur D, Thiberge M, et al. Computed tomography of Marchiafava-Bignami disease. Presented at Proceedings of the 12th Annual Neuroradiologicum Symposium, Washington, D.C., October 10–16, 1982.
177. DeWitt LD, Buonanno FS, Kistler JP, et al. Central pontine myelinolysis: demonstration by nuclear magnetic resonance. Neurology 34:570, 1984.
178. Ingram D, Traub M, Kopelman P, et al. Brain stem auditory-evoked responses in diagnosis of central pontine myelinolysis. J Neurol 223:23, 1986.
179. Sterns RH, Riggs JE, Schochet SS Jr. Osmotic demyelination syndrome following correction of hyponatremia. N Engl J Med 314:1535, 1986.
180. Takeda K, Sakuta M, Saeki F. Central pontine myelinolysis diagnosed by magnetic resonance imaging. Ann Neurol 17:310, 1985.
181. Rippe DJ, Edwards MK, D'Amour PG, et al. MR imaging of central pontine myelinolysis. J Comput Assist Tomogr 11:724, 1987.
182. Okeda R, Kitano M, Sawabe M, et al. Distribution of demyelinating lesions in pontine and extrapontine myelinolysis. Acta Neuropathol (Berl) 69:259, 1986.
183. Price DB, Kramer J, Hotson GC, et al. Central pontine myelinolysis: report of a case with distinctive appearance on MR imaging. AJNR 8:576, 1987.
184. Wolf SM, Schotland DL, Phillips LL. Involvement of nervous systems in Behçet's syndrome. Arch Neurol 12:315, 1965.
185. Kozin F, Haughton V, Bernhard GC. Neuro-Behçet disease: two cases and neuroradiologic findings. Neurology 27:1148, 1977.
186. Willeit J, Schmutzhard E, Aichner F, et al. CT and MR in neuro-Behçet disease. J Comput Assist Tomogr 10:313, 1986.
187. Jacoby CG, Tewfik KK, Blackwelder JT. Cerebellar atrophy developing after cranial irradiation. J Comput Assist Tomogr 6:159, 1982.
188. Haubek A, Lee K. Computed tomography in alcoholic cerebellar atrophy. Neuroradiology 18:77, 1979.
189. Selhorst JB, Kaufman B, Horwitz SJ. Diphenylhydantoin-induced cerebellar degeneration. Arch Neurol 27:453, 1972.
190. Baloh RW, Yee RD, Honrubia V. Late cortical cerebellar atrophy. Brain 109:159, 1986.
191. Brazis PW, Biller J, Fine M, et al. Cerebellar degeneration with Hodgkin's disease. Arch Neurol 38:253, 1981.
192. Koller WC, Glatt SL, Perlik S, et al. Cerebellar atrophy demonstrated by computed tomography. Neurology 31:405, 1981.
193. Brain L, Wilkinson M. Subacute cerebellar degeneration associated with neoplasms. Brain 88:465, 1965.
194. Allen JH, Martin JT, McLain LW. Computed tomography in cerebellar atrophic processes. Radiology 130:379, 1979.
195. Heinz ER, Martinez J, Haenggeli A. Reversibility of cerebral atrophy in anorexia nervosa and Cushing's syndrome. J Comput Assist Tomogr 1:415, 1977.
196. Bentson J, Reza M, Winter J, et al. Steroids and apparent cerebral atrophy on computed tomography scans. J Comput Assist Tomogr 2:16, 1978.
197. Okuno T, Ito M, Konishi Y, et al. Cerebral atrophy following ACTH therapy. J Comput Assist Tomogr 4:20, 1980.
198. Artmann H, Grau H, Adelmann M, et al. Reversible and nonreversible enlargement of cerebrospinal

fluid spaces in anorexia nervosa. Neuroradiology 27:304, 1985.

199. Kohlmeyer K, Lehmkuhl G, Poutska F. Computed tomography of anorexia nervosa. AJNR 4:437, 1983.

200. Enzmann DR, Lane B. Cranial computed tomography findings in anorexia nervosa. J Comput Assist Tomogr 1:410, 1977.

201. Carlen PL, Wortzman G, Holgate RC, et al. Reversible cerebral atrophy in recently abstinent chronic alcoholics measured by computed tomography scans. Science 200:1076, 1978.

202. Carlen PL, Penn RD, Fornazzari L, et al. Computerized tomographic scan assessment of alcoholic brain damage and its potential reversibility. Alcohol Clin Exp Res 10:226, 1986.

203. Artmann H, Gall MV, Hacker H, et al. Reversible enlargement of cerebral spinal fluid spaces in chronic alcoholics. AJNR 2:23, 1981.

204. Smith MA, Chick J, Kean DM, et al. Brain water in chronic alcoholic patients measured by magnetic resonance imaging. (Letter.) Lancet 1:1273, 1985.

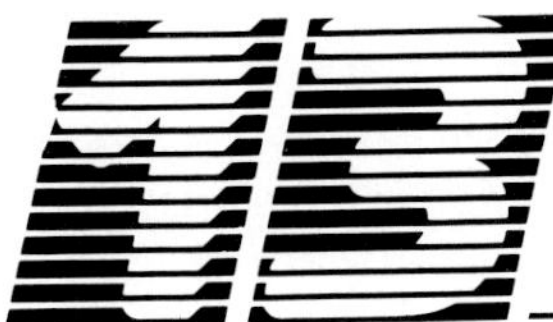

Scott Schlesinger, M.D.

# MRI OF INTRACRANIAL HEMATOMAS AND CLOSED HEAD TRAUMA

## INTRACRANIAL HEMATOMA EVOLUTION

Hematoma evolution on MR is a study of the natural history of intracranial bleeding. Separating and understanding of the pathophysiology of hematoma evolution from the MR appearance are crucial because MR appearances vary depending upon the imaging parameters and field strength used. Review of some basic concepts is necessary as a prelude to understanding the MR appearance of aging blood. Image contrast in MR is dependent upon several basic properties: T1 and T2 relaxation times, proton density, blood flow, and chemical shifts.[26, 30–35, 45, 57, 71, 72] T1, T2, and proton density are the pertinent contrast parameters.

### MR Physics

Protons are contained within a sea of tissue that is exposed to a relatively homogeneous magnetic field ($B_0$). A local tissue magnetic field is induced by the main, static magnetic field ($B_0$). Magnetic susceptibility is the ratio of the magnitude of this induced local field to that of $B_0$. The magnetic susceptibility of a tissue is altered by the addition of ferromagnetic, diamagnetic, and paramagnetic substances. These substances have dipolar properties that cause them to align and polarize when placed in a magnetic field. Ferromagnetic substances (e.g., metallic iron) remain polarized with $B_0$ even after the field is removed.[74] There are no known naturally occurring biologic ferromagnetic substances.[74] Diamagnetic and paramagnetic particles resume their baseline orientation after removal from the influence of $B_0$; however, diamagnetic substances decrease magnetic susceptibility, whereas paramagnetic substances increase magnetic susceptibility.[38, 39, 61]

Knowledge of paramagnetic phenomena is paramount in understanding the MR appearance of aging blood because hemoglobin degradation results in the formation of iron-containing, paramagnetic compounds (Fig. 13–1). Paramagnetic substances interact with surrounding protons in (at least) two ways: (1) *proton-electron dipole-dipole relaxation enhancement* (PEDDPRE) and (2) *preferential T2 proton relaxation enhancement* (PT2PRE).

Proton-electron dipole-dipole relaxation enhancement is the result of dipolar forces that occur between the electrons of a paramagnetic compound and the positively charged surrounding protons. PEDDPRE causes enhancement (shortening) of T1 and T2 relaxation times. The magnitude of these forces is inversely proportional to the sixth power of the distance between the dipoles, and therefore falls rapidly as the distance between the charged particles increases.[83] To have significant T1 and T2 shortening

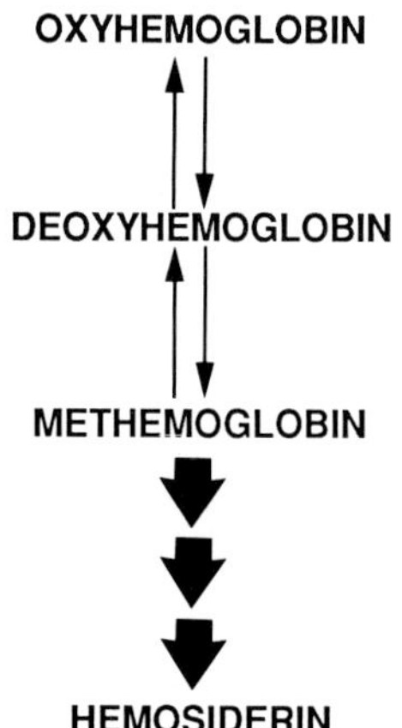


**Figure 13–1.** Hemoglobin degradation.

from dipolar interactions, the electrons in a paramagnetic moiety must be able to approach within approximately 3 Å of aqueous protons.[16, 58, 83] In static magnetic experiments, although oxyhemoglobin has one unpaired electron and is diamagnetic and deoxyhemoglobin has four unpaired electrons and is paramagnetic, neither significantly effects T1 or T2 relaxation times in an aqueous environment because the shape of the molecule precludes aqueous protons' ability to approach these available electrons of iron.[61, 100] In contrast, aqueous protons are able to penetrate into the "inner sphere" of methemoglobin and interact with its five unpaired electrons, causing shortening of T1 and T2 relaxation times.[32] Methemoglobin is the only important hemoglobin degradation product to exhibit significant PEDDPRE (Table 13–1). The magnitude of the PEDDPRE is related to the concentration of paramagnetic centers and to the number of unpaired electron spins per center.[77] At low concentrations similar to those that occur in hematomas, methemoglobin causes significant T1 shortening with substantially less effect on the T2 relaxation time.[79, 236] Because each molecule has five unpaired electrons, its effect is strong. The short T1 of methemoglobin is readily visible at all clinically useful field strengths. In fact, many observations suggest that the short T1 is best visualized at very low field strengths where T1 differences are maximized.[26, 27, 30–35] Thus, in the evolution of a hematoma, methemoglobin interacts with aqueous protons via dipolar interactions to shorten the T1 relaxation time with comparatively little effect on T2, in contrast with the magnetic susceptibility of PT2PRE.

Preferential proton T2 relaxation enhancement, as might be deduced from the name, involves selective enhancement of proton spin dephasing (T2) with no significant effect on T1. Paramagnetic substances alter the magnetic susceptibility around them by causing local field disturbances. In the presence of a static magnetic field, inhomogeneous local magnetic fields are created when a paramagnetic center is inaccessible to water protons.[16, 58, 59] This situation occurs when the paramagnetic substance is insoluble (e.g., hemosiderin) or intracellular, where magnetic gradients are created between the internal and external environments of the cell.[294, 295] As aqueous protons diffuse through these gradients, they lose the phase coherence that was induced by the RF pulse and precess at different frequencies.[77] Since T2 relaxation times are a measure of the time it takes the protons to lose phase coherence and return to their baseline status (before the RF pulse was applied), T2 shortening occurs. Hemosiderin, a large, insoluble polymer containing ferric iron ($Fe^{3+}$), and intracellular deoxyhemoglobin and methemoglobin have been shown to exhibit significant PT2PRE.[16, 63, 100, 296, 299] The magnitude of

**Table 13–1.** PARAMAGNETIC EFFECTS OF HEMOGLOBIN DEGRADATION PRODUCTS

| Compound | Paramagnetic Mechanism | MR Effect |
|---|---|---|
| Intracellular oxyhemoglobin | Minimal PT2PRE | Negligible |
| Free oxyhemoglobin | — | — |
| Intracellular deoxyhemoglobin | PT2PRE | T2 shortening |
| Free deoxyhemoglobin | — | — |
| Intracellular methemoglobin | PT2PRE | T2 shortening |
| Free methemoglobin | PEDDPRE | T1 shortening > T2 shortening |
| Hemosiderin | PT2PRE | T2 shortening |

PT2PRE = Preferential T2 relaxation enhancement (magnetic susceptibility effect).
PEDDPRE = Proton-electron dipole-dipole relaxation enhancement.

PT2PRE is proportional to the square of the concentration of the paramagnetic compound and to the square of the number of unpaired electrons within the substance.[16,77,100] A molecule of oxyhemoglobin has only one unpaired electron, whereas deoxyhemoglobin has four, and methemoglobin and hemosiderin each have five. Thus the magnetic susceptibility of hemosiderin and intracellular deoxyhemoglobin and methemoglobin is high; the PT2PRE from intracellular oxyhemoglobin is insignificant with current imaging techniques (Table 13–1). This spin dephasing is a direct result of magnetic susceptibility from restricted contact of the paramagnetic moiety with surrounding protons. With red cell lysis, intracellular methemoglobin and deoxyhemoglobin are released into solution, and the PT2PRE is lost.

Visualization of the markedly short T2 is highly dependent upon the field strength because the magnitude of PT2PRE is proportional to the square of the strength of $B_0$. At low field strengths (< 0.5 T), using spin-echo (SE) sequences, the PT2PRE from paramagnetic blood breakdown products may not be identifiable (Fig. 13–2); diagnostic capabilities and image specificity are diminished. However, there are imaging sequences that are more sensitive to the presence of paramagnetic compounds and can increase the diagnostic yield with low-field equipment.

Lengthening the TE is a simple way to increase the sensitivity of SE imaging to magnetic susceptibility.[37,63] PT2PRE is due to the spin dephasing of water protons as they tumble through varying magnetic gradients. Lengthening the TE increases the length of time that water protons can tumble prior to the echo. Greater water diffusion results in increased spin dephasing of each proton. The cost of increasing the TE is increased noise; acquisition with TEs longer than 120 msec rapidly becomes noise limited.

Despite a long TE, however, SE imaging remains relatively insensitive to field inhomogeneity. By design, spin echo is relatively insensitive to small variations in magnetic susceptibility. The 180° spin echo refocuses each proton so that it experiences a constant magnetic field that aids in the elimination of untoward effects from variations in field homogeneity. This results in a higher quality image with better signal-to-noise ratio (SNR) and is one of the reasons SE imaging has become so popular. A disadvantage of the refocusing echo is that it indiscriminately diminishes the effects of field inhomogeneity, including those due to the magnetic susceptibility of paramagnetic agents.

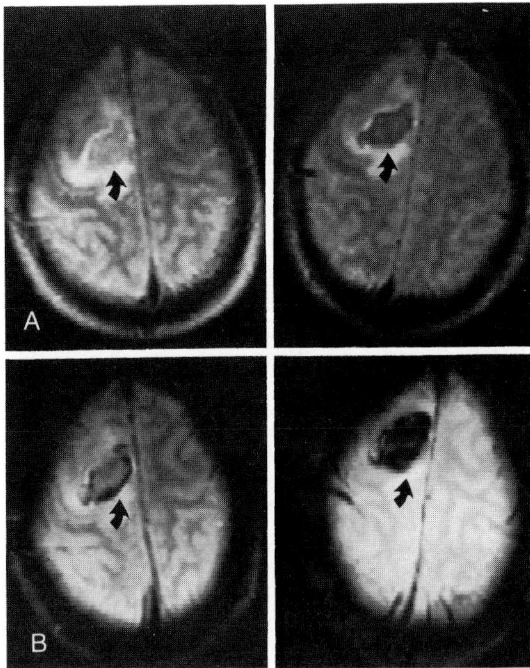


**Figure 13–2. Effect of field strength and gradient echo imaging on magnetic susceptibility (PT2PRE).** *A,* 0.5 T; *B,* 1.5 T. SE T2WI (TR 2500/TE 60), left; gradient echo (TR 430/TE 21, 35° flip angle), right. The hypointense ring, presumably caused by PT2PRE from hemosiderin, is not visible on routine SE imaging at 0.5 T but is appreciated at 1.5 T (*A* and *B,* left). Fast-field imaging at 0.5 T reveals a subtle hemosiderin ring, which becomes strikingly obvious at 1.5 T (*A* and *B,* right). T1WI (not shown) revealed an isointense clot center surrounded by a hyperintense ring of methemoglobin at both 0.5 T and 1.5 T.

Gradient echo sequences use no 180° refocusing echo. They are therefore much more dependent on T2* than on T2 relaxation and are far more sensitive than spin echoes to intravoxel phase shifts (magnetic susceptibility phenomenon). The T2* is inversely proportional to the local magnetic field gradient across the cell membrane, whereas the T2 (measured more by SE) is inversely related to $B_0^2$. Gradient echo imaging therefore helps to counteract the dependence on field strength for visualizing the PT2PRE present in many hematomas. As with spin-echo techniques, a long TE and a long TR produce an image that is T2 weighted, and thus is sensitive to the presence of PT2PRE. Although the TE and TR can be varied, a more effective method to produce either T1 or T2 weighting with gradient echo techniques is to change the tip angle. Large tip angles (e.g., ≥ 60°) produce more T1 weighting, while smaller tip angles (e.g., ≤ 25°) produce more T2 weighting.[36] Decreasing the tip angle results in decreased imaging time, and thus these sequences are commonly referred to as "fast-field" sequences. Fast-field imaging is extremely sensitive to the presence of paramagnetic substances (see Figs. 13–2 and 13–8).[36, 37, 64, 65] The disadvantage of this technique is worsened magnetic susceptibility artifacts and decreased SNR, which decreases as the tip angle is reduced. The lower SNR, however, is partially offset by decreased imaging time and decreased motion artifacts. The tip angle, TE, and TR vary with different imaging equipment, and trial and error unfortunately is necessary to arrive at optimal parameters.

Paramagnetic substances affect T1 and T2 relaxation times via PT2PRE and PEDDPRE and therefore contribute significantly to image contrast on MR. The types of hemoglobin degradation products and their concentration and distribution within intracranial hematomata are time dependent and are the basis for the distinct MR appearances of evolving intracranial blood. This appearance varies, depending upon the field strength and imaging parameters used. Although hematomas (usually) evolve in an orderly pathologic sequence, they do not adhere to strict time coordinates. Their appearance is modified by known physiologic factors such as pH, $PO_2$, temperature, the integrity of the blood-brain barrier, and probably by other factors as yet unknown.[293, 300] However, the vast majority of intracranial hematomas can be relatively accurately classified according to time of appearance. Out of necessity, for ease of discussion, the process of hematoma evolution has been somewhat arbitrarily classified.

## Hyperacute Intracranial Blood
### (Zero to several hours)

Immediately upon release from the intravascular compartment, extravascular blood approximates that of intravascular blood; it is still a solution, the concentration of formed elements (the hematocrit) is unchanged, and hemoglobin is oxygenated, containing predominately ferrous ($Fe^{2+}$) iron.

Because clotting has not occurred, "hyperacute" blood remains a solution and has a long T1 and a long T2 from bulk phase water. The long T1 and T2 are shortened by the addition of proteins and formed elements.[41–43] The unclotted blood is hypointense but of slightly higher signal than CSF on T1-weighted images (T1WI) and near CSF signal intensity on T2-weighted images (T2WI) (Figs. 13–3 and 13–4). Two reports of hyperacute intracranial blood, one of a patient who developed cerebral bleeding during an MR examination (0.15 T) and the second of surgically placed hematomas in monkeys (0.5 T), both demonstrated that hyperacute blood behaves as a proteinaceous solution.[22, 40]

## Acute Intracranial Blood
### (Several hours to three days)

Clot retraction and shift of the hemoglobin molecule from a predominantly oxygenated moiety to a predominantly deoxygenated one are the primary physiologic alterations responsible for the MR appearance of acute intracranial blood. Resorption of low-density serum results in an increase in the concentration of formed elements; the hematocrit may increase from an initially normal value of approximately 45 per cent to as high as 90 per cent in the clot center.[1–3]

As the red cells become hypoxic, hemoglobin becomes progressively deoxygenated. The central portion of the hematoma is the most hypoxic and contains the greatest concentration of deoxyhemoglobin. Early in the acute period, red cells are able to maintain cellular integrity, and the clot consists of intact red cells containing predominantly deoxygenated hemoglobin.[16, 50]

Early on, it was realized that altered magnetic susceptibility from blood made the MR appearance of some intracranial hematomas specific. However, the lack of image specificity of acute blood in studies performed at low field strength using IR or SE sequences in the face of a grossly positive CT was disappointingly common.[20, 24–28, 57]

With high-field imaging (≥ 1 T), acute intracranial blood has a distinctive appear-

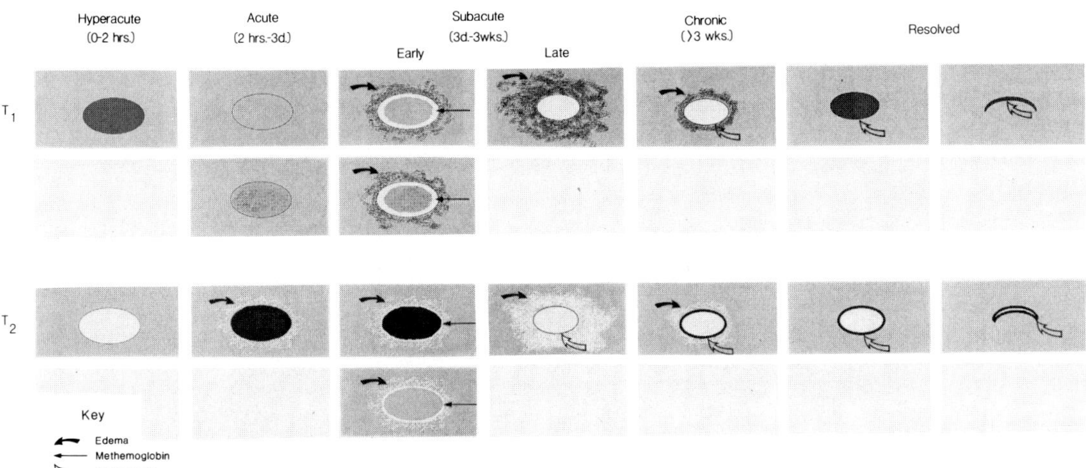


**Figure 13–3. Intracranial hematoma evolution at high field.** *Hyperacute hematoma:* Blood at this stage is unclotted. Still a solution, it has a long T1/T2. The signal is intermediate between CSF and brain on T1WI because the proteins and formed elements shorten the T1.

*Acute hematoma:* The clot has no PEDDPRE and is isointense on T1WI. Extracellular fluid and clot retraction may cause the clot center to appear mildly hypointense. The T2WI reveals the marked hypointensity of the PT2PRE of intracellular deoxyhemoglobin. Mild edema is more conspicuous on the T2WI (curved arrow).

*Early subacute hematoma:* The PEDDPRE of methemoglobin causes a well-developed margin of hyperintensity on T1WI (arrow). The hyperintense margin on T2WI (arrow) is due to the loss of PT2PRE, a result of red cell lysis. It is less developed because red cell lysis lags behind methemoglobin formation. The clot center remains either isointense or slightly hypointense on T1WI, and hypointense on T2WI as centripetally developing peripheral hyperintensity (short T1/long T2) engulfs the clot. Hematomas may also be isointense centrally on both T1WI and T2WI. Early edema formation is hypointense on T1 and hyperintense on T2 (curved black arrows).

*Late subacute hematoma:* The entire clot is hyperintense on T1WI and T2WI owing to the presence of a dilute methemoglobin solution. Early visualization of a hypointense hemosiderin ring (open curved arrow) can be appreciated by this time on T2WI. Edema is maximal 5 to 10 days post-ictus (curved black arrows).

*Chronic hematoma:* The clot becomes somewhat smaller; its methemoglobin-rich center is hyperintense on all sequences, surrounded by a well-formed hemosiderin ring (open curved arrow) that may be evident on the T1WI. Edema has diminished (curved black arrows).

*Resolved hematoma:* The methemoglobin has been resorbed. The underlying healed cavity has a high-bulk water content whose signal may approach that of CSF on T1 (curved arrow). The persisting hemosiderin margin on T2 (curved arrow) may represent the only evidence of prior hemorrhage. The cavity itself may remain relatively isovolumetric, or with resorption of its contents, the walls may fold upon themselves, creating a slitlike cavity.

ance. It is extremely hypointense on T2WI and isointense or hypointense on T1WI (Figs. 13–3 and 13–5). This selective hypointensity on T2WI, which is visible preferentially at high field strengths is an example of spin dephasing from a magnetic susceptibility effect (PT2PRE). Experimentally, PT2PRE results from both intracellular deoxyhemoglobin and intracellular methemoglobin (Table 13–1).[16, 60, 100, 296, 299] Pathologically, deoxyhemoglobin within intact red cells has been found within the center of acute clot; when the cells are lysed, the deoxyhemoglobin becomes free in solution, and the PT2PRE disappears.[16] Thus there is compelling evidence that the distinctive hypointensity of acute intracranial blood on T2WI at high field is due to intracellular deoxyhemoglobin and methemoglobin.

In contrast with the marked hypointensity on T2WI, acute intracranial blood is isointense (Figs. 13–3 and 13–6) or slightly hypointense on T1WI (Figs. 13–3 and 13–5). Since water protons cannot gain access to the unpaired electrons of iron in the aqueous oxyhemoglobin and deoxyhemoglobin molecules, no PEDDPRE occurs. The dense clot is therefore isointense on T1WI. Associated free water as well as extruded serum formed during clot retraction increases the bulk water, causing a long T1,[78] resulting in a mildly hypointense appearance. However, the bulk water causes a long T2 and increased proton density, counteracting the long T1, which may result in an isointense appearance as well.

Because PT2PRE is proportional to the field strength squared, the hypointensity on T2WI that is so characteristic of acute hematomas rapidly becomes less prominent as field strengths decrease. At low field strengths, using SE or IR imaging parameters, acute hematomas are usually isointense with brain on both T1WI and T2WI (Fig. 13–

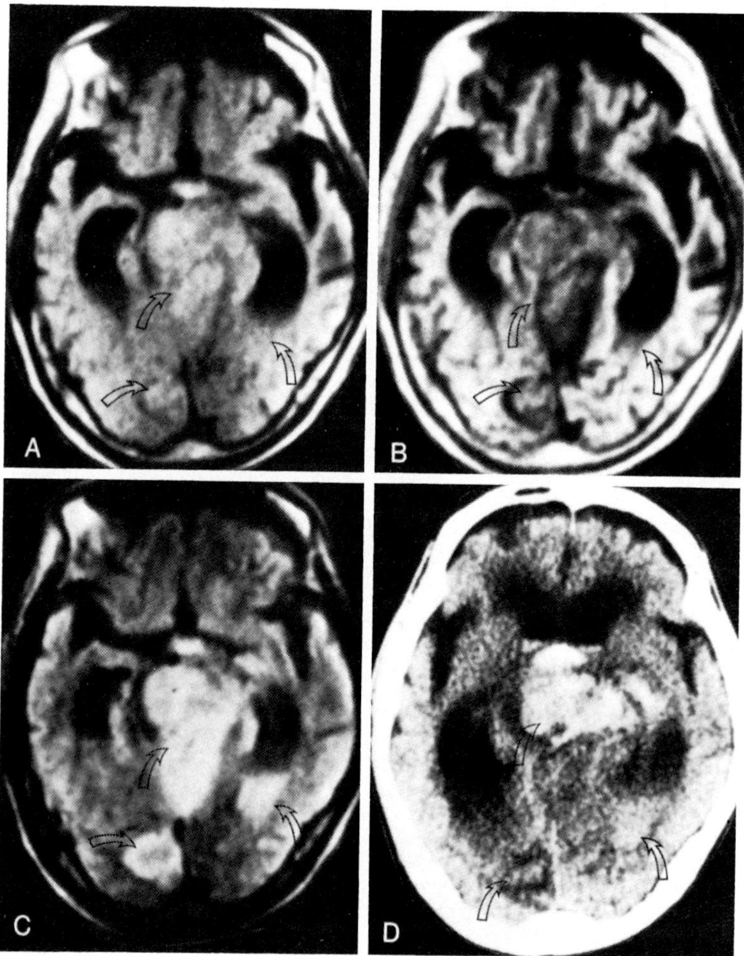


**Figure 13–4. Hyperacute hematoma.** A 78-year-old hypertensive woman who developed an intracerebral hemorrhage while the MR was in progress (0.15 T). *A,* Axial SE T1WI (TR 500/TE 40); *B,* IR T1WI (2000/50); *C,* SE T2WI (TR 2000/40); *D,* noncontrast CT. Abnormal signal in the brain stem, cerebellum, and lateral ventricle (arrows) is low-intermediate (curved arrows) on T1WI (*A* and *B*) and hyperintense (curved arrows) on T2WI *(C).* This nonspecific appearance is consistent with fluid that has a significant component of "bound water " and a high proton density, such as proteinaceous solution. A CT scan *(D)* performed after the MR confirms the presence of hemorrhage. (From Nose T. J Comput Assist Tomogr 11:184, 1987, with permission.)

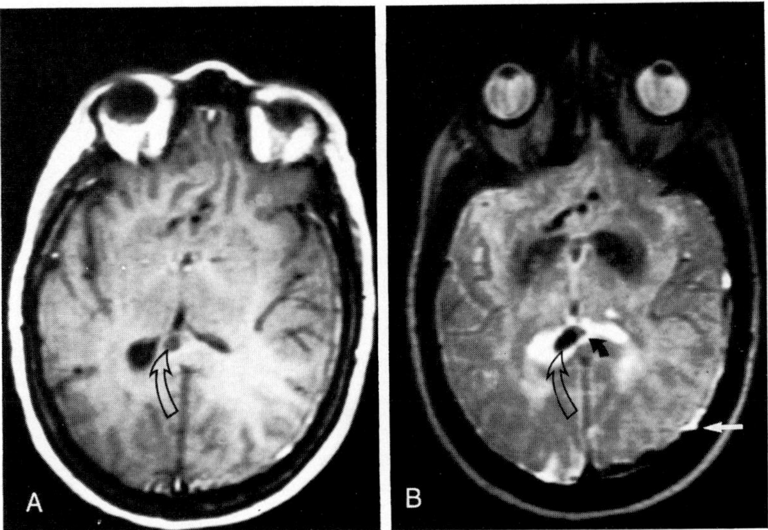


**Figure 13–5. Acute intracranial hematoma (1.5 T).** *A,* Axial SE T1WI (TR 800/TE 20), and *B,* T2WI (TR 2000/TE 80). The focus of abnormal signal in the splenium of the corpus callosum (curved open arrow) is mildly hypointense in *A* and markedly hypointense in *B.* The medial portion of the hematoma is isointense in *A,* but its hypointensity in *B* reveals the true lesion size. The long T2 of surrounding edema (small black arrow) merges with that of CSF in the adjacent ventricles *(B).* Incidentally noted is a "layered" subdural hematoma (white arrow). (Courtesy of Neuroradiology Department, University of Cincinnati, Cincinnati, Ohio.)

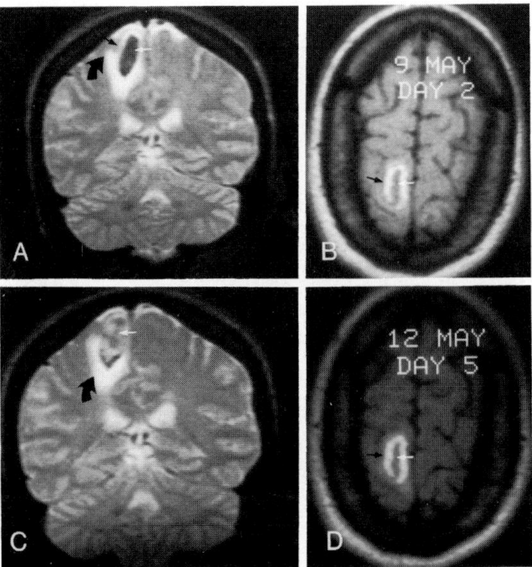


**Figure 13–6. Acute and early subacute hematoma (1.5 T).** *A,* SE T2WI (TR 1800/TE 80), and *B,* T1WI (TR 800/TE 20) day 2. *C,* SE T2WI (TR 1800/TE 80), and *D,* T1WI (TR 800/TE 20) day 5. The acute hematoma center (small white arrow) is hypointense in *A* and isointense in *B.* Peripheral methemoglobin (small black arrow) and the long T2 of surrounding edema (curved black arrow) are present. On day 5, the clot center (small white arrow) remains isointense on T1WI *D* but has become isointense on T2WI *C* as well. Again noted is methemoglobin formation (small black arrow) and edema (curved black arrow). (Courtesy of Neuroradiology Department, University of Cincinnati, Cincinnati, Ohio.)

7) and do not have diagnostically reliable signal characteristics.[20, 24–28, 57] Lengthening the TE with SE imaging or using gradient-echo imaging will increase the diagnostic specificity.

### Subacute Intracranial Blood (Three days to three weeks)

Subacute intracranial blood undergoes several physiologic processes: methemoglobin formation, red cell lysis, and hemosiderin formation. All the systems necessary for red cell survival are present at maturity after release from the bone marrow. Red cells have no nucleus and no mitochondria (no citric acid cycle); red blood cells depend upon glucose and anaerobic glycolysis for ATP production. Methemoglobin contains ferric ($Fe^{3+}$) iron, which is oxidized from ferrous ($Fe^{2+}$) iron in deoxyhemoglobin. Since ferric iron is unable to reversibly bind oxygen, elaborate enzymatic processes protect the cell from oxidants and continually fight the attrition of deoxyhemoglobin by reducing methemoglobin back to deoxyhemoglobin.[80] When red cells become extravascular, glucose supplies are interrupted, and methemoglobin formation is unchecked. With further diminution of ATP, the $Na^+$-

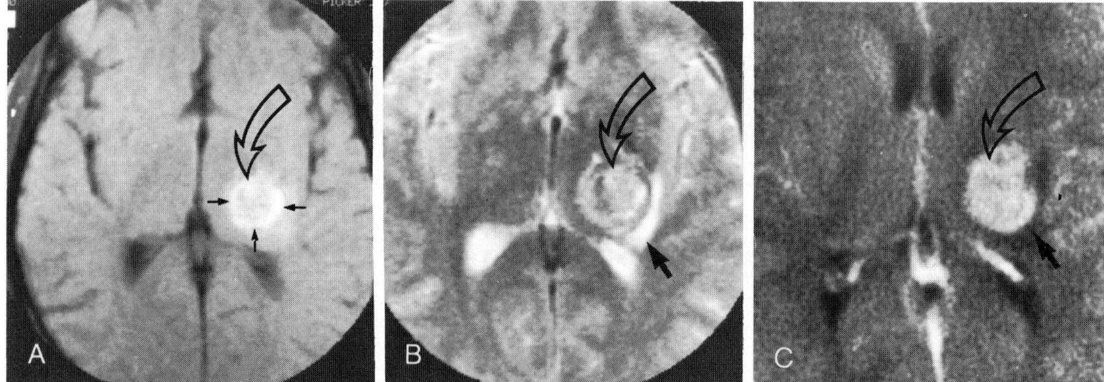


**Figure 13–7. Acute thalamic hematoma.** A 24-year-old patient with paresthesias of the right face and body (0.5 T). *A,* Axial SE T1WI (TR 850/TE 26), and *B,* T2WI (TR 2600/TE 120); *C,* CT *(contrast-enhanced).* The lesion center (curved arrow) is inhomogeneous but predominantly isointense, with gray matter on T1WI and T2WI. Early methemoglobin development (smallest black arrows) is best appreciated in *A.* Surrounding edema is noted (straight black arrow) in *B.* Conspicuously absent is the hypointensity on T2WI so typical of acute hematomas at high field. *C,* The acute intracerebral hematoma (curved arrow) and surrounding edema (black arrow) on CT are identical in distribution to that seen on MR. (Courtesy of Neuroradiology Department, University of Cincinnati, Cincinnati, Ohio.)

$K^+$ pump fails, and the red cells are no longer able to maintain membrane integrity; cell lysis begins. Red cell lysis results in liberation of intracellular hemoglobin degradation products into free solution. These events are responsible for the MR appearances of subacute intracranial blood.

Methemoglobin concentrations reach significant levels three to four days after hematoma formation.[20, 22, 46] Methemoglobin conversion begins at the periphery of the hematoma (Figs. 13–6 and 13–8), advancing centripetally into the center within two to three weeks (Fig. 13–9).[16, 20, 22] Because methemoglobin is formed by oxidation of deoxyhemoglobin and because deoxyhemoglobin is found predominantly in the hypoxic clot center, it should follow that methemoglobin would form preferentially in the central portion of the clot. How can these facts be

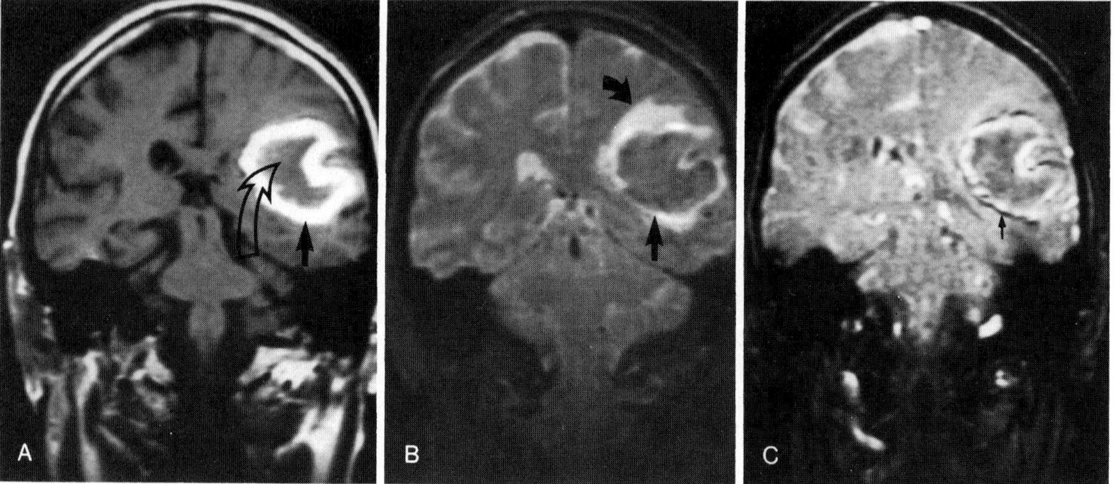


**Figure 13–8. Subacute hematoma (1.5 T).** *A,* Coronal SE T1WI (TR 800/TE 20), and *B,* T2WI (TR 2000/TE 80); *C,* coronal fast-field T2WI (gradient echo TR 21/TE 12, 12° flip angle).

The hematoma center (open curved arrow) is isointense on T1, T2, and fast-field scans. The short T1 from the PEDDPRE of methemoglobin (large straight black arrow) is best appreciated in *A,* owing to the lag in red cell lysis behind methemoglobin formation. Again demonstrated is the increased sensitivity of gradient-echo imaging to PT2PRE *(C).* The hemosiderin ring or susceptibility interface (smallest black arrow) seen in *C* is not of sufficient concentration to be visible by SE techniques, despite high field imaging *(B).* (Courtesy of Neuroradiology Department, University of Cincinnati, Cincinnati, Ohio.)

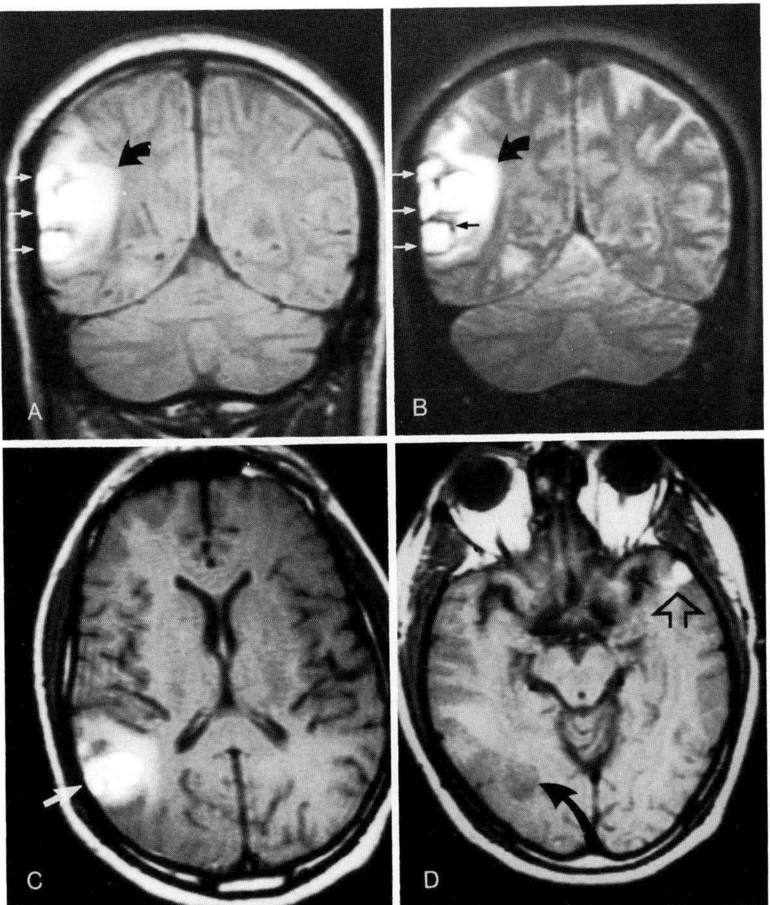


**Figure 13–9. Subacute contusion.** A 60-year-old patient with a seizure who had been struck in the right parietal region with a hammer 10 days earlier (1.5 T). *A* and *B,* Coronal SE N(H)WI and SE T2WI (TR 2000/TE 20/80). *C* and *D,* Axial SE T1WI (TR 800/TE 20). Multiple, well-defined regions of hyperintensity in the right parietal lobe (small white arrows), consistent with hemorrhagic contusions, are present on all sequences. Pericontusional edema (curved black arrow) and thin, hypointense, early hemosiderin rings are present (small black arrow). A contrecoup hematoma in the patient's left temporal tip (open black arrow) is present in *D.* Incidentally noted was a tentorially based mass (large curved black arrow) that was found to be calcified on CT (not shown) and was thought to represent a meningioma. (Courtesy of Neuroradiology Department, University of Cincinnati, Cincinnati, Ohio.)

reconciled? The rate of methemoglobin formation is in part dependent upon $PO_2$.[12–16] Although deoxyhemoglobin is plentiful at low oxygen tensions, the oxidizing substances necessary for the reaction may be in poor supply if $PO_2$ is too low; the conversion is most efficient at low to intermediate $PO_2$ (approximately 20 mm Hg).[13–15, 55] Thus optimal $PO_2$ for methemoglobin production may occur at the interface with brain parenchyma.[16] The PEDDPRE of methemoglobin shortens both T1 and T2 relaxation times, but in dilute solutions such as hematomas, the short T1 predominates.[62, 70, 79, 236]

Early in the subacute phase (three to five days), T1WIs demonstrate a thin, immature, peripheral ring of hyperintensity surrounding an isointense or mildly hypointense hematoma center. Hyperintensity results not only from the short T1 of PEDDPRE of methemoglobin but also from increased proton density and the long T2 of a dilute solution.[234] This is because short TR/TE images are relatively T1-weighted, and T2 relaxation times also contribute to image contrast. T2WIs reveal a similar-appearing peripheral ring of hyperintensity surrounding the clot center, which is hypointense from the PT2PRE of intracellular deoxyhemoglobin and methemoglobin (Figs. 13–3 and 13–6). The development of the high-signal rim on T2WIs (long T2) lags slightly behind the hyperintensity (short T1) which develops on the T1WI. As clot evolution proceeds, the centripetally advancing ring of hyperintensity (short T1/long T2) becomes thicker and more robust (Fig. 13–8), until by two to three weeks the entire clot is hyperintense on all sequences (Fig. 13–9). The lag in peripheral hyperintensity on T2WI is understandable since the processes responsible for the hyperintensity on T1WI (largely a short T1) are different from those that cause the hyperintensity (long T2) on T2WI.

Both intracellular and extracellular methemoglobin shorten T1 relaxation times via PEDDPRE.[100] Initially, methemoglobin is intracellular; as ATP supplies wane, cellular integrity is maintained at all costs, allowing methemoglobin conversion to take place before cell lysis. With red cell lysis, methemoglobin becomes extracellular, and continues to shorten T1 relaxation times. In contrast, on T2WI, prior to red cell lysis, PT2PRE from intracellular deoxyhemoglobin and intracellular methemoglobin causes a very short T2. Therefore, although methemoglobin formation causes peripheral hyperintensity on T1WIs, the clot, including the periphery, remains hypointense on T2WI. With subsequent red cell lysis, the magnetic susceptibility from intracellular deoxyhemoglobin and methemoglobin disappears. In addition to the loss of the PT2PRE of intracellular hemoglobin products, cell lysis results in a dilute solution with significant bulk-phase water. The dominant long T2 of bulk-phase water overrides the negligible T2 shortening from the PEDDPRE of dilute methemoglobin. Thus the appearance of the peripheral high signal on T2WIs generally lags behind that on T1WIs because red cell lysis lags behind methemoglobin formation. Within two to three weeks, though, the entire hematoma is hyperintense on all sequences.

Hemosiderin formation occurs as early as eight days experimentally and has been observed on MR as early as ten days (Fig. 13–9).[50] Late in the subacute phase, the hematoma margin becomes markedly hypointense as a result of the PT2PRE of hemosiderin deposition (see Figs. 13–3 and 13–9).

We have noted several hemorrhagic lesions that have isointense centers on all sequences, including the T2WI (see Figs. 13–6 and 13–8). An underlying pathologic substrate such as a tumor was thought to be present, but surgically proved cases showed only intracranial clot. Figure 13–6 shows the evolution of a clot center that acutely demonstrates a short T2 from magnetic susceptibility of intracellular hemoglobin products, which then become isointense. This is a relatively common phenomenon, and its cause is unsubstantiated. If central red cell lysis occurs during methemoglobin formation instead of lagging behind, the long T2 of bulk water, the increased proton density, and the loss of the PT2PRE of intracellular hemoglobin products that occur with cell lysis, could theoretically negate enough of the short T2 of intact red cells to create an isointense lesion. Indeed, cell lysis occurring predominantly in the clot center has been observed.[50] This appearance has great clinical import, because a hemorrhagic lesion with an isointense center may represent an underlying tumor (Fig. 13–10). However, it is also compatible with a "simple" hemorrhage without underlying pathologic substrate, such as a neoplasm or vascular lesion. The hemorrhagic neoplasms we have seen have either been hyperintense on T2WI or when isointense, they have not been surrounded by a complete methemoglobin rim. That is, the neoplasms tend to bleed nonuniformly (Fig. 13–10).

In summary, at about three to four days on T1WI, intracranial hematomas demonstrate a peripheral thin rim of hyperintensity surrounding an isointense or slightly hypointense center. T2WIs demonstrate a slightly delayed hyperintense rim around a hypointense clot center. By two to three weeks, the entire hematoma is usually hyperintense on all sequences. Hematoma centers may be isointense on both T1WI and T2WI; this appearance does not necessarily indicate the presence of an underlying lesion. The hyperintensity of subacute hematomas is present at all clinically useful field strengths.

### Chronic Intracranial Blood (Over three weeks)

By three weeks, the effects of hematoma resolution become evident. Initially, the clot contains a methemoglobin solution mixed with cellular debris surrounded by an immature hemosiderin ring. Pathologic examination of hematoma cavities at this stage reveals a gelatinous, dark brown material containing large amounts of methemo-

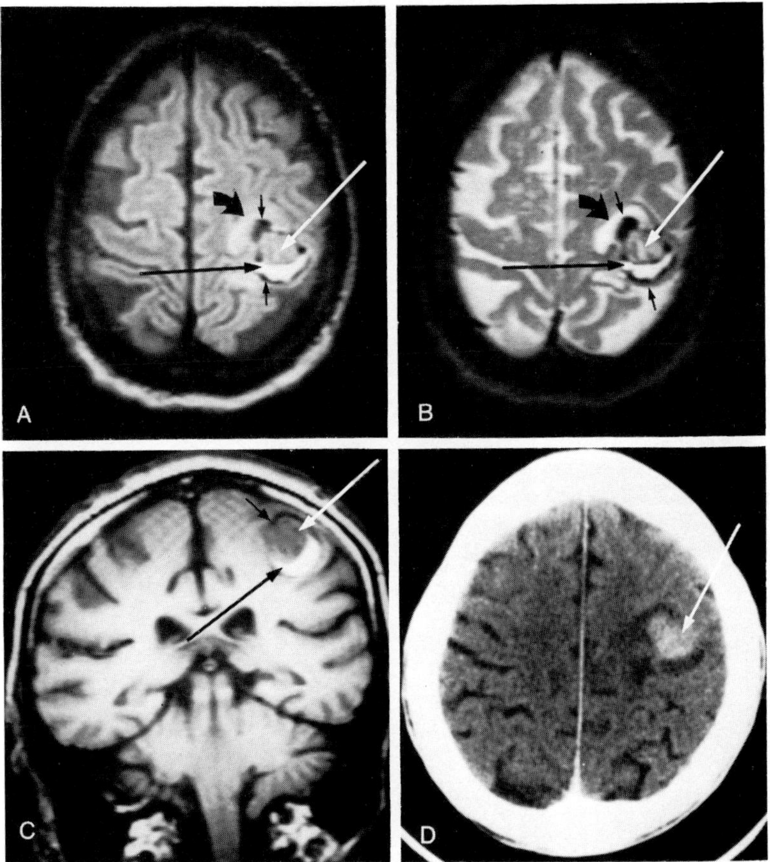


**Figure 13–10. Metastasis with hemorrhage.** A 68-year-old patient with seizures, left-sided weakness, and metastatic adenocarcinoma of the lung (1.5 T). *A* and *B*, Axial SE N(H)WI and T2WI (TR 2000/TE 20/80). *C*, Coronal SE T1WI (TR 500/TE 20). *D*, CT, contrast-enhanced (GE 9800). The metastatic lesion (long white arrows) is isointense on all sequences. It is surrounded by an *incomplete*, irregular ring of hemosiderin (small straight black arrows) and methemoglobin (long black arrows). CT demonstrates the enhancing lesion. Although this lesion is isointense on all sequences, a hematoma (without pathologic substrate) may also be isointense on all sequences (see Figs. 13–6 and 13–8). While differentiation may not always be possible, the incompletely surrounding methemoglobin and hemosiderin suggest the likelihood of an underlying lesion. (Courtesy of Neuroradiology Department, University of Cincinnati, Cincinnati, Ohio.)

globin[67,82] that may persist for years.[16] The length of time that methemoglobin can remain visible on MRI is unknown. Hemosiderin deposition continues to progress as hemoglobin breakdown products are phagocytized by macrophages and converted to hemosiderin. The hemosiderin deposition in the clot periphery may persist for the life of the patient, serving as evidence of previous bleeding.[67,80] The hemosiderin lining is of variable thickness, generally thicker when bleeding is more copious and the pigment burden higher.

High-field MR reveals a hyperintense region of variable size on both T1WI and T2WI (short T1/long T2), surrounded by a prominent hypointense ring on T2WIs (Figs. 13–3 and 13–10). This ring has been attributed to the presence of hemosiderin for several reasons: (1) The location and size of the hypointense ring corresponds to the location and size of hemosiderin deposition identified pathologically.[16,82] (2) Hemosiderin is a large, insoluble molecule containing ferric ($Fe^{3+}$) iron, which causes spin dephasing (PT2PRE) on MR in other organs and disease states, such as in the liver with hemosiderosis.[69,73] (3) The hypointense ring is most prominent on T2WIs and is most noticeable at high field and with gradient echo imaging consistent with PT2PRE.

Continued healing causes gradual resorption of methemoglobin with loss of its PEDDPRE and therefore, gradual loss of its short T1 contribution. The T2 remains long, however, because it is due to the large pro-

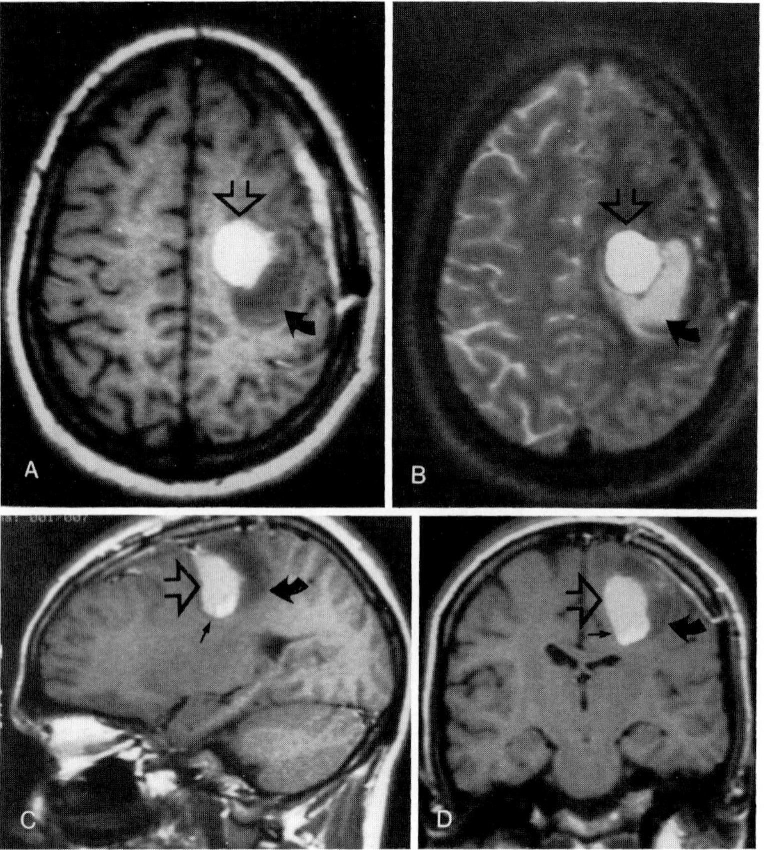


**Figure 13–11. Acute postoperative hematoma.** An 18-year-old patient one day after removal of a low-grade glioma (1.5 T). *A,* Axial SE T1WI (TR 600/TE 20), and *B,* SE T2WI (TR 2000/TE 80). *C* and *D,* Sagittal and coronal SE T1WI (TR 600/TE 20). The postoperative bed contains a well-defined region of hyperintensity on both T1WI and T2WI (open arrow) that is surrounded by the long T1/T2 of edema (curved arrow). A hyperintense supernatant above relatively more hyperintense material in the dependent portion of the hematoma (small arrow) is present (*C* and *D*). (Courtesy of Neuroradiology Department, Children's Hospital Medical Center, Cincinnati, Ohio.)

portion of bulk water in a dilute solution and has little to do with the presence of methemoglobin. Loss of the slight T2 shortening from PEDDPRE will further (minimally) lengthen T2 relaxation times. Thus on T1WI, the signal decreases from hyperintense to intermediate intensity, depending upon the relative proportion of remaining methemoglobin and encephalomalacic brain. If methemoglobin resorption is complete, no residual short T1 contribution will remain. In such cases, the long T1/T2 of encephalomalacia will remain lined with the hypointense hemosiderin ring. This ring identifies the area as an old hemorrhage, enabling a more specific diagnosis of an otherwise nonspecific region of encephalomalacia. Because the magnitude of PT2PRE is proportional to the concentration of paramagnetic foci and the strength of $B_0^2$, high-field MR is extremely sensitive to the presence of even small amounts of hemosiderin. If the hemorrhage was diminutive, only a small amount of hemosiderin will remain in the region of previous bleeding, and a tiny focus of low signal on T2WIs, caused by the spin dephasing from residual hemosiderin, may be the only MR evidence of pathology.

At low field strength, methemoglobin is easily visualized as a region of short T1/long T2 equally well and perhaps better than at high field. If sufficient methemoglobin remains, the hematoma will be hyperintense on all SE sequences. The reliable visualization of methemoglobin at low field strength imaging is in contrast to that of hemosiderin. At low or intermediate field strength, the hemosiderin ring is not reliably identified with SE sequences since the PT2PRE is proportional to the square of the field strength. If there has been complete resorption of all methemoglobin leaving only hemosiderin, no signal abnormalities may be detected, and old blood may not be identified. Again, lengthening the TE or using more sensitive imaging sequences such as gradient echo sequences is helpful.

### Postoperative Hematomas

Although the majority of cases of intracranial and extracranial blood evolve in a manner consistent with the above model, others may follow a somewhat different time course.[82] Acute postoperative intracranial blood is hyperintense (short T1/long T2) on T1WI and T2WI (Fig. 13–11). This is different from the appearance of acute "closed" intracranial hematomas. The short T1/long T2 suggests there has been extensive, precocious methemoglobin conversion and cell lysis, because no PT2PRE is identified. The reasons for this are unproved, but exposure to room air, saline solutions, and direct mechanical trauma subject the red cell to an environment far different from that of a "closed" hematoma. Although hematoma evolution at high-field imaging has been elegantly studied and described,[16, 100] this model does not fully explain all MR appearances. Further investigation into the nature and evolution of aging blood and its MR appearance is needed.

## INTRACRANIAL TRAUMA

Trauma is the number one cause of death between the ages of 1 and 44 and the fourth most common cause of death in the U.S. Head injuries occur most frequently in young adults ages 15–24, and they occur twice as frequently in men. There were 7,560,000 head injuries in 1976 with 1,255,000 classified as "major" head injuries including concussion, contusion, intracranial hemorrhage, cerebral laceration, and crushing injuries. Head injury is responsible for 200–300 hospital admissions per 100,000 population. Because of the young age at which most head trauma occurs, long-term morbidity is of tremendous import. Multiple injuries are common in head injury patients. Associated spine injury (usually cervical) is common and in large series has been reported to occur in 5–17 per cent of fatal head injury patients.[89–92]

### Biomechanics of Closed Head Injury

The biomechanics of head injury are complex and incompletely understood. Two essential types of closed head trauma occur, (1) stationary and (2) moving head injuries, and they produce intracranial damage through three basic forces: compression, shearing, and tensile forces.

Compression is a positive force perpendicularly applied to the brain surface and occurs when the brain impacts with firm, unyielding portions of the skull and dura. The brain is a soft, viscoelastic structure with a high water content, and although it is relatively insensitive to uniform compression, it is exquisitely sensitive to the distortion associated with nonuniform compression.[97–99, 120]

The soft, viscoelastic structure of the brain is also exquisitely sensitive to the distortion from shearing forces.[101] Shearing forces are those applied parallel to the brain surface. They are generated by the inertia from brain movement within the skull during translation (linear movement) and rotation (angular movement) of the head. During acceleration/deceleration experiments, swirling movement of the brain within the cranium has been directly observed.[102]

Tensile forces are negative forces perpendicularly applied to the brain's surface. Although they play a role in head trauma, their importance in the creation of traumatic brain injury is controversial.[93–97]

In this oversimplified working model, closed head trauma can be viewed as a continuum, with pure compression (stationary head injury) at one end and pure inertial trauma at the other. Trauma with a very large inertial component results in shearing injuries. Most closed head trauma lies between these extremes and involves both impact and inertial trauma, producing both compressive and shearing forces that act in concert to produce intracranial pathology.[97, 101, 103] The intracranial pathology produced during blunt head trauma includes focal brain injury (hemorrhagic and nonhemorrhagic contusions, and hematomas) and extracerebral, intracranial fluid collections.

### Focal Cerebral Injury

Focal cerebral injury is an extremely common traumatic intracranial lesion in adults, occurring in as many as 13 per cent to 43 per cent of patients.[10, 19, 297] Multiple parenchymal lesions are common and have been reported in as many as 29 per cent of patients and are associated with extracerebral hematomata in as many as 39 per cent.[10] Lesion location depends upon the mechanism of injury.

Pure compression injuries classically result from a blow to the stationary head; the site of pathology is determined by the site of impact. Cerebral lesions are caused by skull deformation, either bending or fracture, and typically occur in the subjacent cerebral cortex. These are termed *coup* lesions.[101] In contrast, injury on the side opposite the impact force is the rule when significant inertial injury occurs. These are termed *contrecoup* lesions. Contrecoup lesions occur in idiosyncratic locations virtually independent of the specific circumstance of the injury.

Rapid acceleration or deceleration of the head from translation, rotation, or both causes differential inertia between the brain and the cranium. Asynchronous movement results in brain lag with compression of the trailing edge against the skull.[104, 105] Brain movement within the cranium is somewhat analogous to the inertia of passengers within a rapidly decelerating car who are slammed forward. Traumatic cerebral lesions occur at contact points between the brain and the skull's bony ridges and protuberances because compression is more nonuniform and distorting in these locations. The frontal poles impinge upon the rough inner surface of the anterior fossa, and the temporal lobes upon the protuberances of the sphenoid wings. Contrecoup injuries therefore occur most often in the frontal lobes, the "temporal tips," and the lateral temporal lobes, usually the superior or inferior temporal gyri.[19, 110, 111, 297] The uniform surface of the occipital bone and the brain's structural resilience to uniform compression correlate with the relative infrequence of occipital polar injury. As most closed head trauma involves significant head movement, the preponderance of traumatic lesions encountered are contrecoup and are located in the frontal and temporal lobes.

Focal brain injury is a concatenation of pathology that includes variable amounts of neuronal injury, necrosis, ischemia, edema (both cytotoxic and vasogenic), and hemorrhage.[108] Traumatic damage causes cell injury and death and microvascular disruption. Resultant local mass effect causes small vessel compression, local ischemia, and interruption of supplies of vital metabolites. Resulting acidosis and vascular spasm lead to more cell destruction, edema, and further vascular compromise, leading to more neuronal loss.[23, 143] Vascular damage and loss of cerebral blood flow autoregulation result in a variably sized hemorrhagic component.[145]

Although there may be no grossly identifiable hemorrhage, lesions often contain microscopic bleeding. When the degree of bleeding is below the sensitivity of CT or when the high attenuation of hemorrhagic petechial foci mix with low-density edema, causing "isodense" mass effect, "nonhemorrhagic" lesions result. These lesions are often missed on CT.[12, 297, 298] With increasing hemorrhage, the term hemorrhagic contusion may be used. More extensive bleeding and coalescent hemorrhages may be referred to as hematoma.[5, 109] Although the terms *contusion* and *hematoma* are commonly used to describe traumatic brain injury, these lesions really represent varying grades of injury and distinction is difficult but often not clinically important. The hemorrhagic component of both contusions and hematomas is due to rupture of small, oozing parenchymal vessels; rarely is a single, large bleeding source identified.[109] To further complicate matters, contusions may evolve into hematomas.[145–147] The original contusion may not be apparent on the initial CT. These "delayed" hematomas are reported to occur in 3.2 per cent to 8 per cent of head injury patients.[146, 150] Nearly 50 per cent arise after surgical decompression of other traumatic space-occupying lesions, while the rest occur spontaneously, usually within the first 48 hours.[145–147, 150]

### *MR Appearance*

Focal brain injury typically begins in the cortex and extends in a perpendicular fashion into deeper brain substance (see Fig. 3–9). A contusion index has been devised to quantitate the depth and extent of injury.[110] Traumatic lesions may be single or multiple. They are usually round or ovoid and often blend imperceptibly with surrounding edema, causing a poorly defined appearance associated with mass effect.[19] MR is more sensitive than CT in identifying both hemorrhagic and nonhemorrhagic injury.[12, 297, 298]

### *Hyperacute Intracranial Injury*
**(Zero to several hours)**

Hyperacute lesions are those visualized within hours of the traumatic event, while the extravascular blood is still a solution, before significant clot retraction occurs. Hyperacute blood behaves as a protein solution with an intermediately long T1 and T2. The nonhemorrhagic components, cell death and necrosis, surrounding ischemia, and edema, all cause a pathologic increase in bulk water content, resulting in a long T1/T2. At this early stage, the signal characteristics of hyperacute blood are similar to those of the necrosis, ischemia, and surrounding edema and cannot be separated. Hyperacute cerebral injury thus appears as a relatively hypointense region, intermediate between CSF and brain parenchyma on T1WI, whereas on T2WI the region is hyperintense but slightly lower in signal than CSF. The hemorrhagic nature and actual lesion size cannot be defined during the hyperacute stage with current routine imaging techniques. Further delineation can be accomplished by rescanning later in the course of hematoma evolution or by obtaining CT confirmation.

### *Acute Intracranial Injury*
**(Several hours to three days)**

This phase begins with clot retraction. The development of a high-density center and surrounding extracted serum brings an end to the signal characteristics of the hyperacute hemorrhagic solution. The characteristic CT appearance of a high-attenuation center surrounded by low-attenuation vasogenic and cytotoxic edema and extracted serum from clot retraction has its direct counterpart on MRI.[1–3, 17–19, 50] High-field MR reveals a round or oval isointense or slightly hypointense hematoma on T1WI that becomes markedly hypointense on T2WI (Figs. 13–3 and 13–5). Increased bulk water in the surrounding brain causes a variably sized region of long T1 and long T2. Brain edema begins within hours but is generally mild acutely. When edema is slight, it may only be conspicuous on the T2WI (Fig. 13–5).

The marked hypointensity of acute intracranial blood at high field may not always occur in the geometric center of a clot. Layering from a hematocrit effect with higher density elements layering below the less dense supernatant is not uncommon.[4, 293] On CT the dependent high-density layer is higher in attenuation, whereas the supernatant is of lower attenuation. The MR appearance is essentially opposite. The formed elements and red cells containing deoxyhemoglobin separate from the serum, creating a dependent layer that is isointense or slightly hypointense on T1WI and is markedly hypointense on T2WI. The supernatant, largely a proteinaceous fluid, is hypointense or intermediate on T1WI and hyperintense on T2WI.

### *Subacute Brain Injury*
**(Three days to three weeks)**

Early in the subacute period (approximately three to five days), the lesion center is isointense or slightly hypointense on T1WI and extremely hypointense on T2WI. Peripheral methemoglobin formation causes a hyperintense ring that occurs first on T1WI and later on T2WI (see Figs. 13–6 and 13–8). Later in the subacute phase, methemoglobin formation advances centripetally, causing the lesion to appear totally hyperintense on both T1WI and T2WI (see Fig. 13–9). In addition to this classic appearance, we have observed another common appearance of early subacute injury. While peripheral methemoglobin formation is occurring, the hypointense center on T2WI may become isointense before becoming hyperintense (see Figs. 13–6 and 13–8). The reason for this has not been proved but likely is due to concurrent methemoglobin production and erythrocyte lysis within the clot center.

In addition to the changes of the contusion itself, the surrounding cerebral parenchyma undergoes changes of its own. The parenchyma contributes signal changes from edema, hemosiderin formation, and cerebritis. Edema, which began in the acute phase, becomes maximal during the subacute phase, generally between the third and seventh days post ictus. It generally takes two to three weeks before edema begins to diminish. Resolution of edema is related to lesion size; with large hematomas, edema may take four weeks or more to resolve.[19, 50, 149]

An inflammatory process (cerebritis) appears at the hematoma periphery beginning at about three to four days and is characterized by the presence of inflammatory cells

(PMNs), tissue macrophages, microglial cells, fibroblasts, vascular proliferation, and capsule formation.[50, 79, 81] The hematoma margin is often hypointense on both T1WI and T2WI. This has been attributed to the presence of both the fibrous capsule and hemosiderin. The expanding population of macrophages at the hematoma periphery ingests cellular debris, including red cells, and forms hemosiderin from the phagocytized methemoglobin.[66, 67] The hemosiderin ring is markedly hypointense at high field and with gradient echo imaging on T2WI but may be identified on T1WI if enough hemosiderin is present owing to some T2 contribution to the relatively T1-weighted image (see Fig. 13–12). We have seen hemosiderin rings as early as ten days post ictus. Larger hematomas with increased pigment burdens result in larger and thicker hemosiderin rings.[16, 50] The hypointense hemosiderin ring may not be conspicuous at lower field strengths because its magnetic susceptibility (PT2PRE) is proportional to the field strength squared.

### *Chronic Brain Injury* (Over three weeks)

Healing of the surrounding cerebral parenchyma results in re-establishment of autoregulation and further organization of the capsule. The permeable neovascularity of the capsule gradually diminishes, and by four to eight weeks, vascular integrity is generally restored. This correlates with diminished capsular enhancement on CT. On MR restored vascular integrity results in resolving edema, and by six to eight weeks, essentially no discernible edema remains.

Although there is gradual attrition of edema, organization of the injured brain results in increasing hemosiderin formation. The hypointensity of the hemosiderin-containing capsule at the periphery of the traumatized brain has been observed several years post ictus; it may possibly remain indefinitely.[16, 143] This low signal is usually not the smooth rim often schematically depicted, but more often is an irregular peripheral margin, more extensive and heaped in one portion than in another (see Fig. 13–12). Within this hemosiderin-laden capsule, the hematoma has a variable appearance.

Early in the chronic stage, the hematoma becomes smaller and contains a xanthochromic, methemoglobin-rich, proteinaceous fluid. MR reveals a hyperintense region on all sequences (see Fig. 13–12). With increasing resolution, the old blood products are gradually resorbed, leaving a proteinaceous fluid. The hyperintensity on T1WI and T2WI becomes hypointense to intermediate in signal on T1WI and intermediate to hyperintense on T2WI; the clot does not yet behave like CSF because residual protein and debris shorten the T1 and T2 in proportion to their concentration. The MR signal of blood at this stage is similar to that of a hyperacute hematoma because both essentially behave as protein solutions. Unlike

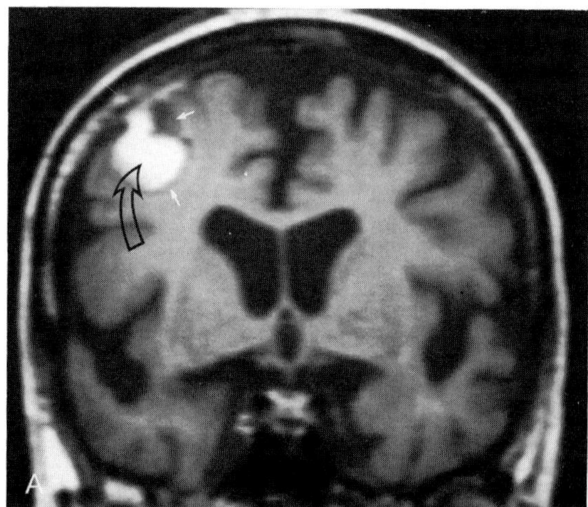


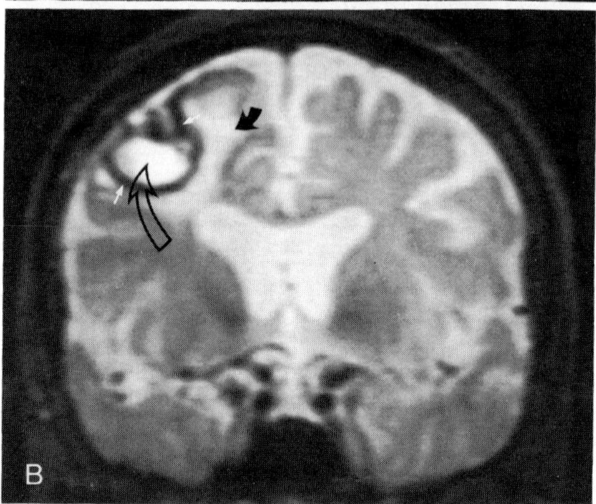


**Figure 13–12. Chronic intracerebral hematoma (1.5 T).** *A*, Coronal SE T1WI (TR 800/TE 20), and *B*, T2WI (TR 2000/TE 80). The hyperintense clot on both images is consistent with the presence of methemoglobin (open curved arrow). The thick, irregular hypointense hemosiderin rim (small white arrows) is prominent on T2WI and also visible on T1WI. White matter edema seen in *B* (black curved arrow) is not conspicuous on T1WI, a not uncommon phenomenon when the degree of edema is mild. (Courtesy of Neuroradiology Department, University of Cincinnati, Cincinnati, Ohio.)

the hyperacute hematoma, however, the conspicuous hemosiderin ring is present in the chronic stage. With further resorption of methemoglobin, protein, and cellular debris, the cavity may contain fluid similar in composition and signal characteristics to CSF, surrounded by a hemosiderin ring on T2WI.

Just as the contents of the cavity vary with the degree of resolution, so too does the shape of the cavity. It may persist as a round or ovoid region or with more complete resorption of contents, may collapse to a slit-like cavity of variable size (see Figs. 13–3 and 13–13). If the clot was initially small, the only clue to its presence may be a punctate region of hypointensity from hemosiderin deposition. Occasionally, the hematoma may rupture into the ventricular system;[148] its contents then evacuate into the ventricle, and the hematoma cavity eventually fills with CSF. This is called a porencephalic cyst. It appears as a variably shaped region of long T1/T2 circumscribed by a hemosiderin ring (see Fig. 13–14). Demonstration of the communication with the ventricle often necessitates careful multiplanar imaging.

It is often clinically desirable to distinguish edema from gliotic brain. However, both have a long T1 and a long T2, and reliable differentiation is not usually possible by signal characteristics alone. The cerebral parenchyma juxtaposed to the contusion reveals local volume loss corresponding to the degree of local tissue destruction. The absence of mass effect and evidence of loss of brain substance, when present, suggest gliosis as the etiology of the abnormal signal. Diffuse atrophy manifested by ventricular expansion and extraventricular CSF space enlargement may be seen when the focal brain injury is part of diffuse, traumatic tissue.[19, 150]

## Shearing Injury (Diffuse Axonal Injury)

Closed head trauma with a significant inertial component may produce differential inertia at interfaces of differing density or fixation with resultant shearing injury at these sites. The gray-white matter junction is a prime example of just such an interface, where differing density and differential fixation among axons, cell bodies, and vessels result in differential inertia, causing distortion of the brain with tearing of axons and vessels.[95, 97–100, 106, 107] Lesions at gray-white interfaces have been consistently produced in nonimpact, acceleration/deceleration experiments.[114, 123–125] The clinical hallmark of diffuse axonal injury is loss of consciousness. Concussion is the prima facie example

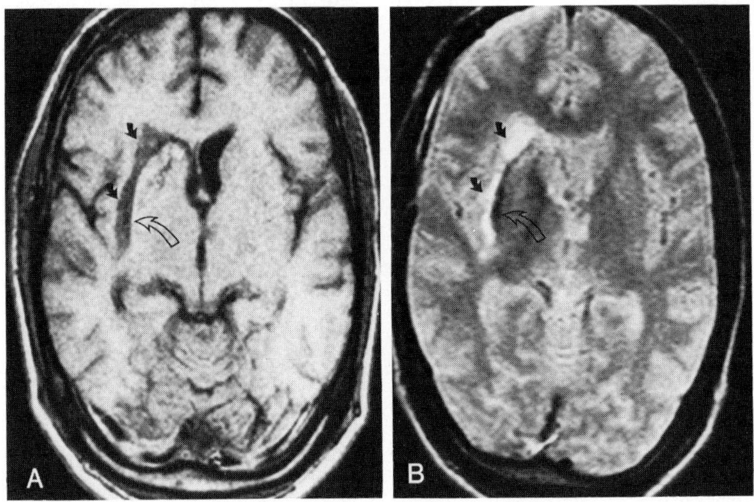


**Figure 13–13. Chronic hematoma (1.5 T).** *A,* Axial SE T1WI (TR 470/TE30) and *B,* axial SE T2WI (TR 2000/TE 80) show a crescentic-shaped region of abnormal signal in the head of the right caudate nucleus and extending along the external capsule. The lateralmost portion (dark arrows) has a long T1/T2 compatible with encephalomacic brain or edema. The medial portion (curved arrow) is isointense in *A* and hypointense in *B* from hemosiderin deposition, indicating previous hemorrhage.

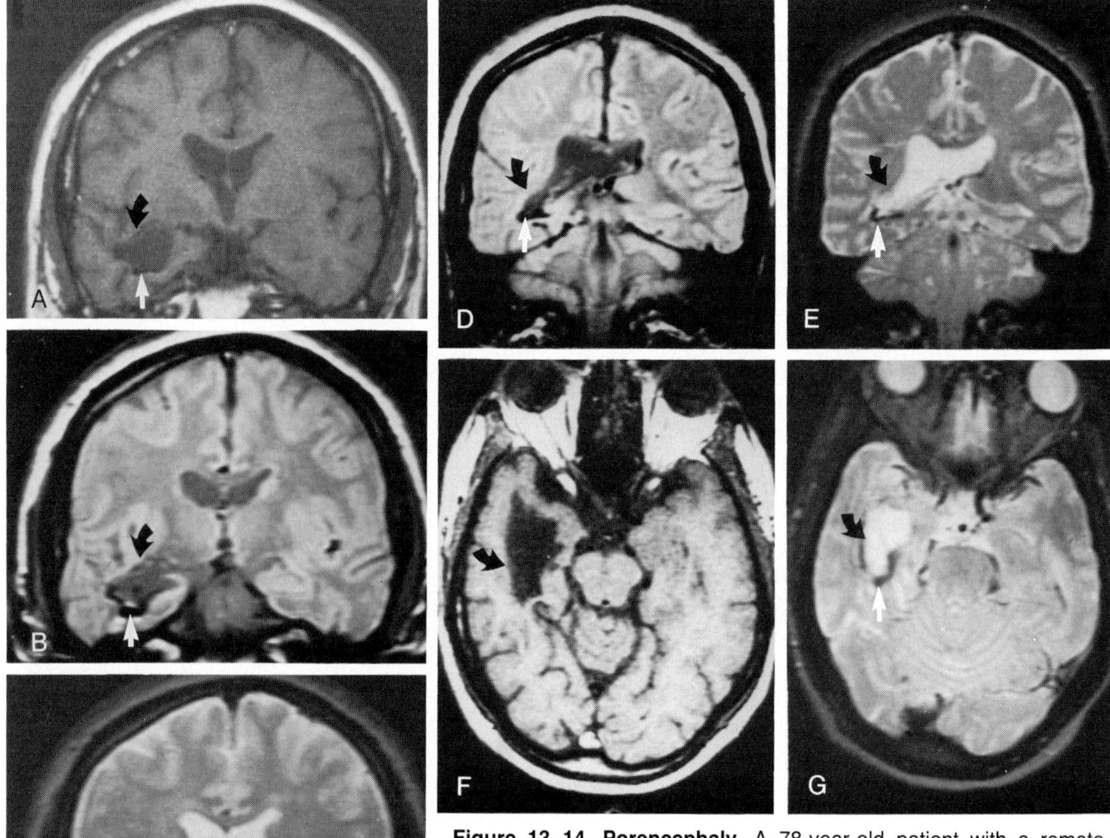


**Figure 13–14. Porencephaly.** A 78-year-old patient with a remote hemorrhage from meningovascular syphilis (1.5 T). *A,* Coronal SE T1WI (TR 600/TE 20); *B* and *C*, Coronal N(H)WI and T2WI (TR 2000/TE 20/80). *D* and *E*, Coronal SE N(H)WI and T2WI (TR 2000/TE 20/80). *F,* Axial SE T1WI. *G,* Axial SE T2WI (TR 2000/TE 80). The abnormal region of CSF signal characteristics (curved black arrow) is surrounded by a hemosiderin ring (small white arrow), that, although subtly visible on T1WI, becomes prominent with increased T2 weighting. Coronal images show the cavity communicates with the ventricle, indicating porencephaly. CT (not shown) revealed a nonspecific area of low attenuation, whereas a comparable MR slice *(G)* demonstrates hemosiderin, indicating its posthemorrhagic nature. (Courtesy of Neuroradiology Department, University of Cincinnati, Cincinnati, Ohio.)

of a shearing injury. Pure shearing injuries generally produce nonlocalized, diffuse neurological deficits.[118] The degree of injury is in large part related to the magnitude of force, and patient presentation varies accordingly, from mild confusion with little or no retrograde amnesia and complete recovery to irreversible brain injury, persistent vegetative state, and death. The literature has popularized the severe end of the spectrum of this type of injury, but less severe injuries are common and may produce clinically important symptoms and sequelae.[6, 11, 113, 119–122, 140] Axonal and synaptic disruption from "minor" head trauma is clinically important, especially in contact sports in which minor head trauma occurs and, in fact, may be the objective. Axonal degeneration has been documented after single concussive injuries in which unconsciousness lasted less than 5 minutes.[141] Abnormal brain stem–evoked potentials, ultrastructural changes, and axonal degeneration have all been demonstrated after "minor" head injury.[125–132] Long-term clinical sequelae such as personality changes, memory deficits, and language and cognitive impairment may develop even after a single concussive episode.[133–136, 142] At the other end of the spectrum, patients with classic, very severe shearing injuries are immediately comatose, and the prognosis is grave; severe disability, persistent vegetative state, or death is the usual outcome.

### MR Appearance

With "minor" injury, shearing lesions are usually limited to the gray-white interfaces.[114] These lesions are typically small and round or ovoid. When ovoid, they tend to be parallel to the direction of white matter tracts.[297, 298] More severe shearing injury may result in lesions of the deep white matter, corpus callosum, and brain stem.[11, 29, 99, 115–117, 138, 139, 297, 298] The pathologic hallmark is axonal disruption. Microscopic manifestations are time dependent. Early changes include "retraction balls" representing extruded axoplasm from the torn axon cylinders. "Microglial stars" appear subacutely and consist of reactive microglial cells around the torn axon cylinders. Chronically, cell death and gliosis are identified. Most lesions are nonhemorrhagic and are associated with increased brain water; therefore they have a long T1 and a long T2. The majority of lesions are microscopic and, although widespread, are below the resolution of CT and MR. In fact, despite widespread diffuse axonal damage, special silver stains with an avidity for synaptic degeneration are often necessary to identify axon cylinder disruption.[137] Larger nonhemorrhagic lesions are however seen on MR as areas of hypointensity on T1WI and hyperintensity on T2WI.

In addition to the widespread axonal damage, vascular disruption from shearing forces causes microscopic or macroscopic hemorrhages. These lesions have the same MR appearance as other hemorrhagic intracranial lesions. Lesion distribution and a history of trauma is the key to the diagnosis. Small superficial subcortical lesions, either hemorrhagic or nonhemorrhagic, indicate a shearing injury (see Fig. 13–15). Recognition of the mechanism of injury is important, as widespread unseen damage may be present. Lesions identified in the deep white matter, corpus callosum, and brain stem imply a grave prognosis.[11, 29] If the patient survives, widespread demyelination and diffuse atrophy with expanded intra- and extra-axial CSF spaces may be seen.

In summary, shearing injuries vary greatly in severity. Hemorrhagic and/or non-hemorrhagic lesion distribution is characteristic. Most of the damage is microscopic and inapparent. The severity of injury extends centripetally beginning in the subcortical gray-white junction. Subcortical lesions may or may not be associated with a good prognosis, but deep-seated lesions indicate a severe injury with a grave prognosis.

## Extracerebral Intracranial Fluid Collections

Closed head trauma commonly results in extracerebral, intracranial fluid collections, including subdural hematomas, epidural he-

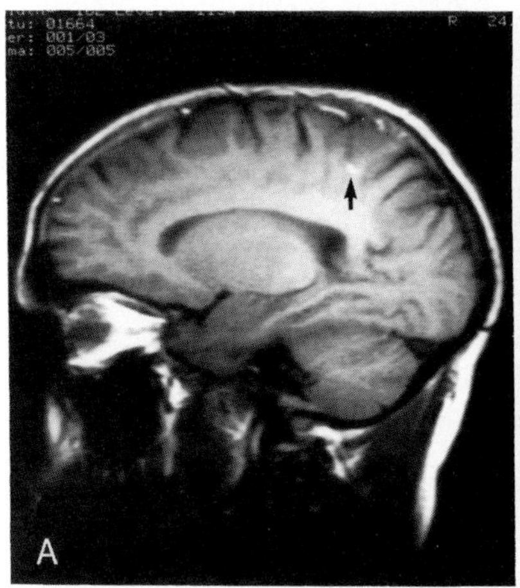

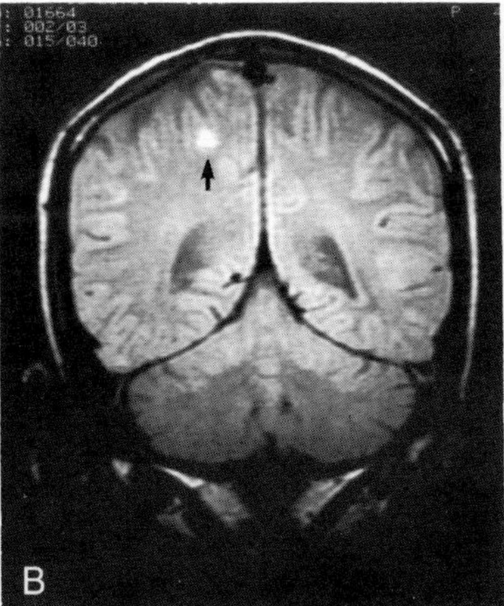

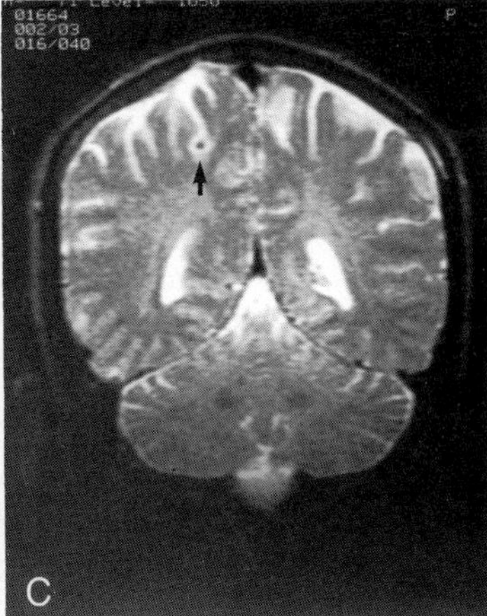


**Figure 13–15. Shearing injury.** A 36-year-old with left-sided weakness two days after a fall from a ladder (1.5 T). *A,* Sagittal SE T1WI (TR 600/TE 20). *B* and *C,* Coronal SE N(H)WI and T2WI (TR 2300/TE 20/100). The focal region of hyperintensity (*A* and *B*) at the gray-white matter interface in the right parietal lobe (arrow), which becomes markedly hypointense on T2WI *(C),* is consistent with a subacute hemorrhagic lesion. The lesion distribution and clinical presentation are typical of a shearing injury. (Courtesy of S. J. Pomeranz, M.D., Christ Hospital, Cincinnati, Ohio.)

matomas, and subdural hygromas. These traumatic sequelae increase morbidity and mortality as a result of their mass effect and distortion of the brain, in addition to any brain injury the patient may already have sustained. Because these collections are amenable to evacuation, early recognition and treatment are imperative.

### *Subdural Hematoma*

Blood in the subdural space, located between the dura and arachnoid, most commonly is due to trauma.[151, 152] Subdural hematoma (SDH) is the most common traumatic lesion requiring neurosurgical intervention,[153, 188] occurring in 1.4 per cent to 5 per cent of all head trauma cases and in 26 per cent to 63 per cent of patients with severe head injury.[5, 12, 156, 157, 246] SDH is most commonly of venous origin, although arterial bleeding rarely occurs.[168, 192, 227–231] As many as 10 per cent of cases have no identifiable bleeding source at surgery.[151] Although SDH is usually post-traumatic, nontraumatic causes are not uncommon and include (1) rapid reduction of increased intracranial pressure, for example, after shunt placement for hydrocephalus, LP, and removal of mass lesions, including hematomas[151, 152, 182–187, 212]; (2) impaired coagulation[151, 152, 155]; (3) bleeding from AVM's and aneurysm rupture[176, 189, 200, 201, 226]; (4) dural metastasis[190, 191]; and (5) spontaneous, or idiopathic, causes.[168, 192]

Traumatic SDH usually results from inertial forces during moving head injury. With the dura firmly attached to the skull and the arachnoid relatively fixed within the convolutions of the brain, a large component of the brain's gliding and swirling motions within the skull occur between the dura and the arachnoid. The resultant shear strains are most pronounced at the junction of the free and tethered portions of the bridging cortical veins as they cross the subdural space to enter the fixed dural sinuses.[151, 152, 154, 202] Tearing of bridging cortical veins within the subdural space is thought to be the most common mechanism of SDH production. Dural sinus tears may occur, usually resulting in an extensive SDH.[151, 152] Additionally, an SDH may arise from direct extension of a cerebral hematoma that ruptures through the arachnoid space[152, 220, 224, 225]; "burst lobe" is the colorful description given to this phenomenon.[152, 220, 224, 225, 246] The magnitude of head trauma associated with an SDH, as with other inertial injuries, is highly variable; minimal and indirect trauma (coughing, straining, whiplash injuries, and falls on the buttocks) may cause subdural collections and are likely responsible for many "spontaneous" SDH.[108, 151–155, 203, 249] Mild trauma is more often associated with slowly enlarging collections, whereas more severe trauma tends to present earlier, either because of the expanding SDH itself or other associated intracranial pathology. Traumatic SDH has been classically, but arbitrarily,[158] grouped according to the time interval between injury and symptom onset.[151, 152, 155, 165, 167] Acute SDH occurs within 3 days; subacute, from 3 to 20 days; and chronic, more than 21 days after injury.[155] Although this information is pathologically useful, it is clinically more useful to divide SDH into acute or subacute and chronic types. Acute and subacute SDHs are usually related to a specific traumatic event, demand more emergent treatment than do chronic subdural hematomas, and are associated with a higher mortality.

**Acute and Subacute Subdural Hematoma.** Acute and subacute SDH can be perceived as one clinical entity. It is a serious complication of head injury because it implies the presence of inertial injury and the likelihood of associated intracranial pathology. The more rapid the evolution and the more severe the neurological deficit, the worse the prognosis. With increasingly severe trauma, associated intracranial pathology becomes increasingly common. Bilaterality occurs in 33 per cent of acute SDHs and 20 per cent of subacute SDHs.[155] The majority of patients with acute SDH have altered consciousness from the moment of injury.[152] Lateralizing findings and focal neurological deficits are found in as many as 70 per cent of patients.[151] A lucid interval is uncommon with an SDH. Headache, usually ipsilateral, is the most common symptom but is usually seen in more slowly accumulating collections such as subacute or chronic SDH. Associated brain injury occurs in as many as 45 per cent of patients and is the main contributing factor to patient mortality.[204, 222] Mortality ranges from 50 per cent to 88 per cent with acute SDH and from 25 per cent to 35 per cent with subacute SDH.[151–153, 155, 158–165, 215–221] Advancing patient age, increasing hematoma size, and delay in hematoma evacuation are independent factors associated with a worse prognosis.[151, 152, 155, 223, 254] In contrast with the poor prognosis associated with an acute SDH, chronic SDH is a separate clinical entity with a much better prognosis.

**Chronic Subdural Hematoma.** Chronic SDH represents a diagnostic challenge. While the majority are post-traumatic, a clear-cut history of trauma is absent in as many as 30 per cent of patients.[153, 155, 243, 250–252] This may lead to misdiagnosis; many patients at autopsy are undiagnosed premortem.[242, 244, 251] The pathogenesis and location of the collections are similar to those of acute and subacute SDHs. Because chronic SDH results from a slow accumulation of blood, the causative head injury is often mild.[108, 151, 152] "Accentuated activities of daily living," such as straining and coughing, may be associated with a chronic SDH and often go unnoticed. Bilaterality occurs in only 10 per cent to 18 per cent of cases, and associated brain injury is uncommon.[155, 243] A preponderance of these collections occur in patients with cortical atrophy, in the elderly, and in alcoholics.[254–256] Theoretically, the atrophic brain rests in a dependent position, putting tension on the superiorly located bridging cortical veins. The stretched, aged veins are thought to be predisposed to rupture. Chronic SDHs have a high recurrence rate because predisposing factors (atrophic brain, anticoagulation status, and brittle, elderly vessels) remain unchanged, and membrane formation as a result of the initial SDH predisposes to rebleeding.

Clinical presentation is, by definition, remote from the head injury. Expanded extra-axial CSF spaces may allow a substantial accumulation of blood in the subdural space before mass effect becomes clinically apparent.[152] Most patients are elderly and present with nonspecific signs and symptoms, the commonest of which include altered mental status, dementia, impaired memory, and headaches.[108, 153–155, 242–244] In contrast with nonchronic SDH, mortality from chronic SDH is low and varies from 0 per cent to 23 per cent.[155, 243, 253] Rebleeding is common, and thus many patients have a "sinusoidal" course with recurrence or aggravation of symptoms.

**MR Appearance.** A subdural hematoma can be characterized by its morphology, mass effect, and signal characteristics. A free and open potential subdural space probably does not exist as such. The dura and arachnoid are attached by interface cells that contain little intercellular collagen and therefore lack coherence.[245] This circumstance allows subdural fluid to spread over large portions of the cerebral hemisphere, limited only by the falx, medially (unless adhesions are present). SDHs are most commonly located in the posterior frontal and temporoparietal region in the center of the hemisphere, often extending into the interhemispheric fissure. Rarely, tearing of interhemispheric or posterior fossa veins or sinuses may occur giving rise to isolated SDH in these areas (Fig. 13–16) or along the tentorium cerebelli (Fig. 13–17).[169–181, 195, 196]

The typical morphology of an acute SDH is that of a convex outer margin and a concave inner margin conforming to brain and calvarium topology, in contrast with an acute epidural hematoma (EDH), which is typically focal, lenticular in shape, and limited by sutural margins.[5, 108, 151–154, 204, 206–214] An SDH is medially limited by the falx and cannot cross the midline, in contrast with

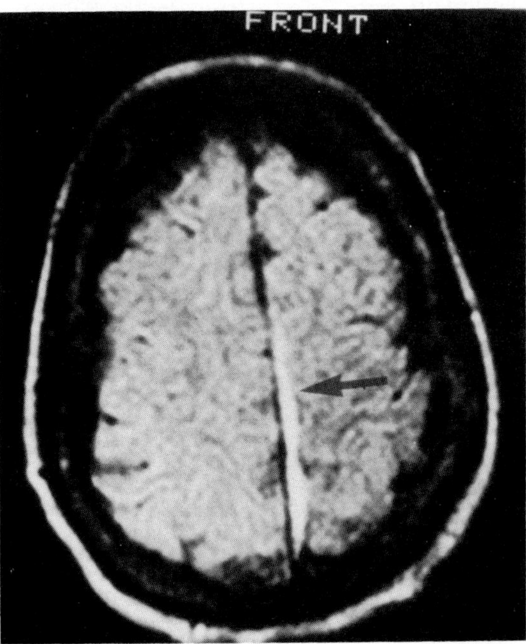


**Figure 13–16. Interhemispheric subdural hematoma (0.35 T).** This T1WI shows an isolated interhemispheric hyperintense extra-axial collection (arrow) consistent with subacute blood. (Courtesy of J. Tobias, M.D., Mount Sinai Hospital, Miami Beach, Fla.)

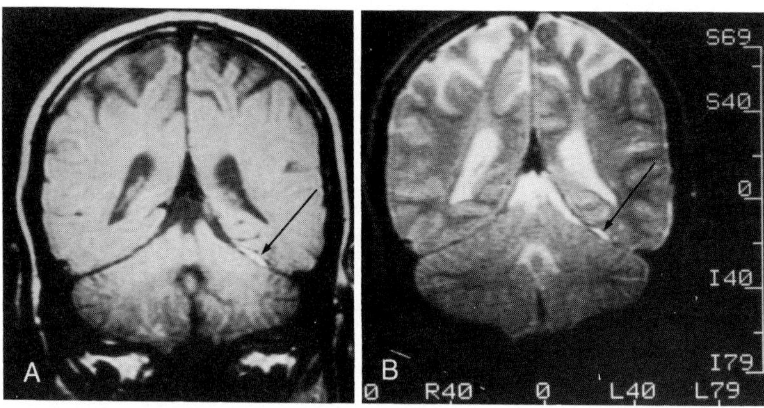


**Figure 13–17. Tentorial subdural hematoma (0.35 T).** A 24-year-old woman with systemic lupus erythematosus. *A,* Coronal SE T1WI (TR 600/TE 20), and *B,* T2WI (TR 1800/TE 80). The extra-axial, tentorial collection is hyperintense on both images (arrow), consistent with late subacute blood. The lesion was not seen on CT. (Courtesy of S. J. Pomeranz, M.D., Christ Hospital, Cincinnati, Ohio.)

an EDH. The classic concave inner border of an SDH may be better appreciated in one imaging plane than another. For instance, an acute SDH may appear lenticular in the axial plane while coronal images show the classic concave inner margin (or vice versa), allowing the correct diagnosis[5, 108, 151–154, 204, 206–214] (Figs. 13–18 to 13–20). Subacutely and chronically, an SDH may maintain its concave inner margin, or with aging and organization, it may evolve to a planar stage or into a final biconvex, lenticular morphology similar to that of an EDH.

Subdural collections usually weigh from 30 to 150 g, although their size is typically described by volume (one half maximum length × width × depth.[247, 248] Because an SDH spreads over large portions of the cerebral hemisphere, the three dimensional volume of the collection may be quite large, while its unidimensional thickness may appear diminutive on an individual slice. In addition, associated cerebral pathology may cause superimposed mass effect. Thus the extra-axial mass effect in association with an SDH is often more extensive than one might expect for its apparent size. Initially, there may be only sulcal effacement (Figs. 13–18 and 13–21).[233] With greater compression, the subjacent gray-white junction is compressed, and the central white matter buckles and thins. Continued compression causes a shift of midline structures, effacement of the ipsilateral lateral ventricle (Fig.

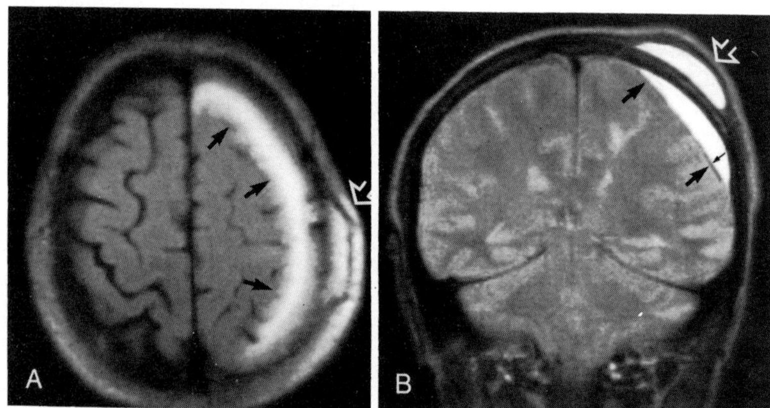


**Figure 13–18. Subacute subdural and subgaleal hematoma.** The patient had a craniotomy 2 weeks prior to the scan (0.5 T). *A,* Axial SE T1WI (TR 850/TE 26), and *B,* coronal T2WI (TR 2000/TE 80). This extra-axial collection is hyperintense on both images and follows brain/calvarial topology. The planar configuration (black arrows) and hypointense membrane (small black arrow) are evidence of organization *(B)*. A subgaleal hematoma is also present (open arrow). (Courtesy of Neuroradiology Department, University of Cincinnati, Cincinnati, Ohio.)

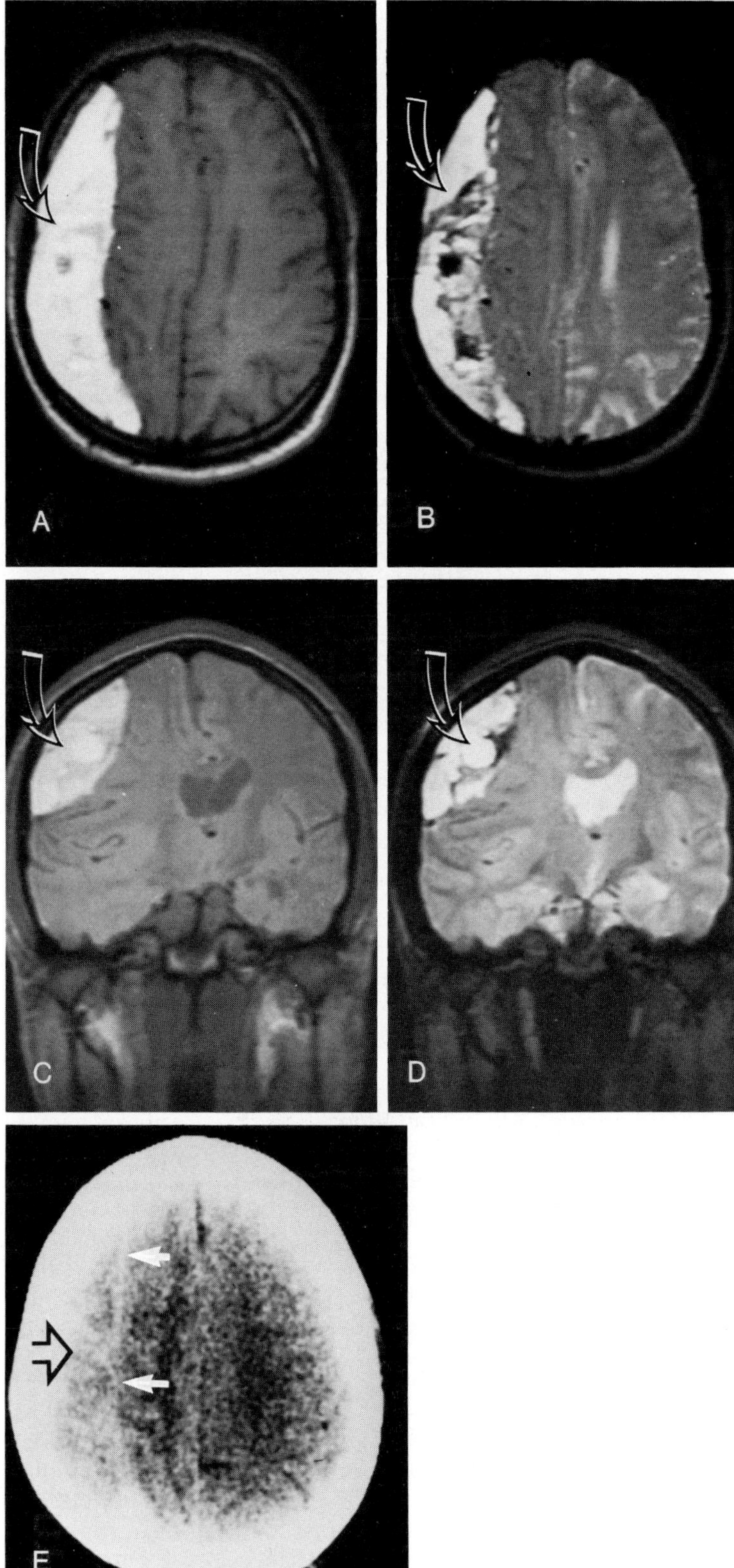


**Figure 13–19. Chronic subdural hematoma (1.5 T).** *A,* Axial SE T1WI (TR 800/TE 20), and *B,* T2WI (TR 2000/TE 80). *C* and *D,* Coronal SE N(H)WI and T2WI (SE TR 2000/TE 20/80). *E,* Contrast-enhanced CT. The biconvex collection with extra-axial mass effect is typical of a chronic SDH. The hyperintense regions on T1WI and T2WI are consistent with the presence of a complex solution containing protein, methemoglobin, or both. Hypointense areas on T2WI are isointense on T1WI, consistent with PT2PRE from either hemosiderin or calcium indicating an old collection, or acute blood, consistent with rebleeding. A contrast-enhanced CT *(E)* shows an enhancing membrane and an isodense collection that was inconspicuous on a noncontrast CT (not shown). (Courtesy of Neuroradiology Department, University of Cincinnati, Cincinnati, Ohio.)

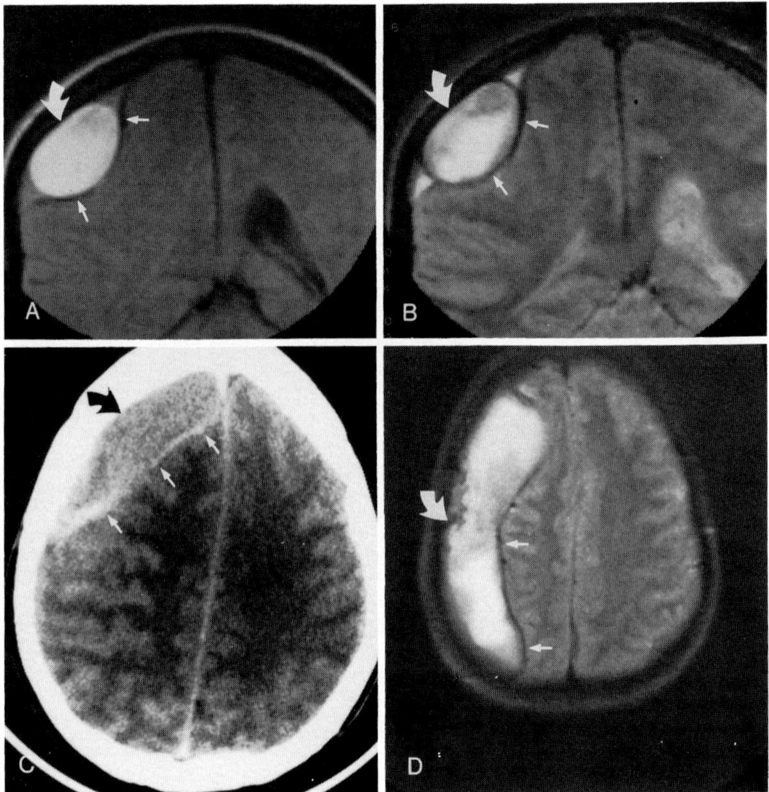


**Figure 13–20. Chronic subdural hematoma (0.5 T).** *A,* Coronal SE N(H)WI(TR 2000/TE 20), and *B,* T2WI (TR 2000/TE 80). *C,* Axial contrast-enhanced CT. *D,* Axial SE T1WI T2WI(TR 2000/TE 80). MR images demonstrate a relatively homogeneous hyperintense lenticular collection (curved white arrow), consistent with a chronic SDH. The enhancing membrane on CT *(C)* is hypointense on MR (small white arrows). (Courtesy of Neuroradiology Department, University of Cincinnati, Cincinnati, Ohio.)

13–19) and eventual herniation. An SDH can be identified not only by its morphology and extra-axial mass effect but also by its signal abnormalities. Signal changes with an SDH from closed head injury are time dependent in a manner similar to but not identical with those of an intracranial hematoma (ICH).

**Hyperacute Subdural Hematoma.** Active bleeding and unclotted blood in acute post-traumatic subdural collections has been described in the CT literature, but their appearance on MR has yet to be reported. An intermediately long T1/T2 similar to that seen with other hyperacute intracranial hemorrhagic collections from high bulk water content is to be expected.

**Acute Subdural Hematoma.** At high field an acute (< three days) SDH is isointense on T1WI and deeply hypointense on T2WI owing to spin dephasing. In contrast with an (ICH), in which vasogenic edema may be hypointense on T1WI, vasogenic edema within extra-axial collections has not been described. Clot retraction with extruded serum, though, does occur and may alter the appearance of an acute SDH such that a margin of water signal (long T1/T2) along the inner or outer border[12] or a diffuse inhomogeneity[206, 207] within the collection occurs. Clot retraction, especially in patients on anticoagulants, may cause a hematocrit effect with a fluid-fluid level.[207] The dependent layer contains intracellular deoxyhemoglobin while the supernatant is essentially serum. At high field, the dependent layer is isointense on T1WI and extremely hypointense on T2WI, while the supernatant has a long T1 and T2 (Fig. 13–22). At low field, an acute SDH may be isointense. Changing imaging parameters as discussed previously may be helpful.

**Subacute Subdural Hematoma** (Three days to three weeks). Subacutely, an SDH is hyperintense at all field strengths and on all SE imaging sequences because of high methemoglobin concentrations. It is at this time

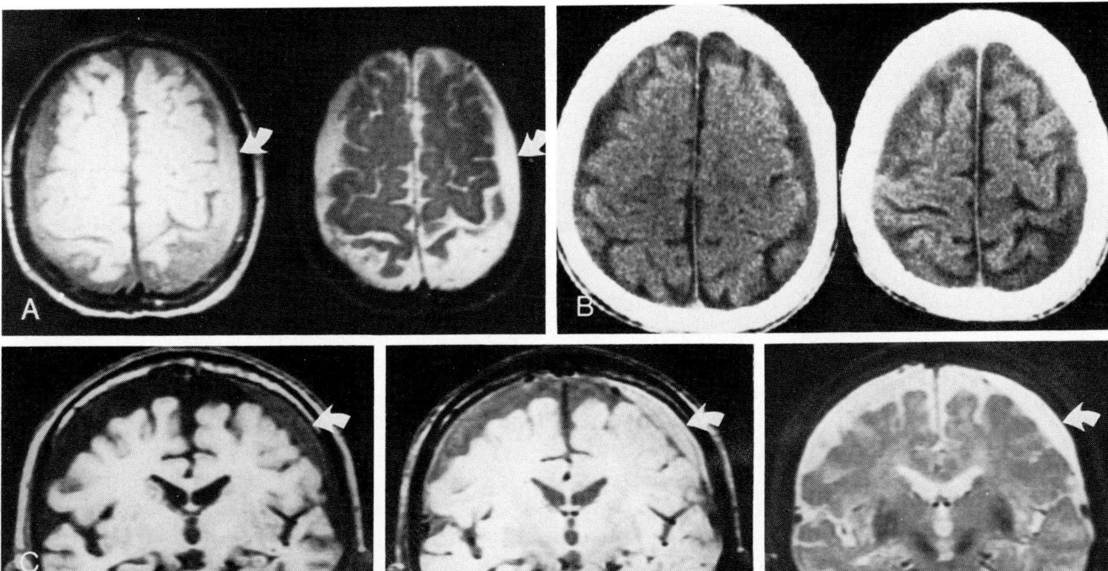

**Figure 13–21. Chronic subdural hematoma (SDH).** An 86-year-old patient with mental status decline and no definite history of trauma (1.5 T). *A,* (L to R) axial SE N(H)WI and T2WI (TR 2000/TE 20/80). *B,* CT, noncontrast. *C,* (L to R) coronal SE T1WI (TR 800/TE 20), N(H)WI and T2WI (TR 2000/TE 20/80). Atrophically expanded CSF spaces are present on both CT and MR; the MR demonstrates a hyperintense subdural collection (arrow). Sulcal effacement is noted on coronal images *(C).* The SDH has a higher signal than surrounding CSF on T1WI, consistent with increased protein, increased methemoglobin, or both. The hyperintensity relative to surrounding CSF on T2WI is thought to result from dampened CSF pulsations. CT shows atrophic changes without sulcal effacement or visualization of the SDH. At surgery, the collection contained protein (800 mg/dl) and old blood. The patient's mental status did not improve postoperatively. (Courtesy of Neuroradiology Department, University of Cincinnati, Cincinnati, Ohio.)

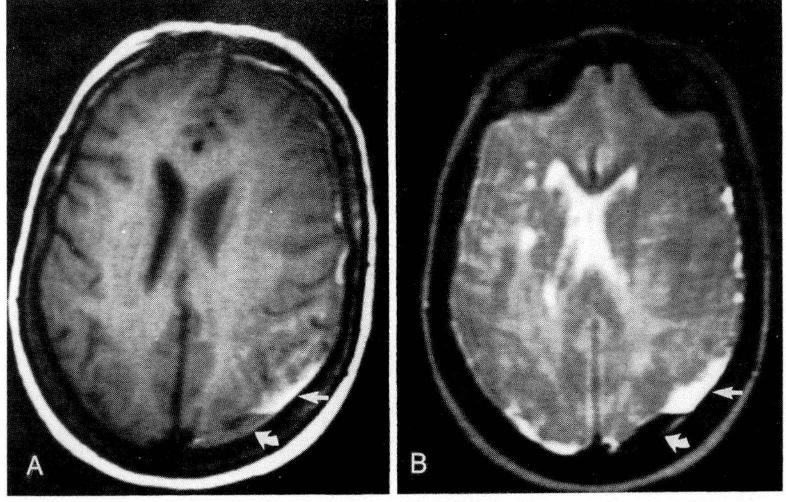

**Figure 13–22. Acute and subacute subdural hematoma.** A middle-aged woman on anticoagulants with multiple episodes of intracranial bleeding. A CT (not shown) was essentially normal (1.5 T). *A,* Axial SE T1WI (TR 800/TE 20), and *B,* T2WI (TR 2000/TE 80). A left posterior subdural hematoma with acute blood layered dependently (curved arrow) is isointense in *A* and hypointense in *B.* The nondependent layer is hyperintense on both the T1 and T2WI, consistent with a dilute methemoglobin solution from earlier bleeding. Also noted is a very small right occipital SDH with similar characteristics. (Courtesy of Neuroradiology Department, University of Cincinnati, Cincinnati, Ohio.)

that lesion contrast is maximal (see Fig. 13–18).[238] SDHs in the subacute period are usually homogeneous, although minimal hypointensity at the inner margin from clot retraction and serum extraction may still be present (see Fig. 13–18). A subacute SDH may maintain its concave inner border, may progress to a planar stage, or may become precociously biconvex, with neomembrane formation and organization.

**Chronic Subdural Hematoma** (Over three weeks). The MR appearance is a result of continued hematoma evolution, membrane formation and its accompanying morphologic changes, and rebleeding. Clot lysis is a continual process, and by three weeks, the collection is usually liquified.[243] It is dark in appearance, resembling crankcase oil, but with continued aging, it gradually becomes a xanthochromic, proteinaceous fluid. Signal abnormalities correlate with the evolutionary changes. The liquified blood has a high methemoglobin concentration, is hyperintense on T1WI and T2WI, and cannot be distinguished from subacute blood. This hyperintensity has been reported to persist for more than four months and can likely remain longer.[169] As hematoma resorption occurs, the collection becomes more of a proteinaceous solution with a decreasing methemoglobin concentration.[108] The T1 becomes longer as a result of increased bulk water and loss of the short T1 from the PEDPRE of the diminishing methemoglobin. The T2 remains long because it is primarily the result of the high bulk water content. Therefore as the chronic SDH ages, its appearance changes from hyperintense on both T1WI and T2WI to intermediately hypointense on T1WI and hyperintense on T2WI. With continued aging, the protein content may decrease and eventually approach that of CSF, making differentiation from a subdural hygroma or an expanded extra-axial space associated with atrophy difficult (Fig. 13–21). Spontaneous resorption of a chronic SDH may also occur.[154, 242]

Chronic SDHs are usually surrounded externally and internally by "neomembranes," which are generally thicker on the dural side and thinner on the arachnoid side.[108] These membranes arise from proliferation of normal dural border cells and collagen formation. Neomembrane formation may be initiated by any process that ruptures the poorly cohesive layer of interface (dural border) cells, separating the dura from the arachnoid.[245] Membrane formation and organization are thought to be responsible for the development of the typical lenticular shape of the chronic SDH. These neomembranes, having extensive collagen components, have few mobile protons and thus are hypointense on T1 and T2WIs (Fig. 13–20).

Fragile capillary sprouting develops on the dural side of the neomembrane and is thought to be responsible for the tendency to rebleed. Rebleeding results in blood in different stages of evolution, often compartmentalized as a result of adhesions and organization (see Fig. 13–19). The time-dependent signal abnormalities of recurrent bleeding are superimposed upon the underlying appearance of the SDH. These regions of rebleeding usually do not mix with the underlying collection but instead flow into allowable spaces as scarring, organization, and compartmentalization permit. Fresh hemorrhages and nests of hemosiderin-laden macrophages are commonly found upon inspection of the membranes.[245] Although no large series has accrued, hypointense regions or margins on T2WIs from hemosiderin deposition may make specific identification of intracellular deoxyhemoglobin from acute rebleeding difficult on MR.

### *Subdural Hygroma*

Classically, a subdural hygroma occurs when a traumatic arachnoid tear allows unidirectional egress of CSF from the subarachnoid space into the subdural space.[151–153, 258] These collections may acutely be identified immediately after injury. They contain pure CSF, are low density on CT, and are devoid of any type of neomembrane.[258–260] Skull fractures may or may not be present. Confusion in terminology arises because CSF-like collections of various antecedents are often referred to as hygromas. Some of these collections are xanthochromic, proteinaceous solutions representing a terminal step in the evolution of a chronic SDH; however, the imaging study is performed remotely and shows only a low-density collection.[257] Some "hygromas" have had membranes at surgery.[257] Inflammatory conditions, especially in children, are known to produce low-density, proteinaceous transudates in the subdural space and are more properly referred to as subdural effusions. Adding to the confusion is that any process that disrupts the dural interface cells and separates the dura from the arachnoid may result in a neomembrane and cause bleeding, transforming what originally begins as a subdural hygroma or effusion into a hemorrhagic collection.[245] Despite the confusing pathophysiology and terminology, the hallmark of a true subdural hygroma is its CSF-like appearance and lack of blood products and membranes.

**MR Appearance.** The collections are of variable constitution, ranging from "pure CSF" to extremely proteinaceous fluid. MR shows a subdural collection with a concave inner margin and a convex outer margin conforming to brain and cranium topology, as occurs with other subdural collections. The fluid has a long T1/T2 because of the high bulk water content. The T1 and T2 may be shortened by the presence of proteins within the collection that cause an intermediately hypointense appearance on T1WI and an intermediately hyperintense appearance on T2WI (Fig. 13–23).

### *Epidural Hematoma*

An epidural hematoma (EDH) is a collection of blood between the skull and the dura. It occurs in approximately 1 per cent to 3 per cent of all head injuries and in 5 per cent to 15 per cent of all fatal head injuries.[151, 152, 261, 262] The majority (70 per cent) of EDHs are localized unilateral hemispheric collections, although bilateral EDHs occur in 2 per cent to 10 per cent of cases.[261, 263, 278, 279, 287] EDHs may also occur in frontal (5 per cent to 10 per cent), occipitoparietal

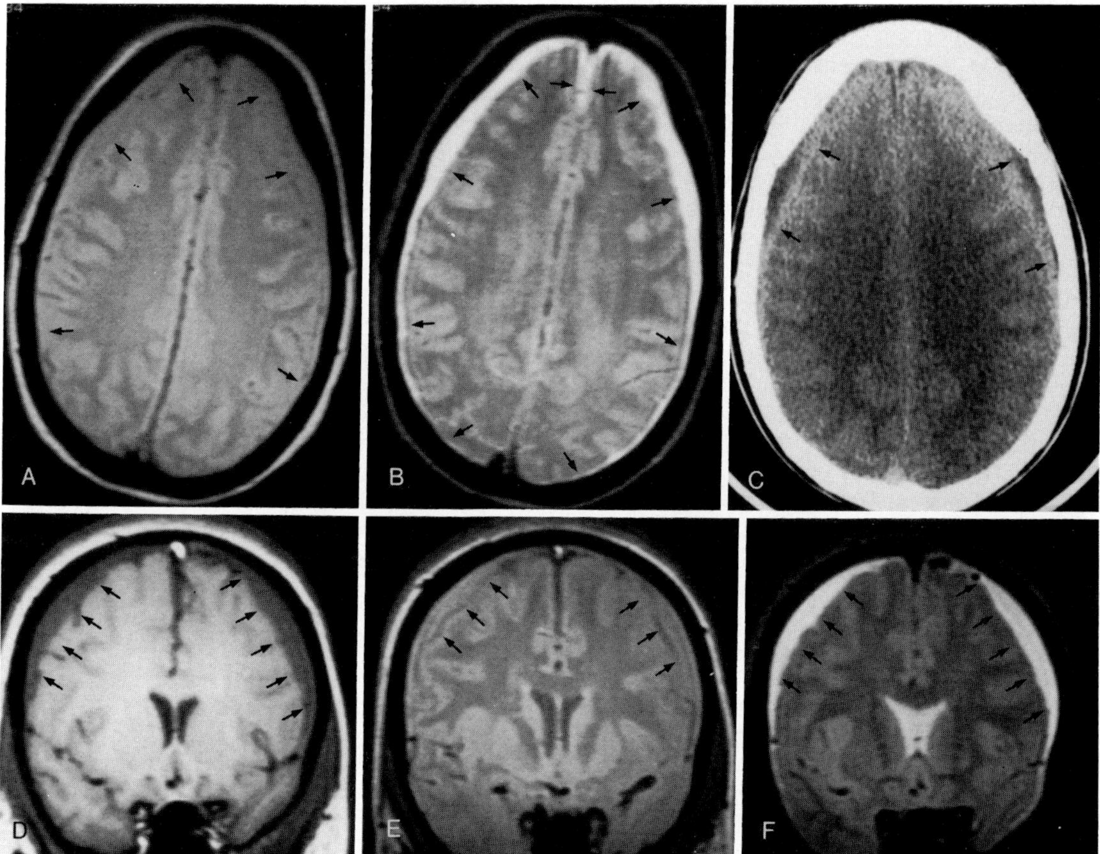


**Figure 13–23. Subdural hygroma.** A 32-year-old patient with headaches in an upright position from CNS hypotension (1.5 T). *A,* Axial N(H)WI (SE TR 2000/TE 20), and *B,* axial T2WI (TR 2000/TE 80). *C,* Noncontrast CT. *D, E,* and *F,* (L to R) coronal SE T1WI (TR 800/TE 20), N(H)WI, and T2WI (TR 2000/TE 20/80). MR images show a subdural fluid collection (arrows) with a long T1/T2. The signal intensity on T1WI is shorter than that of CSF, indicating a solution with either high protein, dilute methemoglobin, or both. The CT demonstrates the typical low density of a subdural hygroma. At surgery, the collections contained $>$ 1000 mg/dl protein and no blood. (Courtesy of Neuroradiology Department, University of Cincinnati, Cincinnati, Ohio.)

(5 per cent to 10 per cent), vertex (8 per cent), or posterior fossa uncommonly.[261, 277]

Unlike an SDH, which is due primarily to inertial trauma, EDH is most often the result of direct impact trauma resulting in a compressive injury. A skull fracture is present in up to 91 per cent of patients.[263, 278, 287] Children and young adults with less brittle, "plastic," skulls sustain an EDH without a fracture much more commonly than do older individuals.[235] The location of the EDH is dependent upon the site of impact.

Because pressures must be high enough to strip the tightly adherent dura from the skull, EDHs usually arise from arterial bleeding, most commonly from laceration of the middle meningeal artery or one of its branches.[152, 153, 261–269] However, an EDH can arise from rupture of the middle meningeal vein.[271, 288]

The presence of an acute EDH is a neurosurgical emergency, requiring immediate evacuation of the expanding mass. Because an EDH is often a result of focal impact trauma as opposed to the inertial trauma with an SDH, associated intracranial injury is less commonly associated with an EDH. Patients with an EDH often respond to surgical evacuation with complete and full recovery or only mild disability, in contrast with patients who incur an SDH.[108] Mortality varies from 6 per cent to 27 per cent and is related both to delay in diagnosis and treatment and to the associated intracranial lesions.[152, 261, 262, 273, 281]

Patient presentation is variable. With an acute EDH, the most common presentation is immediate alteration of consciousness following a well-recognized traumatic event.[274, 275] Rapid increase in mass effect causes increased intracranial pressure. The "classic" lucid interval occurs in less than 50 per cent of patients with acute epidural hematomas.[261, 272, 273]

Nonacute EDHs occur uncommonly.[263, 282, 283, 287] Skull deformation is thought to be the primary event causing separation of the dura from the skull, bleeding from low-pressure sources, such as emissary and diploic veins, and oozing from bone into the void, occurring secondarily.[263, 274, 280–282] Patients may present with insidious onset of nonspecific symptoms, including headache, nausea and vomiting, and alteration of consciousness. Nonacute EDHs may resolve spontaneously.[284–286]

**MR Appearance.** MR appearance is a function of morphology, mass effect, and signal abnormalities. Since it takes significant force to separate the tightly adherent dura from the calvarium, the collection is usually localized. High-pressure arterial bleeding causes the dura to bulge convexly, resulting in a lenticular shape. The focal biconvex extra-axial collection is most commonly unilateral and is usually located over the temporoparietal convexity. The specific location is related to the location of the lacerated arterial branch. Because the dura (periosteum) is the limiting membrane, EDHs are usually limited by sutural margins.[108] Unlike an SDH, an EDH may cross the midline. Extra-axial mass effect is generally proportional to the size of the fluid collection.

Extradural blood undergoes the same evolution as subdural blood.[288] Signal abnormalities from extradural hematomas are time dependent and are the same as those of subdural collections (see previous discussion). An acute EDH is isointense on T1WI and extremely hypointense on T2WI at high field (Fig. 13–24). As the hematoma ages, it becomes hyperintense on all imaging sequences, and chronically, the liquified blood becomes a proteinaceous solution and therefore is intermediate to hypointense on T1WI and hyperintense on T2WI. Hypervascular membrane formation occurs with chronic EDHs as it does with chronic SDHs.[276, 283, 288, 289]

MR differentiation of an EDH from an SDH rests primarily on the basis of morphology, as signal characteristics are similar. Acutely, distinguishing morphologic differences are present, but nonacutely, a lenticular chronic SDH may be exceedingly difficult to distinguish from a chronic EDH.

## CT Versus MR

CT is readily available, noninvasive, quick and relatively easy to perform on acutely injured patients; it has revolutionized the neurosurgical management of head injury. MR is expensive and can be difficult to perform on acutely injured patients requiring mechanical life support systems or traction. In addition, the current long imaging time of MR requires patients to remain motionless for significant periods of time. Although nonferromagnetic halos and traction

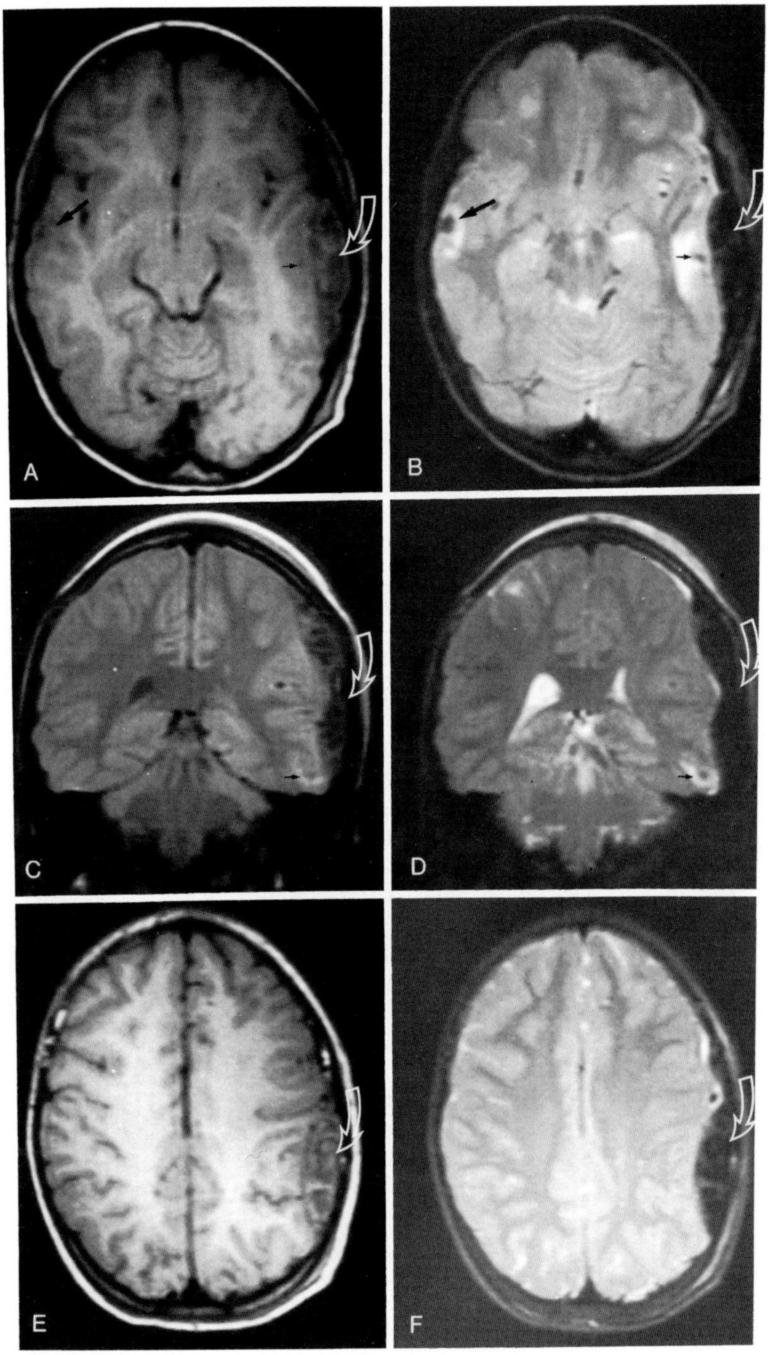

**Figure 13–24. Acute epidural hematoma (EDH).** A child with a left parietal skull fracture after a fall. He was alert with no loss of consciousness. Headaches and vomiting occurred 48 hours later (1.5 T). *A,* Axial SE T1W1 (TR 800/TE 20), and *B,* T2WI (TR 2000/TE 80). *C* and *D,* Coronal SE N(H)WI and T2WI (TR 2000/TE 20/80). *E,* Axial T1WI SE (TR 800/TE 20), and *F,* T2WI (TR 2000/TE 80). A typical lenticular EDH is present (curved arrow) with white matter buckling and compression of the homolateral lateral ventricle. It is inhomogeneous but predominantly isointense on T1WI (*A* and *E*) and markedly hypointense on T2WI (*B, D, F*). Note the small, juxtaposed coup lesion (smallest black arrow) and a contrecoup lesion (black arrow), poorly seen in *A* because it is isointense. (Courtesy of Neuroradiology Department, University of Cincinnati, Cincinnati, Ohio.)

devices are becoming common, MR remains a logistical problem in many acute trauma situations. On the other hand, MR is more sensitive to both hemorrhagic and nonhemorrhagic traumatic intracranial lesions.[12, 56, 142, 290, 297, 298] Judicious use of this new technology requires that MR provide information important to patient management. The issue then becomes, When is the added information clinically important?

In the acute trauma setting, added information from MR does not generally change surgical management.[12, 56] MR better identifies small extra-axial collections, traumatic lesions of the brain stem, posterior fossa and temporal lobe, and associated secondary infarctions.[12] In studies to date, however, acute parenchymal lesions and extra-axial collections large enough to require evacuation have been adequately identified on high-resolution CT scanners. However, an isodense SDH may occur acutely in an anemic patient when the hemoglobin concentration is ≤ 8 g/dl, or when blood is diluted as a result of mixing with CSF from an associated arachnoid tear.[2, 9, 21, 206] MR may play a role in this situation if the CT diagnosis is in doubt. CT remains the initial imaging modality of choice in the evaluation of acute head trauma.

In the nonacute setting, logistic problems are less formidable and the questions to be answered are different; "To operate or not to operate," is no longer the issue. Sensitivity of MR to the presence of parenchymal injuries is particularly advantageous in the diagnosis of the shearing lesions resulting from minor head injury.[12, 142, 297, 298] It is estimated that "minor" and "moderate" head trauma may make up as much as 75 per cent of admissions for head trauma.[290] Neurobehavioral sequelae have important implications in this large group of patients and are manifested by single or multiple focal neurologic deficits, personality changes, learning difficulties, memory impairment, or seizures.[142, 290] "Dementia pugilistica" is but one example of "minor" head injury that is now drawing extensive publicity. MR may satisfy clinical or medicolegal needs to find correlative lesions to explain clinical deficits or both when CT fails.

In addition to identification of parenchymal abnormalities, MR signal characteristics of extra-axial collections may allow identification and characterization when CT is nondiagnostic or nonspecific. The CT density of an SDH varies predictably, according to its globin concentration.[239] As the SDH progresses from a hyperdense to a hypodense collection, it proceeds through an isodense phase that may occur anytime from one week to three months after trauma but typically occurs within two to six weeks.[5, 204, 208, 210, 233, 238, 240, 241] Although current state-of-the-art scanners allow diagnosis of isodense collections more reliably than those used in many of the studies previously referenced, isodense subdural collections, particularly when bilateral, can be diagnostic problems on CT. Fortunately, the diagnosis of extra-axial collections is one of the strengths of MR, particularly subacutely when lesion conspicuity is maximal.

Equally important is the patient who presents on CT with a nonspecific, low-density extra-axial collection that may represent a subdural hygroma, a chronic SDH, a subdural effusion, or even expanded extra-axial CSF spaces secondary to atrophy. MR can demonstrate evidence of hemorrhage long after the CT shows nonspecific, low-density extra-axial fluid. However, there comes a point in time when, after resorption of most of the blood products, the remaining proteinaceous solution has nonspecific signal characteristics on MR as well. Therefore MR has a longer temporal "window" in which to identify the presence of blood; however, a proteinaceous solution or CSF signal characteristics does not exclude previous bleeding.

In conclusion, judicious use of MR technology is paramount. In the acute neurotrauma setting, MR has a limited role, and CT is the initial imaging modality of choice. In the nonacute situation, MR provides valuable information that may aid in clinical management of neurotrauma patients.

## References

1. Bergström M, Ericson K, Levander B, et al. Computed tomography of cranial subdural and epidural hematomas: variation of attenuation related to time and clinical events such as rebleeding. J Comput Assist Tomogr 1:449, 1977.
2. New PFJ, Aronow S. Attenuation measurements of whole blood and blood fractions in computed tomography. Radiology 121:635, 1976.
3. Saul TG, Ducker TB. The role of computed tomography in acute head injury. CT 4:296, 1980.
4. Davis KR, Taveras JM, Roberson GH, et al. Some limitations of computed tomography in the diagnosis of neurological diseases. AJR 127:111, 1976.
5. Merino-deVillasante J, Taveras JM. Computerized tomography (CT) in acute head trauma. AJR 126:765, 1976.
6. New PFJ, Scott WR, Schnur JA, et al. Computerized axial tomography with the EMI scanner. Radiology 110:109, 1974.
7. Messina AV, Chernik NL. Computer tomography: the "resolving" intracerebral hemorrhage. Radiology 118:609, 1976.
8. Kishore PRS, Lipper MH, Becker DP, et al. The significance of CT in the management of patients with severe head injury: correlation with ICP. AJNR 2:307, 1981.
9. Smith WP, Batnitzky S, Rengachary SS. Acute isodense subdural hematomas: a problem in anemic patients. AJNR 2:37, 1981.

10. Zimmerman RA, Bilaniuk LT, Gennarelli T, et al. Cranial computed tomography in diagnosis and management of acute head trauma. AJR 131:27, 1978.
11. Zimmerman RA, Bilaniuk LT, Gennarelli T, et al. Computed tomography of shearing injuries of the cerebral white matter. Radiology 127:393, 1978.
12. Zimmerman RA, Bilaniuk LT, Hackney DB, Goldberg HI, et al. Head injury: early results of comparing CT and high-field MR. AJR 147:1215, 1986.
13. Neill JM. Studies on the oxidation-reduction of hemoglobin and methemoglobin III. The formation of methemoglobin during the oxidation of autoxidizable substance. J Exp Med 41:551, 1925.
14. Neill JM. Studies on the oxidation-reduction of hemoglobin and methemoglobin IV. The inhibition of "spontaneous" methemoglobin formation. J Exp Med 41:561, 1925.
15. Neill JM, Hasting AB. The influence of the tension of molecular oxygen upon certain oxidations of hemoglobin. J Biol Chem 63:479, 1925.
16. Gomori JM, Grossman RI, Goldberg HI, et al. Intracranial hematomas: imaging by high-field MR. Radiology 157:87, 1985.
17. Wolverson MK, Creeps LF, Sundaram M, et al. Hyperdensity of recent hemorrhage at body computed tomography: incidence and morphologic variation. Radiology 148:779, 1983.
18. Butzer JF, Cancilla PA, Cornell SH. Computerized axial tomography of intracerebral hematoma. A clinical and neuropathological study. Arch Neurol 33:206, 1976.
19. Dolinskas CA, Bilaniuk LT, Zimmerman RA, et al. Computed tomography of intracerebral hematomas. I. Transmission CT observations on hematoma resolution. AJR 129:681, 1977.
20. Dooms GC, Uske A, Brant-Zawadzki M, et al. Spin-echo MR imaging of intracranial hemorrhage. Neuroradiology 28:132, 1986.
21. Chakeres DW, Bryan RN. Acute subarachnoid hemorrhage: In vitro comparison of magnetic resonance and computed tomography. AJNR 7:223, 1986.
22. Di Chiro G, Brooks RA, Girton ME, et al. Sequential MR studies of intracerebral hematomas in monkeys. AJNR 7:193, 1986.
23. Dolinskas CA, Bilaniuk LT, Zimmerman RA, et al. Computed tomography of intracerebral hematomas. II. Radionuclide and transmission CT studies of the perihematoma region. AJR 129:689, 1977.
24. Zimmerman RA, Bilaniuk LT, Grossman RI, et al. Resistive NMR of intracranial hematomas. Neuroradiology 27:16, 1985.
25. Sipponen JT, Sepponen RE, Sivula A. Nuclear magnetic resonance (NMR) imaging of intracerebral hemorrhage in the acute and resolving phases. J Comput Assist Tomogr 7:954, 1983.
26. Sipponen JT, Sepponen RE, Tanttu JI, et al. Intracranial hematomas studied by MR imaging at 0.17 and 0.02 T. J Comp Assist Tomogr 9:698, 1985.
27. Sepponen RE, Sipponen JT, Sivula A. Low-field nuclear magnetic resonance imaging of the brain. J Comput Assist Tomogr 9:237, 1985.
28. DeLaPaz RL, New PFJ, Buonanno FS, et al. NMR imaging of intracranial hemorrhage. J Comput Assist Tomogr 8:599, 1984.
29. Diegel JG, Pintar MM. A possible improvement in the resolution of proton spin relaxation for the study of cancer at low frequency. J Natl Cancer Inst 55:725, 1975.
30. Béné GJ. Nuclear magnetism of liquid systems in the earth field range. Phys Report 58:213, 1980.
31. Ling CR, Foster MA, Hutchison JMS. Comparison of NMR water proton T1 relaxation times of rabbit tissues at 24 MHz and 2.5 MHz. Phys Med Biol 25:748, 1980.
32. Koenig SH, Brown RD III, Adams D, et al. Magnetic field dependence of 1/T1 of protons in tissue. Invest Radiol 19:76, 1984.
33. Fullerton GD, Cameron IL, Ord VA. Frequency dependence of magnetic resonance spin-lattice relaxation of protons in biological materials. Radiology 151:135, 1984.
34. Crooks L, Arakawa M, Hoenninger J, et al. Nuclear magnetic resonance whole-body imager operating at 3.5 kgauss. Radiology 143:169, 1982.
35. Bottomley PA, Hart HR Jr, Edelstein WA, et al. Anatomy and metabolism of the normal human brain studied by magnetic resonance at 1.5 tesla. Radiology 150:441, 1984.
36. Buxton RB, Edelman RR, Rosen BR, et al. Contrast in rapid MR imaging: T1-and T2-weighted imaging. J Comput Assist Tomogr 11:7, 1987.
37. Edelman RR, Johnson K, Buxton R, et al. MR of hemorrhage: a new approach. AJNR 7:751, 1986.
38. Abragam A. The principles of nuclear magnetism. Oxford, Clarendon Press, 1961:1–4.
39. Young IR, Khenia DGT, Davis CH, et al. Clinical magnetic susceptibility mapping of the brain. J Comput Assist Tomogr 11:2, 1987.
40. Nose T, Enomoto T, Hyodo A, et al. Intracerebral hematoma developing during MR examination. J Comput Assist Tomogr 11:184, 1987.
41. Koenig SH, Schillinger WE. Nuclear magnetic relaxation dispersion in protein solutions. I. Apotransferrin. J Biol Chem 244:3283, 1969.
42. Saryan LA, Hollis DP, Economou JS, et al. Brief communication: nuclear magnetic resonance studies of cancer. IV. Correlation of water content with tissue relaxation times. J Natl Cancer Inst 52:599, 1974.
43. Brown JJ, van Sonnenberg E, Gerber KH, et al. MR relaxation times of percutaneously obtained body fluids. Radiology 154:727, 1985.
44. Bottomley PA, Foster TH, Argersinger RE, et al. A review of normal tissue hydrogen NMR relaxation times and relaxation mechanisms from 1–100 MHz: dependence on tissue type, NMR frequency, temperature, species, excision, and age. Med Phys 11:425, 1984.
45. Wehrli FW, MacFall JR, Shutts D, et al. Mechanisms of contrast in NMR imaging. J Comput Assist Tomogr 8:369, 1984.
46. Young IR, Burl M, Clarke GJ, et al. Magnetic resonance properties of hydrogen: imaging of the posterior fossa. AJR 137:895, 1981.
47. Hahn EL. Spin echoes. Phys Rev 80:580, 1950.
48. Hoult DI, Lauterbur PC. The sensitivity of zeugmatographic experiment involving human samples. J Magn Reson 34:425, 1979.
49. Lee YY, Moser R, Bruner JM, et al. Organized intracerebral hematoma with acute hemorrhage: CT patterns and pathologic correlations. AJNR 7:409, 1986.
50. Enzmann DR, Britt RH, Lyons BE, et al. Natural history of experimental intracerebral hemorrhage:

sonography, computed tomography, and neuropathology. AJNR 2:517, 1981.
51. Zimmerman RD, Leeds NE, Naidich TP. Ring blush associated with intracerebral hematoma. Radiology 122:707, 1977.
52. Laster DW, Moody DM, Ball MR. Resolving intracerebral hematoma: alteration of the "ring-sign" with steroids. AJR 130:935, 1978.
53. Weisberg LA. Peripheral rim enhancement in supratentorial intracerebral hematoma. Computed Tomography 4:145, 1980.
54. Takasugi S. Cause of ring enhancement in computed tomographic image of intracerebral hemorrhage—an experimental histological study. Neurol Med Chir 20:689, 1980.
55. Bodansky O. Methemoglobinemia and methemoglobin-producing compounds. Pharmacol Rev 3:144, 1951.
56. Snow RB, Zimmerman RD, Gandy SE, et al. Comparison of magnetic resonance imaging and computed tomography in the evaluation of head injury. Neurosurgery 18:45, 1986.
57. Bailes DR, Young IR, Thomas DJ, et al. NMR imaging of the brain using spin-echo sequences. Clin Radiol 33:395, 1982.
58. Bloembergen N, Purcell EM, Pound RV. Relaxation effects in nuclear magnetic resonance absorption. Phys Review 73:679, 1948.
59. Robertson B. Spin-echo decay of spins diffusing in a bound region. Phys Rev 151:273, 1966.
60. Thulborn KR, Waterton JC, Matthews PM, et al. Oxygenation dependence of the transverse relaxation time of water protons in whole blood at high field. Biochim Biophys Acta 714:265, 1982.
61. Pauling L, Coryell C. The magnetic properties and structure of hemoglobin, oxyhemoglobin, and carboxyhemoglobin. Proc Natl Acad Sci USA 22:210, 1936.
62. Bradley WG, Schmidt PG. Effect of methemoglobin formation on the MR appearance of subarachnoid hemorrhage. Radiology 156:99, 1985.
63. Zimmerman RD, Deck MDF. Intracranial hematomas: imaging by high-field MR. Letter. Radiology 159:565, 1986.
64. Bydder GM, Payne AG, Collins AG, et al. Clinical use of rapid T2 weighted partial saturation sequences in MR imaging. J Comput Assist Tomogr 11:17, 1987.
65. Bydder GM, Young IR. Clinical use of the partial saturation and saturation recovery sequences in NMR imaging. J Comput Assist Tomogr 9:1020, 1985.
66. Lindenburg R. Tissue reactions in the gray matter of the central nervous system. In Haymaker W, Adams RD, eds. Histology and Histolopathology of the Nervous System, Vol. 1. Springfield, Ill., Charles C Thomas, 1982:1130.
67. Adams RD, Sidman RL. Introduction to Neuropathology. New York, McGraw-Hill Book Co. 1968:177.
68. Brasch RC, Wesbey GE, Gooding CA, et al. Magnetic resonance imaging of transfusional hemosiderosis complicating thalassemia major. Radiology 150:767, 1984.
69. Bezkorovainy A. Biochemistry of Nonheme Iron. New York, Plenum Press, 1977:207.
70. Dwek RA. Nuclear Magnetic Resonance (NMR) in Biochemistry. Oxford, Clarendon Press, 1973:174.
71. Hinshaw WS, Bottomley PA, Holland GN. Radiographic thin-section imaging of the human wrist by nuclear magnetic resonance. Nature 270:722, 1977.
72. Herfkens R, Davis P, Crooks L, et al. Nuclear magnetic resonance imaging of the abnormal live rat and correlations with tissue characteristics. Radiology 141:211, 1981.
73. Fairbanks VF, Beutler E. Iron metabolism. In Williams WJ, Beutler E, Erslev AJ, et al., eds. Hematology. New York, McGraw-Hill Book Co. 1977:168.
74. Brittenham GM, Farrell DE, Harris JW, et al. Magnetic-susceptibility measurement of human iron stores. N Engl J Med 307:1671, 1982.
75. Singer JR, Crooks LE. Some magnetic studies of normal and leukemic blood. J Clin Eng 3:237, 1978.
76. Mansfield P, Morris PG. NMR Imaging in Biomedicine. New York, Academic Press, 1983:25.
77. Packer KJ. The effects of diffusion through locally inhomogeneous magnetic fields on transverse nuclear spin relaxation in heterogeneous systems: proton transverse relaxation in striated muscle tissue. J Magn Reson 9:438, 1973.
78. Brant-Zawadzki M. NMR imaging: the abnormal brain and spinal cord. In Newton TH, Potts DG, eds. Modern Neuroradiology. Advanced Imaging Techniques, Vol. 2. San Francisco, Clavadel Press, 1983:159.
79. Barnhart JL, Berk RN. Influence of paramagnetic ions and pH on proton NMR relaxation of biologic fields. Invest Radiol 21:132, 1986.
80. Wintrobe MM, Lee GR. Hematologic alterations. In Wintrobe MM, Thorn GW, Adams RD, et al., eds. Principles of Medicine, 7th ed. New York, McGraw-Hill Book Co., 1974:298.
81. Wisniewski H. The pathogenesis of some cases of cerebral hemorrhage (a morphological study of the margins of hemorrhagic foci and areas of the brain distant from the hemorrhage). Acta Med Pol 2:379, 1961.
82. Rubin JI, Gomori JM, Grossman RI, et al. High-field MR imaging of extracranial hematomas. AJR 148:813, 1987.
83. Wolf GL, Burnett KR, Goldstein EJ, et al. Contrast agents for magnetic resonance imaging. In Dressel HY, ed. Magnetic Resonance Annual 1985. New York, Raven Press, 1985:231.
84. U.S. Department of Health, Education, and Welfare. National Center for Health Statistics. Hyattsville, Md, Vital Statistics of the United States: 1975. Washington, D.C., GPO, 1979.
85. Caveness, WF. Incidence of craniocerebral trauma in the United States in 1976 with trends from 1970–1975. Adv Neurol 22:1, 1979.
86. Annegers JF, Grabow JD, Kurland LT, et al. The incidence, causes, and secular trends of head trauma in Olmstead County, Minnesota, 1935–1974. Neurology 30:912, 1980.
87. Kalsbeek WD, McLaurin RL, Harris BSH III, et al. The national head and spinal cord injury survey: major findings. J Neurosurg 53:519, 1980.
88. Bakay L, Glasauer FE. Head Injury. Boston, Little, Brown & Co. 1980.
89. Harris P. Craniospinal injuries. In Head Injuries: Proceedings of an International Symposium. Baltimore, Williams & Wilkins, 1971:321.
90. Maloney AFJ, Whatmore WJ. Clinical and patholog-

ical observations in fatal head injuries—a 5-year survey of 173 cases. Br J Surg 56:23, 1969.
91. Sevitt S. Fatal road accidents. Br J Surg 55:481, 1968.
92. Alcker GJ, Oh YS, Leslie EV. High cervical spine and craniocervical junction injuries in fatal traffic accidents. Orthop Clin North Am 9:1003, 1978.
93. Vogel FS. The anatomy of head trauma. Pathol Annu 6:321, 1971.
94. Gurdjian ES. Cerebral contusions: re-evaluation of the mechanism of their development. J Trauma 16:35, 1976.
95. Strich SJ. Cerebral trauma. In Blackwood W, Corsellis JAN, eds. Greenfield's Neuropathology, 3rd ed. London, Edward Arnold, 1976.
96. Gurdjian ES, Hodgson VR, Thomas LM, et al. Significance of relative movements of scalp, skull, and intracranial contents during impact injury of the head. J Neurosurg 29:70, 1968.
97. Ommaya AK. Mechanisms of cerebral concussion, contusions, and other effects of head injury. In Youmans JR. Neurological Surgery. Philadelphia, W.B. Saunders Co., 1982:1877.
98. Holbourn AHS. The mechanics of brain injuries. Br Med Bull 3:147, 1945.
99. Holbourn AHS. Mechanics of head injuries. Lancet 2:438, 1943.
100. Gomori JM, Grossman RI, Yu-Ip C, et al. NMR relaxation times of blood: dependence on field strength, oxidation state, and cell integrity. J Comput Assist Tomogr 11:684, 1987.
101. Dawson SL, Hirsch CS, Lucas FV, et al. The contrecoup phenomenon. Hum Pathol 11:155, 1980.
102. Pudenz RH, Shelden CH. The lucite calvarium—a method for direct observation of the brain. II. Cranial trauma and brain movement. J Neurosurg 3:487, 1946.
103. Goldsmith W. Biomechanics of head injury. In Fung YC, Perrone N, Anliker M, eds. Symposium on Biomechanics, Its Foundations and Objectives. New York, Prentice-Hall, 1970.
104. Lindenberg R, Freytag E. The mechanism of cerebral contusions. Arch Path 69:440, 1960.
105. Ommaya AK, Grubb RL, Naumann RA. Coup and contrecoup injury: observations on the mechanics of visible brain injuries in the rhesus monkey. J Neurosurg 35:503, 1971.
106. Lindenberg R. Trauma of meninges and brain. In Minckler J, ed. Pathology of the Nervous System. New York, McGraw-Hill Book Co., 1971.
107. Scatliff JH, Williams AL, Krigman MR, Whaley RA. CT recognition of subcortical hematomas. AJNR 2:49, 1981.
108. Zimmerman RA, Bilaniuk LT. Head trauma. In Rosenberg RN. The Clinical Neurosciences, Vol. 4. New York, Churchill Livingstone, 1984:483.
109. Miller JD, Becker DP. General principles and pathophysiology of head injury. In Youmans JR, ed. Neurological Surgery. Philadelphia, W.B. Saunders Co., 1982:1896.
110. Adams JH, Scott G, Parker LS, et al. The contusion index: a quantitative approach to cerebral contusions in head injury. Neuropathol Appl Neurobiol 6:319, 1980.
111. Adams JH, Graham DI, Murray LS, et al. Diffuse axonal injury due to nonmissile head injury in humans. Ann Neurol 12:557, 1982.
112. Winkler ML, Olsen WL, Mills TC, et al. Hemorrhagic and nonhemorrhagic brain lesions: evaluation with 0.35-T fast MR imaging. Radiology 165:203, 1987.
113. Symonds CP. Concussion and its sequelae. Lancet 1:1, 1962.
114. Ommaya AH, Gennarelli TA. Cerebral concussion and traumatic unconsciousness. Correlation of experimental and clinical observations of blunt head injuries. Brain 97:633, 1974.
115. Peerless SJ, Rewcastle NB. Shear injuries of the brain. Can Med Assoc J 96:577, 1966.
116. Lindenberg R, Fisher RS, Durlacher SH, et al. Lesions of the corpus callosum following blunt mechanical trauma to the head. Am J Pathol 31:297, 1955.
117. Gennarelli TA, Thibault LE, Adams JH, et al. Diffuse axonal injury and traumatic coma in the primate. Ann Neurol 12:564, 1982.
118. Gennarelli TA, Thibault LE. Biomechanics of head injury. In Wilkins RH, Rengachary SS, eds. Neurosurgery. New York, McGraw-Hill Book Co., 1985:1531.
119. Strich SJ. Shearing of nerve fibers as a cause of brain damage due to head injury. A pathological study of twenty cases. Lancet 2:443, 1961.
120. Strich SJ. Diffuse degeneration of the cerebral white matter in severe dementia following head injury. J Neurol Neurosurg Psychiatr 19:163, 1956.
121. Jennett B, Plum F. Persistent vegetative state after brain damage. Lancet 1:734, 1972.
122. Jellinger K, Seitelberger F. Protracted post-traumatic encephalopathy. Pathology, pathogenesis and clinical implications. J Neurol Sci 10:51, 1970.
123. Ommaya AK, Hirsch AE. Tolerances of cerebral concussion from head impact and whiplash in primates. J Biomech 4:13, 1971.
124. Ommaya AK, Faas F, Yarnell PR. Whiplash injury and brain damage: an experimental study. JAMA 204:285, 1968.
125. Jane JA, Steward, Gennarelli T. Axonal degeneration induced by experimental noninvasive minor head injury. J Neurosurg 62:96, 1985.
126. Oppenheimer DR. Microscopic lesions in the brain following head injury. J Neurol Neurosurg Psychiatry 31:299, 1968.
127. Parsons LC, Skinner M, Fitzgerald B, et al. Neurofiber degeneration in the brain of rats following a single cerebral concussion. Abstract. Soc Neurosci Abstr 6:12, 1980.
128. Nevin NC. Neuropathological changes in the white matter following head injury. J Neuropathol Exp Neurol 26:77, 1967.
129. Bakay L, Lee JC, Lee GC, et al. Experimental cerebral concussion. Part I: An electron microscopic study. J Neurosurg 47:525, 1977.
130. Brown WJ, Yoshida N, Canty T, et al. Experimental concussion. Ultrastructural and biochemical correlates. Am J Pathol 67:41, 1972.
131. Barth JT, Macciocchi SN, Giordani B, et al. Neuropsychological sequelae of minor head trauma. Neurosurgery 13:529, 1983.
132. Povlishock JT, Becker DP, Cheng CLY, et al. Axonal change in minor head injury. J Neuropathol Exp Neurol 42:225, 1983.
133. Gronwall D, Wrightson P. Cumulative effect of concussion. Lancet 2:995, 1975.
134. Gronwall D, Wrightson P. Delayed recovery of intellectual function after minor head injury. Lancet 2:605, 1974.
135. Rimel RW, Giordani B, Barth JT, et al. Disability caused by minor head injury. Neurosurgery 9:221, 1981.

136. Rimel RW, Giordani B, Barth JT, et al. Moderate head injury: completing the clinical spectrum of brain trauma. Neurosurgery 11:344, 1982.
137. Nauta WJH, Gygax PA. Silver impregnation of degenerating axons in the central nervous system: a modified technique. Stain Technol 29:91, 1954.
138. Adams JH, Mitchell DE, Graham DI, et al. Diffuse brain damage of immediate impact type. Its relationship to "primary brain stem damage" in head injury. Brain 100:489, 1977.
139. Mitchell DE, Adams JH. Primary focal impact damage to the brainstem in blunt head injuries—Does it exist? Lancet 2:215, 1973.
140. Jenkins A, Teasdale G, Hadley MDM, et al. Brain lesions detected by magnetic resonance imaging in mild and severe head injuries. Lancet 2:445, 1986.
141. Pilz P. Axonal injury in head injury. Acta Neurochir 32:119, 1983.
142. Levin HS, Handel SF, Goldman AM, et al. Magnetic resonance imaging after 'diffuse' nonmissile head injury. Arch Neurol 42:963, 1985.
143. Stebhans WE. Pathology of the Cerebral Blood Vessels. St. Louis, C. V. Mosby, 1972:284.
144. Hecht-Leavitt C, Gomori JM, Grossman RI, et al. High-field MRI of hemorrhagic cortical infarction. AJNR 7:581, 1986.
145. Young HA, Gleave JRW, Schmidek HH, et al. Delayed traumatic intracerebral hematoma: report of 15 cases operatively treated. Neurosurgery 14:22, 1984.
146. Ninchoji T, Uemura K, Shimoyama I, et al. Traumatic intracerebral hematoma of delayed onset. Acta Neurochir 71:69, 1984.
147. Fukamachi A, Kohno K, Wakao T, et al. Traumatic intracerebral hematomas. A classification according to dynamic changes on sequential CTs. Neurol Med Chir 19:1039, 1979.
148. Freytag E. Fatal hypertensive intracerebral hematomas. A survey of 393 cases. J Neurol Neurosurg Psychiatr 31:616, 1968.
149. Mutlu N, Berry RG, Alpers BJ. Massive cerebral hemorrhage: clinical and pathologic correlations. Arch Neurol 8:644, 1963.
150. Kishore PRS, Lipper MH, Domingues da Silva AA, et al. Delayed sequelae of head injury. CT 4:287, 1980.
151. Ramamurthi B. Acute subdural haematoma. In Vinken PJ, Bruyn GW, eds. Handbook of Clinical Neurology. Injuries of the Brain and Skull. Part II. Vol. 24. New York, Elsevier Scientific Publishing Co., 1976:275.
152. Bakay L, Glasauer FE. Head Injury. Boston: Little, Brown & Co., 1980:197.
153. Decker DP, Miller JD, Young HF, et al. Diagnosis and treatment of head injury in adults. In Youmans JR, ed. Neurological Surgery, Vol. 4. Philadelphia, W. B. Saunders Co., 1982:1938.
154. Hardman JM. Cerebrospinal Trauma. In Davis RL, Robertson DM, eds. Textbook of Neuropathology. Baltimore, Williams & Wilkins, 1985:842.
155. McKissock W, Richardson A, Bloom WH. Subdural hæmatoma. A review of 389 cases. Lancet 1:1365, 1960.
156. Maloney AFJ, Whatmore WJ. Clinical and pathological observations in fatal head injuries: a 5-year survey of 173 cases. Br J Surg 56:23, 1969.
157. Freytag E. Autopsy findings in head injuries from blunt forces. Arch Path 75:402, 1963.
158. Wintzen AR. The clinical course of subdural hæmatoma. A retrospective study of ætiological, chronological and pathological features in 212 patients and a proposed classification. Brain 103:855, 1980.
159. Echlin FA, Sordillo SV, Garvey TQ, Jr. Acute, subacute, and chronic subdural hæmatoma. JAMA 161:1345, 1956.
160. Rao BD. A critical review of 250 consecutive acute head injuries in Hyderabad. Proc Acad Med Sci 1:122, 1959.
161. Rao BD, Subramaniam MV, Reddy MVR, et al. Mortality in acute head injuries. Neurol India 15:1, 1967.
162. Jain SP, Kankanady VD. A study of 1500 cases of head injury in Delhi. J Indian Med Assoc 52:204, 1969.
163. Kalyanaraman S, Ramamurthi B, Ramamoorthy K, et al. Acute and subacute subdural hematoma. Neurol India 18:18, 1970.
164. Harris P. Acute traumatic subdural hematomas. In Head Injuries. Proceedings of an International Symposium. London, Churchill Livingstone, 1971:321.
165. Rosenørn J, Gjerris F. Long-term follow-up review of patients with acute and subacute subdural hematomas. J Neurosurg 48:345, 1978.
166. Rosenbluth PR, Arias B, Quartetti EV, et al. Current management of subdural hematoma. JAMA 179:756, 1962.
167. Munro D. Cerebral subdural haematomas. A study of three hundred and ten verified cases. N Engl J Med 227:87, 1942.
168. Hesselbrock R, Sawaya R, Means ED. Acute spontaneous subdural hematoma. Surg Neurol 21:363, 1984.
169. Ciembroniewicz JE. Subdural hematoma of the posterior fossa. J Neurosurg 22:465, 1965.
170. Fisher RG, Kim JK, Sachs E Jr. Complications in the posterior fossa due to occipital trauma—their operability. JAMA 167:176, 1958.
171. Miles J, Medlery AV. Posterior fossa subdural hematomas. J Neurol Neurosurg Psychiatr 37:1373, 1974.
172. Tsai FY, Teal JS, Itabashi HH, et al. Computed tomography of posterior fossa trauma. JCAT 4:291, 1980.
173. Vielvoye GJ, Peters ACB, van Dulken H. Acute infratentorial traumatic subdural hematoma associated with a torn tentorium cerebelli in a one-year-old boy. Neuroradiology 22:259, 1982.
174. Glista GG, Reichman H, Brumlik J, Fine M. Interhemispheric subdural hematoma. Surg Neurol 10:119, 1978.
175. Clein LJ, Bolton CF. Interhemispheric subdural hematoma. Case report. J Neurol Neurosurg Psychiatr 32:389, 1969.
176. Fein JM, Rovit RJ. Interhemispheric subdural hematoma secondary to hemorrhage from a callosomarginal artery aneurysm. Neuroradiology 1:183, 1970.
177. Gannon WE. Interhemispheric subdural hematoma. Case report. J Neurosurg 18:829, 1961.
178. Ho SU, Spehlmann R, Ho HT. CT scan in interhemispheric subdural hematoma: clinical and pathological correlation. Neurology 27:1097, 1977.
179. Jacobsen HH. An interhemispherically situated hematoma. Case report. Acta Radiol 43:235, 1955.

180. Sibayan RQ, Gurdjian ES, Thomas LM. Interhemispheric chronic subdural hematoma. Case report. Neurology 20:1215, 1970.
181. Wollschlaeger PB, Wollschlaeger G. The interhemispheric subdural or falx hematoma. AJR 92:1252, 1964.
182. Anderson FM. Subdural hematoma, a complication of operation for hydrocephalus. Pediatrics 10:11, 1952.
183. Davidoff LM, Feiring EH. Subdural hematoma occurring in surgically treated hydrocephalic children. J Neurosurg 10:557, 1953.
184. Foltz EL, Shurtleff DB. Five-year comparative study of hydrocephalus in children with and without operation. J Neurosurg 20:1064, 1963.
185. Becker DP, Nulsen FE. Control of hydrocephalus by valve-regulated venous shunt. Avoidance of complications in prolonged shunt maintenance. J Neurosurg 28:215, 1968.
186. Forrest DM, Cooper DGW. Complications of ventriculoatrial shunts. A review of 455 cases. J Neurosurg 29:506, 1968.
187. Illingworth RD. Subdural hematoma after the treatment of chronic hydrocephalus by ventriculocaval shunts. J Neurol Neurosurg Psychiatr 33:95, 1970.
188. Becker DP, Miller JD, Ward JD, et al. The outcome from severe head injury with early diagnosis and intensive management. J Neurosurg 47:491, 1977.
189. Clarke E, Walton JN. Subdural hæmatoma complicating intracranial aneurysm and angioma. Brain 76:378, 1953.
190. Russell DS, Cairns H. Subdural false membrane or hæmatoma (pachymeningitis interna hemorrhagica) in carcinomatosis and sarcomatosis of the dura mater. Brain 57:32, 1934.
191. Turner DM, Graf CJ. Nontraumatic subdural hematoma secondary to dural metastasis. Case report and review of the literature. Neurosurg 11:678, 1982.
192. McDermott M, Fleming JFR, Vanderlinden RG, Tucker WS. Spontaneous arterial subdural hematoma. Neurosurg 14:13, 1984.
193. Silverstein A. Intracranial bleeding in hæmophilia. Arch Neurol 3:141, 1960.
194. Wiener LM, Nathanson M. The relationship of subdural hematoma to anticoagulant therapy. Arch Neurol 6:282, 1962.
195. Zenteno-Alanis GH, Corvera J, Mateos JH. Subdural hematoma of the posterior fossa as a complication of anticoagulant therapy. Presentation of a case. Neurology 18:1133, 1968.
196. Capistrant T, Goldberg R, Shibasaki H, et al. Posterior fossa subdural hematoma associated with anticoagulant therapy. J Neurol Neurosurg Psychiatr 34:82, 1971.
197. Leonard CD, Weil E, Scribner BH. Subdural hematomas in patients undergoing hæmodialysis. Lancet 2:239, 1969.
198. Zarowny DP, Rose I. Acute subdural hematoma during maintenance hæmodialysis. Can Med Assoc J 103:634, 1970.
199. Schlang HA, Carmichael AH, Freund CJ. Spontaneous subdural hematoma in anticoagulant therapy. Am Pract 13:247, 1962.
200. Schiefer W, Tonnis D. Subdural hæmatoma following hæmorrhage from aneurysms and angiomas. Zbl Neurochir 19:329, 1959, cited in Ramamurthi B. Acute subdural haematoma. In Vinken PJ, Bruyn GW, eds. Handbook of Clinical Neurology. Injuries of the Brain and Skull. Part II. Vol. 24. New York, Elsevier Scientific Publishing Co., 1976:275.
201. King AB. Successful surgical treatment of an intracranial mycotic aneurysm complicated by a subdural hæmatoma. J Neurosurg 17:788, 1960.
202. Gennarelli TA, Bilaniuk LE. Biomechanics of acute subdural hematoma. J Trauma 22:680, 1982.
203. Ommaya AK, Yarnell P. Subdural hematoma after whiplash injury. Lancet 2:237, 1969.
204. Dublin AB, French BN, Rennick JM. Computed tomography in head trauma. Radiology 122:365, 1977.
205. Zimmerman RA, Bilaniuk LT, Gennarelli TA, et al. Cranial computed tomography in diagnosis and management of acute head trauma. AJR 131:27, 1978.
206. Reed D, Robertson WD, Graeb DA, et al. Acute subdural hematomas: atypical CT findings. AJNR 7:417, 1986.
207. Braun J, Borovich B, Guilburd JN, et al. Acute subdural hematoma mimicking epidural hematoma on CT. AJNR 8:171, 1987.
208. Cornell SH, Chiu LC, Christie JH. Diagnosis of extracerebral fluid collections by computed tomography. AJR 131:107, 1978.
209. Forbes GS, Sheedy PF, Piepgras DG, et al. Computed tomography in the evaluation of subdural hematomas. Radiology 126:143, 1978.
210. French BN, Dublin AB. The value of computed tomography in the management of 1000 consecutive head injuries. Surg Neurol 7:171, 1977.
211. Koo AH, LaRoque RL. Evaluation of head trauma by computed tomography. Radiology 123:345, 1977.
212. Lipper MH, Kishore PRS, Girevendulis AK, et al. Delayed intracranial hematoma in patients with severe head injury. Radiology 133:645, 1979.
213. Peyster RG, Hoover ED. CT in head trauma. J Trauma 22:25, 1982.
214. Paxton R, Ambrose J. The EMI scanner. A brief review of the first 650 patients. Br J Radiol 47:530, 1974.
215. Klun B, Fettich M. Factors influencing the outcome in acute subdural hæmatomas. Acta Neurochir 71:171, 1984.
216. Cantore GP, Delfini R, Neri L. Contribution to the surgical treatment of acute supratentorial subdural hæmatomas. Acta Neurochir 41:349, 1978.
217. Hernesniemi J. Outcome following acute subdural hæmatoma. Acta Neurochir 49:191, 1979.
218. Jamieson KG. Extradural and subdural hematoma. J Neurosurg 33:632, 1970.
219. Jamieson KG, Yelland JDW. Surgically treated traumatic subdural hematomas. J Neurosurg 37:137, 1972.
220. McLaurin RL, Tutor FT. Acute subdural hematoma: review of ninety cases. J Neurosurg 18:61, 1961.
221. Richards T, Hoff J. Factors affecting survival from acute subdural hematoma. Surgery 75:253, 1974.
222. Roberson FC, Kishore PRS, Miller JD, et al. The value of serial computerized tomography in the management of severe head injury. Surg Neurol 12:161, 1979.
223. Seelig JM, Becker DP, Miller JD, et al. Traumatic acute subdural hematoma. N Engl J Med 304:1511, 1981.

224. Dolinskas CA, Zimmerman RA, Bilaniuk LT, et al. Computed tomography of post-traumatic extracerebral hematomas: comparison to pathophysiology and responses to therapy. J Trauma 19:163, 1979.
225. Talalla A, Morin MA. Acute traumatic subdural hematoma: a review of 100 consecutive cases. J Trauma 11:771, 1971.
226. Sadik AR, Adachi M, Ransohoff J. Rupture of an intracranial aneurysm within the subdural space in association with trauma. A case report. J Neurosurg 20:609, 1963.
227. Drake CG. Subdural hematoma from arterial rupture. J Neurosurg 18:597, 1961.
228. O'Brien PK, Norris JW, Tator CH. Acute subdural hematomas of arterial origin. J Neurosurg 41:435, 1974.
229. Rengachary SS, Szymanski DC. Subdural hematomas of arterial origin. Neurosurg 8:166, 1981.
230. Shenkin HA. Acute subdural hematoma. J Neurosurg 57:254, 1982.
231. Williams B. Subdural hematoma of arterial origin. Lancet 1:1074, 1971.
232. George AE, Russell EJ, Kricheff II. White matter buckling: CT sign of extraaxial intracranial mass. AJR 135:1031, 1980.
233. Amendola MA, Ostrum BJ. Diagnosis of isodense subdural hematomas by computed tomography. AJR 129:693, 1977.
234. Hackery DB, Atlas SW, Grossman RI, et al. Subacute intracranial hemorrhage: contribution of spin density to appearance on spin-echo MR images. Radiology 165:199, 1987.
235. Zimmerman RA. Massachusetts General Hospital Neuroradiology Review Course. September 1986.
236. Bradley WG. Pathophysiologic correlates of signal alterations. In Brant-Zawadzki M, Norman D, eds. MRI of the Central Nervous System. New York, Raven Press, 1987:23.
237. Young IR, Bydder GM, Hall AS, et al. Extracerebral collections: recognition by NMR imaging. AJNR 4:833, 1983.
238. Moon KL, Brant-Zawadzki M, Pitts LH, et al. Nuclear magnetic resonance imaging of CT-isodense subdural hematomas. AJNR 5:319, 1984.
239. Scotti G, Terbrugge K, Melancon D, et al. Evaluation of the age of subdural hematomas by computerized tomography. J Neurosurg 47:311, 1977.
240. Kim KS, Hemmati M, Weinberg PE. Computed tomography in isodense subdural hematoma. Radiology 128:71, 1978.
241. Möller A, Ericson K. Computed tomography of isoattenuating subdural hematomas. Radiology 130:149, 1979.
242. So SC. Chronic subdural hæmatoma in the elderly. Austr NZ J Surg 46:166, 1976.
243. Richter HP, Klein HJ, Schäfer M. Chronic subdural hæmatomas treated by enlarged burr-hole craniotomy and closed-system drainage: retrospective study of 120 patients. Acta Neurochir 71:179, 1984.
244. Noltie K, Denham MJ. Subdural hæmatoma in the elderly. Age Ageing 10:241, 1981.
245. Friede RL, Schachenmayr W. The origin of subdural neomembranes. II. Fine structure of neomembranes. Am J Pathol 92:69, 1978.
246. Adams JH. Neuropathology of head injuries. In Vinken PJ, Bruyn GW, eds. Handbook of Clinical Neurology. Injuries of the Brain and Skull. Part I. Vol. 23. New York, Elsevier Scientific Publishing Co., 1976:23.
247. Clare FB, Bell HS. Extradural hematomas. JAMA 177:887, 1961.
248. Sachs J, Sachs E Jr. A simple formula for calculating the volume of subdural hematomas. Neurosurgery 1:60, 1977.
249. Van Gijn J, Wintzen AR. Whiplash injury and subdural hæmatoma. Lancet 2:592, 1969.
250. Cameron MM. Chronic subdural hematoma: A review of 114 cases. J Neurol Neurosurg Psychiatr 41:834, 1978.
251. Fogelholm R, Heiskanen O, Waltimo O. Chronic subdural hematoma in adults: influence of patient's age on symptoms, signs, and thickness of hematoma. J Neurosurg 42:43, 1975.
252. Luxon LM, Harrison MJG. Chronic subdural hematoma. QJ Med 48:43, 1979.
253. Loew F, Kivelitz R. Chronic subdural hæmatomas. In Vinken PJ, Bruyn GW, eds. Handbook of Clinical Neurology. Injuries of the Brain and Skull. Part II. Vol. 24. New York, Elsevier Publishing Co., 1976:297.
254. Rashkind R, Glover MB, Weiss SR. Chronic subdural hæmatoma in the elderly: a challenge in diagnosis and treatment. J Am Geriatr Soc 20:330, 1972.
255. Browder J. A resume of the principal diagnostic features of subdural hematoma. Bull NY Acad Med 19:168, 1943.
256. Bender MB. Resolution of subdural hematoma. Trans Amer Neurol Assoc 85:192, 1960.
257. Gannon WE, Cook AW, Browder EJ. Resolving subdural collections. J Neurosurg 19:865, 1962.
258. Winestock DP, Spetzler RF, Hoff JT. Acute, post-traumatic subdural hygroma. Neuroradiology 115:373, 1975.
259. Oka H, Motomochi M, Suzuki Y, et al. Subdural hygroma after head injury. A review of 26 cases. Acta Neurochir 26:265, 1972.
260. Masuzawa T, Kumagai M, Sato F. Computed tomographic evolution of post-traumatic subdural hygroma in young adults. Neuroradiology 26:245, 1984.
261. Jamieson KG, Yelland JDN. Extradural hematoma: report of 167 cases. J Neurosurg 29:13, 1968.
262. McKissok W, Taylor JC, Bloom WH, et al. Extradural hæmatoma. Observations on 125 patients. Lancet 2:167, 1960.
263. Frank E, Berger TS, Tew JM. Bilateral epidural hematomas. Surg Neurol 17:218, 1982.
264. Cordobes F, Lobato RD, Rivas JJ, et al. Observations on 82 patients with extradural hematoma. J Neurosurg 54:179, 1981.
265. Hirsh LF. Chronic epidural hematomas. Neurosurg 6:508, 1980.
266. Jamieson KG. Epidural hæmatoma. In Vinken PJ, Bruyn GW, eds. Handbook of Clinical Neurology. Injuries of the Brain and Skull. Part II. Vol. 24. New York, Elsevier Scientific Publishing Co., 1976:261.
267. Mathur PPS, Dharker SR, Agarwall SK, et al. Fluid chronic extradural hæmatoma. Surg Neurol 14:81, 1980.
268. Parkinson D, Reddy V, Taylor J. Ossified epidural hematoma: case report. Neurosurg 7:171, 1980.
269. Phonprasert C, Suwanwela C, Hongsaprabhas C, et al. Extradural hematoma: analysis of 138 cases. J Trauma 20:679, 1980.

270. Galbraith SL. Age distribution of extradural hæmorrhage without skull fracture. Lancet 1:1217, 1973.
271. Gallagher JP, Browder EJ. Extradural hematoma: experience with 167 patients. J Neurosurg 29:1, 1968.
272. Josephson S. Epidural hæmatoma. A 10-year series. Acta Chir Scand 124:26, 1962.
273. Kvarnes TL, Trumpy JH. Extradural hæmatoma. Report of 132 cases. Acta Neurochir 41:223, 1978.
274. Ford LE, McLaurin RL. Mechanisms of extradural hematomas. J Neurosurg 20:760, 1963.
275. McLaurin RL, Ford LE. Extradural hematoma. Statistical survey of 47 cases. J Neurosurg 21:364, 1964.
276. Iwakuma T, Brunngraber CV. Chronic extradural hematomas. J Neurosurg 38:488, 1973.
277. Borzone M, Gentile S, Perria C, et al. Vertex epidural hematomas. Surg Neurol 11:277, 1979.
278. MacCarty CS, Horning ED, Weaver EN. Bilateral extradural hematoma. J Neurosurg 5:88, 1948.
279. Maurer JJ, Mayfield FH. Acute bilateral extradural hematomas. J Neurosurg 23:63, 1965.
280. Gurdjian ES. Recent advances in the study of the mechanism of impact injury of the head. A summary. Clin Neurol 19:1, 1972.
281. Hooper R. Observations on extradural hæmorrhage. Br J Surg 47:71, 1959.
282. Bullock R, Van Dellen JR. Chronic extradural hematoma. Surg Neurol 18:300, 1982.
283. Pozzati E, Frank F, Frank G, Gaist G. Subacute and chronic extradural hematomas: A study of 30 cases. J Trauma 20:795, 1980.
284. Kemperman CJF, den Hartog MR, Thijssen HOM. Spontaneous resolution of epidural hematomas detected after the first day. Ann Neurol 16:623, 1984.
285. Illingworth R, Shawdon H. Conservative management of intracranial extradural hematoma presenting late. J Neurol Neurosurg Psychiatr 46:558, 1982.
286. Weaver D, Pobereskin L, Jane JA. Spontaneous resolution of epidural hematomas: report of two cases. J Neurosurg 54:248, 1981.
287. Clavel M, Onzain I, Gutierrez F. Chronic epidural hæmatomas. Acta Neurochir 66:71, 1982.
288. Zimmerman RA, Bilaniuk LT. Computed tomographic staging of traumatic epidural bleeding. Radiology 144:809, 1982.
289. Handa J, Handa H, Nakano Y. Rim enhancement in computed tomography with chronic epidural hematoma. Surg Neurol 11:217, 1979.
290. Levin HS, Amparo E, Eisenberg HM, et al. Magnetic resonance imaging and computerized tomography in relation to the neurobehavioral sequelae of mild and moderate head injuries. J Neurosurg 66:706, 1987.
291. Casson IR, Siegel O, Sham R, et al. Brain damage in modern boxers. JAMA 251:2663, 1984.
292. Lampert PW, Hardman JM. Morphological changes in brains of modern boxers. JAMA 251:2676, 1984.
293. Cohen MD, McGuire W, Cory DA, Smith JA. MR appearance of blood and blood products: An in vitro study. AJR 146:1293, 1986.
294. Fabry ME, San George RC. Effect of magnetic susceptibility on nuclear magnetic resonance signals arising from red cells: a warning. Biochemistry 22:4119, 1983.
295. Fabry ME, Eisenstadt M. Water exchange across red cell membranes: II. Measurement by nuclear magnetic resonance $T_1$, $T_2$, and $T_{12}$ hybrid relaxation. The effects of osmolarity, cell volume, and medium. J Membr Biol 42:375, 1978.
296. Fabry ME. Personal Communication. September 1987.
297. Gentry LR, Godersky JC, Thompson B. MR imaging of head trauma: review of the distribution and radiopathologic features of traumatic lesions. AJNR 9:101, 1988.
298. Gentry LR, Godersky JC, Thompson B, et al. Prospective comparative study of intermediate-field MR and CT in the evaluation of closed head trauma. AJNR 9:91, 1988.
299. Gomori JM, Grossman RI, Hackney DB, et al. Variable appearances of subacute intracranial hematomas on high-field spin-echo MR. AJR 150:171, 1988.
300. Zimmerman RD, Heier LA, Snow RB, et al. Acute intracranial hemorrhage: intensity changes on sequential MR scans at 0.5 T. AJR 50:651, 1988.

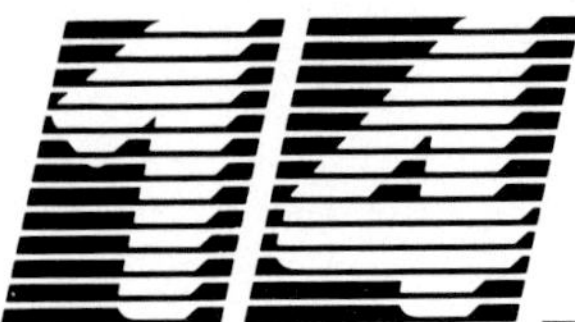

Buckley terPenning, M.D.

# INFLAMMATORY DISEASE OF THE BRAIN AND SPINE

Central nervous system inflammation is still associated with a high degree of morbidity and mortality. Early diagnosis by computerized tomography (CT) and antibiotic administration that is directed by refined culture and sensitivity techniques have done the most to bring about a reduction in mortality to 5% to 10% from 40% to 60% just one decade ago.[1–4] Improvement in the prognosis of CNS inflammation has not changed the incidence of these diseases nor met the increased burden of iatrogenic and acquired immunodeficiency states. Magnetic resonance imaging (MRI) is being investigated as a modality to provide increased sensitivity in the detection of CNS lesions and as a complementary tool to computed tomography.

*Otomastoiditis* is detectable by MR (Fig. 14–1). Normally, mastoid air cells are hypointense and devoid of signal, since they are aerated and air lacks mobile hydrogen protons. The high proton density of proteinaceous fluid and its water content produce intermediate or mildly increased T1-weighted image (T1WI) signal intensity and markedly increased T2-weighted image (T2WI) hyperintensity. CT remains the modality of choice in otomastoid inflammation owing to its superiority in detection of bone involvement or osteomyelitis, cholesteatoma, and status of the fine anatomy of the middle ear.

Inflammatory lesions of the brain, meninges, and associated structures are characterized by T1 and T2 relaxation prolongation

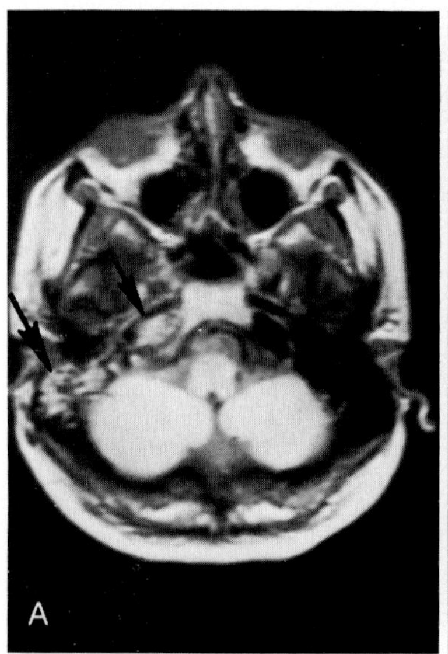



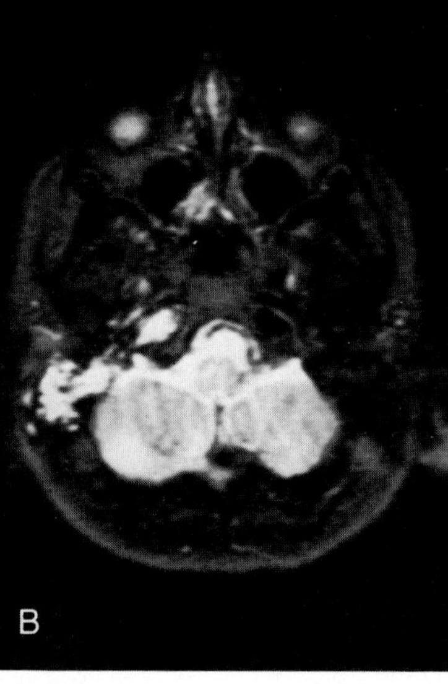



**Figure 14–1. Otomastoiditis and petrositis.** A patient who presented with Gradenigo's syndrome illustrates right-sided serous otitis (large arrow) and apical petrositis (small arrow) (1.5 T). *A,* Axial N(H)WI (TR 2300/TE 20 msec). The mastoid air cells are normally hypointense owing to proton-deficient air; proton-rich fluid has accumulated in this patient's mastoids as a result of inflammation. The mastoid fluid is also hyperintense to CSF seen in basal cisterns. This suggests a shorter T1 than that of CSF, implying that the fluid is moderately proteinaceous. *B,* T2WI (TR 2300/TE 100 msec) shows the similar intensity of the T2 signal of the collection with CSF. (Courtesy of S. J. Pomeranz, M.D., Christ Hospital, Cincinnati, Ohio.)

on MR, seen as hypointensity on T1WI and hyperintensity on T2WI. This appearance is analogous to inflammation elsewhere in the body and has been correlated with blood-brain barrier (BBB) disruption and influx of both intracellular and extracellular fluid. Hemorrhagic inflammatory lesions, not uncommon, are an exception to this rule. Acute or subacute hemorrhage may shorten T1 and T2 relaxation times, thereby making a lesion more hyperintense on T1WI and more hypointense on T2WI.[5] In addition, spin density, N(H)WI, MR images may miss inflammatory lesions since the bright T2 and darker T1 signal contributions cancel out. The extent of signal alteration, and in many cases tissue reaction, depends on the immunocompetency of the patient. Immunocompromised patients do not manifest the same degree of inflammation seen in immunocompetent individuals with the same degree of CNS infection.[6]

Almost any mass effect or extra-axial collection seen on CT can be visualized with MR. This is particularly true at the skull base and cerebral convexities, where beam hardening obscures brain parenchymal visualization on CT. The superior contrast resolution of MR may provide earlier detection of inflammatory foci when compared with CT. In addition, retardation of normal myelination of the brain can be seen in MR of young children with encephalitis or meningitis.[7] Nonetheless, a major disadvantage of MR is its limited capability to detect calcification. Most calcifications appear hypointense on MR owing to their low mobile proton content. This hypointensity is more conspicuous on T2WI or fast-field MR. Calcification is a marker and frequent sequela of inactive chronic inflammatory disease.

## INFECTIONS

### Bacterial Infections

Epidural empyema is most often caused by paranasal sinusitis and also often results from mastoiditis. In this condition, pus formed beneath the inner table of the skull strips away the dural membrane from its adherence to the bone as the abscess grows between the two. The frontal pole is the most frequent location. Subdural empyema, in contrast, most frequently occurs over the convexity of one or both hemispheres 80% of the time, with interhemispheric and basal collections occurring less frequently. The route of subdural infection is most likely to be retrograde progression through emissary veins, often from paranasal sinusitis.[5–8]

CT reveals both types of empyemas as lenticular low-density areas surrounded by an enhancing rim. Medial rim enhancement is likely to be thick in the case of epidural empyema since the inflamed meninges bordering the medial aspect of the abscess readily enhance and are contrasted by two neighboring low-attenuation areas, empyema and cerebrospinal fluid (CSF). The overlying skull may show erosions. Subdural empyema is less likely to have an enhancing border; the enhancing meninges are adherent to high attenuation bone, and the underlying brain tissue may appear normal unless infected. Occasionally, subdural empyema may assume a crescentic shape. Mass effect upon adjacent parenchyma and ventricles is greater in subdural than in epidural empyema since the dura compresses the collection of epidural abscess.[9] Fluid or soft tissue may fill neighboring osseous sinus in both instances. The variability of these often subtle findings has prompted some to assert that there are no clear distinguishing features between subdural and epidural empyema on CT.[8]

The lenticular shapes of epidural and subdural empyema are also apparent on MRI.[4, 10] The pus collections in epidural and subdural empyema both appear dark on T1 and bright on T2 images compared with neighboring brain tissue. However, signal intensity is usually not as hypointense on T1 or as hyperintense on T2 images as CSF because the cellular debris in abscess cavities in general shortens relaxation values with respect to CSF.[10] This difference allows empyemas to be distinguished from CSF collections in most cases. Still, an epidural empyema may have signal characteristics quite similar to CSF (Fig. 14–2). The brain underlying empyema may lose corticomedullary definition: MRI has demonstrated reduced contrast between subjacent gray and white matter on T1WI in two published cases of subdural empyema; this is believed to be due to edema of brain parenchyma neighboring the subdural empyema with resultant diminution of the T1 difference between gray and white matter.[4]

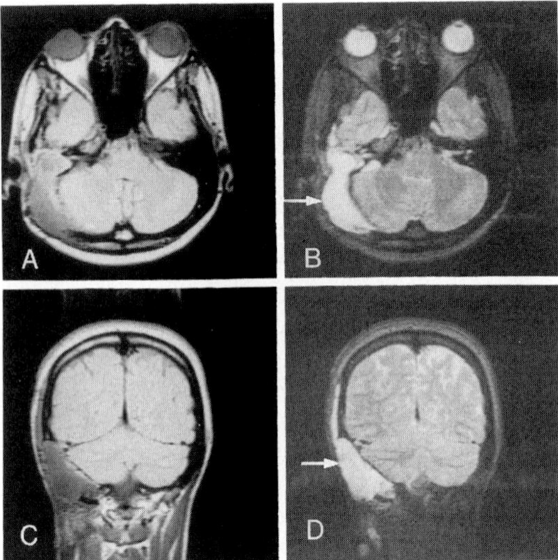


**Figure 14–2. Epidural empyema.** Epidural empyema (arrow) occurred at the site of a posterolateral craniectomy (1.5 T). *A* and *B*, Axial N(H)WI (TR 2200/TE 20 msec) and T2WI (TR 2200/TE 100 msec). The abscess is not confined by bone and is bulging the soft tissues outward. *C* and *D,* Coronal N(H)WI and T2WI show mass effect upon the subjacent cerebellum with no evidence of parenchymal inflammation. The lesion (arrow) has similar but not identical signal intensity to that of CSF within cisterns on all acquisitions. (Courtesy of S. J. Pomeranz, M.D., Christ Hospital, Cincinnati, Ohio.)

Suppurative meningitis is the most frequent cause of meningeal inflammation. In the early stages, inflammation is limited to the membranes, and CT may be normal, may show increased contrast enhancement of meninges, or may show gyral enhancement of subjacent cortex. Advanced disease may lead to diffuse brain swelling, focal edema, cerebral infarct owing to thrombosis, hydrocephalus, or cerebritis. The late stages are usually seen on CT as focal or diffuse ventricular dilatation, mass effect, or focal or diffuse parenchymal low attenuation due to infarct or edema caused by vasculitis. Subdural effusions are common in *Haemophilus influenzae* meningitis.[6, 11]

N(H)WI images of infectious meningitis show a thin rim of high signal arising from the inflamed leptomeninges (Fig. 14–3). Meningeal carcinomatosis would have a similar MR appearance and exhibits T1WI signal hyperintensity with CEMR. Subarachnoid hemorrhage exhibits bright signal on N(H)WI but would also appear hyperintense on T1WI in subacute or chronic stages, whereas the T1-weighted images of infectious meningitis are often unremarkable or hypointense.[12, 13] Image acquisition technique is important in any suspected meningeal disease because of the need to discriminate the bright T2 signal of inflamed leptomeninges from the overpowering T2 signal of the adjacent CSF. This is efficiently accomplished through judicious selection of TE and TR parameters. N(H)WI images may allow discrimination between edematous tissue and CSF. The signal contributions to N(H)WI images have been discussed in detail.[14]

Cerebral inflammation may appear as focal cerebritis, diffuse encephalitis, or as abscess. Abscesses occur more commonly than subdural or epidural empyemas, and they are frequently found in young males; their peak incidence is in the third decade.[1, 17] Abscesses develop from necrotic areas of cerebritis, most commonly caused by direct extension (usually venous) but also from penetrating trauma or from arterial seeding. A recent series of 26 cases of CSF empyema reported concomitant cerebral abscesses, proven in 23% of patients and suspected in another 3%. Predisposing sinusitis was present in 50% and otitis in 15%.[8] One large series reported a predominance of temporal lobe abscesses with otitis media, a common

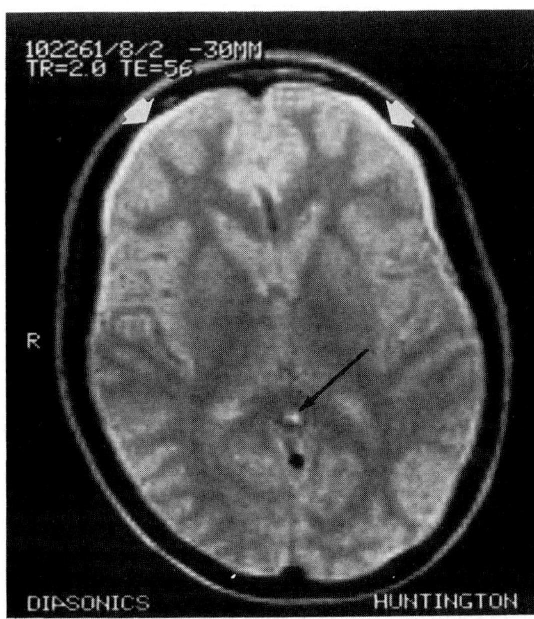


**Figure 14–3. Infectious meningitis.** Intermediate T2WI (TR 2000/TE 56 msec). A thin rim of high signal arises from the leptomeninges that surround the frontal lobes (white arrows), cerebellum, and brain stem. The pineal cistern also appears involved (long black arrow). Meningeal carcinomatosis would have a similar appearance. (From Bradley WG. Neurol Res 6:91–106, 1984, with permission.)

predisposing infection. In frontal lobe abscesses, one third of cases had underlying sinusitis.[15]

Arterial seeding often occurs at the corticomedullary junction, whereas venous seeding often involves subcortical white matter, which is relatively hypovascular. This supports the theory that a necrotic nidus is often the matrix for abscess development.[15, 16] Arterial seeding most often results from cyanotic heart disease with right to left shunting, and usually produces a solitary abscess, whereas all other causes of arterial seeding most frequently result in multiple abscesses.[16]

Abscesses appear on nonenhanced CT to have low-attenuation centers with a rim of slightly higher attenuation than surrounding uninvolved brain; the rim markedly enhances on contrast-enhanced CT (CECT) while the center remains lower density. The center often shows enhancement on delayed images. The rim-enhancing characteristic can also appear in the late cerebritis stage before an abscess cavity is present histologically. The rim is usually thin, uniform, and attenuated on its white matter origin, a finding that is sometimes useful in differentiating abscess from neoplasm. Mass effect is seen in the presence of both cerebritis and abscess, and may help differentiate the inflammatory process from cortical infarct on CT. Besides abscess, the CT appearance of enhancing rings with low to isointense centers may be seen in cerebral hematoma, infarct, or neoplasm.

Ventriculitis or ependymitis is the inflammation of the ventricular mural tissue and can be due to rupture of a periventricular abscess, ascending inflammation from basal cisterns to the fourth ventricle, or ventricular catheterization (Fig. 14–4). Unenhanced CT images may appear normal if ventricular debris and hydrocephalus are absent. Thin, uniform enhancement of ventricular lining is often seen on CECT images. Purulent or necrotic material is seen as medium attenuation within the posterior ventricles in a CECT tomogram taken during the acute phase of ventriculitis. The signal from intraventricular debris will stand out starkly against normal CSF signal on both T1WI and T2WI. The inflamed ventricular membranes show hyperintense T2 signal intensity.

The CT appearance of encephalitis is most often a subtle, poorly defined area of low attenuation. Encephalitis may appear on CECT as irregular patchy areas of both gray and white matter enhancement in the areas involved.[17] Both appearances are nonspecific but have served as an early localization for further diagnostic evaluation. In the past, this has been radionuclide imaging, angiography, or electroencephalography, but current practice is to obtain MRI if the patient's condition permits.

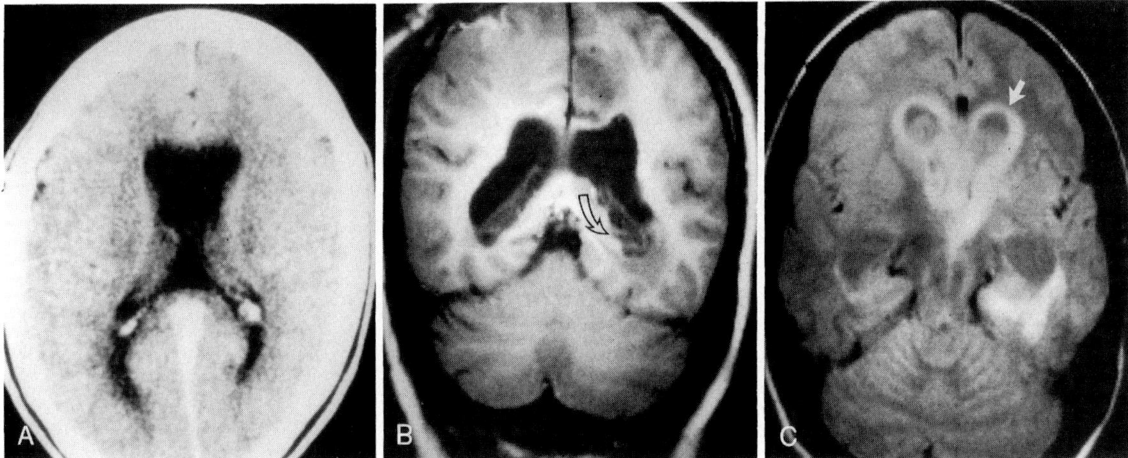


**Figure 14–4.** ***Proteus* ventriculitis.** *A,* Axial CECT shows intermediate attenuation in the posterior aspect of the lateral ventricles in a middle-aged woman who developed headache and fever following Omaya reservoir placement. *B,* Coronal T1WI illustrates intermediate signal layering in the dependent portion of the lateral ventricular atria (curved arrow). *C,* Axial T2WI demonstrates an intraventricular signal that differs from the normal homogeneous hyperintensity of CSF with an adjacent ependymal and periventricular signal hyperintensity (arrow). (Courtesy of S. Schlesinger, M.D., New York University Hospital, New York, N.Y.)

The brain abscess cavity appears on T1WI as an area of low or rarely isointense signal with respect to brain (Figs. 14–5 and 14–6).[18–20] The signal characteristics are similar to those of empyema.[4] The surrounding brain parenchyma has diminished T1 signal owing to edema. The increased T2 signal in the surrounding brain parenchyma is more

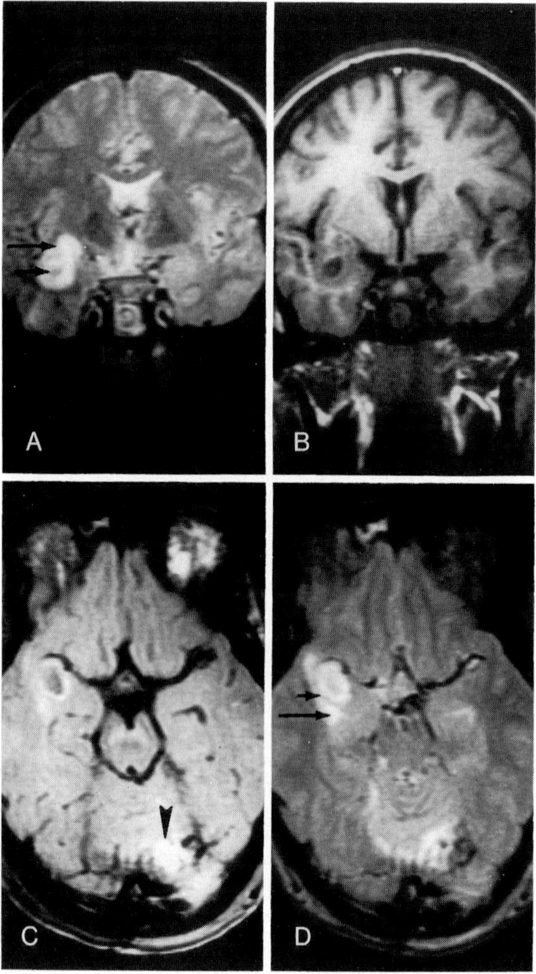

**Figure 14–5. Temporal lobe abscess.** A young man with severe sphenoid sinusitis after instrumentation (1.5 T). *A*, Coronal T2WI (TR 2200/TE 80 msec). An abscess cavity is present (short arrow) in the right temporal lobe with surrounding parenchymal edema (long arrow). *B*, T1WI (TR 600/TE 20 msec) shows better anatomic definition of the lesion. *C*, Axial N(H)WI (TR 2000/TE 20 msec) shows hypointense T1 signal from the central cavity and hyperintense signal from the wall of inflammatory tissue. *D*, T2WI (TR 2000/TE 80 msec) shows surrounding edema (long arrow) delineated from the abscess cavity by a thin ring of lower signal (short arrow). Posterior fossa hemorrhage appears as increased signal from the tentorium on both images (arrowhead). (Courtesy of C. Pleatman, M.D., University of Cincinnati Hospital, Cincinnati, Ohio.)

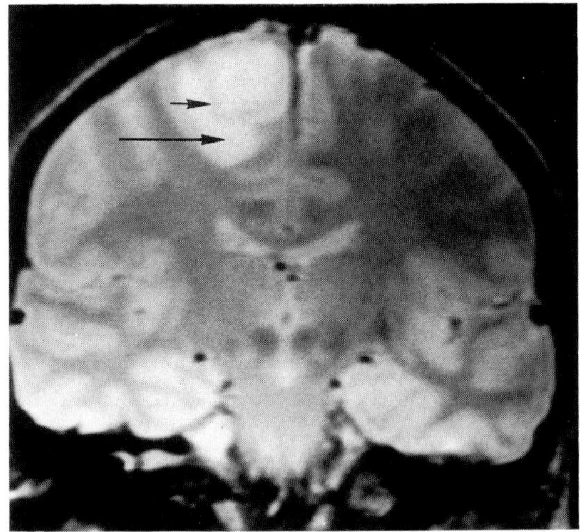

**Figure 14–6. Anaerobic brain abscess.** A patient with progressive left lower extremity weakness six months following dental surgery (1.5 T). Coronal T2WI (TR 2000/TE 100 msec). The right parasagittal frontal cortex shows high T2 signal with a thin ring of homogeneous thickness. Low signal (short arrow) demarcates the lesion wall from surrounding high signal of parenchymal edema (long arrow). (Courtesy S. Pomeranz, M.D., Christ Hospital, Cincinnati, Ohio.)

extensive on MRI than the area of contrast enhancement on CT, suggesting that changes in T2 relaxation times are a more sensitive indicator of cerebral edema than is blood-brain barrier breakdown.[11, 18] The same T2 sensitivity allows detection by MRI of developing abscesses while they are still in the early stage of cerebritis, an advantage over CT. MRI sensitivity to edema obscures delineation of the abscess cavity from surrounding edematous brain on T2WIs, but T1WIs show good resolution of the anatomic pathology in our experience, despite published reports to the contrary.[10, 18, 21]

The intravenous administration of the paramagnetic contrast agents gadolinium-DTPA and nitroxide stable free radicals have been used in experimental MRI to enhance the definition of the abscess cavity from surrounding edema and to increase the sensitivity of MRI to the initial stage of cerebritis.[19, 21, 22] Contrast MRI has been reported to both increase the area of abnormal signal around an already apparent cerebritis and to enhance an area of cerebritis that is not apparent in the early stage.[21, 22] Whether or not an abscess cavity is subsequently formed, cerebritis appears as an area of elongated T2 relaxation, and swelling may be present.[23] The clinical utility of enhancing MRI in cerebral abscess has not been established.

## Viral Infections

Viral encephalitis is most often caused by herpes simplex virus type 1. Herpes simplex virus type 2 causes congenital neural lesions. Type 1 often causes diffuse, severe necrotizing cerebritis with hemorrhage, characteristically in the deep frontal and temporal lobes. Mass effect occurs in about half of reported cases. CT discloses a poorly defined area of low attenuation and mass effect. A variety of contrast-enhancement patterns are described that appear to depend upon the vagaries of blood flow, infarct, and blood-brain barrier state.[24]

MRI discloses pronounced decrease in T1 and increase in T2 signal in the presence of herpetic encephalitis (HE) (Fig. 14–7). The

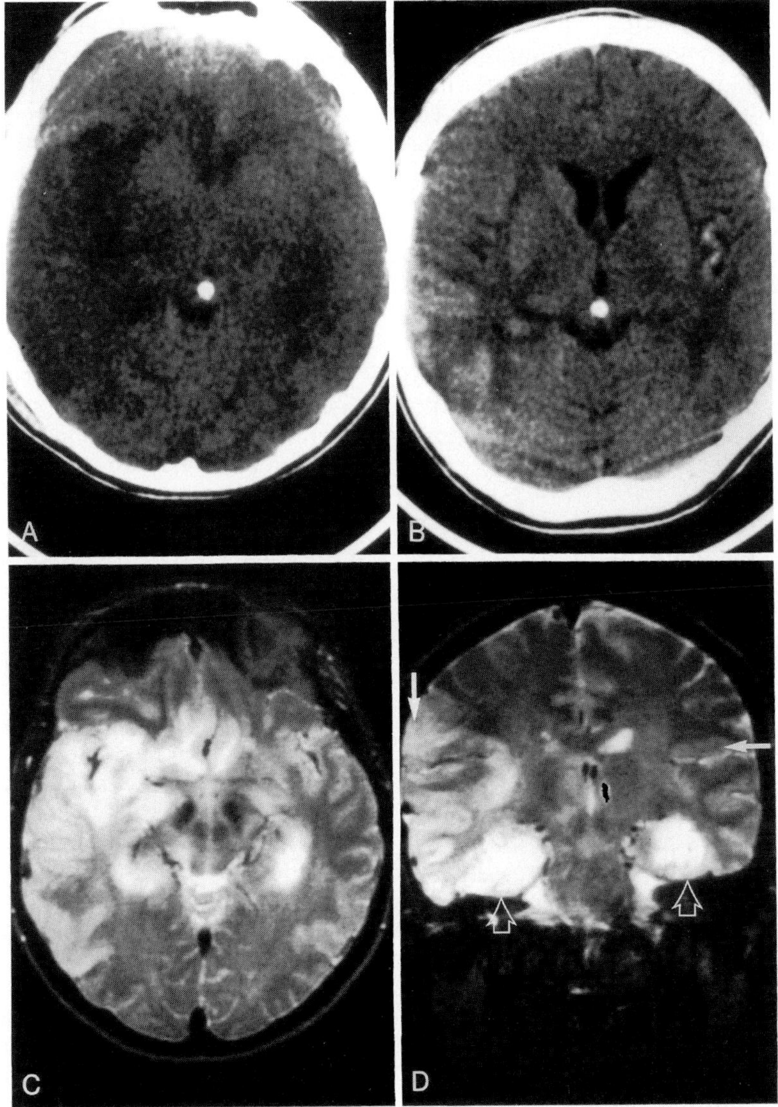


**Figure 14–7. Herpetic encephalitis.** A young woman with seizures and fever (1.5 T). *A,* Axial NCCT shows an ill-defined low attenuation area in the right temporal lobe with deep left temporal and parasagittal frontal lobe involvement. *B,* Enhanced axial CT shows gyriform enhancement in the right corticomedullary area and cortical enhancement in the left perisylvian region. *C,* Axial T2WI (TR 2000/TE 100 msec) at a similar level shows the greater extent of hyperintense inflammatory and edematous foci in the right and left temporal lobes. *D,* Coronal T2WI shows the most pronounced hyperintense inflammatory change in both inferior (uncal) temporal lobes (open arrows) with suprasylvian extension on the right (arrow) and perisylvian on the left (arrow). (Courtesy of L. Eynon, M.D., Mercy Hospital, Fairfield, Ohio.)

signal abnormality has been reported to include a more extensive area of brain than revealed by concomitant CT imaging.[25, 26] MRI has demonstrated temporal lobe localization in two cases of HE and one case of rubella.[7] MRI of the temporal lobes is superior to CT since the temporal fossa is often obscured on CT by artifact from petrous and sphenoid bones. Bilateral asymmetric temporal lesions were a common MRI appearance in one series.[10, 24]

Progressive multifocal leukoencephalopathy (PML) similarly shows lesions characterized by prolonged T1 and T2 relaxation with greater extension and better differentiation on MRI than in the corresponding low-attenuation areas seen on CT images. The occipitoparietal location of the lesions seen on MRI are in a characteristic location for PML, but the signal changes are nonspecific.[12, 27]

Areas of demyelination seen in postinfectious disseminated encephalomyelitis appear as focal or patchy areas of prolonged T1 and T2 signal identical to the appearance of cerebritis or encephalitis. MRI appears to be more sensitive than CT for detecting the involvement and resolution of this postviral childhood disorder.[28]

### Fungal Infections

Pulmonary fungal infection is the most common source of fungal meningitis and encephalitis. Gastrointestinal and intravenous routes have been implicated in CNS candidiasis.[29] Candidiasis, aspergillosis, cryptococcosis, and coccidioidomycosis are the most frequent types of CNS fungal infections.[29, 30] The two former diseases are more commonly seen as CNS abscesses, whereas the two latter more commonly occur as meningitis.[31] All four causative organisms can incite a vasculitis with resultant cerebral infarction. *Aspergillus* is characteristically angioinvasive.

Fungal infection appears similar to bacterial infection on CT. Nonspecific focal or diffuse white matter lucencies with variable enhancement continue to produce a diagnostic dilemma: septic, viral, fungal, or vascular disease. A cerebritis-like picture of diffuse low attenuation white matter lesions with mild mass effect and slight enhancement is often present. Cisternal spaces are more likely to be inflamed and congested with thickened exudate. The aqueduct may be occluded, accounting for the prevalence of hydrocephalus. Signs of diffuse leptomeningitis, such as deformed or enhancing cisterns are often present, especially in coccidioidomycosis, along with the earlier-mentioned strokelike lesions. Multiple brain abscesses are not uncommon in CNS candidiasis; the central areas of candidal abscess are likely to display higher attenuation than those of bacterial abscess. Mass effect is likely to be mild, if present at all. Mass effect is commonly seen around nocardial abscesses.[29, 30, 32–34]

MRI of an immunocompromised child with a fungal abscess revealed an area of inhomogeneously elongated T1 in the left occipital lobe. A T2WI demonstrated a low-signal center surrounded by high signal. Three months following abscess drainage, the surrounding area of long T1 and T2 had become much smaller.[35] The area corresponding to the abscess cavity had hypointense T2 signal, unlike that reported for bacterial abscesses. Further study of fungal abscesses is required before it is learned if there is any significant association with shorter T2 relaxation from the fungal abscess cavity. Hypointense T2WI signal and hyperintense T1WI signal may be attributed to either subacute hemorrhage or hemosiderin within the abscess cavity.

### Tuberculous Infections

Tuberculous meningitis or cerebritis is seeded by hematogenous dissemination from systemic infection, although the primary infection may be silent. Granuloma formation in the meninges or the brain is common, as is a generalized meningitis with thickened exudate that may cause ventricular obstruction. Meningitis typically occurs about the base of the brain, in the interpeduncular fossae. Abscess formation, distinct from caseating tuberculomas, is rare. Arteritis is a more common finding in granulomatous than in purulent meningitis.[11]

Tuberculous meningitis usually demonstrates hydrocephalus on CT scan owing to obstruction of basal cisterns and ventricles by inflamed meninges and purulent exudate. The inflamed membranes often enhance. Tuberculomas within brain parenchyma are less common and may exhibit low- to high-attenuation density on CT. Ring enhancement is commonly seen but is also variable. The attenuation of the tuberculoma within the enhancing ring is often denser than the surrounding brain. Edema or mass effect is often present in the early stages but is usually absent in the later stages of parenchymal tuberculosis. A similar appearance may occur in metastatic squamous cell carcinoma from lung. Irregular high-attenuation masses are sometimes seen on CT and are believed to be several coalesced ring lesions.[36, 37]

Early MRI studies reported hypointense T1 signal from areas where tuberculous abscesses had been demonstrated on CT. Follow-up in one study showed partial resolution of MRI findings after therapy.[38] Multiple infarctions have been reported as an indirect, nonspecific MRI finding in granulomatous meningitis.[10, 11] MRI has an adjunctive role to CT in detecting early changes and the extent of peripheral cortical involvement in cerebral infarction.[10, 24, 38] In one case, MRI disclosed an internal carotid aneurysm at the site of meningoencephalitis that was probably tuberculous.[4]

## Parasitic Infections

*Toxoplasma gondii* infection of the adult CNS has become more common since the increase in both iatrogenic and acquired immunosuppression. All areas of the brain are likely to be infected with a tendency to involve periventricular and corticomedullary areas.[39] The CT appearance overlaps with parasitic, viral, bacterial, fungal infections, and septic emboli. The imaging appearance of toxoplasmosis depends upon the form of the disease, which in turn depends upon the host's immune response. Brain abscesses are seen in relatively immunocompetent individuals and may appear similar to pyogenic abscesses. Ring enhancement is common and may be smooth or irregular, thick or thin. Surrounding edema and mass effect are often seen with abscesses, since these individuals can mount an immune response. Multiple, active granulomata are also found in relatively immunocompetent patients. These also are associated with calcification, surrounding edema, and mass effect; they enhance predominantly in a nodular pattern, but a thick ring pattern may also be seen. Poorly defined areas of low attenuation occur in patients too immunocompromised to suppress and wall-off the infection. Gyral enhancement is reported in about half of these cases. Double contrast examination is suggested to increase the sensitivity of the examination.[34, 39]

MRI of toxoplasmosis shows scattered lesions usually displaying elongated T1 and T2 relaxation times, occasionally associated with hypointense areas of calcification.[4, 40] However, low central signal on T2WI is also reported with concomitant high signal on T1WI, indicating shortened relaxation times. This unusual appearance for inflammatory foci can occur in both untreated active and treated chronic lesions.[41] The low signal on T2WI may possibly be due to hemosiderin from prior hemorrhage within a proteinaceous liquefaction that maintains a shortened T1 relaxation. Another report describes subependymal elongated T2 and shortened T1 relaxations, likely due to hemorrhage in the germinal matrix.[4] MRI shows better sensitivity to toxoplasma lesions than does CT, but the trade-off of poor discrimination from surrounding edema and poor resolution of neighboring lesions is present in toxoplasmosis as it is in other inflammations (Figs. 14–8 and 14–9).[40, 41] Post and co-workers report that the activity of toxoplasma lesions can best be assessed by the degree of contrast enhancement on CT, since the MRI signal does not appear to discriminate activity; however, diminution of lesions and edema with treatment could be followed by both CT and MRI.[41] Toxoplasma lesions are usually necrotic and often hemorrhagic owing to the vasculitis incited by toxoplasma endothelitis. The prevalence of hemorrhagic signal alterations in T2WI of toxoplasma abscesses is suggestive of hemosiderin contribution. Correlative histopathology will provide much needed information into the MRI appearance of parasitic and fungal CNS inflammation.

Cysticercosis is one of the more prevalent parasitic CNS diseases worldwide, and its incidence in the United States is increasing. Infection involves the CNS in 60% to 92% of cases.[42, 43] Meningeal and cerebral infections are most common. Ventricular cysticerci are usually viable and freely mobile. They may therefore elicit little, if any, immune reaction and seldom calcify. The thin walls and CSF-like cyst fluid may make

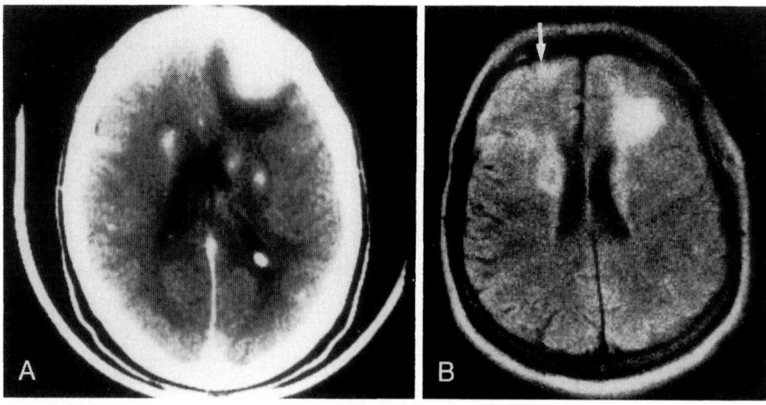

**Figure 14–8. Cerebral toxoplasmosis.** A 28-year-old Haitian with AIDS (0.35 T). *A,* CECT shows multiple enhancing lesions with surrounding edema and mass effect. *B,* Axial N(H)WI (TR 1500/TE 35 msec) MR image through a similar level does not discriminate individual lesions from edema and from each other as well as CT, but absence of a beam-hardening artifact uncovers left frontal lesions and right frontal involvement (arrow). (Courtesy of J. Sheldon, M.D., Mt. Sinai Hospital, Miami Beach, Fla.)

ventricular cysticerci transparent even to MRI, but the living larvae may be seen as a mural nodule of intermediate signal if thin sections are obtained (Fig. 14–10). Mass effect upon ventricular walls or choroid plexus may be seen. The fourth ventricle is most often involved, with lateral ventricle, foramen of Monro, third ventricle, and aqueduct of Sylvius involvement, in descending order.[44, 45]

A cysticercus in the subarachnoid CSF space degenerates into a nonviable, multilobular racemose cyst. Although sterile, the wall can grow, and the cyst may block CSF flow. Lacking a larva, they do not calcify. Racemose cysts may have different signal intensity than parenchymal forms, being isointense with CSF.[46] The intracisternal location of these forms may therefore be well-concealed, and their presence may only be inferred by subtle expansion of the CSF spaces (Fig. 14–10*D*). The cyst wall is only about 0.1mm thick and would not be expected to give sufficient signal of its own, but contiguous, reactive glial brain tissue may give off sufficient signal, since a reactive arachnoiditis is not uncommon.[43, 46]

There is great variability in the reported incidence of parenchymal, ventricular, and meningobasal forms of cystercercosis. The latter two forms appear to be over-reported by series dependent upon contrast ventriculography, whereas the parenchymal form may be over-reported by CT studies.[34, 42–47] MRI also selectively shows parenchymal forms to advantage but has the promise of surveying all forms of the disease with improved sensitivity through optimal use of imaging flexibility and careful observation.

## Syphilis

Parenchymatous neurosyphilis is the most common form of this disease; it is usually asymptomatic, but can give rise to tabes

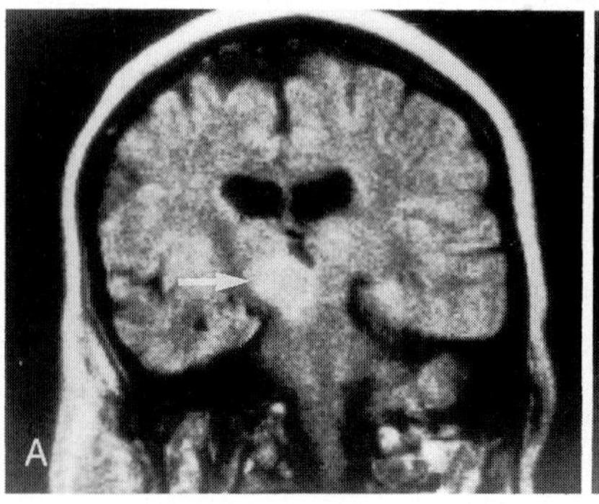

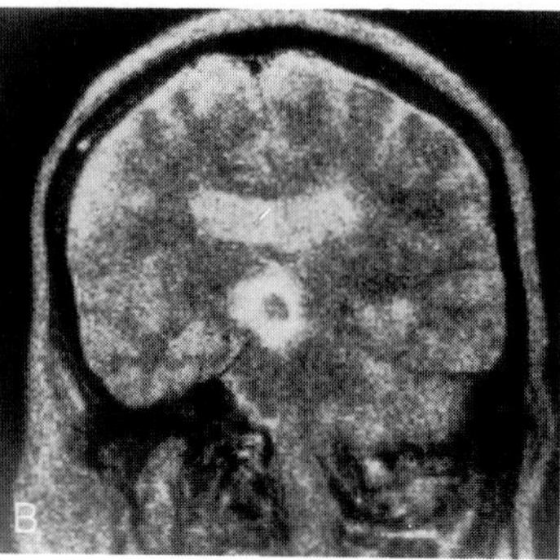

**Figure 14–9. Cerebral toxoplasmoma.** Patient with seizures, left hemiparesis, and known AIDS (0.35 T). *A,* Coronal N(H)WI (TR 1500/TE 35 msec) of right cerebral peduncle shows hyperintense signal from lesion and surrounding edema (arrow). *B,* T2WI (TR 1500/TE 70 msec) shows an area of central hypointensity with surrounding edema and mild mass effect. (Courtesy of J. Sheldon, M.D., Mt. Sinai Hospital, Miami Beach, Fla.)

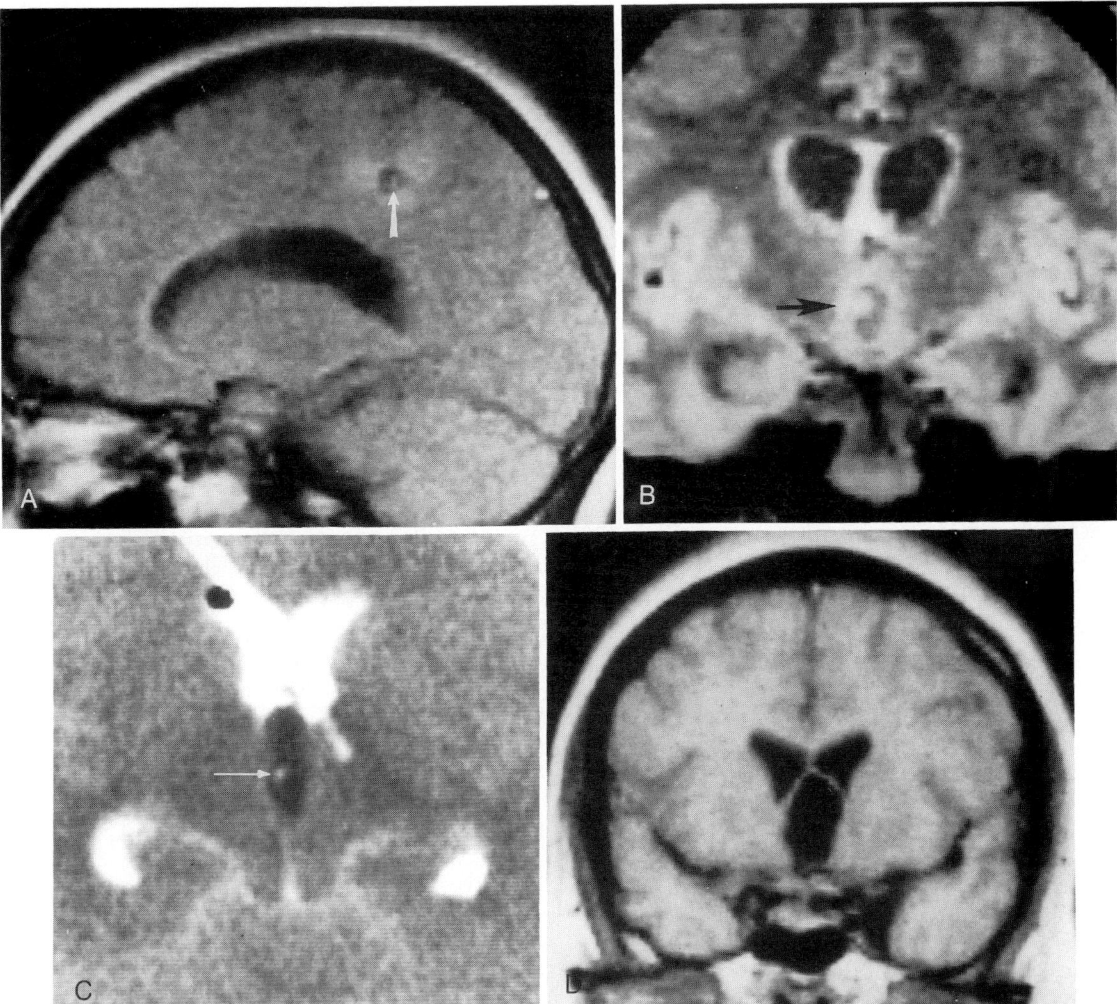


**Figure 14–10. Cysticercosis** (0.35 T). *A,* Sagittal T1WI (TR 500/TE 56 msec) shows a homogeneously hypointense T1-signal cyst surrounded by higher parenchymal signal owing to shorter T1 relaxation and higher proton density. The cysticercus scolex appears as a point of bright signal (arrow). Mild ventriculomegaly is present. *B,* Coronal N(H)WI (TR 500/TE 56 msec) through the third ventricle identifies the scolex of an interventricular cyst (arrow) as an eccentric point of high signal contrasted by a lower intracystic fluid signal. The cyst is surrounded by high signal, suggesting reactive inflammation of the third ventricle lining. *C,* Coronal CT ventriculography outlines the cyst seen in *B.* The scolex nodule is enhanced (arrow), suggestive of metrizamide absorption. *D,* A coronal T1WI (TR 500/TE 28 msec) through the third ventricle of a different patient shows disproportionate enlargement of the third ventricle with superior displacement of the fornices. No scolex or inflammatory signal is present. (From Suss, R. A., et al. AJNR, 7:235–242, 1986, with permission.)

dorsalis or general paresis.[48] The less common form of the disease is meningovascular neurosyphilis, named for the meningitis and vasculitis that are present.[49]

Syphilitic gummas may be seen on CT as homogeneously enhancing masses in parenchymatous neurosyphilis, whereas syphilitic arteritis appears as acute or chronic changes of cerebral ischemia or infarction in meningovascular syphilis. Chronic atrophic changes appear on CT predominantly as decreased attenuation throughout white matter, with sparing of gray matter zones, especially basal ganglia.

Both loss of gray matter and peripheral infarction have been reported from MR images of the brain with neurosyphilis.[38] MRI of meningovascular neurosyphilis discloses areas of prolonged T2 signal that correspond to low attenuation areas seen on CT images, giving an image identical to that of acute infarction. Small foci of bright T2 signal are seen in the perivascular white matter, not apparent on CT imaging and similar in appearance to chronic cerebrovascular infarction.[50] Peripheral infarcts on T1- and T2-weighted images may be the sole manifestation of this disease (Fig. 14–11).

## IDIOPATHIC DISEASES

### Neurosarcoidosis

Systemic sarcoidosis involves the CNS in 5% to 15% of cases. There is a female predominance, and involvement in both sexes peaks during the third and fourth decades of life. Hydrocephalus is a common finding on CT, since granulomatous leptomeningitis is the most frequent form of this disease. Less commonly, single or multiple noncaseating granulomata may involve the brain, usually the basal structures, such as pituitary stalk, hypothalamus, floor of third ventricle, or optic chiasm, or at higher levels, they may be adjacent to the ventricles (Fig. 14–12).[51–53] The lesions are closely related to vasculature and proliferate along Virchow-Robin spaces.[54, 55] Granulomata usually appear as either isointense or high-attenuation areas on CT, with homogeneous enhancement upon contrast administration. A single granuloma may therefore be difficult to distinguish from a dense, enhancing neoplasm such as meningioma, medulloblastoma, or oligodendroglioma. Minimal surrounding edema characterizes granulomata of sarcoidosis.[53, 55]

### Behçet's Disease

Behçet's disease is a vasculitis of unknown origin that involves the CNS in about 10% to 33% of cases with reported incidence as high as 49%.[56–58] Peak incidence is at about age 30 years but ranging from 15 to 45 years. Pediatric cases are occasionally reported. The disease has increased prevalence among Mediterranean, near-eastern, and Asian populations. Vasculitis commonly affects heart, lungs, intestines, eyes, and skin, usually involving medium-sized veins. In the CNS, vasculitis frequently causes a leptomeningitis, but most often brain stem and basal ganglia are involved.[57, 59] Also affected are internal capsule, palladium, and brain stem at about the levels of the decussations of the brachia. The early lesion is a collection of inflammatory cells around vessels, progressing to a chronic vasculitis with perivascular tissue softening, hemorrhage, and infarction. Grossly, necrosis crossing the corticomedullary junction can be seen.[56] Patients often present with generalized neurological signs of headache, seizure, or psychosis.

Patients with Behçet's disease have demonstrated a symmetric signal increase on T2WI in both cerebral peduncles at lower field strengths in two cases we have encountered (Fig. 14–13). T1WIs were unremarkable. Another reported case of neuro-Behçet's disease similarly had high signal on T2WI, whereas the T1WI appeared normal. The area involved was similar, left midbrain and inferior thalamus.[57] The value of these im-

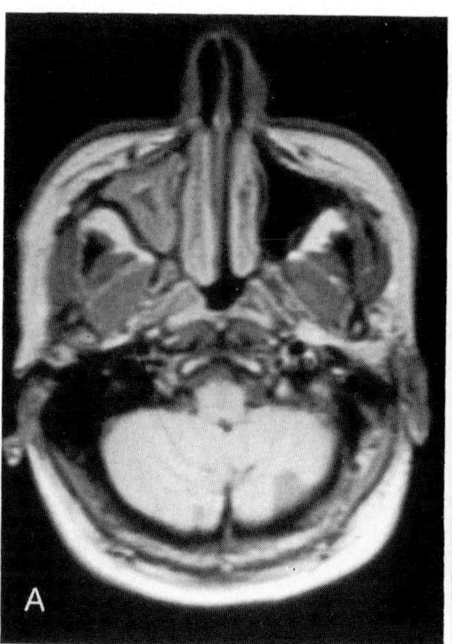


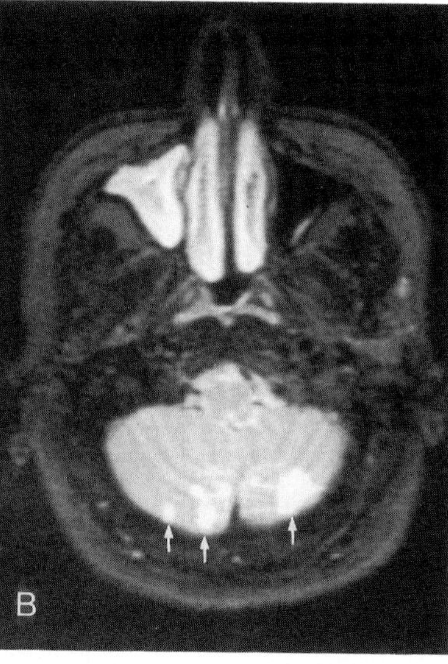


**Figure 14–11. Syphilitic vasculitis.** A 22-year-old woman with ataxia and positive CSF antibody titers (1.5 T). *A,* Axial T1WI (TR 2300/TE 20 msec) reveals low signal from peripheral chronic cerebellar infarcts (arrows). *B,* The infarcted areas are hyperintense on T2WI (TR 2300/TE 80 msec). Right maxillary sinus disease is incidentally noted. (Courtesy of S. J. Pomeranz, M.D., Christ Hospital, Cincinnati, Ohio.)

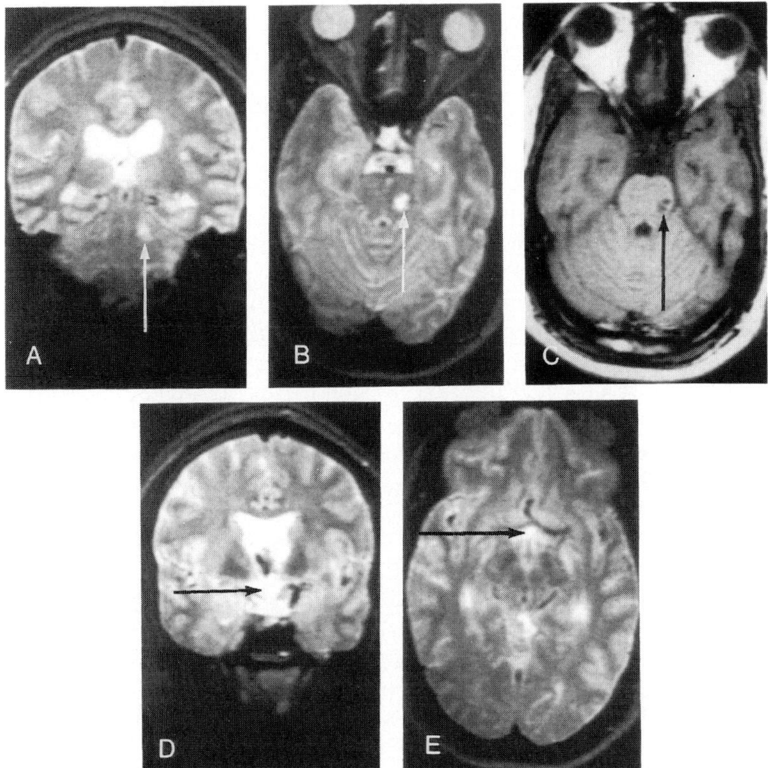

**Figure 14–12. Neurosarcoidosis.** A 25-year-old male presented with worsening frontal and occipital headaches and one episode of obtundation. A two and one-half year history of pulmonary and uveal sarcoidosis was present (1.5 T). *A* and *B,* Coronal and axial T2WI (TR 2000/TE 80 msec), respectively, show a hyperintense focus of signal in the left brain stem (arrows). *C,* An axial T1WI (TR 650/TE 20 msec) through the same level as *B* shows abnormally hypointense signal from the lesion (arrow). *D* and *E,* Coronal and axial T2WI, respectively, show a second lesion in the hypothalamus (arrows) that was isointense on T1WI. (Courtesy of A. Chambers, M.D., University of Cincinnati Hospital, Cincinnati, Ohio.)

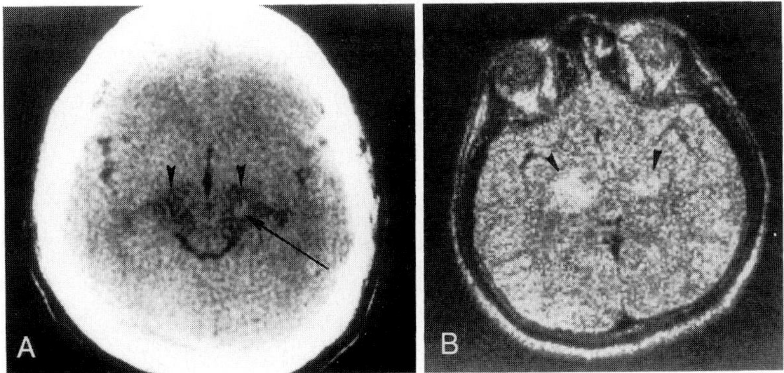

**Figure 14–13. Neuro-Behçet's disease.** Woman with recurrent meningitis and uveitis (0.35 T). *A,* Axial NCCT through the basal ganglia shows bilateral low attenuation in the cerebral peduncles (arrowheads) with a focus of central normal attenuation on the left (arrow). *B,* A T2WI (TR 1500/TE 70 msec) through the approximate area discloses increased signal from the peduncles (arrowheads), corresponding to the CT changes in *A.* (Courtesy of S. Pomeranz, M.D., Christ Hospital, Cincinnati, Ohio.)

ages is their ability to localize such lesions at an early stage for further workup. For this purpose, MRI has increased sensitivity over CT.

## Radiation Changes

Changes in the brain parenchyma following a series of radiation treatments may be as subtle as atrophy with no evident histopathology. More pronounced damage, such as microangiopathy with dystrophic calcification, may be present, or changes may be as severe as a pervasive leukoencephalopathy. Grossly, CT may show low attenuation areas of ventricular leukoencephalopathy, cortical atrophy, ventriculomegaly, and high attenuation areas of acute hemorrhage or calcification from remote hemorrhage. Often, the pattern of the affected areas may suggest the field of radiation exposure.

T2WI show a unique appearance to the cerebral hemispheres that strongly suggests radiation injury over other inflammatory etiologies (Fig. 14–14). The white matter damage is often periventricular; there is a scalloped appearance to the white matter margins that is not noticeable in other demyelinating conditions and is not smooth or uniform in appearance as is the transependymal absorption of CSF seen in hydrocephalus. The increased signal often extends all the way to the corticomedullary junction. There may be normal-appearing white matter intervening between periventricular and subcortical areas of increased T2 change. All other white matter tracts can be involved, but the corpus callosum is reportedly spared.[60] Ventricular enlargement and cortical atrophy are usually present.[61] N(H)WIs and T2WIs show the extent of degeneration, whereas T1WIs provide little if any information (Fig. 14–15). Areas of calcification and hemosiderin deposition may occur owing to microangiopathy (see Chap. 15) and usually appear as signal hypointensity, but posthemorrhagic calcifications can exhibit T1 hyperintensity.

As yet, postradiation MR images have not been interpreted taking into account the radiation dose, concurrent chemotherapy, the type and extent of tumor, or the patient's age. Cytotoxic drugs increase the risk and possibly the severity of brain damage.[62] In a study of 11 patients who had received varying regimens of brain irradiation and chemotherapy, the extent of demyelination correlated in a purely qualitative clinical assessment with the degree of neurologic impairment.[62] Both CT and MRI cannot discriminate recurrent or residual brain tumor from radiation brain necrosis (Fig. 18–13).[63]

Radiation changes of the spine consist of fatty replacement of marrow that gives an increased signal on both T1 and N(H)W images. There is no obvious signal change in vertebrae on T2WI. The appearance is characteristic if both T1WI and T2WI are compared. Often, the abrupt transition of the bright T1 signal is a clue that the change corresponds to a radiation port. Spinal involvement by tumor conversely produces a hypointense T1 signal in vertebral bodies

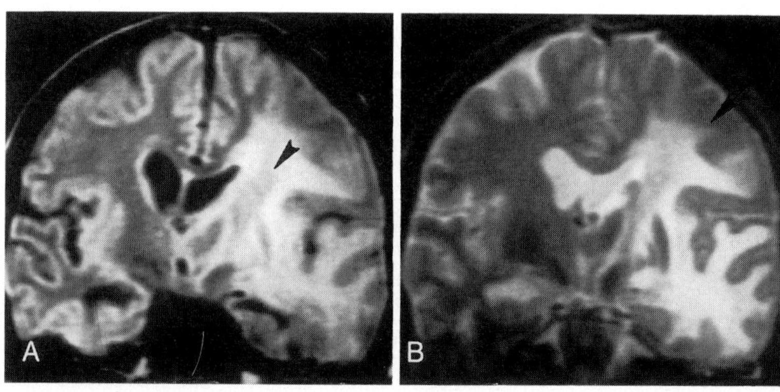


**Figure 14–14. Central coagulation necrosis and radiation effect without recurrent tumor—biopsy proven.** A 47-year-old woman, post 40-gray whole brain and 10-gray left temporoparietal irradiation following resection of a left parietal metastasis (1.5 T). *A*, N(H)WI shows global mild atrophy and mixed signal that appears hypointense centrally (arrowhead) and hyperintense peripherally. *B*, T2WI shows periventricular hyperintense signal with scalloped margins that may represent radiation change or edema extending into the temporal lobe. (Courtesy of R. Lukin, M.D., University of Cincinnati Hospital, Cincinnati, Ohio.)

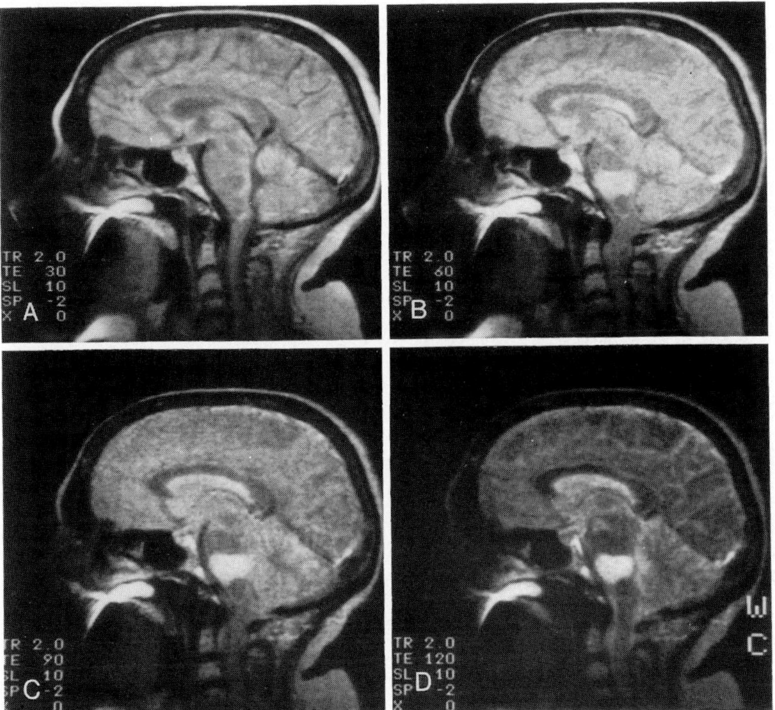


**Figure 14–15. Pontine necrosis/postirradiation.** *A* to *D,* An echo train (TR 2000/TE 30, 60, 90, 120 msec) illustrates elongated T1 *(A)* and T2 (*B* to *D*) relaxation that formed after therapeutic radiation to a brain stem astrocytoma (1.5 T). (Courtesy of S. J. Pomeranz, M.D., Christ Hospital, Cincinnati, Ohio.)

(Fig. 14–16).[64] In comparison, both skeletal radiation effect and sclerotic metastases appear hyperdense on CT.

## SPINAL INFECTIONS

### Vertebral Osteomyelitis and Diskitis

Vertebral osteomyelitis occurs primarily by hematogenous spread of infection and accounts for 3% of all osteomyelitis.[65] *Staphylococcus aureus* has supplanted *Mycobacterium tuberculosum* as the most frequent causative organism of osteomyelitis.[66] Intravenous drug abuse has become a common predisposing factor, although spread from primary sites of infection also occurs from urinary tract infection and furunculosis.[66–68]

Inflammatory changes involving disks alone are not unusually seen in adults owing to the avascular nature of the disk, but isolated inflammation of the vascular disk in children is reported.[69] Diskitis is seen in children owing to hematogenous spread, but blood channels are present in disk tissue for only the first three decades of life.[66] Diskitis occurs in adults postoperatively due to contamination. Both of these infections are most often caused by *S. aureus*.[68]

Plain film changes do not appear before three to four weeks of diskitis and most often appear as narrowing of the disk space and fraying of the adjacent end-plates. Disk space narrowing and a paraspinous soft tissue bulge are the most frequent findings on plain films in osteomyelitis and diskitis.[70] The infection spreads to paraspinous soft tissue in about 20% of cases. CT may show patchy osteopenia within the vertebral body, erosion of the cortex, or both. Loss of tissue planes and swelling may be apparent in the surrounding soft tissues due to edema.

T1WI of the spine show good anatomic resolution. Cortical bone and ligaments, along with CSF, give the lowest signals on T1WI, whereas fat-containing vertebral marrow and especially epidural fat gives the brightest signals. The latter provides excellent contrast from the contained nerve or nerve root and facilitates evaluation of nerve course, caliber, and impingement. The T1 appearance of the vertebral disk is of intermediate signal. Vertebral osteomyelitis and

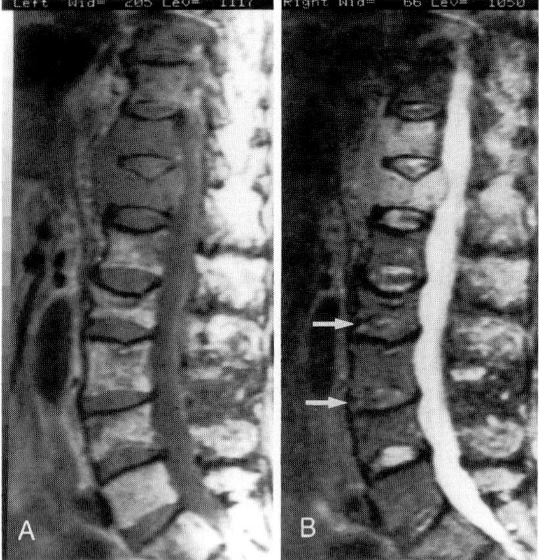


**Figure 14–16. Vertebral metastases and radiation effect.** A man with prostatic carcinoma metastatic to the thoracolumbar spine (1.5 T). *A,* N(H)WI (TR 1800/TE 20 msec). Increased T1 signal is apparent in vertebrae T12 through L5; this is due to increased yellow marrow due to radiation. Low T1 signal emanates from vertebral bodies T10 and T11, involved by tumor. *B,* A T2WI (TR 1800/TE 80 msec) illustrates normal T2 signal from the irradiated vertebral bodies, whereas the metastatic vertebrae produce increased T2 signal. Also noted are hypointense T2 signal intensities from degenerated intervertebral disks (arrows) in the field of radiation. (Courtesy of T. Tomsick, M.D., University of Cincinnati Hospital, Cincinnati, Ohio.)

diskitis can be seen as a diffuse decrease in T1 signal of vertebral bodies and disk spaces with obliteration of margins between disk and adjacent vertebral end-plates (Fig. 14–17).[71] Decrease in T1 signal accompanies a lengthening in T1 relaxation that occurs with edema or inflammation. However, we and others have observed both increased and diminished T1 signal changes in vertebral bodies adjacent to degenerated, noninfected vertebral disks (Fig. 14–18).[72]

T2WIs display brightest signal from CSF and the central portion of the disk. These images provide "MR myelography," in which an extradural defect can be seen as a low-signal invagination against the hyperintense subarachnoid CSF signal (Fig. 14–16B). The central disk region contains bright signal owing to the long T2 inherent in the hydrated state. Degenerative disk disease is seen as relatively low disk intensity on T2WI and is believed to be due to desiccation.[72] Concomitant disk space narrowing is observed, as well. A frequent normal finding on T2W spinal images is a dark line bisecting the bright disk transversely. This has been termed the *intranuclear cleft* and appears to be a normal finding in the lumbar spine after the third decade.[73] A recent study of 53 subjects found clefts in 93% of normal lumbar disks on MRI.[74] Disappearance of this cleft and increased signal from the intervertebral disk can be the earliest signs of diskitis. Disk space narrowing in association with an absent intranuclear cleft is strongly suggestive of diskitis, and high T2 signal from adjacent vertebral bodies may provide further support. Furthermore, disk hyperintensity relative to normal disks on T2WI should arouse suspicion of infection. Vertebral osteomyelitis may have similar findings since inflammation can involve the adjacent disk (Fig. 14–17).

Normal disk signal in the presence of vertebral body changes is most often seen in metastatic disease to the spine, with rare exceptions. However, normal disks have been described in early vertebral osteomyelitis that had subsequently progressed to involve the disk space.[75,76] The reappearance of the cleft or of a central area of decreased signal corresponding to degeneration is a

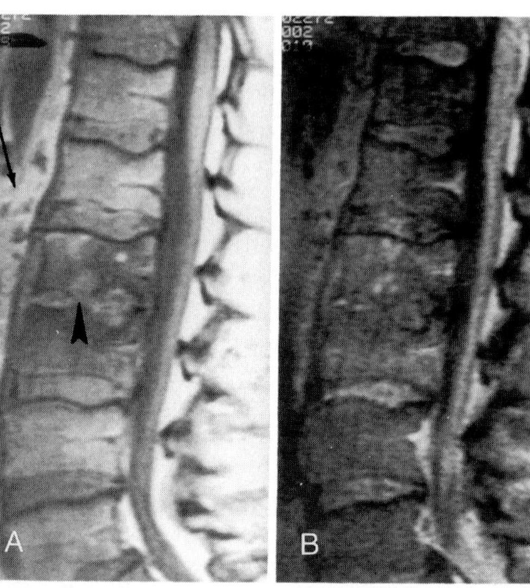


**Figure 14–17. Diskovertebral osteomyelitis—*Mycobacterium tuberculosis* and *Propionibacterium*.** A 29-year-old man with low back pain and night sweats (1.5 T). *A,* Sagittal N(H)WI (TR 2000/TE 20 msec). *B,* T2WI (TR 2000/TE 80 msec). In both images, loss of the vertebral end-plate (arrowhead) is evident, along with thickening and indistinctness of the prespinal soft tissues (arrow). (Courtesy of S. J. Pomeranz, M.D., Christ Hospital, Cincinnati, Ohio.)

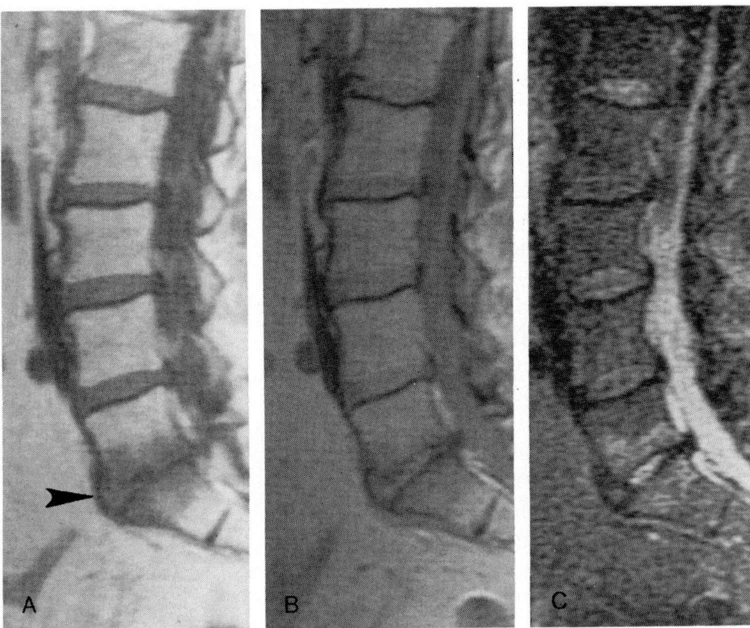


**Figure 14–18. Degenerative disk disease simulating diskitis.** *A,* T1WI (TR 600/TE 20 msec) shows hypointense signal in vertebral bodies adjacent to a degenerated L5–S1 disk (arrowhead) (1.5 T). *B,* Bony signal changes are subtle on N(H)WI (TR 1800/TE 20 msec). *C,* Hyperintense signal arises from disk and adjacent L5–S1 vertebral bodies on T2WI (TR 1800/TE 80 msec). There was no clinical evidence of diskitis. (Courtesy of S. J. Pomeranz, M.D., Christ Hospital, Cincinnati, Ohio.)

good indicator of resolution of inflammation and may provide an indication of therapeutic efficacy.[14]

Using the criteria of diminished T1 signal, increased T2 signal in vertebral bodies and disks, and disk space configurational change, MRI was 96% sensitive, 93% specific, and 94% accurate in diagnosing 37 patients with suspected vertebral osteomyelitis; administration of antibiotics during the acute phase did not alter the MR appearance of the disease.[71] Similar signal changes are also seen in tuberculous spondylitis with increased paravertebral extension of inflammation, a hallmark of spinal tuberculosis (TB). When the paraspinous extent of tuberculous spondylitis becomes extensive, T1 and T2 changes clearly delineate the spread within soft tissues.[77] In one case report, intravenous gadolinium-DTPA administration significantly shortened the T1 signal of vertebral and paravertebral components of the tuberculous inflammatory tissue, as well as the infected vertebral body.[78] However, the clinical utility of Gd-DTPA for vertebral osteomyelitis has not been established.

## Postoperative Changes

Until recently, the problem of recurrent prolapse of the disk space versus postoperative scar had best been studied by contrast-enhanced CT. However, MR has recently demonstrated signal differences between scar and reprolapsed disk. Scar, being the product of granulation tissue, is often hyperintense to degenerated disk on T2WI and hypointense to fat on T1WI.[79] Subacute scar and fibrosis give an intermediate T2 signal that may be distinguishable from the signal of recurrent disk.[70] Scar is brighter than disk on T1WI; this is the predominant finding throughout the literature but by no means the rule.[80] One study differentiated recurrent herniation from postsurgical scar by using the opposite criterion: their subjects' disks were of higher T2 or N(H)WI signal than epidural scar.[81] Difficulty arises when the reherniation is acute and the nucleus has a T2 signal of similar to or of greater intensity than scar. Unfortunately, this is quite common. The T2 intensity of an extruded or herniated disk fragment depends upon the age of the reprolapse. The time course of surgery and symptom recurrence must be considered in the evaluation of postsurgical spinal MRI. Discrimination between disk and scar by MRI can be difficult in the acute period and is best performed after two to three months have elapsed.

The following criteria, based on a combination of 96 postoperative disk reprolapse cases examined at Christ Hospital with MR in conjunction with published reports, have been developed for diagnosing disk reprolapse.[70, 79, 80, 82] Sagittal N(H)WIs and T2WIs (TR 1800/TE 20 and 80 msec at 1.5 T) and additional axial images are obtained through suspected levels. Contiguity of disk prolapse margins with the disk space, isointensity or hyperintensity of the fragment to the disk itself, and a polypoid-shaped protrusion all support the diagnosis of reprolapse. In addition, the prolapsed disk fragment becomes more conspicuous with increased T2 weighting, whereas scar decreases in conspicuity with T2WI and blends with the CSF signal in the thecal sac (Figs. 14–19 and 14–20; see also Figs. 18–28 to 18–30). CEMR in the axial and sagittal projections using T1WI show disk reprolapse as nonenhancing intermediate signal and scar as enhancing hyperintense signal. In this setting, MRI shows greater discrimination between reprolapsed disk and scar than does contrast-enhanced CT and has become the test of choice for differentiating disk reprolapse from postoperative scar.

## Inflammation of Cord and Membrane

Inflammation of the dura, the leptomeninges, and the cord itself are rare today. The inflammations classically are manifested as radicular pain, since they tend to be focal. Parathesias develop distal to the involved level as nerve roots become compressed acutely by inflammatory tissue and subsequently by fibrosis. If left untreated, cord compression develops and produces myelopathy in the severest cases. Subtle variations in neurologic signs formerly were the primary means of localizing the lesion. Now, conventional and CT myelography are primarily relied upon to localize spinal canal infections, and MRI promises to provide superior localization of some inflammations and complementary information for other focal inflammations.

### *Arachnoiditis*

Arachnoiditis is the most common spinal inflammation.[83] It may occur after subdural

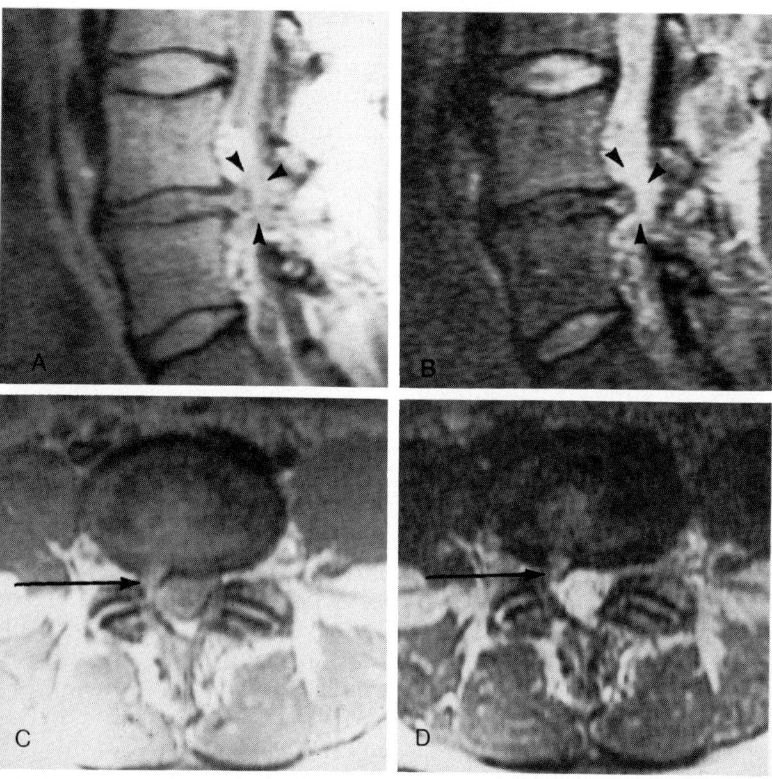


**Figure 14–19. Disk reprolapse and postoperative scar—L4-L5.** Rightward radiculopathy in a 29-year-old man 16 weeks postdiskectomy (1.5 T). *A* and *B,* Sagittal N(H)WI and T2WI (TR 1800/TE 20/80 msec). A crescentic scar (arrowheads) lies just posterior to a herniated degenerated disk. Signal contrast between disk and scar is more conspicuous on T2WI. *C* and *D,* Similar acquisitions in the axial plane show herniated disk (arrows). (Courtesy of S. J. Pomeranz, M.D., Christ Hospital, Cincinnati, Ohio.)

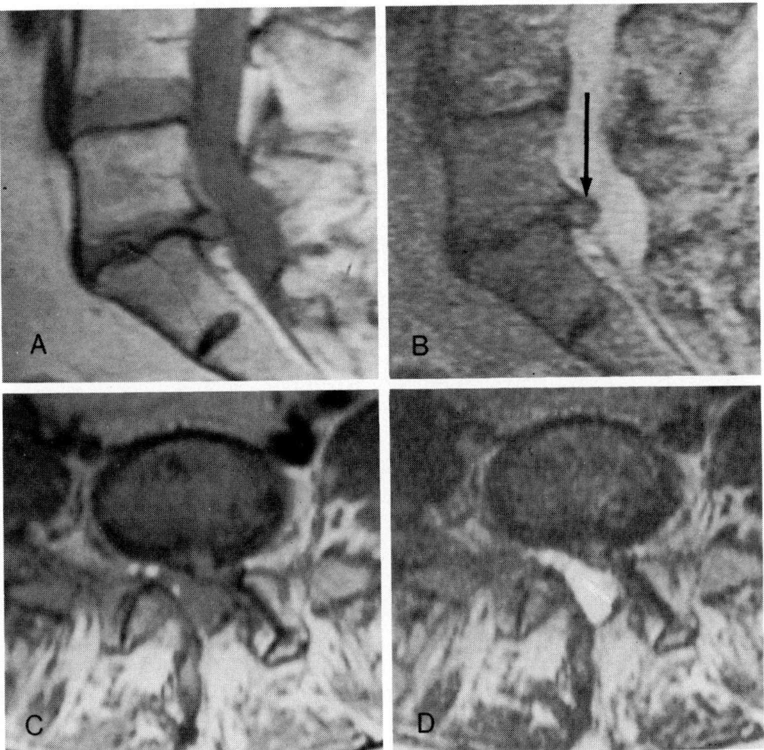


**Figure 14–20. Disk reprolapse—L4-L5.** A 37-year-old man with leftward radiculopathy 11 months following diskectomy (1.5 T). *A* to *D*, Sagittal and axial N(H)WI (TR 1800/TE 20 msec) and T2WI (TR 1800/TE 80 msec) illustrate the polypoid appearance of the reprolapsed disk (arrow), demonstrating contiguity and isointensity with disk space. Reprolapse is more conspicuous on T2WI. (Courtesy of S. J. Pomeranz, M.D., Christ Hospital, Cincinnati, Ohio.)

hemorrhage, Pantopaque insertion, or it may be the result of therapeutically resistant meningitis, usually granulomatous meningitis such as tuberculosis, cryptococcosis, sarcoid, and, formerly, syphilis.[5, 84, 85] Direct extension of staphylococcal osteomyelitis to the meninges is rare.[5, 31] Arachnoiditis may have a varied clinical presentation despite its local nature. Distal paresis and atrophy may occur if the cauda equina is involved. Arachnoiditis causes opacification, thickening and adhesion of membranes, and obliteration of the arachnoid space by connective tissue. The adhesions vary in severity; they may distort the dural sac and may deform and compress nerve roots. Pantopaque myelography was one common cause of arachnoiditis in the past (Fig. 14–21).

Myelography has been the imaging modality of choice for arachnoiditis, and CT myelography a valuable adjunct. Early thickening of nerve roots is first seen as blunting of axillary root sleeves on myelography. Later, clumping and dural adhesion of nerve roots appear on both conventional and CT myelography.[85] Stenosis or complete block of the spinal canal may be demonstrated by myelography, depending upon the severity of the adhesions.

The very long T1 and T2 relaxation times of the CSF allow a wide, dynamic range of signal strengths to be imparted to the fluid by the varied selection of acquisition protocols. Almost any lesion, therefore, can be made to contrast starkly against the CSF background. A useful technique to image arachnoiditis in the caudal sac is to use a T1WI to delineate the higher signal nerve roots against the low signal of the CSF contained within the sac.[70]

When imaging the cord itself, most prefer a T2WI that produces a bright CSF myelographic image and shows cord impingement and CSF flow irregularities to advantage. Bizarre flow-void phenomena on T2WI MR may occur secondary to intercalated septation and scar formation in arachnoiditis. Nerve root clumping, adherence of nerves to the thecal sac periphery, and pseudoconus formation appear on T2WI MR. Despite its

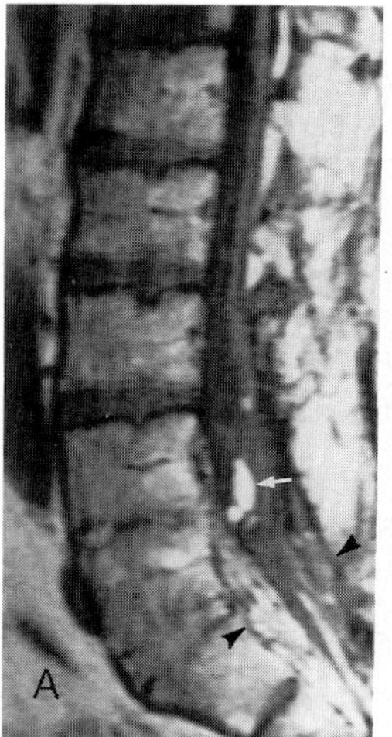
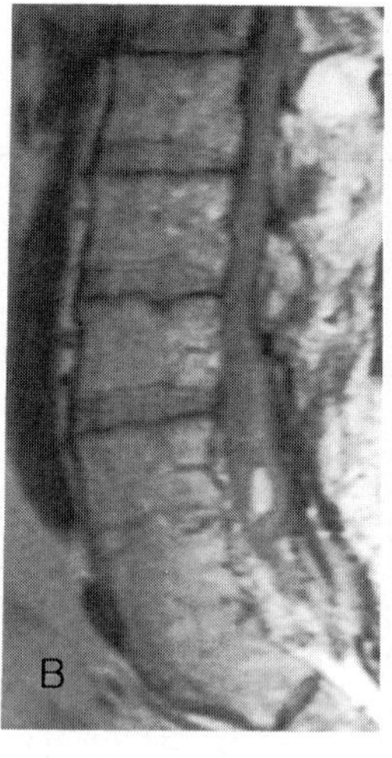
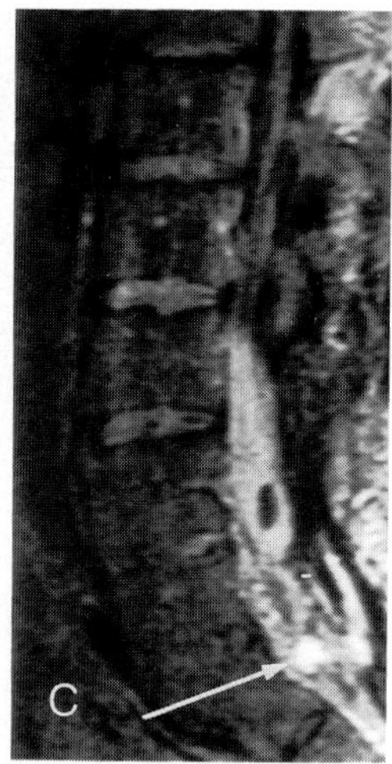

**Figure 14–21. Pantopaque arachnoiditis.** A 52-year-old man with chronic back pain and prior pantopaque myelography (1.5 T). *A* to *C*, Sagittal T1WI (TR 600/TE 20 msec), N(H)WI (TR 1800/TE 20 msec), and T2WI (TR 1800/TE 80 msec), respectively, show mixed signal from fibrosis (between black arrowheads) with clumped nerve roots. Pantopaque signal is hyperintense on T1WI (short arrow), hypointense on T2WI. Hyperintense signal on T2WI may occur secondary to absence of flow from trapped CSF (long arrow). (Courtesy of S. J. Pomeranz, M.D., Christ Hospital, Cincinnati, Ohio.)

multiplanar capability, good contrast, and resolution similar to postmyelographic CT, MRI has not replaced the complementary myelography/CT studies for arachnoiditis at most centers, since cord thickening and clumping is well demonstrated by myelography.

### *Epidural and Subdural Abscesses*

Epidural and subdural spinal abscesses are rare. The most common cause of epidural or subdural abscess is hematogenous spread from intravenous drug abuse, or a *Staphylococcus aureus* urinary tract infection (UTI), furunculosis, or osteomyelitis.[83, 87] Epidural abscess can follow vertebral osteomyelitis by direct extension, but subdural abscess from this cause is rare. Intramedullary spinal abscesses are rare.[84]

Contrast-enhanced CT imaging of epidural abscess may show a low attenuation mass with enhancing rim compressing the sac. CT myelography with subarachnoid contrast may disclose complete block or filling defect.[87, 88] Epidural or prevertebral abscess signal may appear similar to that of neighboring CSF on MR imaging and may be hidden unless a soft tissue component (Fig. 14–22) is present.[72] T2WIs have disclosed a paraspinal abscess cavity with a sinus tract extending to the epidural space.

### *Transverse Myelitis*

Acute transverse myelitis often follows a viral infection somewhere else in the body. The localized cord swelling produces neurologic symptoms that are indistinguishable from spinal cord compression, similar but

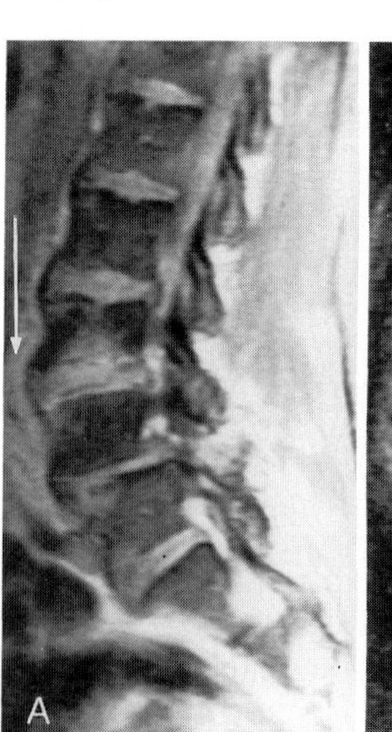
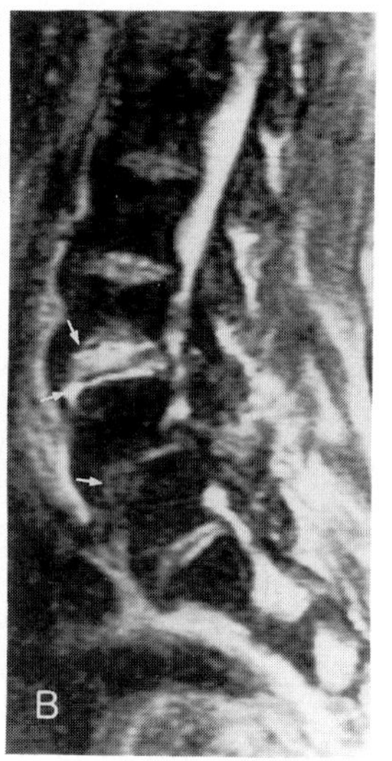

**Figure 14–22. Diskovertebral osteomyelitis with prespinal abscess.** A 68-year-old woman on hemodialysis with low back pain (1.5 T). *A,* N(H)WI (TR 1800/TE 20 msec). Prevertebral soft tissue mass (arrow) is present. *B,* T2WI (TR 1800/TE 80 msec) reveals hyperintense prevertebral signal. The L3-L4 disk space, the end-plate, and part of the L4-L5 disk space (arrows) show foci of hyperintense signal. (Courtesy of S. J. Pomeranz, M.D., Christ Hospital, Cincinnati, Ohio.)

more pronounced than the findings of the foregoing extramedullary focal segmental inflammations. Although trauma is the most common cause of transverse myelopathy, transverse myelitis is believed to be most commonly caused by multiple sclerosis.

High-resolution CT provides a good view of the spinal column, thecal sac, and nerve roots, but intraspinal soft tissues are only occasionally visualized, and the obligatory axial orientation may not display a gradual longitudinal swelling of the spinal cord. Angled coronal and direct sagittal images of the spine provide optimal delineation of cord swelling. T2W "myelographic" images allow the cord to stand out in relief against the brighter signal of the CSF, maximizing boundary contrast of the cord perimeter (Figs. 14–23 and 14–24). Distinction of cord from thecal sac is facilitated with T2WI electrocardiographic-gated MR or images that utilize flow compensation software. These images usually show the extent of intramedullary signal alterations as areas of hyperintensity within the expanded cord. The extension of lesions shown on MRI usually exceeds their visualization on CT. Acquisition of multiple images with different TE values during one scanning sequence that uses a long TR interval (usually 1800 to 3000 msec) provides a series of differently T2-weighted images that assists in discrimination between fat, blood, cord, fluid, and edema.

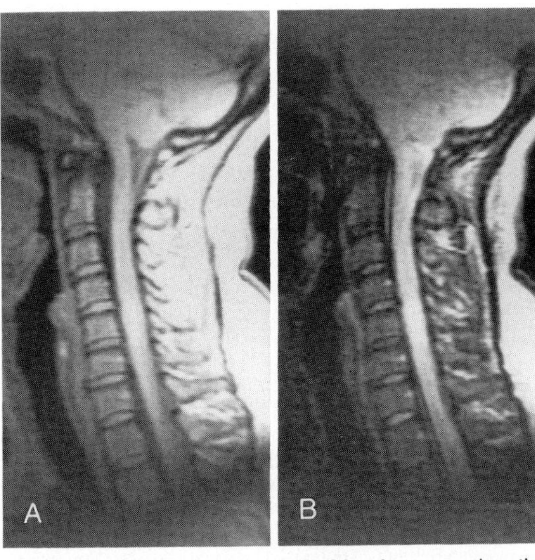


**Figure 14–24. Transverse myelitis.** Acute myelopathy in a 22-year-old woman with flu-like symptoms (1.5 T). *A,* Sagittal N(H)WI (TR 1800/TE 20 msec). Mild cord expansion and subtle, poorly defined hyperintense signal is seen at C5. *B,* T2WI (TR 1800/TE 80 msec) shows subtle signal hyperintensity to advantage. (Courtesy of S. J. Pomeranz, M.D., Christ Hospital, Cincinnati, Ohio.)

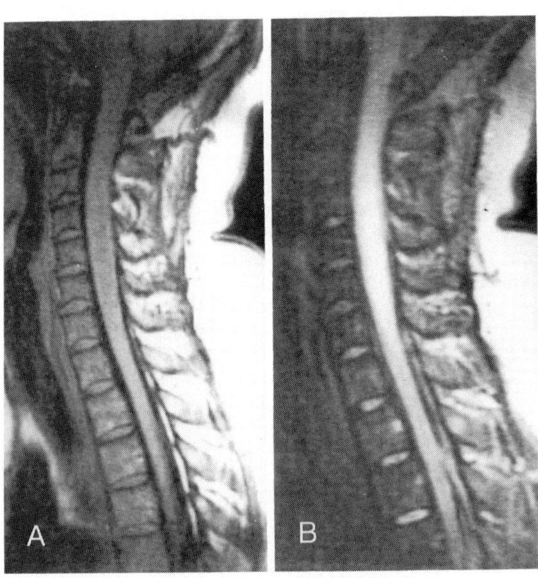


**Figure 14–23. Myelitis, etiology unknown.** Sudden myelopathy that subsided with steroid therapy (1.5 T). *A,* Sagittal N(H)WI (TR 1800/TE 20 msec). Cord is expanded through the C3-C7 level and is slightly hypointense to normal cord caudal to C7. *B,* T2WI (TR 1800/TE 80 msec) illustrates hyperintense signal at the site of cord enlargement. (Courtesy of T. Tomsick, M.D., University of Cincinnati Hospital, Cincinnati, Ohio.)

## Summary

Investigation of CNS inflammation is proceeding at a slower pace than other MRI applications owing to the intensive care required by such patients and the need to adapt life-support equipment to high magnetic fields. Even the modest number of investigations to date have suggested that MRI has several primary and complementary roles in evaluating the patient with suspected CNS inflammation.

The decrease in morbidity and mortality of cerebritis and cerebral abscess partly attributed to early diagnosis by CT promises to decline further if patients suspected of such disease have access to MR imagers with their greater sensitivity for soft tissue inflammation. Early evaluation of herpes encephalitis is one example of MR's diagnostic benefit. The major antecedents of CNS infection, sinusitis and otitis, although best evaluated with CT, are often present and are also well demonstrated by MRI.

MRI is assuming a greater role in the primary evaluation of inflammatory spinal disease. While arachnoiditis is still best diagnosed with myelography/CT, entities such as transverse myelitis, extra-axial abscess, diskitis, osteomyelitis, and postoperative scar formation may be best evaluated with MR and CEMR.

## References


1. Kaplan K. Brain abscess. Med Clin North Am 69:345–360, 1985.
2. Gomori JM. Intracranial hematomas: imaging by high-field MR. Radiology 157:87–93, 1985.
3. Enzmann DR, Brant-Zawadzki M, Britt RH. CT of central nervous system infections in immunocompromised patients. AJNR 1:239–243, 1980.
4. Davidson HD, Steiner RE. Magnetic resonance imaging in infections of the central nervous system. AJNR 6:449–504.
5. Walton JN, ed. Brain's Diseases of the Nervous System, 9th ed. New York, Oxford University Press, 1985.
6. Grinker RR, Sahs AL. Neurology, 6th ed. Springfield, Ill, Charles C Thomas, 1966.
7. Silverberg AL, DiNubile MJ. Subdural empyema and cranial epidural abscess. Med Clin North Am 69:345–360, 1985.
8. Moseley IF, Kendall BE. Radiology of intracranial empyemas, with special reference to computed tomography. Neuroradiology 26:333–345, 1984.
9. Kaufman D, Leeds NE. CT in the diagnosis of intracranial abscesses. Neurology 27:1069–1073, 1977.
10. Bydder GM. Nuclear magnetic resonance imaging of the brain. Br Med Bull 40:170–174, 1984.
11. Sawar M, Falkoff G, Naseem M. Radiologic techniques in the diagnosis of CNS infections. Neurol Clin 4:41–68, 1986.
12. Bradley WG. Magnetic resonance imaging of the central nervous system. Neurol Res 6:91–106, 1984.
13. Wong WS, Tsuruda JS, Kortman KE, et al. Practical Magnetic Resonance Imaging: a case study approach. Rockwell, Md, Aspen Publishers, Inc., 1987.
14. Modic MT, Pavlicek W, Weinstein MA, et al. Magnetic resonance imaging of intervertebral disk disease. Radiology 152:103–111, 1984.
15. Nielsen H. Cerebral abscess. Dan Med Bull 32:170–178, 1985.
16. Rowland LP, ed. Merritt's Textbook of Neurology, 7th ed. Philadelphia, Lea & Febiger, 1984.
17. Post MJVD, Hoffman TA. Cerebral inflammatory disease. In Rosenberg RN, ed. The Clinical Neurosciences, Vol. 4, New York, Churchill Livingstone, 1983.
18. Brant-Zawadski M, Enzmann DR, Placone RC Jr., et al. NMR imaging of experimental brain abscess: comparison with CT. AJNR 4:250–253, 1983.
19. Grossman RI, Joseph PM, Wolf G, et al. Experimental intracranial septic infarction: magnetic resonance enhancement. Radiology 155:649–653, 1985.
20. Grossman RI, Wolf G, Biery D, et al. Gadolinium-enhanced nuclear magnetic resonance images of experimental brain abscess. Comput Assist Tomogr 8:204–207, 1984.
21. Runge VM, Clanton JA, Price AL, et al. Evaluation of contrast-enhanced MR imaging in a brain-abscess model. AJNR 6:139–147, 1985.
22. Brasch RC, Nitecki DE, Brant-Zawadzki M, et al. Brain nuclear magnetic resonance imaging enhanced by a paramagnetic nitroxide contrast agent: preliminary report. AJR 141:1019–1023, 1983.
23. Furman JM, Brownstone PK, Baloh RW. Atypical brainstem encephalitis: magnetic resonance imaging and oculographic features. Neurology 35:438–440, 1985.
24. Bailes DR, Young IR, Thomas DJ, et al. NMR imaging of the brain using spin-echo sequences. Clin Radiol 33:395–414, 1982.
25. Schroth G, Gawehn J, Thron A, et al. Early diagnosis of *Herpes simplex* encephalitis by MRI. Neurology 37:179–183, 1987.
26. Neils E, Lukin R, Tomsick T, et al. Magnetic resonance and computerized tomography of *Herpes simplex* encephalitis. J Neurosurg. In press.
27. Gulleux M-H, Steiner RE, Young IR. MR imaging in progressive multifocal leukoencephalopathy. AJNR 7:1033–1035, 1986.
28. Dunn V, Bale JF, Zimmerman RA. MRI in children with postinfectious disseminated encephalomyelitis. Magn Reson Imaging 4:25–32, 1986.
29. Parker JC Jr., McCloskey JJ, Lee RS. The emergence of candidosis. The dominant postmortem cerebral mycosis. Am J Clin Pathol 70:31–36, 1978.
30. Lipton SA, Hickey WF, Morris JR, et al. Candidal infection in the central nervous system. Am J Med 76:101–108, 1984.
31. Schochet SS Jr. Infectious Diseases. In Rosenberg RN, ed. The Clinical Neurosciences, Vol. 3. New York, Churchill Livingstone, 1983.
32. Beal MR, Kleinman GM, Ogemann RG, et al. Aspergillosis of the nervous system. Neurology 32:473–479, 1982.
33. Dublin AB, Phillips HE. Computerized tomography of disseminated cerebral coccidioidomycosis. Radiology 135:361–368, 1980.
34. Enzmann DR. Imaging of infections and inflammations of the central nervous system: computed tomography, ultrasound, and nuclear magnetic resonance. New York, Raven Press, 1984.
35. Johnson MA, Pennock JM, Bydder CM, et al. Clinical NMR imaging of the brain in children: normal and neurologic disease. AJR 141:1005–1018, 1983.
36. Price HI, Danziger A. Computed tomography in cranial tuberculosis. AJR 130:769–771, 1978.
37. Rovira M, Romero F, Torrent O, et al. Study of tuberculous meningitis by CT. Neuroradiology 19:137–141, 1980.
38. Bydder GM, Steiner RE, Young IR, et al. Clinical NMR imaging of the brain. AJR 139:215–236, 1982.
39. Post MJD, Chan JC, Henslet GT, et al. Toxoplasma encephalitis in Haitian adults with acquired immunodeficiency syndrome: a clinical-pathological CT correlation. AJNR 4:155–162, 1983.

40. Levy RM, Rosenbloom S, Perret LV. Neuroradiologic findings in AIDS: a review of 200 cases. AJR 147:977–983, 1986.
41. Post MJD, Sheldon JJ, Hensley GT, et al. Central nervous system disease in acquired immunodeficiency syndrome: prospective correlation using CT, MR imaging, and pathologic studies. Radiology 158:141–148, 1986.
42. Latovitzki N, Abrams G, Clark C, et al. Cerebral cysticercosis. Neurology 28:838–842, 1978.
43. Zee CZ, Segall HD, Miller C, et al. Unusual neurological features of intracranial cysticercosis. Radiology 137:397–407, 1980.
44. Madrazo I, Garcia-Renteria JA, Sandoval M, et al. Intraventricular cysticercosis. Neurosurgery 12:148–152, 1983.
45. Madrazo I, Garcia-Renteria JA, Paredes G, et al. Diagnosis of intraventricular and cisternal cysticercosis by computerized tomography with positive intraventricular contrast medium. J Neurosurg 55:947–951, 1981.
46. Suss RA, Marvalla KR, Thompson J. MR imaging of intracranial cysticercosis: comparison with CT and anatomo-pathologic features. AJNR 7:235–242, 1986.
47. Rodriguez-Cabajal J, Salgago P, Gutierrez-Alvarado R, et al. The acute encephalitic phase of neurocysticercosis: computed tomographic manifestations. AJNR 4:51–55, 1983.
48. Clark EG, Danbolt N. The Oslo study of the natural course of untreated syphylis. Med Clin North Am 48:613–623, 1964.
49. Merritt H, Adams R, Solomon H. Neurosyphilis. New York, Oxford University Press, 1946.
50. Holland BA, Perrett LA, Mills CM. Meningovascular syphilis: CT and MR findings. Radiology 158:439–442, 1986.
51. Brooks BS, El Gammal T, Hungerford GD. Radiologic evaluation of neurosarcoidosis: role of computerized tomography. AJNR 3:513–521, 1982.
52. Kumpe DA, Rao KCVG, Garcia JH, et al. Intracranial neurosarcoidosis. Comput Assist Tomogr 3:324–339, 1979.
53. Bahr AL, Krumholz A, Kristt D. Neuroradiological manifestations of intracranial sarcoidosis. Radiology 127:713–717, 1978.
54. Harriman DGF. Bacterial infections of the central nervous system. In Blackwood W, Corsellis JAN, eds. Greenfield's Neuropathology, 3rd ed. London, Edward Arnold, Ltd., 1976.
55. Post MJD, Quencer RM, Tabei SZ. CT demonstration of sarcoidosis of the optic nerve, frontal lobes, and falx cerebri: case report and literature review. AJNR 3:523–526, 1982.
56. Lindberg R, Haymaker W. Tissue reactions in the grey matter of the central nervous system. In Haymaker W, Adams RD, eds. Histology and histopathology of the nervous system, Vol. 1. Springfield, Ill, Charles C Thomas, 1982.
57. Willeit J, Schmutzhard E, Aichner U, et al. CT and MR imaging in neuro-Behçet's disease. Comput Assist Tomogr 10:313–315, 1986.
58. O'Duffy JD, Goldstein NP. Neurological involvement in seven patients with Behçet's disease. Am J Med 61:170–178, 1976.
59. Rubinstein LJ, Ulrigh H. Meningoencephalitis of Behçet's disease. Brain 86:151–160, 1963.
60. Curves JT, Lester DW, Ball MR, et al. MRI of radiation injury to the brain. AJR 147:119–124, 1986.
61. Tsuruda JS, Kortman KE, Bradley WG, et al. Radiation effects on cerebral white matter: MR evaluation. AJNR 8:431–437, 1987.
62. Packer RJ, Zimmerman RA, Bilaniuk LT. Magnetic resonance imaging in the evaluation of treatment-related central nervous system damage. Cancer 58:635–640, 1986.
63. Doom GC, Hecht S, Brant-Zawadzki M, et al. Brain radiation lesions: MR imaging. Radiology 158:149–155, 1986.
64. Ramsey RG, Zacharias CE. MR imaging of the spine after radiation therapy: easily recognizable effects. AJNR 6:247–251, 1986.
65. Goldman AB, Freiberger RW. Localized infectious and neuropathic diseases. Semin Roentgenol 14:19–32, 1979.
66. Kelly PJ. Infections of the spine. In Ruga D, Wiltse LL, eds. Spinal disorders: diagnosis and treatment, 1st ed. Philadelphia, Lea & Febiger, 1977.
67. Fang HSY, Ong GB. Direct approach to the upper cervical spine. J Bone Joint Surg 44A:1588–1604, 1962.
68. Batson OV. The vertebral vein system: Caldwell lecture 1956. AJR 78:195–212, 1957.
69. Norris S, Ehrlich MG, Keim DE, et al. Early diagnosis of disc-space infection using gallium-67. J Nucl Med 19:384–386, 1978.
70. Berger PE, Atkinson D, Wilson WJ, et al. High resolution surface coil magnetic resonance imaging of the spine: normal and pathologic anatomy. Radiographics 6(4):573–602, 1986.
71. Modic MT, Feiglin DH, Piraino DW, et al. Vertebral osteomyelitis: assessment using MR. Radiology 157:157–166, 1985.
72. Modic MT, Masaryk T, Paushter D. Magnetic resonance imaging of the spine. Radiol Clin North Am 24:229–245, 1986.
73. Modic MT, Weinstein MA, Pavlicek W, et al. Magnetic resonance imaging of the cervical spine: technical and clinical observations. AJR 141:1129–1136, 1983.
74. Aguila LA, Piraino DW, Modic MT, et al. The intranuclear cleft of the intervertebral disk: magnetic resonance imaging. Radiology 155:155–158, 1985.
75. Resnick D, Niwayama G. Intervertebral disc abnormalities associated with vertebral metastasis: observations in patients and cadavers with prostatic cancer. Invest Radiol 13:182–190, 1978.
76. Norman A, Kambolis CP. Tumors of the spine and their relationship to the intervertebral disk: a roentgenographic-anatomic correlation. AJR 92:1270–1274, 1964.
77. Wagle V, Melanson D, Etthier R, et al. MR in spinal tuberculous abscess. AJNR 8:175–176, 1987.
78. de Ross A, van Meerten ELvP, Bloem JL, et al. MRI of tuberculous spondylitis. AJR 147:79–82, 1986.
79. Chafetz NI, Genant HK, Moon KL, et al. Recognition of lumbar disk herniation with NMR. AJR 141:1153–1156, 1983.
80. Paushter DM, Modic MT, Masaryk TJ, et al. Magnetic resonance imaging of the spine. Radiol Clin North Am 23:551–561, 1985.
81. Mikhael MA, Ciric IS, Kudrna JC, et al. Recognition of lumbar disc disease with magnetic resonance imaging. Comput Radiol 9:213–222, 1985.

82. Maravilla KR, Lesh P, Weinreb JC, et al. Magnetic resonance imaging of the lumbar spine with CT correlation. AJNR 6:237–245, 1986.
83. D'Angelo CM, Whistler WW. Bacterial infections of the spinal cord and its coverings. In Vinken PJ, Bruyn GW. Handbook of Clinical Neurology, Vol. 33. New York, Elsevier-North Holland Publishing Co., 1978.
84. Epstein BS. The Spine: a Radiological Text and Atlas, 4th ed. Philadelphia, Lea & Febiger, 1976.
85. Adams RD, Victor M. Principles of Neurology. New York, McGraw-Hill Book Co., 1981.
86. Baleriaux-Waha D, Soeur M, Stadnik T, et al. CT of the adult spine with metrizamide. In Post MJD, ed. Radiographic evaluation of the spine. New York, Masson Publishing USA, Inc., 1980.
87. Wehlan MA, Schonfeld S, Post JD, et. al. Computed tomography of nontuberculous spinal infection. Comput Assist Tomogr 9:180–187, 1985.
88. Chafetz NI, Genant HK, Mani JR. Computed tomography of the spine. In Moss AA, Gamsu G, Genant HK. Computed Tomography of the Body. Philadelphia, WB Saunders Co., 1983.

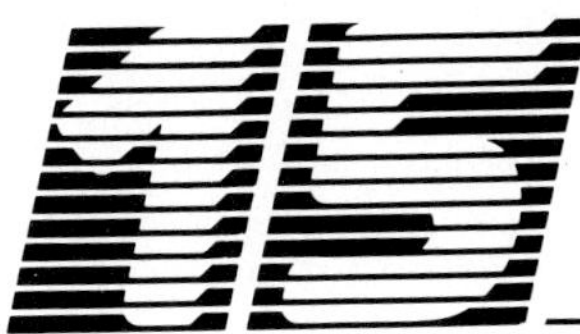

Kalevi P. Soila, M.D.

# MRI OF DEMYELINATING AND OTHER WHITE MATTER DISEASES

The sensitivity and clinical value of magnetic resonance imaging (MRI) in detecting subtle changes in the structure of water in tissues were first proved in the evaluation of white matter. A study conducted at Hammersmith Hospital in London, published 1981, proved the superior capability of MRI over computer-assisted tomography (CT) scanning in detecting demyelinating plaques in the brains of patients with multiple sclerosis.[1]

Since then several studies conducted with technically more advanced equipment have confirmed this initial observation. The accuracy of MRI has been quantitated and projected against CT scanning and a battery of clinical tests; the weaknesses have also been charted.[2–6]

An ever-increasing amount of knowledge is accumulating concerning numerous other causes of signal abnormalities in the white matter of the central nervous system. Some diseases lead to changes that closely mimic the findings seen with multiple sclerosis, and careful clinical correlation is needed for differentiation. Others, especially when followed over a period of time, evolve in a characteristic manner and allow a more specific diagnosis.

## DEFINITIONS

**Demyelination:** Refers to the removal of normal myelin from axons of the central and peripheral nervous systems. Within the lesions, a *selective loss of myelin with relative sparing of axons* is seen.[7, 8] The most common member of the group and the archetype is multiple sclerosis. The component diseases are linked by an acquired (usually viral) etiology, white matter lesions or "plaques" that possess a prominent perivenous inflammatory response, and at least some evidence of an autoimmune pathogenesis.[7] A controversial practice is to refer to the demyelinating diseases just defined as *primary* demyelinating diseases and to the loss of myelin that follows parenchymal destruction in a wide spectrum of neuropathologic states as *secondary* demyelination.[7] A more correct definition of *secondary* demyelination would be *diseases causing myelin loss.*

**Myelinoclastic:** Adjective used to describe the demyelinating diseases defined above; it is falling into disfavor owing to its redundancy.[7]

**Dysmyelination:** Indicates deficient development of myelin during its formation. This can be caused by a number of abnormalities of different types in the metabolism related to the formation and maintenance of white matter.

**Leukodystrophies:** Also called *hereditary dysmyelinating diseases,* a heterogeneous group of disorders that have in common extensive degenerative changes of the white matter. As the underlying abnormalities are elucidated, these diseases are constantly being reclassified.[7]

## CLASSIFICATION OF DEMYELINATING AND OTHER WHITE MATTER DISEASES

Various classifications for this heterogeneous group of diseases have evolved with time. In this presentation the principles previously mentioned are applied.

A. Demyelinating diseases of the CNS
   1. Chronic multiple sclerosis
   2. Variants of multiple sclerosis
      a. Acute multiple sclerosis
      b. Neuromyelitis optica
      c. Concentric sclerosis
   3. Acute disseminated encephalomyelitis
      a. Postinfectious encephalomyelitis
      b. Postvaccinal encephalomyelitis
   4. Acute hemorrhagic leukoencephalopathy
   5. Progressive multifocal leukoencephalopathy
B. Metabolic diseases affecting white matter
   1. Leukodystrophies, which can be subdivided into the following categories:
      a. Metabolic diagnosis
         (1) Metachromatic leukodystrophy
         (2) Krabbe's disease
         (3) Adrenoleukodystrophy
      b. Pathologic diagnosis
         (1) Alexander's disease
         (2) Canavan's disease
         (3) Pelizaeus-Merzbacher disease
         (4) Cockayne's disease
         (5) Sudanophilic leukodystrophies
      c. Other leukodystrophies
   2. Storage disorders
      a. Lipidoses
      b. Mucopolysaccharidoses
      c. Mucolipidoses
      d. Generalized glycogenoses
   3. Other metabolic disorders
      a. Disorders of amino acid metabolism
      b. Hyperammonemia
      c. Metabolic acidosis
      d. Hypoglycemia
      e. Copper metabolism
      f. Lesch-Nyhan syndrome
C. Other conditions causing white matter abnormalities
   1. Inflammatory diseases
   2. Tumor-related causes
   3. Hydrocephalus
   4. Trauma
   5. Anoxic injury
   6. Radiation- and chemotherapy-induced conditions
   7. Toxins
   8. Other generalized conditions

## NORMAL WHITE MATTER

### Structure

The normal appearance of the brain on an MR scan depends on the age of the patient and on the pulse sequence used.[9]

The changes in the intensity of white matter during normal maturation and those related to demyelinating diseases are better understood if one is familiar with the microscopic structure of normal white matter and myelin.

The myelin sheath around an axon consists of tightly packed layers of paired proteolipid protein membranes draped around the axons (Fig. 15–1). This sheath is produced by interfascicular oligodendrocytes that have several cell processes to different axons. These flat processes spiral around the axons numerous times, and as the cytoplasm within the processes retreats, the tightly proximated membranes remain and fuse on the cytoplasmic, "inner" side, to form the myelin "insulation" around the axon.[7]

The protons in tightly bound lipid molecules in the bilayered membranes are considered to give little if any contribution to the image in proton MR imaging,[10–12] although this concept has been recently challenged in reference to immature myelin, which contains much shorter chains of fatty acids in the phosphatides of the myelin molecule.[13] The signal of mature white matter arises from tissue water protons.

Relaxation times of water protons in biologic tissues are a reflection of their interaction and collisions with surrounding macromolecules, membranes, and cell organelle surfaces.[10, 14] The tissues with the shorter relaxation times contain an abundance of surfaces, primarily in the form of membranes or large macromolecular surfaces.

In the white matter, the glial cells, myelin and axonal membrane surfaces, and the axoplasm constitute macromolecular environments and barriers for the tissue water protons.

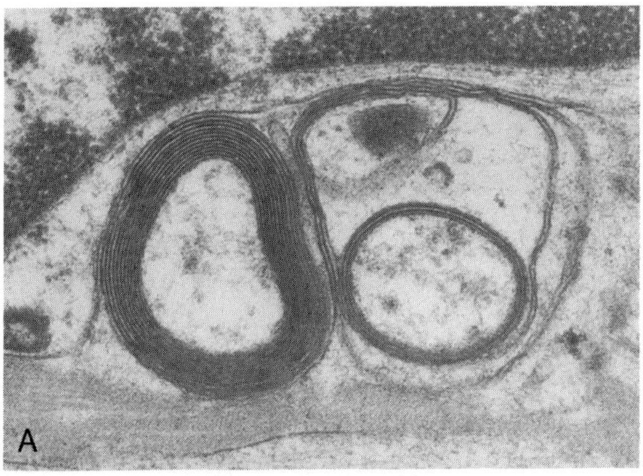


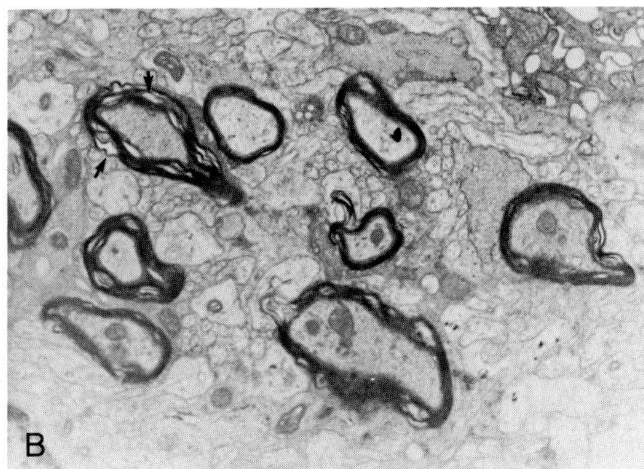


**Figure 15–1. Structure of normal myelin.** *A*, Electron micrograph demonstrating the normal structure of myelin sheath in a peripheral nerve. *B*, A disrupted myelin sheath allows more free water between the bilayered membranes (arrows), resulting in T2 and T1 prolongation.

The gradual shortening of T1 and T2 values observed during maturation of the white matter is due to a decrease in the amount of free water and to more structure around the water molecules secondary to the decreasing water content, rapid proliferation of glial cells, and the process of myelination.[15]

## Normal Maturation

The normal maturation of white matter consists of gray-white matter differentiation and myelination. These processes take place simultaneously, advancing myelination following progressive gray-white matter differentiation. This differentiation, which is seen associated with a decrease in brain water, may be a prerequisite for myelination; however, a causal relationship has not been proved.[15] These changes are also paralleled by decreasing ventricle-brain ratio and by decreasing size of the extracerebral subdural space.[16]

This development proceeds at a predictable rate and in preterm infants reaches a level equal to full-term development at 38 to 42 weeks if no complicating factors exist.[15, 36]

In the normal full-term newborn brain, the T1 and T2 relaxation values of the white matter are longer than those of the gray matter. The brain is relatively featureless on moderately T2-weighted images (T2WI), but on heavily T2WI, excellent differentiation of the gray and white matter can be obtained, the white matter showing higher intensity than the gray matter (Fig. 15–2*A*).[11, 12, 36]

Gray-white differentiation is seen as decreasing intensity of the white matter on T2WI. At approximately six to eight months, the white matter is isointense to gray matter, as its T1 and T2 shorten, and it subsequently becomes hypointense in relation to gray matter. Nearly adult level T2 relaxation values are reached by age two years. A small decrease in T2 values continues until early adolescence (Fig. 15–2*B* and *C*).[11]

On T1-weighted images (T1WI), the unmyelinated white matter in the newborn is hypointense in relation to gray matter owing to its longer T1 relaxation time.[11, 17] The T1 values in the unmyelinated white matter decrease with diminishing water content causing increasing intensity on T1WI. The progressing myelination introduces additional T1 shortening of the white matter and on T1W inversion recovery (IR) images, the myelinated areas are strikingly hyperintense.[12, 17, 18]

On T2WI, myelination can also be observed, although the contrast is not as striking as on heavily T1WI. It leads to further regional decrease in intensity in addition to the generalized decrease described above.[11, 13]

The regional T1 and T2 shortening in the white matter caused by myelination allows precise following of this process on MR images (Fig. 15–3).[11, 12, 17–19, 36]

In a full-term infant, myelin is seen in the brain stem in the entire pons and around the fourth ventricle. In the cerebellum, it extends to the medullary substance. It extends through the posterior limb of the internal capsule to the central portion of the corona radiata.[11, 15, 19, 36]

Myelination of the subcortical white mat-

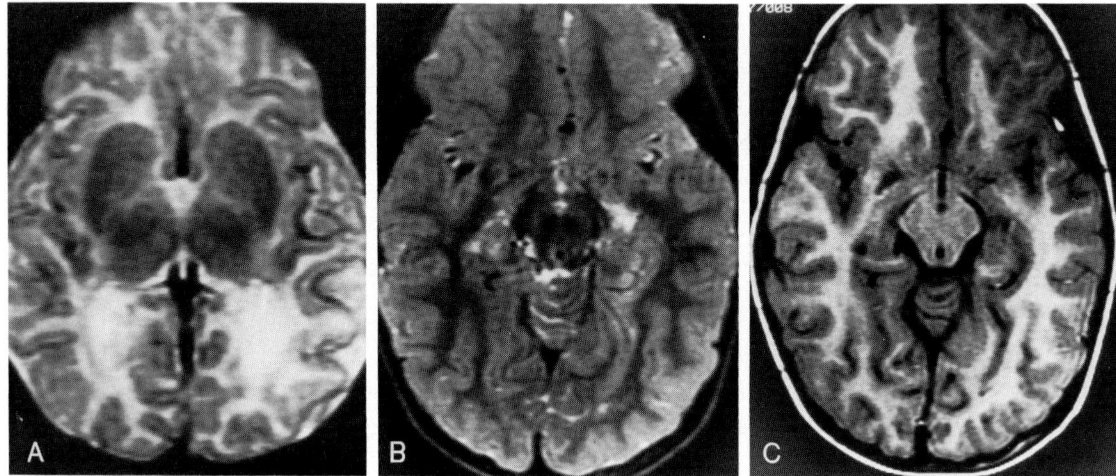

**Figure 15–2. Normal maturation of white matter (1.5 T).** *A,* A 2-month-old infant. Axial T2WI (SE TR 2000/TE 100) demonstrates high intensity in the unmyelinated, immature posterior white matter. Gray matter is less intense. Myelinated white matter seen at the level of basal ganglia is nearly isointense with gray matter. *B,* A 10-month-old baby. Axial T2WI (SE TR 2500/TE 100) demonstrates how maturation and myelination decreases the T2 of the white matter. It is less intense than gray matter. *C,* Axial T1WI (SE TR 400/TE 25) at the same anatomic level as in *B*. The areas of high intensity in the white matter show the extent of myelination.

ter proceeds from the corona radiata, first extending posteriorly toward the calcarine cortex by the fourth postnatal month and subsequently toward the association areas of the parietal, temporal, and frontal convexity. On MR images, nearly adult appearance is reached by two years of age, and after that only quantitative measurements of T1 and T2 will demonstrate the changes of maturation. Myelination is completed during the second decade.[11, 36]

Arcuate ("U") fibers are subcortical fibers at the margin of gray and white matter. Occasionally, they can be seen on T2WI at 1.5 T in normal individuals as a ribbon of decreased signal intensity, owing to higher iron (ferritin) concentration in the arcuate fibers compared with cerebral gray or white matter. Their diagnostic importance concerns the sparing or involvement in various pathologic processes and may improve diagnostic specificity in the evaluation of white matter disorders.[20]

In the mature brain, focal areas of in-

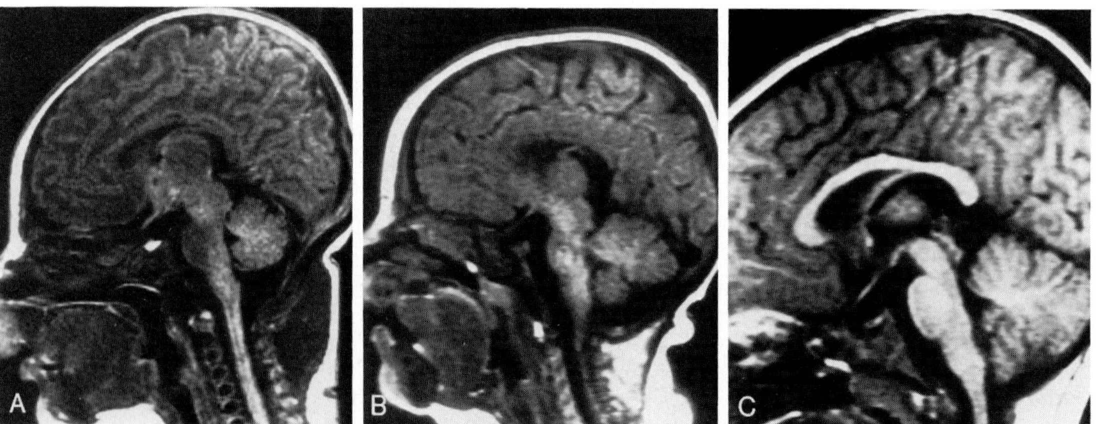

**Figure 15–3. Normal progression of myelination in the brainstem (1.5 T).** *A,* One-week-old infant. A sagittal T1WI (SE TR 600/TE 20) demonstrates higher intensity in myelinated areas in the spinal cord, medulla, pons, and cerebellum, around the fourth ventricle and extending to the midbrain. Unmyelinated white matter is hypointense in relation to supratentorial cortical gray matter. *B,* A two-month-old infant. A sagittal T1WI (SE TR 400/TE 25) demonstrates increased myelination (hyperintensity) in the pons, midbrain, and cerebellum. *C,* A one-year-old infant. A sagittal T1WI (SE TR 400/TE 25) demonstrates increased myelination of the entire brainstem, cerebellar white matter, and corpus callosum, extending to the cerebral hemispheres. The cortex now is less intense than the white matter.

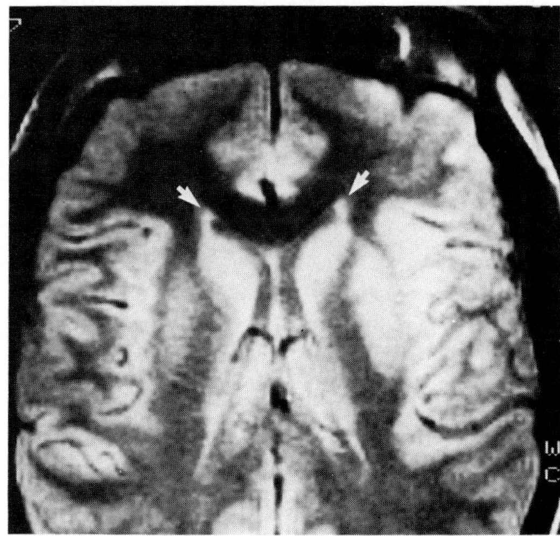

**Figure 15–4. Ependymitis granularis (1.5 T).** Axial moderately T2WI (SE 2000/TE 28) demonstrates high intensity foci at the tip of the frontal horns, a normal finding (arrows).

creased T2 are often seen anterior to frontal horns (Fig. 15–4). This circumstance is due to a change in the water balance at this site owing to "ependymitis granularis." This is a normal finding, may be asymmetric, and is not to be confused with pathologic demyelination; but careful clinical correlation is needed.[21]

With increasing age, periventricular signal abnormalities are seen that may mimic changes related to various white matter diseases. As much as 30% of clinically asymptomatic people may have these abnormalities in the sixth and the seventh decades, and differentiation from pathologic changes may be impossible.[22] This finding could be considered similar to other age-related involutional changes that develop in the CNS, such as atrophy. However, histologic analysis of these subclinical lesions reveals that these signal abnormalities are related to arteriosclerosis and associated white matter changes such as gliosis, cystic rarefaction, and necrosis. The severity of these findings increases with cerebral vascular risk factors. The sensitivity of MR probably allows identification of a prolonged preclinical stage of ischemic white matter disease.[23]

In a study of carefully selected 59- to 71-year-old normal volunteers with absolutely no ischemic risk factors, the appearance of the white matter was normal in 18 of 20 subjects; one showed a single lesion; and only one, multiple foci of T2 prolongation.[24] Careful clinical correlation is needed to exclude underlying pathology.[9, 24, 25] Ischemia and hydrocephalus are such causes and are addressed in Chapter 12. Other differential diagnostic possibilities are discussed in this section.

## IMAGING TECHNIQUES

### Routine Examination

#### *The Mature Brain*

Screening the mature brain for white matter disease should start with T1W scout views in the midline sagittal projection, in order to quickly determine the level for further axial double-echo T2WI, which have proven to be most sensitive, and the need to obtain a view of the anatomy in the sagittal plane.[5, 26–28] The sagittal view is of primary importance in the region of the foramen magnum, the fourth ventricle, and the sylvian aqueduct (Fig. 15–5).

In addition to the axial images, coronal T2W double-echo images should be obtained. They are helpful in determining whether small focal lesions are truly in the white matter, are the result of averaging, or are artifactual (one of the numerous MR "pitfalls"; see Chap. 16). Also, precise periventricular localization along the upper and

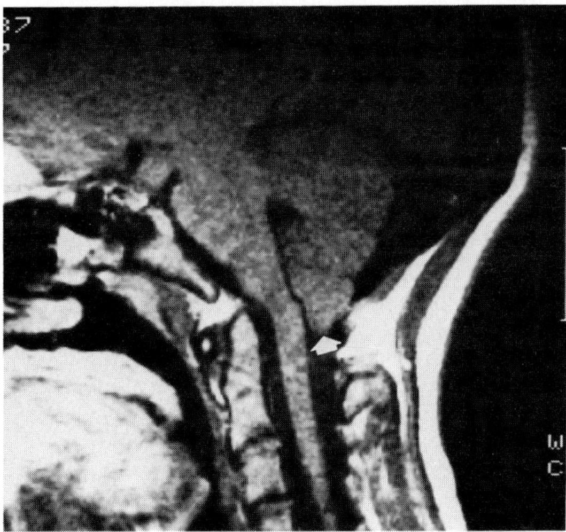

**Figure 15–5. Tonsillar herniation.** Sagittal T1WI SE (TR 500/TE 16). This 30-year-old female presented with symptoms suggestive of multiple sclerosis (1.5 T). The midline sagittal image demonstrates cerebellar tonsillar herniation (arrow) consistent with Arnold-Chiari type 1 malformation.

lower surfaces of the ventricular system can be obtained. Often subtle mass effect is best seen in the contour of the ventricles in the coronal view.

Inversion recovery T1WI are useful in special situations; lesions in the brain stem are better seen, and periventricular and other lesions can be evaluated for their T1 morphology.[29, 30]

### The Immature Brain

T2WI of an immature brain should be obtained with sufficiently long repetition times to avoid effect of T1 in the white matter decreasing its intensity and causing isointensity between gray and white matter. At higher field strengths (1.0 to 1.5 T), TR of 1.8 to 3.5 sec combined with sufficiently long echo delay (TE 80 to 160 msec) gives excellent gray-white differentiation. Exact scanning parameters for the time of physiologic crossover in the relaxation values of gray and white matter around eight months of age are not precisely known and may be slightly different for each individual, depending on the normal variations in the rate of development.[12]

T1WI with short TE and TR spin-echo or IR sequence show progressive myelination and also give the best CNS to CSF demarcation in coronal, axial, and sagittal planes.[1, 13, 15, 18, 19]

## Special Techniques

### Contrast Enhancement

The role of contrast enhancement in evaluation of white matter abnormalities is twofold; it assists in differential diagnosis and allows evaluation of activity and severity of white matter lesions, particularly in multiple sclerosis (MS).[31, 32] In many instances, there is no documentation as to its role in a given entity, which therefore must be projected from known results in CT scanning.

### Short Inversion Time IR Scan (STIR)

Improved lesion detection has been reported in the optic nerve by using STIR sequence.[33] This improvement is due to the suppression of signal from the orbital fat surrounding the optic nerve. On spin-echo images, the adipose signal masks subtle signal differences within the optic nerve.[29, 33]

Other techniques for fat-water signal separation could probably also be used for detection of lesions in the optic nerve to obtain similar results.

### Motion Compensation Gradients

Motion compensation gradients are used in high-field imaging to decrease artifacts from motion, including CSF pulsations, particularly in detection of lesions at the level of basal cisterns. Contrast-to-noise ratio is improved between lesions and normal white matter and between gray and white matter; signal-to-noise ratio in white matter is also improved. The combined use of refocusing gradients and low bandwidth techniques will probably be routinely applied at high field strength imaging in diagnosing white matter diseases.[34]

### Narrow Flip Angle Sequences

Little experience has been obtained on the use of fast-imaging sequences that combine the narrow flip angle with gradient echoes in the evaluation of white matter. Discouraging results in the evaluation of multiple sclerosis have been reported.[35] Although relative intensities among gray matter (GM), white matter (WM), and CSF are equal to those obtained by T2W spin-echo images, the detectability of MS plaques was less or was totally lacking. It was concluded that further work is needed to explain this phenomenon and to evaluate whether some added specificity could be obtained from the use of such sequences.

### The Role of CT Scanning

The contrast differences between unmyelinated and myelinated brain and normal and abnormal white matter are significantly less on CT than on MR images obtained with proper pulse sequence. Therefore CT is most useful in detecting patterns of calcification and in confirming the presence of acute hemorrhage and gas and thus providing information for differential diagnostic purposes.

# PATHOLOGY

## Demyelinating Diseases of the CNS

### *Chronic Multiple Sclerosis*

The "classic" form of multiple sclerosis is characterized by a sudden or gradual onset of neurologic dysfunction of various systems and a remitting and relapsing but progressive course that gradually results in mild to severe deficits or even death. The etiology is unknown. Age of onset is usually the second to fourth decade but may occur from the first to seventh decade. There is a female predominance.[7, 37]

Often the diagnosis is difficult. The deficits may be subtle or initially focal and may mimic various other neurologic conditions, including tumors or vascular disorders.[38] The patient may undergo numerous tests before the correct diagnosis is made.[37, 39–42] The lack of specificity of findings even in typical cases mandates careful clinical correlation before a *definite* diagnosis is made.

Criteria for a *definite* diagnosis are the following: (1) a history of neurologic symptoms with relapses and remissions, (2) evidence of two or more anatomically separate lesions documented by clinical examination, evoked responses, or imaging techniques, (3) evidence of an immunologic disturbance in the central nervous system revealed by a demyelinative spinal fluid profile.

Diagnosis is *probable* in patients with two or more lesions if either of the other two criteria is met. The diagnosis is *possible* if there is evidence of one lesion and only one of the other criteria is fulfilled.[43]

Histologically, the active lesions (plaques) show inflammation, demyelination and edema, and indistinct margins. Chronic inactive plaques show persisting demyelination and fibrillary gliosis with marked disruption of normal architecture of the white matter. The surviving axons demonstrate shrinkage and oligodendroglial depletion is severe.[7]

**Paraclinical Tests.** Presently, the paraclinical tests used in conjunction with history and physical examination are visual, auditory, and somatosensory evoked potentials. Clinically silent lesions can be detected but cannot be accurately localized. In cases of definite MS, the abnormalities are found in approximately 65% to 75%, although one study reported as high as 90.5% in cases of possible MS.[37, 41, 43–45]

Laboratory analysis of CSF for MS profile gives additional evidence for the diagnosis; it is positive in 54% to 74% of cases of proven MS.[37, 41, 44]

**Imaging Studies.** A significant function of diagnostic imaging studies in the workup of suspected MS is to exclude other pathologies such as midline tumors or Arnold-Chiari malformations, which can present with similar symptoms and signs (Fig. 15–5). Once this goal has been obtained, attention is then directed to findings associated with MS. The success of MR lies not only in its superiority over CT in detecting MS lesions but also in its ability to better detect most types of CNS abnormalities.[6]

**CT.** Before the invention of MRI, the only modality able to show characteristic MS lesions in the CNS was CT. However, owing to the limited soft tissue contrast derived from alterations in the electron density in the MS lesions, CT often is normal even in cases of definite MS, or when results are positive, CT shows fewer lesions. With CT scanning, the best results are obtained with the double-dose, delayed technique in which active plaques are seen as enhancing lesions.[37, 40] Positive scan is obtained in 29% to 62% of definite cases.[37, 40, 44, 46] As intravenous contrast enhancement becomes routine in MR imaging, the role of CT will diminish in the evaluation of MS patients.[31]

Nonenhancing lesions are seen as ill-defined hypodensities in the white matter that cause irregularity of the ventricular margins. In relatively long-standing cases, atrophy is seen.

**MRI**

**APPEARANCE OF LESIONS IN THE BRAIN.** Often, the appearance of MS on MRI is characteristic, with bilateral high intensity lesions of varying size and shape on T2WI in the periventricular location and also deeper in the white matter (Fig. 15–6). Some lesions are seen in the cerebellum and brain stem.[2, 37, 39–42, 47] However, the appearance of MS lesions on MR images can be extremely variable.

The number of lesions varies from one to innumerable.The size ranges from millimeters to large contiguous lesions along lateral ventricles. Only rarely do giant plaques involve the entire centrum semiovale and demonstrate mass effect.

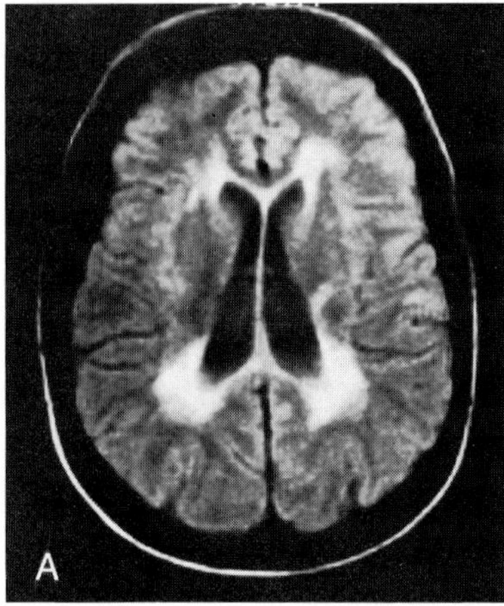


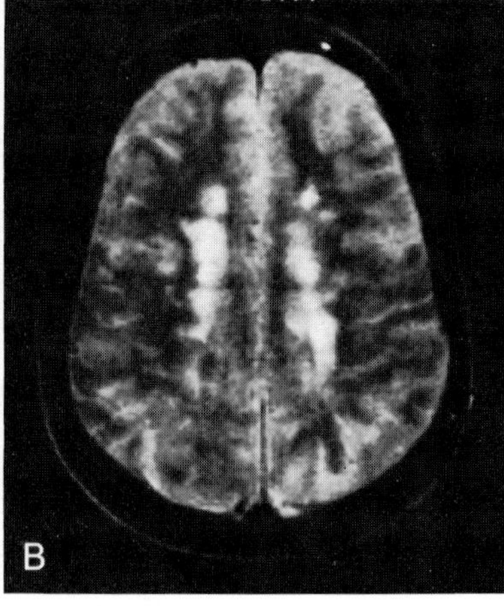


**Figure 15–6. Chronic multiple sclerosis (0.5 T).** *A,* An axial N(H)WI (SE TR 2000/TE 35) demonstrates characteristic periventricular lesions most prominent around the atria of the lateral ventricles. *B,* Axial T2WI (SE 2000/TE 80) at the level of the centrum semiovale demonstrates numerous periventricular hyperintense plaques. More lesions are also seen scattered in the white matter.

The smallest lesions are punctate in shape. When several lesions are present, they may be round, angular, oblong, linear, confluent, or "lumpy and bumpy."[42] It has been suggested that a "right-angle demyelination" lesion (round on axial image and linear in coronal image, with orientation perpendicular to the lateral ventricle) is more specific (84%) for MS.[48] These lesions correspond anatomically to perivenular plaques (Dawson's fingers) (Fig. 15–7).[7, 48] Linear lesions have been described in the inner aspect of the corpus callosum (CC), seen as increased signal intensity on T2WI and an irregular, low-intensity band on T1WI. In 40% associated atrophy of the CC is seen (Fig. 15–8*A*).

The most common location of the plaques is along the lateral ventricles, especially the atria and occipital horns, and also scattered in the supratentorial white matter.[39, 40–42, 50] In one study, 84% were found in this location, and 8% involved the gray matter, 5% in midbrain, and 2% in the cerebellum (Fig. 15–8*B*).[37]

In patients with isolated brain stem syndrome the most common location of brain stem lesions is the floor of the fourth ventricle and in the sylvian aqueduct.[51] Of these patients, 77% have associated supratentorial lesions if the symptoms have persisted three months or less; 70%, if symptoms are more long-standing (over nine months). The location of lesions in the brain stem correlates well with the clinical symptoms[51] as opposed to lesions of the supratentorial white matter, where the correlation is poor.[39–42, 44, 50]

The appearance of the lesions varies with different pulse sequences owing to differences in the inherent T1 and T2 values and in proton density. Chronic plaques demonstrate low intensity on T1WI and high intensity on the less T2-weighted "spin density" images and show relative increase in intensity on the more T2-weighted second-echo images of a double-echo sequence.[39–42, 50] Some lesions are seen only on T2WI, and the lesions with long T1 tend to appear

**Figure 15–7. Right-angle demyelination (0.5 T).** A coronal N(H)WI (SE TR 2000/TE 35) illustrates the linear shape of a plaque perpendicular to the lateral ventricle (arrows). Other periventricular lesions, atrophy causing enlargement of the fourth ventricle, and involvement of the gray matter (arrowhead) are demonstrated.

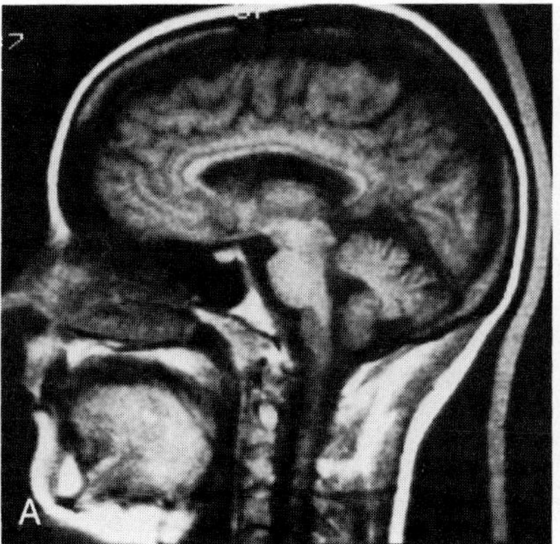


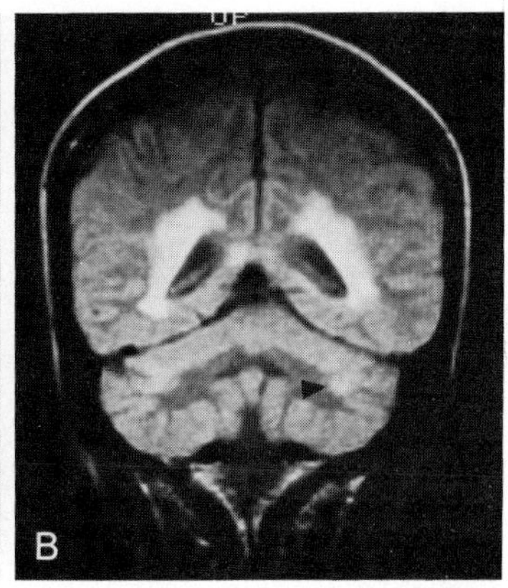


**Figure 15–8. Chronic multiple sclerosis (MS)** (0.5 T). *A,* Atrophy of the corpus callosum. A sagittal T1WI (TR 300/TE 17) with marked atrophy of the corpus callosum due to chronic MS. Periatrial and cerebellar plaques. *B,* coronal N(H)WI (SE TR 2000/TE 35) demonstrates characteristic prominent periatrial plaques and a peripheral white matter lesion in the left cerebellar hemisphere (arrowhead).

larger on T2WI (Fig. 15–9). They have a peripheral zone of T2 abnormality only.[42, 50] This appearance reflects a more extensive disruption of the neuropil with complete demyelination of the core of the lesions, which causes an increase in the free- to bound-water ratio.[7, 50, 52] T1 prolongation correlates in a more direct manner with the increase in bulk water. The T2 value is sensitive to the more subtle changes in the molecular environment and shows the earlier and less extensive damage in the intracellular and intercellular structures.[50]

Arcuate fibers at the gray-white junction are often partially involved by the more peripheral MS lesions, an observation that can assist in the differential diagnosis in some cases.[20]

Relaxation time measurements of the MS lesions have not consistently helped in the differentiation of active from chronic plaques, nor have they shown specific values.[40, 52, 53] However, T1 and T2 prolongation in the gray matter and T2 or T1 and T2 prolongation in the visibly unaffected white matter have been reported.[53, 54]

Although location of the lesions often does not correlate well with the clinical symptoms, as stated previously, in careful clinical studies a significant relationship has been found between severity of disease shown on MRI and the clinical disease.[47]

In more long-standing cases, cerebral atrophy develops. It is seen in up to 45% of patients with clinically definite MS. The most common abnormality reported on CT, it probably develops owing to demyelination and gliosis with wallerian degeneration of the axons.[4, 39, 49, 55]

On the MR images, manifestations of atrophy are well demonstrated on T1WI. In the midline sagittal plane especially, atrophy of the corpus callosum, an area which has been difficult to evaluate on CT scanning, can be depicted.[55]

Change in the intensity of thalamus and putamen on T2WI in patients with definite MS is an important observation recently

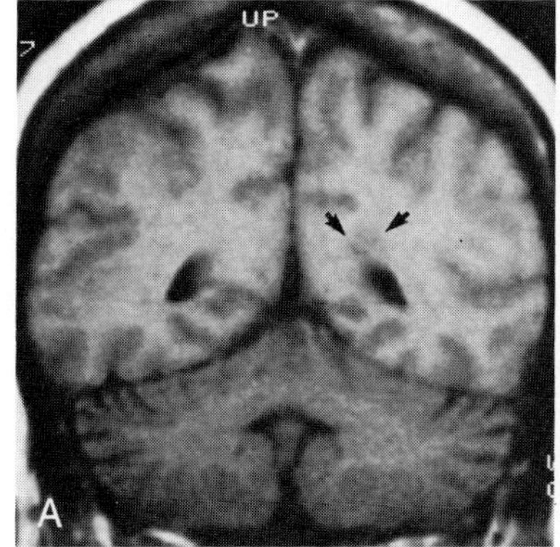


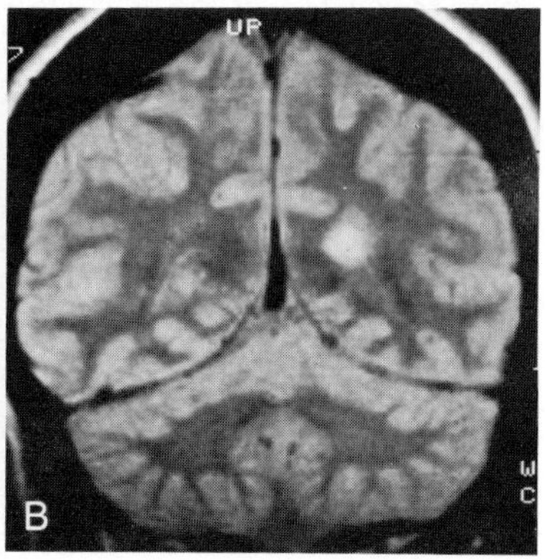


**Figure 15–9. TI and T2WI of multiple sclerosis plaque (1.0 T).** *A,* Coronal TIWI (SE TR 500/TE 17) of a periatrial plaque demonstrating an ill-defined area of patchy T1 prolongation (arrows). *B,* Coronal N(H)WI (SE TR 2500/TE 28), the plaque demonstrates high intensity and larger size than on the T1W image.

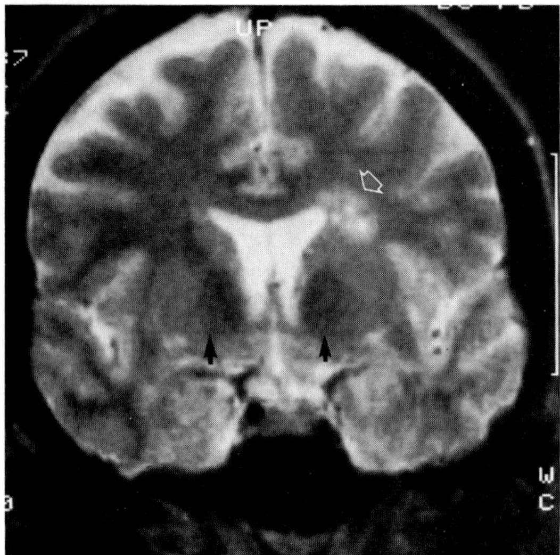

**Figure 15–10. Chronic multiple sclerosis (MS) with normal globus pallidus iron.** There is decreased intensity in the globus pallidus (1.0 T). Coronal T2WI (SE TR 2500/TE 80) demonstrates the normal decreased intensity commonly seen (arrows) in globus pallidus owing to ferritin deposits. Increased basal ganglia iron can occur in chronic MS. Chronic periventricular MS plaque is seen on the left (open arrow).

published.[56] This change is seen at high field strength and correlates with increased ferritin, which causes local magnetic field inhomogeneities and thus shortens T2. In abnormal cases, the intensity of the globus pallidus is equal to or less than that in the putamen and the caudate and is minimally more prominent than or equally prominent as that in the thalamus (Fig. 15–10). The prominence of the decreased signal intensity directly correlates with the extent and number of white matter lesions. The underlying mechanism of this finding remains speculative.

**Serial Studies.** The lesions of MS may remain stable, may progress, or may regress in follow-up studies.[39] The appearance of new lesions and enhancement of the lesions correlate with relapses.[31] New lesions may appear or previous ones may become larger (Fig. 15–11).

When comparison with previous studies is made, careful attention must be given to technique and positioning to avoid misdiagnosis of artifactual changes.

**Contrast Enhancement.** Enhancement of MS lesions has proved more distinct on MRI than on CT scans. The patterns of enhancement of the lesions can be nodular or ring shaped. Some lesions may be less evident following enhancement, owing to the timing of the scan after contrast administration.

Noncontrast T2WIs demonstrate more lesions than T1WIs with enhancement, as enhancement correlates with activity of the plaques. Enhancing lesions tend to correlate with localized symptoms, as opposed to the lesions on T2WI, which often are clinically silent, particularly in the supratentorial brain.[32, 39–42, 50, 57]

In evaluation of patients with optic neuritis, enhancement may be helpful in detecting active lesions in the intracranial portion of the optic nerve and the chiasm.[58]

Corticosteroid administration may have an effect on size of lesions during a relapse, but it does not consistently affect them. Many lesions continue to enlarge in size, others may regress and disappear, whereas most remain unchanged.[59]

**Spinal Cord.** In as much as 70% of patients with definite MS, lesions are demonstrated in the spinal cord (mostly in the cervical but also in the thoracic cord).[60, 61] Only studies of high technical quality visualize these le-

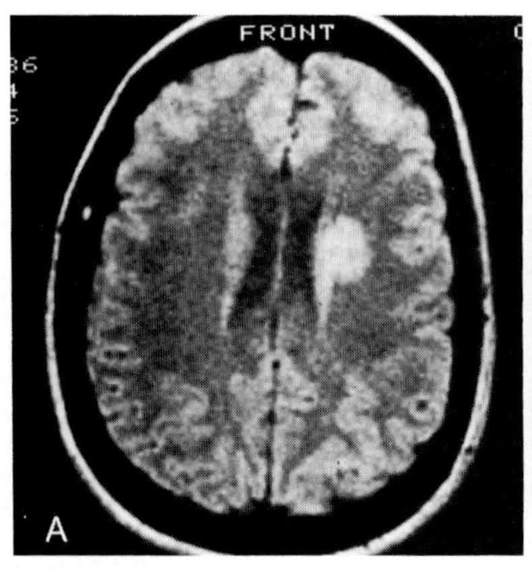


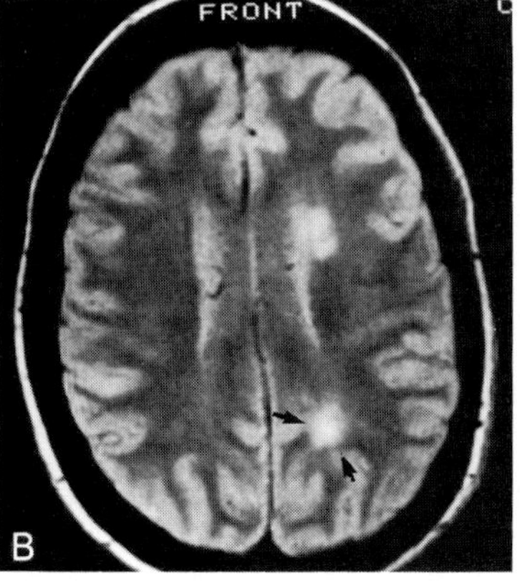


**Figure 15–11. Serial examinations in multiple sclerosis (MS) (0.5 and 1.0 T).** *A,* Axial N(H)WI (SE TR 2000/TE 35) demonstrates a prominent periventricular MS plaque on the left. *B,* On a follow-up study nine months later, on a N(H)WI (SE TR 2500/TE 28) the periventricular lesion shows decrease in size, but a new lesion has appeared in the posterior parietal region. Note involvement of the subcortical arcuate fibers (arrows).

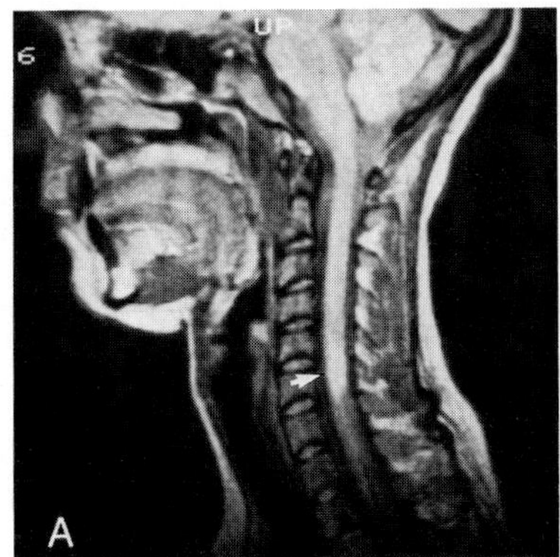


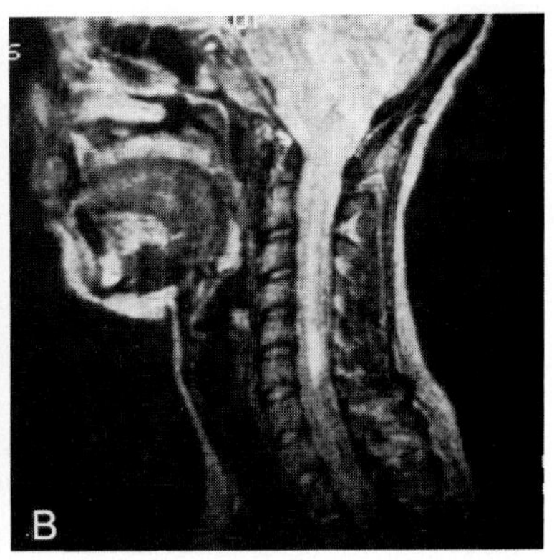


**Figure 15–12. MS plaque in the cervical spinal cord (0.5 T).** *A*, Sagittal N(H)WI (SE TR 2500/TE 45) demonstrates an area of increased signal intensity within the cord (arrow). *B*, On the T2W (SE TR 2500/TE 90) second-echo image, the relative intensity of the lesion increases, and the oblong shape is better delineated.

sions.[62] Although a common pathologic finding, spinal cord lesions have not been successfully demonstrated on imaging studies other than MRI.[60, 63] A characteristic lesion has an elongated configuration over a distance of several centimeters. During the acute stage, focal expansion of the cord, which resolves on serial follow-up studies, can be seen.[60, 61] The lesions do not correspond to fiber tracts and do not respect gray-white matter boundaries. They preferentially occur in the dorsal and lateral segments (Fig. 15–12).[63]

The majority of patients with cord symptomatology have lesions in the brain.[41, 43, 60, 63] These may be asymptomatic.[43] Some of the patients that present clinical findings consistent with MS but manifest no lesions in the brain most likely have involvement of the cord alone. In these patients, careful scanning of the cord is indicated and may successfully demonstrate the lesions to support the diagnosis.

**Optic Neuritis.** Isolated optic neuritis may be a manifestation of MS. It may be the presenting symptom or the only symptom with clinically silent MS lesions in the white matter. The percentage of patients with optic neuritis who have MS lesions in the brain has been reported to range from 50% to 89%.[41, 64] Only some of these will later develop other clinical manifestations of MS, although this risk may be up to 75%.[58, 64]

The optic nerve lesion usually is not seen on standard spin-echo sequences but can be detected in up to 75% of cases with STIR.[33, 37, 40, 58] Visual evoked potentials can be used in the negative cases to document the presence of optic nerve lesions, and MRI of the brain will allow a more specific diagnosis when the characteristic brain lesions are seen.[65]

### *Variants of Multiple Sclerosis*

*Acute multiple sclerosis* is a variant of MS that resembles acute encephalomyelitis and is invariably fatal. Absence of documentable infection or immunization helps in the differentiation. Clinical manifestations are headache, vomiting, brain stem signs, and spinal cord and optic nerve involvement.

Scattered white matter lesions are seen with a distribution comparable to that of chronic multiple sclerosis. Brain stem lesions are common.[7]

*Neuromyelitis optica* (Devic's disease) is a variant characterized by an acute onset of partial or complete blindness and signs of myelopathy occurring successively within an interval of several weeks or less. It is rare in western countries but more common in India and in the Far East. Lesions in the optic nerves, chiasm, and the cord should be sought. Other regions of the CNS may also show involvement.[7]

On MRI, swelling of the entire cord has been described in a patient with subsequent severe atrophy five months later. No associated brain lesions were seen.[66]

*Concentric sclerosis* is a rare, curious form of MS that is diagnosable only at autopsy. Clinical features include acute onset in a young individual, early symptoms suggestive of a space-occupying lesion, and marked motor symptoms or psychic syndromes. The survival period may be three to five years; the disease has a monophasic course and death occurs as a result of some intercurrent cause. The pattern of involvement is multifocal, as in MS, but u fibers and gray matter are spared.[7]

Most of the cases referred to as *Schilder's disease* have been in young males with classic adrenoleukodystrophy. The remainder probably had some variant of multiple sclerosis. Because of this fact, and because Schilder's original cases did not constitute a uniform group, the term *Schilder's disease* should not be used.[7]

### Acute Disseminated Encephalomyelitis

Acute disseminated encephalomyelitis (ADE) is an uncommon, acute, demyelinating disease of the central nervous system. The postinfectious form typically occurs following childhood viral infections but also occurs in adults following a nonspecific viral upper respiratory illness.

This disease may also occur spontaneously or after vaccination against rabies, diphtheria, smallpox, tetanus, or typhoid. A latent period of four days to three weeks is seen prior to onset of severe symptoms, differentiating ADE from encephalitis. The clinical course is monophasic. Fever, headache, and meningeal signs are seen followed by seizures, coma, papilledema, ataxia, and motor deficits.[67] In 15% to 20% of patients, the disease has been fatal.[7, 67] The mechanism of white matter damage is believed to be vascular damage secondary to circulating immune complex deposition and complement activation. With early steroid therapy, remarkable reversal of symptoms can occur.[68]

ADE is demonstrated on T2WI as multifocal, often confluent, white matter lesions of increased intensity in cerebrum, brain stem, and cerebellum, consistent with T2 prolongation (Fig. 15–13*A* and *B*). Lesions can be asymmetric and are less often periventricular than in MS.[69] Segmental involvement of gray-white junction is often seen, including the arcuate fibers. Spinal cord involvement is common. Lesions are usually nonhemorrhagic, asymmetric, and correlate well with clinical symptoms and signs. Some lesions show T1 prolongation and may have mass effect. Enhancement of the lesions probably is more uniform than in MS since all lesions in ADE are active.[67]

With successful steroid therapy, follow-up scans show resolution of the lesions, or persistent but less extensive lesions may be seen.[53, 67, 68]

CT scanning occasionally shows poorly demarcated lesions but is often negative.

### Acute Hemorrhagic Leukoencephalopathy

Acute hemorrhagic leukoencephalopathy is most often seen in childhood and in males more often than in females. Onset is frequently preceded by a viral infection. The condition probably is a hyperacute form of ADE and is characterized by an abrupt onset of headache, fever, motor and sensory dis-

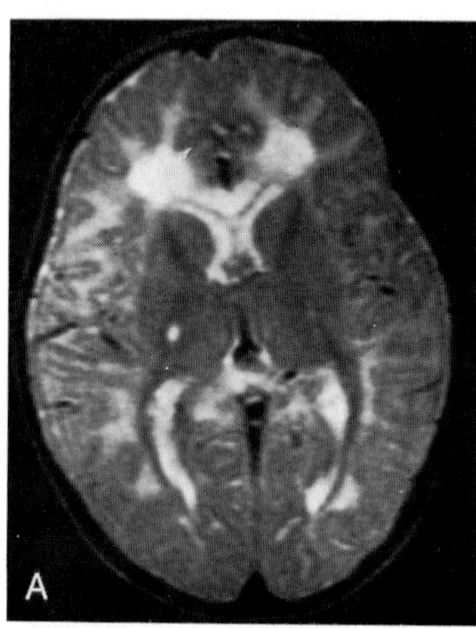


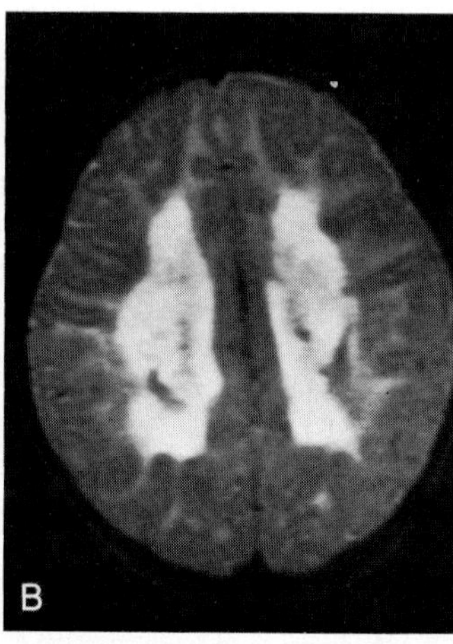


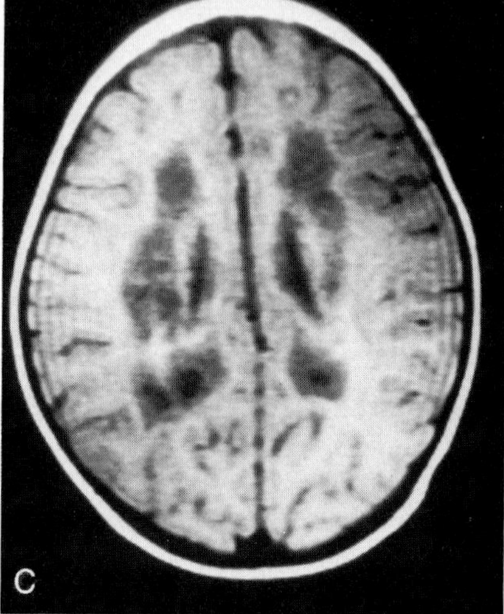


**Figure 15–13. Acute disseminated encephalomyelitis, postvaccinal.** One-year-old girl, vaccinated against mumps, measles, and rubella days before the onset of symptoms (1.5 T). *A,* T2WI (SE TR 2500/TE 100) at the level of atria shows bilateral, quite symmetric, periventricular and deep white matter involvement. *B,* A more cephalad image showing extensive bilateral involvement of white matter. *C,* Axial TIWI (SE TR 800/TE 200) at the same level as *B* demonstrates T1 prolongation, particularly in the center of some of the lesions. (Courtesy of Radiology Department, Children's Hospital Medical Center, Cincinnati, Ohio.)

turbances, and lethargy. These signs rapidly progress to stupor and coma, with a fatal outcome in one to six days.

Pathologic changes include widespread or localized, prominent involvement of white matter, small petechial hemorrhages, or large confluent zones of hemorrhage and necrosis. The pathogenesis probably results from a hyperacute reaction resulting from sensitization to myelin antigens or from myelin damage as a secondary, bystander event during viral white matter involvement. Cerebrum, cerebellum, and brain stem are equally vulnerable. The basal ganglia, cortex, and spinal cord are usually spared.[7, 67]

On high-field MRI, acute hemorrhagic leukoencephalopathy can be differentiated from ADE by noting the presence of various stages of hemorrhage superimposed on areas of demyelination.[67]

### *Progressive Multifocal Leukoencephalopathy*

Progressive multifocal leukoencephalopathy (PML) conforms poorly to the criteria stated in the definition of the demyelinating diseases. It has a known infectious cause (papovavirus), a marked predilection for white matter, and shows sparing of axons. In future classifications, it may well be considered a neoplastic condition.[7]

Clinically progressive multifocal leukoencephalopathy is a rare, fatal disease of adults; onset is usually between 40 and 60 years of age. The male to female ratio is 3:2. It develops most frequently against a background of lymphoproliferative disease, although it is also linked both to acute and chronic myelocytic leukemia, to carcinomatosis, and to benign diseases of the reticuloendothelial system.

A precipitating factor is immunosuppression (irradiation, cytotoxic agents or adrenocorticosteroids or both, and acquired immunodeficiency syndrome [AIDS]). Some cases occur without associated disease.[70]

Cerebral signs predominate; slightly less often are cerebellar signs manifested. The brain stem and cord can also be involved. Motor, mental, and visual disturbances are the most common symptoms. Also seen are sensory deficits, incontinence, ataxia and bulbar signs, terminal paraparesis, and coma.[7]

MRI shows multiple, asymmetric long T1 and long T2 lesions in the white matter. Initially, the lesions are small and either round or oval. Later they become confluent and large. The disease begins in the subcortical white matter then spreads to the deeper areas. Cortical gray matter is usually spared. The involvement is most often asymmetric. Mass effect is absent or scant, vascular territories are crossed, and lesions usually are not periventricular (Fig. 15–14).[70]

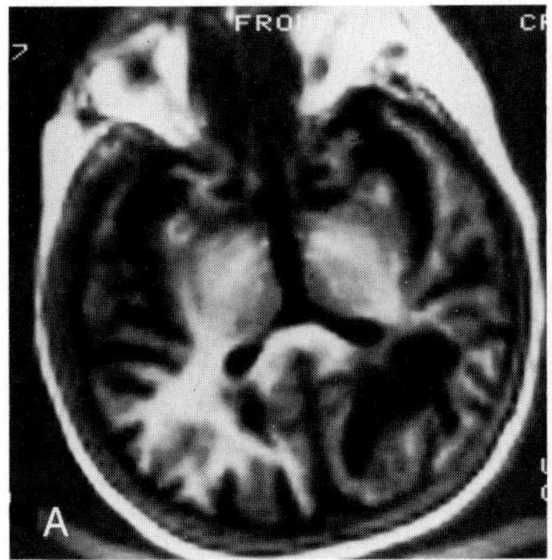


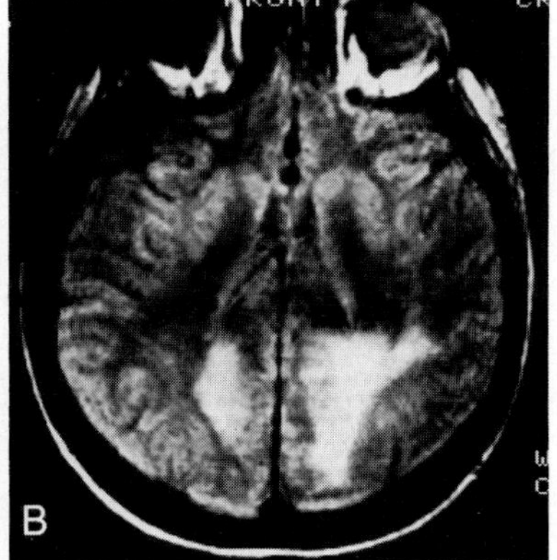


**Figure 15–14. Progressive multifocal leukoencephalopathy.** A 67-year-old woman with decreased white count at the time of admission but no other risk factors. *A,* Axial TIWI (IR TR 2500/TI 600/TE 28) demonstrates hypointense areas of T1 prolongation in the parietal white matter, more pronounced on the patient's left. There is sparing of the splenium of corpus callosum. *B,* A T2WI (SE TR 2500/TE 28) demonstrates T2 prolongation in the same regions. No additional lesions were noted on T2W images.

## METABOLIC DISEASES AFFECTING WHITE MATTER

At present only scattered reports concerning associated white matter changes on MR images related to some disease entities in this category have been published. However, projecting from detailed descriptions in neuropathology texts and findings on CT scans, a spectrum of findings varying from normal appearance to severe destruction of the white matter can be hypothesized.

Considering ongoing clinical research, characteristic MR findings in all probability will soon be described for most of these entities.

### Leukodystrophies

#### *Metabolic Diagnosis*

**Metachromatic Leukodystrophy.** Metachromatic leukodystrophy (MLD) is a group of autosomal recessive genetic diseases characterized by deficient arylsulfatase A, leading to the accumulation of metachromatic granules and diffuse demyelination of the central and peripheral nervous system. MLD can also be classified as a storage disorder in the subgroup of sphingolipidoses. It may present in late infantile, juvenile, adult and multiple sulfatase deficiency types.[7]

The late infantile form appears clinically between one and two years of age with motor signs of peripheral neuropathy followed by intellect, speech, and coordination deterioration that is often rapid. Within two years of onset, there is evidence of severe, diffuse white matter dysfunction, decerebrate posturing, quadriplegia, and blindness.[7]

CT shows marked symmetric, bilateral white matter hypodensity. The ventricles are moderately enlarged; cortex is spared.[71] The presence of peripheral neuropathy may help in differential diagnosis.

The bilateral, widespread white matter abnormalities with sparing of the cortex are clearly depicted on T2-weighted MR images (Fig. 15–15).

There is a continuum in the ages at onset of clinical signs and symptoms of MLD from neonatal period through later adulthood. Cases commencing between 3 and 21 years of age are considered the juvenile form of MLD. Clinically, it is manifested as learning difficulties, problems with concentration, emotional instability, and motor impairment. Initially, peripheral neuropathic signs are not common.[7]

On CT, diffuse, confluent bilateral involvement in the white matter of the centrum semiovale is seen. The lesions are nonenhancing. A scalloped, lateral border with sparing of arcuate (U) fibers and gray matter is noted.[72]

In the adult form, the earliest clinical symptoms are gradual onset of personality changes and behavioral disturbances as well as gradual worsening and dementia over the course of years. It is a rare disorder; however, the true incidence has probably been underestimated, as only a small minority of cases were correctly diagnosed before autopsy.[73]

The CT findings in the adult forms differ from earlier forms in that the white matter

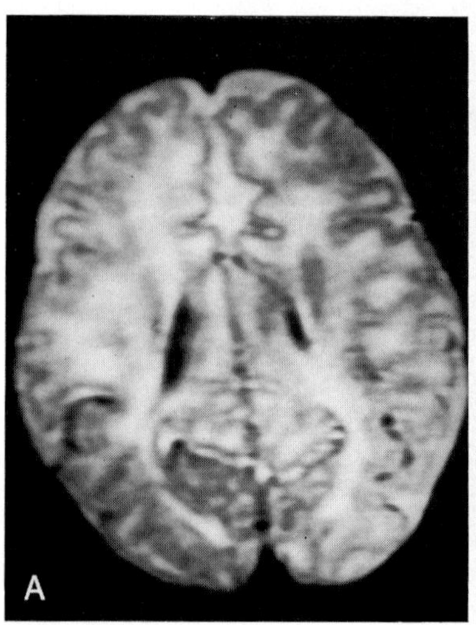


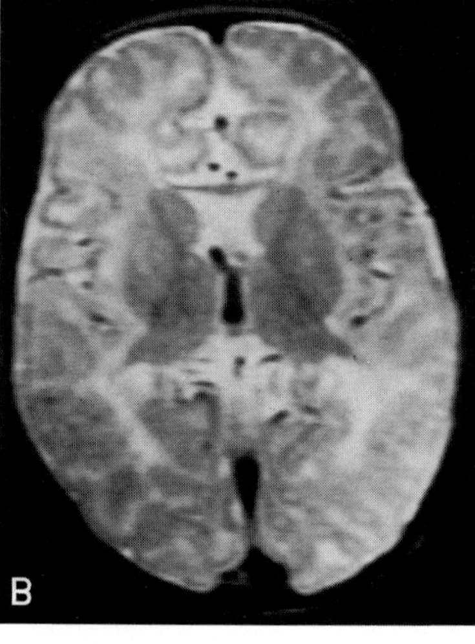


**Figure 15–15. Late infantile metachromatic leukodystrophy.** An eight-month-old girl with deteriorating neurologic status and positive blood tests and urinalysis. *A,* Axial T2WI (SE TR 2000/TE 100) demonstrates widespread bilateral abnormal increased signal intensity in the white matter inappropriate for age with sparing of the cortex. *B,* At the level of the atria, the hyperintense lesions merge with the high signal from CSF. (Courtesy of Radiology Department, Children's Hospital Medical Center, Cincinnati, Ohio.)

abnormalities show moderate frontal predominance and are less intimately coupled with neurologic symptoms. Central atrophy with prominence of basal cisterns is seen early, followed by cortical atrophy. No contrast enhancement is seen.[74–76]

MR findings have been described in adult onset MLD. Bilateral, confluent, symmetric periventricular T2 prolongation in the white matter in characteristic frontal and parieto-occipital regions with associated ventricular enlargement has been noted. As with other white matter diseases, the extent visible on MR is much broader than the subtle hypodensities seen on CT. On T1WI, central and cortical atrophy with mild frontal dominance is clearly depicted. Atrophy in the posterior fossa may be prominent.[73, 76]

**Krabbe's Disease.** Krabbe's disease, or globoid cell leukodystrophy, is a rare autosomal recessive leukodystrophy. It is the result of deficiency of β-galactocerebrosidase activity. Clinical manifestations appear at two to six months of age, after which the affected infants rapidly lose previously attained developmental skills. Fever, irritability, myoclonic seizure, blindness, spasticity, and quadriparesis follow. Optic atrophy is common. Size of the head remains small. Death occurs within the first two years.[7, 77] A late juvenile form has been described.

Histologically, very little myelin is present, but it is normal, probably having been formed before the enzyme deficiency was fully manifested biochemically.[7]

CT and MR findings are characteristic. Initially, CT reveals discrete and symmetric dense areas in the thalami, corona radiata, and body of caudate nuclei and later in the cerebellum, brain stem, and subcortical white matter. These are of unknown histologic etiology. White matter hypodensities representing demyelination and associated edema are seen. Atrophy subsequently develops.[78]

On MR symmetric, high-intensity white matter abnormalities are seen on T2WI owing to increased water content in the cerebrum with relative sparing of subcortical U fibers. Low-intensity lesions on T2WI (0.35 T), correlating to the high-density areas on CT, are seen. Possible paramagnetic substance accumulation has been hypothesized to be the cause. The lesions are not well seen at this field strength on T1WI. Global atrophy is also demonstrated (Fig. 15–16).[77]

**Adrenoleukodystrophy.** Adrenoleukodystrophy (ALD) is inherited as an X-linked recessive disorder and manifests in four clinically recognizable forms: (1) classic ALD, (2) adrenomyeloneuropathy (AMN), (3) neonatal adrenoleukodystrophy, and (4) symptomatic heterozygotes. Central nervous system demyelination and abnormalities of the adrenal glands are the hallmarks of this group of diseases.

*Classic ALD* usually manifests during the first decade of life. Duration from onset to death is one to nine years; the course is steadily progressive, although relapses and remissions have been described. Behavioral disturbances, seizures, visual loss, and corticospinal tract involvement progressing to quadriparesis are seen.

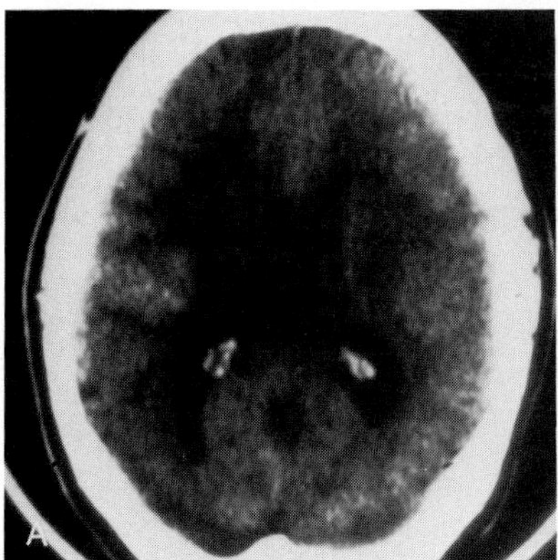

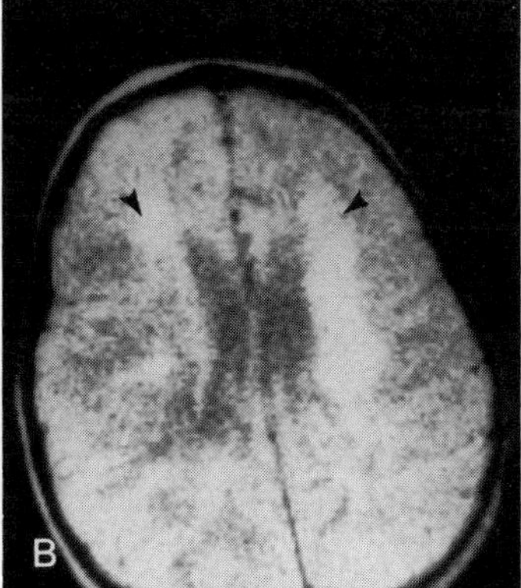

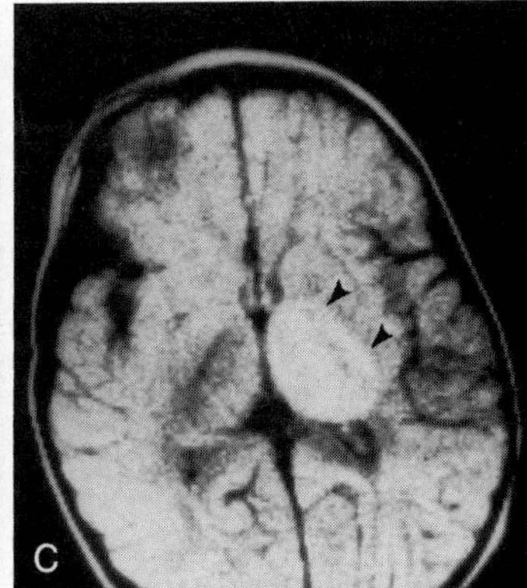


**Figure 15–16. Krabbe's disease.** A three-year-old boy with bizarre nystagmus and deteriorating neurologic status (0.35 T). *A*, Axial CT scan shows bilateral white matter hypodensities and areas of increased density in the subcortical white matter. *B*, Axial N(H)WI (SE TR 1500/TE 35) demonstrates bilateral, in this case asymmetric, white matter lesions (arrowheads). *C*, Asymmetric involvement of the patient's left thalamus (arrowheads) is also noted.

CT scanning is less sensitive to the extent of white matter damage than MRI. The involvement of areas other than the centrum semiovale and the occipitoparietal region is not consistently demonstrated. In some instances, calcifications are seen at the level of atria. A zone of enhancement is often seen surrounding the hypodense central portion of abnormal white matter, and this is presumed to represent an area of active demyelination. This zone is less obvious on the nonenhanced MR images (Fig. 15–17*A*).[79]

On MR, T2WIs clearly demonstrate the distribution of the abnormalities in the brain. They are seen in the white matter and are usually most severe in the occipital, parietal, and posterior temporal lobes, rarely occurring in the frontal lobes. Results of secondary atrophy can be seen in the pyramidal tracts, the posterior limb of the internal capsule, the lateral cerebral peduncles, the basis pontis, the pyramids, and the lateral corticospinal tracts. The cerebellar white matter is variably involved. Main involvement in the brain stem is wallerian degeneration of the corticospinal tract, and in cases with dentate nuclear involvement, the superior cerebellar peduncles may be similarly affected.[7, 26, 79]

Regional distribution is demonstrated in superb detail in coronal and axial images. With proper clinical correlation, these images allow a specific diagnosis to be made. Precise correlation with anatomic pathways and the extent of white matter abnormalities is seen in patients with impaired hearing or vision (Fig. 15–17*B* and *C*).[79]

*Adrenomyeloneuropathy* is a variant manifesting in adulthood as peripheral polyneuropathy and myelopathy. Adrenal insufficiency and hypogonadism are associated. In the brain, loss of axons and myelin from the corticospinal tracts throughout the brain stem and spinal cord and from the fasciculus gracilis is seen.[7]

MR depicts increased signal intensity on

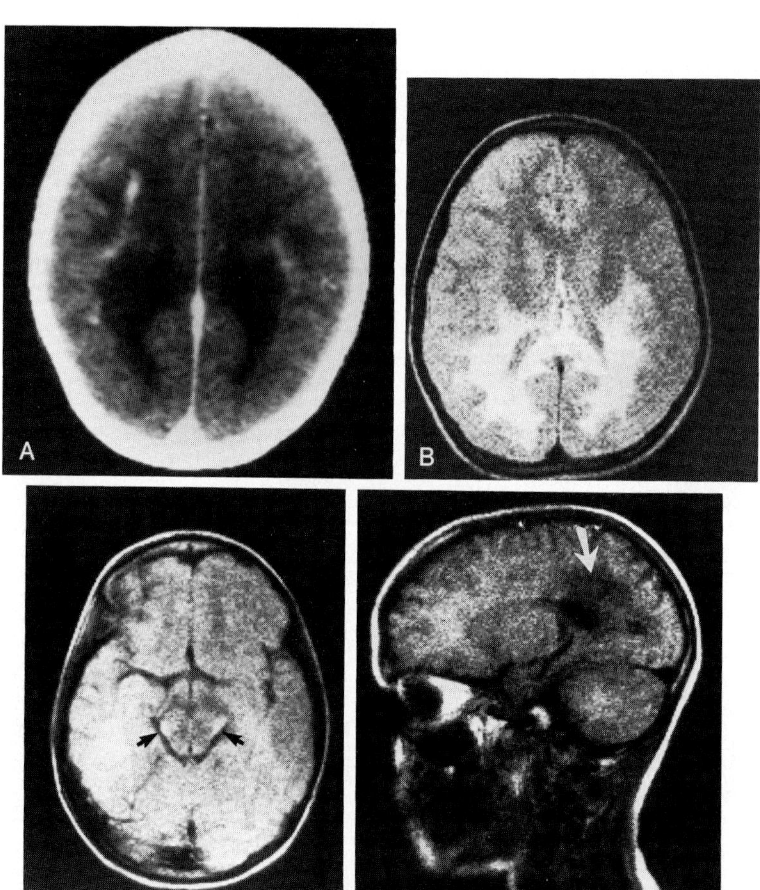


**Figure 15–17. Adrenoleukodystrophy.** A ten-year-old boy whose uncle has adrenoleukodystrophy (0.35 T). *A,* A contrast-enhanced CT scan demonstrates bilateral posterior parietal white matter hypodensities and zones of enhancement in the periphery of the hypodense areas. *B,* Axial T2WI (SE TR 1500/TE 70) demonstrates bilateral abnormal high-intensity areas in parietal white matter. *C,* Axial N(H)WI (SE TR 1500/TE 35) shows characteristic bilateral involvement in the topography of the lateral aspect of cerebral peduncle, lateral lemniscus, and brachium of the inferior colliculus (arrows). *D,* Sagittal T1WI (SE TR 300/TE 35) demonstrates T1 prolongation (arrow) in the involved white matter.

T2WI in the white matter around the trigones of the lateral ventricles, in the posterior limb of the internal capsule, in the dorsal corpus callosum, and in the pons. On T1-weighted IR images, these areas show low intensity. The resulting atrophy is seen as compensatory enlargement of the adjacent lateral ventricle.[7, 80] CT shows the atrophy but not the parenchymal changes.

*Neonatal adrenoleukodystrophy* occurs early in infancy with failure to thrive and seizures that begin during the first week of life. Heritance is autosomal recessive; there is no sex predilection. Psychomotor retardation and adrenocortical failure develop, and death occurs between two and seven years. Loss of myelin is seen in the centrum ovale, brain stem, and cerebellum. Craniofacial abnormalities may co-exist. Cerebral cortex in some cases is polymicrogyric.[7, 79]

A *symptomatic heterozygote* form has been reported in two families. It manifests both in males and in females. Clinical findings include primary adrenal insufficiency, hypogonadism, and neurologic abnormalities.[7]

### *Pathologic Diagnosis*

**Alexander's Disease.** Alexander's disease is a progressive disorder in infants, juveniles, and adults with a probable autosomal recessive inheritance.

The infantile form is characterized clinically by psychomotor retardation, spasticity, seizures, and rapidly increasing megalencephaly. The average age of onset is six months, but symptoms may appear at birth. Histologically, there is diffuse demyelination of variable severity. Innumerable Rosenthal's fibers are dispersed throughout the neuropil, with greatest concentration in the subpial, subependymal, and perivascular zones. Cause of demyelination is not clear.[7, 81–83] Patients with the juvenile form show spasticity, bulbar signs, and mental deterioration.

Megalencephaly and ventricular dilatation are common findings in Alexander's disease. The exact etiology remains uncertain. Findings on CT in the infantile form are extensive, and it is anticipated that MR will yield even further information.

On CT the earliest change in the white matter is increased density, perhaps owing to hyperemia. Subsequently, this progresses to bilateral, symmetric, moderately well-demarcated zones of reduced density in the frontal and temporal lobes, external capsules, and extreme capsules, with relative sparing of the internal capsules. The changes are most severe in the centrum semiovale of the frontal lobes and in the external and extreme capsules. There is associated enlargement of the lateral ventricles with frontal predominance.[81–83] Also, the third ventricle is enlarged. The abnormal white matter lucency extends peripherally to affect the subcortical arcuate fibers.[81]

Areas of increased density are seen subependymally and in the optic chiasm and optic radiations, in the columns of the fornices, in the corpus striatum, and in the proximal portions of the forceps minor. This distribution, with frontal predominance, is helpful in differentiating Alexander's disease from Canavan's disease, which also causes megalencephaly, but with a more even distribution of the white matter abnormality.[81, 82] Brain stem and cerebellar involvement is inconsistently reported on CT and probably will be much more obvious on MRI.[81]

Enhanced CT shows striking enhancement of those regions that are dense on the prior noncontrast CT, and these areas can also be expected to enhance with Gd-DTPA on MRI.[81, 83] When the disease is studied in subsequent years, the white matter lesions are more sharply demarcated, and neither enhancement nor dense zones is seen.[81–83] The appearance, in general, is less specific at this later stage.[78]

Atypical distribution has been reported on MRI of biopsy-proven cases of Alexander's disease. Patterns with focal periventricular distribution of lesions or predominantly cerebellar involvement were visible.[84]

In the juvenile form, marked dilatation of the lateral and third ventricles and diffuse, symmetric, low-density areas within the white matter are described on CT.[81] In the adult form, megalencephaly is absent, and the progression is very slow, simulating MS.[83]

**Canavan's Disease.** Canavan's disease, or spongy degeneration, is an autosomal recessive condition occurring most often in Jewish infants. The onset is typically in the first six months of life. Apathy, loss of motor activity, and hypotonia are noted. Blindness and optic atrophy ensue, followed by spasticity, decerebration, myoclonus, and seizures by one year of age. Megalencephaly is conspicuous. The biochemical basis is unknown. A rare juvenile form in non-Jewish children older than five years with no megalencephaly or mental retardation has been reported.[7]

In classic infantile spongy degeneration, white matter involvement is extensive, showing soft gelatinous texture with marked vacuolization under microscopy, often involving the cortex, although the cortex may be spared.[85, 86]

CT scanning shows bilateral, symmetric, hypodense white matter involvement (Fig. 15–18*A*) without increase in the ventricular size.[85–87] The globus pallidus is severely involved, with the spinal cord and brain stem less affected. The cerebellum is atrophic.[7]

Quite extensive signal abnormalities can be predicted in the white matter on MRI owing to the histopathologic picture. Cortical and U fiber involvement are helpful in excluding other leukodystrophies, as is the rather symmetric bilateral involvement.

**Pelizaeus-Merzbacher Disease.** Peli-

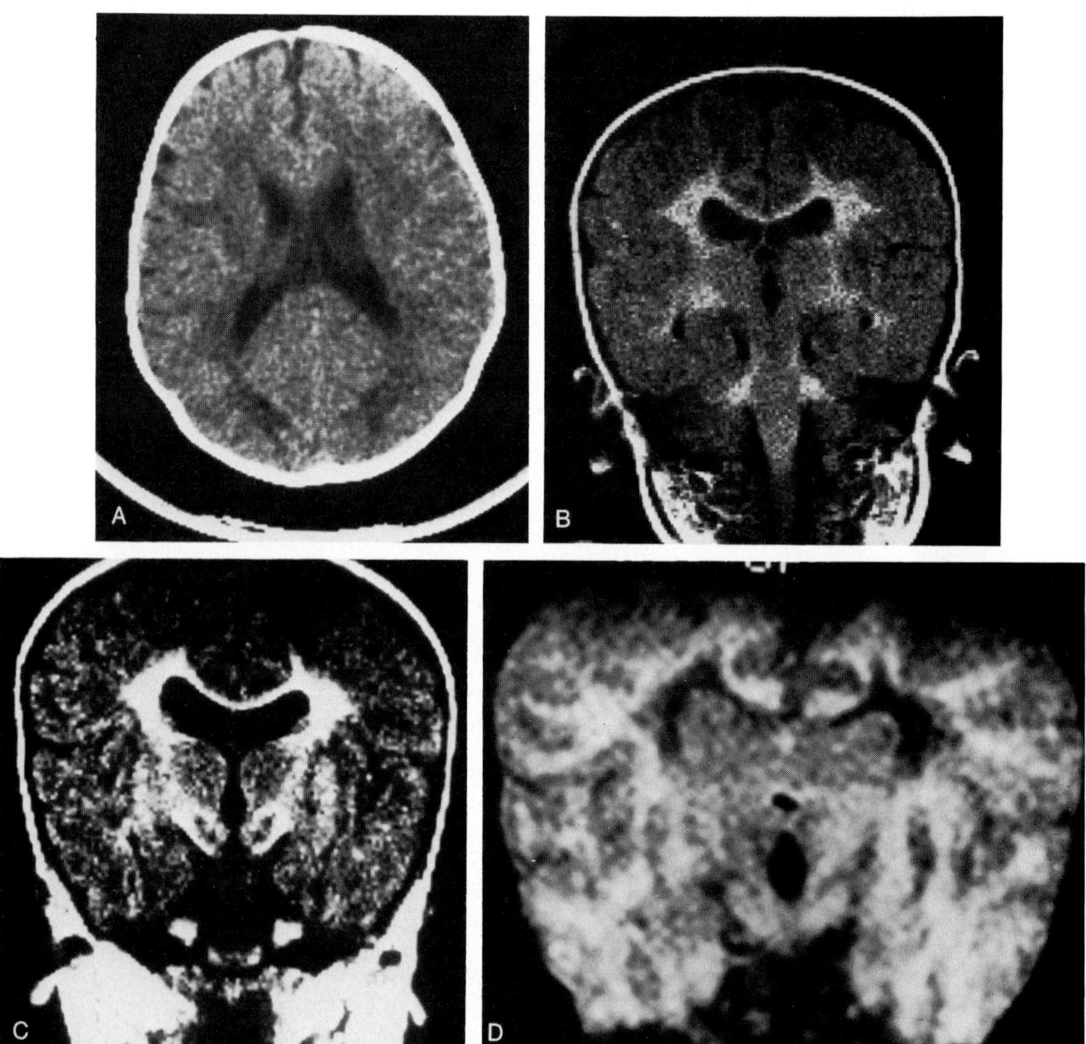


**Figure 15–18. Canavan's disease.** A 13-month-old boy with markedly delayed development and megalencephaly (0.35 T). His twin sister is also affected. *A,* A CT scan demonstrates symmetric, diffuse, white matter hypodensity and no evidence of hydrocephalus. *B,* Coronal T1WI (SE TR 300/TE 35) image demonstrates delayed myelination and megalencephaly. *C,* Follow-up study nine months after *B*: Coronal T1WI (SE TR 300/TE 35) demonstrates complete arrest in myelination; no further myelination has taken place in the interim. *D,* Coronal T2WI (SE TR 1500/TE 35) shows the arrested myelination as a low intensity area, and immature white matter with high intensity appears in the periphery.

zaeus-Merzbacher disease (PMD) is a rare, slowly progressive, sex-linked dysmyelinating disorder primarily affecting males but occasionally occurring in females. Classification has been controversial. Three subtypes can be recognized.

In the infantile form, nystagmus, extrapyramidal signs, and complete failure of psychomotor development are seen. Neuropathologic findings consist of an atrophic brain with a striking and diffuse absence of myelin.[7]

The juvenile form is the classic type, and the findings on CT and MR are known from the literature.[88–90] This form is clinically manifested in the first decade of life—in some cases, immediately after birth. Progression is very slow. Nystagmus, intermittent shaking movements of the head, ataxia, choreoathetoid movements, and psychomotor retardation are clinical features.

CT is essentially normal during the first decade and the beginning of the second, despite severely incapacitating neurologic signs. Eventually, as the disease progresses, enlargement of the ventricles occurs, and symmetric, patchy, low-density areas are seen in the periventricular white matter and in the centrum semiovale and the cerebellar hemispheres. Diffuse cerebellar and cortical atrophy develops.[89, 90]

MRI clearly shows the extension of abnormality in the entire supratentorial white matter on T2WI. Involvement is bilateral and symmetric. There is reversal of the normal intensity patterns of gray and white matter; all the white matter shows higher intensity than the gray matter, owing to increased water content and dysmyelination. The thalami and lentiform nuclei have been reported to have decreased signal intensity of indeterminate etiology on T2WI (0.35 T). Abnormal iron accumulation has been a speculative cause of this finding.[88, 89]

T1WI best show the atrophic changes. The white matter abnormality is not obvious on T1WI at an earlier stage; this is consistent with less severe changes in the white matter than in many other demyelinating diseases and also explains why CT is negative at this stage.

The adult form is inherited as an autosomal dominant trait. Psychotic features, together with corticospinal tract involvement, ataxia, and speech difficulties, are characteristic. The brain tends to be mildly atrophic with severe demyelination, associated with astrogliosis. The U fibers are spared.[7]

**Cockayne's Syndrome.** The main features of Cockayne's syndrome are autosomal recessive inheritance, onset in late infancy, dwarfism, deafness, photosensitive dermatitis, optic atrophy, retinal pigmentation, thickened skull, mental deficiency, and peripheral neuropathy. The pathogenesis is unknown.

Pathologically, the white matter shows patchy "tigroid" demyelination, and extensive calcification is seen in the walls of capillaries and arteries in the basal ganglia. The brain is small; leptomeninges are thickened. The optic nerves and the cerebellum are atrophic. The U fibers are not spared.[7]

On CT scanning, characteristic discrete calcifications in the putamina are seen. Lateral ventricles show mild dilatation. Dorsal kyphosis, osteopenia, and squared appearance of the pelvis are associated radiographic findings.[91] MR should have prominent findings, although no complete reports are yet available.

**Sudanophilic Leukodystrophies.** The term *sudanophilic leukodystrophies* (SLD) is applied to leukodystrophies that cannot be classified as inflammatory demyelinating disease, those without metachromatic substances or other distinguishing neuropathologic features. Histologically, these are characterized by sudanophilic, lipid-laden macrophages associated with widespread myelin loss.

The onset in different forms varies from the perinatal period to adulthood.[7]

**Other Leukodystrophies.** A number of other leukodystrophies, some with characteristic neuropathologic features, have been described; others have been incompletely described and cannot be adequately categorized.

*Congenital muscular dystrophy* with associated leukodystrophy presents extensive bilateral white matter abnormalities. There is T1 and T2 prolongation in the abnormal white matter.[17, 26, 92] The area of abnormality appears to be more extensive on T2WI than on T1WI.[36]

*Polycystic lipomembranous osteodysplasia* is of interest to radiologists. It occurs in adults and is associated with cysts in the bones of the extremities and with diffuse brain demyelination.

*Dermatoleukodystrophy, SLD with menin-*

*geal angiomatosis*, and *pigmented glial cell type of leukodystrophy* are some of the better-defined, rare leukodystrophies.[7]

### Storage Disorders

Storage disorders are characterized by genetically determined enzymatic defects. The defect, such as a specific lysosomal enzyme in lysosomal storage disease, results in storage of undigested material, which eventually leads to CNS damage. Some disorders have a defect in more than one enzyme. The main groups are lipidoses, mucopolysaccharidoses, mucolipidoses, and generalized glycogenoses.[7]

MRI findings in some of the mucopolysaccharidoses (MPS) have been described and include hydrocephalus or moderate ventricular dilatation, mild cortical atrophy, multifocal symmetric deep white matter abnormalities (Fig. 15–19), deposition of mucopolysaccharides along the dura and dens, and spinal stenosis and cord compression.[17, 93–95] MRI is ineffective in demonstrating leptomeningeal and dural thickening. Delayed myelination has been documented.[96] Gray-white contrast is poor.[95]

The extent of deep white matter abnormalities on T2WI correlates well with the extent of clinical disease. These abnormalities probably correspond to extensive cribriform and cavitary changes of the subcortical white matter and the presence of abnormal viscous fluid and mononuclear cells in the enlarged periadventitial spaces around the cerebral blood vessels, as seen on autopsy studies in patients with MPS.[93]

Bone marrow transplantation is used as a method of therapy in the MPS with resultant improvements in the clinical and biochemical features of the diseases. The effects of therapy can be monitored by MRI. Improvement in gray-white matter contrast, progressive increase in myelination, and less prominent periventricular T2 abnormality are seen, whereas the size of the ventricles and cortical sulci remains unchanged. On CT the parenchymal changes cannot be seen.[17, 95]

### Other Metabolic Disorders

A wide spectrum of metabolic disorders affects the nervous system to diverse degrees by a variety of mechanisms. Vacuolation of areas undergoing myelination and delayed or arrested myelination can be seen. In some disorders such as *Fabry's disease, Menke's disease,* and *homocystinuria,* the vasculature can be altered sufficiently to initiate thrombosis and cerebral infarction. In others, liver dysfunction may cause the encephalopathy. In still others, mental retardation is seen without neuropathologic changes that would explain the neurologic dysfunction.[7]

To what extent the alterations are reflected on MR images is still largely unknown except for anecdotal reports. Some of the examples that are available demonstrate varying combinations of findings that together with clinical information may allow a more specific diagnosis.

The MRI findings of some aminoacidopathies and metabolic acidoses are summarized as follows.

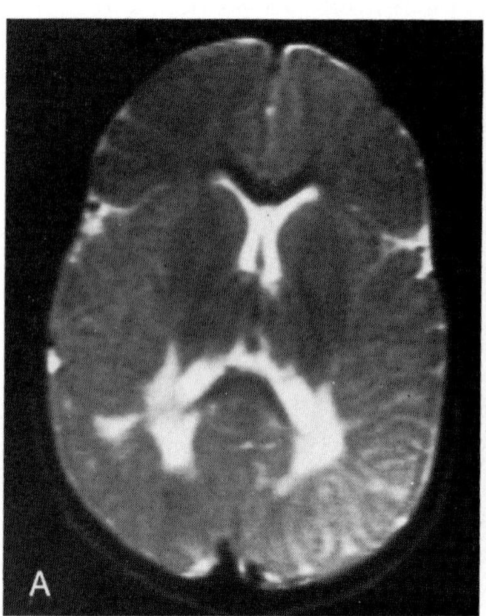


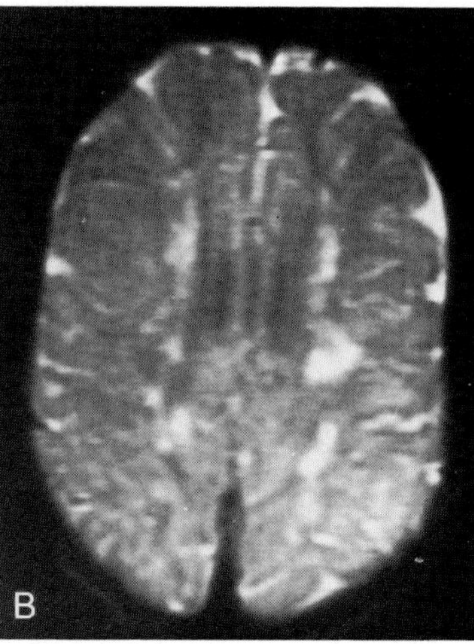


**Figure 15–19. Hurler's disease.** A two-year-old girl with dysmorphic facies (1.5 T). *A,* Axial T2WI (SE TR 2000/TE 100) at the level of the atria demonstrates bilateral patchy areas of increased signal. *B,* At the level of the centrum semiovale and forceps major there are quite extensive patchy hyperintense lesions in both hemispheres. (Courtesy of William Ball, M.D., Radiology Department, Children's Hospital Medical Center, Cincinnati, Ohio.)

*Nonketotic hyperglycemia*, which belongs to the group of aminoacidopathies, was found to cause abnormal myelination, deep gray matter signal abnormalities, and atrophy, whereas in *Hartnup's disease*, also an aminoacidopathy, MRI was normal.

Of the metabolic acidoses, *proprionic acidemia* was found to cause atrophy, diffuse white matter, and deep gray matter abnormality without regional changes to suggest abnormal myelination. In *lactic acidemia*, atrophy and some white matter abnormality were seen. *Methylmalonic aciduria* was characterized by deep gray matter signal abnormalities with some white matter involvement but normal myelination for age.[36, 99]

*Leigh's disease* (subacute necrotizing encephalopathy) also is a metabolic acidosis. A detailed description of the MR appearance has been given.[97] It is an autosomal recessive disease of infancy and childhood, causing encephalopathy with metabolic acidosis. Occasionally, it has an adult onset. Clinically hypotonia, ataxia, bulbar paresis, nystagmus, visual disturbances, and regressive psychomotor development are seen. The precise metabolic defect is unknown. Vaculation of neuropil, demyelination, and gray matter involvement are characteristic.

On CT a characteristic finding, although not always present, is hypodensity of the putamina. Atrophy, nonenhancing white matter lucencies with focal extension to the gray matter, and involvement of the caudate nuclei can also be seen.[98]

MR shows focal areas of increased signal intensity on T2WI in the striate nuclei, caudate nuclei, centrum semiovale, cerebral cortex, midbrain, and pons. More lesions are depicted on MR than on CT. On T2WI, the predilection of these lesions for gray matter, particularly in the brain stem, is striking. T1 and T2 prolongation is seen in these focal lesions. Lesions progress over the course of months, and eventually severe atrophy develops.

*Loewe's syndrome*, or oculocerebrorenal syndrome (OCRS), is an aminoaciduria with X-linked recessive heritance. A defect in the renal tubular transport causes metabolic acidosis, aminoaciduria proteinuria, and hypophosphatemic rickets. Pathologic descriptions are not consistent. Atrophy, generalized and concentrated in superior temporal gyrus, splenium, and lemnisci, as well as poor myelination and absence of any neuropathologic findings have been observed.[7, 100]

Clinically, ocular abnormalities, including cataracts in infancy, are seen, followed by progressive neurologic deterioration.

The CT findings are helpful in setting a specific diagnosis. Marked scalloping of the calvarial bones is seen, especially in the occipital regions. The brain does not have specific findings. However, mild atrophy and periventricular hypodensities are often present.

MR shows patchy bilateral periventricular increased signal on T2WI. These lesions were not demonstrated on T1W SE images with TR 0.8/TE 40 sequence timing.[100]

## OTHER CONDITIONS CAUSING WHITE MATTER ABNORMALITIES

With ongoing clinical research, new observations are constantly made on the numerous causes for abnormalities in the white matter. In some instances, the cause is evident on the images; in others, it must be sought in the history, findings on physical examination, and other criteria.

Those related to trauma, hydrocephalus, vascular diseases, inflammatory and neoplastic diseases are discussed in greater detail elsewhere in the text. A brief summary of these with various other causes is included.

*Inflammatory diseases* directly affect the white matter in the presence of encephalitis or an abscess. Patterns may suggest the etiology, as in the case of herpes encephalitis.[101] In slow viral involvement, such as subacute sclerosing panencephalitis (SSSP), the symptoms and slow progression may be misleading for an infectious etiology and the parenchymal white matter lesions could mimic other white matter diseases.[102]

When mass effect is present, differentiation from tumor-related changes is difficult, particularly on T2WIs. Intravenous Gd-DTPA contrast enhancement on T1WIs may be helpful in differentiating tumors and abscesses.[57]

*Hydrocephalus* leads to varying degrees of signal increase in the periventricular white matter. This usually is seen as a

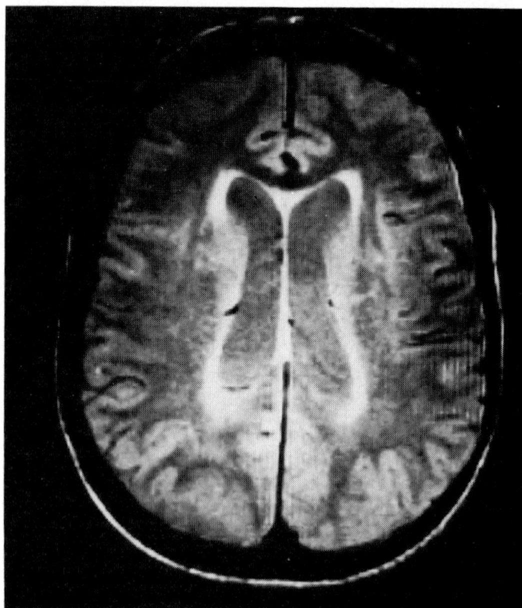

**Figure 15–20. Transependymal (CSF migration—communicating hydrocephalus.** A 64-year-old female with communicating hydrocephalus resulting from abundant oily myelographic contrast in the basal cisterns (1.5 T). Axial T2WI (SE TR 2500/TE 28) demonstrates smooth, symmetric periventricular zone of increased signal associated with hydrocephalus.

smooth, confluent band of increased signal on T2WI, quite evenly distributed (Fig. 15–20). However, patchy areas may be associated should another condition, such as Binswanger's disease, co-exist.[103]

*Trauma* to the brain can lead to focal areas of edema and later myelin loss in typical locations: near the bony ridges at the base of the brain and at the poles.[104] Shear-type injuries are better seen with MR than with CT. They involve white matter and may resemble MS plaques. U fibers are spared (Fig. 15–21).

*Ischemic-anoxic injury* causes delayed myelination in infants. Regional differences in sensitivity to ischemia lead to characteristic patterns of involvement.[105] Localized signal abnormalities in the external capsule-lentiform nucleus region are seen. Also watershed-type ischemic lesions in the hemispheric white matter and global edema are well demonstrated on MRI.[17]

*Vasculitides* may cause lesions that fully mimic patterns of white matter abnormalities seen with MS.[106, 107] Clinical presentation may be quite similar, including transverse myelitis and optic neuritis. Behçet's disease, systemic lupus erythematosus, and polyarteritis nodosa have been reported with this pattern (see Chap. 14). Cortical involvement, infarcts, and collateral vessels (moyamoya) may help in differentiation from MS.[53, 108, 109] Successful steroid therapy may reverse the progression of lesions, and the foci of T1 and T2 prolongation may return to normal.[110]

Vasculitis is considered the cause of white matter lesions in patients with Sjögren's syndrome; 50% of these patients have neuropsychiatric and cognitive dysfunction without focal neurologic disease but demonstrate abnormalities on MR scan of the brain. Supratentorial and infratentorial high intensity

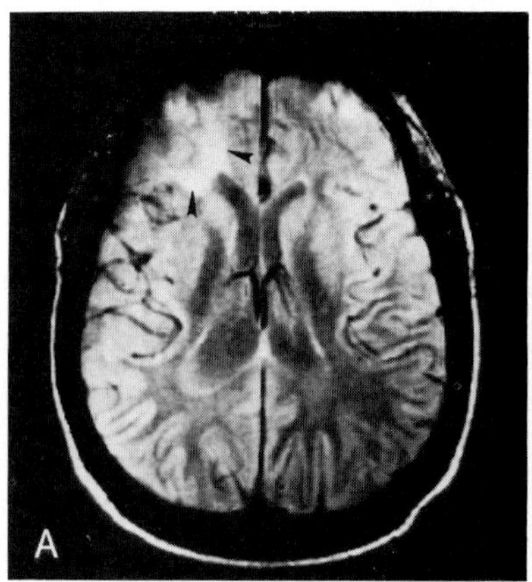


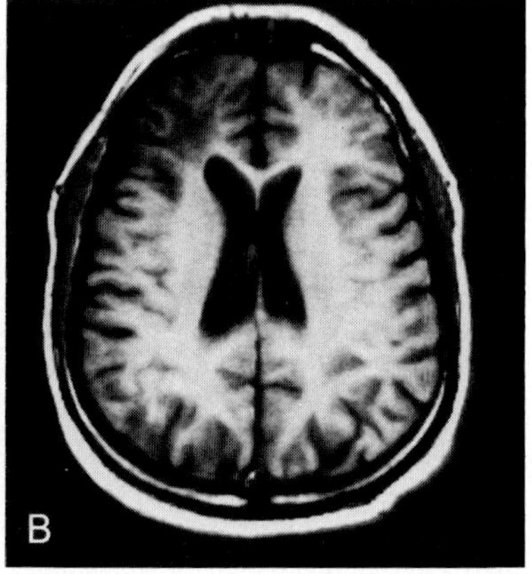


**Figure 15–21. Post-traumatic leukomalacia.** A 40-year-old man with a history of trauma to the head six years before the scan (1.5 T). *A,* Axial T2WI (SE TR 2500/TE 28) demonstrates an area of T2 prolongation in the white matter in the right frontal lobe (arrowheads). Note the sparing of the U-fibers. *B,* T1WI (SE TR 500/TE 17) demonstrates T1 prolongation in the corresponding area, and associated mild, ex vacuo enlargement of the adjacent frontal horn is seen.

lesions on T2WI are seen in 90% of patients with focal neurologic deficits.[111]

*Sickle cell disease* leads to small vessel occlusions and also to larger branch occlusions in the brain. MRI shows unilateral or bilateral white matter, lacunar, and cortical infarcts.[112, 113]

*Migraine* can cause ill-defined white matter lesions with prolonged T2 relaxation. These are most often bilateral. Lesions involving the U fibers, gray matter, and the posterior fossa also occur. The lesions frequently have no associated focal neurologic deficit. Mild atrophy may accompany these findings.[114–116]

*Sarcoidosis* causes patchy white matter lesions by invading the blood vessel walls and causing stenosis or occlusion of the lumen. In hydrocephalus resulting from granulomatous meningitis, high signal intensity of the basal meninges and intracerebral medullary nodular or suprasellar mass lesions (see Fig. 14–12) are helpful differential diagnostic features.[117–119]

*Toxic agents* in chronic exposure or in acute, larger doses related to industrial accidents or suicide attempts can cause leukoencephalopathy. In some instances, the distribution is characteristic for the noxious agent.

Carbon monoxide, cyanide, hydrogen sulphide, and ethylene glycol (antifreeze) cause bilateral symmetric lesions in the globus pallidi with high intensity on T2WI. In addition, symmetric confluent areas of increased signal in the white matter of the temporal occipital and posterior parietal lobes has been described (Figs. 15–22 and 12–30).[120–123] Signal increase on T2WI may occur in the brain stem periaqueductal gray. Lesions are potentially reversible with hyperbaric $O_2$ therapy.

Methanol intoxication typically causes cortical blindness. On MRI the bilateral symmetric involvement of the occipital lobes, not detectable on CT, is seen together with lesions that appear on both modalities in the putamina of basal ganglia.[122, 123]

*Alcoholism* can lead to a variety of abnormalities in the brain.

In the gray and white matter, raised T1 values are seen during alcohol exposure. During abstinence there tends to be reduction in T1 over 7 to 21 days, particularly in the gray matter. This is consistent with the hypothesis that the brain becomes excessively hydrated during chronic alcohol consumption, and abstinence results in subsequent dehydration.[124]

In addition to cortical and cerebellar atrophy, multiple rounded white matter lesions have been documented in a group of chronic alcoholics in which other risk factors were excluded.[125]

*Wernicke's encephalopathy* is known to cause lesions in the thalamus, most often in the dorsal medial nucleus. Prominent atrophy of the mamillary bodies develops.[7] Nonenhancing bilateral hypodensities have been reported on CT and likely will be demonstrated on MR images with greater contrast.[126]

*Marchiafava-Bignami disease* is due to toxic demyelination of the corpus callosum in severe alcoholism. Clinically, decreased levels of consciousness, hemiparesis, and interhemispheric disconnection syndrome can be seen. An acute form leads to rapid death; the chronic form can last for several years. CT can demonstrate the focal lesions in the corpus callosum, most often located in the genu, but the lesions are far better demonstrated on T1W sagittal MR images.

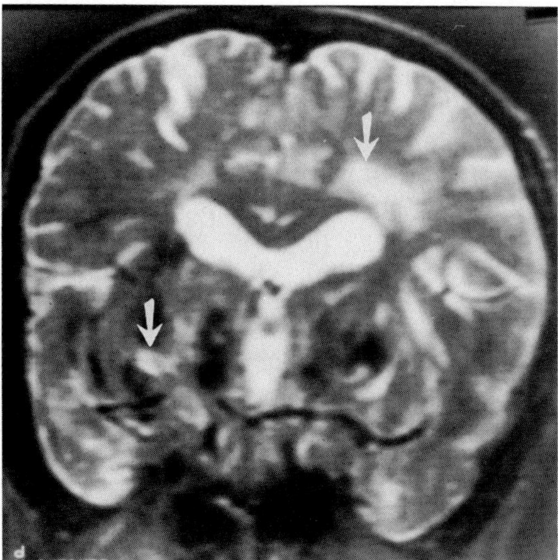

**Figure 15–22. Carbon monoxide poisoning.** A 38-year-old woman with a history of carbon monoxide exposure in a garage three days earlier (1.5 T). Coronal T2WI (SE TR 2300/TE 100) demonstrates a rather patchy pattern of abnormal increased signal in the basal ganglia and deep in the white matter (arrows). Lesions resolved with hyperbaric oxygen therapy, and clinical improvement occurred. (Courtesy of S. J. Pomeranz, M.D., Christ Hospital, Cincinnati, Ohio.)

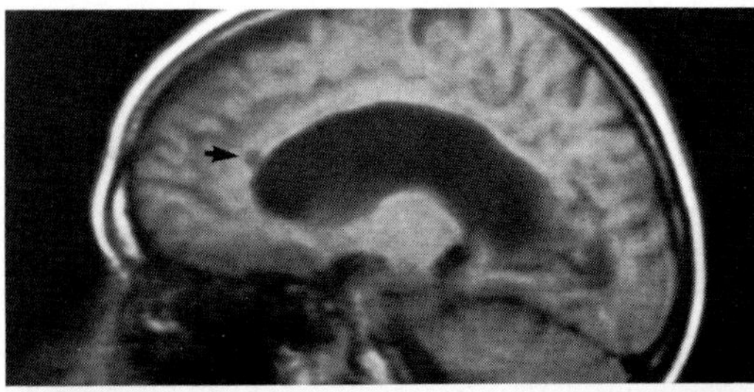

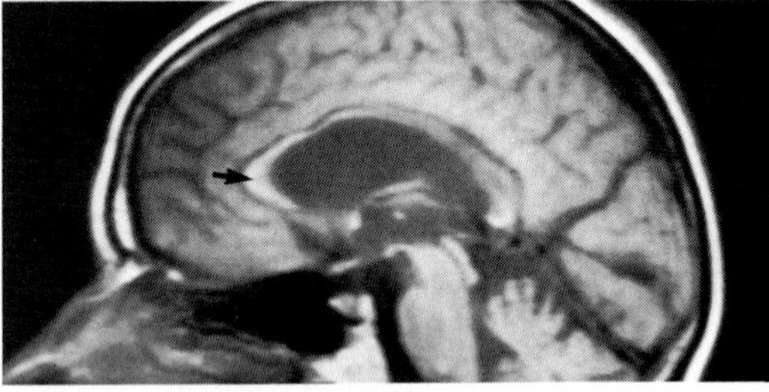

**Figure 15–23. Marchiafava-Bignami disease.** A 32-year-old man with a history of long-standing alcohol (moonshine) abuse (1.5 T). Sagittal T1WI (SE TR 600/TE 20) demonstrate a focal disruption with long T1 relaxation in the genu of the corpus callosum (arrows). Atrophy is also present. (Courtesy of S.J. Pomeranz, M.D., The Christ Hospital, Cincinnati, Ohio.)

Hypointense lesions represent necrotic areas in the corpus callosum (Fig. 15–23).

In the acute form, extensive hypodense areas in the hemispheric white matter have been reported on CT scans and will probably be even more obvious on MRI.[127]

*Central pontine myelinolysis* (*CPM*) is seen associated with hypernatremia or correction of hyponatremia caused by alcohol abuse. The term *osmotic demyelination syndrome* has been used synonymously.[128] As the entity has become better understood, it is evident that numerous conditions may be the cause of the sodium imbalance. Milder cases of CPM found at autopsy are clinically undetected. Typical clinical presentation is some initial neurologic improvement with electrolyte normalization, followed by development of quadriparesis and lower cranial nerve palsies.[130]

CT is often normal, especially early in the disease. A nonenhancing low-density lesion without mass effect located in the basis pontis is the characteristic finding.

On MRI a symmetric pontine low intensity region is seen on T1WI; however, in the early stages of the disease only focal symmetric or asymmetric lesions may be present (see Fig. 12–49, in Chap. 12). Even with larger lesions, sparing of pontine tegmentum and a peripheral rim of ventral pontine tissue is present. A three-pointed, trident-shaped configuration is characteristic. On T2WI the abnormal area shows increased intensity. The corticospinal tracts appear relatively spared. Associated extrapontine lesions in the thalami are frequent.[128–130]

*Radiation treatment* causes capillary endothelial damage that leads to breakdown of blood-brain barrier and vasogenic edema. Cerebral blood flow may be reduced owing to heterogeneous endothelial hyperplasia, fibrinoid necrosis of the penetrating arterioles, and atherosclerotic-like changes in the larger arteries. Animal studies have shown focal demyelination with associated proliferation of glial elements and mononuclear cells weeks or months after completion of radiotherapy.[7, 131]

Clinically, the patients may be asymptomatic or have signs of neurotoxicity characterized by varied degrees of irreversible dementia, confusion, ataxia, and psychomotor retardation. In general, the patients with the most severe forms of neurologic compromise have the most extensive changes. Focal neurologic findings often correlate with regions of focal signal change.

On CT scanning, periventricular hypodensities and atrophic changes can be demonstrated. CT is less sensitive in demonstrating white matter abnormalities.[131] Sometimes calcifications develop as a result of radiotherapy, most commonly subcortical.[132]

On T2WI, MRI shows symmetric, confluent, high-signal foci in the deep periventricular white matter within five to nine months from the time of the treatment (Fig. 15–24).[131–135] T1 changes in the white matter are much less common.[134] The areas most often involved are adjacent to the frontal horn tip, occipital horn tip, lateral aspect of the ventricular body, lateral aspect of the occipital and temporal horns, and centrum semiovale. The U fibers are frequently involved.[20] There is relative sparing of the posterior fossa, basal ganglia, and internal capsules. Areas of coarse calcification are seen as signal void. The involvement may be equally severe in the contralateral hemisphere and is seen remote from the tumor. Minimal mass effect is seen related to the areas of abnormal signal. Once this type of lesion has developed, it remains stable.

With increasing age, the lesions are more

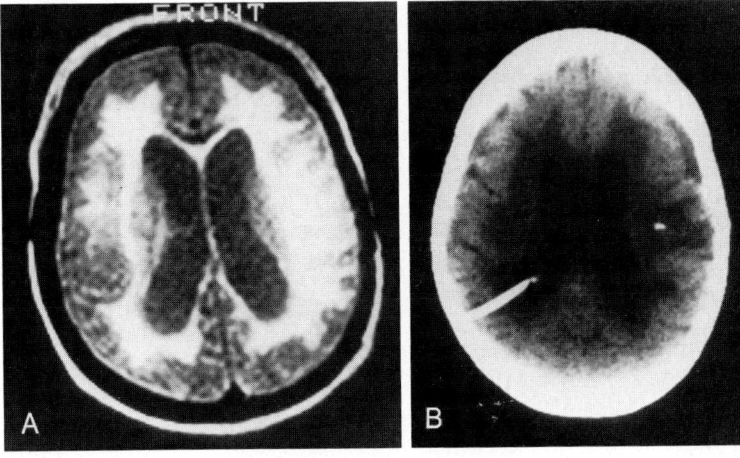


**Figure 15–24. Radiation leukomalacia.** A 63-year-old woman with a history of irradiation for glioma three years earlier (0.35 T). *A,* Axial T2WI (SE TR 1500/TE 70) demonstrates extensive white matter abnormalities in both hemispheres. Ventricular enlargement is consistent with central atrophy or hydrocephalus. *B,* A CT scan following shunt placement. Hypodensities in the white matter are seen. Calcification at the site of the tumor was not seen on MR images.

common and widespread. This is probably due to existing age-related small vessel disease that becomes significant owing to the additional damage from the radiation.

Sometimes white matter develops small necrotic foci, vacuolation, and petechial hemorrhage months to several years following radiotherapy (Fig. 15–25). The focal abnormalities frequently occur in areas that have received the highest dose of irradiation. Enhancement has been demonstrated on CT.[131] Atrophy is commonly noted. Depending on the severity of these changes, patient age, and total irradiation dose, these lesions may partially resolve, stabilize, or progress over a protracted course of several months to several years. Eventually, this may lead to widespread, potentially fatal brain destruction characterized by coagulation necrosis.[7, 131] The appearance on MRI varies, depending on the stage of the disease, with long T1 in necrotic areas and short T1 or T2 or both in areas of hemorrhage in a characteristic pattern (Chap. 14). Mass effect may be present, and coagulation necrosis (see Fig. 14–14, in Chap. 14) may mimic intracranial neoplasm.

Hydrocephalus may develop owing to damage to the arachnoid resorption mechanism (Fig. 15–24).

Disseminated necrotizing leukoencephalopathy (DNL) describes the severe changes in the white matter that develop secondary to combined irradiation and intrathecal che-

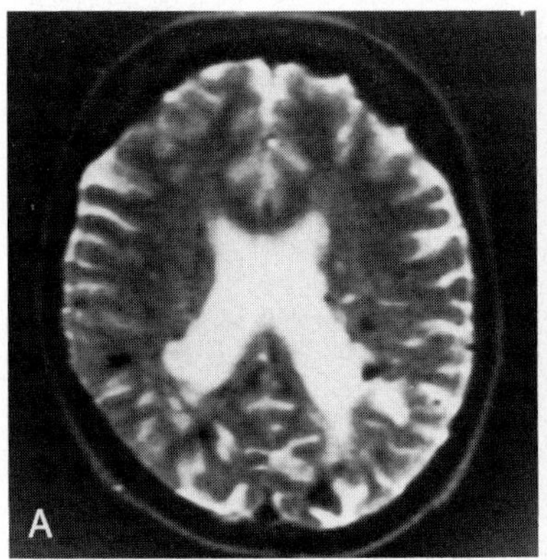


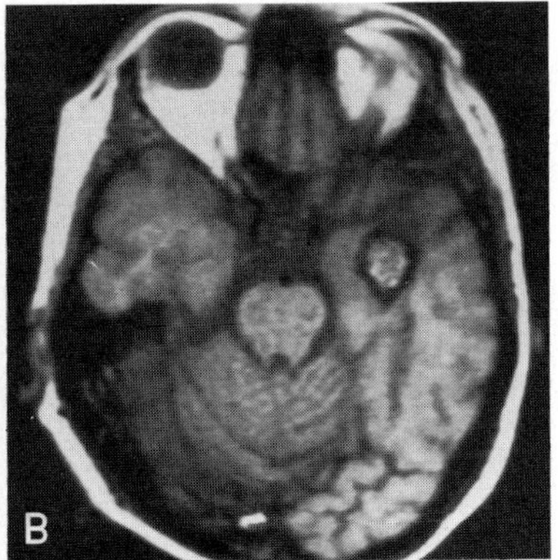


**Figure 15–25. Radiation leukomalacia with remote hemorrhage.** A 41-year-old woman with a history of radiation treatment several years ago who developed bizarre neurologic deficits and choreoathetotoid movements (1.5 T). *A,* Axial T2WI (SE TR 2000/TE 80) shows demyelinative periventricular lesions with increased signal, but also punctate foci of decreased signal intensity representing remote hemorrhage. *B,* Axial T1WI (SE TR 400/TE 25) demonstrates short T1 focus in the temporal lobe with a hypointense rim consistent with chronic or remote hemorrhage. Hyperintense lesion was calcified on CT. (Courtesy of S. J. Pomeranz, M.D., Christ Hospital, Cincinnati, Ohio.)

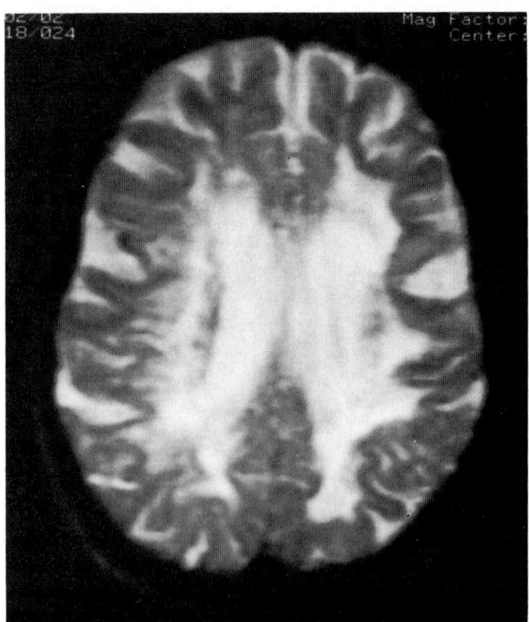


**Figure 15–26. Disseminated necrotizing leukoencephalopathy.** A 47-year-old woman with rapidly deteriorating neurologic status following combined radiation and intrathecal methotrexate therapy (1.5 T). Axial T2WI (SE TR 2000/TE 100) demonstrates the extensive white matter abnormalities in both hemispheres.

motherapy, particularly with methotrexate. Demyelination, axonal damage, and areas of coagulation necrosis with absence of inflammatory cellular response in the scattered white matter lesions are characteristic (Fig. 15–26).[7, 133]

*Fahr's disease* is a familial disorder characterized by intracranial calcification without abnormalities in the serum calcium or phosphate levels. The clinical presentation varies from asymptomatic to choreo-athetoid movements in childhood and general progressive mental deterioration in adulthood. Pathologically, the calcifications occur in vessel walls and in the perivascular spaces of arterioles, capillaries, and veins. Mucopolysaccharides and zinc, phosphorus, chlorine, iron, aluminum, magnesium, and potassium are present.[7, 136]

On CT scan, the symmetric, dense, homogeneous calcifications are seen in a characteristic distribution in the dentate nucleus, caudate, putamen, globus pallidus and in the white matter of the centrum semiovale (Fig. 15–27*A*).[136, 137]

There is hyperintense signal on MR T2WI (0.5 T) in the white matter of the centrum semiovale that arises from the noncalcified elements. In the basal ganglia, low-signal intensity is seen, probably owing to the heavier calcification displacing the signal-giving elements or paramagnetic effects of iron. The dentate nuclei show intermediate signal intensity (Fig. 15–27*B* and *C*).

*Progressive supranuclear palsy* is a neurodegenerative disorder. Characteristic clinical findings are supranuclear ophthalmoparesis, pseudobulbar palsy, parkinsonian signs without tremor but with axial rigidity, broad gait, and postural instability. Dementia develops later in the disease. Men are affected twice as often as women. Onset is

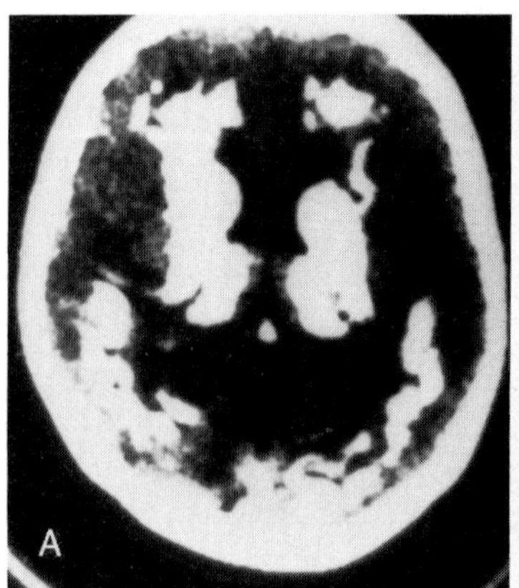


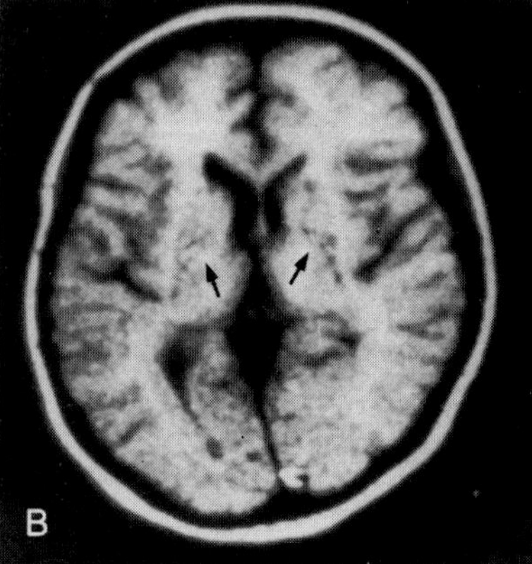


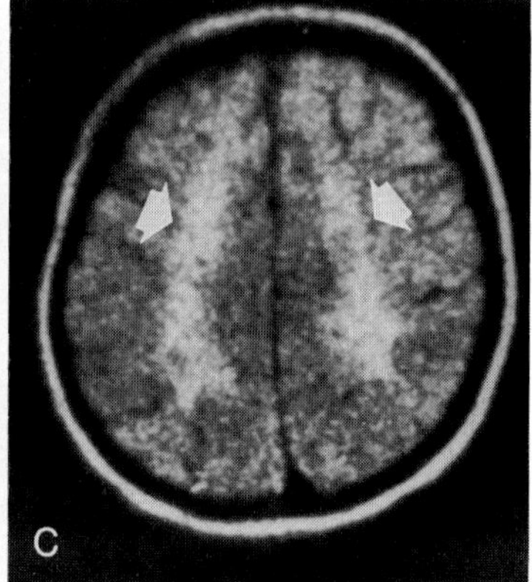


**Figure 15–27. Fahr's disease.** An eight-year-old patient with a bizarre movement disorder (0.35 T). *A,* Axial NCCT shows diffuse confluent calcification in the basal ganglia, thalami, caudate nucleus, and posterior subcortical white matter. *B,* Axial T1WI (SE TR 300/TE 35) demonstrates foci of signal decrease in the region of the basal ganglia (arrows) likely related to calcification. *C,* Axial T2WI (SE TR 1500/TE 70) demonstrates unsuspected evidence of diffuse white matter signal hyperintensity (white arrowheads) involving both corona radiata.

gradual, usually beginning between the fifth and seventh decades, and leads to death in five to ten years.[7, 138, 139]

On high resolution CT and MRI, striking atrophy is seen in the midbrain (see Fig. 12–45), with widening of interpeduncular cistern and prominent perimesencephalic cisterns (see Chap. 12). Less atrophy is seen in the pons.[138, 139] MRI shows hyperintense periventricular lesions both bilaterally and deeper in the white matter of the frontal lobes.[138]

## References


1. Young IR, Hall AS, Pallis CA, et al. Nuclear magnetic resonance imaging of the brain in multiple sclerosis. Lancet 2:1063, 1981.
2. Poser CM, Kleefield J, O'Reilly GV, et al. Neuroimaging and the lesion of multiple sclerosis. AJNR 8:549, 1987.
3. Lukes SA, Crooks LE, Aminoff MJ, et al. Nuclear magnetic resonance imaging in multiple sclerosis. Ann Neurol 6:592, 1983.
4. Noseworthy JH, Paty DW, Ebers GC. Neuroimaging in multiple sclerosis. Neurol Clin 2:759, 1984.
5. Runge VM, Price AC, Kirshner HS, et al. Magnetic resonance imaging of multiple sclerosis: a study of pulse-technique efficacy. AJR 143:1015, 1984.
6. Huynen C, Ruijs S. The superiority of MRI over CT scanning in diseases of brain and cervical spine. Presented at The Society of Magnetic Resonance in Medicine Annual Meeting, London, August 19–23, 1985.
7. Davis RL, Robertson DM. Textbook of Neuropathology. Baltimore, Williams & Wilkins Co., 1985.
8. Okazaki H. Fundamentals of Neuropathology. New York, Igaku-Shoin, 1983:141.
9. Zimmerman RD, Fleming CA, Lee BCP, et al. Periventricular hyperintensity as seen by magnetic resonance: prevalence and significance. AJR 146:443, 1986.
10. Jolesz FA, Polak JF, Adams DF, et al. Myelinated and nonmyelinated nerves: comparison of proton MR properties. Radiology 164:89, 1987.
11. Holland BA, Haas DK, Norman D, et al. MRI of normal brain maturation. AJNR 7:201, 1986.
12. Nowell MA, Hackney DB, Zimmerman RA, et al. Immature brain: spin-echo pulse sequence parameters for high-contrast MR imaging. Radiology 162:272, 1987.
13. Valk J, van der Knaap MS. The role of T2W images in the assessment of progress of myelination in infants and children. Presented at The Society of Magnetic Resonance in Medicine Annual Meeting, New York, August 17–21, 1987.
14. Koenig SH, Brown RD. The importance of the motion of water for magnetic resonance imaging. Invest Radiol 20:297, 1985.
15. McArdle CB, Richardson CJ, Nicholas DA, et al. Developmental features of the neonatal brain: MR imaging. Part I. Gray-white matter differentiation and myelination. Radiology 162:223, 1987.
16. McArdle CB, Richardson CJ, Nicholas DA, et al. Developmental features of the neonatal brain: MR imaging. Part II. Ventricular size and extracerebral space. Radiology 162:230, 1987.
17. Pennock JM, Bydder GM, Dubowitz LMS, et al. Magnetic resonance imaging of the brain in children. Magn Reson Imag 4:1, 1986.
18. Johnson MA, Pennock JM, Bydder GM, et al. Serial MR imaging in neonatal cerebral injury. AJNR 8:83, 1987.
19. Martin E, Kikinis R, Boesch C, et al. Investigation of early brain maturation in neonates, infants, and age-matched anatomical preparations: improved spatial resolution with high-field MRI (2.35 T). Presented at The Society of Magnetic Resonance in Medicine Annual Meeting, New York, August 17–21, 1987.
20. Drayer PB, Johnson PC, Hodak JA, et al. Imaging of the arcuate (subcortical "u") fibers. Presented at The Society of Neuroradiology Annual Meeting, New York, May 10–15, 1987.
21. Sze G, De Armond SJ, Brant-Zawadzki M, et al. Foci of MRI signal (pseudo lesions) anterior to the frontal horns: histologic correlations of a normal finding. AJR 147:331, 1986.
22. Brant-Zawadzki M, Fein G, Van Dyke C, et al. MR imaging of the aging brain: patchy white-matter lesions and dementia. AJNR 6:675, 1985.
23. Heier LA, Farrar J, Morgello S, et al. White matter lesions of the aging brain: pathologic correlation with MR imaging. Presented at The Radiological Society of North America Annual Meeting, Chicago, November 29–December 4, 1987.
24. Manelfe C, Mark AS, Marc-Vergnes JP, et al. MRI of the aging brain. Presented at The Society of Neuroradiology Annual Meeting, New York, May 10–15, 1987.
25. Hayman LA, Kirkpatrick JB. White-matter lesions in MR imaging of clinically healthy brains of elderly subjects: possible pathologic basis. Radiology 162:509, 1987.
26. Young IR, Randell CP, Kaplan PW, et al. Nuclear magnetic resonance (NMR) imaging in white matter disease of the brain using spin-echo sequences. J Comput Assist Tomogr 7:290, 1983.
27. Brant-Zawadzki M, Norman D, Newton TH, et al. Magnetic resonance of the brain: the optimal screening technique. Radiology 152:71, 1984.
28. Crooks LE, Hoenninger J, Arakawa M, et al. High-resolution magnetic resonance imaging. Radiology 150:163, 1984.
29. Bydder GM, Young IR. MR imaging: clinical use of the inversion recovery sequence. J Comput Assist Tomogr 9:659, 1985.
30. Young IR, Burl M, Bydder GM. Comparative efficiency of different pulse sequences in MR imaging. J Comput Assist Tomogr 10:271, 1986.
31. Miller DH, Rudge P, MacManus DG, et al. Serial MRI studies with gadolinium-DTPA in acute relapsing multiple sclerosis. Presented at The Society of Magnetic Resonance in Medicine Annual Meeting, New York, August 17–21, 1987.
32. Grossman RI, Gonzalez-Scarano F, Atlas SW, et al. Multiple sclerosis: gadolinium enhancement in MR imaging. Radiology 161:721, 1986.
33. Miller DH, Johnson G, McDonald WI, et al. Detection of optic nerve lesions in optic neuritis with magnetic resonance imaging. Lancet 1:1490, 1986.
34. Runge VM, Wood ML, Kaufman DL. Motion-compensating gradients in the study of multiple sclerosis. Presented at The Radiological Society of

North America Annual Meeting, Chicago, November 29–December 4, 1987.
35. Kanal E, Brunberg JA, Prorok R. Low flip angle gradient-recalled echo imaging of multiple sclerosis. Presented at The Society of Neuroradiology Annual Meeting, New York, May 10–15, 1987.
36. Johnson MA, Pennock JM, Bydder GM, et al. Clinical NMR imaging of the brain in children: normal and neurological disease. AJR 141:1005, 1983.
37. Stewart JM, Houser OW, Baker HL, et al. Magnetic resonance imaging and clinical relationships in multiple sclerosis. Mayo Clin Proc 62:174, 1987.
38. Rudick RA, Schiffer RB, Schwetz KM. Multiple sclerosis: the problem of incorrect diagnosis. Arch Neurol 43:578, 1986.
39. Tobias JA, Sheldon JJ, Soila KP, et al. Magnetic resonance imaging of multiple sclerosis—a review. RIR 11:143, 1986.
40. Jackson JA, Leake DR, Schneiders NJ, et al. Magnetic resonance imaging in multiple sclerosis: results in 32 cases. AJNR 6:171, 1985.
41. Sheldon JJ, Siddharthan R, Tobias J, et al. MR imaging of multiple sclerosis: comparison with clinical and CT examinations in 74 patients. AJR 145:957, 1985.
42. Runge VM, Price AC, Kirshner HS, et al. The evaluation of multiple sclerosis by magnetic resonance imaging. RadioGraphics 6:203, 1986.
43. Edwards MK, Farlow MR, Stevens JC. Cranial MR in spinal cord MS: diagnosing patients with isolated spinal cord symptoms. AJNR 7:1003, 1986.
44. Scotti G, Scialfia G, Biondi A, et al. Magnetic resonance in multiple sclerosis. Neuroradiology 28:319, 1986.
45. Giesser BS, Kurtzberg D, Vaughan HG, et al. Trimodal-evoked potentials compared with magnetic resonance imaging in the diagnosis of multiple sclerosis. Arch Neurol 44:281, 1987.
46. Spiegel SM, Vinuela F, Fox AJ, et al. CT of multiple sclerosis: reassessment of delayed scanning with high doses of contrast material. AJR 145:497, 1985.
47. Edwards MK, Farlow MR, Stevens JC. Multiple sclerosis: MRI and clinical correlation. AJR 147:571, 1986.
48. Davis KA, Stears JC, Franklin GM, et al. Right-angle demyelination in multiple sclerosis. Presented at The Radiological Society of North America Annual Meeting, Chicago, November 29–December 5, 1986.
49. Simon JH, Holtas SL, Schiffer RB, et al. Corpus callosum and subcallosal-periventricular lesions in multiple sclerosis: detection with MR. Radiology 160:363, 1986.
50. Jacobs L, Kinkel WR, Polachini I. Correlations of nuclear magnetic resonance imaging, computerized tomography, and clinical profiles in multiple sclerosis. Neurology 36:27, 1986.
51. Ormerod IEC, Bronstein A, Rudge P, et al. Magnetic resonance imaging in clinically isolated lesions of the brain stem. J Neurol Neurosurg Psychiatr 49:737, 1986.
52. Barnes D, Johnson G, McDonald WI, et al. The quantitative MRI characteristics of lesions in multiple sclerosis. Presented at The Society of Magnetic Resonance in Medicine Annual Meeting, New York, August 17–21, 1987.
53. Miller DH, du Boulay GH, Kendall BE, et al. Differentiation of multiple sclerosis from other inflammatory multifocal central nervous system diseases: an MRI study. Presented at The Society of Magnetic Resonance in Medicine Annual Meeting, New York, August 17–21, 1987.
54. Larsson HBV, Kjoer L, Frederiksen JL, et al. In vivo determination of T1 and T2 in the brain of patients with severe but stable multiple sclerosis. Presented at The Society of Magnetic Resonance in Medicine Annual Meeting, New York, August 17–21, 1987.
55. Cobb SR, Mehringer CM. Wallerian degeneration in a patient with Schilder disease: MR imaging demonstration. Radiology 162:521, 1987.
56. Drayer B, Burger P, Hurwitz B, et al. Reduced signal intensity on MR images of thalamus and putamen in multiple sclerosis: increased iron content. AJNR 8:413, 1987.
57. Brant-Zawadzki M, Berry I, Osaki L, et al. Gd-DTPA in clinical MR of the brain: 1. Intra-axial lesions. AJR 147:1223, 1986.
58. Gadolinium-DTPA enhanced MRI of the brain and orbits in patients with clinically isolated optic neuritis. Presented at The Society of Magnetic Resonance in Medicine Annual Meeting, New York, August 17–21, 1987.
59. Uhlenbrock D, Herbe E, Beyer HK. One-year follow-up of patients with MS. Presented at The Radiological Society of North America Annual Meeting, Chicago, November 29–December 5, 1987.
60. DeLaPaz R, Floris R, Enzmann D, et al. High field MRI of spinal cord multiple sclerosis. Presented at The Society of Neuroradiology Annual Meeting, New York, May 10–15, 1987.
61. DeLaPaz RL, Floris R, Norman D, et al. High field MRI of spinal cord multiple sclerosis. Presented at The Society of Magnetic Resonance in Medicine Annual Meeting, New York, August 17–21, 1987.
62. Patel SC, Sanders W, Haggar AL, et al. Prevalence of unsuspected intracranial demyelination in spinal form of multiple sclerosis. Presented at The Society of Magnetic Resonance in Medicine Annual Meeting, New York, August 17–21, 1987.
63. Maravilla KR, Weinreb JC, Suss R, et al. Magnetic resonance demonstration of multiple sclerosis plaques in the cervical cord. AJR 144:381, 1985.
64. Jacobs L, Kinkel PR, Kinkel WR. Silent brain lesions in patients with isolated idiopathic optic neuritis: a clinical and nuclear magnetic resonance imaging study. Arch Neurol 43:452, 1986.
65. Yedavally S, Pernicone J, Kaufman D. MRI demonstrates that a higher percentage of patients with acute optic neuritis have multiple sclerosis than has previously been documented. Presented at The Society of Magnetic Resonance in Medicine Annual Meeting, New York, August 17–21, 1987.
66. Tashiro K, Ito K, Maruo Y, et al. MR imaging of spinal cord in devic disease. J Comput Assist Tomogr 11:516, 1987.
67. Atlas SW, Grossman RI, Goldberg HI, et al. MR diagnosis of acute disseminated encephalomyelitis. J Comput Assist Tomogr 10:798, 1986.
68. Dunn V, Bale JF, Bell WE, et al. MRI in children with postinfectious disseminated encephalomyelitis. Magn Reson Imag 4:25, 1986.
69. Dunn V, Bale JF, Bell WE, et al. MRI in children with postinfectious disseminated encephalomyelitis. Presented at The Society of Magnetic Resonance in Medicine, Annual Meeting London, August 19–23, 1985.
70. Guilleux MH, Steiner RE, Young IR. MR imaging in

progressive multifocal leukoencephalopathy. AJNR 7:1033, 1986.
71. Buonanno FS, Ball MR, Laster DW, et al. Computed tomography in late-infantile metachromatic leukodystrophy. Ann Neurol 4:43, 1978.
72. Carlin L, Roach ES, Riela A, et al. Juvenile metachromatic leukodystrophy: evoked potentials and computed tomography. Ann Neurol 13:105, 1983.
73. Waltz G, Harik SI, Kaufman B. Adult metachromatic leukodystrophy: value of computed tomographic scanning and magnetic resonance imaging of the brain. Arch Neurol 44:225, 1987.
74. Schipper HI, Seidel D. Computed tomography in late-onset metachromatic leukodystrophy. Neuroradiology 26:39, 1984.
75. Finelli PF. Methachromatic leukodystrophy manifesting as a schizophrenic disorder: computed tomographic correlation. Ann Neurol 18:94, 1985.
76. Reider-Grosswasser I, Bornstein N. CT and MRI in late-onset metachromatic leukodystrophy. Acta Neurol Scand 75:64, 1987.
77. Baram TZ, Goldman AM, Percy AK. Krabbe disease: specific MRI and CT findings. Neurology 36:111, 1986.
78. Kwan E, Drace J, Enzmann D. Specific CT findings in Krabbe disease. AJR 143:665, 1984.
79. Kumar AJ, Rosenbaum AE, Naidu S, et al. Adrenoleukodystrophy: correlating MR imaging with CT. Radiology 165:497, 1987.
80. Bewermeyer H, Bamborschke S, Ebhardt G, et al. MR imaging in adrenoleukomyeloneuropathy. J Comput Assist Tomogr 9:793, 1985.
81. Trommer BL, Naidich TP, Dal Canto MC, et al. Noninvasive CT diagnosis of infantile Alexander disease: pathologic correlation. J Comput Assist Tomogr 7:509, 1983.
82. Farrell K, Chuang S, Becker LE. Computed tomography in Alexander's disease. Ann Neurol 15:605, 1984.
83. Holland IM, Kendall BE. Computed tomography in Alexander's disease. Neuroradiology 20:103, 1980.
84. Nowell MA, Grossman RI, Goldberg HI, et al. Magnetic resonance imaging of pediatric white matter disease. Presented at The Society of Magnetic Resonance in Medicine Annual Meeting, New York, August 17–21, 1987.
85. Rushton AR, Shaywitz BA, Duncan CC, et al. Computed tomography in the diagnosis of Canavan's disease. Ann Neurol 10:57, 1981.
86. Patel PJ, Koawole TM, Mahdi AH, et al. Sonographic and computed tomographic findings in Canavan's disease. Br J Radiol 59:1226, 1986.
87. Andriola MR. Computed tomography in the diagnosis of Canavan's disease. Ann Neurol 11:323, 1982.
88. Penner MW, Li KC, Gebarski SS, et al. MR imaging of Pelizaeus-Merzbacher disease. J Comput Assist Tomogr 11:591, 1987.
89. Journel H, Roussey M, Gandon Y, et al. Magnetic resonance imaging in Pelizaeus-Merzbacher disease. Neuroradiology 29:403, 1987.
90. Statz A, Boltshauser E, Schinzel A, et al. Computed tomography in Pelizaeus-Merzbacher disease. Neuroradiology 22:103, 1981.
91. Levinson ED, Zimmerman AW, Grunnet ML, et al. Cockayne syndrome. J Comput Assist Tomogr 6:1172, 1982.
92. Levene MI, Whitelaw A, Dubowitz V, et al. Nuclear magnetic resonance imaging of the brain in children. Br Med J 285:774, 1982.
93. Andrew JL, Jonas AJ, Williams JC, et al. Craniocervical manifestations of mucopolysaccharidoses by MR imaging. Presented at The Society of Magnetic Resonance Imaging Annual Meeting, San Antonio, Texas, February 28–March 4, 1987.
94. Lund G. MRI findings in children with psychomotor retardation. Presented at The Society of Magnetic Resonance in Medicine Annual Meeting, New York, August 17–21, 1987.
95. Johnson MA, Desai S, Hugh-Jones K, et al. Magnetic resonance imaging of the brain in Hurler syndrome. AJNR 5:816, 1984.
96. Johnson MA, Pennock JM, Bydder GM, et al. Magnetic resonance imaging studies of the brain in infants and children. Presented at The Society of Magnetic Resonance in Medicine Annual Meeting, New York, August 17–21, 1987.
97. MR of Leigh's disease (subacute necrotizing encephalomyelopathy). AJNR 8:71, 1987.
98. Paltiel HJ, O'Gorman AM, Meagher-Villemure K, et al. Subacute necrotizing encephalomyelopathy (Leigh disease): CT study. Radiology 162:115, 1987.
99. Glass RF, Press GA, Hesselink JR, et al. Magnetic resonance imaging of neurodegenerative disorders. Presented at The Society of Magnetic Resonance in Medicine Annual Meeting, New York, August 17–21, 1987.
100. O'tuama LA, Wayne Laster D. Oculocerebrorenal syndrome: case report with CT and MR correlates. AJNR 8:555, 1987.
101. Schroth G, Gawehn J, Thron A, et al. Early diagnosis of herpes simplex encephalitis by MRI. Neurology 37:179, 1987.
102. Krawiecki NS, Dyken PR, El Gammal T, et al. Computed tomography of the brain in subacute sclerosing panencephalitis. Ann Neurol 15:489, 1984.
103. Brant-Zawadzki M, Fein G, Van Dyke C, et al. MR imaging of the aging brain: patchy white-matter lesions and dementia. AJNR 6:675, 1985.
104. Reider-Grosswasser I, Grosswasser Z, Machtey Y, et al. MRI in the follow-up of craniocerebral injured patients. Presented at The Society of Magnetic Resonance in Medicine Annual Meeting, New York, August 19–22, 1986.
105. Taylor SB, Quencer RM, Holzman BH, et al. Central nervous system anoxic-ischemic insult in children due to near-drowning. Radiology 156:641, 1985.
106. Aisen AM, Gabrielsen TO, McCune WJ. MR imaging of systemic lupus erythematosus involving the brain. AJNR 6:197, 1985.
107. Vermess M, Bernstein RM, Bydder GM, et al. Nuclear magnetic resonance (NMR) imaging of the brain in systemic lupus erythematosus. J Comput Assist Tomogr 7:461, 1983.
108. Miller DH, Ormerod IEC, Gibson A, et al. MR brain scanning in patients with vasculitis. Neuroradiology 29:226, 1987.
109. Fujisawa I, Asato R, Nishimura K, et al. Moyamoya disease: MR imaging. Radiology 164:103, 1987.
110. Willeit J, Schmutzhard E, Aichner F, et al. CT and MR imaging in neuro-Behçet disease. J Comput Assist Tomogr 10:313, 1986.
111. Kumar AJ, Rosenbaum AE, Wang H, et al. Magnetic

resonance imaging in Sjögren's syndrome. Presented at The Society of Neuroradiology Annual Meeting, New York, May 10–15, 1987.
112. Gammal TE, Adams RJ, Nichols FT, et al. MR and CT investigation of cerebrovascular disease in sickle cell patients. AJNR 7:1043, 1986.
113. Zimmerman RA, Gill F, Goldberg HI, et al. MRI of sickle cell cerebral infarction. Neuroradiology 29:232, 1987.
114. Soges LJ, Cacayorin ED, Ramachandran TS, et al. Migraine: evaluation by MRI. Presented at The Society of Neuroradiology Annual Meeting, New York, May 10–15, 1987.
115. Kemp S, Grossman RI, Goldberg HI, et al. MRI in the evaluation of migraine headache. Presented at The Society of Neuroradiology Annual Meeting, New York, May 10–15, 1987.
116. Kuhn MJ, Davis KR, Shoukimas GM, et al. Magnetic resonance imaging of migraine: comparison with CT. Presented at The Society of Neuroradiology Annual Meeting, New York, May 10–15, 1987.
117. Greco A, Steiner R. Magnetic resonance imaging in neurosarcoidosis. Magn Reson Imag 5:15, 1987.
118. Sherman JL, Hayes WS, Stern BJ, et al. MR evaluation of intracranial sarcoidosis: comparison with CT. Presented at The Society of Neuroradiology Annual Meeting, New York, May 10–15, 1987.
119. Ketonen L, Oksanen V, Kuuliala I. Preliminary experience of magnetic resonance imaging in neurosarcoidosis. Neuroradiology 29:127, 1987.
120. Horowitz AL, Kaplan R, Gunseli S. Carbon monoxide toxicity: MR imaging in the brain. Radiology 162:787, 1987.
121. Davis PD. The magnetic resonance imaging appearance of basal ganglia lesions in carbon monoxide poisoning. Magn Reson Imag (4):489, 1986.
122. Dooms GC, Mathurin P, Cornelis G, et al. MR imaging and CT in methanol intoxication. Presented at The Radiological Society of North America Annual Meeting, Chicago, November 29–December 4, 1987.
123. Nelson DL, Batnitzky S, McMillann JH, et al. The CT and MRI features of acute toxic encephalopathies. Presented at The Society of Neuroradiology Annual Meeting, New York, May 10–15, 1987.
124. Smith MA, Chick J, Kean DM, et al. Changes in brain water during withdrawal of alcohol in chronic alcohol patients. Presented at The Society of Magnetic Resonance in Medicine Annual Meeting, New York, August 19–23,1985.
125. Gallucci M, Amicarelli I, Di Cesare E, et al. MR imaging identification of white matter lesions in uncomplicated alcoholism. Presented at The Radiological Society of North America Annual Meeting, Chicago, November 29–December 4, 1987.
126. McDowell JR, LeBlanc HJ. Computed tomography findings in Wernicke Korsakoff syndrome. Arch Neurol 41:453, 1984.
127. Clavier E, Thiebot J, Delangre T, Hannequin D, Samsom M, Benozio M. Marchiafava-Bignami disease: a case studied by CT and MR imaging. Neuroradiology 28:376, 1986.
128. Rippe DJ, Edwards MK, D'Amour PG, et al. MR imaging of central pontine myelinolysis. J Comput Assist Tomogr 11:724, 1987.
129. DeWitt LD, Buonanno FS, Kistler JP, et al. Central pontine myelinolysis: demonstration by nuclear magnetic resonance. Neurology 34:570, 1984.
130. Price DB, Kramer J, Hotson GC, et al. Central pontine myelinolysis: report of a case with distinctive appearance on MR imaging. AJNR 8:576, 1987.
131. Tsuruda JS, Kortman KF, Bradley WG, et al. Radiation effects on cerebral white matter: MR evaluation. AJR 149:165, 1987.
132. Davis PC, Hoffman JC Jr., Pearl GS, et al. CT evaluation of effects of cranial radiation therapy in children. AJR 147:587, 1986.
133. George AE, Stylopoulos LA, De Leon MJ, et al. MRI features of necrotizing leukoencephalopathy following irradiation of malignant glioma. Presented at The Society of Neuroradiology Annual Meeting, New York, May 10–15, 1987.
134. Packer RJ, Zimmerman RA, Bilaniuk LT. Magnetic resonance imaging in the evaluation of treatment-related central nervous system damage. Cancer 58:635, 1986.
135. Semmler W, Gademann G, Niendorf HP, et al. Follow-up in brain tumors after high-dose external stereotactic irradiation: correlation of stereotactic biopsies and radiation field with contrast-enhanced MRI. Presented at The Society of Magnetic Resonance Imaging Annual Meeting, San Antonio, February 28–March 4, 1987.
136. Scotti G, Scialfia G, Tampieri D, et al. MR imaging in Fahr disease. J Comput Assist Tomogr 9:790, 1985.
137. Friedman L, Dubowitz B, Papert B, et al. Computed tomographic findings in Fahr's disease. S Afr Med J 70:704, 1986.
138. Patel S, Sanders W, Haggar A, et al. Progressive supranuclear palsy: magnetic resonance imaging at 1.5 T. Paper presented at Society of Magnetic Resonance Imaging Annual Meeting, San Antonio, Texas, February 28–March 4, 1987.
139. Masucci EF, Borts FT, Smirniotopoulos JG, et al. Thin-section CT of midbrain abnormalities in progressive supranuclear palsy. AJNR 6:767, 1985.

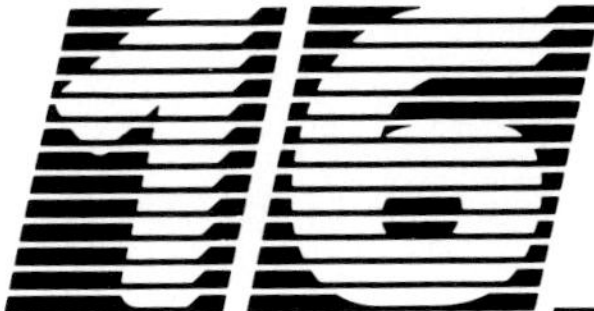

**Stephen J. Pomeranz, M.D.**

# PITFALLS IN CRANIOSPINAL MR

Magnetic resonance (MR), because of its contrast properties, produces unique appearances of normal structures and unusual pitfalls not typical of other imaging modalities.[1–3] We have divided these pitfalls into the following categories: normal variants; pitfalls related to head canting, head tilting, or volume averaging; and MR artifacts. Flow-related pitfalls are discussed in Chapter 2 of this text.

## NORMAL VARIANTS

*The crista galli, falx cerebri, and dorsum sella* may contain normal amounts of hyperintense marrow or fat signal (Fig. 16–1) on T1-weighted images (T1WI). The crista galli fat should not be confused with subfrontal hemorrhage, and the falx marrow signal, present in 5% to 10% of patients, is occasionally mistaken for intrafalcine subdural hematoma, sinus thrombosis, or perifalcine intra-axial hematoma on T1WI. These normal fat collections diminish in signal intensity on T2-weighted images (T2WI) in a manner similar to normal subcutaneous adipose tissue. Unfortunately, acute thromboses and hemorrhages may also appear hypointense at high field strengths on T2WI. A midline location and hypointense "cortical" rim in the axial and coronal planes permit identification of normal falcine marrow signal. Hyperintense T1 signal approximating fat may also be observed in the posterior pituitary gland.

*The posterior pituitary signal,* separate from fat in the posterior clinoids (Fig. 16–2), has been labeled by some as a pituitary "fat pad" and is made more conspicuous by chemical shift misregistration effect.[4–6] No focal fat collections have been pathologically identified in the pituitary fossa by visual inspection. This "bright spot" corresponds anatomically to the posterior neurohypophysis.[7] It appears to represent intracellular lipid droplets identified histologically in the posterior pituitary pituicytes and becomes more prominent with increasing glandular hormonal activity.[8, 9]

Other normal structures or variants on MR that may simulate disease include the red nuclei, suboccipital veins, pacchionian granulations, xanthogranulomata, medullary clava, pineal cysts, and asymmetrically aerated anterior clinoid processes.[1, 10]

*Red nuclei,* because of their iron content, produce characteristic midbrain signal hypointensity on T2WI (Fig. 16–3). They should not be confused with infarct or tumor in the sagittal plane when particularly prominent.

*Suboccipital veins* are quite noticeable on MR (Fig. 16–4) since their characteristic flow-void signal contrasts sharply with adjacent soft tissue and fat. These may be quite bulbous in configuration but should not be incorrectly labeled as cortical or subcortical varices, rare entities.[11]

*Pacchionian granulations,* when large, may simulate calvarial metastases. Size less than 2 to 3 cm, a parasagittal location, and a sessile configuration in the sagittal or coronal plane suggest their true identity (Fig. 16–5). In addition, contiguity to a dural sinus, sharp margins, and a grapelike or clustered appearance assist in distinction from pathologic processes.[12]

*Xanthogranuloma,* a benign incidental finding, is not infrequent on MR and involves the choroid plexus glomera. Foci of T2WI signal hyperintensity (Fig. 16–6) averaging 5 mm but up to 20 mm in size may be observed in the choroid plexus in 15% of

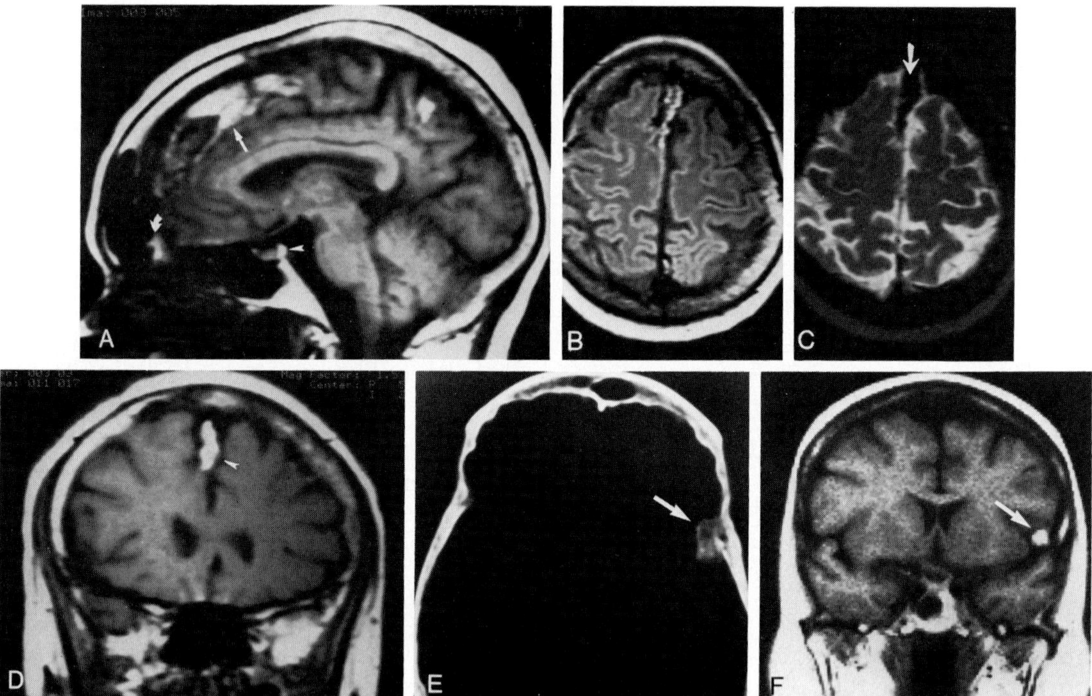

**Figure 16–1. Multiple examples of intracranial "fat" signal.** A 22-year-old man with head trauma. *A,* Sagittal midline T1WI demonstrates irregular anterior hyperintensity (arrow). Also note the normal fat signal in the dorsum sella (arrowhead) and the crista galli (curved arrow). *B* and *C,* Axial multiecho N(H)WI and T2WI shows a midline signal increase that becomes hypointense on T2WI (arrow). Its signal is similar to intradiploic fat (arrow). This represents normal fat-containing marrow in the falx and is occasionally confused with subacute sagittal sinus thrombosis or interhemispheric subdural hematoma at high-field strengths. *D,* Coronal T1WI of falcine marrow fat. Exact midline location, central hyperintensity, and circumferential hypointensity are typical (arrowhead).

*E* and *F,* Ossified pterion lesion containing fat (0.35 T). *E,* CT (noncontrast). *F,* Coronal T1WI (TR 300/TE 16). An ossified inner table lesion (arrow) exhibits signal intensity similar to subcutaneous fat or marrow in the intradiploic space on T1WI and T2WI (not shown). The lesion's osseous nature is best appreciated on CT. (*E* and *F,* Courtesy of J. Tobias, M.D., Radiology Department, Mount Sinai Hospital, Miami Beach, Fla.)

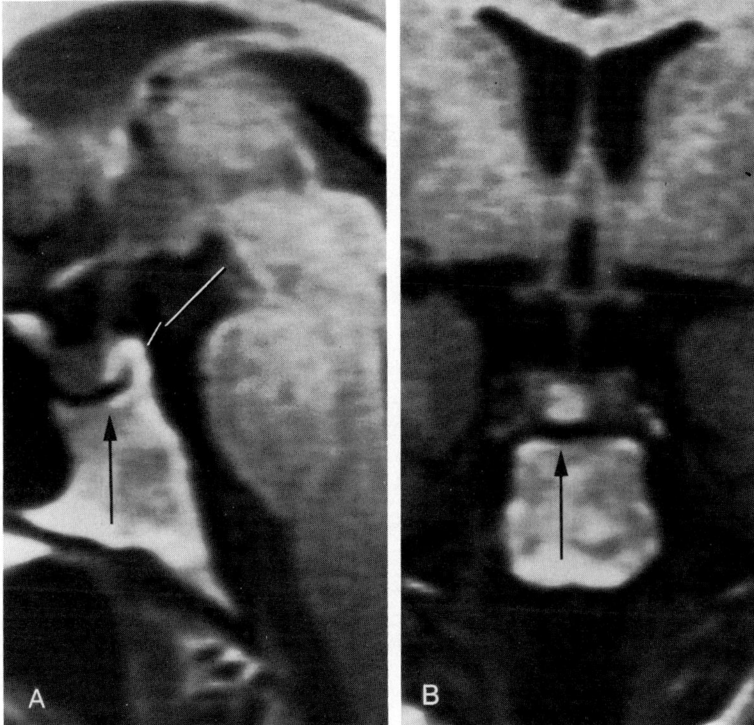


**Figure 16–2. Retrasellar and intrasellar "fat."** *A* and *B,* Axial and coronal 3-mm T1WI show how the normal hyperintensity of the posterior neurohypophysis (arrow) may simulate a pituitary lesion (Rathke's cyst) in the coronal plane (arrow). The hyperintense signal in the adjacent dorsum sella (arrowhead) is a normal finding.

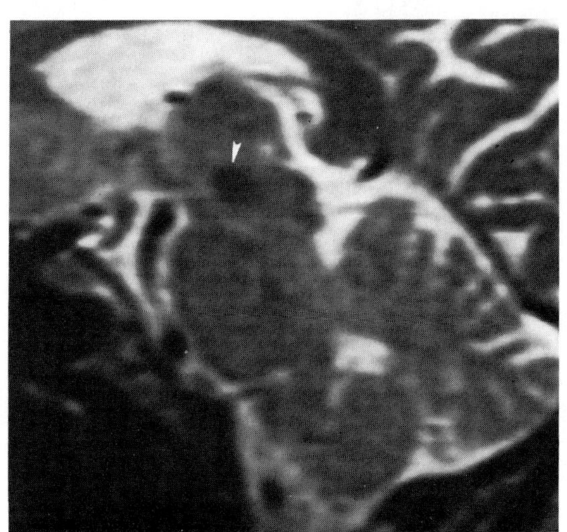

**Figure 16–3. Red nucleus.** Sagittal T2WI shows prominent, rounded, hypointense signal (arrowhead) in the midbrain. This corresponds to normal iron in the red nucleus, shortening its T2 relaxation.

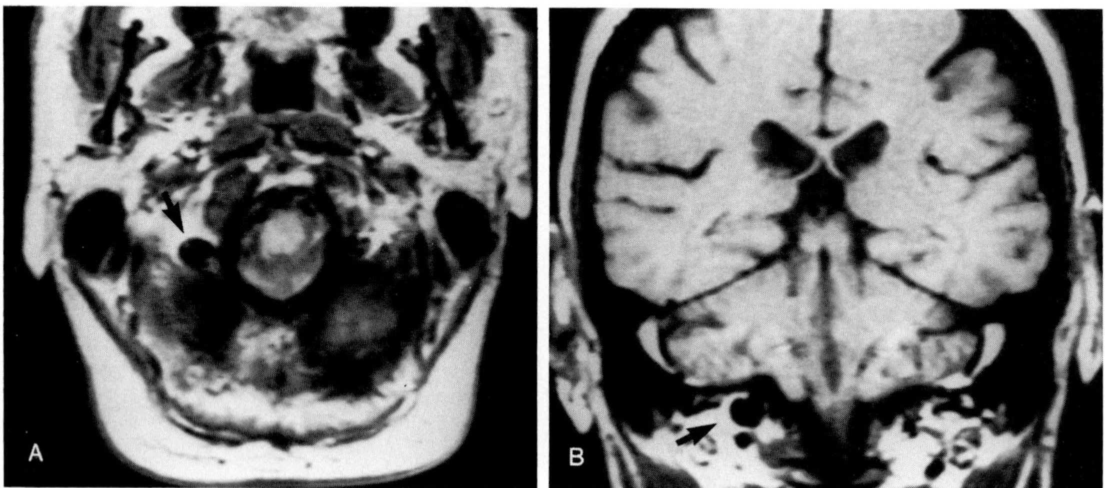


**Figure 16–4. Suboccipital vein.** *A* and *B,* Axial and coronal T1WI. Rounded signal void is located adjacent to the foramen magnum (arrow). This normal, prominent suboccipital draining vein should not be misconstrued as an aneurysm or a varix.

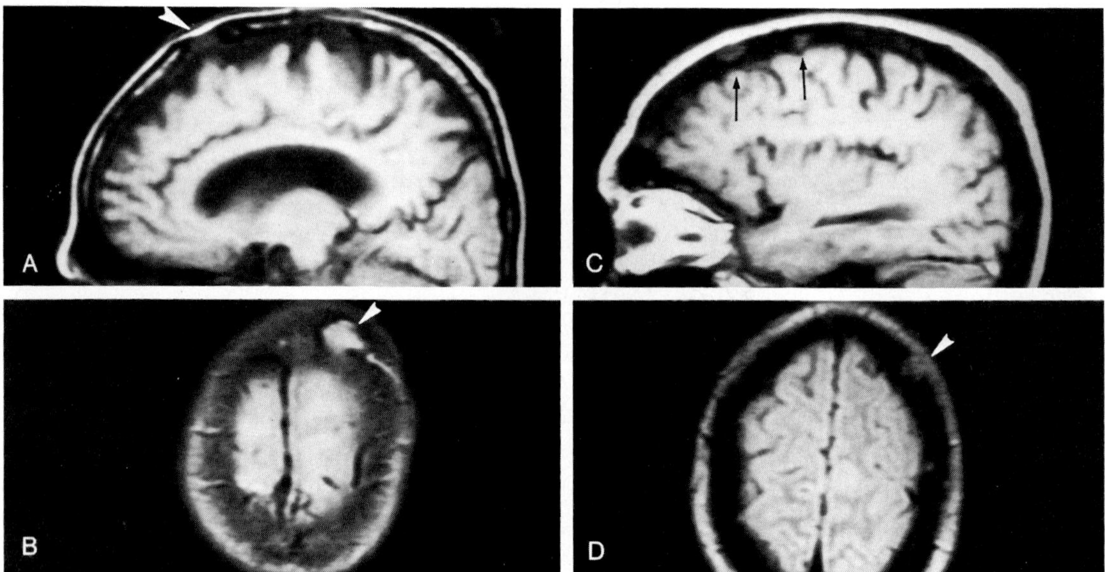


**Figure 16–5. Two patients with lung carcinoma.** *A* and *B,* Sagittal T1WI and axial N(H)WI show apparent intradiploic signal alteration (arrowheads) that appear masslike on N(H)WI. Proximity to midline, triangular shape, and signal merging with adjacent CSF on T1WI confirm this as a pacchionian granulation. *C* and *D,* Sagittal and axial images utilizing the same pulsing parameters. Lesion multiplicity, rounded shape (arrows), peripheral eccentric location (arrowhead), and signal not consistent with CSF confirm these as calvarial metastases.

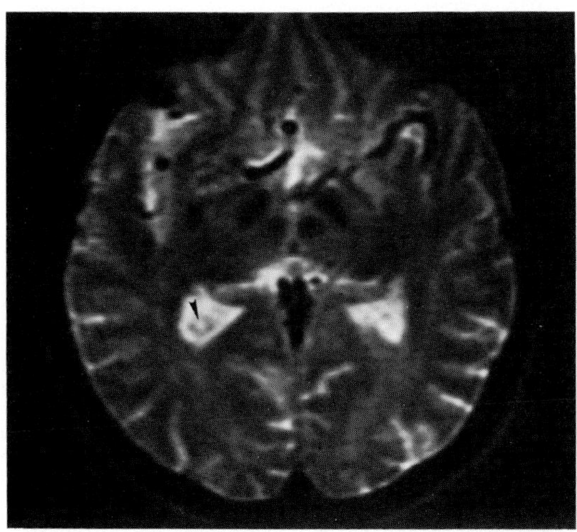

**Figure 16–6. Xanthogranuloma.** (1.5 T). Axial T2WI shows punctate focus of signal hyperintensity (arrowhead) in the right atrial choroid plexus. A size less than 2 cm, absence of hydrocephalus, and frequency as an incidental finding identify this as a normal variant derived from sloughed neuroepithelial stroma.

patients. These correspond to accumulated lipid deposits and small neuroepithelial cysts derived from degenerated epithelial stroma, typical of xanthogranulomata. These xanthogranulomata do not produce ventricular horn obstruction and correspond to foci of low attenuation, but not to fat attenuation, on computed tomography (CT.)[13] They do not enhance with Gd-DTPA or iodinated conventional contrast agents.

*The claval pseudotumor,* a posterior medullary protrusion harboring the nucleus cuneatus and gracilus (Fig. 16–7), may appear prominent in normals. A posterior cervicomedullary contour alteration may also occur in those with cervicomedullary junction anomalies, including Arnold-Chiari malformation. Confusing these protrusions with brain stem neoplasm is eliminated when its isointensity with remaining brain stem anatomy on multiple pulsing sequences is recognized.

*Pineal cysts,* developmental in origin, produce signal hyperintensity in normal-sized pineal glands on T2WI (Fig. 16–8). They are nonenhancing and are more frequently observed in the pediatric population. Some may attain sizes of up to 1 cm.

*Spinal medullary skeletal fat* signal may assume many varied appearances depending on age and nutritional status. Some of these variations are depicted in Chapter 17. Focal areas of fat deposition in vertebral marrow may produce local areas of T1WI signal hyperintensity.[14] These may appear rounded (Fig. 16–9) and may occur in the center of the vertebral body. In fact, a peculiar but normal pattern of spinal marrow consists of central signal hyperintensity on T1WI at all levels (see Fig. 17–16*A*). Not uncommonly, at vertebral end-plates adjacent to degenerated disks, linear or rectangular focal fat deposition occurs. Conversely, signal hypointensity on T1WI is observed along end-plates of degenerated disks. Age-related vertebral marrow alterations have been reviewed extensively in Chapter 17 and must be understood so overdiagnosis is avoided when assessing the spine for metastases.[15] The prepubescent population and those with excessive axial skeletal hematopoietic (red) marrow exhibit lower vertebral T1 signal intensity (diminished adipose/yellow marrow).[16, 17] With aging, cachexia, and systemic debilitation, adipose marrow is replaced by fibrous tissue becoming less cellular and producing poorly defined irregular foci of diminished signal on T1WI that simulate diffuse metastases (Fig. 16–10). These areas of T1WI signal hypointensity are poorly defined and are rarely associated with extremes in their T1 or T2 relaxation characteristics. When extensive, this pattern may be difficult to differentiate from diffuse myelomatosis (Fig. 16–11), skeletal carcinomatosis (prostate), or other sclerotic bone diseases. However, most diffuse sclerotic bone processes produce more marked signal hypointensity on T1WI. A rule of thumb on most T1WI, even when diffuse disease exists, is that the hyperintense vertebral bodies are the normal ones. Occasionally, the reader is presented with a single hyperintense vertebral body, and the remaining axial skeleton is hypointense. It is tempting to single out the hyperintense vertebra as abnormal when, in fact, this is rarely the case (lipoma of bone or hemangioma) on T1WI (Fig. 16–12). We have only encountered one case of metastatic spinal neoplasm hyperintense in signal relative to the uninvolved marrow (Fig. 16–13) on T1WI. Most often it is the hypointense vertebral bodies that are pathologic on T1WI.

*The Schmorl's node* is another normal structure potentially simulating metastatic disease if its normal appearance is unfamiliar in the sagittal plane (Figs. 16–14 [and Fig. 16–15]). These end-plate herniations of

*Text continued on page 498.*

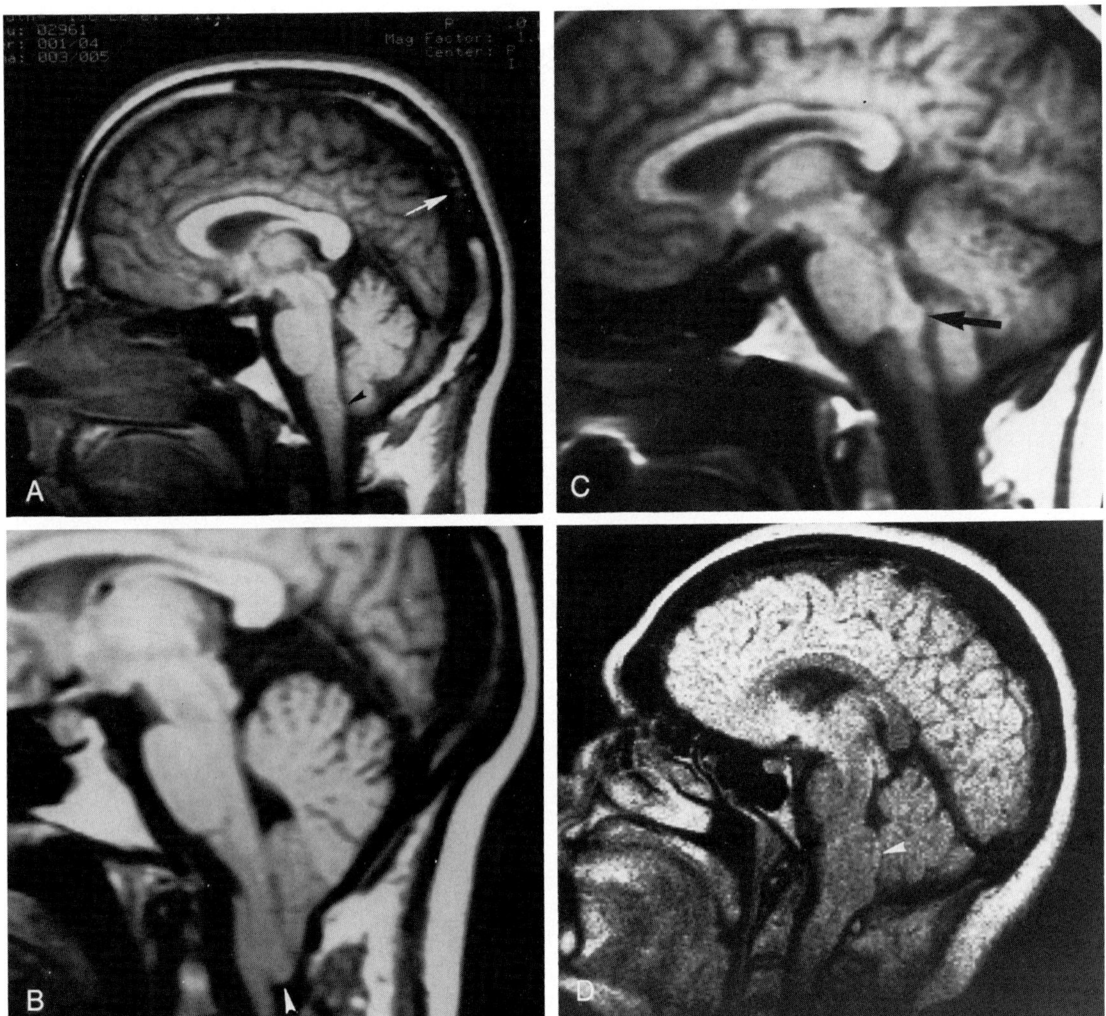


**Figure 16–7. Claval pseudotumors (*A* and *B*) and tumors (*C* and *D*).** Four different patients evaluated for posterior fossa symptoms. *A,* Sagittal T1WI. Subtle posterior contour of the brain medulla (arrowhead) is a normal structure, the clava. It is isointense on all pulsing sequences. Incidental averaging of the sagittal suture interrupts the normally hyperintense intradiploic signal (arrow) and simulates calvarial metastasis. *B,* Sagittal T1WI. Pseudotumor (arrowhead) mimicking the clava is created by dural adhesions and traction on the brain stem in Arnold-Chiari malformation. Tonsillar ectopia suggests the correct etiology of this protrusion. *C,* Sagittal T1WI. The clava is hyperintense and appears enlarged (arrow). Diagnosis: claval metastasis. *D,* Sagittal N(H)WI. Enlargement of the clava is apparent (arrowhead), but it is isointense with the brain stem. Lesion is hyperintense on T2WI (not shown). Diagnosis: Claval glioma.

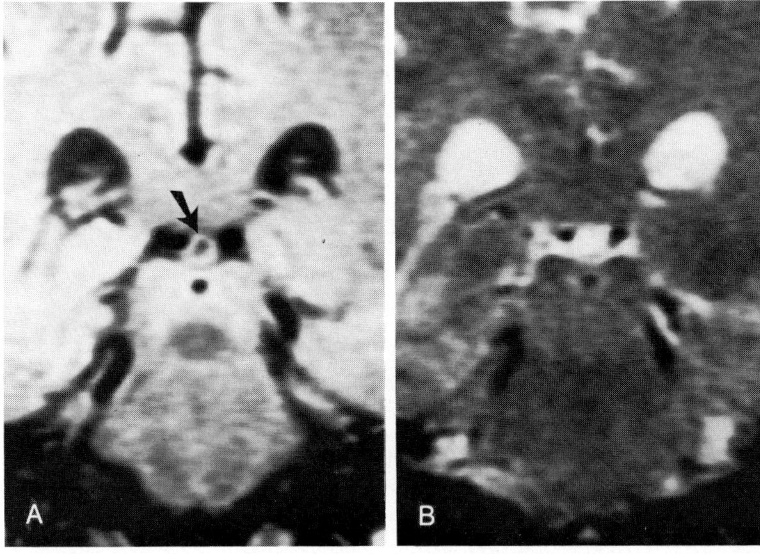


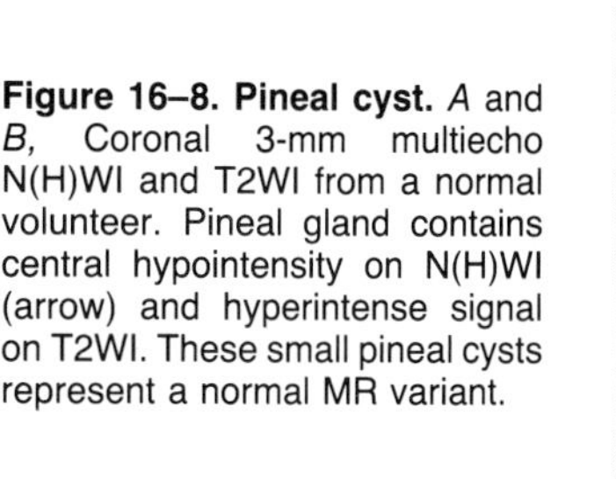

**Figure 16–8. Pineal cyst.** *A* and *B,* Coronal 3-mm multiecho N(H)WI and T2WI from a normal volunteer. Pineal gland contains central hypointensity on N(H)WI (arrow) and hyperintense signal on T2WI. These small pineal cysts represent a normal MR variant.

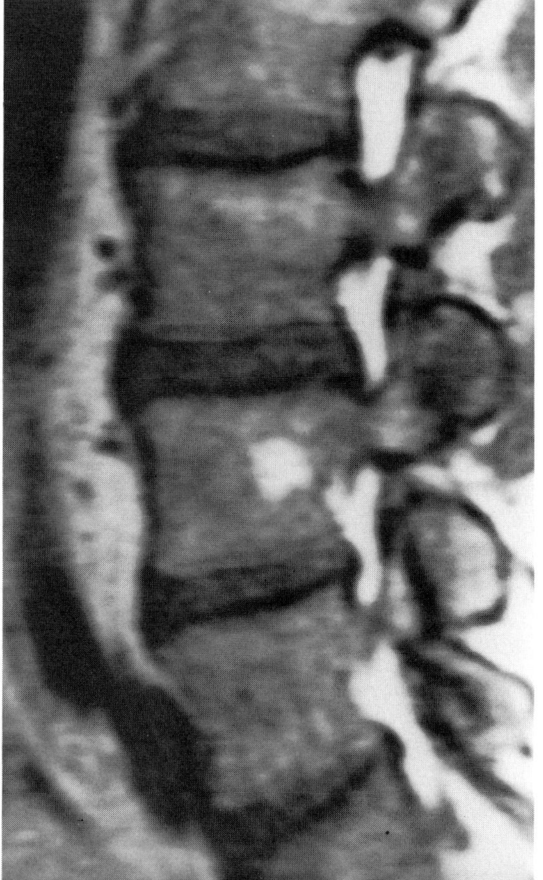

**Figure 16–9. Focal vertebral "bright spot."** Sagittal N(H)WI (1.5 T). Focal vertebral hyperintensity is a normal variant and can result from axial skeletal fat deposition, hemangioma, or large venous channels. Recognition averts misdiagnosis as neoplasm, although lipoma may also exhibit this appearance.

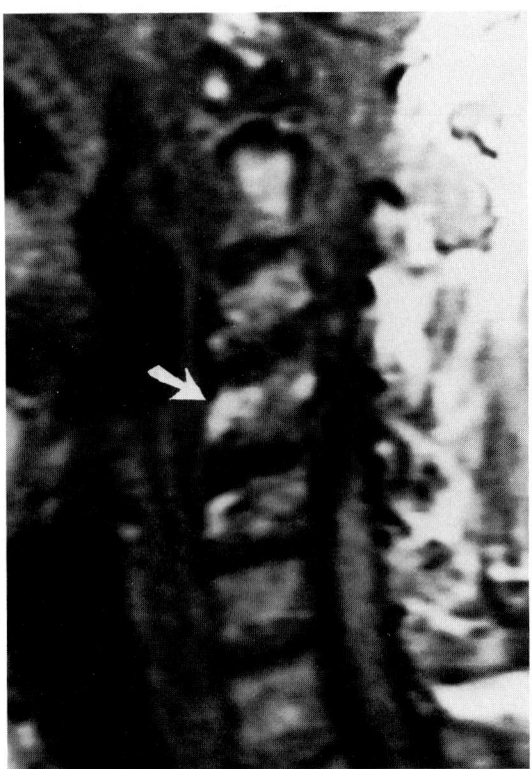

**Figure 16–10. Degenerative marrow signal.** A 62-year-old man with spondylosis and neck pain. Sagittal cervical spine T1WI (TR 600/TE 20 msec) shows marked irregular and diffuse hypointensity of vertebral marrow signal due to degenerative disease. Islands of residual hyperintense marrow persist (arrow) and should not be mistaken for neoplasm.

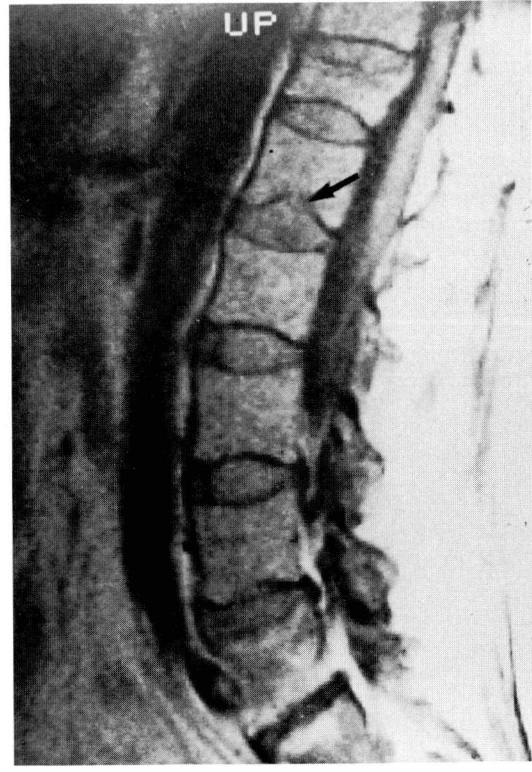


**Figure 16–11. A 47-year-old male with diffuse myelomatosis.** (0.35 T). Sagittal T1WI (TR 300/TE 35 msec). End-plate softening (arrow) is present. The vertebral marrow signal is diffusely more hypointense than expected for a patient this age on T1WI, but this is a subtle finding. (Courtesy of J. Tobias, M.D., Radiology Department, Mount Sinai Hospital, Miami Beach, Fla.)

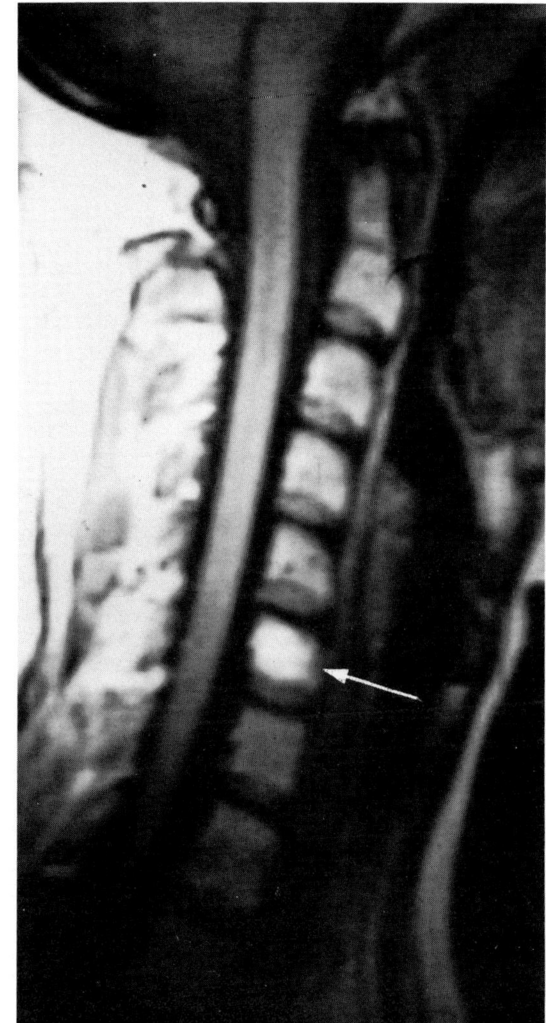

**Figure 16–12. Vertebral lipoma.** Sagittal T1WI (0.5 T). The solitary hyperintense vertebral body (arrow) could represent a lipoma, hemangioma, large venous channel, or hemorrhage.

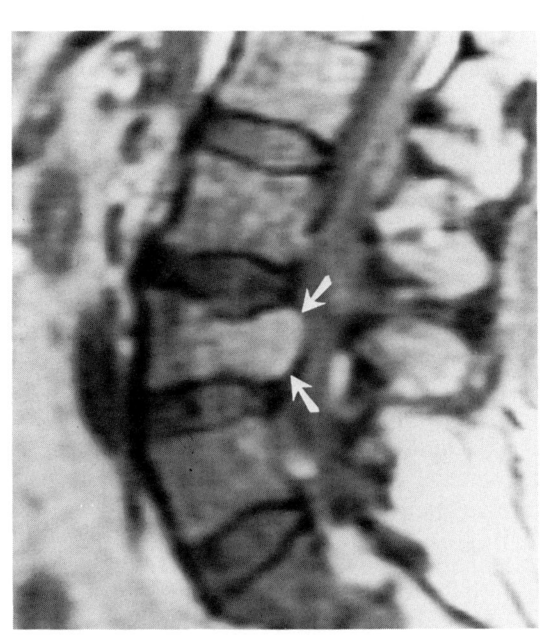

**Figure 16–13. Metastasis, breast carcinoma.** A 66-year-old woman (1.5 T). Sagittal T1WI shows a mass extending posteriorly (arrows) with signal hyperintense relative to normal marrow. Metastases are usually hypointense relative to marrow signal on T1WI.

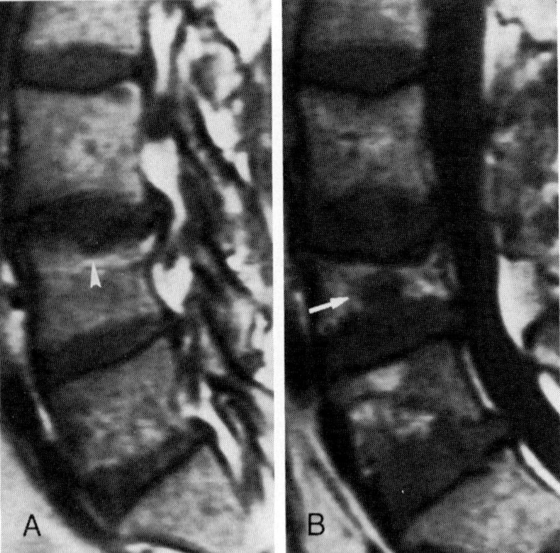


**Figure 16–14. *A* and *B*, A 52-year-old woman with breast carcinoma (1.5 T).** Adjacent sagittal T1WI (TR 600/TE 20 msec) sections illustrate the difference between a Schmorl's node (arrowhead) and juxta–end-plate metastasis (arrow). Schmorl's node exhibits obtuse margins and contiguity with the disk space, unlike neoplasm, forming acute angles with the disk space. T2WI will assist in separating the signal of neoplasm from the adjacent disk.

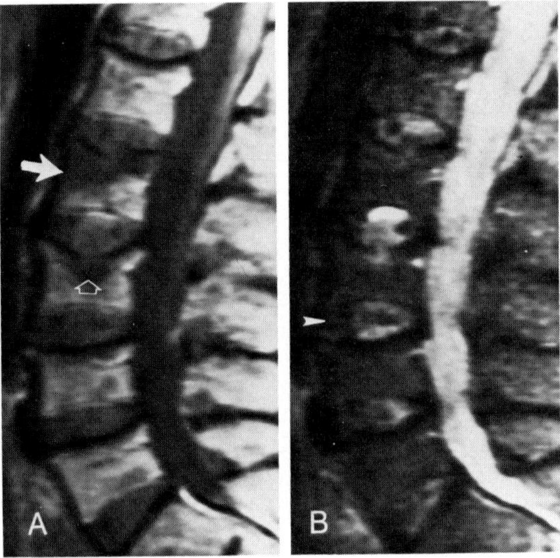


**Figure 16–15. A 41-year-old woman with breast carcinoma and back pain (1.5 T).** *A* and *B*, Sagittal multiecho N(H)WI and T2WI (TR 1800/TE 20/80 msec). Hypointensity (large arrow) at L2 has a linear caudal margin compatible with degenerative end-plate disease, not neoplasm. Minimal signal increase occurs on T2WI. Schmorl's node (open arrow) at L3 is contiguous with disk space on N(H)WI and T2WI. Also note normal intranuclear cleft (arrowhead) on T2WI.

disk material exhibit obtuse margins compatible with their "extra-axial" invaginating nature and yield a signal isointense with adjacent normal disks on multiple pulsing sequences. They are hypointense relative to normal medullary fat. Conversely, juxta–end-plate metastases are often rounded, exhibit acute angles relative to the disk endplate, and do not match the normal disk space signal intensity on multiple pulsing sequences.

*The intranuclear cleft,* located in the anterior portion of the intravertebral disc, is a well-recognized normal structure unique to sagittal MR (Fig. 16–15).[18] Its disappearance has been suggested as an early, but nonspecific, finding of diskitis.[19]

## HEAD CANTING, VOLUME AVERAGING, AND OTHER PITFALLS

Volume averaging artifacts may be accentuated and produced by asymmetric head or spine positioning. Obliquely oriented sections owing to head rotation produce confusing appearances. Because of the unusual contrast properties of magnetic resonance, these artifacts and pitfalls are unique and unlike CT.

Volume averaging in thin-section MR of the sagittal spine may produce several confusing appearances. Parasagittal spinal sections are a typical example of this effect. The false impression of disk degeneration or dessication occurs when the hypointense lateral disk margin instead of the more hyperintense nucleus pulposus is imaged on T2WI.

*Pseudosyringes* are of three types: (1) parasagittal vertebral artery averaging (hypointense) and (2) artifacts due to truncation errors, or (3) averaging of central cord gray matter.[20, 21] Subtle, intra-axial, linear signal hypointensity, or "pseudosyrinx," may be produced, on T1 or spin-density images N(H)WI. Conversely, T2WI sagittal sections often produce a linear, thin, hyperintense signal (Fig. 16–16). If the pseudosyrinx extends cranially toward the obex, averaging of central gray matter is the likely culprit. However, if no obex communication is apparent, a truncation artifact is responsible. This linear truncation, or edge-ringing artifact (Gibb's phenomenon) is discussed later in this section. It occurs at sharp edges,

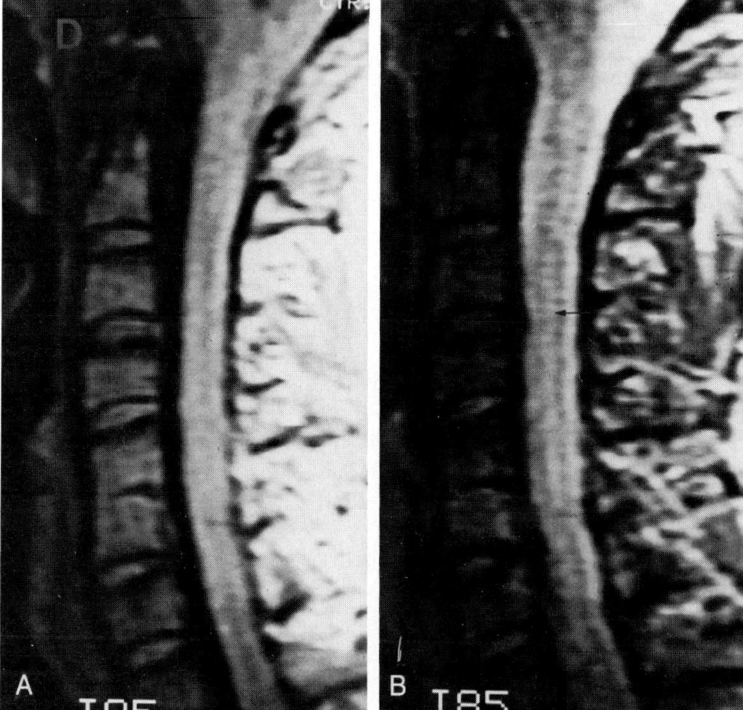


**Figure 16–16. Gibbs truncation or edge-ringing effect (see text).** *A* and *B,* A 20-year-old man evaluated for possible syrinx. (1.5 T). Sagittal 3-mm multiecho N(H)WI and T2WI (TR 2000/TE 20/80 msec). Longitudinal white line in cord (arrow) is normal and is seen only on T2WI. It represents Gibb's truncation or edge-ringing effect (see text).

where there are large changes in signal intensity resulting in striations of alternating signal intensity that may project over the cord as thin hyperintense or hypointense lines. This effect is most commonly observed perpendicular to the phase-encoded direction. Parasagittal averaging of the vertebral artery in the craniocervical region is another cause of pseudosyrinx (Fig. 16–17). It results in a linear hypointense signal that appears intra-axial. However, an anterosuperior course above the foramen magnum and persistent signal hypointensity (flow-void) on all sequences suggests the correct diagnosis. Axial images through the spinal cord will be normal in such cases.

*Petroclival marrow fat* (hyperintense) and cortical (hypointense) bone may produce confusion on MR when head canting or tilting occurs. Unilateral averaging of the petrous bone arcuate eminence may simulate an intra-axial temporal lobe hypointense mass (Fig. 16–18). This pseudomass of cortical bone may increase slightly in signal on T2WI since adjacent CSF and dura are also averaged. Petroclival marrow, exhibiting the expected signal hyperintensity of fat on T1 and spin-density, or N(H)WI, images, may be averaged as part of the acoustic nerve complex in either the axial or coronal projection (Fig. 16–19). This pseudomass is particularly common when section thickness exceeds 3 mm. These signal characteristics (hyperintense on T1WI) would be unusual for acoustic neuroma or cerebellopontine angle masses other than lipoma. Multiple-projection, thin-section (3-mm) imaging helps to avert misdiagnosis in this region. Like the petrous marrow, clival marrow may be coronally averaged, simulating pituitary macroadenoma or hemorrhage on T1WI. Similarly, marrow in the dorsum sella may create the impression of a hyperintense "pseudoadenoma" of the pituitary on T1WI (see Fig. 16–2).

*The sellar, suprasellar, and hypothalmic regions* may produce several unusual signal patterns. Parasagittal sellar averaging of CSF, carotid artery, and dura may produce central pituitary signal hypointensity on sagittal T1WI (Fig. 16–20). Protruding subfrontal gray matter gyri may be sagittally averaged on T1 or N(H)WI creating a pseudomass, anterior to the rostrum of the corpus callosum in the sagittal projection (Fig. 16–21).

Averaging of the splenium of corpus callosum due to head rotation during a sagittal acquisition may create the false impression of a peripheral mass (Fig. 16–22). Likewise, assymmetric volume averaging of differen-

*Text continued on page 504.*

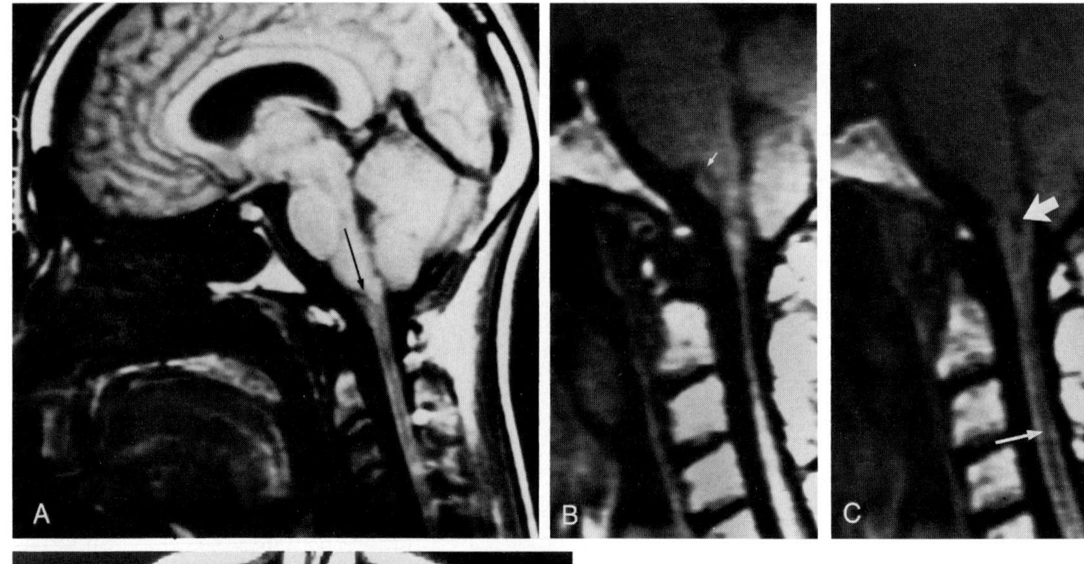


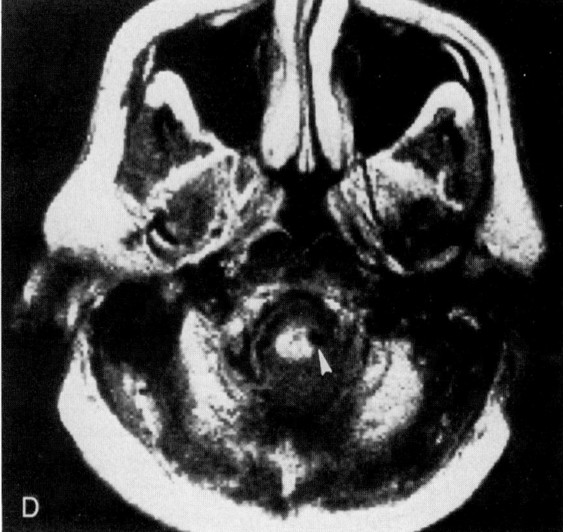


**Figure 16–17. Pseudosyrinx, parasagittal vertebral artery averaging, normal volunteers.** *A,* Sagittal T1WI scout. Linear signal hypointensity in the cord courses anterosuperiorly (arrow) at the brain stem level, the expected course of the vertebral artery. *B* and *C,* Sagittal 3-mm T1WI from another patient demonstrates a proven cord cyst (short arrow, *C*) extending into the medulla (thin arrow) in *C*. This contrasts with the linear signal hypointensity of the vertebral artery coursing anteriorly on an adjacent section *(B)* from the same patient (arrow). *D,* The axial section demonstrates the proximity of the vertebral artery (arrowhead) with respect to cord and medulla, so that parasagittal sections may average this structure.

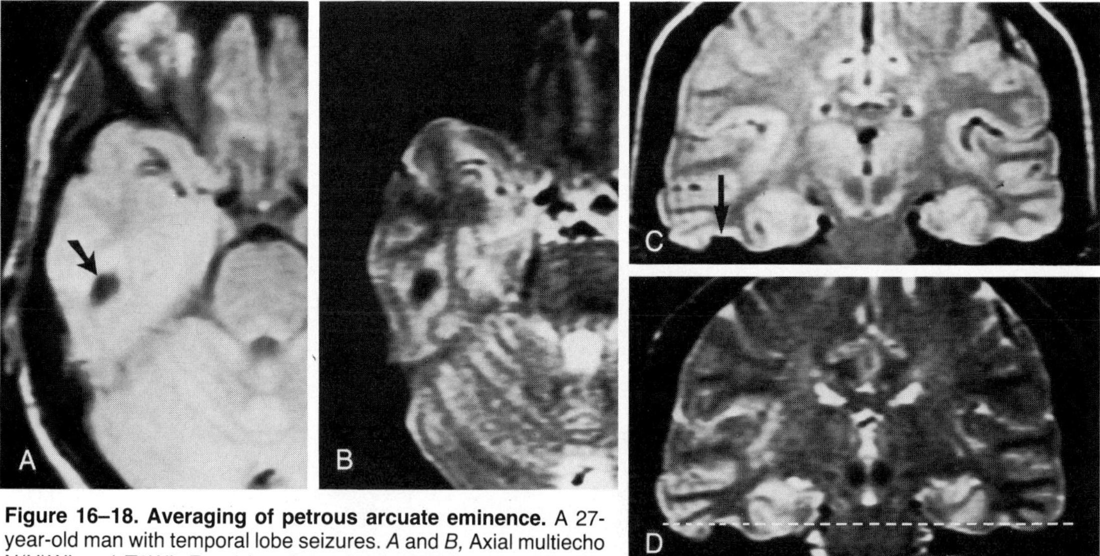


**Figure 16–18. Averaging of petrous arcuate eminence.** A 27-year-old man with temporal lobe seizures. *A* and *B,* Axial multiecho N(H)WI and T2WI. Focal hypointensity (arrow) is present in the right temporal lobe. *C* and *D,* Coronal N(H)WI and T2WI demonstrate how head canting or asymmetric size of the petrous arcuate eminence (arrow) may be averaged in the axial plane to create this temporal lobe defect.

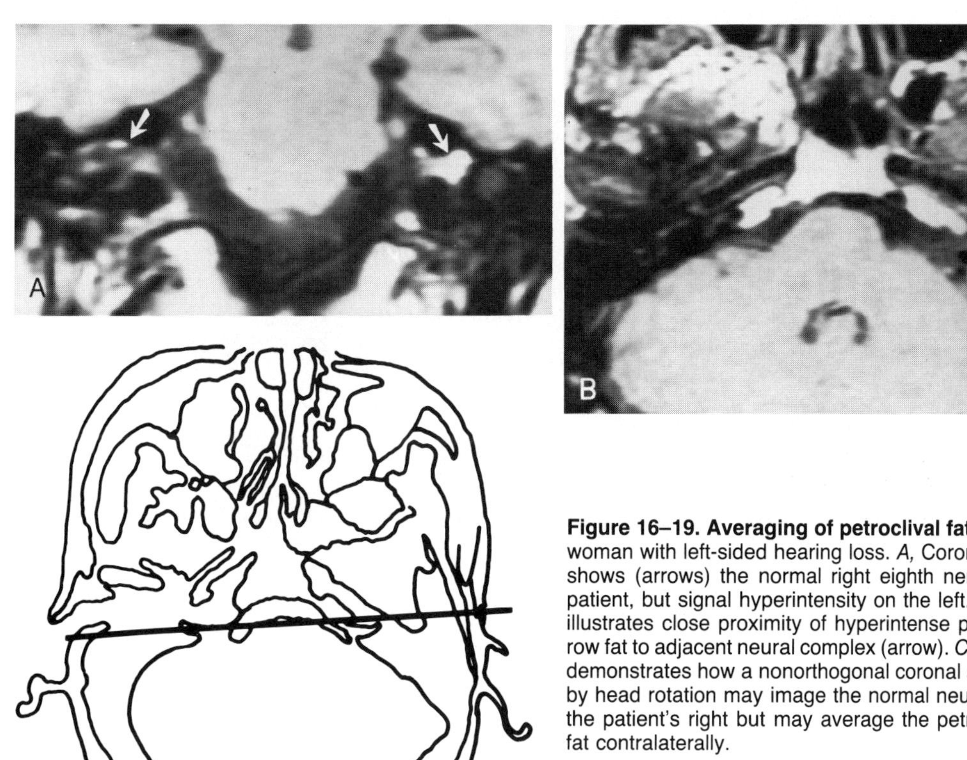


**Figure 16–19. Averaging of petroclival fat.** A 33-year-old woman with left-sided hearing loss. *A,* Coronal 3-mm T1WI shows (arrows) the normal right eighth nerve complex of patient, but signal hyperintensity on the left. *B,* Axial T1WI illustrates close proximity of hyperintense petrous tip marrow fat to adjacent neural complex (arrow). *C,* A line drawing demonstrates how a nonorthogonal coronal section created by head rotation may image the normal neural complex on the patient's right but may average the petroclival marrow fat contralaterally.

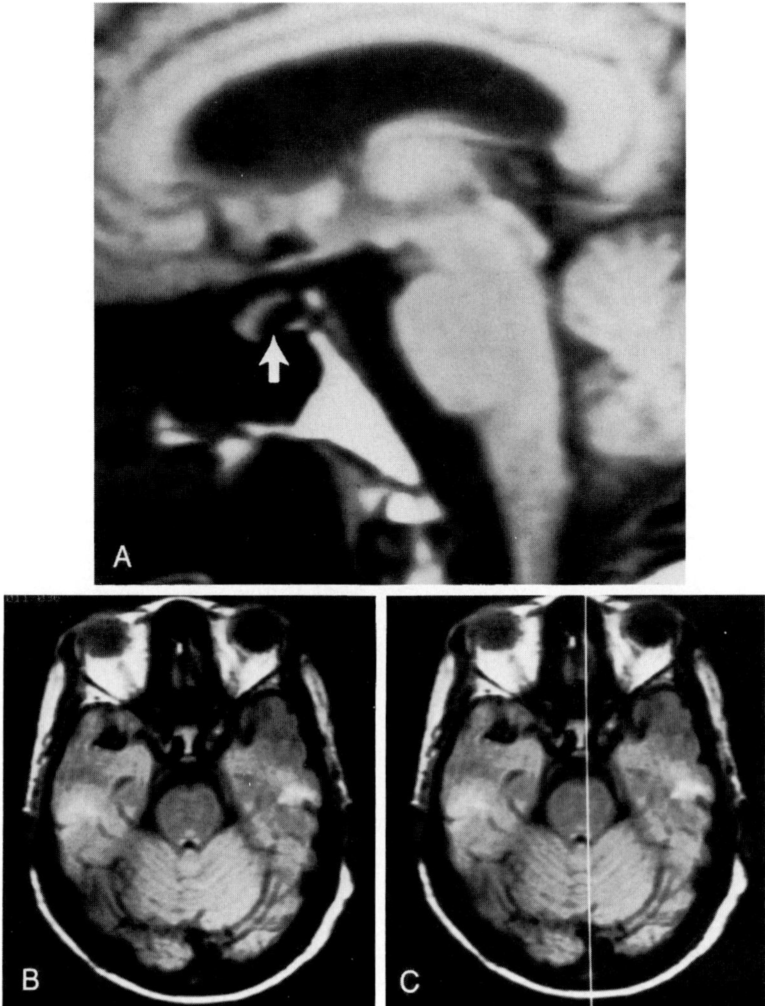


**Figure 16–20. Parasellar carotid artery averaging.** *A,* Sagittal 3-mm T1WI demonstrates focal hypointensity in the posterior aspect of the pituitary gland (arrow). *B* and *C,* The hypointense parasellar carotid arteries lie in close apposition along the lateral sellar margins. Parasagittal averaging of the adjacent carotid vasculature, as illustrated (white line), is responsible for this appearance.

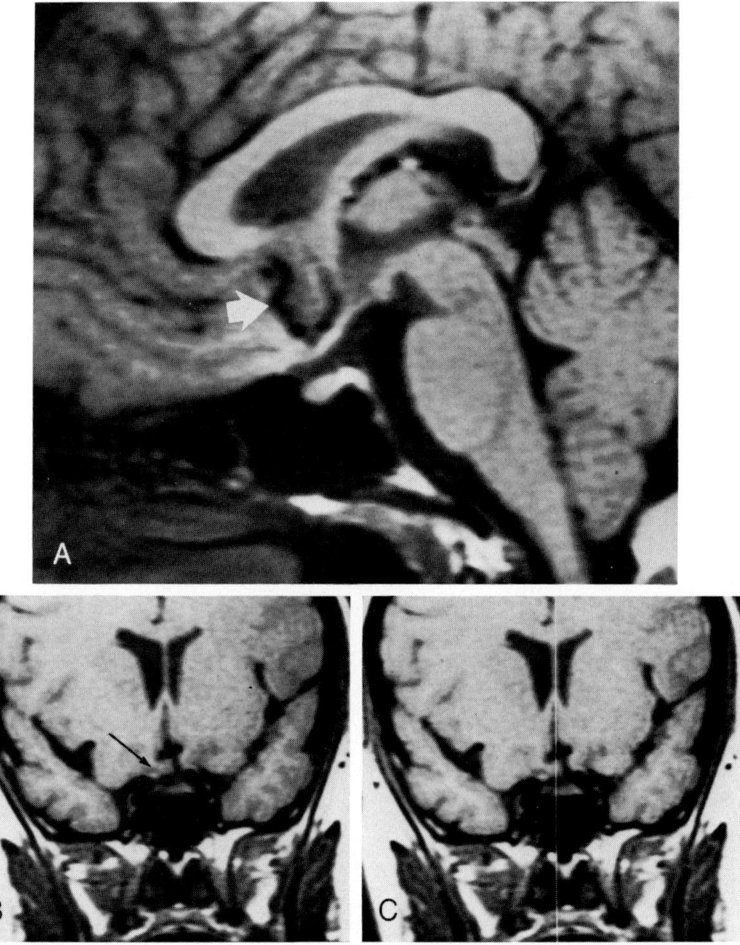


**Figure 16–21. Suprasellar pseudomass.** A 35-year-old man evaluated for visual disturbance. *A,* Sagittal T1WI. Suprasellar pseudomass (arrow) located above the optic chiasm on scout sequences represents averaging of a subfrontal cerebral gyrus owing to its asymmetric protrusion or nonorthogonal head positioning in the MR gantry. *B* and *C,* Coronal T1WI shows how sagittal section (line) bisects the protruding gyrus (arrow), creating the pseudomass in *(A).*

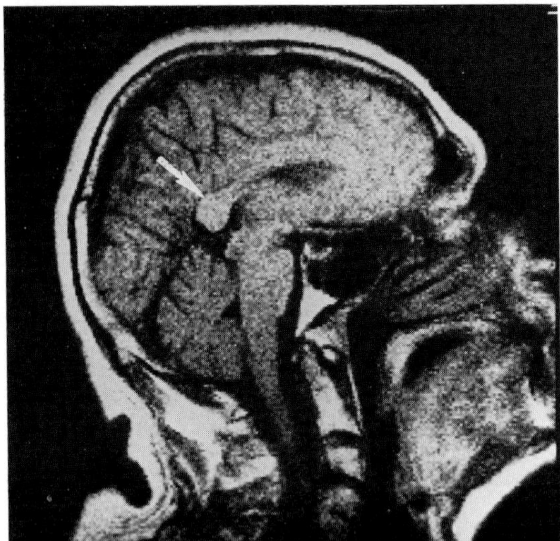

**Figure 16–22. Asymmetric corpus callosum averaging.** Sagittal T1WI (0.35 T). Pseudomass of the corpus callosum splenium (arrow) resulting from parasagittal averaging of this structure. An oblique section is created by nonorthogonal head positioning in the MR gantry. (Courtesy of Mount Sinai Hospital, Radiology Department, Miami Beach, Fla.)

tially aerated anterior clinoid processes may simulate a mass effacing the intracanalicular optic nerve in the axial projection (Fig. 16–23).

*Cortical sulci and gyri* are common sources of problematic signal averaging in the coronal and axial evaluation of multiple sclerosis (MS). The signal produced depends on the structures being averaged. If a sulcus and its cerebrospinal fluid are involved, then T1 signal hypointensity and T2 signal hyperintensity are produced. Lacunar infarction or focal encephalomalacia may be simulated. If cortical gray matter is averaged (Fig. 16–24), no abnormality is apparent on T1WI, but punctate signal hyperintensity, simulating MS, is produced on N(H)WI and T2WI. This signal increase is more apparent than real. Identification of these as pseudoplaques rather than true MS plaques is made on the following bases: signal intensity on N(H)WI that actually matches normal cortex; peripheral juxtasulcal location, nonvisualization on T1WI, and the inability to identify these pseudoplaques in another projection time. MS plaques are hyperintense on both N(H)WI and T2WI but are properly identified by utilizing the criteria listed above.

## ARTIFACTS

MR artifacts have been reviewed in detail in the literature.[22] Their physical bases are not described here in detail. The following are examples of selected common MR artifacts.

*Aliasing, also called foldover or "wraparound,"* occurs when a field of view (FOV) too small for the body part examined is selected. The image actually appears wrapped around itself, a phenomenon that primarily occurs in the phase-encoded direction (Fig. 16–25). Reduction of the analog filter bandwidth minimizes wraparound in the frequency-encoded direction. This can be adjusted manually. A software "trick" is employed by some manufacturers (for example, "no-phase wraparound" (General

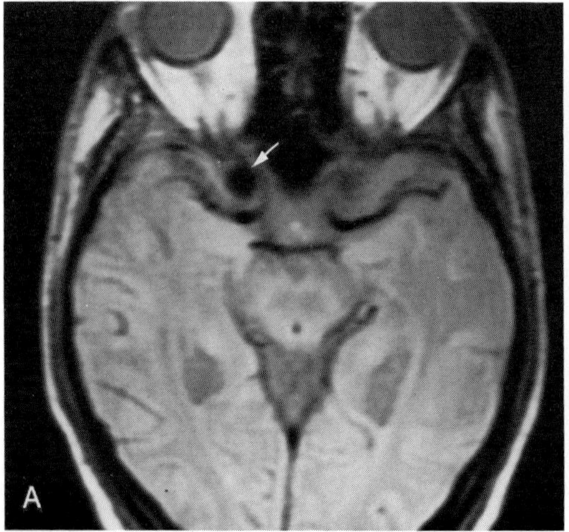


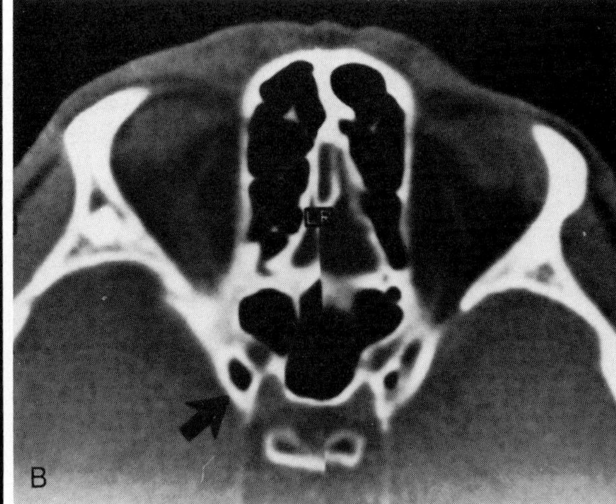


**Figure 16–23. Arterial clinoid pseudomass.** *A* and *B,* Axial N(H)WI shows focal hypointensity (arrow) adjacent to the right intracanalicular optic nerve simulating a mass. Axial CT illustrates normal asymmetric anterior clinoid aeration (arrow).

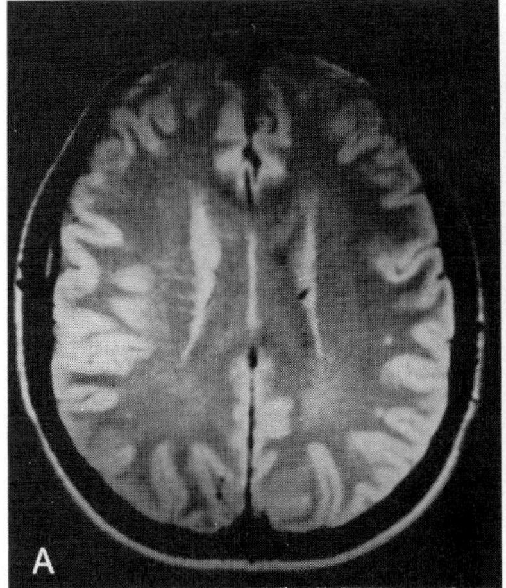


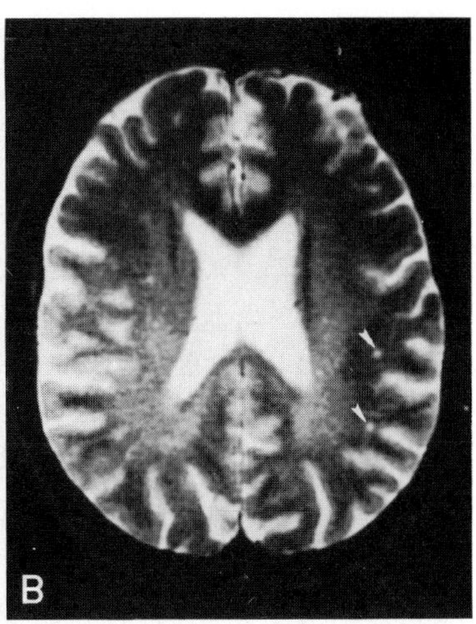


**Figure 16–24. Multiple sclerosis pseudoplaques.** A 37-year-old woman evaluated for possible multiple sclerosis. *A* and *B,* Axial N(H)WI and T2WI. Hyperintense foci (arrowheads) on T2WI mimic MS plaques. The following points identify these foci as pseudoplaques rather than true MS plaque: (1) peripheral location, (2) isointensity with gray matter on N(H)WI (true plaques are hyperintense on N(H)WI), and (3) alignment with sulci.

Electric, Milwaukee, Wisconsin) to reduce foldover effects. The operator selects the desired FOV and matrix. The FOV and matrix are automatically doubled so that pixel sizes are held constant but aliasing is avoided. To maintain constant imaging/acquisition time, the averages or excitations are halved. The image is then displayed showing the region-of-interest or FOV originally selected by the operator. Software aliasing correction is available in both the phase and frequency encoded dimensions. An artifact similar to aliasing occurs when one data channel fails during acquisition and an image is reflected in both the phase- and frequency-encoded directions—"double-wrap-around."

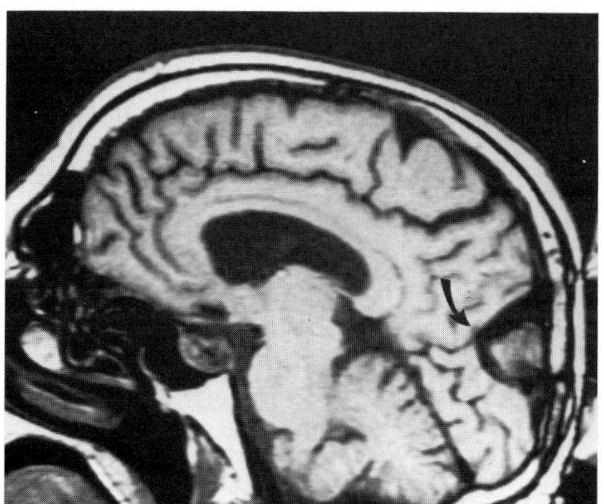

**Figure 16–25. Aliasing, wraparound, or foldover artifact.** The patient's nose (arrow) is "wrapped around" into the occipital lobe. This form of spatial selected misregistration is more common in the phase-encoding dimension and occurs with anatomy lying outside the field-of-view (FOV). Aliasing is minimized with bandpass filters in the frequency-encoded direction, increasing the pixel numbers (pixel dimensions constant) in the phase-encoded dimension, or by utilizing larger FOVs. Foldover may be offset from a region of interest by utilizing "off-axis" FOV. Foldover in the image periphery is eliminated by interpolated magnification before photography.

*The "zipper" artifact* occurs when there is contribution of 180° pulses acting as 90° pulses outside the true selected slice. This phenomenon occurs with one-excitation imaging and simulates a zipper, parallel to the frequency-encoded or readout gradient. Similar artifacts may occur in the phase-encoded axis when the direct current level of each phase-encoded step is not constant. These artifacts may result in a point of signal hyperintensity when all views have the same direct current offset. This is particularly troublesome in the brain stem region where lacunar infarct is simulated.

*Radio frequency (RF) interference* artifacts may take several forms, both intrinsic and extrinsic.[23] A line across an image perpendicular to the frequency-encoded direction, the "RF zinger" or zipper artifact, is one common type. This occurs when extrinsic RF energy sources (flourescent lights, motors, television, or radio) produce radio frequency interference in the receiver coil of the scanner. The distance of this artifactual line from the center of an image is proportional to the difference between the magnet's center frequency and the extraneous signal. Another common RF interference pattern, the "herringbone," results from transient alterations in the system's intrinsic hardware function (Fig. 16–26).

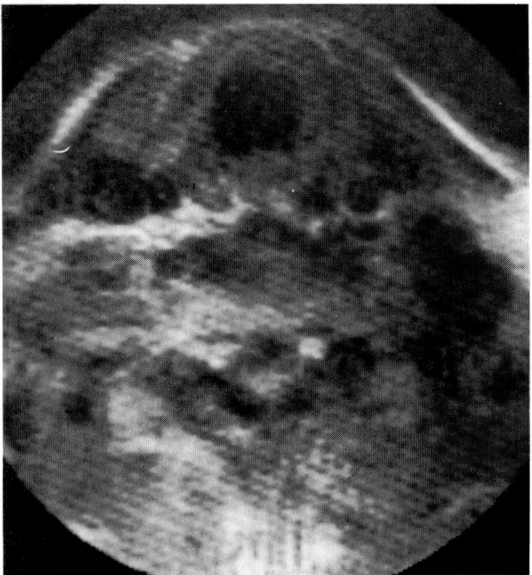

**Figure 16–26. "Herringbone" pattern of radio frequency (RF) interference.** RF interference may also appear as a band or line in the frequency-encoded direction. It may result from hardware malfunction or extrinsic sources that utilize similar bandwidths, or frequencies, to function. (Courtesy of Wellington Diagnostics, Cincinnati, Ohio.)

*Data clipping* occurs if the peak MR signal lies outside the computation range of computer and software used in image reconstruction. Data clipping refers to the fact that large numbers, lying outside allowable limits, are made small, and information is distorted or unrecoverable. Data clipping may also occur if a patient moves when the signal attenuator is set. A ghostlike image resembling data clipping may occur when a patient moves during central view acquisition (view 128 of 256 phase-encoded steps) of an actual scan.

*Image shading* is a common MR problem. Static magnetic field inhomogeneity may produce regions of signal hyperintensity or hypointensity during whole-volume imaging. Shim coils attempt to reduce these inhomogeneities. Various quality control manuevers, including daily phantom assessment, have been employed to evaluate these "hot spots." In addition, uniform distribution of an RF pulse throughout the scan slice may not occur since each patient's electrical and magnetic properties are unique.[24] This is particularly true with a linear drive RF excitation technique and main field inhomogeneities accentuate these RF problems. An RF penetration problem is created, producing a change in signal intensity even in tissue of uniform composition. This depends on the location of the tissue in the imaging plane.

During surface coil imaging, image shading also occurs (Fig. 16–27). Tissues close to and centrally positioned under the coil exhibit greater signal intensity than eccentric or deeply positioned structures.[25] These forms of asymmetric signal distortion, one intentional (surface coil) and the other unintentional (whole volume), differ from geometric field distortion.

*Aspect ratio, or geometric field distortion,* occurs most often in the frequency-encoded direction and arises from macroscopic imperfections in the magnetic field that may be produced by static field inhomogeneity or the presence of a magnetic substance in a constant field. In addition, if time-varying magnetic field gradients in the x (frequency) or y (phase) direction are not proportionally adjusted together, the aspect ratio, or height and width of the image, is distorted (Fig. 16–28). Therefore, artifactual image expansion (barrel) or contraction (pincushion) distortion occurs. Degradation of spatial resolution may result.

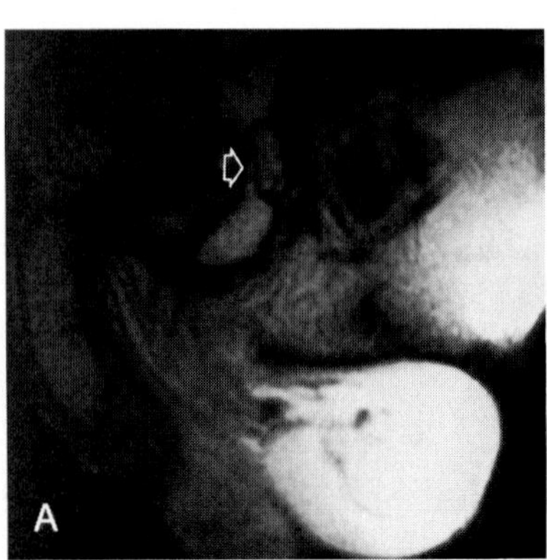


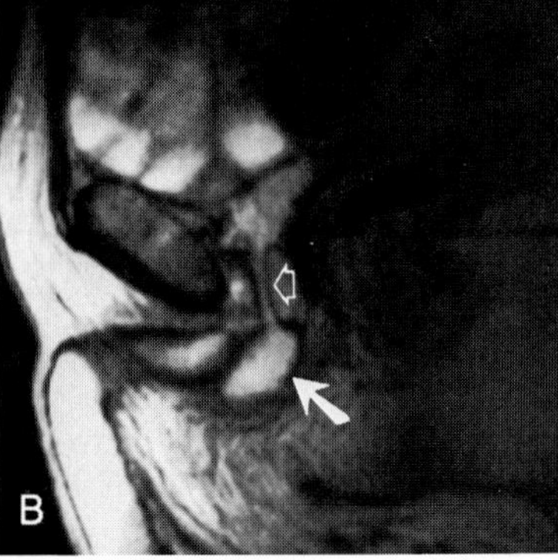


**Figure 16–27. Image shading with surface coil MR.** *A,* Sagittal N(H)WI (TR 1800/TE 20)-coil positioned posteriorly. *B,* Sagittal N(H)WI (TR 1800/TE 20)-coil positioned anteriorly. A perineal abscess (arrow) with fistulization (open arrow) to the prostatic bed is present. Because of the signal fall-off with increasing depth from the coil surface, the signal is barely adequate to demonstrate the pathology when the coil is positioned posteriorly. However, proper coil centering and anterior position over the symphysis pubis *(B)* allows optimal visualization of the fistula.

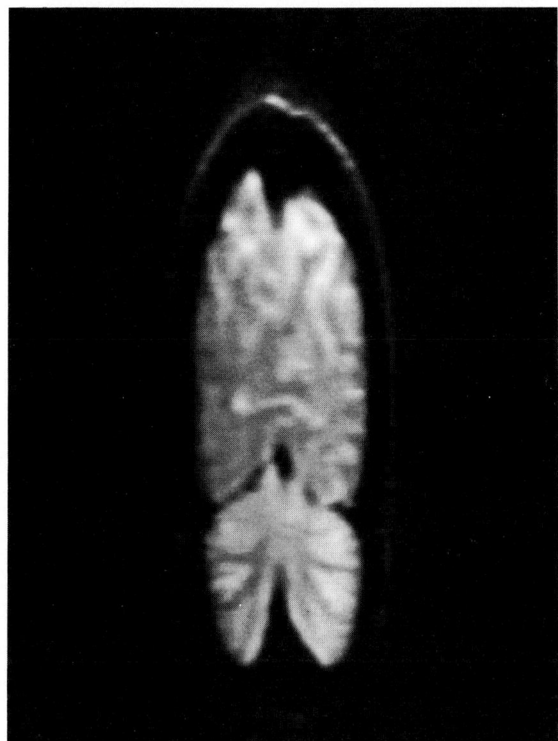

**Figure 16–28. 1.5 T. Coronal T2WI shows artifactual geometric image distortion and elongation in the frequency (craniocaudad) direction (see text).** The height and width of the image become imbalanced if time-varying gradients in the x and y directions are not adjusted together. Diagnosis: aspect-ratio distortion.

*Ferromagnetic/diamagnetic and nonferromagnetic* metallic objects also produce field distortion (Fig. 16–29). The size, shape, and ferromagnetic/diamagnetic susceptibility of an object determine the size of the artifact. Nonferromagnetic metallic objects, particularly when bent or twisted, may produce less extensive distortions owing to induction of local eddy currents generated by changing magnetic gradients.[26] The direction of misregistration is determined by the direction of the readout gradient. The characteristic appearance is a low-intensity region surrounded by regions of signal hyperintensity. This may occur at craniotomy and laminectomy sites in the absence of radiographically demonstrable metal density. Deposition of metallic drill bit fragments is the suggested cause of this phenomenon. Most surgical clips are nonferromagnetic, poorly visualized, and, in fact, a myriad of clips on plain film have gone virtually undetected with MR. Patients with Harrington's rods exhibit local field distortion, but the anterior spinal canal and disk margins are often visualized even at high field strengths utilizing T1WI. These are distinct advantages over CT.

*Chemical shift* is an artifact unique to MR (Fig. 16–30). The x coordinates of an MR image are determined by the linear variation in proton resonant (Larmor) frequency as induced by the readout gradient coil. This linear frequency spectrum is a direct function of the gradient's strength. The computer records this frequency spectrum during spin-echo sampling. The micromagnetic environments of fat and water differ, so that a proton-resonant frequency shift of approximately 3 to 5 parts per million (ppm) exists. This shift is directly proportional to the main magnetic field strength and is more pronounced at higher field. The result is that images obtained at high field strengths experience pixel shift of fat relative to water in the read only, or x, dimension.[27] Unfortunately, the computer and the Fourier transform reconstruction algorithm cannot distinguish frequency shifts induced by the readout gradient and those produced by the tissue influence of fat and water on each other.

At high field strengths, the ratio of chemical shift in frequency (3 to 5 ppm for fat and water) to the bandwidth per pixel is large. The resulting pixel shifts are most visible at interfaces between hydrated and fat-containing structures, where signal void occurs on one margin and signal hyperintensity on the contralateral margin. This phenomenon is of little consequence in the brain, where there are few direct fat-water interfaces. This misregistration effect is more conspicuous in the orbit and spine. Its recognition in the craniospinal axis is helpful in identifying lesions such as lipoma or dermoid tumor as fat-containing rather than hemorrhagic.

Depending on the manufacturer, the read or frequency gradient may be situated in any orientation. "Swapping" the orientations of the phase and frequency directions, or placing the patient in the MR gantry in a different position (feet first instead of head first) will reverse or alter the direction of chemical shift–induced artifact.

*Motion* degrades image resolution and increases coherent image noise (Fig. 16–31). Noise propagated in the phase-encoded di-

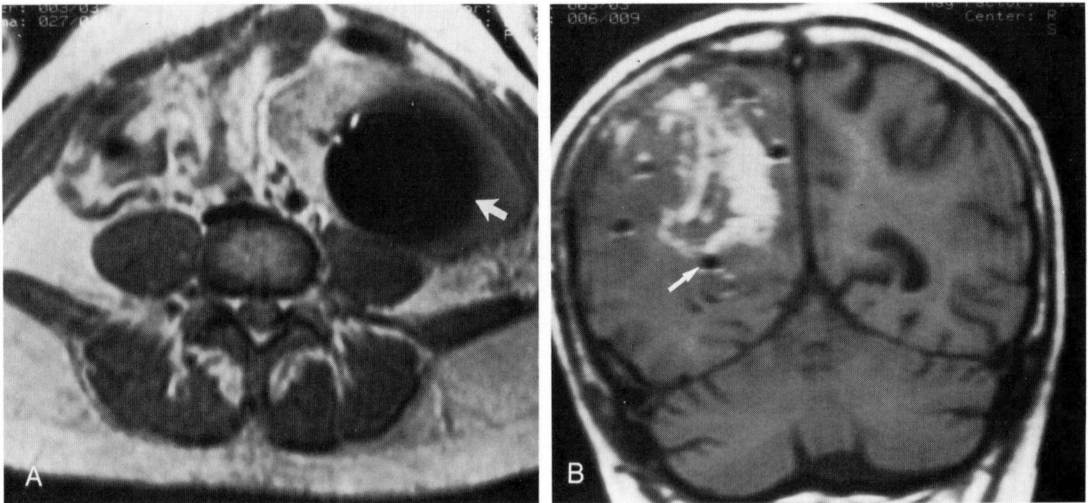

**Figure 16–29.** ***A*, Ferromagnetic artifact (arrow) due to intravascular coil placement.** Artifact size depends on object mass and degree of ferromagnetism. Central signal hypointensity with bizarre peripheral hyperintensity is typical. *B*, Nonferromagnetic radiotherapy seed implants produce less marked signal hypointensity (arrow) than ferromagnetic counterparts and minimal geometric, or signal distortion. Nonferromagnetic objects may induce some distortion artifact, particularly when bent or twisted.

rection from bowel peristalsis, respiration, cardiac activity, blinking, or by the patient's swallowing, talking, or chewing may adversely affect spinal or even cranial MR. The sensitive 2DFT algorithm is not equipped to handle phase errors associated with the above. These motion-induced phase errors result in blurring or banding, propagated in the y or phase dimension. Naturally, movement diminishes resolution owing to both motion unsharpness and to coherent noise.

Flow artifacts from vessels, particularly the caroticojugular vessels, and from CSF are frequently seen. These, too, are oriented in the phase, or y, dimension regardless of direction of flow. They are more apparent during surface coil acquisition because of improved signal to noise ratio (SNR). These artifacts may be redirected over a less critical portion of an image by operator selection of the phase-encoded direction. While surface coils make flow-related artifacts more con-

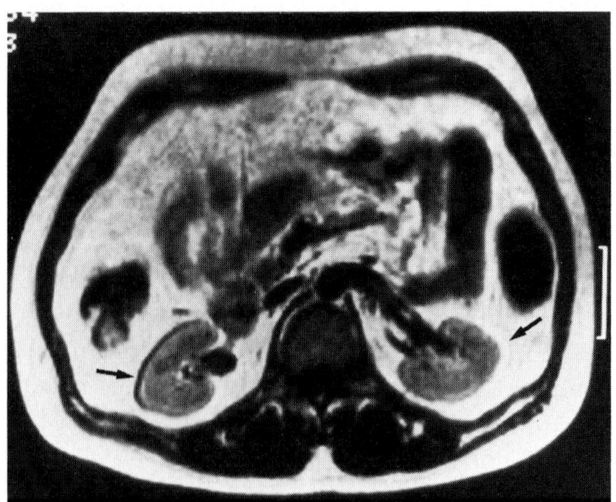

**Figure 16–30. Chemical shift artifact (see text). Misregistration and pixel shift in the frequency-encoded direction.** At fat-water interfaces, this pixel shift appears as signal hypointensity on one margin and hyperintensity on the other (arrows). High field strength accentuates this phenomenon.

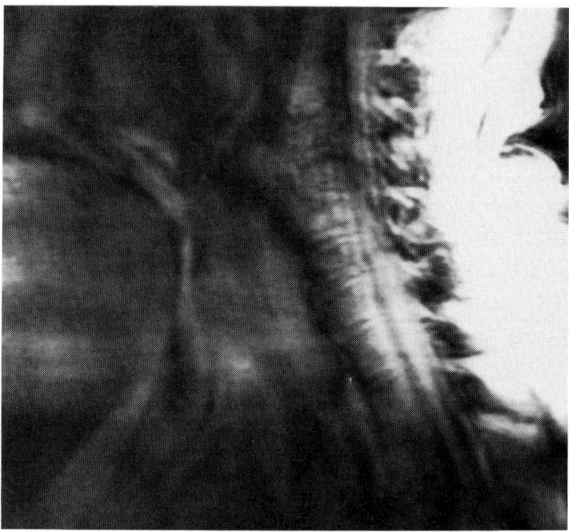

**Figure 16–31. Coherent noise.** Sagittal T1WI, cervical spine. Coherent noise due to patient coughing is propagated in the phase-encoding dimension. This appearance may mimic the data-clipping artifact (see text).

spicuous, they may be positioned to only receive signal from nonmoving tissue.[28] When the spine is imaged, coherent noise contribution from respiration or peristalsis is minimized with surface coils. Glucagon is occasionally used to reduce peristaltic noise contribution.

The periodic phase-oriented artifacts from respiration become more widely separated with increased respiratory rate or prolonged repetition time (TR). Respiratory amplitude increase accentuates blurring of original and ghost image.[29–31] Multiple excitations (6) or averages (4 or 8) with selection of shorter repetition times may reduce these artifacts. Unfortunately, techniques such as respiratory gating may increase scan times two- or fourfold. Phase-encoded smearing and the periodicity of respiratory motion may be minimized utilizing centrally ordered phase-encoding (COPE), respiratory ordered phase-encoding (ROPE), or other motion artifact suppression techniques (MAST).[32, 33] Image quality improvement is more conspicuous at higher field strengths.[34] Image reconstruction times may be slightly prolonged with some of these methods. Some have advocated routine cardiac gating to either the R wave of the QRS complex or to the peripheral pulse; however, cardiac gating does not correct for either aperiodic motion or periodic motion that is asynchronous with the cardiac cycle.[35] Various forms of nongated flow correction software, including gradient-moment nulling (flow compensation) or presaturation pulses have been implemented by some manufacturers and are described in Chapter 2 of this text.

*The Gibbs phenomenon—truncation, or edge-ringing artifact*—is not motion-related but does resemble the periodic ghosting at image margins that results from patient motion. It results from imprecise Fourier transformation data reconstruction at sharp boundary interfaces of markedly differing contrast.[36] Only a finite set of data is available to calculate an image with a mathematical formula using an infinite data set. Instead of a reproducible sharp interface, an oscillatory interface with alternating waves of increased and decreased signal intensity occurs (Fig. 16–32; see also Fig. 16–13). These fade as their distance from the interface increases and are most frequently seen perpendicular to the phase-encoding dimension. The appearance of truncation artifacts depends on the size of the object imaged and the pixel size. Edge-ringing effects can be made less conspicuous by employing smaller pixel sizes or by increasing the field of view. "Swapping" the phase and frequency directions of matrix acquisition will

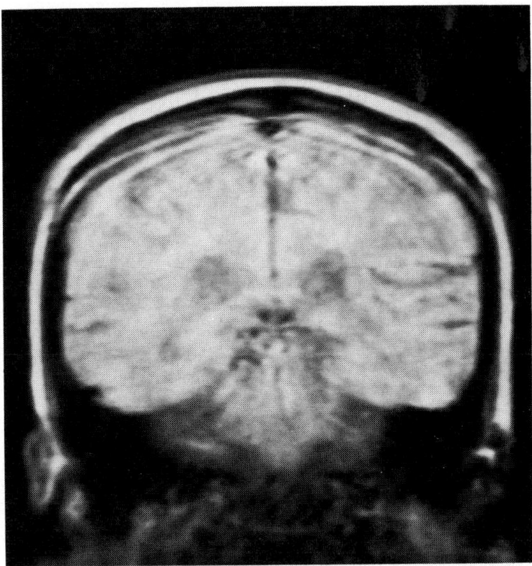

**Figure 16–32. Gibb's edge effect.** This occurs from imprecise data acquisition and object contrast reproduction. It results in oscillatory signal and image blurring at high-contrast interfaces (see text).

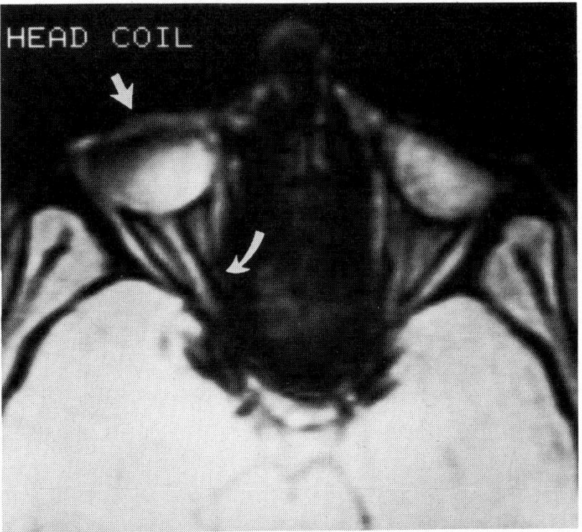


**Figure 16–33. Susceptibility artifact.** Axial fast-scan (flip angle 50°/TR 30/TE 12). Abrupt interface between tissues of differing susceptibility, such as the fluid-filled vitreous and air anterior to it (arrow) or orbital cone, bone, and adjacent sinus (curved arrow), has resulted in an artifact or signal void. Susceptibility reflects the willingness of a tissue to undergo magnetization. Susceptibility differences result in an artifact on sequences that accentuate susceptibilty effects, namely, fast-scan techniques.

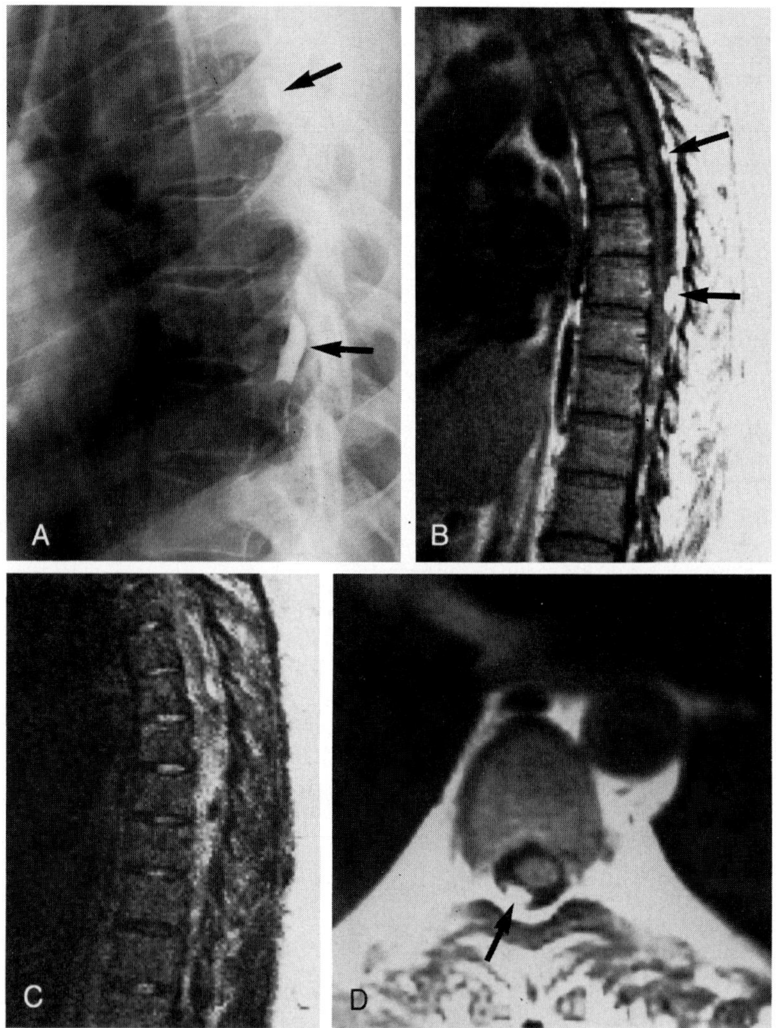


**Figure 16–34. Pantopaque artifact.** *A,* Lateral radiograph, thoracic spine. *B,* Sagittal T1WI (TR 500/TE 17). *C,* Sagittal T2WI (TR 2500/TE 90. *D,* Axial T1WI (TR 500/TE 17). Residual Pantopaque is visible on conventional radiograph along the dorsal aspect of the thoracic spinal canal (arrows). Pantopaque exhibits hyperintense signal on T1WI in *B* and *D* but becomes hypointense on T2WI *(C)* because these oily droplets have short T1 and T2 relaxations. (Courtesy of J. Tobias, M.D., Radiology Department, Mount Sinai Hospital, Miami Beach, Fla.)

alter the direction and appearance of the truncation artifact.

*The susceptibility artifact* is another product of imprecise data interpretation of differing interfaces (Fig. 16–33). Susceptibility simply represents the extent to which tissues are magnetized when exposed to an external magnetic source. The effective field created may exaggerate (paramagnetic susceptibility) or weaken (diamagnetic susceptibility) the applied external field. When two tissues differ markedly in susceptibility (air and water), the effective field their nuclei experience differs markedly. At their interface, a field gradient is created that induces rapid dephasing. Dephasing is counteracted in conventional spin-echo by the applied 180° pulse. Many fast-scan techniques employ gradient echoes rather than a 180° pulse. Therefore, dephasing is accentuated, and signal loss occurs at air-tissue interfaces.[37] Recognition of this artifact, or effect, can be useful in identifying hemorrhage with gradient-echo techniques. Susceptibility-induced signal loss may occur at the boundary between paramagnetic methemoglobin in hemorrhage and normal tissue.[38]

Pantopaque artifact produces signal alterations in the brain or spine that may simulate subacute hemorrhage at high field, lipoma, fat graft or other fat-containing lesions (Fig. 16–34). Residual Pantopaque, an oily substance, when left in the neural axis exhibits hyperintensity on T1WI and hypointensity relative to CSF on T2WI, not unlike subcutaneous fat.[39, 40] Correlation with and visualization of Pantopaque on conventional radiographs eliminates any diagnostic confusion.

## References


1. Pomeranz SJ, Soila K. Pitfalls in cranial magnetic resonance imaging. In MRI: Update Series, Vol. 2, pt. 1 (1 & 2). Princeton, 1986.
2. Pomeranz SJ. Pitfalls in magnetic resonance imaging: sella, internal auditory canals, and petromastoid regions. In MRI: Update Series, Vol. 2, pt. 6 (11 & 12). Princeton, 1986.
3. Vogler JB III, Helms CA, Callen PW. Normal Variants and Pitfalls in Imaging. Philadelphia, W. B. Saunders, 1986.
4. Mark L, Pech P, Daniels D, et al. The pituitary fossa: a correlative anatomic and MR study. Radiology 153:453, 1984.
5. Bilaniuk LT, Zimmerman RA, Wehrli FW, et al. Magnetic resonance imaging of pituitary lesions using 1.0 to 1.5 T field strength. Radiology 153:415, 1984.
6. Babcock EE, Brateman L, Weinreb JC, et al. Edge artifacts in MR images: chemical shift effect. J Comput Assist Tomogr 9:252, 1985.
7. Nishimura K, Fujisawa I, Togashi K, et al. Posterior lobe of the pituitary: identification by lack of chemical shift artifact in MR imaging. J Comput Assist Tomogr 10:899, 1986.
8. Sze G, Pardo F, Kucharczyk W, et al. The posterior pituitary gland: MR correlation with anatomy and function. Presented at The American Society of Neuroradiology 25th Annual Meeting, New York, May 10–15, 1987.
9. Kucharczyk W, Kucharczyk J, Berry I, et al. Chemical nature and functional significance of the posterior pituitary "bright spot." Presented at The American Society of Neuroradiology 25th Annual Meeting, New York, May 10–15, 1987.
10. Mamourian HC, Towfighi J. Pineal cysts: MR imaging. AJNR 7:1081, 1986.
11. Tanohata K, Tadayuki M, Noda M, et al. Isolated cerebral varix of superficial cortical vein: CT demonstration. J Comput Assist Tomogr 10:1073, 1986.
12. Pressman BD, Lotysch MJ. MR of pacchionian granulations. Presented at the American Society of Neuroradiology 25th Annual Meeting, New York, May 10–15, 1987.
13. Hinshaw DB Jr, Miller J, Peckham N, et al. The bright choroid plexus: MRI, CT and pathologic appearance of lateral ventricular choroid plexus xanthogranulomata. Presented at The American Society of Neuroradiology 25th Annual Meeting, New York. May 10–15, 1987.
14. Baker LL, Hajek PC, Goobar JE, et al. Focal fat deposition in axial bone marrow: diagnostic considerations and distinction from pathology by MR imaging. Radiology 161(P):132, 1986.
15. Dooms GC, Fisher MR, Hricak H, et al. Bone marrow imaging: magnetic resonance imaging related to age and sex. Radiology 155:429, 1985.
16. Yoshida H, Isamu M, Yashiro N, et al. MR imaging of bone marrow disorders. Radiology 161(P):23, 1986.
17. Steiner RE, Bydder GM, Young IR. MR distinction between red and yellow bone marrow: normal and abnormal. Radiology 161(P):24, 1986.
18. Aguila LA, Piraino DW, Modic MT, et al. The intranuclear cleft of the intervertebral disc: magnetic resonance imaging. Radiology 155:155, 1985.
19. Modic MT, Feiglin DH, Piraino DW, et al. Vertebral osteomyelitis: assessment using MR. Radiology 157:157, 1985.
20. Levy LM, Di Chiro G, Brooks RA, et al. Spinal cord artifacts from truncation errors during MR imaging. Radiology 166:479, 1988.
21. Bronskill MJ, McVeigh ER, Kucharczyk W, et al. Syrinx-like artifacts on MR images of the spinal cord. Radiology 166:485, 1988.
22. Bellon EM, Haake EM, Coleman PE, et al. MR artifacts: a review. AJR 147:1271, 1986.
23. Schenck JF, Hart HR Jr, Foster TH, et al. High resolution magnetic resonance imaging using surface coils. In Kressel HY, ed. Magnetic Resonance Annual: 1986. New York, Raven Press, 1986.
24. Glover GH, Hayes CE, Pelc NJ, et al. Comparison of linear and circular polarization for magnetic resonance imaging. J Magnetic Resonance 64:255, 1985.
25. Ehman RL. MR imaging with surface coils. Radiology 157:549, 1985.
26. New PFJ, Rosen BR, Brady TJ, et al. Potential hazards and artifacts of ferromagnetic and nonferromagnetic surgical and dental materials and devices in nuclear magnetic resonance imaging. Radiology 147:139, 1985.
27. Soila KP, Viamonte M, Starewicz PM. Chemical shift misregistration effect in magnetic resonance imaging. Radiology 153:819, 1984.
28. Edelman RR, McFarland E, Stark DD, et al. Surface coil MR imaging of abdominal viscera. Part I. Theory, technique, and initial results. Radiology 157:425, 1985.
29. Haacke EM, Patrick JL. Reducing motion artifacts in two-dimensional Fourier transform imaging. Magn Reson Imag 4:359, 1986.
30. Wood ML, Henkelman RM. MR imaging artifacts from periodic motion. Med Phys 12:143, 1985.
31. Schultz CL, Alfidi RJ, Nelson AD, et al. The effect of motion on two-dimensional Fourier transformation magnetic resonance images. Radiology 152:117, 1984.
32. Bailes DR, Gilderdale DJ, Bydder GM, et al. Respiratory ordered phase encoding (ROPE): a method for reducing respiratory motion artifacts in MR imaging. J Comput Assist Tomogr 9:835, 1985.
33. Haacke EM, Patrick JL, Bond CK, et al. Correction for motion artifacts based on a linear expansion model. (Abstract). Presented at The Society of Magnetic Resonance in Medicine Annual Meeting, London, August 19–23, 1985.
34. Quencer RM, Pattany PM, Horen H, et al. T2 brain MR with in-view rephased magnetization. Presented at The American Society of Neuroradiology 25th Annual Meeting, New York, May 10–15, 1987.

35. Elster AD, Moody DM, Moeser PM, et al. Use of a motion artifact suppression technique (MAST) for improved cranial and spinal MR imaging. Presented at The American Society of Neuroradiology 25th Annual Meeting, New York, May 10–25, 1987.
36. Wood ML, Henkelman RM. Truncation artifacts in magnetic resonance imaging. Magn Reson Med 2:517, 1985.
37. Wehrli FW. Introduction to Fast-Scan Magnetic Resonance. Milwaukee, Wis., General Electric Medical Systems, 1986.
38. Edelman RR, Johnson K, Buxton R, et al. MR of hemorrhage: a new approach. AJNR 7:751, 1986.
39. Mamourian AC, Briggs RW. Appearance of Pantopaque on MR images. Radiology 158:457, 1986.
40. Braun IF, Malko JA, Davis PC. The behaviour of Pantopaque on MR: in vivo and in vitro analyses. AJNR 7:997, 1986.

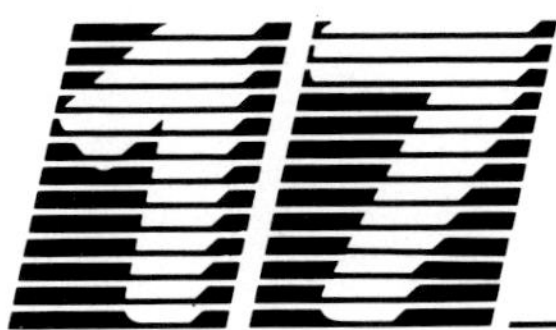

**Stephen J. Pomeranz, M.D.**

# NEOPLASMS OF THE SPINE

Magnetic resonance (MR) has rapidly become the modality of choice in evaluation of primary and secondary spine neoplasm. The following advantages of MR make it the examination of choice over computed tomography (CT) in spinal neoplasm assessment: (1) intrathecal contrast is not required to assess cord size and the shape and extent of tumor; (2) MR may differentiate pure cord cysts from solid neoplasm, myelomalacia, hematomyelia, and other causes of cord enlargement; (3) beam-hardening artifacts are absent on MR; (4) artifacts from Pantopaque or metal are negligible; and (5) thoracic lesions with motor signs, difficult to localize at a specific clinical level, are less likely to be missed with sagittal MR than axial CT.[1, 2]

Intraspinal tumors of the cord, meninges, nerve roots, or vasculature are most often found in adults 30 to 60 years of age. Tumor predilection based on gender (females, 4:1) is found only in meningioma. A racial predilection occurs exclusively in Chinese with neurinomas. Lesions in adults favor a thoracic spine location. Neurilemmoma, meningioma, and glioma account for almost 80% of spinal neoplasms.[3] Extramedullary intradural neoplasms (55%) are more common than extradural (30%) or intramedullary (15%) tumors. Ependymomas (55%) and astrocytomas (25%) account for the bulk of intramedullary lesions. Approximately 10% of lesions are "dumbell shaped," involving extradural and extramedullary intradural compartments.[4]

Some authors still recommend water-soluble contrast myelography (WSCM) or CT for neoplastic evaluation because extent and degree of cord enlargement can be assessed.[5] We utilize MR in two imaging planes as the first and often the only imaging modality to evaluate possible spinal neoplasm (Table 17–1) in all compartments.[6] When complete block or myelopathy is apparent, MR is the examination of choice.[7] T2-weighted images (T2WI) produce an "intrathecal contrast effect," with high-signal CSF bathing the lower signal intensity cord. Compartmental localization of spinal masses (intra-axial versus extra-axial) should only be attempted with both sagittal and axial MR, never with sagittal series alone.

## INTRAMEDULLARY NEOPLASMS

### Glioma

Gliomas are the most common intramedullary neoplasms, ependymomas accounting for the majority (55% to 65%).[8] Ependymomas occur in the third through sixth decades, exhibit slight male predominance, and are particularly vascular in the filum terminale. The papillary forms exhibit a propensity toward acute subarachnoid hemorrhage (Fincher's syndrome). Filum lesions may attain large size prior to detection, producing canal widening in 25%. Although papillary, cellular, epithelial, and mixed types have been described histologically, myopapillary forms favor the filum. Extradural filum terminale externum lesions occur in 3% of patients.[9] Cavity or cyst formation in intramedullary neoplasm is most likely to occur in ependymoma (45%).[10]

Astrocytomas, like ependymomas, exhibit slight male predominance, affecting individuals in the third through fifth decades. Unlike ependymoma, they are more extensive, less well defined, favor a thoracic location, affect multiple levels, and account for 25%

**Table 17–1.** DIFFERENTIAL DIAGNOSIS OF SPINAL NEOPLASIA

| Tumor/Compartment | Age/Sex | Location | T1 and T2 Relaxation | | Incidence | Cyst | Miscellaneous |
|---|---|---|---|---|---|---|---|
| | | | T1 | T2 | | | |
| ***Intramedullary*** | | | | | ***15% of IST***[+] | | |
| Ependymoma | 30–60 | Filum/conus | + | ++ | 55% of IMT[++] | 45% | Hemorrhagic; especially myxopapillary form |
| Astrocytoma | 30–50 | Thoracic | + | ++ | 25% of IMT | 38% | Low malignancy potential hyperintense T2 |
| Hemangioblastoma* | 30–40 | Thoracic (50%) Cervical (40%) | ++ | ++ | <10% of IMT 80% solitary | 40% | Mural nodule; FVS** of dilated vessels |
| Metastases | 50–70 | Thoracolumbar | = | ++ | <5% of IMT | — | Lung, breast, melanoma |
| ***Intradural*** | | | | | ***55% of IST*** | | |
| Meningioma | 40–60 | Thoracodorsal (F)*** (80%) Ventral (M)**** | = | =/+ | 25% of IST | | $Ca^{+}$ 40%; sessile; male distribution, cervicothoracic and ventral |
| Neurinoma | 20–40 | Lumbar; AL[+++] | +/= | ++ | 25% of IDT[a] | | Ovoid, round; not associated w. neurofibromatosis |
| Neurofibroma | 10–40 | Cervicothoracic | +/= | ++ | | | Neurofibromatosis[++]; central low signal intensity on T2WI |
| Lipoma (isolated) | 20–40 | Thoracic (40%) Cervicothoracic (30%) | - | - | <2% of IST | | 40% extradural with skeletal anomalies in dysraphic type |
| Metastases | | Conal/lumbar; amputated sac–like appearance | + | ++ | <2% of IST | | Drop lesions; pineal; germinoma; medullo/ependymoblastoma |
| ***Extradural*** | | | | | ***30% of IST*** | | |
| Metastases | 50–70 | Thoracic (T4-T11) | ++ | ++ | 25% of IST | | Hypointense marrow T1 foci; ovoid; round |
| Teratoma | 0–10 | Cervicothoracic | =/— | +/= | <1% of IST | | $Ca^{+}$ frequent; sinus tract; midline locale |
| Epidermoid | | Lumbar | ++ | ++ | <1% of IST | | Iatrogenic; adherent to nerve root/arachnoid |
| Lymphoma | 30–60 | Thoracolumbar | + | ++ | <3% of IST | | Osseous signal 30%; insinuates; infiltrates; epidural T1 fat signal decreased |

| | | | | | | |
|---|---|---|---|---|---|---|
| Lipomatosis | 20–40 | Cervicothoracic | - | - | | Dorsally located; assoc. obesity or steroid use |
| Lipoma dysraphic type | 0–15 | Lumbar | - | - | <1% of IST | Assoc. myelomeningocele; tethering, etc. |
| ***Other*** | | | | | | |
| Chordoma | 50–70 | Sacral (50%)<br>Clival (25%)<br>Cervical C2 | + + | + + | | Tumor signal in contiguous disk; $Ca^{+}$ 20%; predilection, C2 |
| Arachnoid cyst | 20–40 | Thoracic, intra- or extradural | + + + | + + + | | Arise posteriorly; CSF signal match; 40% communicate w. thecal sac |
| Hematomyelia | | Thoracolumbar | - | + + | | Signal~chronicity |
| Syringomyelia | | Cervicothoracic | + + | + +/- | | T2 signal varies with CFVS |
| Pseudotumor | | Cervical | = | =/— | | Location about dens; hx of RA, DJD, or trauma; no T2 signal increase |

AI: anterolateral spinal canal.
CFVS: CSF flow-void sign related to CSF movement and transmitted cardiac pulsation, reducing T2 image signal intensity.
IDT: intradural tumors.
IMT: intramedullary tumors.
IST: intraspinal tumors.
*Intramedullary 60%; intradural 40%.
**FVS: flow-void signal owing to hypertrophied feeding vessels.
***F: female sex predominance.
****M: male sex predominance.
— Short proton relaxation time (hyperintense T1 signal; hypointense T2 signal intensity).
- Very short proton relaxation time.
+ Long proton relaxation time (hypointense T1 signal; hyperintense T2 signal intensity).
+ + Very long proton relaxation time.
= intermediate proton relaxation (isointense or intermediate signal intensity).

of intramedullary neoplasms. Cyst formation occurs in 38%, and lower grade lesions are seen in 75% of cases.[11, 12]

MR findings of ependymoma and astrocytoma may be indistinguishable, but a lumbar/conus location heavily favors the former, whereas a cervicothoracic location (Fig. 17–1) favors the latter. The normal conus on T2-weighted axial images is 5 to 8 mm in anteroposterior and 8 to 11 mm in transverse dimension. A ventromedian fissure at T11 and posterior midline eminence with straight posterolateral margins at T12/L1 are normally seen.[13] Cord enlargement ("cigar-shaped"), distortion of normal anatomy, and elongated foci of T2 relaxation prolongation with variable T1 relaxation occur.[14] Signal alteration around the central canal favors ependymoma. Local tumor recurrence or spread from the posterior fossa may present as diffusely increased thecal sac signal on T1 or spin-density images, a subtle finding.[15] A more obvious form of recurrence produces intramedullary, nodular drop metastases that exhibit multifocal increased signal on T2WI (Fig. 17–2). Since delayed (6 to 24 hours) water–soluble contrast CT may demonstrate intra-axial enhancement in areas of cystic neoplasm, syringomyelia/hydromyelia, or cord damage, MR is an important diagnostic tool to help differentiate simple from neoplastic cord cyst. On MR simple cyst formation produces homogeneous intra-axial foci of T1 and T2 prolongation without surrounding hyperintense T2 edema.[16–19] When cysts transmit the normal CSF pulsations or exhibit fluid phase shifts (CSF flow-void sign [CFVS]), the expected T2 signal hyperintensity may not occur. Hypointensity of cyst relative to cord results on T2WI.[20–23] CFVS may be less common in neoplastic than in non-neoplastic cord cyst. Absence of CFVS may be a sign of successful syringotomy or shunt.

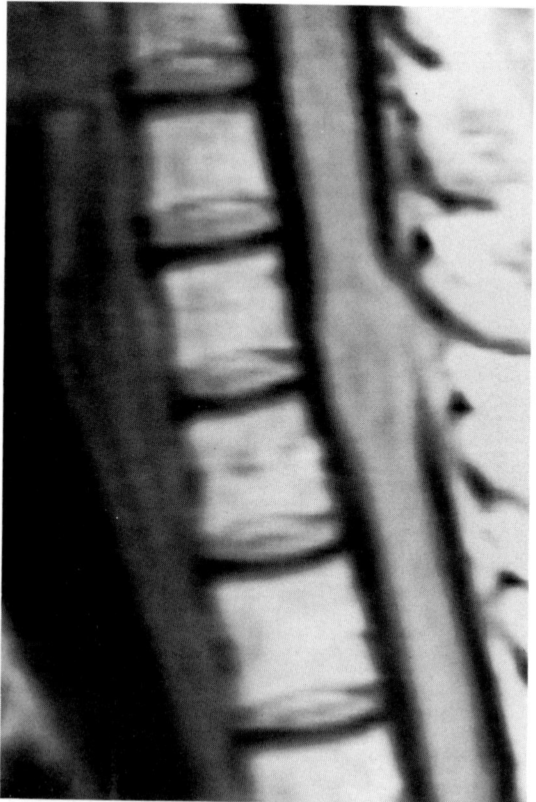

**Figure 17–1. Glioma.** A 22-year-old woman with neurofibromatosis and myelopathy (1.5 T). Sagittal T1WI (TR 600/TE 20 msec) shows a focal cord contour abnormality.

A myelomalacic cord exhibits increased T2 signal without discrete or confluent hypointense T1WI signal. Cord atrophy rather than enlargement is usually present. Cystic neoplasm (Fig. 17–3) may demonstrate focal, or elongated foci of, prolonged T1 or T2 relaxation (the cyst) and also surrounding regions of increased signal on T2WI.[24] The edema and solid tumor may remain hyperintense on the first echo of a double echo sequence while cyst contents decrease in signal. Focal tumor containing regions of T2 prolongation that are not cystic may be on T1WI, but the presence of cord enlargement favors neoplasm. Unfortunately, foci of T2 signal hyperintensity at margins of large non-neoplastic cysts may occur secondary to reactive gliosis, myelomalacia, or edema (Fig. 17–4).[25, 26] Cysts that are poorly marginated and whose signals poorly match normal CSF likely are neoplastic.[27] Gd-DTPA–enhanced spinal MR may prove useful in such cases.[28–30]

Two types of cysts associated with neoplasm are recognized. The first is truly intratumoral and is surrounded by solid neoplasm. These cysts may appear only as ill-defined inhomogeneous regions of diminished signal within the tumor mass on T1WI. Poor tissue contrast between this intratumoral cyst and tumor or cord may occur owing to protein elevation and byproducts of prior hemorrhage, shortening its T1 relaxation. Others have reported varied T1 and T2 relaxations (hyper-, iso- or hypointense) of these cysts for similar reasons.[31] The sec-

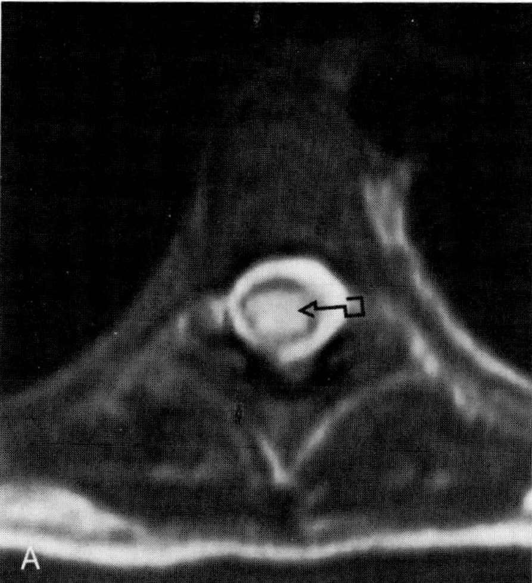

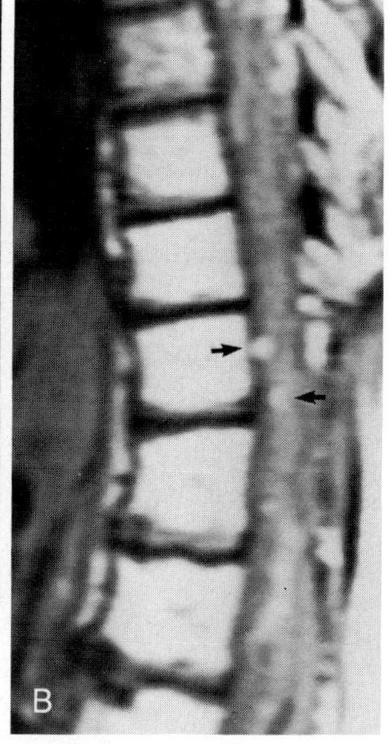

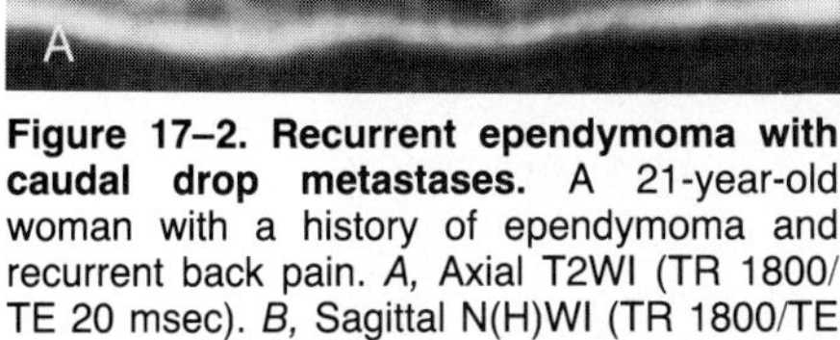

**Figure 17–2. Recurrent ependymoma with caudal drop metastases.** A 21-year-old woman with a history of ependymoma and recurrent back pain. *A,* Axial T2WI (TR 1800/TE 20 msec). *B,* Sagittal N(H)WI (TR 1800/TE 20 msec). Axial T2WI at the mid-thoracic level demonstrates cord enlargement and intramedullary cord hyperintensity compatible with intramedullary tumor recurrence (arrow). Sagittal N(H)WI depicts rounded drop metastases (arrows) in the thoracolumbar region.

ond type, caudal or rostral cysts, occurs along the superior or inferior solid tumor margins, is not truly tumorous histologically, and is well defined on MR (long T1/T2).[32] The CFVS sign is more likely to occur in this cyst subtype, in large cavities without septations and in communicating syringomyelia. It is important to recognize the two neoplastic cyst types because the solid tumor and intratumoral cysts must be removed but marginal cysts may only require decompression, a cord-sparing procedure. It is

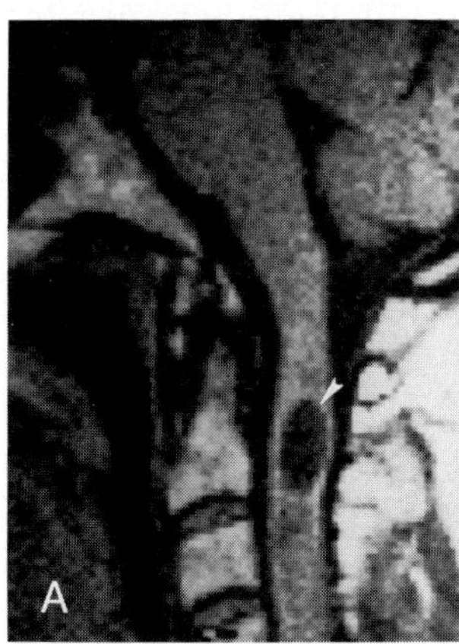

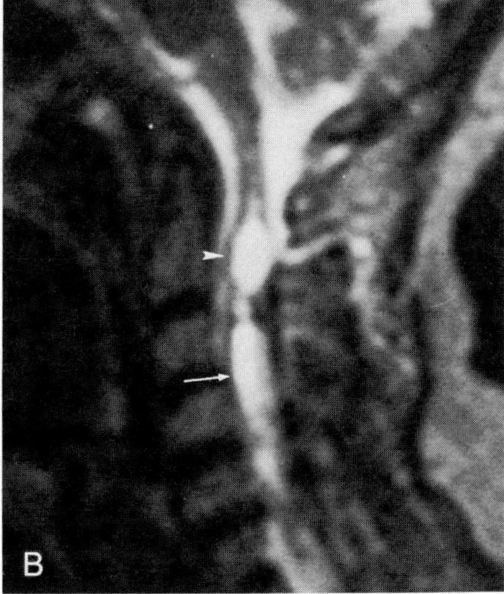

**Figure 17–3. Astrocytoma with marginal cyst.** *A,* Sagittal (0.35T) T1WI (TR 300/TE 35 msec). Hypointense cyst (arrowhead) identified in cord. *B,* Sagittal T2WI (TR 1500/TE 200) echo pulse train (only fourth echo shown). Hyperintense cyst is identified (arrowhead). Hyperintense intramedullary signal below (arrow) is not cystic on T1WI and represents a solid neoplasm. (Courtesy of J. Tobias, M.D., Radiology Department, Mount Sinai Hospital, Miami Beach, Fla.)

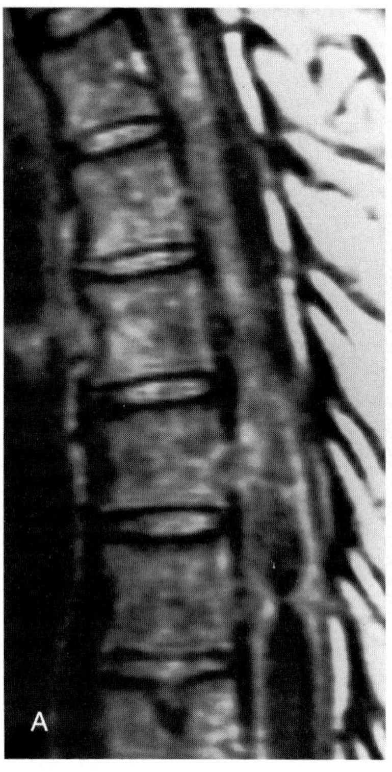


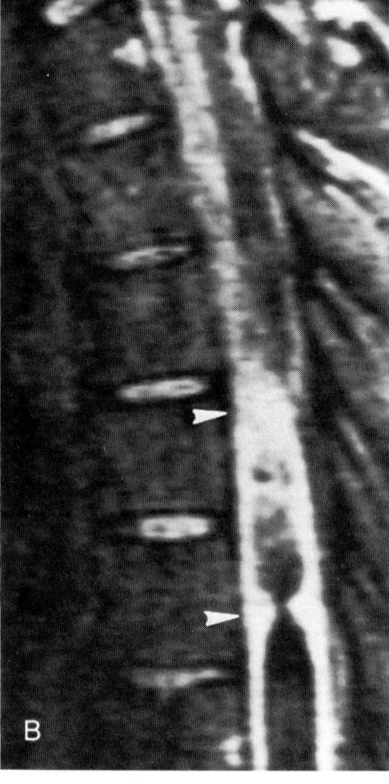


**Figure 17–4. Syringohydromyelia with gliosis.** A 32-year-old man with weakness and abnormal gait (1.5 T). 20 *A* and *B*, Sagittal multiecho N(H)WI and T2WI (TR 1800/TE/80 msec). Syringohydromyelia involves the lower thoracic cord and is hypointense owing to flow-void of pulsatile CSF. Focal nodularity and masslike hyperintensity of cord at two levels (arrowheads) suggests tumor, but none was found.

also important to recognize cyst septation since multiple syringotomies may be required.[33]

The differential diagnosis of cord syrinx includes trauma, radiation, and intra-axial neoplasm. A small syrinx may rarely occur at the margins of intradural extramedullary masses.[34] Hematomyelia often yields short T1/long T2 intramedullary signal[35, 36] or acutely (see Fig. 19–1), at high field strengths, short T2 relaxation.[35, 36] Myelitis often precedes the development of radiation-induced cord cyst and a clinical history of radiation exposure is often present.

### Hemangioblastoma

Hemangioblastoma accounts for 2% of all cord tumors. Most occur in the dorsal portion of the cord; 60% of these are intramedullary and 40%, extramedullary and intradural.[37] These neoplasms are manifested in the fourth decade, and one third of patients have von Hippel-Lindau disease. A thoracic location occurs in 50% and cervical distribution in 40%. Lesions are single in 80%, and 40% are associated with syrinx or cord cyst.

MR findings in cord hemangioblastoma have been described. The diagnosis is suggested by an intramedullary mass with foci of T1 and T2 relaxation prolongation (cord cyst, 40%), focal hyperintense or intermediate signal nodule on T2WI, and minimal cord edema (Fig. 17–5). Nidus localization, either intramedullary or intradural, is possible with MR.[38] Linear foci of signal void on T1 and T2WI due to flow in dilated feeding vessels may be present. Depiction of all these findings may require both axial and sagittal T2WI.[39]

## INTRADURAL EXTRAMEDULLARY NEOPLASMS

### Neurinoma

Neurinomas are one of the most common spinal neoplasms (25%–30%) and account for 25% to 30% of extramedullary intradural lesions. Radiculopathy rather than myelopathy is the usual clinical presentation. Lesions are usually single, occurring in the second through fourth decades with a slight lumbar predilection.[40] Neurinomas are not

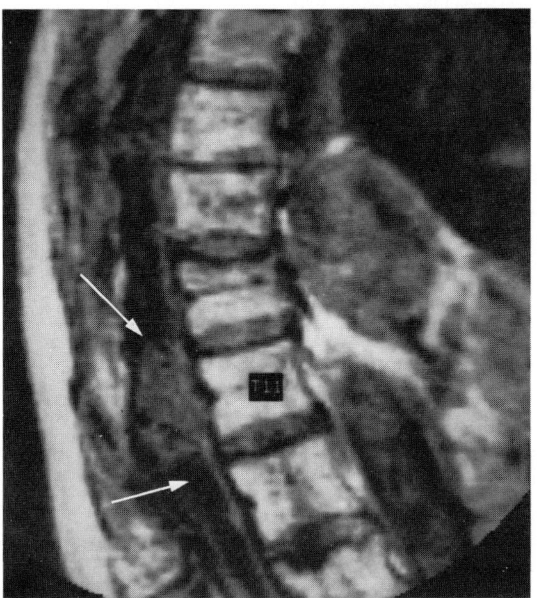


**Figure 17–5. Hemangioblastoma and cord syrinx.** Sagittal (0.5 T) T1WI (TR 800/TE 30 msec). Solid intramedullary nodular (long arrow) marginated cranially and caudally (arrow) by hypointense cord cyst. (Courtesy of R. Lukin, M.D., Wellington Diagnostics, Cincinnati, Ohio.)

sessile, more often involve posterior roots, and are positioned in the anterolateral portion of the spinal canal. Calcification is rare. Intradural location (67%) is most common, followed by dumbell-shaped intradural/extradural (17%), and extradural (17%) sites. Intramedullary lesions are rare and may arise from small perforating arterial vessels. Intraosseus neurinomas are quite rare.

Moderate or increased T1 and increased T2 relaxation is typical of the neurinoma (70%). Since lesions are firm and well-encapsulated, they are frequently round or ovoid and displace adjacent thecal sac or cord. Adjacent skeletal medullary signal abnormality is unusual. Widening or extension into the neural foramina is typical. Thin (3- or 5-mm) section T2 multiecho sagittal and axial images are often required to demonstrate the ipsilateral arachnoid space expansion with contralateral cord displacement so characteristic of intradural abnormalities.

Differentiation of neurinoma from other spinal masses is often possible. Neurofibromas located outside the craniospinal axis are slightly hyperintense relative to muscle on T1WI but have signal intensity (hypointense T1/hyperintense T2) similar to neurinomas in the spine. Neurofibromas are more often multiple, may be less well defined (plexiform neurofibroma), and are always associated with neurofibromatosis. In addition central stellate foci of signal hypointensity, corresponding to fibrous tissue histologically, may be present in neurofibromas. In contrast, meningiomas are sessile in contour, are more often dorsally located, and may be hypointense, isointense, or hyperintense compared with gray matter on T2WI. Arachnoid cysts, meningoceles, and dural ectasias demonstrate markedly prolonged T1 and T2 relaxations and are often isointense with adjacent thecal sac. Metastases are more frequently multifocal with adjacent vertebral foci of diminished T1 signal. Detection of bone signal abnormality owing to metastasis has been most accurate with MR as the primary imaging modality in our experience and in early reports.[41]

## Meningioma

Meningiomas arise from meningothelial arachnoidal cells in close proximity to nerve roots. Unlike cranial meningiomas, the distribution of spinal lesions does not follow arachnoid cells. Accounting for 25% of spinal tumors, a posterolateral canal location predominates in women, in whom 82% of lesions are thoracic (cervical, 17%; lumbar, 1.5% to 7%).[42, 43] An almost equal cervical (41%) and thoracic (47%) distribution is found in men. It is men in whom anterior meningiomas are more frequently located, particularly in the foramen magnum region. Rare metastatic spinal meningioma has been reported.[44]

Like their intracranial counterparts, these lesions frequently affect women (4:1) and may present with long tract signs as opposed to radiculopathy produced by neural tumors. Most meningiomas are intradurally positioned; however, combined intradural/extradural (7%) and rare extradural meningiomas do occur.[45] Multiplicity occurs in 1% to 2% and suggests underlying neurofibromatosis. Histologic classification may be simplified into two basic types, meningothelial and fibroblastic, with an overlap of these two, the mixed variety. No prognostic significance is assigned to any of these histologic subtypes.[46]

MR diagnosis of meningioma is suggested by a sessile or broad-based thoracic or a cervical intradural mass (Fig. 17–6) that often lies in the posterolateral spinal canal. Lesion isointensity or subtle hyperintensity on T2WI relative to gray matter was most common in our series of over 35 craniospinal meningiomas. Less than 20% of meningiomas exhibited absolute hypointense signal on T2WI relative to cord gray matter. Over 90% of lesions are hypointense or isointense on T1WI. Signal inhomogeneity in adjacent medullary bone (hypointense T1/isointense or hyperintense T2) may be reactive and is rarely related to actual tumoral involvement.[47, 48] Calcification is present in one third of patients. Meningiomas are firm; therefore deformation of adjacent structures is common and lesion pliability is unusual. As a variant of the "en plaque" meningioma, a circumferential mass surrounding the spinal cord often affecting the cervical region may exhibit isointensity with neural parenchyma on multiple pulsing sequences (Fig. 17–7). Neural tumors, unlike meningiomas, are rounded in shape and more anteriorly located. They are not broad-based; they exhibit T2 prolongation and may be "dumbell-shaped," extending into neural foramina. "Dumbell-shaped" meningioma is rare.

## Neurofibromatosis

Many intrinsic spinal cord lesions are associated with neurofibromatosis, including ependymoma, astrocytoma, syringomyelia, hamartoma, and central neurinoma. Like neurinomas, neurofibromas arise from Schwann's cells and are most often extramedullary in location. Unlike neurinomas, they contain fibroblasts and nerve cells, and all patients have neurofibromatosis. Familial dominant genetic transmission occurs in 50% of patients, and 50% of neurofibromatosis cases arise by spontaneous mutation. Peripheral neurofibromas occur in 59% of patients with this condition, whereas bony spinal dysplasia is less frequent (47%). Neurinomas do not undergo malignant degeneration, but 4% to 11% of neurofibromas do so.[49] Of patients with malignant nerve sheath tumors, 40% have neurofibromatosis. Patients with neurofibromatosis and neurofibrosarcoma are more often female, whereas no sex predominance occurs in solitary malignant neurofibrosarcoma. Malignancies associated with neurofibromatosis are more centrally located and aggressive, with frequent local recurrences. After local recurrences, 75% metastasize, usually to the

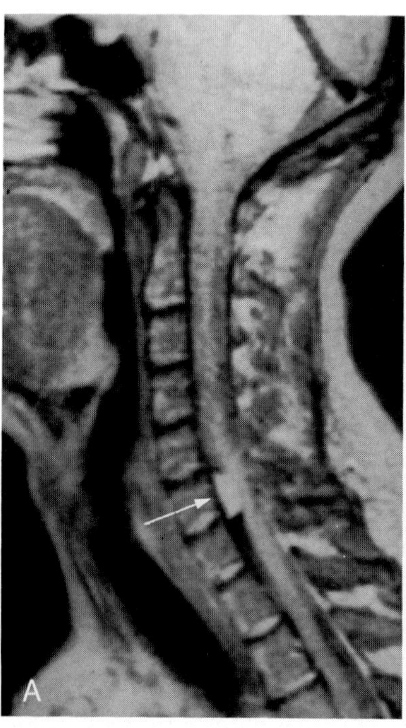


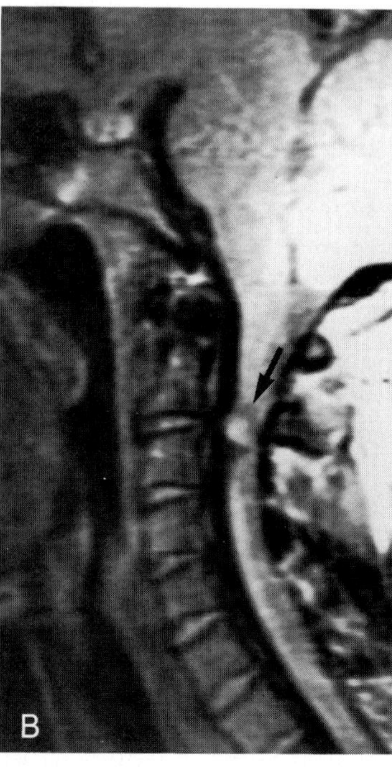


**Figure 17–6. *A,* Meningioma; *B,* neurinoma.** Two different patients with two different diagnoses exhibit similar lesions. *A,* Sagittal N(H)WI (TR 2000/TE 25 msec). *B,* Sagittal N(H)WI (TR 2000/TE 25 msec). Patient *A* demonstrates a slightly hyperintense mass with a broad, anterior, dural-based margin (arrow) that displaces the cord posteriorly and widens the hypointense subarachnoid space below. Patient *B* demonstrates a mass that assumes a more rounded contour (black arrow) as would be expected with neurinoma. (*A,* Courtesy of A. Chambers, M.D., Neuroradiology Department, University Hospital, Cincinnati, Ohio. *B,* Courtesy of S. Weinberg, M.D., Medi-Center North, Bethesda North Hospital; Cincinnati, Ohio.)

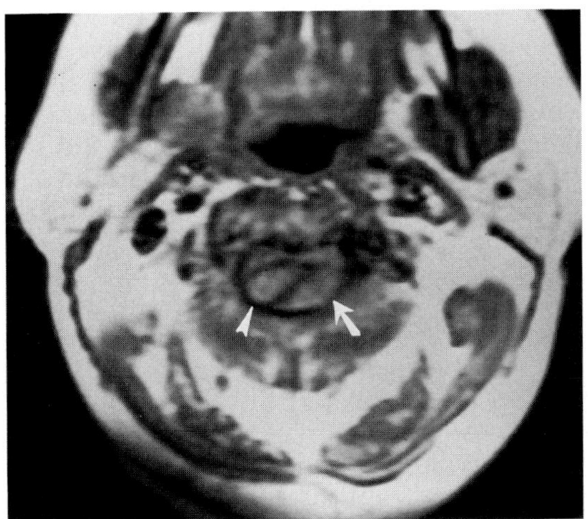

**Figure 17–7. Infiltrative foramen magnum meningioma.** A 59-year-old man with progressive myelopathy (1.5 T). Axial T1WI (TR 600/TE 20 msec). An infiltrative mass (arrow) surrounds and compresses the thecal sac into a teardrop shape (arrowhead).

**Figure 17–8. Neurofibroma.** A 25-year-old woman with neurofibromatosis and radiculopathy (1.5 T). Axial T1WI (TR 700/TE 20 msec). Mass (arrow) expands the right neural foramen. On T1WI, signal is similar to cord, not hypointense as in meningocele CSF. (Courtesy of T. Seward, Medi-Center North, Cincinnati, Ohio.)

lungs. Malignant nerve sheath tumors may occur at sites of prior irradiation with a 14-year median time to manifestation.[50]

Signal intensities of neurofibroma and neurinoma in the central skeleton are similar (long T1/T2) (Figs. 17–8 and 17–9).[51] Lesion multiplicity and history assist in differentiation. Neurofibromas are often sausage shaped and have slightly higher signal intensity than skeletal muscle on T1WI. This is due to relative T1 shortening produced by large mucopolysaccharide molecules of myxoid tissue interacting with tissue water. Increased T2WI signal with central foci of hypointensity corresponding to fibrous tissue in neurofibromas may assist in differ-

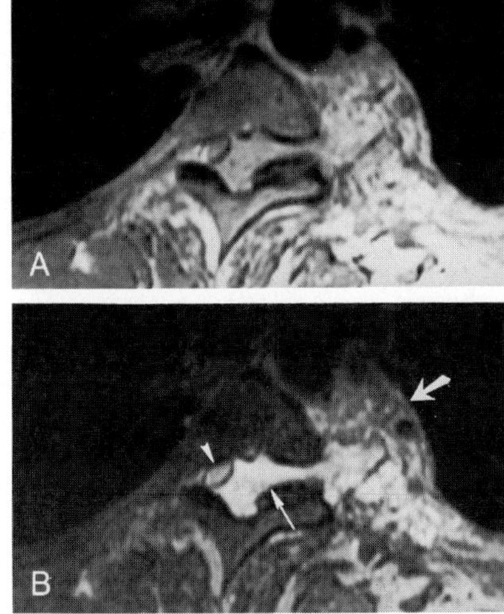


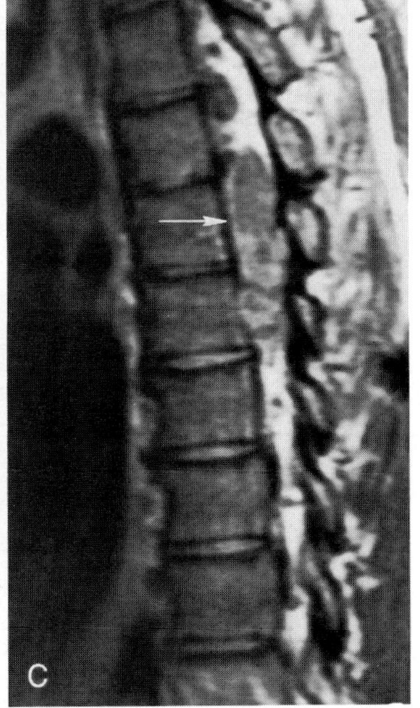


**Figure 17–9. Plexiform neurofibromatosis.** A 26-year-old man with kyphoscoliosis and lower extremity weakness (1.5 T). *A* and *B,* Axial multiecho N(H)WI and T2WI (TR 1800/TE 20/80 msec). Irregular paraspinal mass (arrow) invading spinal canal (thin arrow) and compressing spinal cord (arrowhead). *C,* Sagittal T1WI (TR 600/TE 20 msec) shows craniocaudad extent of mass (arrow) in the lateral recess.

entiation from the homogeneous signal of meningocele.[52] The T1WI signal of meningocele is less than that of skeletal muscle. It is of interest that dense acellular collagenous lesions such as aggressive fibromatosis produce T1WI and T2WI signal hypointensity.[53]

Malignant neurofibrosarcoma may produce heterogeneous T2WI signal corresponding to pathologic necrosis, unlike the more uniform or target-like appearance of benign lesions.[54] Since excessive radiation does produce risk of malignancy, MR is an ideal method of serial evaluation. The signal intensity of lateral or anterior meningocele (homogeneous and isointense with adjacent thecal sac/long T1 and T2) permits differentiation from neural tumor. Associated conditions and anomalies of neurofibromatosis, kyphoscoliosis, spinal dysplasia and neoplasms of the craniospinal axis (cranial neuroma; meningioma; optic pathway dysplasia; choroid plexus hamartoma/glioma) are easily assessed with MR.[55–57]

## CONGENITAL SPINAL NEOPLASMS

Lipomas account for 1% of spinal tumors. Some report them to be the most common filum terminale neoplasm.[58] They are usually associated with dysraphic states and are rarely isolated. Lumbosacral dysraphism usually occurs in patients who present in the first decade. Patients of any age may exhibit cutaneous hemangioma, dermal sinus, hair tuft, cafe-au-lait spot, or subcutaneous lipoma. As isolated phenomena, these lesions are usually thoracic (40%), cervico-thoracic (30%), or cervical (15%) in location. Approximately 60% of isolated lesions are intradural, whereas 40% are extradural. Intradural lesions may appear intramedullary owing to their inward growth.[59] Lipomas exhibit short T1 relaxation[60, 61] and match subcutaneous fat in signal intensity on multiple pulsing sequences (Fig. 17–10).[60, 61] They are usually dorsally located. Cord tethering and other associated anomalies are discussed in Chapter 6.

Spinal teratomas occur in the first decade of life and are usually midline in the cervical or thoracolumbar region. One half are associated with spinal anomalies. True teratomas have three histologic germ (trigerminal) layers while those with two layers (bigerminal) may be referred to as "teratoid" lesions. Smoker and co-workers reported that most teratomas are extradural, however 20 intradural lesions and 3 intramedullary lesions have also been identified.[62] These authors illustrated a teratoma with layering cystic (long T2) and solid (short T2) components. A pathologically proven spinal teratoma exhibited the following characteristics on MR: (1) a tumor head or nidus (intermediate T1/long T2) surrounded by fat (short T1/T2 and (2) a body composed of keratin (mild T1 hyperintensity relative to CSF/isointense on T2 relative to CSF).[63]

Intraspinal epidermoid cysts are rare, and 40% are iatrogenically produced.[64, 65] These lesions are posterior and are closely adherent to arachnoid and nerve roots. Inhomogenous and serpiginous T1 and T2 signal prolongation is typical. In our series of cranial epidermoids and in those proved in the literature, only one lesion was hyperintense on T1WI, despite the presence of cholesterin in all lesions.[66, 67] Diffuse hyperintensity on T1WI should suggest other diagnoses (dermoid, lipoma, hemorrhage).

## EXTRADURAL NEOPLASMS

### Metastases

Extradural neoplasms are usually due to metastatic disease or lymphoma. Excluding dysraphic states, ependymoma of the external filum, isolated lipomas, and rare extradural neurinomas or meningiomas account for the remaining epidural tumors. Lung, breast, renal, thyroid, and prostate primaries are the most frequent.[68, 69] The thoracic spine is most often affected, particularly T4 and T11. Vertebral body collapse is often present but is less frequent in osteoblastic metastases.[70] Direct vertebral invasion and cord compression may occur in oat cell carcinoma.

Approximately 5% of metastases produce cord compression. A gradual clinical syndrome or an abrupt one resulting from superimposed ischemia may occur. Patients present with local or radicular pain, bilateral when thoracic and unilateral when cervical or lumbar. Weakness is the second most frequent symptom complex. Paraplegia of more than 12 hours has a poor prognosis, and only 20% of patients recover motor

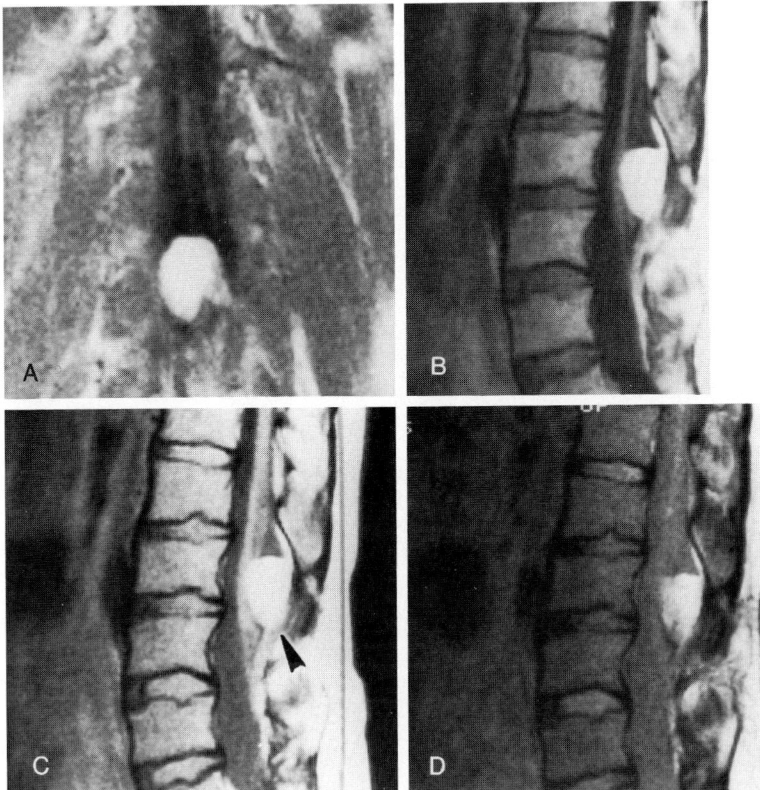


**Figure 17–10. Lipoma with cord tethering.** Patient with gait disturbance; MR was performed at 0.35 T. *A,* Coronal T1WI (IR TI 400/TR 2100/TE 35). *B,* Sagittal T1WI (TR 500/TE 30). *C,* N(H)WI (TR 1700/ TE 35). *D,* T2WI (TR 1700/TE 70). A mass with hyperintense signal on T1WI (arrowhead) is dorsally located behind the conus. The signal matches subcutaneous fat in intensity; therefore hemorrhage is excluded. Signal hypointensity relative to CSF would occur more heavily on T2WI. Conventional radiographs would eliminate the possibility of residual Pantopaque as the cause of this signal abnormality. (Courtesy of J. Tobias, M.D., Radiology Department, Mount Sinai Hospital, Miami Beach, Fla.)

function after treatment for complete neoplastic thoracolumbar block.

Direct intradural metastases do occur with melanoma and occasionally with lung, breast, or lymphomatous tumors, but most are a result of direct seeding ("drop metastases") from various cerebral neoplasms.[71] Most drop metastases result from medulloblastoma, ependymoblastoma, pineal germinoma, and less commonly from high-grade astrocytomas, mature ependymomas, malignant choroid plexus papillomas and angioblastic meningiomas.[72, 73] These are nodular or sheetlike in configuration and are dorsally located; occasionally, they may aggregate about the distal dural sac, producing an "amputated sac" appearance.

Intramedullary (intra-axial) metastases are most often from lung (small cell and non–small cell) or breast carcinoma.[74–76] Melanoma and lymphoma metastasize to the spinal cord with greater regularity than to the epidural space.[77] Intramedullary metastases resulting from direct extension of posterior fossa neoplasms such as medulloblastoma do occur.[78] Although some authors suggest that cord edema is indistinguishable from intramedullary metastasis, we have not found this to be true in a majority of cases.[79] Focal rather than gradual cord enlargement, increased cord signal, and central intermediate signal intensity suggest cord metastasis (Fig. 17–11). Any focal cord contour and T2WI signal increase should be considered metastatic in patients with known neoplasm elsewhere. Small intramedullary lesions may be missed with T1WI only and are best detected with T2WI. Detection on MR of intramedullary metastases, despite negative CT, scintigraphy, and myelography does occur.[80]

MR is the modality of choice in evaluating possible metastatic spine disease in the following instances: abnormal nuclear scintigraphy and normal or equivocal conventional radiograph, myelopathy or suspected complete block, compression fracture of unknown etiology, patients with known cancer and new back pain, neurologic deficit and normal CT or myelography, and differentiation of radiation sclerosis (short T1 relaxation) versus sclerotic metastases (long T1 relaxation) (Fig. 17–12).[81, 82] The shortened T1 relaxation following radiation exposure

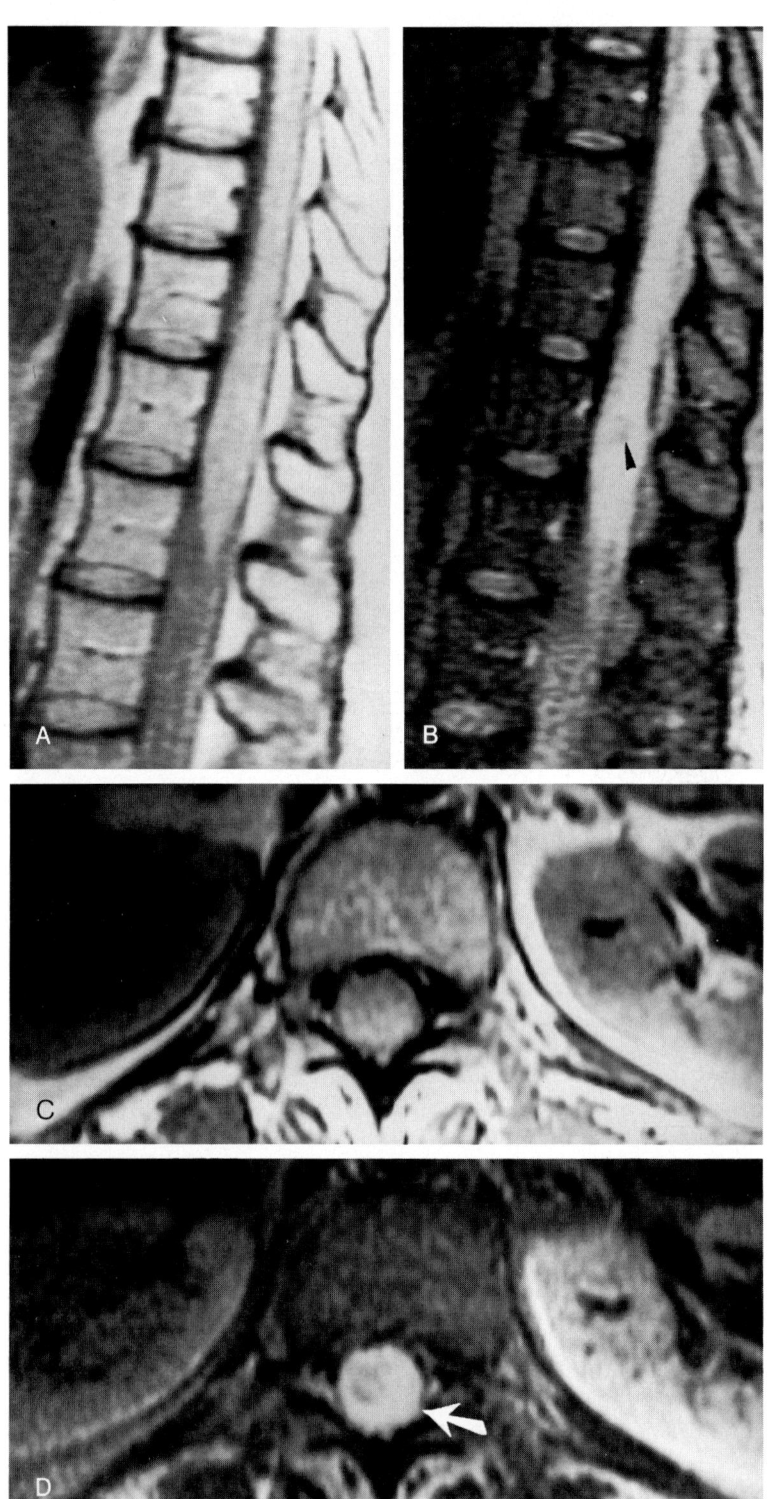


**Figure 17–11. Conus metastasis and conus edema.** A 36-year-old woman with breast carcinoma and progressive paraparesis (1.5 T). *A* and *B,* Sagittal multiecho N(H)WI and T2WI (TR 1800/TE 20/80 msec). The conus is enlarged and hyperintense on T2WI. It contains an intermediate signal intensity nodule (arrowhead). *C* and *D,* Axial N(H)WI and T2WI show the conus hyperintense on T2WI (arrow), filling spinal canal. Intermediate signal metastasis is again apparent.

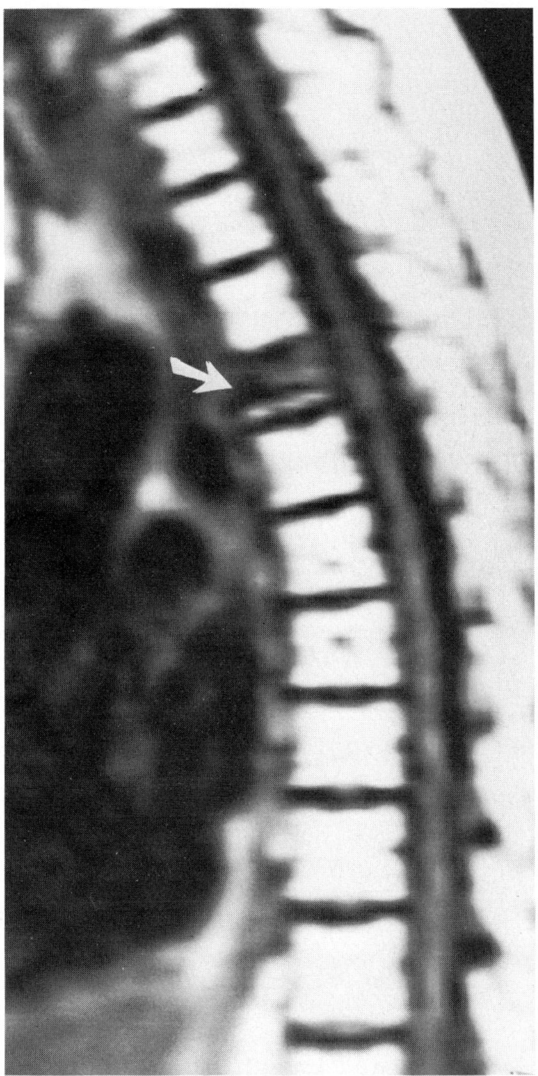

**Figure 17–12. Thoracic vertebral metastasis.** A 46-year-old woman with lung carcinoma, back pain, and positive bone scintigraphy (1.5 T). Sagittal T1WI shows homogeneous vertebral hypointensity (arrow).

results from an increased marrow ratio of yellow to red (Fig. 17–13).

Metastases appear as rounded foci of well-demarcated signal hypointensity (long T1) relative to hyperintense vertebral fatty marrow on T1WI (Fig. 17–14). Care should be taken not to confuse tumor with Schmorl's node formation, degenerative vertebral end-plate sclerosis (Fig. 17–15), and fibrotic changes related to the "aged" spine. Schmorl's nodes are hypointense relative to marrow but are contiguous and isointense with disk. Unlike metastases, they have obtuse margins compatible with their extravertebral origin. Degenerative sclerosis or end-plate bone infarction often has linear margins, may be extensive, but abuts the end-plate. The vertebrae may demonstrate spurring or vertebral body collapse. Linear foci of hyperintensity or hypointensity on T1 or T2 images may occur. Hypointensity on T1WI and hyperintense juxta–end-plate T2WI signal may occur in active degenerative disk disease. Focal areas of hyperintense T1 signal may be produced by normal focal fat deposition (Fig. 17–16). The prevalence of this finding increases with age at sites of osseous stress and in patients with degenerative disease.[83] Rounded or angled shape, lesion multiplicity, acute sharp margins, and soft tissue or extradural mass (Fig. 17–17) support a neoplastic rather than degenerative cause of signal alteration. If these signal alterations are absent in the collapsed vertebra of an oncology patient, a non-neoplastic etiology is likely (Fig. 17–18).

Lesion contrast depends upon T1 relaxation of vertebral marrow. Young patients have more hematopoietic vertebral marrow that exhibits longer T1 relaxation than adipose marrow. Therefore it appears more hypointense on T1WI, like tumor signal intensity. Elderly patients exhibit fibrosis, sclerosis, and yellow marrow involution, also producing the same effect on T1WI.[84] Lesions may appear less conspicuous in these patients. Pathologic studies have shown that hyperplastic marrow as in thalassemia increases and hypoplastic marrow decreases T1 relaxation.[85, 86] Diffusely diminished T1 vertebral signal may be seen with osteopetrosis, extensive sclerotic prostate metastases (Fig. 17–19), or myeloma.[87] Therefore knowledge of normal age-related signal variations is essential.

The T2 appearance of metastases is variable, but lesion isointensity or hyperintensity (80%) is often demonstrated relative to normal skeletal signal (Fig. 17–20). Lesion isointensity or "hiding" may occur with spin density (N[H]WI), or rarely with T2WI.[88] Occasionally, foci of increased T2 may surround a central hypointense region in early sclerotic metastases, whereas advanced sclerotic tumor may exhibit hypointensity on both T1 and T2 images.[89] T2WI are useful in assessing cord or sac compromise, since block is likely present when the hyperintense signal of intradural circumferential

*Text continued on page 530*

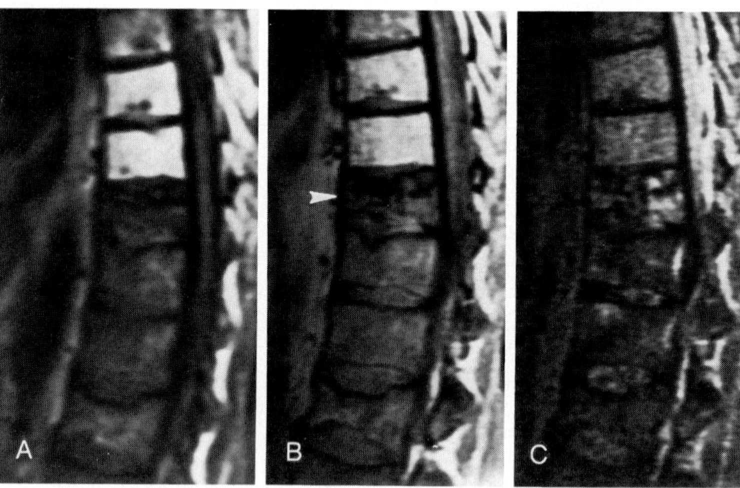


**Figure 17–13. Radiation change; metastasis, solitary.** A 72-year-old woman with breast carcinoma and back pain. *A* and *B,* Sagittal T1WI (TR 600/TE 20) and N(H)WI (TR 2000/TE 20 msec). Vertebral body labeled (arrowhead) contains proven tumor not appreciated on these sequences. Levels above are hyperintense owing to prior irradiation and levels below are hypointense owing to fatty marrow degeneration. *C,* Sagittal T2WI depicts tumor signal hyperintensity in the posterior aspect of the vertebra labeled in *B*. When fatty marrow becomes more fibrous or hypointense, metastases are more easily detected on T2WI instead of T1WI. Lesions in medullary bone are commonly "hidden" on N(H)WI.

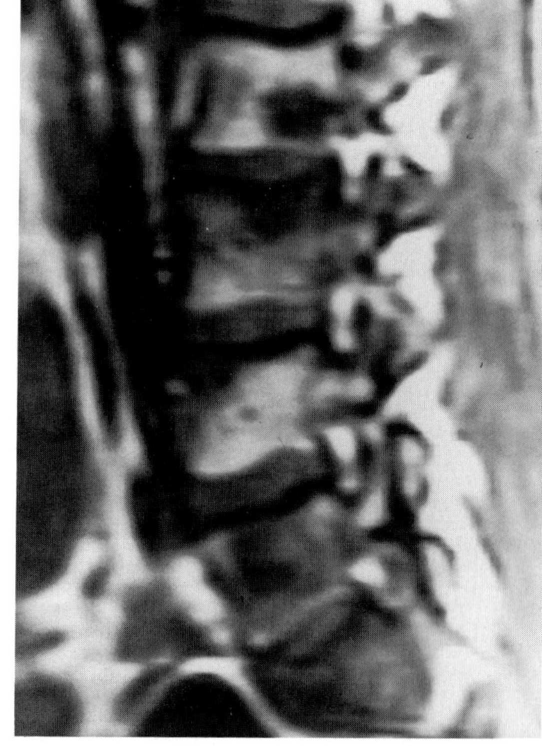

**Figure 17–14. Multifocal vertebral metastases (prostate).** A 49-year-old man presents with low back pain (1.5 T). Sagittal T1WI shows signal hypointensity rounded at L2, oblique in shape at L4, and irregular but diffuse at L3/L5.

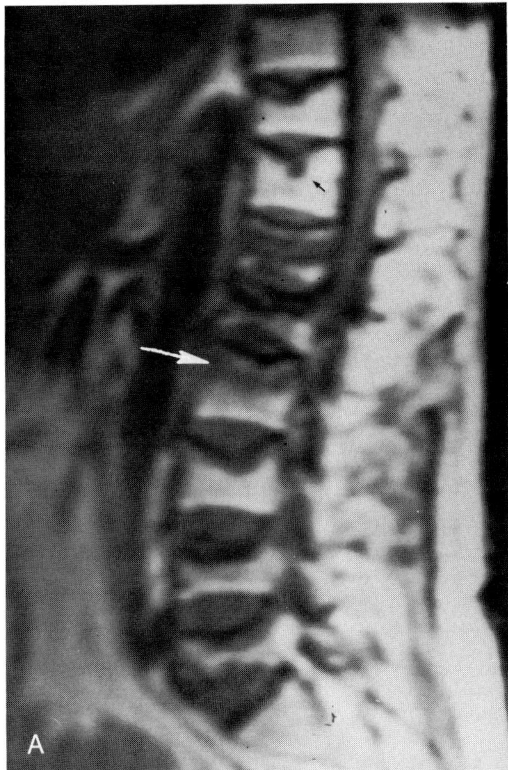

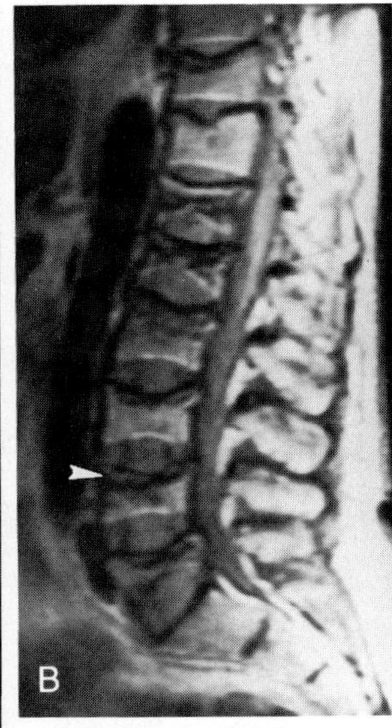

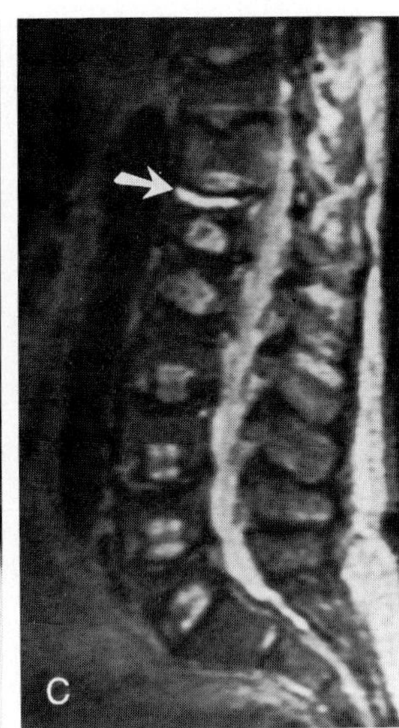

**Figure 17–15. Nonpathologic compression fractures (linear pattern).** A 37-year-old woman with breast carcinoma and back pain (1.5 T). *A,* Sagittal T1WI. Linear pattern of hypointensity (arrow) observed in nonpathologic compression fractures due to end-plate edema, sclerosis, or both. Note hypointense Schmorl's node at T11 superior endplate (black arrow). *B* and *C,* Sagittal N(H)WI and T2WI shows end-plate linear signal interface (arrow and arrowhead) due to hemorrhage resulting from recent compression.

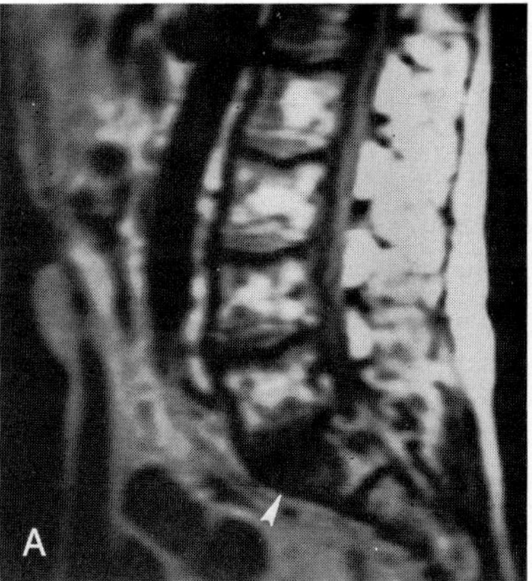

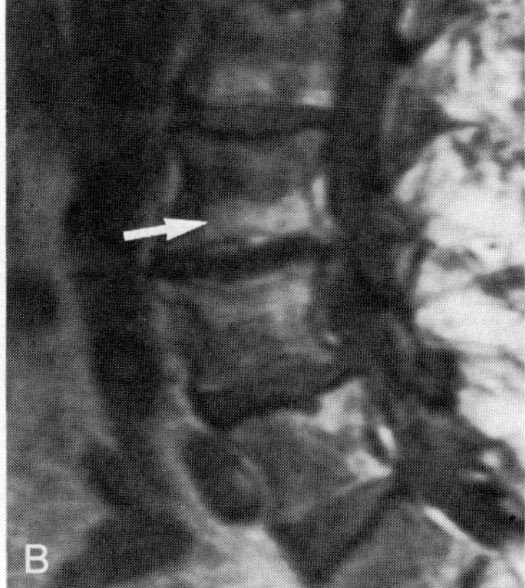

**Figure 17–16. Two middle-aged men with known primary neoplasms and back pain (1.5 T).** *A,* Sagittal T1WI (TR 600/TE 20 msec). Central signal hyperintensity at each vertebral body level represents an unusual pattern of normal axial skeletal white marrow distribution and should not be misconstrued as tumor. Hypointense sacral metastasis is present (arrowhead). *B,* Sagittal T1WI demonstrates a juxta–end-plate pattern of hyperintense marrow signal (arrow) alternating with marrow hypointensity in degenerative disease of the spine. Pattern recognition helps avert misdiagnosis of neoplasm.

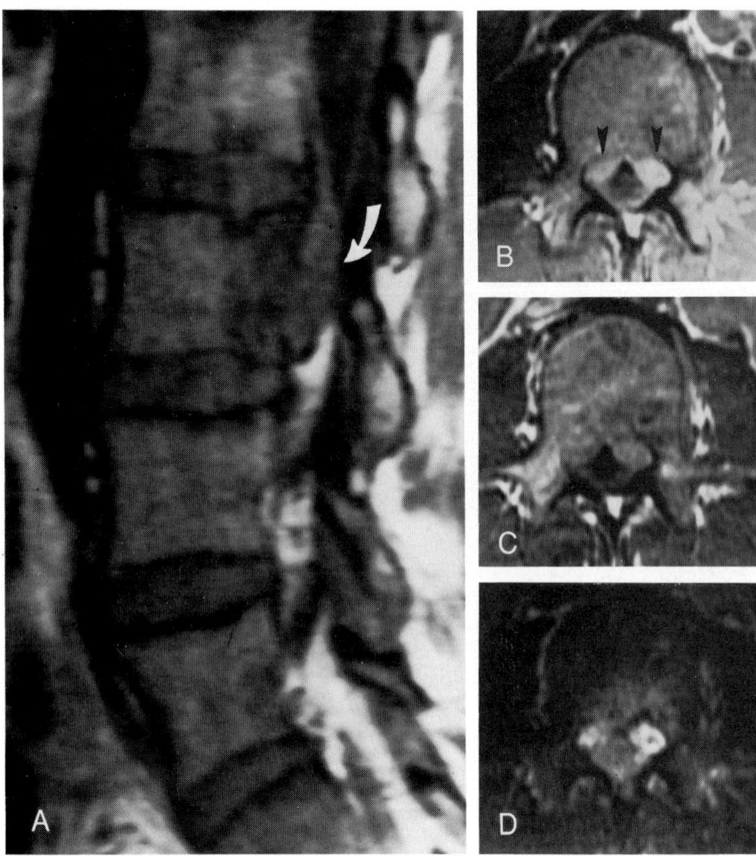


**Figure 17–17. Metastatic extradural choriocarcinoma.** A 23-year-old woman four months post partum with back pain and persistent chorionic gonadotropin (hCG) elevation (1.5 T). *A,* Sagittal T1WI (TR 600/TE 20 msec). An elliptical mass abuts the L2 vertebral body (arrow). A subtle signal hypointensity of the adjacent vertebral body suggests bone involvement. *B, C* and *D,* Axial T1WI and multiecho N(H)WI and T2WI show bilobed extradural mass (arrowheads). The thecal sac deforms the mass centrally, suggesting lesion pliability.

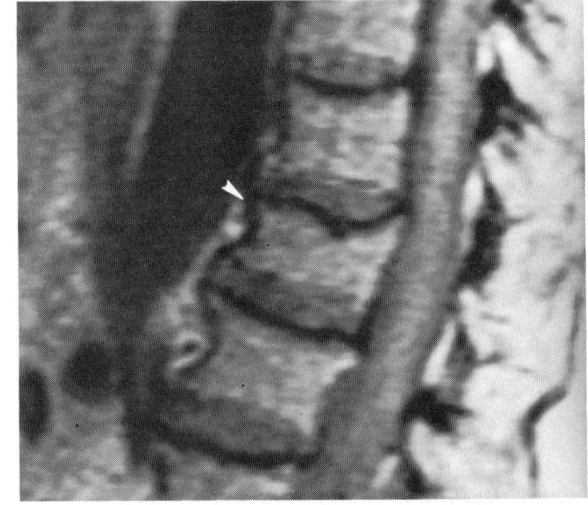

**Figure 17–18. Nonpathologic vertebral collapse (proved).** A 42-year-old woman with breast carcinoma, back pain, and positive bone scintigraphy. Sagittal T1WI shows vertebral body (arrowhead) height loss with a superior end-plate Schmorl's node. Signal matches other normal vertebrae.

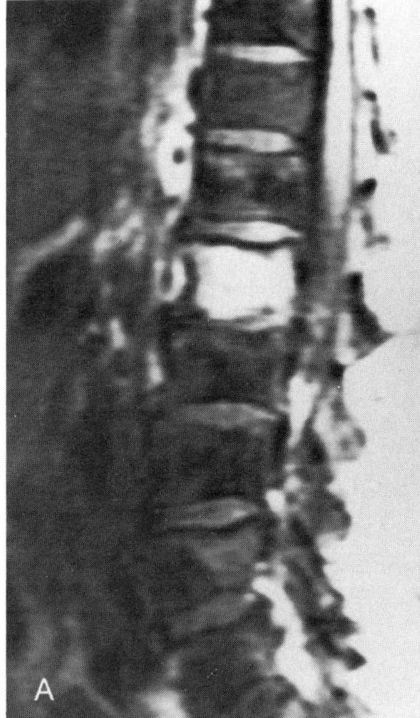


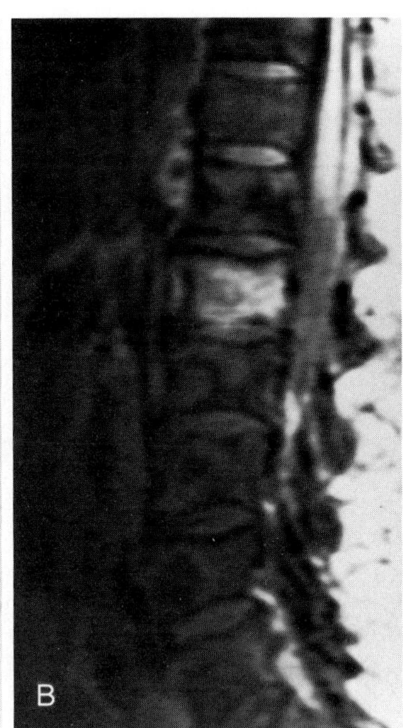


**Figure 17–19. Diffuse prostate metastases.** A 57-year-old man with prostate carcinoma (1.5 T). *A* and *B,* Sagittal T1WI (TR 600/TE 20 msec) and T2WI (TR 1800/TE 80). The solitary hyperintense vertebral body is the only one not involved by tumor. The marrow signals in the remaining hypointense vertebrae on T1WI are replaced by neoplasm.

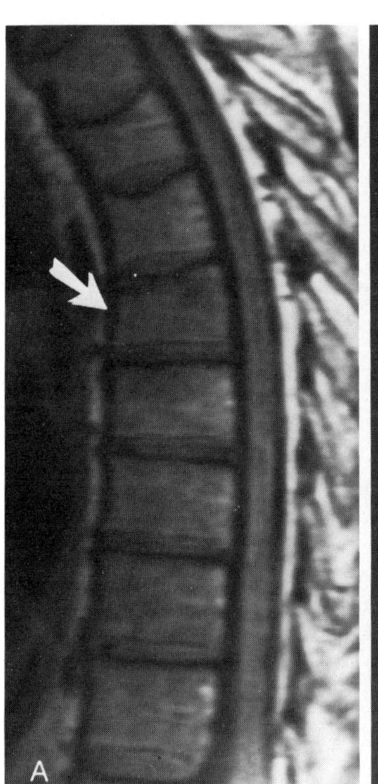


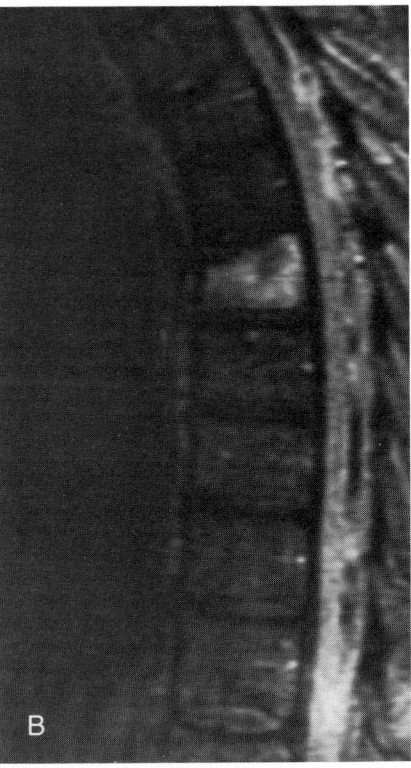


**Figure 17–20. Metastatic colon carcinoma.** A 39-year-old woman with back pain, normal conventional radiography, and abnormal bone scintigraphy (1.5 T). *A* and *B,* Sagittal multiecho N(H)WI and T2WI (TR 1800/TE 20/80 msec). As is often the case, pathology in medullary bone is "hidden" on N(H)WI (arrow) while lesion hyperintensity is present on T2WI.

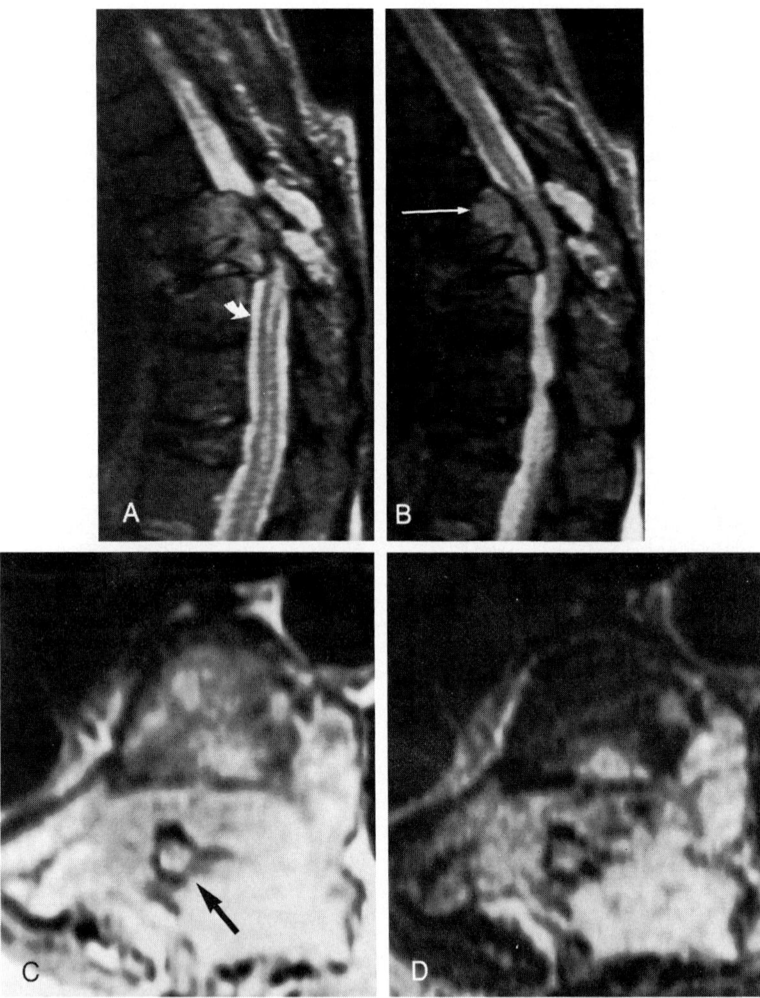


**Figure 17–21. Vertebral and extradural metastasis with MR complete block.** A 62-year-old man with lung carcinoma (1.5 T). *A* and *B*, Sagittal T2WI (TR 1800/TE 80 msec). The intermediate signal cord is displaced posteriorly by a mass (arrow). Hyperintense thecal sac CSF (curved arrow) is absent at the level of the neoplasm. *C* and *D*, Axial multiecho N(H)WI and T2WI. Cord and surrounding hypointense dura (arrow) is circumscribed by neoplasm. No hyperintense CSF is apparent at this level on T2WI. Notice the hyperintense CSF signal on sagittal T2WI obtained without flow compensation suggestive of high-grade obstruction and dampened CSF pulsations.

CSF is absent or "choked" from a given level (Fig. 17–21). Only the intermediate signal intensity of spinal cord surrounded by isointense or hyperintense solid tumor is demonstrated at the blocked level. The presence of homogeneous CSF signal hyperintensity on sagittal T2WI without the use of flow compensation techniques suggests that pulsatile CSF flow effects have been dampened and high-grade obstruction is present. We no longer perform myelography for evaluation of metastatic tumor-induced spinal block.

## Lymphoma

Approximately 0.5% to 15% of patients with lymphoma exhibit extradural spinal involvement. A bulky soft tissue mass insinuating itself into foramina, extending over multiple segments, and producing less skeletal involvement than expected for lesion size are tipoffs to the correct diagnosis (Figs. 17–22 and 17–23).[90] A similar MR appearance may occur with intraspinal extension of neuroblastoma.[91] Spinal osseous involvement occurs in 30%.[92] As in most neoplasms, T1 and T2 prolongation are present in lymphoma, with lesions hyperintense relative to cord on T2WI.[93] Extradural lesions that require differentiation from metastases and lymphoma include epidural hematoma (short T1) or abscess (long T1/T2), extradural veins (signal void), chronic scar (intermediate or short T2, history of surgery or myelography), synovial cyst (short T1/long T2 and juxta-articular location), posterior disk her-

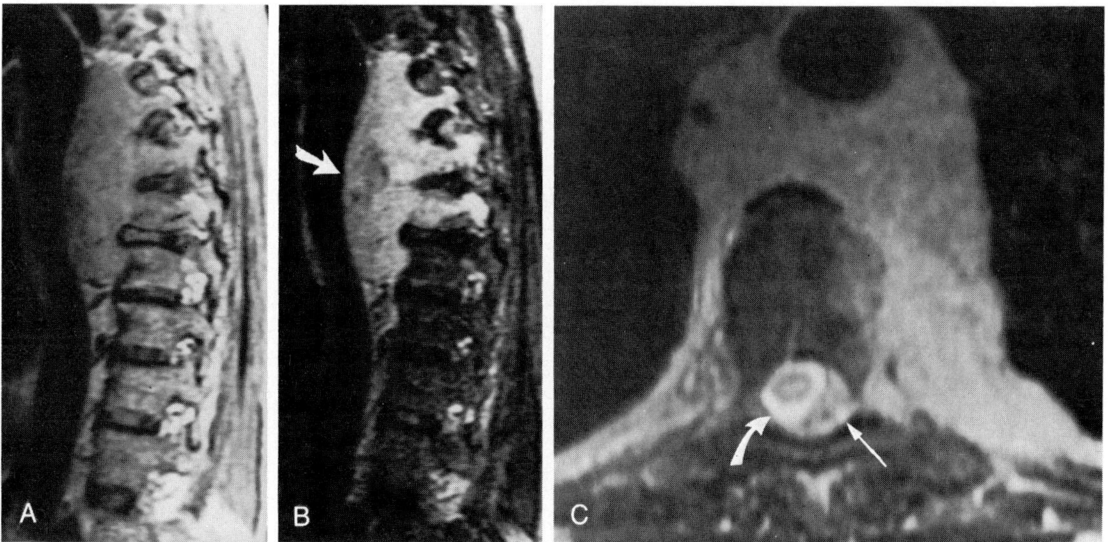

**Figure 17–22. Lymphoma.** A 37-year-old man with back pain (1.5 T). *A* and *B,* Sagittal multiecho N(H)WI and T2WI (TR 1800/TE 20/80 msec). A prespinal mass (arrow) with extension into foramina at multiple levels is seen. Relative skeletal sparing is present. *C,* Axial T2WI. The mass has grown into the spinal canal (arrow) and compresses the hyperintense thecal sac (curved arrow). A displaced intermediate signal cord is also identified.

niation, and posterior longitudinal ligament calcification (linear T2 signal hypointensity).

## PSEUDOTUMORS ON MR

The most frequently recognized pseudotumor on MR occurs at the craniocervical junction and is composed of pannus or fibrous tissue. Some have suggested that this occurrence results from chronic subluxation of C1 and C2 from any cause. The nonneoplastic etiology of these masses is suggested by their signal hypointensity on T2WI, compatible with a fibrous origin. Conventional radiographic changes of subluxation, degeneration, or arthritis, particularly

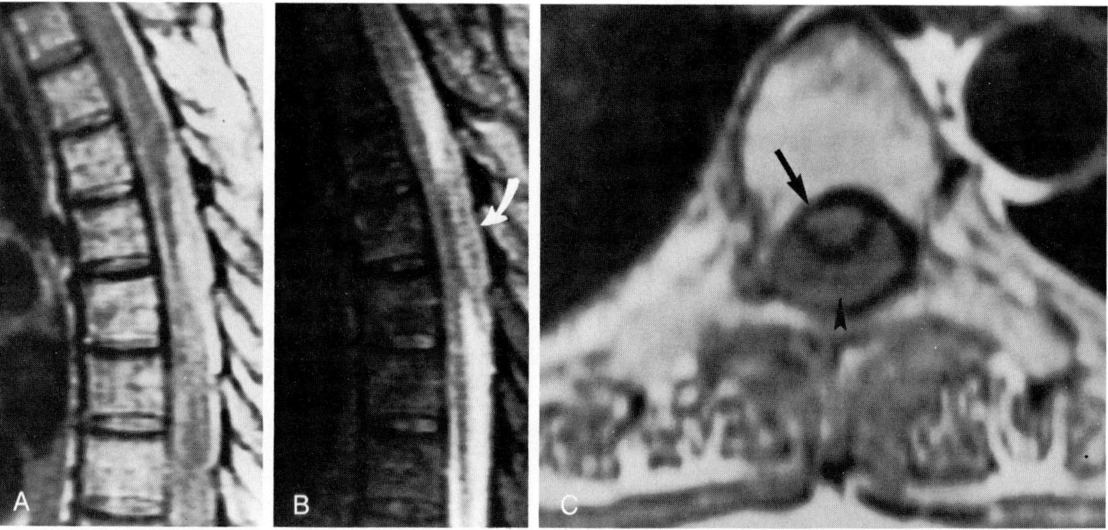

**Figure 17–23. Extradural lymphoma.** A 58-year-old woman with back pain and Lhermitte's sign (pain with neck flexion) (1.5 T). *A* and *B,* Sagittal multiecho N(H)WI and T2WI. An extradural mass (arrow) displaces the cord anteriorly and effaces the hyperintense thecal sac on T2WI. The mass is isointense with the cord on T2WI. The signal suggests meningioma, but the extradural location is atypical. *C,* Axial T1WI. The cord is displaced anteriorly (arrow) by a homogeneous mass (arrowhead).

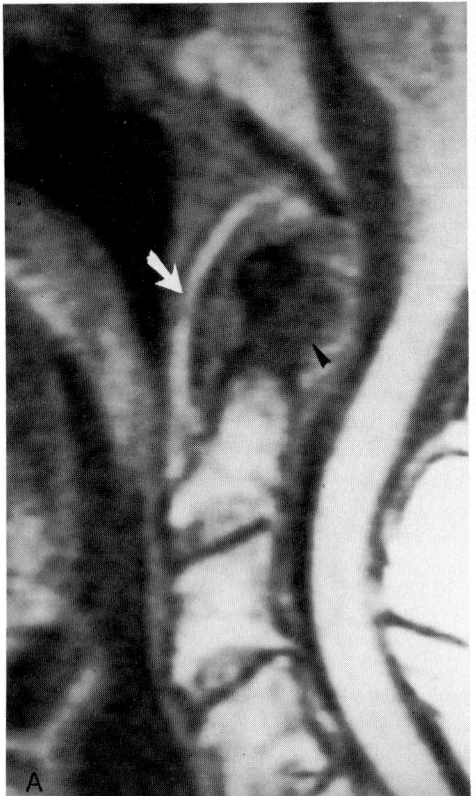


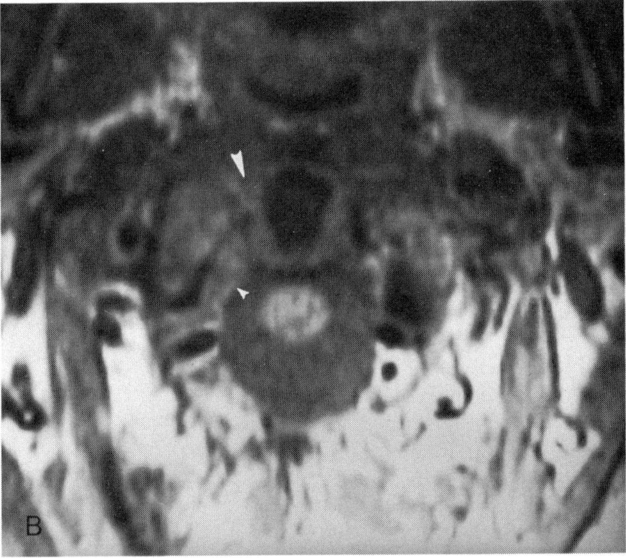


**Figure 17–24. Pseudotumor C2 with synovial proliferation.** A 47-year-old man with history of prostate carcinoma and abnormal screening bone scintigraphy at C2 (1.5 T). Sagittal and axial T1WI shows hypointensity (arrowhead) of the dens (a normal variant) and anterior displacement of preligamentous fat (arrow) by a mass. Axially, the mass circumscribes the dens in the distribution of atlantodental synovium (arrowheads).

**Figure 17–25. C1, C2 fusion and assimilation.** Sagittal (0.5T) T1WI (TR 800/ TE 30 msec). A hyperintense contour abnormality involves the dens tip and simulates a mass. (Courtesy of A. Chambers, M.D., Wellington Diagnostics, Cincinnati, Ohio.)

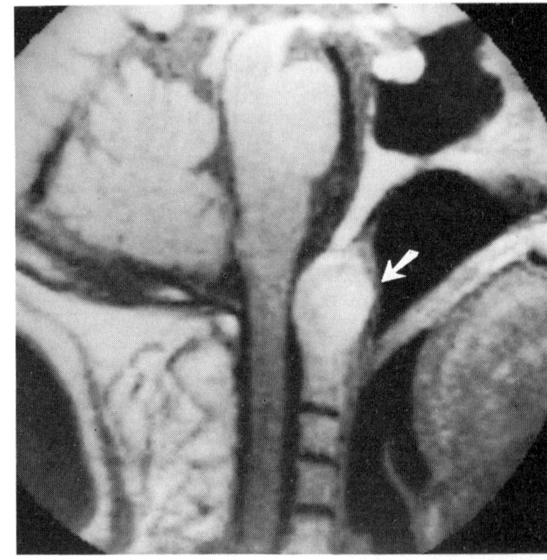

rheumatoid, add further support. Associated cervicomedullary compression and basilar invagination can be evaluated with sagittal MR with or without flexion or extension positions.[94–97] Differentiation from small chordomas (hyperintense T2) or meningiomas (iso-, hypo-, or hyperintense T2) may be difficult using signal intensity criteria alone. Attention to location is helpful. The typical pseudotumor is located between the following areas: the dens and anterior arch of C1; the dens and transverse ligament; or between the lamina, spinous processes, and facet joints (Fig. 17–24).[98] Rarely are meningiomas solely extradural, and the epicenter of cervical chordoma appears at the dens tip or clival base in many instances. Other tumorlike lesions seen on MR include the bony spur of diastatomyelia, various craniocervical fusions, spontaneous cervical hematoma, excessive epidural fat, gouty tophi, villonodular synovitis, elastofibroma, tumoral form of calcium pyrophosphate deposition disease, and os odontoideum (Fig. 17–25).[99–106]

## ARACHNOID CYSTS AND RELATED CONDITIONS

Arachnoid cysts are diverticula that connect in ball-valve fashion with the subarachnoid space through a narrow neck and account for 1% of spinal space-occupying lesions. Lesions are more often congenital than acquired and may produce complete block. They may communicate with the subarachnoid CSF (40%) and may remain intradural or may squeeze extradurally.[107] Most intradural cysts arise near the septum posticum, whereas extradural lesions are found in either the dorsal midline, at the junction of dura with dorsal root sleeve and along the root sleeve itself. Perineurial cysts are intraradicular subperineurial cysts distal to the junction of dorsal root with spinal ganglion. Unlike arachnoid cysts, they always contain nerve fibers or ganglion cells and are rarely symptomatic unless large and located in the sacrum. A meningocele is a protrusion, redundancy, or diverticulum of both dura and arachnoid.

The MR findings of spinal arachnoid cysts (and meningoceles or Tarlov's cysts) include a mass of homogeneous signal intensity, with marked T1 and T2 relaxation prolongation similar to CSF in signal intensity (Fig. 17–26).[108, 109] Differentiation of these three lesions may be made on the basis of size, location, and clinical history. Usually, sagittal and axial T2WI demonstrate a multilobulated mass that displaces cord anteriorly and expands the spinal canal. Occasionally, pronounced anterolateral canal erosion with central sparing may simulate the spur of diastatomyelia with associated intraspinal meningocele.[110] Dural ectasia is a similar abnormality that exhibits CSF signal intensity, allowing differentiation from neural tumors in patients with neurofibromatosis (Fig. 17–27).

## CHORDOMA AND OTHER PRIMARY VERTEBRAL NEOPLASMS

Chordoma is a locally destructive neoplasm of notochordal origin with little metastatic potential. Females in the fifth through seventh decades are most often affected.[111] Approximately 50% of chordomas are sacrococcygeal, 35% clival, and 15% cervical.[112] A propensity for the C2 level in the cervical spine exists. Although CT was previously appreciated as the modality of choice for lesion staging,[113] it misses soft tissue extension.[113, 114] We believe MR will replace CT because it provides more accurate assessment of nerve root status. If three sacral nerves ipsilaterally and two contralaterally can be preserved with sacral chordoma resection, normal bowel and bladder function can be maintained. Direct coronal, sagittal, and axial MR provide superior contrast of lesion to medullary bone (T1WI) and soft tissue (T2WI).[115, 116] The T2 signal hyperintensity of these lesions is not unlike the signal of nucleus pulposus (Fig. 17–28).[117] To optimize detection of foraminal or presacral involvement and maximize spatial resolution, small FOV (12- or 16-cm) 3-mm surface coil T1 and T2WI are utilized. Involvement of multiple vertebral levels, disk space destruction, and soft tissue mass suggest the diagnosis. A "frondlike" or "cauliflower shape" is typical of cervical chordomas in the sagittal projection. It is this projection that also allows assessment of airway, brain stem, and cord compromise.

Other primary osseus spinal lesions are likely best evaluated with CT and conven-

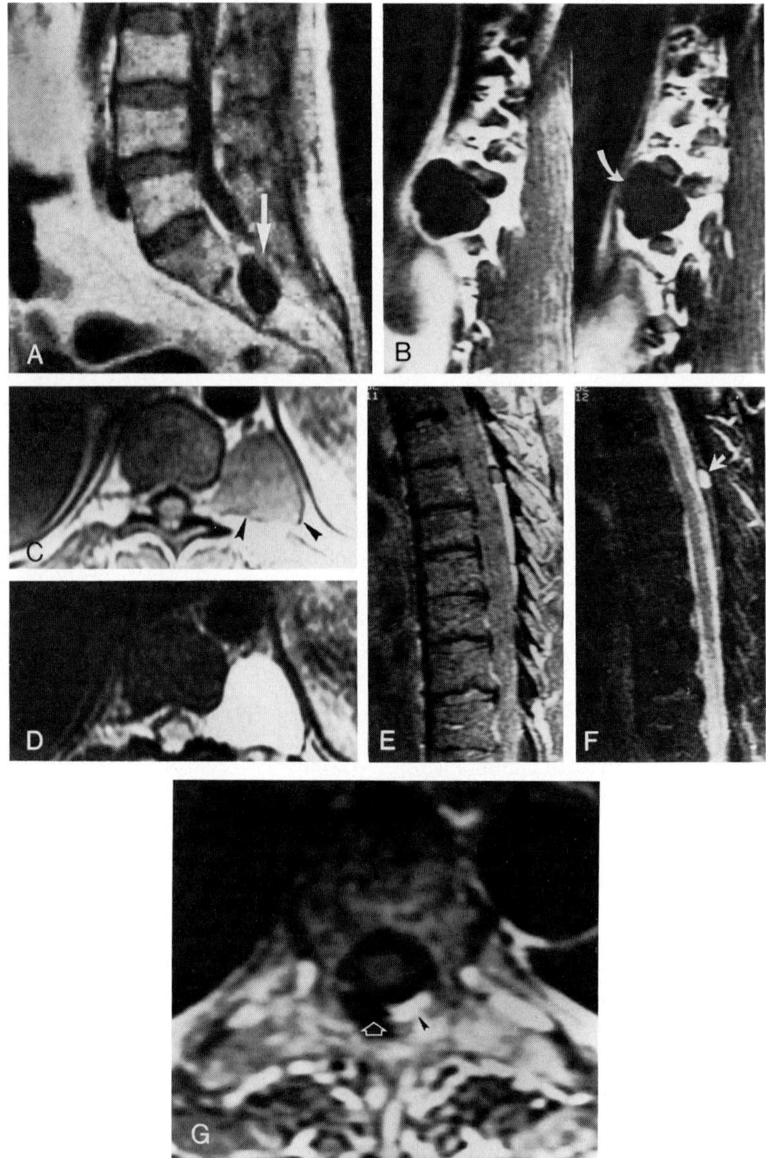


**Figure 17–26. *A,* Intradural arachnoid cyst; *B* to *D,* lateral thoracic meningocoele *E* to *G,* extradural thoracic arachnoid cyst.** Cystic lesions from three different patients. *A,* Sagittal T1WI in a 42-year-old man with difficulty voiding (0.35 T). Sagittal T1WI *(B),* axial N(H)WI and T2WI *(C* and *D)* in a 21-year-old man, who was asymptomatic (1.5 T). Sagittal N(H)WI and T2WI *(E* and *F),* axial T1WI *(G)* in a 65-year-old patient with chronic back pain (1.5 T). The signals of the sacral mass in *A* (arrow) and the thoracic masses in *B* (curved arrow) and *G* (open arrow) are hypointense on T1WI, virtually matching normal CSF signal. The mass effaces epidural fat (arrowhead) in *G.* Notice the homogeneous signal match of mass with CSF on N(H)WI (arrowhead) in *C* and T2WI (short arrow) in *F.*

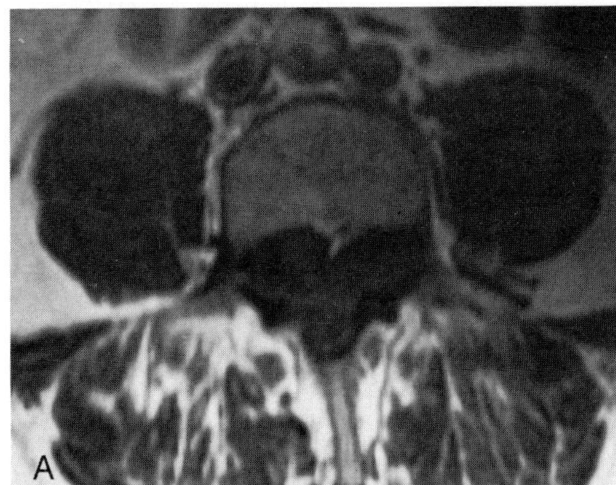


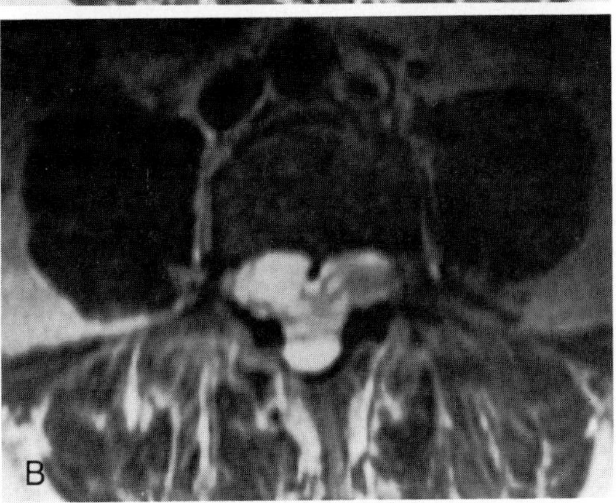


**Figure 17–27. Dural ectasia.** *A* and *B*, Axial (1.5) T1WI (TR 800/TE 20 msec) and T2WI (TR 1800/TE 80). A homogeneous signal, hypointense on T1WI and hyperintense on T2WI, is compatible with a fluid-filled structure. (Courtesy of A. Chambers, M.D., Neuroradiology Department, University Hospital, Cincinnati, Ohio.)

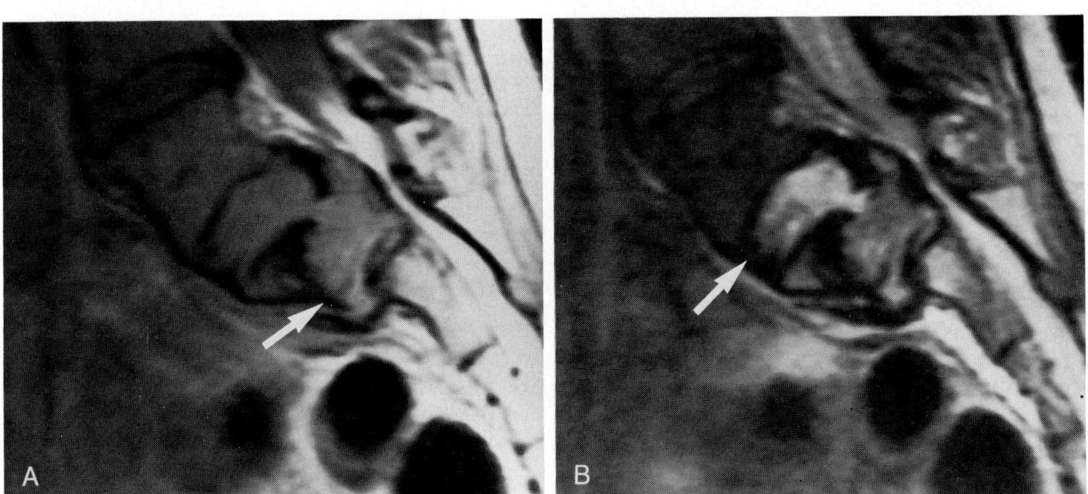


**Figure 17–28. Chordoma.** A 32-year-old woman with incontinence. *A* and *B,* Sagittal (1.5 T) multiecho N(H)WI and T2WI (TR 1800/TE 20/80 msec). A mass involves the sacrum (arrow). Origin from the L5-S1 disk space is inferred by expansion and hyperintensity of the disk on T2WI (arrow).

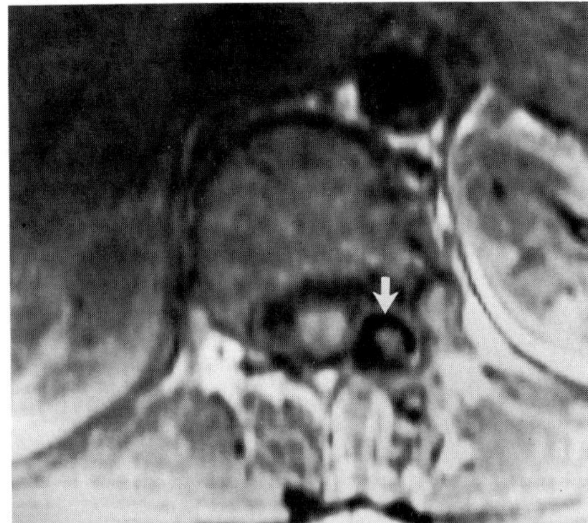

**Figure 17–29. Osteoid osteoma.** An 18-year-old man with back pain. Axial N(H)WI shows leftward (to reader's right) thoracic pedicular mass (arrow) with a hypointense cortical rim and a central signal nidus.

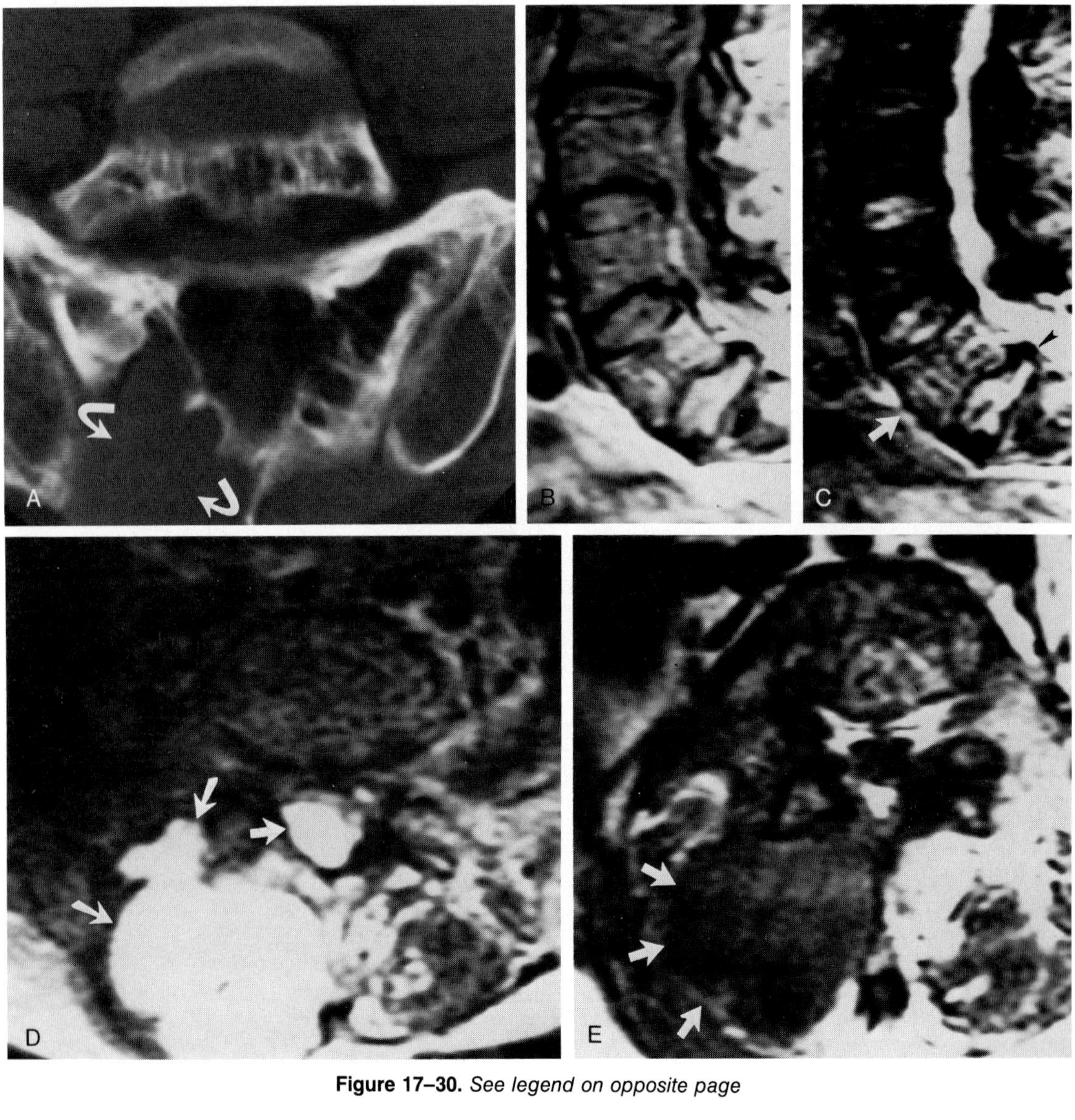

A B C D E

**Figure 17–30.** *See legend on opposite page*

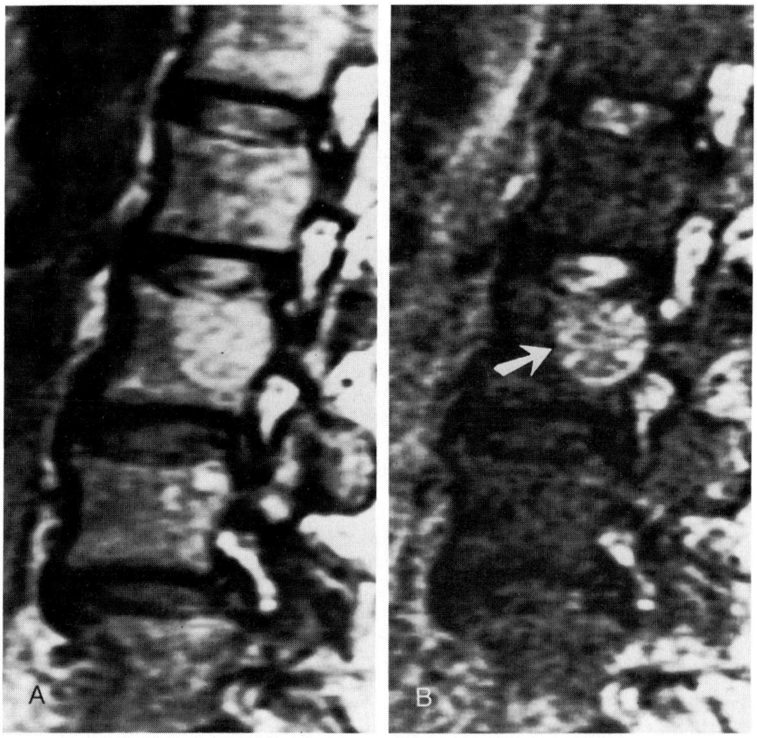

**Figure 17–31. Hemangioma.** A 57-year-old woman. *A* and *B,* Sagittal N(H)WI and T2WI (TR 1800/TE 20/80). A rounded, focal signal alteration at L-3 is hyperintense on both N(H)WI and T2WI (arrow). Lesion was hyperintense on T1WI (not shown) and its "starburst" or "speckled" appearance is characteristic. Hyperintensity on more T1-weighted images may be related to fat content within this lesion.

tional radiography unless myelopathy is present. The MR findings of lesions such as aneurysmal bone cyst, osteoblastoma, giant cell tumor, Ewings sarcoma, and eosinophilic granuloma are not specific. However, the appearance of osteoid ostema may be specific.[118–121] Rimlike hypointensity and central hyperintensity is often present (Fig. 17–29).

Diffusely diminished T1 signal with occasional end-plate sparing occurs in myeloma. Pagetoid bone exhibits diffuse T1 and T2 prolongation with the expected vertebral body enlargement (Fig 17–30).

Hemangiomas of bone yield variable signal intensities on T1 and hyperintense signal on T2WI. A characteristic MR appearance of vertebral hemangioma consisting of a hyperintense mottled or "starburst" signal on T1 and T2WI in the osseous portion of the tumor has been suggested (Fig. 17–31). If an extradural component is present, T1WI hyperintensity does not occur in this portion of the tumor. The areas of signal increase on T1WI are related to the presence of adipose tissue.

## References


1. Mamourian AC, Briggs RW. Appearance of Pantopaque on MR images. Radiology 158:457, 1986.
2. Braun IF, Malko JA, Davis PC, et al. The behavior of Pantopaque on MR: in vivo and in vitro analyses. AJNR 7:997, 1986.
3. Cheng MK. Spinal cord tumors in the People's Republic of China: a statistical review. Neurosurg 10:22, 1982.
4. Shapiro R. Myelography. Chicago, Year Book Medical Publishers, 1975.
5. Baker RA. In Taveras JM, Ferruci JT, eds. Radiol-


**Figure 17–30. Paget's disease with cystic dedifferentiated chondrosarcoma.** A 62-year-old man with diffuse Paget's disease and severe back pain (1.5 T). *A,* Axial NCCT, bone window setting. *B* and *C,* Sagittal N(H)WI and T2WI. *D,* Axial T2WI. *E,* Axial T1WI. CT shows the coarsened trabeculae of Paget's disease at L5-S1 level, with a rightward posterolateral soft tissue mass (curved arrows). Sagittal MR shows coarsened, striated signal hyperintensity in Pagetoid vertebral body (arrow). Symptomatic disk herniation was also present (arrowhead). Axial T1WI and T2WI shows cystic mass within and posterior to spinal canal (arrows). Notice the speckled appearance of the vertebral body on axial T1WI.

ogy: Diagnosis, Imaging and Intervention, Vol. 3. Philadelphia, J. B. Lippincott Co., 1987.
6. Claussen C, Treisch J, Massih M, et al. MR imaging and CT of intraspinal tumors. Radiology 161(P):33, 1986.
7. Hackney DB, Wismer GL, Edelman R, et al. Magnetic resonance imaging of the spine: noninvasive evaluation of spinal block. Abstract. Proceedings of the American Society of Neuroradiology. AJNR 6:476, 1985.
8. Slooff JL, Kernohan JW, MacCarty CS. Primary Tumors of the Spinal Cord and Filum Terminale. Philadelphia, W. B. Saunders, 1964.
9. Morantz RA, Kepes JJ, Batnitzky S, et al. Extraspinal ependymomas. Report of three cases. J Neurosurg 52:383, 1979.
10. Kopelson G, Lingood RM, Kleinman GM, et al. Management of intramedullary spinal cord tumors. Radiology 135:473, 1980.
11. Epstein F, Epstein N. Surgical treatment of spinal cord astrocytomas of children. A series of 19 patients. J Neurosurg 52:685, 1982.
12. Alter M. Statistical aspects of spinal cord tumors. In Viaken PJ, Bruya AW, eds. Handbook of Clinical Neurology, Vol. 19. New York, Elsevier Scientific Publishing, 1975.
13. Grogan JP, Daniels DL, Williams AL, et al. The normal conus medullaris: CT criteria for recognition. Radiology 151:661, 1984.
14. Han JS, Benson JE, Yoon YS. Magnetic resonance imaging in the spinal column and craniovertebral junction. Radiol Clin North Am 22:805, 1984.
15. Pomeranz SJ. Magnetic resonance imaging of the spine. NMR: Update Series. 10:1, 1985.
16. De La Paz RL, Brady TJ, Buonanno FS, et al. Nuclear magnetic resonance (NMR) imaging of Arnold-Chiari type I malformation with hydromyelia. J Comput Assist Tomogr 7:126, 1983.
17. Yeates A, Brant-Zawadski M, Norman D, et al. Nuclear magnetic resonance imaging of syringohydromyelia. AJNR 4:234, 1983.
18. Lee BCP, Zimmerman RL, Manning JJ, et al. MR imaging of syringomyelia and hydromyelia. AJNR 6:221, 1985.
19. Pojunas K, Williams AJ, Daniels DL, et al. Syringomyelia and hydromyelia: magnetic resonance evaluation. Radiology 153:679, 1984.
20. Enzmann DR, O'Donohue J, Shuer L, et al. CSF pulsations within nonneoplastic spinal cord cysts. Radiology 161(P):251, 1986.
21. Sherman JL, Citrin CM, Gangarosa RE, et al. The MR appearance of CSF pulsations in the spinal canal. AJNR 7:879, 1986.
22. Sherman JL, Citrin CM. Magnetic resonance imaging of normal CSF flow. AJNR 7:3, 1986.
23. Enzmann DR, O'Donohue JO, Rubin JB, et al. CSF pulsations within nonneoplastic spinal cord cysts. AJR 149:149, 1987.
24. Di Chiro GD, Dopman JL, Dwyer AJ, et al. Tumors and arteriovenous malformations of the spinal cord: assessment using MR. Radiology 156:689, 1985.
25. Sherman JL, Barkovich AJ, Citrin CM. The MR appearance of syringomyelia: new observations. AJNR 7:985, 1986.
26. Gebarski SS, Maynard FW, Gabrielson TO, et al. Posttraumatic progressive myelopathy. Radiology 157:379, 1985.
27. Williams AL, Haughton VM, Pojunas KW, et al. Differentiation of intramedullary neoplasms and cysts by MR. AJR 149:159, 1987.
28. Bydder GM, Brown J, Niendorf HP, et al. Enhancement of cervical intraspinal tumors with intravenous gadolinium-DTPA. J Comput Assist Tomogr 9:847, 1985.
29. Brant-Zawadski M, Berry I, Osaki L, et al. Gd-DTPA in clinical MR of the brain: 1. Intraaxial lesions. AJR 147:1223, 1986.
30. Slasky BS, Bydder GM, Niendorf HP, Young IR. MR imaging with gadolinium-DTPA in the differentiation of tumor, syrinx, and cyst of the spinal cord. J Comput Assist Tomogr 11:845, 1987.
31. Halimi PH, Sigal R, Blas C, et al. High-field MR imaging of spinal cord tumors. Radiology 161(P):251, 1986.
32. Goy AMC, Pinto RS, Raghavendra BN, et al. Intramedullary spinal cord tumors: MR imaging, with emphasis on associated cysts. Radiology 161: 381, 1986.
33. Barkovich AJ, Sherman JL, Citrin CM, et al. MR of postoperative syringomyelia. AJNR 8:319, 1987.
34. Quencer RM, Gammal TE, Cohen G. Syringomyelia associated with intradural extramedullary masses of the spinal canal. AJNR 7:143, 1986.
35. Modic MT, Masaryk T, Paushter D. Magnetic resonance imaging of the spine. Radiol Clin North Am 24:229, 1986.
36. Naseem M, Zachariah SB, Stone J, et al. Cervicomedullary hematoma: diagnosis by MR. AJNR 7:1096, 1986.
37. Kendall B, Russell J. Haemangioblastomas of the spinal cord. Br J Radiol 39:817, 1986.
38. Blas C, Halimi Ph, Sigal R, et al. High-field MR imaging of spinal cord vascular lesions. Radiology 161(P):33, 1986.
39. Rebner M, Gebarski SS. Magnetic resonance imaging of spinal cord hemangioblastoma. AJNR 6:287, 1985.
40. Rubinstein LJ. Tumors of the Central Nervous System. Atlas of Tumor Pathology, 2nd series, fascicle 6. Bethesda, Md, Armed Forces Institute of Pathology, 1972.
41. Daffner RH, Lupetin AR, Dash N, et al. MRI in the detection of malignant infiltration of bone marrow. AJR 146:353, 1986.
42. Levy WJ, Bay J, Dohn D. Spinal cord meningiomas. J Neurosurg 57:804, 1982.
43. Wood JB, Wolpert SM. Lumbosacral meningiomas. AJNR 6:450, 1985.
44. Dastur KJ, Raji MR, Smith WI Jr. Pulmonary metastasis from intraspinal meningioma. AJNR 5:483, 1984.
45. Hallpike JF, Stanley P. A case of extradural spinal meningioma. J Neurol Neurosurg Psychiatr 31:195, 1968.
46. Okazaki Haruo. Fundamentals of Neuropathology. New York, Igaku-Shoin, 1983.
47. Zimmerman RD, Fleming CA, Saint-Louis LA, et al. Magnetic resonance imaging of meningiomas. AJNR 6:149, 1985.
48. Spagnoli MV, Goldberg HI, Grossman RI, et al. Intracranial meningiomas: high-field MR imaging. Radiology 161:369, 1986.
49. Brasfield RD, Das Gupta TK. Von Recklinghausen's disease: a clinicopathologic study. Ann Surg 175:86, 1972.

50. Sordillo PP, Helson L, Hajdu SI, et al. Malignant schwannoma—clinical characteristics, survival, and response to therapy. Cancer 47:2503, 1981.
51. Chi-Zing Z, Segall HD, Boswell WD, et al. MR imaging in the diagnosis of spinal schwannomas and neurofibromas. Radiology 157(P):149, 1985.
52. Burk LD Jr, Brunberg JA, Kanal E, et al. Spinal and paraspinal neurofibromatosis: surface coil imaging at 1.5 T. Radiology 162:797, 1987.
53. Aisen AM, Martel W, Braunstein EM, et al. MRI and CT evaluation of primary bone and soft-tissue tumors. AJR 146:749, 1986.
54. Horvath K, Fink I, Patronas NJ, et al. MR characterization of neurofibromas and neurofibrosarcomas. Radiology 153(P):307, 1984.
55. Pomeranz SJ. MR imaging of the visual pathways in neurofibromatosis. Radiology 153(P):328, 1985.
56. Bilaniuk LT, Zimmerman RA, Kemp S, et al. MR imaging of phakomatosis. Radiology 153(P):212, 1985.
57. Kuhn JP, Cohen ML, Duffner PK, et al. MR imaging of the brain in neurofibromatosis. Radiology 161(P):202, 1986.
58. Epstein BS. The Spine, 4th ed. Philadelphia, Lea & Febiger, 1976.
59. Wood BP, Harwood-Nash DC, Berger P, et al. Intradural spinal lipoma of the cervical cord. AJR 145:174, 1985.
60. Han JS, Kaufman B, El Yousef SJ, et al. NMR imaging of the spine. AJR 141:1137, 1983.
61. Modic M, Weinstein MA, Pavlicek W, et al. Nuclear magnetic resonance of the spine. Radiology 148:757, 1983.
62. Smoker WRK, Biller J, Moore SA, et al. Intradural spinal teratoma: case report and review of the literature. AJNR 7:905, 1986.
63. Monajati A, Spitzer RM, Wiley JL, et al. MR imaging of a spinal teratoma. J Comput Assist Tomogr 10:307, 1986.
64. Donoghue V, Chuang SH, Chilton SJ, et al. Intraspinal epidermoid cysts. J Comput Assist Tomogr 8:143, 1984.
65. Manno NJ, Uihlein A, Kiernohan JW. Intraspinal epidermoids. J Neurosurg 19:754, 1962.
66. Kortman KE, Van Dalsem WJ, Bradley WG, et al. MR imaging of epidermoid tumors. Radiology 157:71, 1985.
67. Hershey B, Grossman RI, Goldberg HI, et al. MR imaging of epidermoids. Radiology 157(P):71, 1985.
68. Gilbert RW, Kim JH, Posner JB. Epidural spinal cord compression from metastatic tumor: diagnosis and treatment. Ann Neurol 3:40, 1978.
69. Livingston KE, Perrin RG. The neurosurgical management of spinal metastases causing cord compression. J Neurosurg 49:839, 1978.
70. Green BA, Diaz RD, Post JD. In Post JD, ed. Computed Tomography of the Spine. Baltimore, Waverly Press, Inc, 1984:676.
71. Shapiro R. Myelography, 4th ed. Chicago, Year Book Medical Publishers, 1984.
72. Banna M, Gryspeerdt GL. Intraspinal tumors in children (excluding dysraphism). Clin Radiol 22:17, 1971.
73. Dorwart RH, Wara WM, Norman D, et al. Complete myelographic evaluation of spinal metastases from medulloblastoma. Radiology 139:403, 1981.
74. Murphy KC, Feld R, Evans WK, et al. Intramedullary spinal cord metastases from small cell carcinoma of the lung. J Clin Oncol 1:99, 1983.
75. Smaltino F, Bernini FP, Santoro S. Computerized tomography in the diagnosis of intramedullary metastases. Acta Neurochir (Wein) 52:299, 1980.
76. Costigan DA, Winkelman MD. Intramedullary spinal cord metastases. A clinicopathological study of 13 cases. J Neurosurg 62:227, 1985.
77. Edelson RN, Deck MDF, Posner JB. Intramedullar spinal cord metastases. Clinical and radiographic findings in nine cases. Neurology 22:1222, 1972.
78. Deutsch M, Reigel DH. The value of myelography in the management of childhood medulloblastoma. Cancer 45:2194, 1980.
79. Post MJD, Quencer RM, Green BA, et al. Intramedullary spinal cord metastases, mainly of nonneurogenic origin. AJNR 8:339, 1987.
80. Pomeranz SJ, Brown OL, Masters JM, et al. Intramedullary metastases: MR findings with normal CT, myelography and scintigraphy. Unpublished.
81. Smoker WRK, Godersky JC, Knutzon RK, et al. The role of MR imaging in evaluating metastatic spinal disease. AJNR 8:901, 1987.
82. Ramsey RG, Zacharias CE. MR imaging of the spine after radiation therapy: easily recognizable effects. AJR 144:1131, 1985.
83. Baker LL, Hajek PC, Goobar JE, et al. Focal fat deposition in axial bone marrow: diagnostic considerations and distinction from pathology by MR imaging. Radiology 161(P):132, 1986.
84. Dooms GC, Fisher MR, Hricak H, et al. Bone marrow imaging: magnetic resonance studies related to age and sex. Radiology 155:429, 1985.
85. Moon KL, Genant HK, Helms CA, et al. Musculoskeletal applications of nuclear magnetic resonance. Radiology 147:161, 1983.
86. Yoshida H, Isamu M, Yashiro N, et al. MR imaging of bone marrow disorders. Radiology 161(P):23, 1986.
87. Rao VM, Dalinka MK, Mitchell DG, et al. Osteopetrosis: MR characteristics at 1.5 T. Radiology 161:217, 1986.
88. Krol G, Heier L, Becker R, et al. MR imaging of primary or metastatic tumors of the spine: contribution of T1 and T2 weighting and multiple echo sequences. Radiology 161(P):220, 1986.
89. Utz J, Herfkens RJ, Fram EK, et al. MR imaging of vertebral metastases. Radiology 161(P):278, 1986.
90. Beres J, Pech P, Berns TF, et al. Spinal epidural lymphomas: CT features in seven patients. AJNR 7:327, 1986.
91. Siegal MJ, Jamroz GA, Glazer HS, et al. MR imaging of intraspinal extension of neuroblastoma. J Comput Assist Tomogr 10:593, 1986.
92. Rao TV, Narayanasswamy KS, Shankar SK. "Primary" spinal epidural lymphomas. A clinico-pathologic study. Acta Neurochir (Wein) 62:307, 1982.
93. Holtas SL, Kido DK, Simon JH. MR imaging of spinal lymphoma. J Comput Assist Tomogr 10: 111, 1986.
94. Algra PR, Breedveld FC, Vielvoye GJ, et al. MR imaging of the cervical spine in rheumatoid arthritis. Radiology 161(P):365, 1986.
95. Bewermeyer H, Dreesback HA, Hundermann B, et al. MR imaging of familiar basilar impression. J Comput Assist Tomogr 8:953, 1984.

96. Han JS, Huss RG, Benson JE, et al. MR imaging of the skull base. J Comput Assist Tomogr 8:944, 1984.
97. Smoker WRK, Menezes AH, Harnsberger R, et al. MR imaging in the evaluation of rheumatoid arthritis of the craniovertebral junction. Radiology 161(P):181, 1986.
98. Kudo H, Iwano K, Yoshizawa H. Cervical cord compression due to extradural granulation tissue in rheumatoid arthritis. J Bone Joint Surg (Br) 66:426, 1984.
99. Han JS, Benson JE, Kaufman B, et al. Demonstration of diastatomyelia and associated abnormalities with MR imaging. AJNR 6:215, 1985.
100. Haykal HA, Wang A-M, Zamani AA, et al. Computed tomography of spontaneous acute cervical hematoma. J Comput Assist Tomogr 8:229, 1984.
101. Badami JP, Hinck VC. Symptomatic deposition of epidural fat in a morbidly obese woman. AJNR 4:664, 1982.
102. Guegan Y, Fardoun R, Launois B, et al. Spinal cord compression by extradural fat after prolonged corticosteroid therapy. J Neurosurg 58:580, 1982.
103. Leaney BJ, CAlvert JM. Tophaceous gout producing spinal cord compression. J Neurosurg 58:580, 1983.
104. Kleinman GM, Dagi TF, Poletti CE. Villonodular synovitis in the spinal canal. J Neurosurg 52:846, 1980.
105. Prete PE, Henbest M, Michalski JP, et al. Intraspinal elastofibroma. Spine 8:800, 1983.
106. Smoker WRK, Keyes WD, Dunn VD, et al. MRI versus conventional radiographic examinations in the evaluation of the craniovertebral and cervicomedullary junction. Radiographics 6:953, 1986.
107. Naidich TP, McLone DG, Harwood-Nash DC. Arachnoid cysts, paravertebral meningocoeles, and perineurial cysts. In Newton TH, Potts DG, eds. Computed Tomography of the Spine and Spinal Cord, Vol. 1. San Anselmo, Calif., Clavadel Press, 1983:383.
108. Sundaram M, Awwad EE. Magnetic resonance imaging of arachnoid cysts destroying the sacrum. AJR 146:359, 1986.
109. Keyes WD, Gentry LR, Smoker WRK, et al. Intradural spinal arachnoid cysts: MR, CT, and myelogrpahic imaging pitfalls. Radiology 161(P):150, 1986.
110. Grivegnee A, Delince P, Ectors P. Comparative aspects of occult intrasacral meningocoele with conventional x-ray, myelography and CT. Neuroradiology 22:33, 1981.
111. Hertzanu Y, Glass RBJ, Mendelsohn DB. Sacrococcygeal chordoma in young adults. Clin Radiol 34:327, 1983.
112. Mindell ER. Chordoma. J Bone Joint Surg (Am) 63:501, 1981.
113. Krol G, Sundaresan N, Deck M. Computed tomography of axial chordomas. J Comput Assist Tomogr 7:286, 1983.
114. Hudson TM, Galceran M. Radiology of sacrococcygeal chordomas: difficulties in detecting soft tissue extension. Clin Orthop 175:237, 1983.
115. Rosenthal DI, Scott JA, Mankin HJ, et al. Sacrococcygeal chordoma: magnetic resonance imaging and computed tomography. AJR 145:143, 1985.
116. Mapstone TB, Kaufman B, Ratcheson RA. Intradural chordoma without bone involvement: NMR appearance. J Neurosurg 59:535, 1983.
117. Pettersson H, Hudson D, Hamlim K, et al. Magnetic resonance imaging of sacrococcygeal tumors. Acta Radiol Diagn 26:161, 1985.
118. Zimmer WD, Berquist TH, Sim FH, et al. Magnetic resonance imaging of aneurysmal bone. Mayo Clin Proc 59:633, 1984.
119. Brady TJ, Gebhardt MC, Pykett IL, et al. NMR imaging of forearms in healthy volunteers and patients with giant-cell tumor of bone. Radiology 144:549, 1982.
120. Zimmer WD, Berquist TH, McLeod RA, et al. Bone tumors: magnetic resonance imaging versus computed tomography. Radiology 155:709, 1985.
121. Graif M, Pennock JM. MR imaging of histiocytosis X in the central nervous system. AJNR 7:21, 1986.

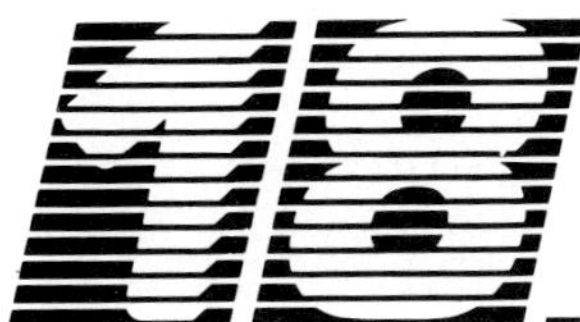

**Susan Weinberg, M.D.**
**Thomas Seward, M.D.**

# DISK DISEASE, SPONDYLOSIS, AND RELATED DISORDERS

Back pain afflicts 60% of Americans each year. Disk degeneration, protrusion, herniation, extrusion, spinal stenosis and postlaminectomy scarring are all potential causes of disabling pain.

Until recently, computed tomography (CT), with or without intrathecal contrast, has been the primary spinal imaging modality. The multiplanar capability of magnetic resonance (MR) and its superior contrast resolution, absence of ionizing radiation, and improving spatial resolution with high field strength surface coil images has altered the diagnostic approach to neck and back pain. An overview of the role of MR in assessment of disk disease, its benefits and disadvantages, and an algorithmic approach to degenerative spine lesions is presented.

## TECHNICAL CONSIDERATIONS

### Pulse Sequence and Image Plane Selection

The selection of a proper MR pulse sequence and imaging plane depends on the pathology in question and size of the area to be covered. Suggested standard screening techniques for the cervical, thoracic, and lumbar spine are summarized in the appendices of this text. These guidelines can be applied to most MR scanners.

Several authors have suggested that a combination of T1- and T2-weighted images (T1WI and T2WI) are required for spine evaluation.[1] For pure evaluation of disk disease or herniation, some have advocated only T1WI images with image interpretation based on anatomy rather than signal alterations.[2] T1 images provide poor tissue contrast between ligaments, fibrous tissue, and cortical bone, making evaluation of osteophytes difficult.[3] Most examinations begin with a localizer, or "quick" scout image (1 excitation [nex] or ½ average [av], TR 200-600/TE 20-40 msec). Many obtain the scout image in a coronal orientation; however, a sagittal scout, centering on midline structures is acceptable. Thoracic spine scout series may require large fields of view (FOV) or minimal zoom factor so that exact vertebral levels can be counted. Knowledge of the following anatomical relationships facilitates level localization (and surface coil placement): thyroid cartilage, C4; suprasternal notch, T2; sternal angle, T4; inferior scapular angle, T7; xiphiosternal junction, T9; and superior mesenteric artery (SMA), T12 or L1.

After an initial localizer sequence, T1WIs are performed (Figs. 18–1 and 18–2). Two or four excitations (1 or 2 av) are used, depending on the signal quality seen on the scout image. The repetition time (300 to 600 msec) utilized depends on slice thickness and distance to be covered. The shortest echo time (TE) available is selected. The sagittal scout image with 2 nex (1 av) may be used as a diagnostic T1 sequence if one obtains the midline slice by centering on the nasion or the symphysis pubis. T1WIs provide excellent contrast between medullary bone pathology (hypointense) and normal vertebral marrow (hyperintense); cord or roots (moderate intensity) and epidural fat (hyperintense); and cord or conus (moderate intensity) versus thecal sac CSF (hypointense). Although disks are best visualized on

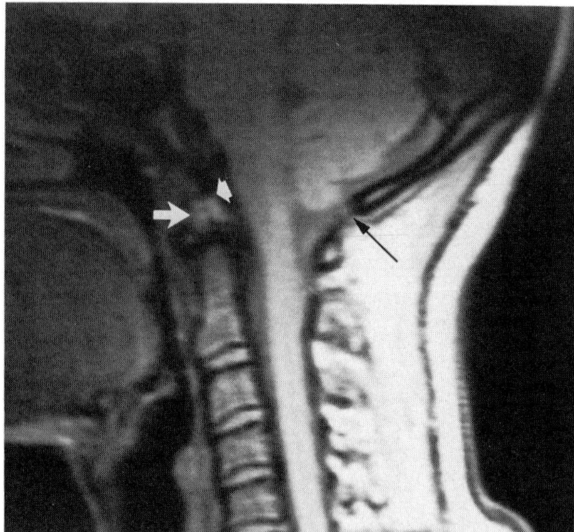

**Figure 18–1. Normal mid-sagittal T1WI (TR 600/TE 20), upper cervical spine (1.5 T).** Demarcating the foramen magnum is the hypointense signal of posterior occipital cortical bone (black arrow), whereas the hyperintense signal of fat (white arrow) lying cephalad to the dens is used by some as the anterior foramen magnum margin. An alternative and more cephalad anterior foramen magnum margin is located at the junction of the fat collection and the cortical bone of the caudad clival tip (short arrow).

spin-density images, or N(H)WI, T1WI provide adequate disk visualization. Images with very short parameters (TR 200/TE 15 msec) have been advocated by some and are discussed later.[4] High-signal intervertebral foraminal fat is easily contrasted with nerve roots (Fig. 18–3) on T1WI, and nerve root encroachment is evident on these images.

If one has chosen to perform the examination with only T1 images, then an axial T1WI with TR 400 to 1000 msec and the shortest available TE is completed. The TR is determined by the slice thickness and the number of disk levels to be covered.

T2WI are necessary for evaluation of spinal neoplasm, the postoperative back, trauma, and most conditions other than simple disk disease or spondylosis. If the decision is made to continue an examination with multiecho T2WI, then spin-echo sagittal, and if necessary, axial images are performed (TR 1500-2000/TE 15 to 35 and 56 to 100 msec [2 or 4 nex]) after the scout series. Flow compensation, gradient moment nulling, or motion artifact suppression is utilized in the sagittal projection. Presaturation pulses can be used in one, or usually two, planes with axial T1WI. Gradient moment nulling is only occasionally used with multiecho axial T2WI, since it markedly reduces the number of obtainable slices for a given TR. The TR selected depends on the length of area to be covered, slice thickness, number of excitations chosen, patient cooperation, and the quality of signal/noise ob-

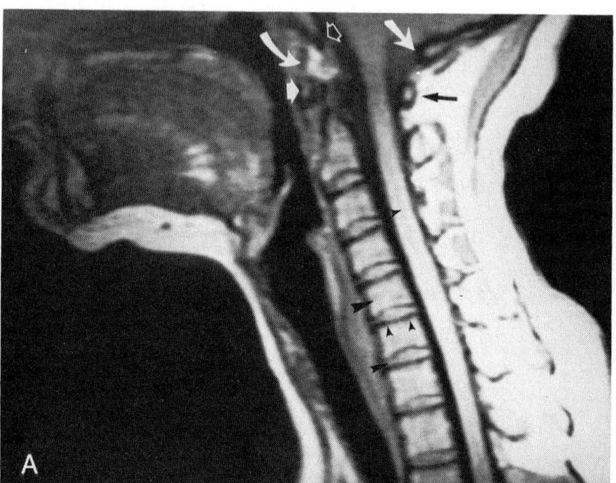


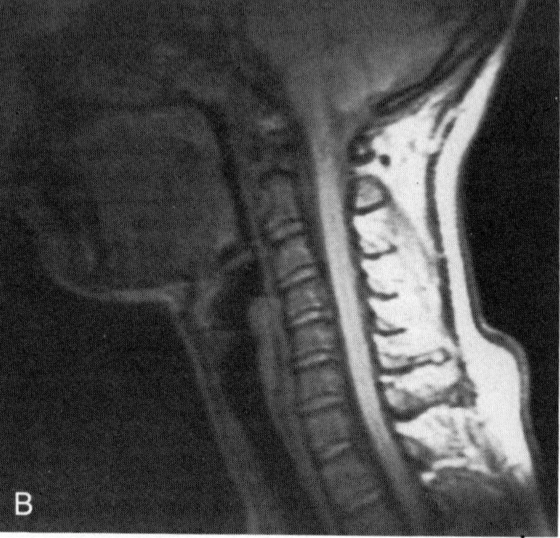


**Figure 18–2. Normal sagittal cervical anatomy.** (1.5 T) *A,* Sagittal T1WI (TR 600/TE 20). *B,* Sagittal N(H)WI (TR 1800/TE 20). Surface-coil image of a normal cervical spine on T1WI shows hyperintense marrow-filled vertebral bodies (large arrowhead). Hypointense CSF surrounds the intermediate signal intensity cord (small arrowhead). Identified are the intervertebral disk (medium-sized arrowhead) and hypointense linear signal of vertebral cortical bone/end-plate and outer cortical annular fibers of disk (paired small arrowheads). The anterior (short white arrow) and posterior (black arrow) arches of C-1 are identified. Normal hyperintense fat (curved arrow) is present above the dens. Delineating the foramen magnum is a line drawn from the posterior hypointense cortical margin of the occipital bone (white arrow) to the cortical bone of the inferior clival tip (open arrow). Note that on N(H)WI, imaged vertebral bodies diminish in signal intensity, whereas disks increase in signal intensity.

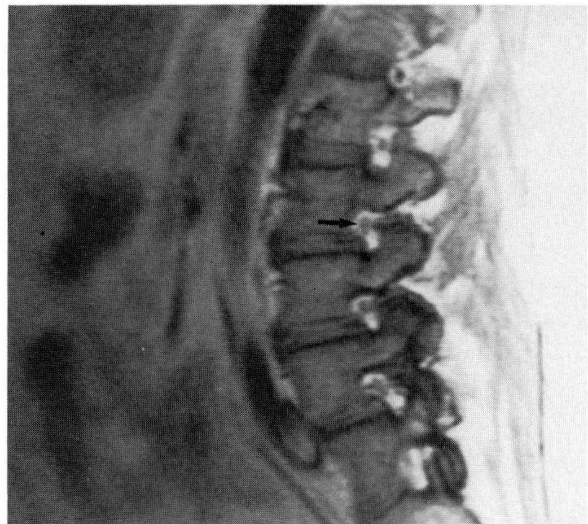

**Figure 18–3. Orthogonal sagittal 5-mm section through the lumbar neural foramen.** Sagittal N(H)WI (TR 2000/TE 20) (1.5 T) demonstrates an hourglass foraminal shape that contains hyperintense fat and intermediate signal intensity nerve roots (arrowhead). At this level, the roots are subpedicular.

served on the scout series. A patient yielding poor signal on a scout image may require longer TR or more excitations to improve image signal. Image signal to noise can be markedly (30%) improved by opting for single-echo rather than multiecho technique. Large FOV and thicker sections also improve image signal but at the price of larger voxel size (subsequently addressed).

T2 images (Fig. 18–4) provide an "intrathecal contrast" appearance to the intraspinal contents. The hyperintense CSF and isointense cord are separated from the extradural anatomy (see Fig. 18–1). T2-weighted axial images are useful in distinguishing disk herniation from adjacent thecal sac when epidural fat is obliterated and lost as a landmark on T2WI. This imaging sequence also helps identify the hypointense epidural venous anatomy when confusion over masses in this region arise. T2 sagittal images are important in the assessment of disk dessication (Fig. 18–5) and fast-scan axial sequences helpful in assessing cervical radiculopathy since the hyperintense CSF signal bathes exiting dorsal and ventral nerve roots (Fig. 18–6). Balanced or proton density images (Figs. 18–2, 18–4, 18–6) provide several advantages. Contrast between thecal sac or nerve roots and epidural fat can be maintained with excellent disk visualization and optimal signal/noise characteristics. Excellent axial and sagittal visualization of ventral and dorsal nerve roots or ganglia is achieved.

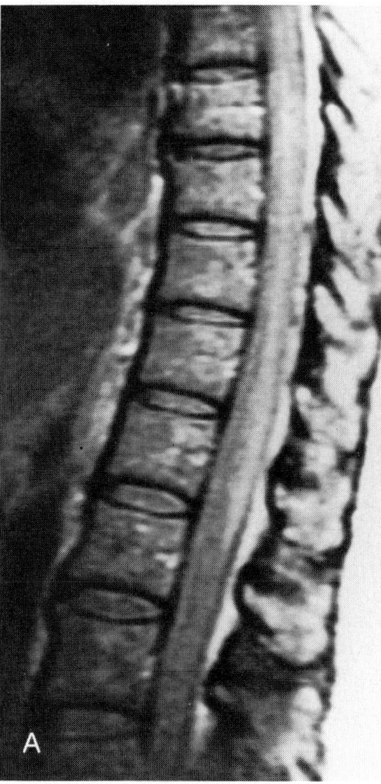


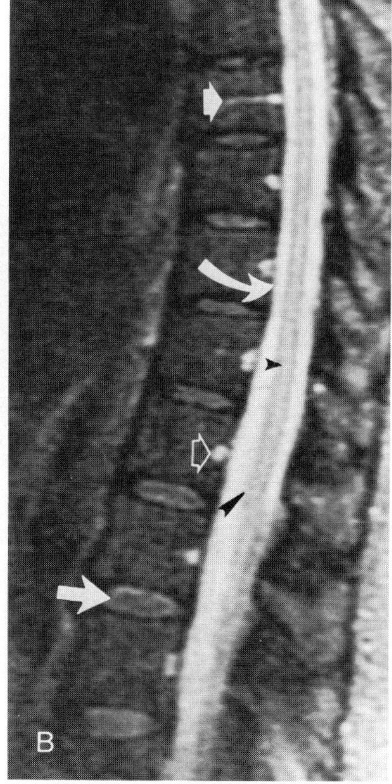


**Figure 18–4. Normal sagittal thoracolumbar anatomy.** (1.5 T) *A* and *B,* Sagittal multiecho N(H)WI and T2WI (TR 1800/TE 20/80). High-resolution protocol for examination of the thoracic spine utilizes a 24-cm field of view (FOV) and visualizes eight vertebral bodies. This multiecho protocol is repeated more cephalad to examine the remainder of the thoracic spine. Utilized are 3-mm sections, two or four excitations, and gradient moment nulling providing flow compensation. Lower resolution protocols employ one sagittal series and > 32-cm FOV. Normal structures demonstrated include intervertebral disk and cleft (arrow), hyperintense thecal sac (curved arrow), linear (short white arrow) and rounded (open arrow) appearance of basivertebral plexus, distal spinal cord and conus (arrowhead), and normal central gray hyperintense signal (small arrowhead). (Courtesy of S. J. Pomeranz, M.D., The Christ Hospital, Cincinnati, Ohio.)

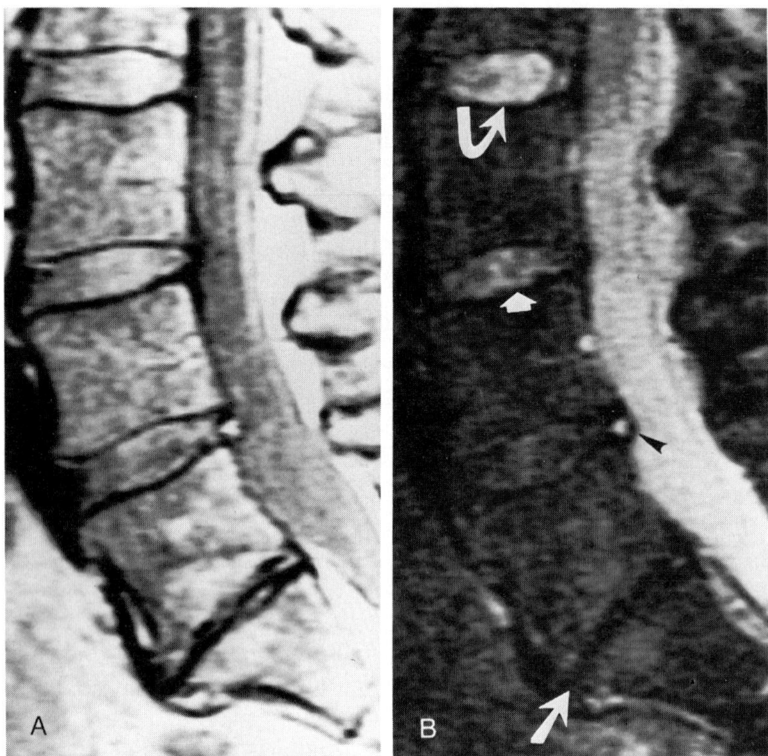


**Figure 18–5. Varying degrees of disk degeneration and desiccation.** Sagittal multiecho N(H)WI and T2WI (TR 2000/TE 20/80), lumbar spine (1.5 T). Progressive levels of disk desiccation are present in the caudal direction. The L2-L3 disk demonstrates normal T2 signal (curved arrow) hyperintensity. The less hydrated L3-L4 disk (short white arrow) is less hyperintense. Progressive hypointensity of L4-L5 due to disk desiccation has resulted from prior diskectomy, and a normal posterior hyperintensity (arrowhead) following diskectomy is apparent. Severest disk space narrowing, disk desiccation, and signal loss (white arrow) is present at L5-S1. (Courtesy of S. J. Pomeranz, M.D., The Christ Hospital, Cincinnati, Ohio.)

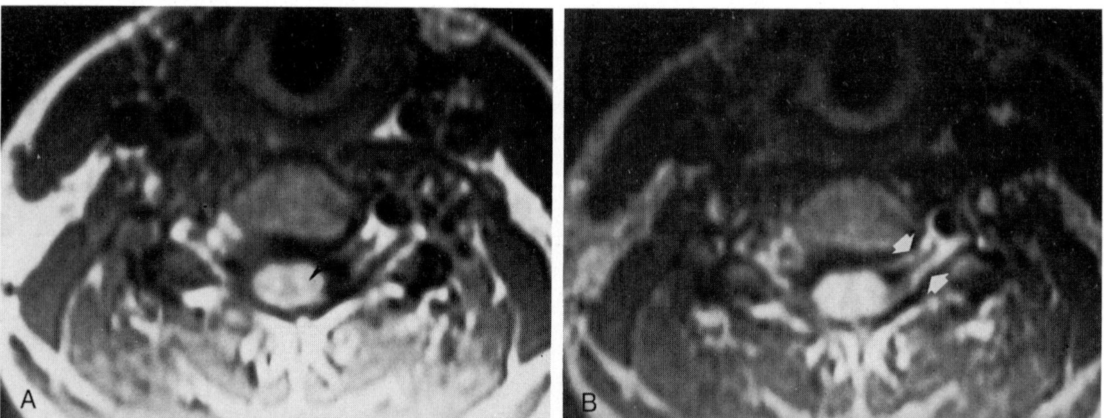


**Figure 18–6. Normal axial cervical anatomy.** *A,* Axial N(H)WI (TR 2000/TE 20) (1.5 T). *B,* Axial T2WI (TR 2000/TE 80). Ventral and dorsal exiting nerve roots are of intermediate signal intensity but become hyperintense on T2WI (short arrows) owing to surrounding CSF. Cervical cord (arrowhead) and its gray and white matter components are identified on axial N(H)WI.

### Slice Acquisition

Developing acceptable MR technique requires many compromises. Factors such as patient cooperation, matrix size, number of excitations or averages, slice thickness, repetition time, and number of pulsing sequences desired must be weighed. With unlimited scanning time and no patient motion, a scan utilizing 6 excitations, prolonged TR, 512 x 512 matrix and contiguous thin sections would be ideal. However, there are other considerations.

Most sequences are acquired with a 128 x 256 matrix size. The 256 matrix is acquired in the read only, or x direction, with no time penalty. Doubling the matrix in the y, or phase direction, from 128 to 256 doubles imaging time. Some decrease in pixel size or increased spatial resolution will occur at a cost of increased image noise. Therefore, large matrix sizes are only desirable when optimal signal-to-noise ratio (SNR) is present and very detailed resolution is required in a cooperative patient.

Slice thickness and gap selection are determined by the size of pathology sought and the length of area to be covered. High–field strength magnets and surface coils (large SNR) may be needed to counteract the higher noise level of thin sections. Most sequences are obtained with 3-mm or 5-mm sections and 0.6-, 1-, or 2-mm gap. If contiguous or overlapping coverage is desired, then two imaging sequences will be necessary. A suboptimal situation is the attempt to obtain thin sections with short repetition time, few excitations, and long echo times. All these factors exacerbate the poor SNR of small voxels.

The number of excitations selected depends on SNR characteristics of the pulsing sequence chosen or the inherent SNR generated from each patient. The number of excitations or averages is directly proportional to the imaging time. Image SNR is proportional to the square root of the averages. With the exception of a single excitation scout, 4 or less commonly, 2 excitations are enforced on most pulsing sequences. This choice depends on the quality of signal observed on the localizer scan, repetition time, FOV, slice thickness, patient cooperation, and coil type utilized. When factors that reduce SNR are utilized, at least 4 excitations (2 av) are necessary.

Field of view chosen depends on the size of an area of interest and the desired spatial resolution (pixel size). When surface coils are utilized, depth of pathology from the coil itself is relevant. Objects extremely superficial or deep may be missed with very small FOVs. When surface coils are implemented, 24-cm FOV is most commonly utilized. Larger FOV defeats the purpose of surface coil MR, which is the reduction of pixel size. Occasionally, when good SNR characteristics exist, 20-cm and 16-cm FOVs are employed. Important disadvantages of smaller FOVs are that they reduce image signal by the square of the FOV reduction and may produce aliasing artifact in the phase or y direction.

Certain special considerations deserve mention in this section. Surface coils allow smaller fields of view which reduce pixel dimensions when matrix is held constant. These coils should be utilized in the cervical, thoracic, and lumbar spine. Occasionally, it may be necessary to image the entire thoracic spine. Whole-volume body coil or larger FOV surface coil (>24) may be used in this instance. Butterfly, circular, or rectangular coils are available from most manufacturers.

Undesirable signal alteration may occur in the thoracolumbar spine from adjacent respiratory, abdominal peristaltic, vascular phase-shift, or pulsatile CSF flow artifacts. These may be overcome with respiratory or flow compensation and/or cardiac (peripheral pulse) gating. Cardiac gating increases acquisition time. Centrally-ordered phase encoding (COPE) or respiratory-ordered phase encoding (ROPE) are phase-reordering methods that reduce periodic respiratory artifacts degrading spinal MR.[5, 6] They do not significantly prolong scanning or image reconstruction times. Placement of the phase-encoding mechanism from left to right in the axial projection (x direction) and cephalocaudad (z direction) in the sagittal projection reduces motion artifact from bowel or abdominal wall motion affecting the spine. Surface coils themselves reduce the contribution of noise related to motion that is produced outside an area of interest.[7]

Nonorthogonal, or oblique, MR is routinely used in our spinal MR examinations, particularly in the axial plane. The early prototype of multisection oblique MR is the MAVIN method of disk evaluation. This multiple-angle, variable-interval, nonorthogonal technique allowed independent selection of slice angle and position of each image in a multislice sequence. This resulted in a tremendous reduction in imaging time with axial sections tangent to each disk space.[8] This technique, coupled with fields of view producing pixels of less than 1 mm$^2$, voxels less than 5 mm in thickness, and pulsing sequences modified as described above seem ideal and are now possible.

Some have advocated cervical foraminal evaluation with direct oblique, or nonorthogonal, images.[9] Oblique sagittal MR views are performed when radiculopathic symptoms are unresolved with routine axial or sagittal images and differentiation of "soft" disk from hard disk has not been possible with the standard protocols.[10]

## NORMAL ANATOMY

The spine is a series of vertebral bodies separated by intervertebral disks. T1-weighted images produce a homogeneous MR vertebral marrow signal hyperintense relative to adjacent disk. The T1 signal intensity of the odontoid is less than the remaining vertebral bodies. Young patients with active axial hematopoietic marrow rather than yellow marrow exhibit a less intense vertebral body signal.[11] Older patients often have poorly defined inhomogeneous regions of alternating signal intensity.[12] Occasionally, these may be manifested as relatively central foci of signal hyperintensity at each vertebral level.[13] Vertebral end-plate foci of axial focal fat deposition (hyperintense T1) or discogenic end-plate sclerosis (hypointense T1, hyperintense T2) may occur.[14] These patterns are likely related to the distribution of marrow fat and fibrous marrow change, unique to each patient. An appreciation for the normal variation of these patterns is vital.

Sagittal T1WI delineate the foramen magnum. Its anterior margin is represented either by a fat pad that lies superior to the odontoid process (Fig. 18–1) or by the signal void produced by cortical bone of the clival tip. Its posterior margin is delineated by the caudal aspect of the occipital bone, which most often appears as a tapered region of absent signal representing cortical bone. The spinal cord exhibits intermediate signal intensity on the sagittal T1 image. It is bathed by hypointense CSF (long T1), which may become isointense with cord on spin-density images. CSF hyperintensity relative to cord (long T2) when T2 weighting and flow compensation is utilized produces the "myelogram effect" (Fig. 18–4). Using larger FOVs, the cord and conus are visualized routinely on T1 and heavily T2-weighted images.

Epidural fat yields a hyperintense signal on T1WI and provides excellent soft tissue contrast with hypointense CSF and intermediate intensity of cord and nerve roots. Epidural veins and intravertebral venous plexi may appear either hypointense (flow-related signal void) or hyperintense (flow-related enhancement). The latter is more frequent with short TE, partial saturation sequences.

The intervertebral disk has a central gel-like nucleus pulposus and peripheral laminar fibers composing the annulus fibrosus. The normal disk exhibits intermediate signal intensity on T1WI. A black line occurs at an interface between the vertebral end-plate and disk. This line is composed of end-plate cortical bone, peripheral annular fibers, and in some cases, chemical shift artifact.[15] When images are obtained with repetition times less than 200 msec and echo times less than 20 msec, the annulus and nucleus may become isointense, leaving only a thin dark line of vertically oriented collagen fibers.[8] A central region of signal hyperintensity is seen in the intervertebral disk on T2WI (Fig. 18–7 and Fig. 18–8). It was initially thought this region corresponded to the well-hydrated nucleus while a peripheral black rim corresponded to the less well-hydrated annulus.[16] Recent work suggests that this distinction between nucleus and annulus may not be real.[12] A cleft is present in most adult disks on T2WI. The cleft is a thin line of low signal that indents the anterior and mid portion of the higher signal intervertebral disk (Fig. 18–8). The cleft may communicate posteriorly in 80% of cases. The cleft is absent in the infant spine, appears in the adult spine after the third decade, and likely represents normal invagination of annular material into the nuclear matrix.[17] The cleft is a useful anatomic landmark and can be obliterated in pathological processes such as disk-space infection.[18] In the axial projection, the normal disk is concave posteriorly (Figs. 18–9 and 18–10), but may exhibit slight posterior convexity from L5 to S1.

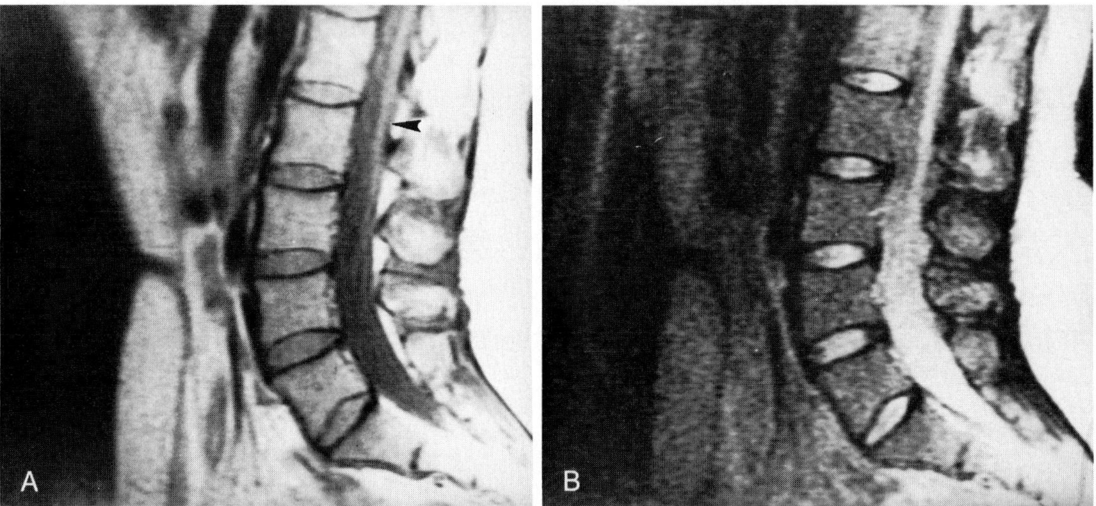


**Figure 18–7. Normal sagittal lumbar anatomy.** *A* and *B,* Multiecho sagittal lumbar N(H)WI and T2WI (TR 2000/TE 20/80) (1.5 T). Disks become hyperintense proceeding from N(H)WI to T2WI image, whereas vertebral marrow signal decreases. Without flow compensation, as in this case, distinction between cauda equina nerve roots (arrowhead) and CSF is more easily made on N(H)WI than T2WI image. With flow compensation, the converse is true.

**Figure 18–8. Normal sagittal vertebral cleft.** Mid-sagittal T2WI surface coil, lumbar spine. The normal intervertebral cleft is seen as a thin line of signal hypointensity that indents the anterior to mid portion of the hyperintense intervertebral disk (arrowhead).

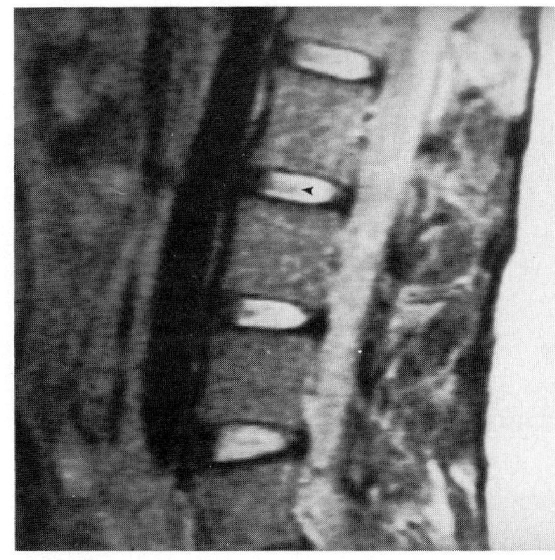

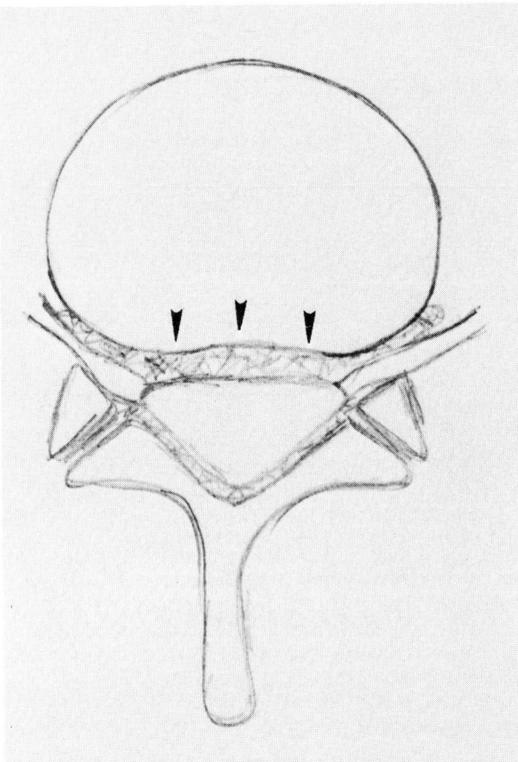

**Figure 18–9. Axial schematic of a normal intervertebral disk.** The central, gel-like, nucleus pulposus is surrounded by laminar fibers of the annulus fibrosus. The normal concave margin of the disk is identified (arrowheads), although at L5-S1, a convex posterior margin may be present. The outer annular fibers contribute to the peripheral hypointense signal of disk margins on MR.

## THE ABNORMAL INTERVERTEBRAL DISK

(Table 18–1)

MR of intervertebral disks requires knowledge of T1 and T2 characteristics of the normal and degenerated disk. The nucleus pulposus of the normal disk is 85% to 90% water in the first two decades of life and decreases to 70% with age and degeneration. Water content of the normal annulus is 78% and decreases to 70% with age. The nucleus cannot truly be separated from the annulus on T2WI. The normal hyperintense disk signal diminishes with disk degeneration or dessication on T2-weighted images (Fig. 18–5).[19] All herniated disks eventually degenerate and dessicate, but MR has shown that many asymptomatic dessicated disks are not herniated.

The nucleus pulposus may lose its usual turgor. The adjacent annulus becomes less elastic and bulges beyond the posterior margin of adjacent vertebral body. The posteriorly bulging disk usually develops a convex margin but may occasionally retain a midline concavity in the axial projection (Fig. 18–11). The sagittal appearance of annular bulges is less familiar to most radiologists. Extension of disk signal posterior to the posterior vertebral body margin on virtually every sagittal image is apparent. An-

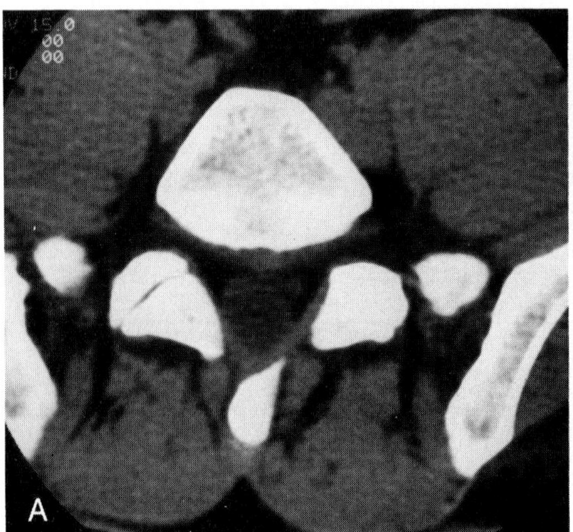


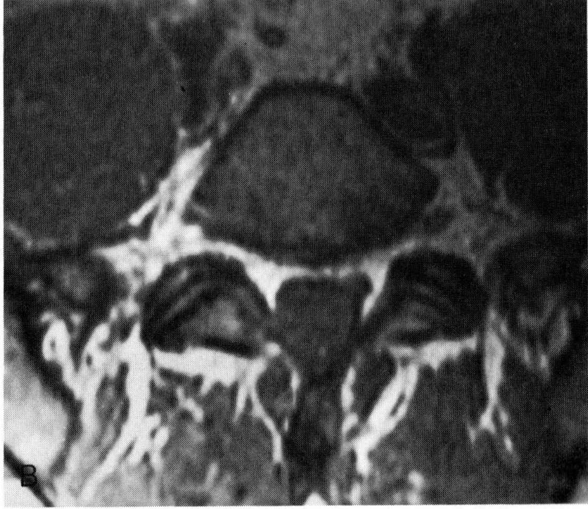


**Figure 18–10. Normal axial lumbar anatomy.** *A,* Axial CT (L5-S1). *B,* Axial T1WI (TR 600/TE 20) (L5-S1). The posterior disk margin is slightly convex. The hypodense epidural fat on CT is hyperintense on T1WI MR. Nerve roots and thecal sac are hypointense and of identical signal intensity on T1-weighted MR. Superior contrast resolution of MR allows clear distinction of anatomy in the anterior spinal canal.

**Table 18–1.** DIFFERENTIAL DIAGNOSIS OF DISK DISEASE BY MR

| Entity | Location | T1 Signal | T2 Signal | Additional Findings |
|---|---|---|---|---|
| Disk herniation | Anterior or lateral | +/− | ++ | Contiguity with disk material in sagittal plane; posterior displacement of hyperintense epidural veins and fat |
| Postoperative scar/ fibrosis | Posterior posterolateral +/− anterior | Chronic +/− acute + | Chronic − acute ++ | Not contiguous with disk space, poor signal match with disk in the sagittal projection; clumped nerve roots, axial projection; "twisted rope" appearance, sagittal projection |
| Pseudodisk spondylolisthesis | Anterior broad L4/L5 | +/− | ++ | Posterior margin of disk does not protrude posterior to the dorsal margin of the vertebral body below in the sagittal plane |
| Epidural veins | Anterior | +/− or − | − | Paucity of mass effect; largest in thoracic spine; T1 signal may vary owing to flow phenomena |
| Metastasis | Anterior> posterior | +/− | ++/+++ | Focal skeletal marrow signal hypointensity on T1 image |
| Dysraphism, lipoma | Posterior, anterior | +++ | +/− | Associated myelomeningocoele, thickened filum, tethered cord, dural band, skeletal anomalies |
| Neuroma | Lateral foraminal | +/− or − | +++ | Multiplicity; associated with nerve root; no contiguity with disks in sagittal plane |
| Ossified posterior logitudinal ligament (PLL) | Anterior | − | −− | +/− Associated with DISH; central and retrovertebral sagittal linear signal void; skip areas; cervical most severely affected |
| Epidural abscess | Posterior> posterolateral> anterior | +/− | + | Most often thoracolumbar; may be associated diskitis or paravertebral mass |
| Meningocele or pseudomeningocele | Posterior | − | +++ | Smooth contour, matches CSF in signal intensity; may scallop vertebral bodies |
| Epidural hemorrhage | Posterior | ++ | +++ | Thoracic most common; hematoma of the ligamentum flavum most common |
| Spur/osteophyte | Anterior | − to + | − | T1 signal intensity of osteophyte depends on amount of medullary bone within; correlation of sagittal projection with plain film necessary; ?CT required |
| Spur/diastematomyelia | Anterior | +/− | − | Associated hemicords; duplicated sac +/− associated skeletal change |
| Pantopaque | Posterior> anterior | ++ | − | Conventional radiographic correlation diagnostic |
| Lymphoma | Variable | +/− | ++ | Insinuates into foramina; paucity of skeletal signal alteration for lesion size |
| Conjoined nerve root | Anterolateral | +/− | + | Isointense with cord/sac; hyper intense T2 rim corresponds to CSF root sleeve; L5-S1 common |
| Arteriovenous malformation | Posterior> anterior | −− | −− | Characteristic flow-void in hypertrophied vessels |
| Root avulsion | Lateral | − | +++ | MR positive only with pseudomeningocele formation |

+ = increased signal.
− = decreased signal.

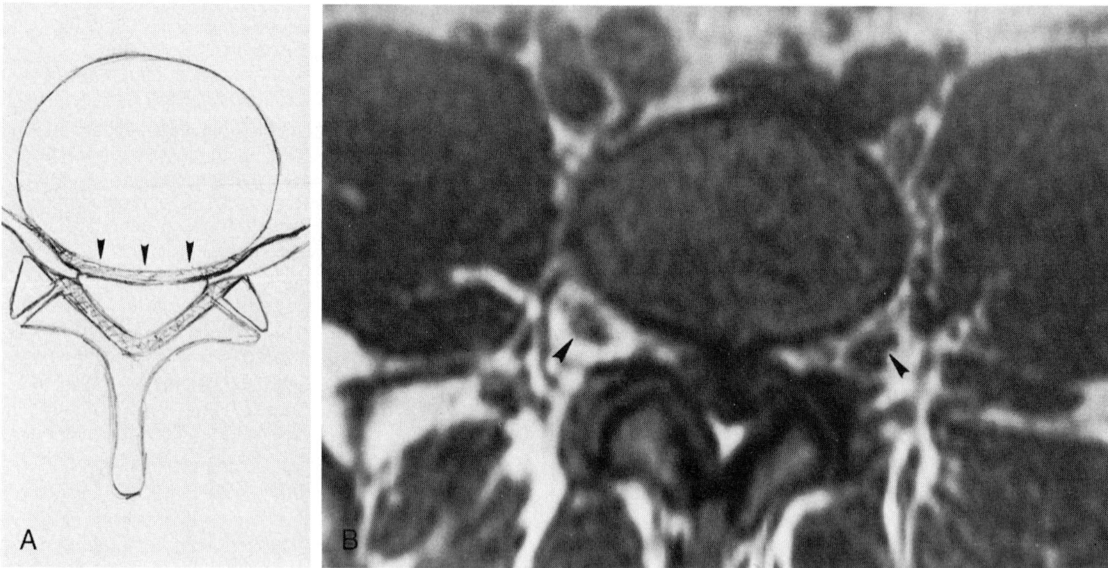


**Figure 18–11. Lumbar disk bulge: axial projection.** *A,* Axial line drawing. *B,* Axial T1WI (1.5 T). Axial schematic demonstrates a diffuse, smooth, disk bulge with a convex posterior margin of the disk space (arrowheads). Similar configuration is noted on T1WI MR. Nerve roots in *B* (arrowheads) are spared. Mild effacement of the thecal sac is present. On sagittal images, a disk bulge will appear to protrude beyond the posterior margin of adjacent vertebral bodies on multiple sections.

terior disk protrusion has been suggested as a sign favoring disk bulge over herniation in the sagittal projection; however, we have not found this sign helpful in distinguishing the two.

Nuclear material may herniate through a defect in the annulus, usually through its thinner posterior or posterolateral margin.[20] The herniated disk and its effect on thecal sac and nerve roots are appreciated on both sagittal and axial images (Figs. 18–12 to 18–19). The observer must become accustomed to identifying disk signal and nerve roots in the lateral recesses or foramina in the sagittal projection. Occasionally, it may be difficult to distinguish "hard disk" or osteophyte (Figs. 18–20 to 18–21), from soft disk herniation, since calcification and cortical bone is poorly identified on MR. We routinely interpret MR of the spine for disk disease with conventional radiographs.

A technically satisfactory MR is reportedly equivalent to CT and myelography in disk disease and spinal stenosis.[21] Therefore MR has become a complementary screening modality. This occurs despite a paucity of extradural fat in these regions and is related to superior contrast resolution and multiprojectional capability of MR. As a rule, CT or myelography or both is utilized when spondylosis is present on conventional radiographs. Otherwise, MR is the initial screening modality.

A free fragment occurs when nuclear material passes through the posterior longitudinal ligament into the epidural space (Figs. 18–16 and 18–18). MR is superior to CT in the assessment of the extruded free fragment. The sagittal images routinely available with MR alert the observer to the level at which an extruded fragment has been found. The resolution of sagittal reformatted CT is far inferior to MR. Axial images on MR delineate the extruded fragment and possible thecal sac, cord, and nerve root compromise (Fig. 18–18). Acute disk herniations may be isointense with the signal of normal disks. Chronicity may reduce the signal in disk and adjacent end-plate.[22] Although most herniated disks are of intermediate signal intensity relative to epidural fat, we, together with others, have observed signal hyperinstensity in postoperative disk reprolapse and in sequestered disks.[23] Disk signal on T2WI likely depends on disk size, age, and water content. One must be careful not to confuse true disk signal increase from displacement of adjacent epidural fat or epidural veins. These veins may exhibit flow-related signal increase facilitated by posterior disk effacement and are particularly apparent in the sagittal projection (Fig. 18–12).[24]

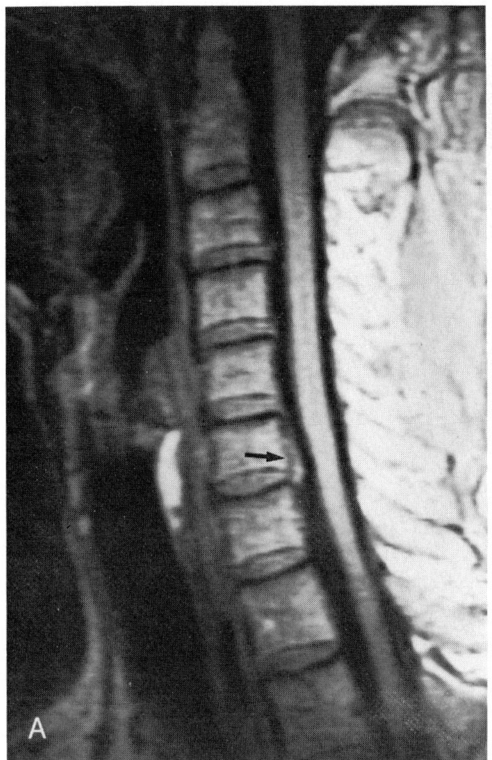


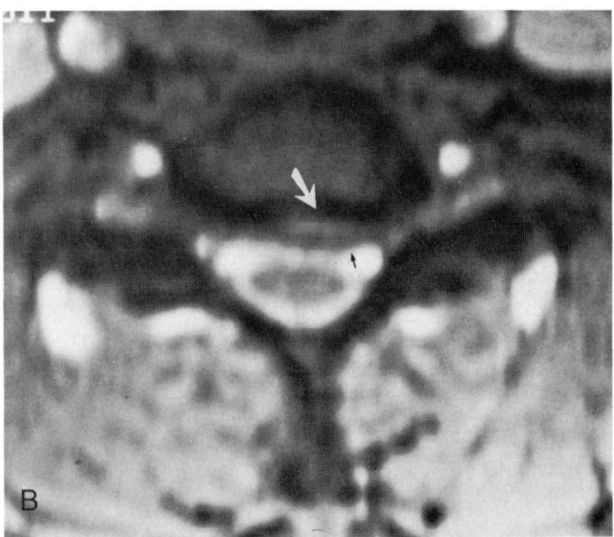


**Figure 18–12. Central and leftward C6-C7 soft disk herniation.** A 58-year-old man with left arm pain (1.5 T). *A,* Sagittal T1WI (TR 600/TE 20). *B,* Axial fast-scan (flip angle 12°/TR 30/TE 13). Sagittal T1WI shows a hyperintense flow effect in an anterior epidural vein (arrow), an indirect sign of mass effect anteriorly from spur or disk. Axial fast-scan confirms the presence of central and leftward soft disk (black arrow), which differs in signal from the margin of the anterior vertebral body and disk space (white arrow). (Courtesy of S. J. Pomeranz, M.D., Christ Hospital, Cincinnati, Ohio.)

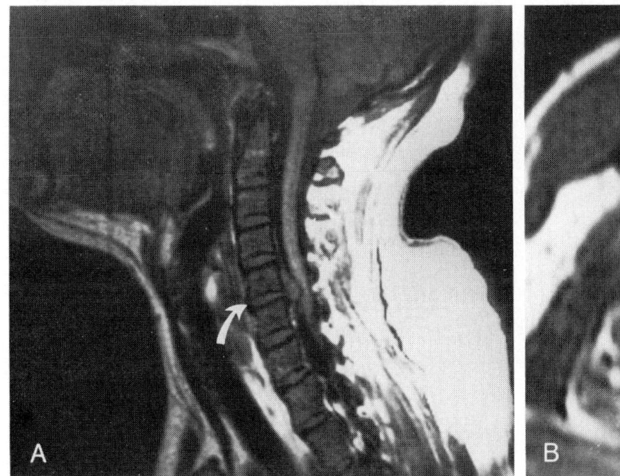


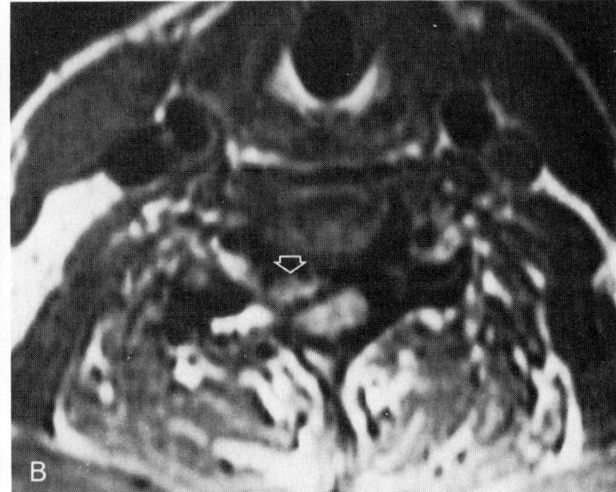


**Figure 18–13. Herniated cervical disk.** *A,* Sagittal T1WI (1.5 T). *B,* Axial N(H)WI. At the C5-6 level (curved arrow) a focal, rounded, extradural mass effaces the intermediate signal intensity spinal cord and the hypointense thecal sac. This mass appears slightly more hyperintense (open arrow) on the axial N(H)WI image and displaces the cord posteriorly and leftward.

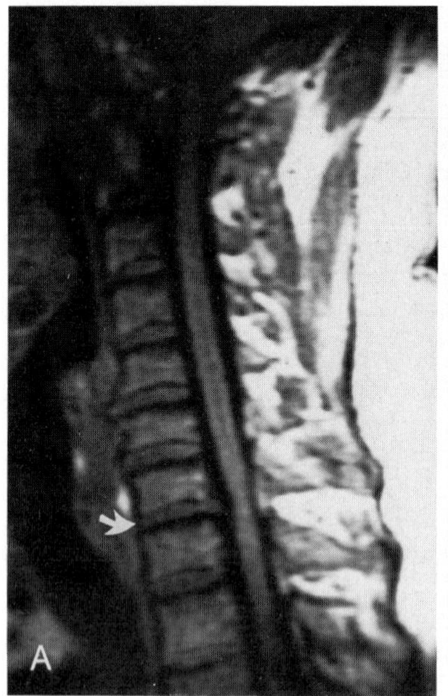


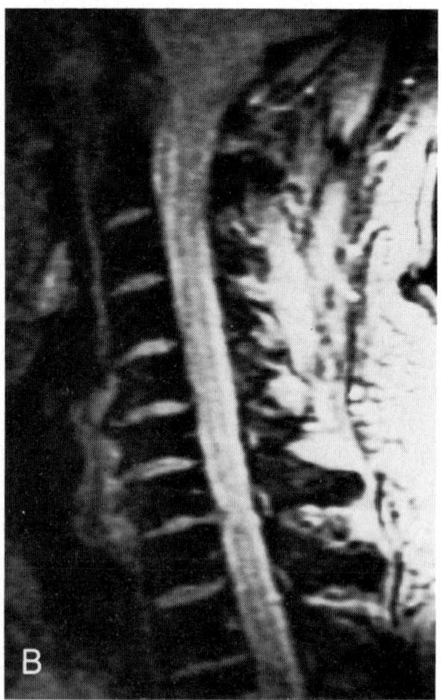


**Figure 18–14. Soft disk herniation.** A 27-year-old man with rightward C7-T1 radiculopathy (1.5 T). *A,* Sagittal T1WI (TR 600/TE 20). *B,* Fast-scan (TR 30/TE 12/flip 13°). Focal posterior disk exhibits intermediate signal intensity on fast-scan image and T1 (arrow) at C7-T1. With hard disk or spur, hypointense signal of bone would cover disk signal above and below on fast-scan. (Courtesy of S. J. Pomeranz, M.D., Christ Hospital, Cincinnati, Ohio.)

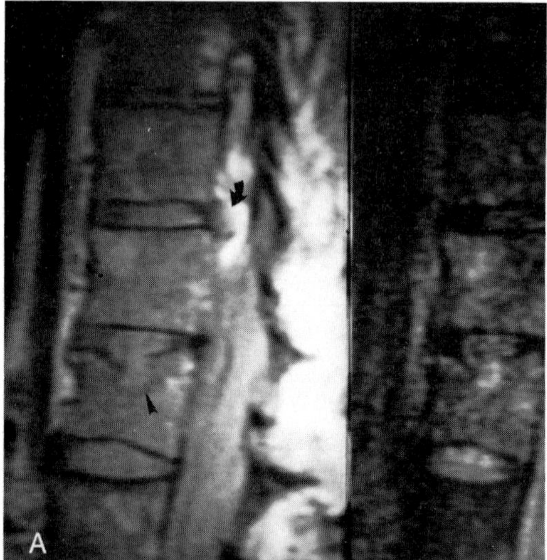


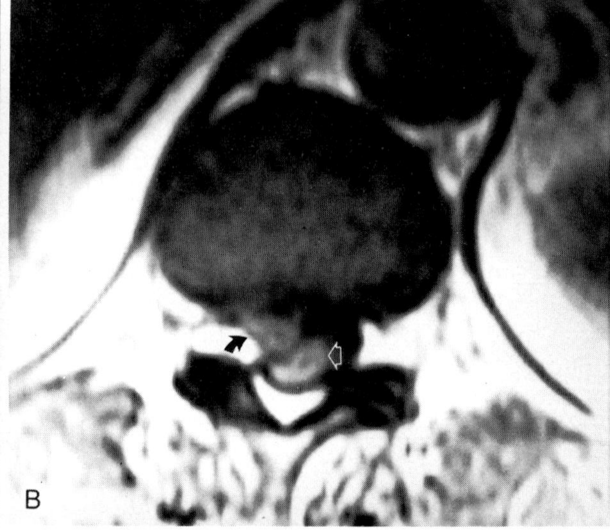


**Figure 18–15. Herniated thoracic disk.** *A,* Sagittal T1WI (TR 600/TE 20) (1.5 T). *B,* Axial T1WI. Extradural mass at the T8–T9 level has occurred rightward and posteriorly (curved arrows). It effaces the hypointense thecal sac and intermediate signal intensity cord (open arrow) leftward. An incidental Schmorl's node one level below is demonstrated (arrowhead). (Courtesy of S. J. Pomeranz, M.D. Christ Hospital, Cincinnati, Ohio.)

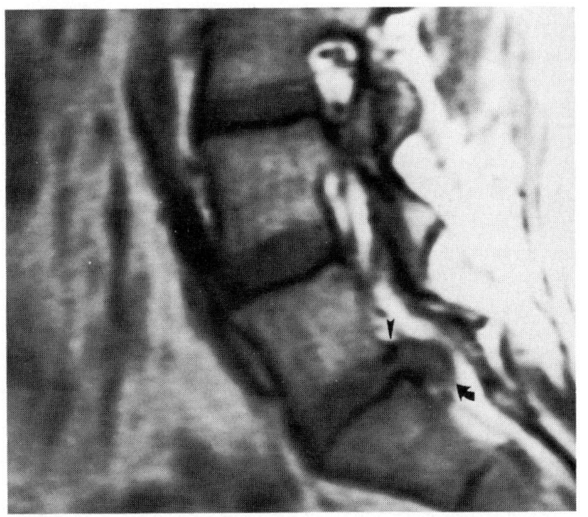

**Figure 18–16. Extruded L5-S1 disk fragment.** A 32-year-old woman with sudden onset of left leg and back pain (1.5 T). Sagittal T1WI (TR 600/TE 20). Intermediate signal intensity disk is extruded (arrow) into the lateral recess fat at the L5-S1 level. The point where the hypointense ligament (arrowhead) has ruptured is apparent on its superior margin. (Courtesy of S. J. Pomeranz, M.D., Christ Hospital, Cincinnati, Ohio.)

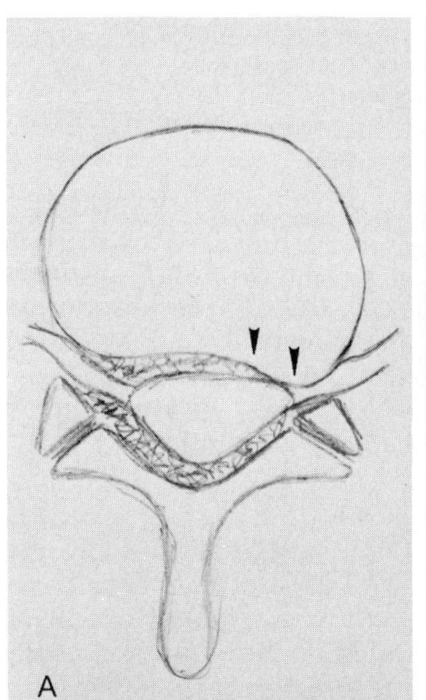


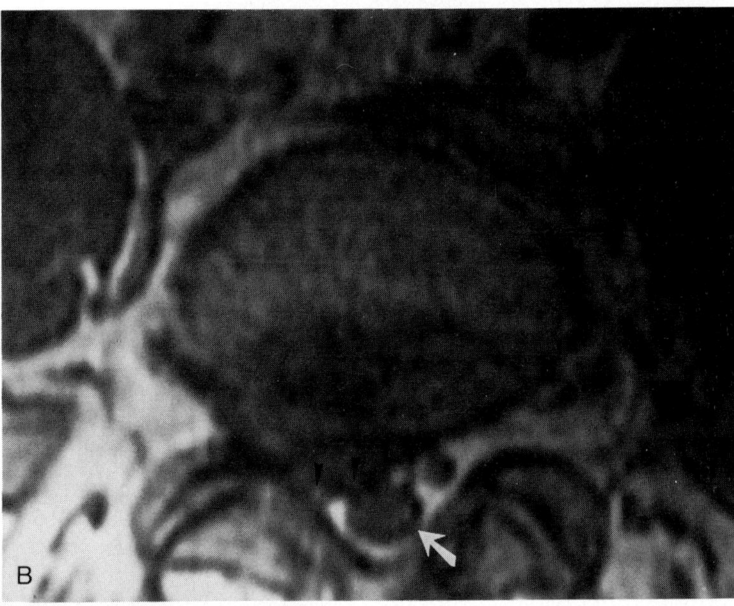


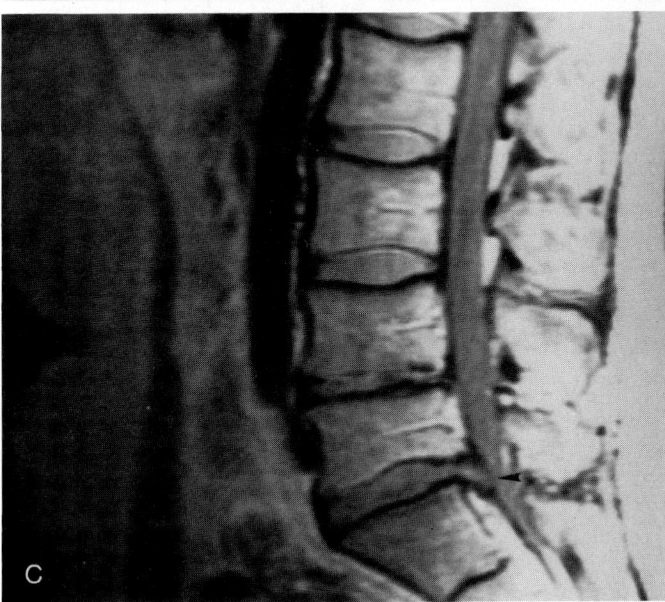


**Figure 18–17. Lumbar disk herniation.** *A,* Axial line diagram. *B,* Axial T1WI (1.5 T). *C,* Sagittal N(H)WI. Axial schematic illustrates focality of posterolateral disk herniation (arrowheads) effacing the ipsilateral nerve roots. Actual rightward herniation on T1WI demonstrates focal disk herniation and effacement of the ipsilateral nerve root. The thecal sac (arrow) is virtually spared. Sagittal MR shows posterior displacement of disk material (arrowhead) beyond the posterior margins of adjacent vertebral bodies. Disk above is degenerated and exhibits diminished disk height. Herniation on sagittal images is inferred by focality, i.e., the abnormality is present on only one or two sections, and the disk position returns to normal on other adjacent sections.

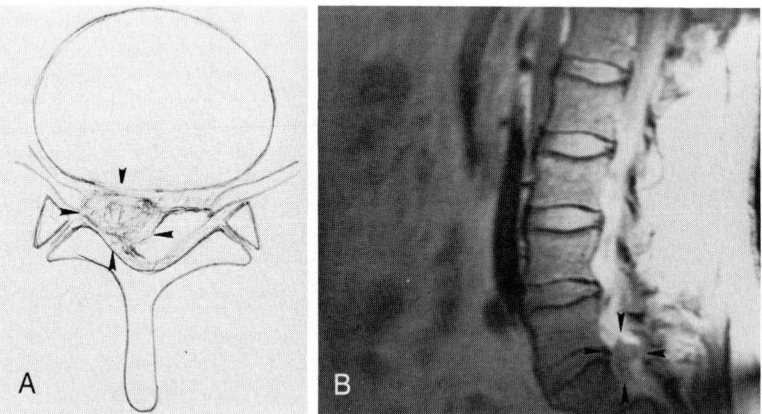


**Figure 18–18. Extruded lumbar disk.** *A,* Axial line drawing. *B,* Sagittal N(H)WI (TR 2000/TE 20) (1.5 T). Axial schematic shows how an extruded disk fragment positioned posteriorly and beyond the posterior longitudinal ligament appears "free floating" (arrowheads). Sagittal MR shows fragment lying separate from the L5-S1 disk itself and surrounded by the hyperintense epidural fat of the right lateral spinal recess (arrowheads).

## Spondylosis and Radiculopathy

CT without intrathecal contrast has been disappointing in the diagnosis of soft disk herniation in the cervicothoracic spine. CT is still superior in the evaluation of bony foraminal and recess stenosis since both hard and soft disk disease are difficult to diagnose with MR in these lateral regions. With regard to affected foramina, oblique views may be helpful. Therefore, in patients with excessive hypertrophic bone formation on plain film, CT is more accurate in patients with radiculopathic symptoms. Patients without excessive spondylitic disease on conventional radiographs are examined with MR first (Fig. 18–22). Only when MR is equivocal do we proceed with noncontrast high resolution CT. The combination of multiplanar, thin-section, multiecho, surface coil MR and noncontrast CT is as accurate as water-soluble myelogaphy followed by CT.[25] MR is often selected as the first and only examination in thoracic spine evaluation. MR is the preferred examination in almost all cases of myelopathy, including those related to bony cord compromise.

The contrast resolution of MR permits visualization of dorsal and ventral nerve roots as they exit from the cervical cord and course laterally to the neural foramen.[26] This anatomy is particularly well demonstrated on N(H)WI and T2WI (see Fig. 18–6). Hyperintense fat in the neural foramen is seen anteriorly but not posteroinferiorly to nerve roots. T2-weighted axial high-resolution images illustrate high signal CSF that bathes the cord and nerve roots. Effacement of these structures is readily apparent in the axial projection. The spinal facets are well delineated in the axial projection, and joint fluid resulting from facet arthropathy is visualized with MR, not CT.[27] We now routinely use fast-scan MR T2WI spin-echo in axial cervical spine evaluation to obtain a T2 effect.

The changes that accompany the aging spine and the degenerative spine have already been discussed (Fig. 18–23). Focal poorly defined regions of diminished vertebral body signal (fibrous marrow involution) and increased signal (focal fat deposition) are part of these processes.[28] With disk degeneration or dessication, these signal alterations may be positioned at disks and end-plates, simulating diskitis or other pathology. One must avoid diagnosing disk dehydration on parasagittal sections because volume averaging may produce hypointense disk signal.[29] Schmorl's node formation is identified in the sagittal projection by its contiguity and similar signal intensity with adjacent disk (Fig. 18–23). These Schmorl's nodes exhibit obtuse margins with the vertebral end-plate, further assisting in their differentiation from entities such as eccentric vertebral body metastases.

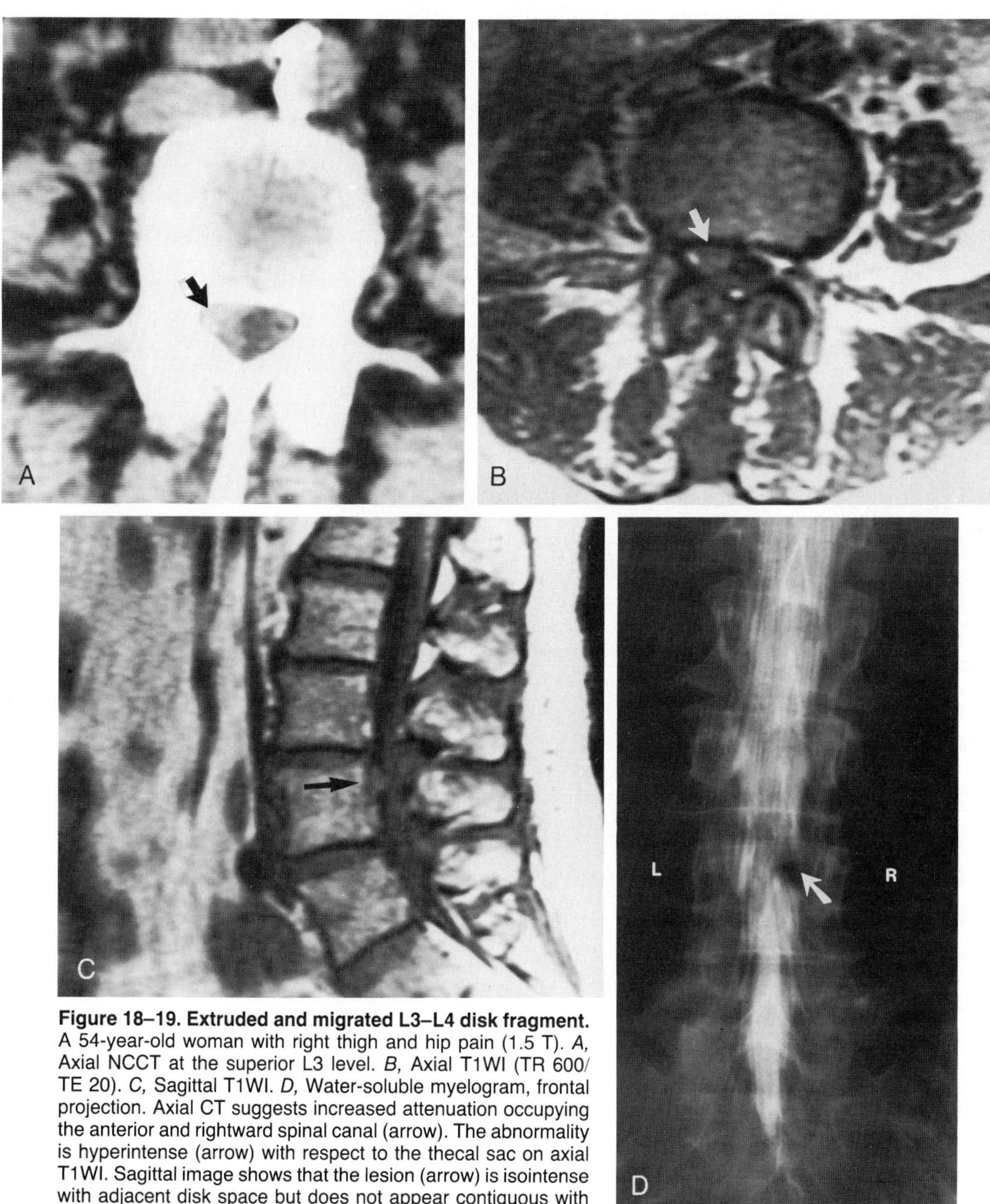


**Figure 18–19. Extruded and migrated L3–L4 disk fragment.** A 54-year-old woman with right thigh and hip pain (1.5 T). *A,* Axial NCCT at the superior L3 level. *B,* Axial T1WI (TR 600/TE 20). *C,* Sagittal T1WI. *D,* Water-soluble myelogram, frontal projection. Axial CT suggests increased attenuation occupying the anterior and rightward spinal canal (arrow). The abnormality is hyperintense (arrow) with respect to the thecal sac on axial T1WI. Sagittal image shows that the lesion (arrow) is isointense with adjacent disk space but does not appear contiguous with it. Eccentric myelographic defect is apparent (white arrow). (Courtesy of S. J. Pomeranz, M.D., Christ Hospital, Cincinnati, Ohio.)

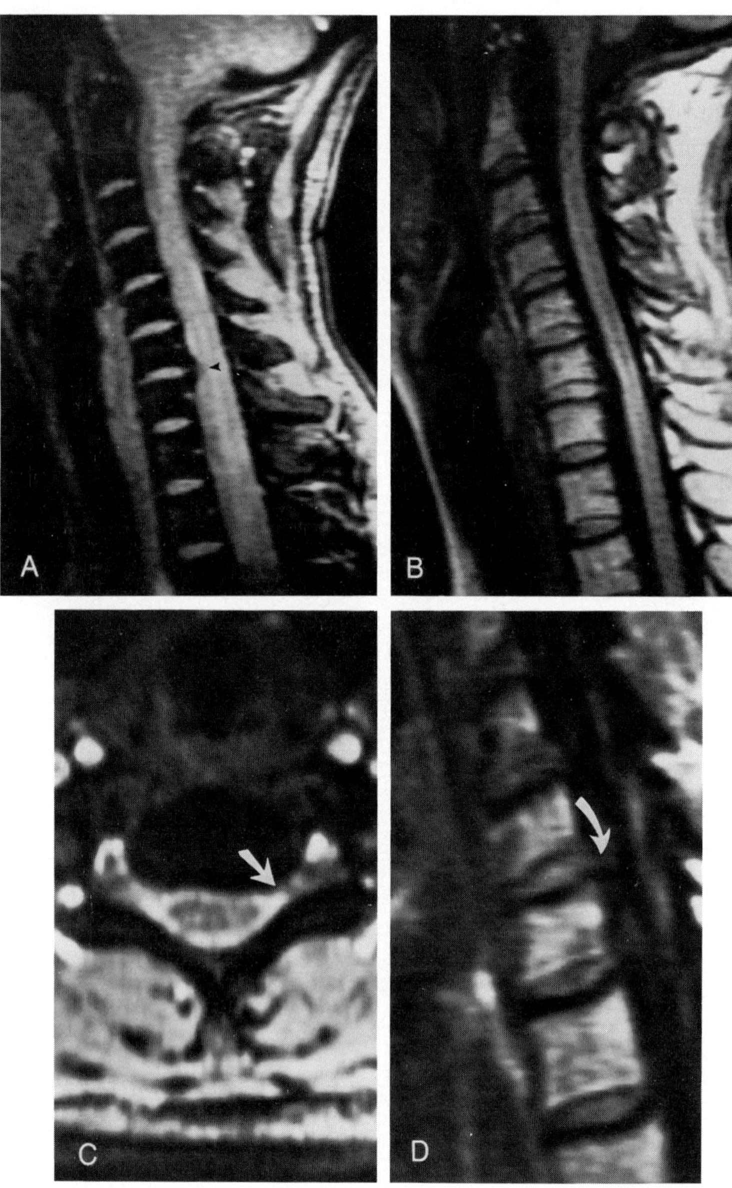


**Figure 18–20. "Hard disk," or calcified spur.** A 39-year-old man with left-sided neck pain (1.5 T). *A,* Sagittal fast-scan (TR 25/TE 12.5/flip angle 15°). B, T1W1 (TR 600/TE 20). *C,* Nonorthogonal axial fast-scan (TR 30/TE 13/Flip angle 12°). *D,* Sagittal T1WI. Focal contour alteration (arrowhead) at C6–7 appears covered above and below by hypointense spurs. Axial image shows central and leftward thecal sac effacement by signal (arrow) that matches normal hypointense bone and correlates with eccentric spur (curved arrow). (Courtesy of S. J. Pomeranz, M.D., Christ Hospital, Cincinnati, Ohio.)

## Spinal Stenosis

Spinal stenosis occurs when there is narrowing of the spinal canal, lateral recesses, or intervertebral foramina, The narrowing may be produced by soft tissue or bone and may be congenital, acquired, or both. Measurements of the normal anteroposterior, transverse, and cross-sectional areas of the spine are available in the literature.[30] Routine strict application of these measurements is discouraged since normal anatomic variation may make application difficult in many cases. Rather than evaluating the size of a bony canal, it is more important to evaluate the relationship of roots, cord, or thecal sac to the canal.

Magnetic resonance is an effective method of evaluating patients for spinal stenosis, particularly in the cervicothoracic region, where a paucity of extradural fat exists. Axial T2WIs or fast-scans provide an intrathecal contrast effect that is useful and noninvasive. Spin-density images of a multiecho sequence outline the bony anatomy. Compromise of hyperintense CSF bathing cord and roots is readily appreciated on T2WI (Fig. 18–24). Since cortical bone pro-

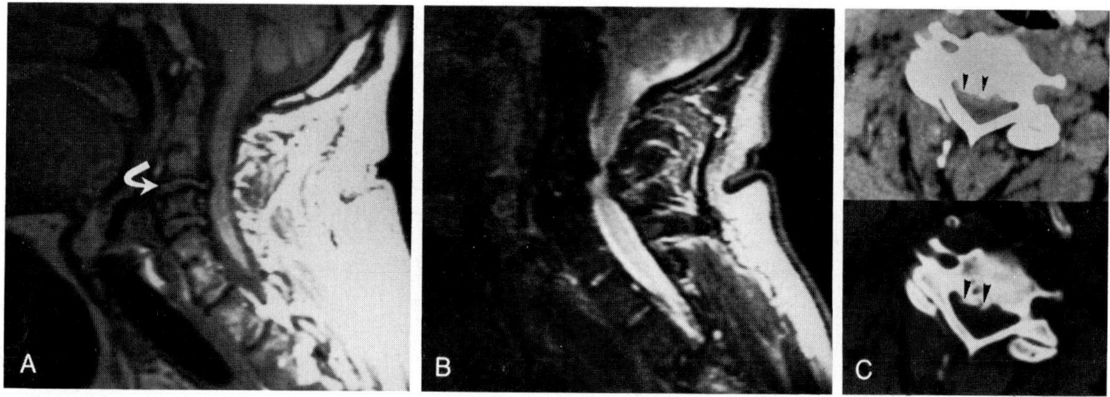


**Figure 18–21. Cervical "hard disk," or spur.** *A* and *B*, Sagittal multiecho N(H)WI and T2WI (TR 2000/TE 20/80) (1.5 T). *C*, Axial soft tissue and bone window setting CT (C3-4). Sagittal MR shows posterior relationship of disk material to the adjacent vertebral bodies and associated cord effacement. However, on T2WI the C3-4 disk space is uniformly hypointense. Axial CT confirms that the abnormality represents "hard disk," or spur. This case emphasizes the need to interpret sagittal MR with axial sections and lateral conventional radiographs or even with axial CT in selected patients.

vides no signal, examinations should be interpreted with conventional radiographs. Nevertheless, ossific structures such as posterior longitudinal ligament calcification are recognized as linear longitudinal retrovertebral signal hypointensity, well demonstrated on T2 sagittal images. Correlative CT without intrathecal contrast may be required to adequately define general bony anatomy, and we prefer high-resolution CT for bony stenosis in the lumbar spine. Compromise of spinal contents by soft tissue structures such as bulging or herniated disk, ligamentous hypertrophy or any combination of these may be delineated on T1, or proton-density, images alone (Fig. 18–25).

## Synovial Cyst

Synovial cysts are usually a manifestation of osteoarthritis of the synovial-lined apophyseal joint. Along with joint space narrowing, sclerosis, and hypertrophic spur formation, hyperplasia of the synovial membrane and resultant cyst formation can be seen. Most patients exhibit high-signal interfacet fluid on T2WI. The cyst itself appears as a posterior eccentric extradural mass exhibiting intermediate or even short T1 (hyperintense) and long T2 relaxation. These signal characteristics most likely relate to the high protein content of these lesions (Fig. 18–26).

## Arachnoiditis

Arachnoiditis is a cause of pain in 5% to 15% of postoperative patients.[31] Etiologies include infection, intrathecal steroids or anesthesia, trauma, surgery and hemorrhage.[32] The MR appearance of arachnoiditis (Fig. 18–27) is not too dissimilar from CT. T1- or heavily T2-weighted axial images will demonstrate either nerve root clumping, a

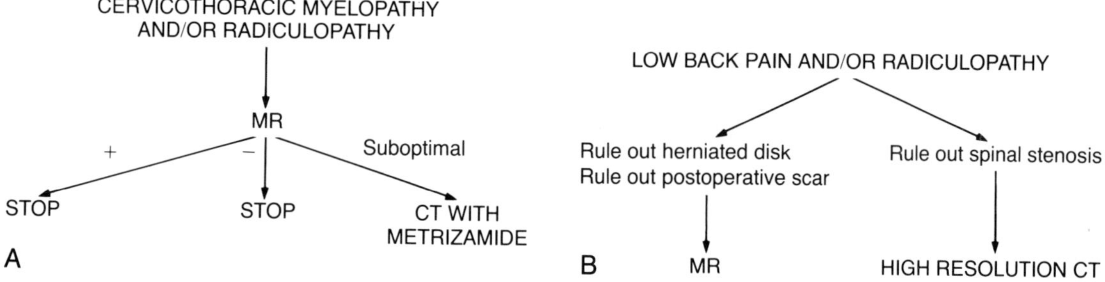


**Figure 18–22.** General imaging algorithm for spinal diagnosis. (*A* and *B*).

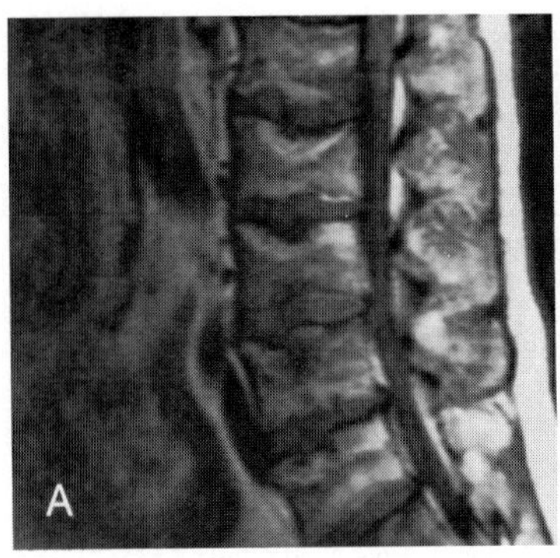

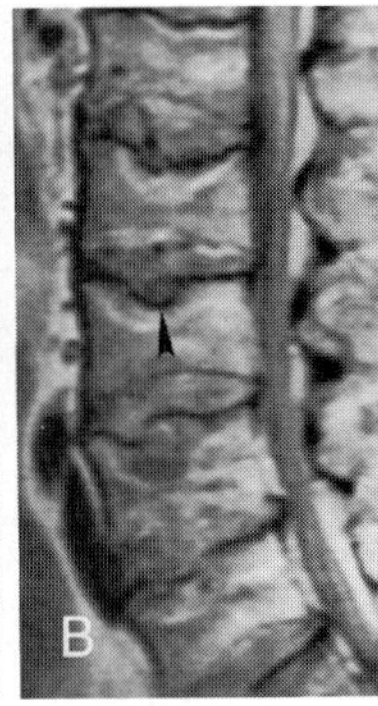

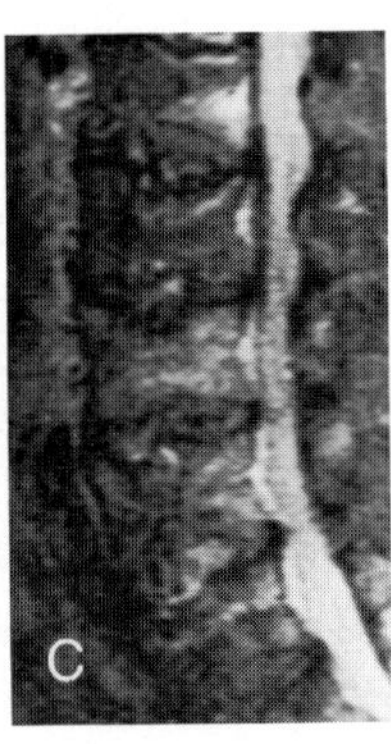


**Figure 18–23. Scheuermann's disease.** A 22-year-old man with back pain (1.5 T). *A,* Sagittal T1WI. *B* and *C,* Sagittal multiecho N(H)WI and T2WI. Schmorl's node formation (arrowhead) at every end-plate level is apparent, with a linear pattern of focal juxta–end-plate signal hyperintensity compatible with premature degenerative change and focal axial fat deposition. (Courtesy of S. J. Pomeranz, M.D., Christ Hospital, Cincinnati, Ohio.)

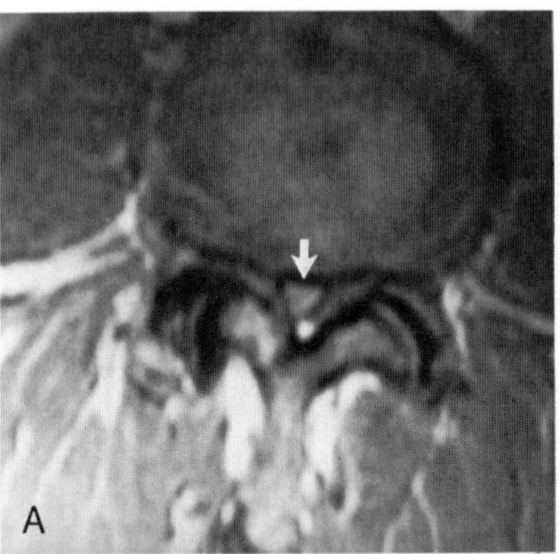

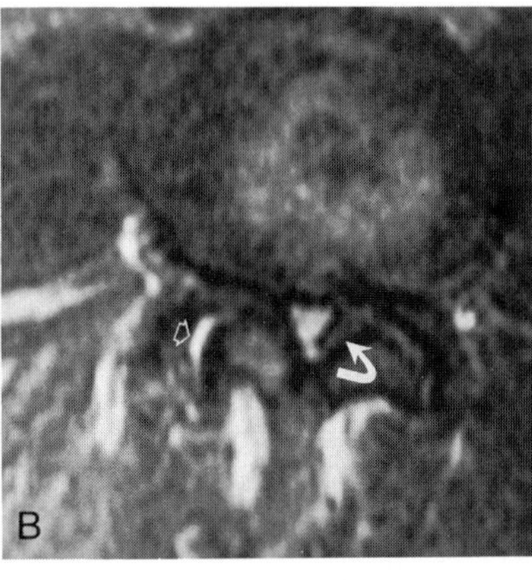

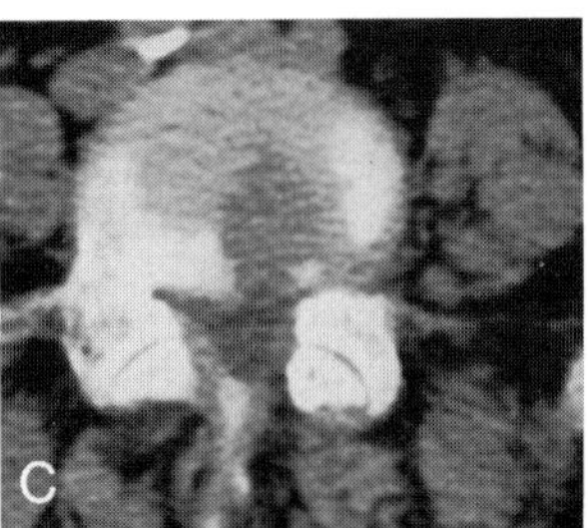


**Figure 18–24. Central lumbar canal stenosis.** *A,* Axial N(H)WI (TR 2000/TE 20) (1.5 T). *B,* Axial T1WI (TR 2000/TE 80). *C,* Axial noncontrast CT. Axial MR images at L4-5 show central canal stenosis, but the contribution of bony elements, ligamentum flavum (curved arrow), and disk bulge is difficult to determine. Thecal sac (arrow) and fluid in the right facet joint (clear arrow) are identified. CT more accurately allows assessment of contribution by facets, ligaments, and disk bulge.

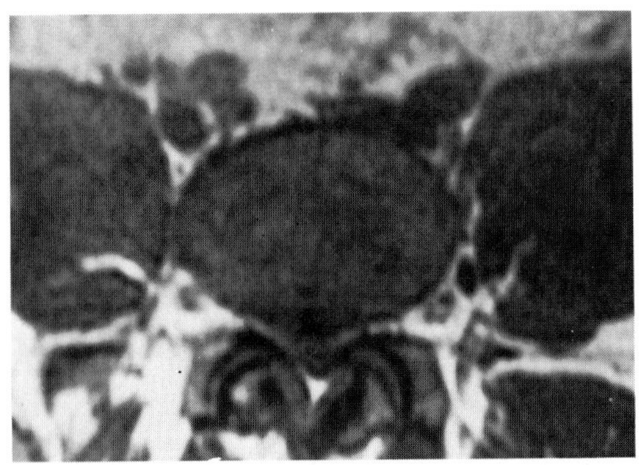

**Figure 18–25. Lumbar canal stenosis; subligamentous disk herniation L4–L5.** A 42-year-old man with rightward radiculopathy (1.5 T). Axial T1WI. Rightward subligamentous disc herniation and facet hypertrophy has compromised the spinal canal area.

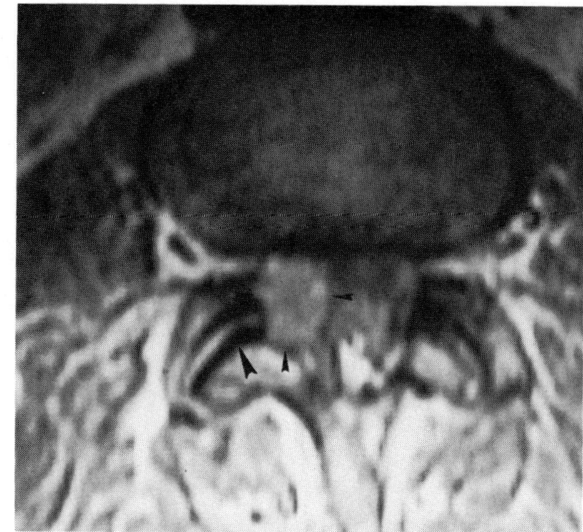

**Figure 18–26. Synovial cyst.** A 62-year-old woman with right-sided radiculopathy (1.5 T). Axial N(H)WI (TR 1800/TE 20) shows an extradural mass at the L4-5 level. The mass (arrowheads) is hyperintense relative to the adjacent disk space and lies virtually contiguous to the adjacent right facet joint (large arrowhead). Lesion hyperintensity may reflect high protein and mucin contents. (Courtesy of S. J. Pomeranz, M.D., Christ Hospital, Cincinnati, Ohio.)

nondependent nerve root position, or a peripheral orientation around the thecal sac margins.[33, 34] Familiarity with a normal appearance of nerve roots at various levels on sagittal and axial MR is crucial.[35] With axial projections at the L2 and L3 levels, nerve roots layer in the dependent position. However, as one progresses caudally, the L4 and L5 levels allow identification of individual nerve roots, some of which may be peripherally oriented in the thecal sac.

A "twisted rope" appearance of nerve

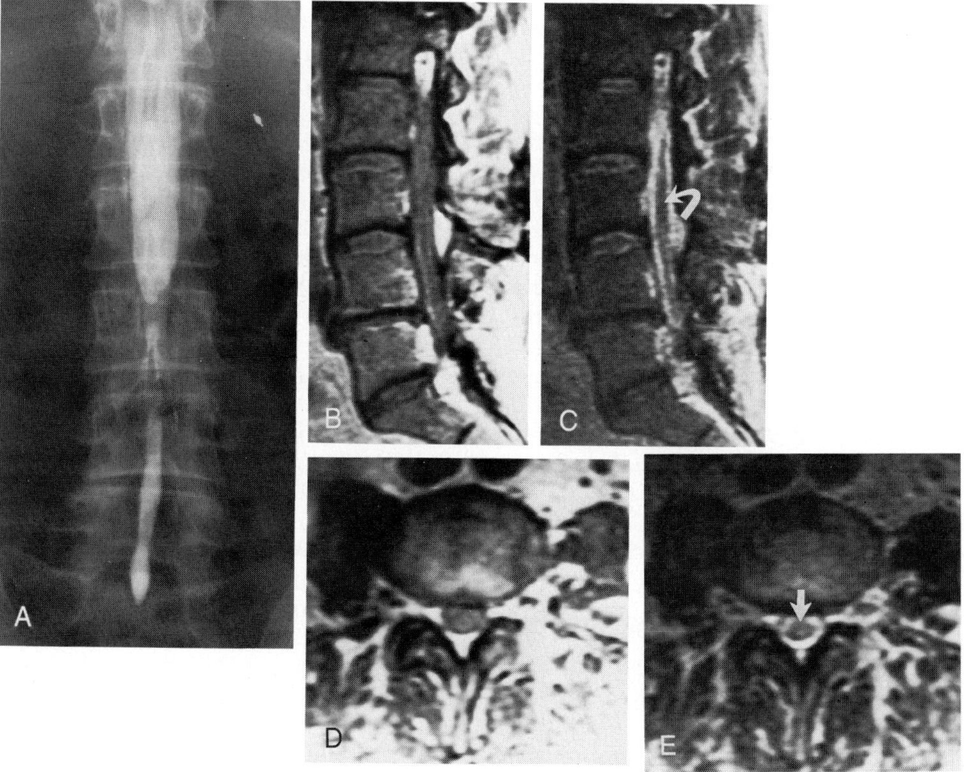


**Figure 18–27. Arachnoiditis.** A 31-year-old woman with chronic back pain and lower extremity weakness. *A,* Water-soluble myelogram, frontal projection. *B* and *C,* Sagittal N(H)WI and T2WI (TR 1800/TE 20/80). *D* and *E,* Axial N(H)WI and T2WI. Thecal sac tapering is present from L-3 through S-1 on the myelogram. Intermediate signal intensity nerve roots are clumped (curved arrow) on sagittal T2WI. "Pseudocord" due to nerve root clumping is apparent on axial T2WI at the L-3 level (arrow). (Courtesy of S. J. Pomeranz, M.D., Christ Hospital, Cincinnati, Ohio.)

roots may appear in the sagittal orientation in those patients who have received accidental subdural Pantopaque injection or patients with other forms of severe arachnoidits.[36] Extradural scar is a frequent accompanying feature of the spine with arachnoiditis. The signal intensity of scar is variable and is discussed subsequently. On MR the most severe form of arachnoiditis appears as a soft tissue mass of intermediate signal in the subarachnoid space. Nerve roots and even CSF signal may not be identifiable. Bizarre CSF flow phemenona may occur adjacent to and around areas of septation or scar. In these cases, complete block may be present myelographically. Foci of hyperintense signal on T1WI may represent trapped residual Pantopaque from prior examinations. The diagnosis of arachnoiditis on MR should never be undertaken from one axial image. Both T1- and T2-weighted axial and sagittal images are helpful in this regard.

### Chymopapain

The disk space narrows, and degenerative changes are accelerated on plain film, CT, or MR following chymopapain injection.[37] In some but not all cases, there is reduction or encroachment by disk on adjacent subarachnoid space. Reduction in disk size and symptomatic improvement correlate poorly; however, patients who exhibit symptomatic improvement can demonstrate diminished disk height and width or increased signal intensity around the disk margin.[38] MR imaging has shown that in nearly 25% of injected intervertebral discs, T2WI demonstrate adjacent end-plate hyperintensity and T1 hypointensity. This signal alteration may result from chymopapain-induced inflammation or end-plate edema. These changes may mimic those occurring in disk space infection, a complication present in 2.5% of chemonucleation patients.[39] Occasionally, end-plate signal hyperintensity on T1WI may result from focal marrow fat deposition.

The progressive signal hypointensity of the disk itself, which is produced on the T2WI following chymopapain instillation is likely related to a combination of diminished mucopolysaccharide content and water loss. Acutely, disk spaces exhibit signal hyperintensity on T2WI. Not infrequently, MR coincidentally demonstrates the hyperintense signal of a sequestered disk fragment in the postchemonucleolysis patient.[40] Sequestered disk fragment is a major cause of chymopapain failure.

### The Postoperative Spine

The spectrum of failed back surgery syndrome includes reprolapse (15%), spinal stenosis (50%), arachnoiditis (10%), and epidural fibrosis (7%).[41] Limitation of function and intractable pain may occur in 10% to 40% of postoperative spine cases. Postoperative laminectomy is easily recognized by the absence of normal cortical bone, signal void, and absence of hyperintense marrow on T1WI. With laminotomy, only absence of the ligamentum flavum may denote previous surgery. The thecal sac may protrude into the laminectomy defect. Immediately in the postoperative state, intermediate signal is present anterior to the thecal sac at the surgical site. This soft tissue merges smoothly with the posterior disk margins on sagittal T1WI but exhibits signal hyperintensity on T2WI. Mass and adjacent disk together may appear as large as the original disk herniation. This signal and contour alteration progressively decreases over time. The normal hypointense rim representing the posterior longitudinal ligament and outer posterior annular fibers are interrupted at the diskectomy site on T2WI sagittal MR in the acute postoperative phase. This finding becomes less apparent over time. At the curettage site, a linear tract of signal hyperintensity extending into the nucleus is apparent on axial T2WI. Progressive diminution in disk space occurs over time, and diminished signal may later be seen on sagittal T2WI. With simple diskectomy, a minority of patients will eventually exhibit signal hypointensity on T1WI and hyperintensity on T2WI at adjacent end-plates. At a foraminotomy site, intermediate signal intensity surrounding the nerve root may be present on T1WI and hyperintense signal may appear on T2WI. Sagittal images are most helpful in distinguishing this soft tissue process from lateral disk reprolapse.

Additional iatrogenic factors following back surgery require description on MR.[42] Bone fusions may have a variable appearance. Allografts tend to show diminished signal on T1WI and T2WI, whereas autografts exhibit signal hyperintensity on T1WI because they contain yellow marrow. Old, solid, bony fusion masses exhibit confluent foci of signal hypointensity on T1WI and T2WI but may also contain foci of hyperintensity on T1WI owing to the presence of marrow.

The presence of soft tissue signal with hyperintensity on T1WI and T2WI should arouse suspicion of soft tissue hemorrhage. The signal intensity of epidural scar is variable and depends on its age and degree of hemorrhagic component. Most acute scars are intermediate on T1WI and hyperintense on T2WI. With time, progressive decrease in signal intensity occurs on both T1 and T2WI unless a hemorrhagic component is present. Differentiation of scar from disk is subsequently discussed. Quite commonly, posterior fluid collections or pseudomeningocele formation may occur. Homogeneous T1 and T2 relaxation prolongation is appreciated and may differ slightly from the normal CSF in the subarachnoid space owing to the absence of transmitted pulsations in the extraspinal fluid collection. Free fat grafts are easily identified by their signal intensity matching adjacent subcutaneous fat. Frequently, these exhibit a circular pseudocapsule and lie posterior to the thecal sac. The fat grafts may be surrounded by foci of intermediate signal intensity scar. Metallic artifacts frequently accompany prior spinal surgery even when no metal is appreciated on conventional radiographs. These artifacts may be related to flakes or shavings from the metallic drill bits that are used to improve surgical exposure in this region.

The postoperative findings of arachnoiditis have already been addressed. The presence of exuberant scar with soft tissue, intermediate signal replacing the thecal sac, an "empty" sac, or clumped nerve roots should raise suspicion of this diagnosis. Frequently, hyperintense signal on T1WI and hypointense signal on T2WI may be located at sites of postoperative arachnoiditis or simple postoperative diskectomy and represent residual Pantopaque from prior examination. Gelfoam (absorable gelatin sponge) is frequently placed at postoperative surgical sites and exhibits hypointense signal on both T1WI and T2WI. With time, progressive diminution in size of this hypointense focus often occurs. Similarly, methyl methacrylate exhibits hypointense signal on both T1WI and T2WI.[43] The superiority of CT for imaging cortical bone makes this the modality of choice when assessing the stability, position, and status of neural elements after fusion.

Disk reprolapse, unlike postoperative scar, is said not to enhance following high-dose intravenous contrast CT.[44] However, even bolus intravenous CT is not consistently helpful in distinguishing postoperative disk and scar. We believe MR is the examination of choice in this circumstance and distinguishes these two entities in over 80% of patients (Fig. 18–28).[45] We have found sagittal MR to be most useful in the distinction between disk reprolapse and postoperative scar (Fig. 18–29). We have employed the following criteria to make this diagnosis: (1) a polypoid protrusion emanating from the disk space itself; (2) signal intensity protruding into the thecal sac that blends with the disk and becomes more apparent as T2-weighting is increased in contrast with scar, which tends to blend in signal with the thecal sac and becomes less apparent as T2-weighting is increased; (3) contiguity of mar-

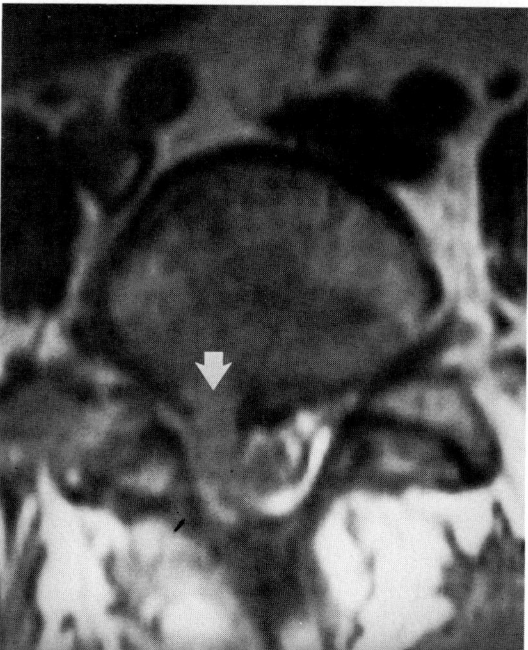

**Figure 18–28. Disk reprolapse.** Axial N(H)WI at the L5-S1 level seven months following diskectomy. A signal hyperintense relative to the thecal sac emanates from the prior curettage site (arrow), confirming disk rather than scar etiology. Frequently, the curettage tract can be traced as a linear hyperintense signal on N(H)WI and, particularly, on T2WI axial sections. (Courtesy of S. J. Pomeranz, M.D., Christ Hospital, Cincinnati, Ohio.)

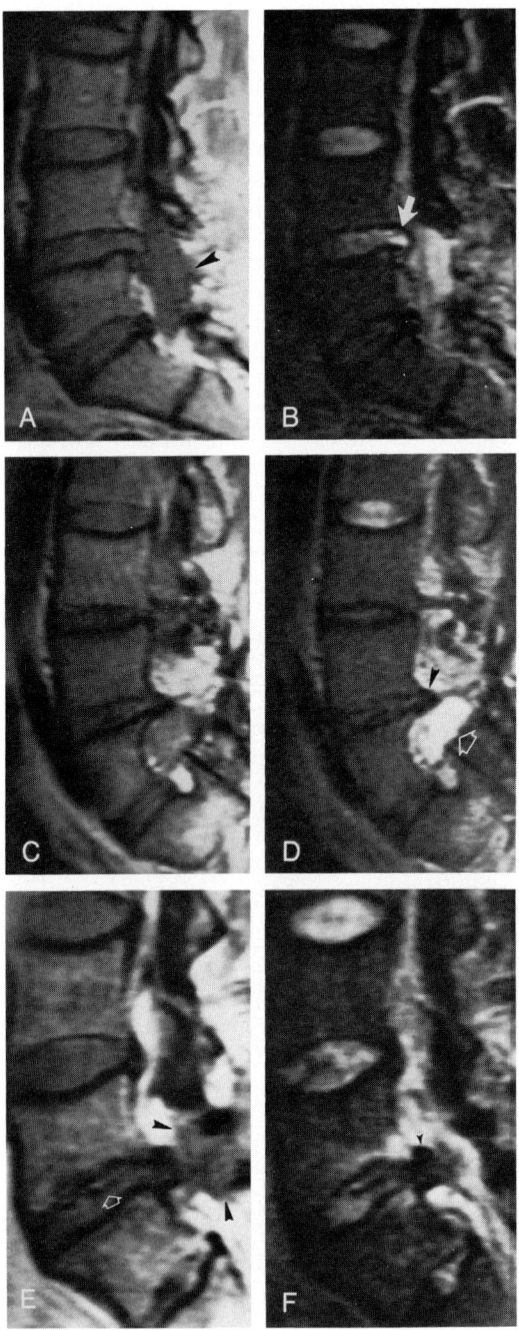


**Figure 18–29. Sagittal images from three different patients following L4-5 diskectomy at, respectively, one week, three months, and one year following surgery.** *A* and *B,* Sagittal N(H)WI and T2WI one week postoperation. *C* and *D,* Sagittal N(H)WI and T2WI three months postoperation. *E* and *F,* Sagittal N(H)WI and T2WI one year postoperation. In the acute postoperative state (*A* and *B*), the posterior portion of the disk is often hyperintense. This does not necessarily reflect disk reprolapse (white arrow). Over time, shrinkage of this posterior disk protrusion was observed. Granulation tissue or soft tissue edema is separable from disk on N(H)WI (arrowhead) and T2WI. *C* and *D,* Patient three months postoperation shows persistent L4-5 disk prolapse posteriorly (arrowhead). The intermediate/hypointense disk signal is easily separable from adjacent hyperintense scar (open arrow) on T2WI. *E* and *F,* Patient one year postoperation shows intermediate signal intensity scar on N(H)WI (arrowheads). Note that the scar blends with the remainder of the thecal sac and fat on T2WI and is virtually undetectable, whereas the disk reprolapse (small arrowhead) becomes more apparent. Disc reprolapse is polypoid in appearance, and its margins blend imperceptibly with the adjacent disk space. A linear hypointense vacuum phenomenon is present within the disk (open arrow). (Courtesy of S. J. Pomeranz, M.D., Christ Hospital, Cincinnati, Ohio.)

gin with the disk itself; and (4) variable signal intensity when compared with that of adjacent normal disks. There are several reasons why signal intensity cannot be used as a valid criteria to differentiate disk reprolapse from scar. As stated, scar has a variable appearance, depending upon its hemorrhagic component and age. Long-standing scar may be hypointense on all pulsing sequences. In contrast, sequestered disk herniations may exhibit focal signal hyperintensity on T2WI. In addition, in the acute postoperative stage, the posterior disk margin may exhibit increased signal intensity without reprolapse being present. Last, acute postoperative scar may exhibit signal hyperintensity relative to disk, particularly when a hemorrhagic component in the scar is present (Fig. 18–30).[46] All these factors may make the diagnosis of recurrent disk herniation more acutely difficult. Often, rescanning the patient in six to eight weeks, using the criteria stated earlier will help to improve diagnostic specificity. We and others have observed that with MR it is easier to distinguish postoperative scar and disk reprolapse by following this protocol.[47] Some have advocated the use of T1WI Gd-DTPA to selectively enhance postoperative fibrosis. In addition, image subtraction from noncontrast T1WI may be performed.[48] These maneuvers are rarely necessary when high-resolution, multiecho, T2WI nonorthogonal MR (see also Figs. 14–19 and 14–20) is available. We primarily use sagittal and axial multiecho MR alone to evaluate the failed back syndrome.

In summary, we utilize MR and will use CEMR as the primary and only modalities in assessing failed back syndrome. When a question of bony stenosis arises, CT is often performed as an adjunctive examination. MR is useful in assessing the patient with postoperative diskovertebral osteomyelitis. However, when soft tissue abscess or infection is suspected, we still prefer CT as the primary diagnostic modality.

## Spondylolysis, Spondylolisthesis, and Scoliosis

Spondylolysis is not well assessed with MR since cortical bone is poorly demonstrated. However, sagittal MR has an important role in evaluating spondylolisthesis since the extent of cord compromise is easily determined while the "pseudodisk" of spondylolisthesis is concomitantly distinguished from true disk herniation (Fig. 18–31). The posterior margin of true disk herniations will project beyond the posterior margins of the vertebral bodies above and below the slippage. "Pseudodisk" related to slippage does not project dorsal to the posterior margin of the vertebral body below.

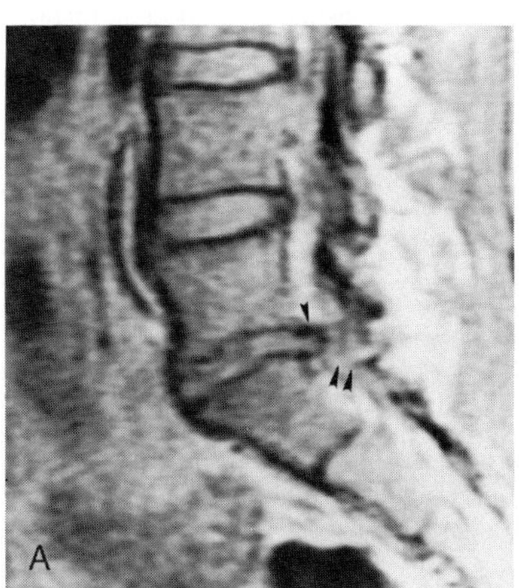


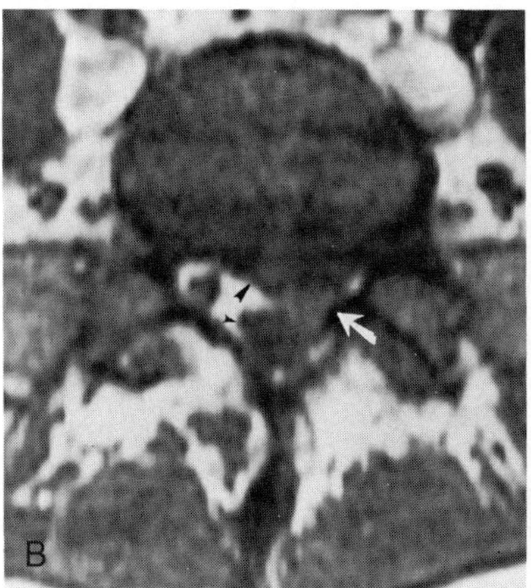


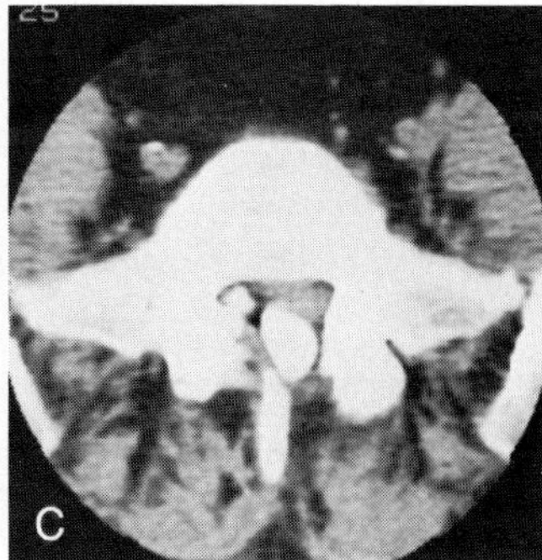


**Figure 18–30 Disk reprolapse and hemorrhagic scar.** A 27-year-old woman, three months postdiskectomy, at L5-S1, with leftward radiculopathy (1.5 T). *A,* Sagittal N(H)WI. *B,* Axial T1WI. *C,* Axial CT-IV contrast. Disk protrudes posteriorly (single arrowhead) and is easily separable from the scar (paired arrowheads) in the sagittal projection. The scar is hyperintense (white arrow) in the axial projection on T1WI, and a hemorrhagic component to the scar was demonstrated pathologically. Also identified in *B* are recurrent disk (large arrowhead) prolapse and thecal sac (small arrowhead). Disk and scar are inseparable on CT. (Courtesy of S. J. Pomeranz, M.D., Christ Hospital, Cincinnati, Ohio.)

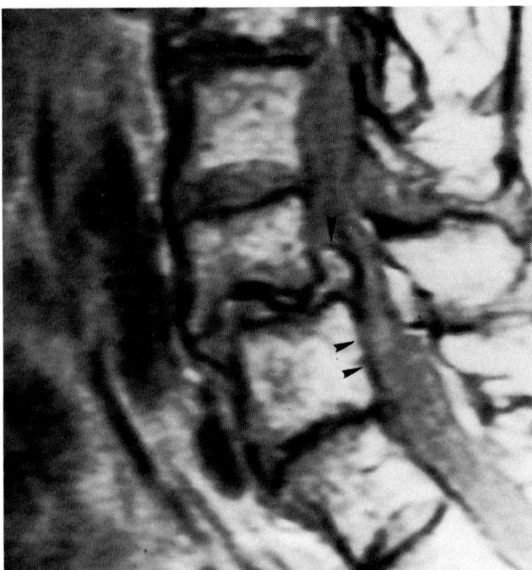

**Figure 18–31. Spondylolisthesis with disc herniation.** A 32-year-old man with bilateral leg pain (1.5 T). Sagittal T1WI. Disk (single arrowhead) protrudes dorsal to the posterior margin of the vertebral body below (arrowheads) confirming the presence of true disk herniation rather than pseudoherniation of spondylolisthesis. The spinal canal is narrowed. In pseudoherniation, disk does not protrude posterior to the posterior margin of the vertebra below. (Courtesy of S. J. Pomeranz, M.D., Christ Hospital, Cincinnati, Ohio.)

Scoliosis presents an obvious technical difficulty in MR evaluation of the spine. When disk evaluation is crucial, axial or compound nonorthogonal paraxial images must be relied upon. If long-segment cord evaluation is necessary, coronal or paracoronal images may be useful. Contiguous thin sections may offset some of these inherent difficulties. MR is the modality of choice to exclude underlying spinal pathology in the scoliotic spine of patients with neurofibromatosis.

## References


1. Modic MT, Weinstein MA, Pavlicek W, et al. Magnetic resonance imaging of intervertebral disc disease—clinical and pulse sequence considerations. Radiology 152:103, 1984.
2. Norman D. Magnetic resonance imaging of the spine. In Brant-Zawadski M, Norman D, eds. Magnetic Resonance Imaging of the Central Nervous System. New York, Raven Press, 1986.
3. Modic MT, Masaryk T, Boumphrey F, et al. Lumbar herniated disc disease and canal stenosis: prospective evaluation by surface coil MR, CT, and myelography. AJNR 7:709, 1986.
4. Reicher MA, Gold RH, Halbach VV, et al. MR imaging of the lumbar spine: anatomic correlations and the effects of technical variations. AJR 147:891, 1986.
5. Haacke EM, Patrick JL. Reducing motion artifacts in two-dimensional Fourier transform imaging. Magn Reson Imag 4:359, 1986.
6. Bailes DR, Gilderdale DJ, Bydder GM, et al. Respiratory ordered phase encoding (ROPE): a method for reducing respiratory motion artifacts in MR imaging. J Comput Assist Tomogr 9:835, 1985.
7. Axel L. Surface coil magnetic resonance imaging. J Comput Assist Tomogr 8:381, 1984.
8. Reicher MA, Lufkin RB, Smith S, et al. Multiple-angle variable-interval non-orthogonal MRI. AJR 147:363, 1986.
9. Edelman RR, Stark DD, Saini S, et al. Oblique planes of section in MR imaging. Radiology 159:807, 1986.
10. Modic MT, Masaryk TJ, Ross JS, et al. Cervical radiculopathy: value of oblique MR imaging. Radiology 163:227, 1987.
11. Steiner RE, Bydder GM, Young IR. MR distinction between red and yellow bone marrow: normal and abnormal. Radiology 161:24, 1986.
12. Dooms GC, Fisher MR, Hricak H, et al. Bone marrow imaging: magnetic resonance studies related to age and sex. Radiology 155:429, 1985.
13. Richardson ML, Helms CA. Artifacts, normal variants, and imaging pitfalls of musculoskeletal magnetic resonance imaging. Radiol Clin North Am 24:145, 1986.
14. Sobel DF, Zyroff J, Thorne RP. Diskogenic vertebral sclerosis: MR imaging. J Comput Assist Tomogr 11:855, 1987.
15. Pech P, Haughton VM. Lumbar intervertebral disc: correlative MR and anatomic study. Radiology 156:699, 1985.
16. Modic MT, Weinstein MA, Pavlicek W, et al. Magnetic resonance imaging of intervertebral disc disease—clinical and pulse sequence considerations. Radiology 152:103, 1984.
17. Aguila LA, Piraino DW, Modic MT, et al. The intranuclear cleft of the intervertebral disc: magnetic resonance imaging. Radiology 155:155, 1985.
18. Modic MT, Feiglin DH, Piraino DW, et al. Vertebral osteomyelitis: assessment using MR. Radiology 157:157, 1985.
19. Berger PE, Atkinson D, Wilson WJ, et al. High resolution surface coil magnetic resonance imaging of the spine: normal and pathologic anatomy. Radiographics 6:573, 1986.
20. Harris RI, Macnab I. Structural changes in the lumbar intervertebral discs. J Bone Joint Surg (Br) 36:304, 1954.
21. Modic MT, Masaryk T, Boumphrey F, et al. Lumbar herniated disk disease and canal stenosis: prospective evaluation by surface coil MR, CT, and myelography. AJNR 7:709, 1986.
22. Han JS, Benson JE, Yoon YS. Magnetic resonance imaging in the spinal column and craniovertebral junction. Radiol Clin North Am 22:805, 1984.
23. Masaryk TJ, Ross JS, Modic MT, et al. High-resolution MR imaging of sequestered lumbar intervertebral discs. Radiology 161:220, 1986.
24. Flannigan BD, Lufkin RB, McGlade C, et al. MR imaging of the cervical spine: neurovascular anatomy. AJNR 8:27, 1987.
25. Modic MT, Masaryk TJ, Mulopulos GP, et al. Cervical radiculopathy: prospective evaluation with surface coil MR imaging, CT with metrizamide, and metrizamide myelography. Radiology 161:753, 1986.

26. Daniels DL, Hyde J, Kneeland JB, et al. The cervical nerves and foramina: local-coil MR imaging. AJNR 7:129, 1986.
27. Yu S, Sether L, Wagner M, et al. Spinal facet joints: correlative MR and anatomic study. Radiology 161:132, 1986.
28. Baker LL, Hajek PC, Goobar JE, et al. Focal fat deposition in axial bone marrow: diagnostic considerations and distinction from pathology by MR imaging. Radiology 161:132, 1986.
29. Vogler JB III, Helms CA, Callen PW. Normal Variants and Pitfalls in Imaging. Philadelphia, W. B. Saunders Co., 1986:614.
30. Ullrich CG, Binet EF, Saneeki MG, et al. Quantitative assessment of the lumbar spinal canal by computed tomography. Radiology 134:137, 1980.
31. Burton CV, Kirkaldy-Willis WH, Yong-Hing K, et al. Causes of failure of surgery on the lumbar spine. Clin Orthop 157:191, 1981.
32. Quiles M, Marchisello PJ, Tsairis P. Lumbar adhesive arachnoiditis, etiologic and pathologic aspects. Spine 3:45, 1978.
33. Edelman RR, Shoukimas GM, Stark DD, et al. High-resolution surface coil imaging of lumbar disc disease. AJNR 6:479, 1985.
34. Ross JS, Masaryk TJ, Modic MT, et al. MR imaging of lumbar arachnoiditis. AJNR 8:885, 1987.
35. Monajati A, Wayne WS, Rauschning W, et al. MR of the cauda equina. AJNR 8:893, 1987.
36. Tobias JA. Personal communication, 1986.
37. Brown BM, Stark EH, Dion G, et al. Computed tomography and chymopapain chemonucleolysis: preliminary findings. AJNR 6:51, 1985.
38. Huckman MS, Clark JW, McNeill JW, et al. Chemonucleation and changes observed on lumbar MR scan: preliminary report. AJNR 8:1, 1987.
39. Deeb ZL, Schimel S, Daffner RH, et al. Intervertebral disk-space infection after chymopapain injection. AJNR 6:55, 1985.
40. Masaryk TJ, Boumphrey F, Modic MT, et al. Effects of chemonucleolysis demonstated by MR imaging. J Comput Assist Tomogr 10:917, 1986.
41. Burton CV, Kirkaldy-Willis WH, Yong-Hing K, et al. Causes of failure of surgery on the lumbar spine. Clin Orthop 157:191, 1981.
42. Ross JS, Masaryk TJ, Modic MT, et al. Lumbar spine: postoperative assessment with surface-coil MR imaging. Radiology 164:851, 1987.
43. Heindel W, Friedman G, Bunke J, et al. Artifacts in MR imaging after surgical intervention. J Comput Assist Tomogr 10:596, 1986.
44. Yang PJ, Seeger JF, Dzioba RB, et al. High-dose IV contrast in CT scanning of the postoperative lumbar spine. AJNR 7:703, 1986.
45. Pomeranz SJ, Brown OLB, Masters JM, et al. MR of postoperative disc and fibrosis: a review of ninety-six cases. (In press.)
46. Chafetz N, Genant HK, Moon KC. Recognition of lumbar disc herniation with NMR. AJR 141:153, 1986.
47. Ross JS, Modic MT, Masaryk TT, et al. MR imaging of the postoperative spine. Radiology 161:220, 1986.
48. Maas R, Kooijman H, Langkowski J, et al. Value of MR imaging with Gd-DTPA for differentiation of scar and reprolapse after lumbar disc operations. Radiology 161:309, 1986.

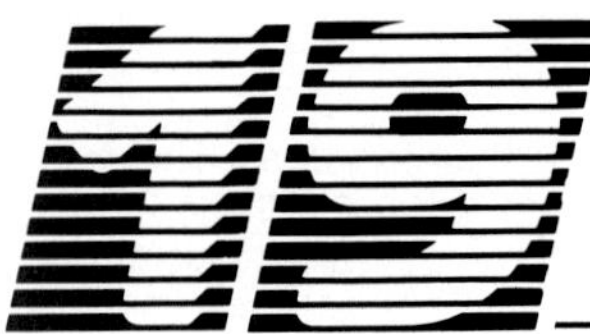

Scott Schlesinger, M.D.

# MRI OF SPINAL TRAUMA

With improved accident scene care and early retrieval from the "field," as many as 45 per cent of patients with spinal cord trauma have an incomplete neurologic injury. Early surgical intervention in the acutely injured patient is directed toward preserving or restoring function. Knowledge of the specific nature and level of the cord injury is paramount to proper neurosurgical care. Magnetic resonance (MR) has the ability to directly image the spine and the cord in multiple planes. MR is noninvasive and can be performed on patients in traction, patients with cardiac monitoring devices, and those on respirators, even at high field.[2, 100] MR is now being used routinely in several centers for neuroradiologic evaluation of cord injury. Traumatic neurologic cord dysfunction can be conveniently divided into medullary and extramedullary pathology.

## POST-TRAUMATIC MYELOPATHY

### Acute

Cord damage from trauma may acutely occur upon impact or may chronically evolve over a longer period of time. Acutely, a spectrum of changes from concussion to complete cord transection may take place. Experimental cord injury causes consistent pathologic changes.

Concussion is a functional deficit manifested by a reversible loss of conduction for a variable period of time (usually hours or days) thought to be due to membrane damage.[8] Contusion, on the other hand, results in anatomic derangements.

The spinal cord reacts to trauma quickly and dynamically. There are three basic destructive processes involved: an initial mechanical insult, hemorrhage and enzymatic cord destruction, and superimposed vascular insult.[1, 20] Increasing compression results in a progression of injury through three basic types of lesions: type A—predominant gray matter cavitation; type B—white matter large fiber destruction predominates, and type C—severe, combined gray and white matter lesion in a connective tissue scar.[7]

Type A lesions are direct injuries to central gray matter cell bodies with immediate release of lysosomal enzymes. Edema follows and leads to further rupture and necrosis of cell bodies and further edema. The small intramedullary vessels within the gray matter are particularly susceptible to contussive injury and rupture easily. Petechial hemorrhages appear within minutes.[7] The central cord syndrome is the prime clinical example of a type A injury. The syndrome is caused by a hyperextension injury, usually without associated fracture, and is characterized by disproportionate upper extremity weakness, bladder dysfunction (usually retention), and variable sensory loss.[8] The degree of recovery is related to the amount of reversible edema versus irreversible destruction and hemorrhage, ranging from complete recovery to total destruction, ascending hematomyelia, and death.[7–9, 14]

Type B injury results in white matter cavitation in addition to the gray matter lesion. There is selective destruction of the large-diameter myelinated fibers in accordance with Laplace's law.[10] Because the unmyelinated and smaller myelinated fibers remain intact, the cord is not transected.[11] However, damage to large fibers leads to profound consequences. Within hours, the damaged ends of the fibers begin to swell and fill with axoplasm.[13] As swelling continues, microcysts are formed. At one day post injury, these microcysts rupture; axoplasm is spilled, and cavity formation begins. Lysosomal enzyme activation results in autolysis and liquefactive necrosis, which is usually complete in approximately three weeks.[7, 12]

A type C lesion is essentially a cord transection or maceration. In addition to the central gray matter and large-fiber white matter injury, the small fibers in the white matter are also damaged, resulting in loss of cord integrity. An outpouring of axoplasm, tissue debris, red cells, neutrophils, and fibroblasts occurs. The transection site is subsequently transformed into a connective tissue scar.[7] Liquefactive necrosis and cavitation are therefore part of the natural reparative process of the spinal cord.[16]

Traumatic cord injuries are concatenations of edema, necrosis, and variable amounts of hemorrhage. In addition to direct mechanical injury, vascular damage, vasospasm with resultant thrombosis, and hemorrhage occur. Compromise of cord circulation results in further loss of integrity of the blood-brain barrier and progressive edema. A vicious cycle results, and in the presence of an intact, inelastic pial membrane, may cause further tamponade, vascular insult, and more edema.[18–22, 31–33] The amount of hemorrhage is usually small and part of an overall picture of hemorrhagic necrosis of cord parenchyma. Uncommonly, if the hemorrhage is large and confluent, a space-occupying hematomyelia may occur.

### *MR Appearance*

The main advantage of MR is its ability to show the cord itself and its relationship to surrounding structures. Cord edema and hemorrhage frequently occur after spinal trauma. MR has a high sensitivity for detecting edema and hemorrhage in the brain and has been shown to be superior to CT in the visualization of the spinal cord and the detection of cord injury.[2, 25, 99] MR changes vary depending on the relative proportions of edema, cell injury, and hemorrhage. Cord edema begins within minutes of injury and may last for as long as 20 days.[33] Changes observable on MR consist of a change in size and an alteration of signal.[23, 24, 99] Cord edema may cause focal cord enlargement and an abnormally long T1/T2 because of increased bulk water content (see Figs. 19–3 and 19–4). As T2WIs are more sensitive to the presence of edema, focal enlargement with a hyperintense region on T2WI without signal changes on T1WI may also be seen. The abnormal signal extends for a variable distance rostrally and caudally from the site of injury, often in a cone-shaped fashion, into the central gray matter.[24] This correlates well with experimental evidence of the increased susceptibility of gray matter to injury. In addition to the long T1/T2 of cord edema, loss of normal landmarks in an enlarged cord with inhomogeneous signal has also been reported, reflecting the fact that, pathologically, most cord lesions represent a mixture of edema, necrosis, and hemorrhage.[23, 99]

Limited experience suggests that hemorrhage within the cord evolves in a manner similar to that of an intracerebral hematoma (see Chap. 13).[2, 23–25, 99] At high field strengths, an acute hematomyelia is isointense on T1WI and hypointense on T2WI (Fig. 19–1), and a subacute or chronic hematomyelia (Fig. 19–2) is hyperintense on both T1WI and T2WI with a surrounding hypointense ring on T2WI, similar to the findings with intracranial hematomas. However, we have encountered signal alterations in spinal blood outside the cord that behave differently from intracranial hemorrhage (see Figs. 19–1, 19–10, and 19–11). Clinically, it may be important to differentiate an edematous cord from hematomyelia. Although usually treated conservatively, cord hematomas may respond to evacuation.[2–6, 15] MR differentiation of cord hemorrhage from edema is possible. In the acute situation, edema may not be separable from blood on the T1WI as both may be hypointense or isointense, but on T2WI the long T2 of edema contrasts markedly with the short T2 of acute blood. Edema can be identified at the perimeter of the hematomyelia as surrounding regions of long T1/T2 (see Fig. 19–1). In the nonacute situation, both blood and edema have a long T2, but the long T1 of edema is easily separable from the short T1 of nonacute blood. Although these signal abnormalities are discernible in a relatively intact cord, with severe cord damage, as with maceration and transection, specific signal abnormalities may be difficult to identify.

Cord maceration and transection represent the most severe spectral end of cord injury. Cord maceration involves abnormal signal involving the entire cord width from wide-

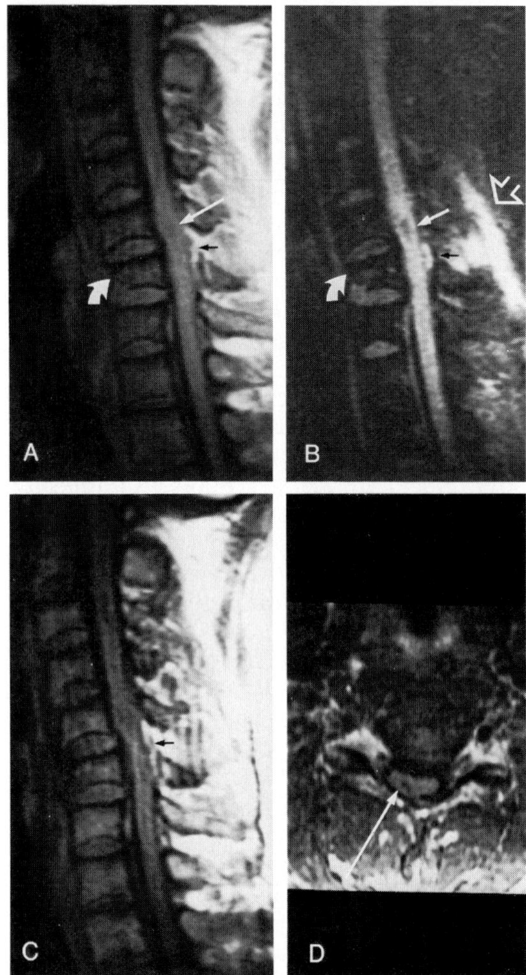


**Figure 19–1. Acute hematomyelia.** *A,* Sagittal N(H)WI (SE TR 1800/TE 20). *B,* Sagittal T2WI (SE TR 1800/TE 80). *C,* Sagittal T1WI (SE TR 600/TE 20). *D,* Axial T1WI (SE TR 600/TE 20).

A wedge compression fracture of C6 is present, surrounded by an ill-defined region of hyperintensity (curved white arrow) in the midportion of the body on T2WI *(B).* Acute blood within the spinal cord (straight white arrow) is hypointense in *B,* minimally hypointense in *A,* and not visualized in *C.* Surrounding long T2 consistent with cord edema is present on the T2WI. Thecal sac and cord compression are present on all images, but only *D* accurately defines the degree of compression (long white arrow). A small spinal epidural hematoma (small black arrow) is hyperintense on all sequences. A single traumatic event has resulted in blood that has two different MR appearances at the same time. Also note the paraspinal muscle injury (open white arrow) and traumatic C6-C7 disk morphology. (Courtesy of Neuroradiology Department, University of Cincinnati, Cincinnati, Ohio.)

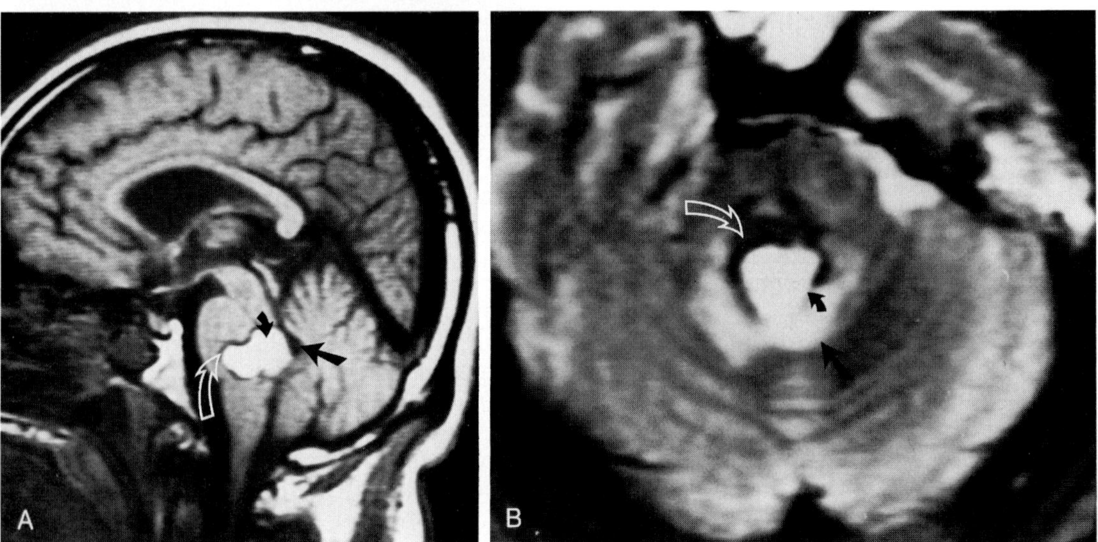


**Figure 19–2. Chronic hematobulbia.** This 50-year-old man was found unconscious (1.5 T). The MR was done three weeks post-ictus. *A,* Sagittal T1WI (SE TR 800/TE 20). *B,* Axial T2WI (SE TR 2000/TE 80).

There is a large region of hyperintensity (short T1/long T2) in the posterior pons (curved black arrow) with mass effect and mild compression of the fourth ventricle (straight black arrow). A thin, extremely hypointense rim of hemosiderin that becomes more prominent on the T2WI (open white arrow) is present in *A.* Mild T2 contribution to image contrast on the relatively T1WI is the reason for the visibility of hemosiderin in *A.* (Courtesy of L. Eynon, M.D., Mercy Hospital, Cincinnati, Ohio.)

spread edema and necrosis, usually manifested by prolonged T1 and T2 relaxation (Fig. 19–3). Cord transection is suggested by the absence of discernible neural tissue (Fig. 19–4). Volume averaging and cord displacement by fracture fragments and hematomas can create the appearance of transection with seeming absence of the cord on sagittal scans, making thin-section axial images helpful for confirmation. Routine SE sagittal and axial T1WI have a high signal-to-noise ratio (SNR) and provide excellent anatomic detail. Routine spin-echo (SE) T2WI may be too noisy for the demonstration of small cord lesions. We have found cardiac-gated or flow-compensated sagittal SE T2WI to be superior to routine SE T2WI, because CSF pulsation artifacts and ghosting (phase-shift) artifacts are diminished.[25–28] In addition, fast-field, low tip angle axial images may also be helpful when axial T2WI are necessary.

Signal abnormalities, especially the long T1/T2 within a traumatic cord lesion, may disappear, and neurologic function may return wholly or partially.[99] The signal abnormalities in these cases apparently represent edema, not irreversible cell destruction. With current surface coil technology and imaging strategies, edema and necrosis have a similar appearance on MRI. Studies to date have not been able to reliably differentiate edema from necrosis; thus, currently, the relative amount of reversible damage to the cord is difficult to discern.

### Chronic

Patients who have sustained spinal cord injury may later undergo clinical deterioration of neurologic function. These patients have a potpourri of large cysts, small cystic regions, variable-sized regions of gliosis, edema, and loss of neuronal substance (atrophy); any of these elements may predominate.[54]

Post-traumatic progressive myelopathy may be segregated into large cystic (syringomyelia) and noncystic myelopathy

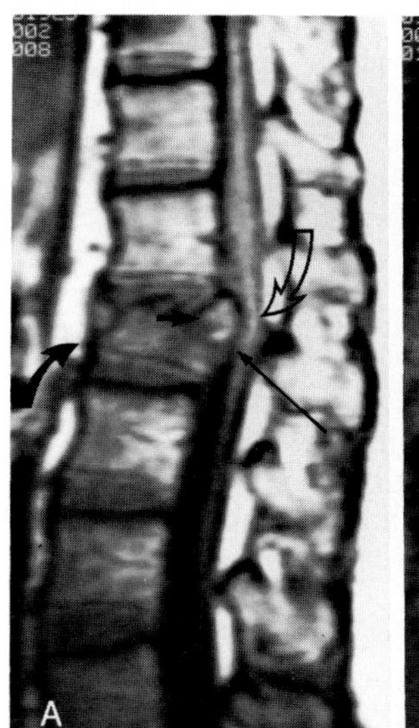

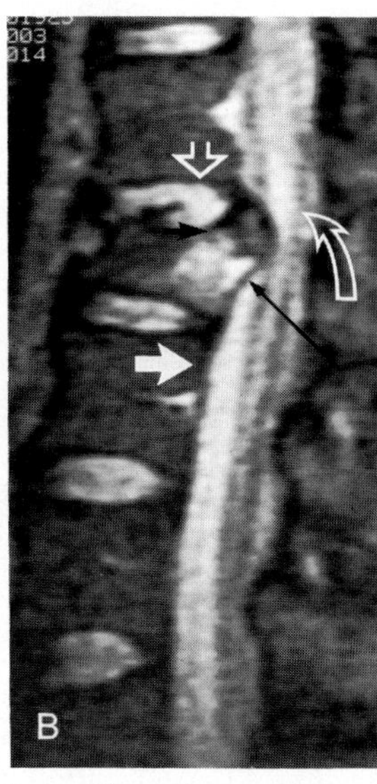

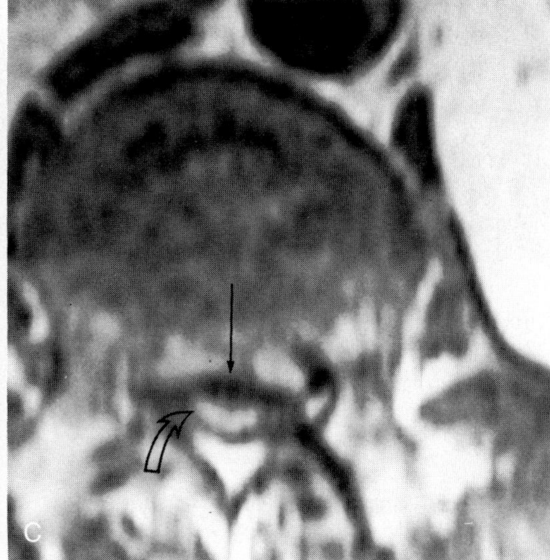


**Figure 19–3. Acute burst fracture with cord maceration and near-complete block (1.5 T).** *A,* Sagittal T1WI (SE TR 600/TE 20). *B,* Sagittal T2WI (SE TR 1800/TE 80). *C,* Axial T1WI (SE TR 600/TE 20) through the burst fracture.

A comminuted fracture of the vertebral body of L2 (curved black arrow) is manifested by a well-defined hypointense line best seen in *A*. A retropulsed fragment (small black arrows) compresses the thecal sac and cord. The intact low signal line posteriorly, representing cortical bone, posterior ligament complex, and dura indicates that the retropulsed fragment is extradural. Disk trauma (open straight white arrow) with annular rupture and extension of hydrated nuclear material into the superior end-plate of L2 is seen in *B*.

The conus is hyperintense in *B,* indicating cord edema (open curved white arrow). Cord compression (open curved black arrow) is suggested on sagittal images and confirmed axially *(C)*. Compare with Figure 19–10, where the sagittal view suggests compression, whereas axial images show the cord is actually displaced. High-grade stenosis is present, manifested by a relative increase in hyperintensity of CSF on T2WI (closed white arrow) from dampened CSF flow dynamics. (Courtesy of S. Pomeranz, M.D., Christ Hospital, Cincinnati, Ohio.)

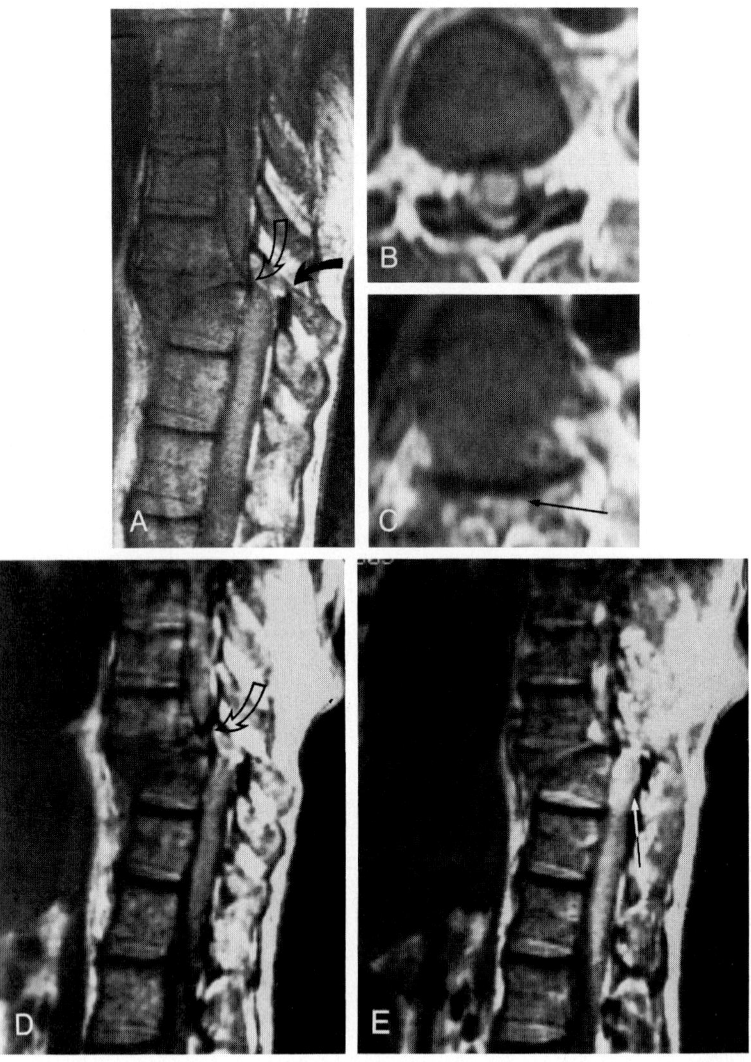


**Figure 19–4. Cord transection (1.5 T).** *A,* Sagittal T1WI (SE TR 500/TE 20) demonstrates a fracture-dislocation through a midthoracic vertebra. A laminar fracture is present (curved black arrow). No discernible cord tissue is identified at the site of injury (curved open black arrow). Inferiorly, the cord is widened owing to edema, better seen in *E. B,* Axial T1WI (SE TR 500/TE 20) above the transection site shows normal relations between the cord and vertebral body. *C,* Axial T1WI (SE TR 500/TE 20) at the level of the transection shows no visible cord. Low signal cortical bone abuts the epidural fat posteriorly (long black arrow). *D,* Sagittal N(H)WI (SE TR 2000/TE 20) again shows the cord transection (open curved black arrow). *E,* Sagittal T2WI (SE TR 2000/TE 20) demonstrates cord edema inferior to the transection site (long white arrow) (Courtesy of Neuroradiology Department, University of Cincinnati, Cincinnati, Ohio.)

(myelomalacia). Distinction is paramount because the former may respond to decompression whereas the latter unfortunately is not currently treatable.[39, 40, 42, 54, 55]

## Post-Traumatic Syringomyelia

Post-traumatic cystic myelopathy has been well-described.[34–43] The prevalence of clinically important post-traumatic cyst formation varies from 0.3 per cent to 3.2 per cent.[34–40] These data are based on retrospective studies using myelography, surgery, or early CT for diagnosis. With the advent of MR, delayed metrizamide CT scanning, and intraoperative sonography, the prevalence of post-traumatic syringomyelia (PTS) appears higher than previously assumed. Motor vehicle accidents, diving accidents, falls, stab and gunshot wounds, spinal anesthesia, spinal surgery, vertebral osteomyelitis, and disk protrusions have all been reported as causes of PTS.[37]

Cyst formation is the natural end-product of lysosomal digestion, edema, ischemia, and liquefaction of traumatic cord injury (see previous discussion).[43, 44] Syrinxes may also result from lacerations (fissures) of the cord, which result in a direct communication of the subarachnoid space with the damaged cord. Theoretically, adhesions and tethering occur, allowing CSF to penetrate into the cord.[96] If this penetration occurs in a ball-valve fashion, ensuing enlargement of the cord defect may create an associated cyst.[97, 98] The myelographic-CT hallmark of a fissure is the immediate, direct passage of intrathecal contrast medium into the cyst cavity.

Spinal cord cysts vary in size from the microscopic to the involvement of nearly the whole length of the cord. The cysts also vary in number. Gliosis is usually present at the leading edge of the syrinx.[46, 47] Associated arachnoidal adhesions are nearly always present and may or may not cause a block. With the exception of a single series in which 7.9 per cent of patients with complete tetraplegia developed PTS, neither the level nor the severity of injury has been found to be predictive of the eventual development of PTS or its time of onset.[34] The onset of symptoms and signs of PTS may develop as quickly as 2 months or as late as 23 years following the injury.[37] The most common presenting symptom is pain, usually unilateral, which may be precipitated by coughing, straining, or exercise. Sensory loss, predominantly spinothalamic, is the second most frequent presenting complaint. Progression to motor deficits, and signs of autonomic dysfunction such as hyperhidrosis or piloerection are less frequent presenting complaints. The natural history is usually one of rapid or slow progression to severe disability. If untreated, sensory loss and motor weakness become bilateral and ascend, occasionally as cephalad as the brain stem.[37] Surgical decompression in symptomatic patients is the treatment of choice, and PTS is more responsive to decompression than other forms of syringomyelia.[40] Pain is the most responsive symptom to shunting; motor weakness and sensory deficits are less responsive.[35, 39, 40] The progressive, disabling nature of PTS and its correctible course makes its diagnosis of utmost importance; MR is the initial imaging modality of choice.[54, 55, 60–65, 75]

### MR Appearance

The cavities in PTS are fluid-filled and therefore have fluid characteristics (long T1/T2). Cord cysts, despite a higher average protein content than pure CSF, generally behave like CSF unless complicated by other pathology (Fig. 19–5).[33, 39] The syrinxes vary in length and width from focal cystic structures (Fig. 19–6) to long cavities taking up virtually the entire length and breadth of the cord (Fig. 19–7). They can be single, multilocular, or multiple. Multilocular cavities may occur in side-by-side arrangements or juxtaposed one above the other.[1, 101] This circumstance indicates the need for thin sagittal and selective thin axial images with a surface coil to optimize resolution and signal-to-noise ratio (SNR) and reduce volume-averaging problems.[54, 58, 79, 80] Axial images help determine (1) the number of cavities, as side-by-side arrangement may appear unilocular on sagittal images; (2) the syrinx

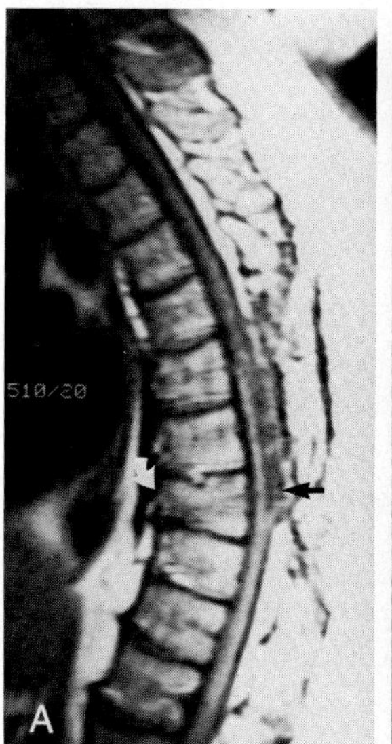

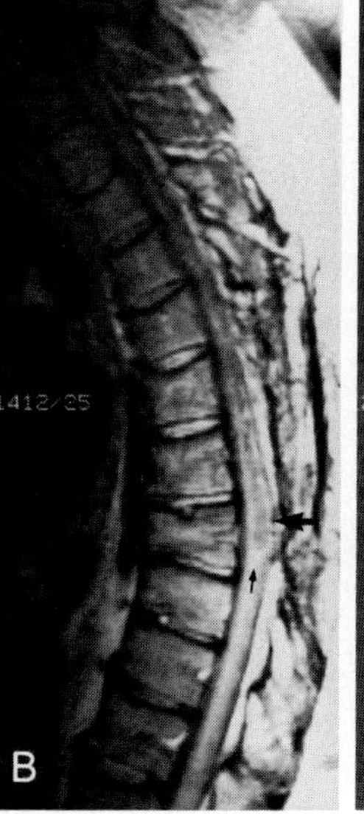

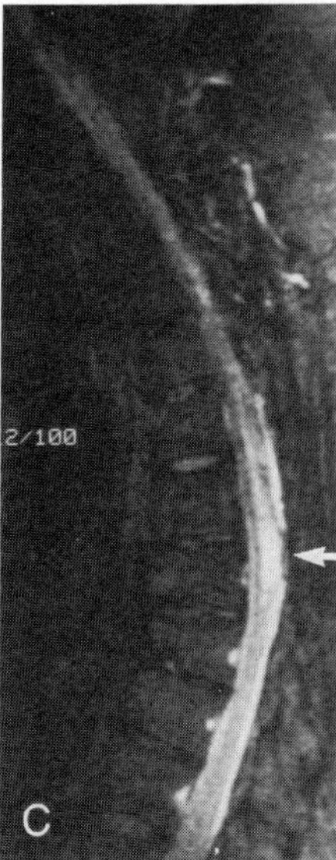


**Figure 19–5. Post-traumatic syrinx, cardiac-gated (1.5 T).** *A,* Sagittal T1WI (SE TR 510/TE 20). *B,* Sagittal N(H)WI, cardiac-gated SE TR 1412/TE 25). *C,* Sagittal T2WI, cardiac-gated (SE TR 1412/TE 100). A wedge compression fracture of a mid-thoracic vertebral body is present (curved arrow). The cord is mildly enlarged, with a syrinx in its midportion (straight arrows). CSF/fluid behavior of the cyst is demonstrated by the long T1 (hypointensity) in *A* and long T2 (hyperintensity) in *C*. In *B*, a thin, peripheral region of hyperintensity (small black arrow) represents surrounding myelomalacia. Intraparenchymal bulk water (edema and myelomalacia) converts to high signal at a shorter TE than does CSF. Notice in *C* that when the TE is increased, the CSF converts to high signal, incorporating the regions of myelomalacia and making the syrinx appear larger. (Courtesy of Neuroradiology Department, University of Cincinnati, Cincinnati, Ohio.)

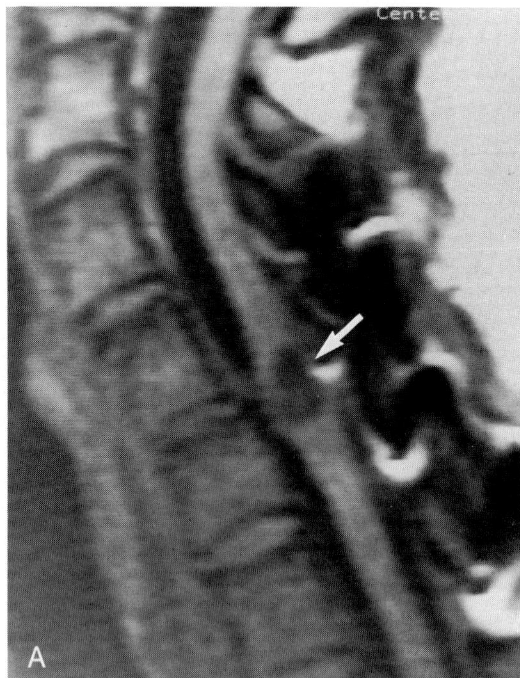

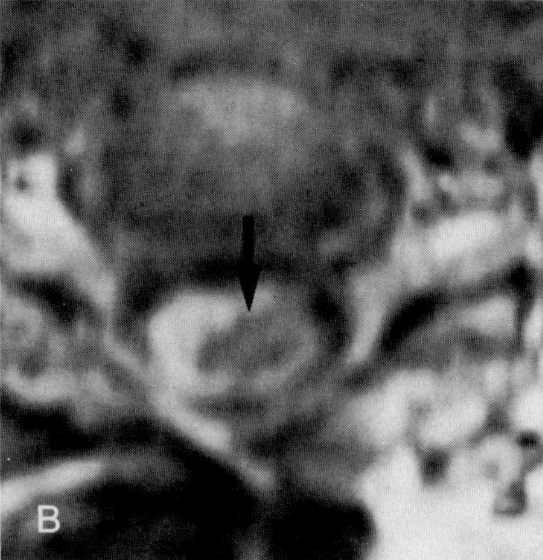

**Figure 19–6. Post-traumatic syrinx (1.5 T).** *A,* Sagittal T1WI (SE TR 600/TE 20). *B,* Axial T1WI (SE TR 600/TE 20). Focal cord enlargement is noted on both sagittal and axial images. A localized region of long T1 is present (white arrow) consistent with syrinx. The cyst occupies nearly the entire cord width. Ferromagnetic artifact in the posterior paraspinal soft tissues from previous wire fusion is manifested by an ill-defined region of signal void (Courtesy of S. J. Pomeranz, M.D., Christ Hospital, Cincinnati, Ohio.)

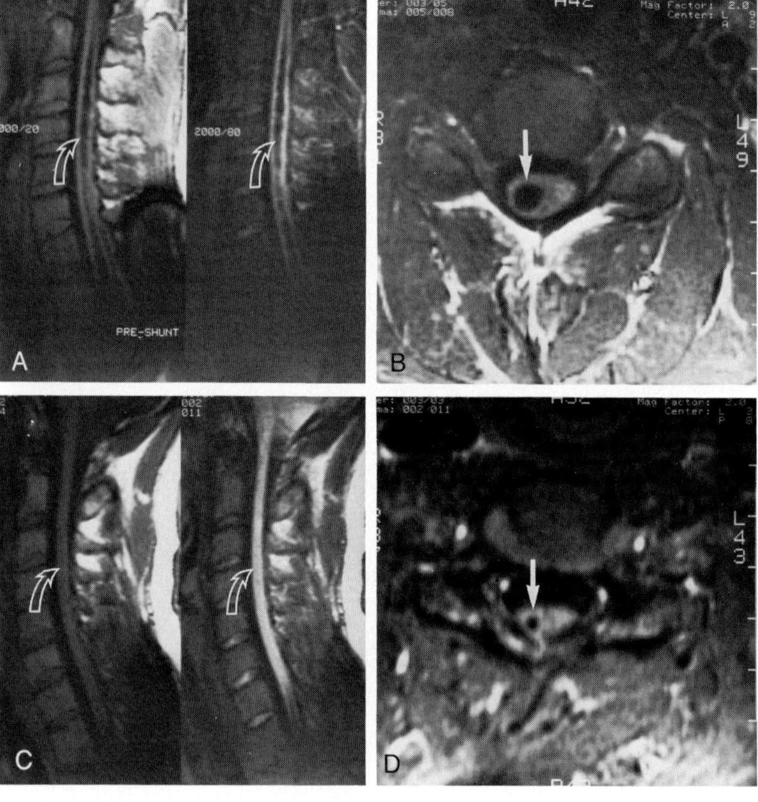

**Figure 19–7. Post-traumatic syrinx, pre- and postdecompression (1.5 T).** *A,* Preoperative sagittal multiecho N(H)WI and T2WI (TR 2000/TE 20/80) demonstrate a diffusely enlarged cervical cord with a central syrinx throughout (curved arrows), extending into the thoracic cord. Note that on the T2WI, the fluid within the syrinx has the signal flow void typical of large syringes. The walls of the syrinx are beaded, and may indicate gliotic banding. *B,* Preoperative axial T1WI (TR 600/TE 20) demonstrates the relative size and position of the syrinx (arrow). *C,* Postoperative sagittal multiecho N(H)WI and T2WI (TR 2000/TE 20/80) demonstrate reduction in syrinx size (arrows). The cord is diffusely atrophic. Consequently, the subarachnoid space is excessively capacious, resulting in flow void, making the CSF hypointense. *D,* Postoperative mid-cervical axial T1WI (TR 600/TE 20) demonstrates that the syrinx persists (arrow), but is much smaller. Cord atrophy is present as evidenced by the diminutive cord volume and expanded CSF space anteriorly. (Courtesy of Neuroradiology Department, University of Cincinnati, Cincinnati, Ohio.)

width; and (3) the location of the syrinx within the cord, as its position may have a bearing on the surgical procedure. The syringomyelic cord may be small, normal, or enlarged.[42]

The extent of the cavity or cavities is seen best on sagittal T1WI as longitudinally arranged intramedullary regions of low signal comparable to that of CSF. Because of higher SNR and less ghosting and motion artifact, the axial T1WI is the best sequence on which to determine the arrangement of the cavity or cavities within the cord. A simple cavity will convert to high signal similar to that of CSF on T2WI. This "fluid behavior" within a well-defined intramedullary lesion is the sine qua non of syringomyelia. This appearance may be modified by nonfluid substances within the cyst, such as hemorrhage, protein, infection and cellular debris, and CSF flow dynamics. Solutes diminish the amount of bulk water, shortening both the T1 and T2, causing an increase in signal on T1WI and diminished signal on T2WI.[66, 67]

Pulsatile flow within cavities is thought to result from cardiac pulsations, and intrathoracic and intra-abdominal pressures transmitted by epidural veins and surrounding CSF.[35, 39, 50, 51] Larger cysts generally have greater and more turbulent flow, which results in signal loss from spin dephasing on both T1 and T2WI.[48–51] Because of image contrast, signal loss is more conspicuous on T2WI. The cavity or portions of the cavity affected by flow void generate less signal than usual on T1WI and remain hypointense on T2WI (Fig. 19–7). When T2 contrast is needed to characterize lesions, cardiac-gated T2WI are often helpful, as signal loss and motion artifacts from CSF flow are diminished, resulting in better resolution than routine SE T2WI (see Fig. 19–5). The long T2 of the cyst may be more apparent with gated images, making identification more specific.

A disadvantage of cardiac-gated studies is the loss of some physiologic information gleaned by the presence of flow void. Signal loss from CSF pulsations can be useful information. Surgical decompression of a septated cyst may require separate shunts or conversion of the multiloculated, septated cavity to a unilocular cavity. A beaded appearance with septations from gliotic bands traversing the cavity raises the possibility of a multiseptated cyst (see Fig. 19–5). Absence of flow void in a large cyst or the presence of flow void in one portion of a cyst and its absence in another portion suggests the possibility of multiloculation,[50] and may herald the need for intraoperative sonography. MR is an excellent way to follow patients with PTS postoperatively after cyst decompression (Fig. 19–7). Collapse of the cyst and absence of flow void suggest adequate treatment.[65]

Cord gliosis (myelomalacia) and edema are frequently present at the cyst margins.[36, 37, 42] Gliosis and edema both have an intermediate to long T1/T2 and cannot currently be separated on MR. Thus the amount of reversible edema cannot be separated from irreversible myelomalacia. A heavily T2WI (TE $>$ 60 msec/TR 2000 msec) results in loss of conspicuity of the peripheral myelomalacia or edema, the signal of which may merge with that of cyst fluid, making the cyst appear larger. An image with a shorter TR, shorter TE (often called a spin-density image), or both may help delineate the true extent of the cyst, because free fluid has a longer T2 than the surrounding myelomalacia (see Fig. 19–5).[54, 59, 79] Direct noninvasive visualization of the cord and syrinx and the ability to determine the presence or absence of flow within the syrinx makes MR ideal in the diagnosis and follow-up of post-traumatic syringomyelia.[54, 55, 60–65]

## Noncystic Post-Traumatic Myelopathy

Patients who come to clinical attention because of progressive neurologic dysfunction after cord injury may not have large cysts that may respond to decompression. Evaluation is performed primarily to exclude a treatable cause, especially PTS. "Noncystic" is a practical division of post-traumatic myelopathy and includes myelopathy with small cysts, noncystic myelomalacia, and cord atrophy. This heterogeneous group of disorders represents a spectrum of chronic changes that do not generally respond to shunting.[39, 40, 42, 54–55]

### *MR Appearance*

The appearance of myelomalacic cord tissue corresponds to the pathology. Spinal cord size may be large, normal, or small. Small cysts are variably sized foci of long T1/T2, surrounded by myelomalacia (gliosis and edema) (Fig. 19–8). Because of their small size, these cysts do not exhibit appreciable signal loss from flow void. Myelomalacic foci contribute long T1/T2 because of increased free water content. The relative proportion of interspersed normal cord tissue with the myelomalacic foci varies. If a cord segment is essentially completely myelomalacic (a cord maceration), MR will predominantly display the long T1/T2 of increased water. However, with increasing interspersed normal neural tissue, the signal becomes intermediate between CSF and normal cord on both T1WI and T2WI.[55] With extreme T2 weighting, myelomalacic cord signal may merge with that of CSF. A spin-density image can separate myelomalacic cord from CSF and small cysts, since myelomalacia has a shorter TE than the free fluid in cysts and CSF.

Cord atrophy (loss of neuronal substance) is present to some degree after any significant injury; however, cord atrophy may be the dominant pathology.[69–74] Three basic patterns have been identified on metrizamide CT: diffuse (transverse myelopathy), hemiatrophy (Brown-Sequard syndrome), and anterior (anterior spinal artery) spinal atrophy.[69]

Transverse myelopathy is manifested by cord of diminutive size, which also is often flattened and misshapen (see Fig. 19–7).[6] The subarachnoid space is expanded because of small cord volume and has a greater tendency to exhibit CSF flow void (Fig. 19–7).[51] An atrophic cord may assume complex shapes, especially when associated with arachnoiditis. Cord atrophy is typically localized to several segments. If cord damage is severe enough to cause extensive wallerian degeneration or if there is associated vascular compromise and cord ischemia, diffuse atrophy of nearly the entire cord length may be seen.[71, 74] Although hemiatrophy may result from blunt trauma it is usually a result of penetrating trauma.[76, 77] The Brown-Sequard syndrome is clinically manifested by ipsilateral flaccid paralysis below the lesion and contralateral spinothalamic (pain and temperature) loss. Loss of cord substance in one half of the cord with an intact anterior median fissure has been found with metrizamide CT.[69] Anterior atrophy is usually caused by disease of the anterior spinal artery and is only rarely traumatic in origin. MR experience in identification and subtyping of cord atrophy is limited; however, cord morphology is easily discernible with current surface coil technology and high-resolution techniques.

MR may identify either abnormal cord morphology or signal or both. The atrophic

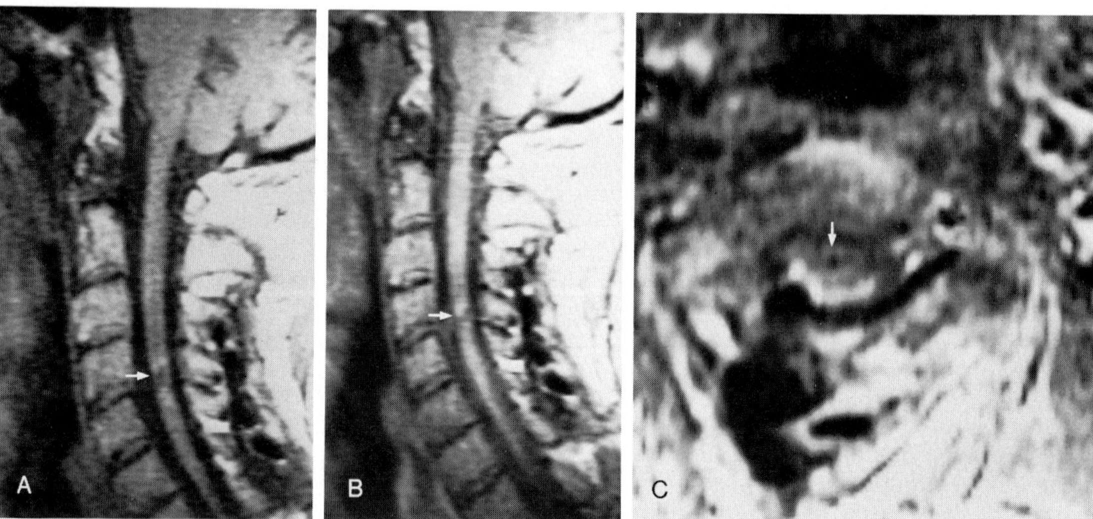


**Figure 19–8. Myelomalacia.** *A,* Sagittal T1WI (SE TR 600/TE 20) shows a small focus of inhomogeneous signal hypointensity (arrow). *B,* Sagittal N(H)WI (SE TR 1800/TE 30) demonstrates that the lesion becomes hyperintense with increased TR. *C,* Axial T1WI (SE TR 600/TE 20) shows that the cervical cord is slightly atrophic. A small well-defined focus of hypointensity is present in the cord center. This lesion represents microcyst formation edema, gliosis, or any combination of the three. These myelomalacic components cannot be separated on the basis of the MR and, in fact, usually coexist. (Courtesy of S. J. Pomeranz, M.D., Christ Hospital, Cincinnati, Ohio.)

cord is diminutive by definition. The distribution of loss of cord substance is most easily identified on axial images and may be missed on sagittal scans alone. The small cord may be of normal signal or reflect a variably sized component of gliosis or myelomacia.[78] The atrophic cord is easiest to identify on T1WI because of contrast with the low-signal CSF. Cord displacement and volume averaging make axial images necessary. T1WI, because of increased subject contrast and SNR, have yielded the best anatomic resolution, although we are now obtaining diagnostic axial T2WI with a high SNR and anatomic resolution with fast-field images using a low flip angle.

## EXTRAMEDULLARY CORD COMPROMISE

Extramedullary cord compromise (spinal cord compression) in acute trauma is a result of mass effect. Post-traumatic masses include displaced bony fragments, herniated disk material, ruptured ligaments, fluid collections such as epidural and subdural hematomas, and penetrating objects. Subacutely or chronically, compression may also result from pseudomeningoceles, epidural abcesses, arachnoiditis, and synovial cysts.

### Fractures

Spinal cord injury is usually associated with fractures and/or dislocations of the spine. Approximately 10 to 14 per cent of fracture-dislocations are associated with neurologic damage, although cord injury accompanies 85 per cent of bilateral locked facets,[83] and thoracolumbar fractures are likely to produce neurologic damage because of the small subarachnoid space and tight fit of the cord within the canal as well as the tremendous force necessary to fracture these large vertebrae.[95] Cord injury accompanies 85 per cent of bilateral locked facets.[83]

Burst fractures warrant special mention. These are among the most disruptive types of injury to the vertebral column and neurologic injury is "the rule."[85, 86] Multiple, noncontiguous fractures are not uncommon occurring in 4.5 per cent of cases.[87] Approximately 10 per cent of spinal cord injuries have no associated fractures; these are primarily hyperextension injuries in elderly patients with spondylosis.

#### *MR Appearance*

Fracture lines are identified as either low signal or high signal relative to either bone marrow or cortical end-plate.[88] Fracture lines through marrow are variably well-defined linear regions of low signal interrupting the normal fatty marrow signal (Fig. 19–9; also see Figs. 19–3 and 19–4) and are seen best on T1WI, where contrast between the high fat signal of the marrow and the low signal of the fracture line is maximal. Fractures extending through the cortex are manifested by well-defined high signal interruptions and malalignments of the bony cortex. One must be careful not to mistake the basivertebral venous plexus for a fracture (Fig. 19–9). Associated findings include variable amounts of edema (Fig. 19–9) and hemorrhage around the fracture line (Fig. 19–9; also see Fig. 19–3). Vertebral body and posterior element fractures can be identified on MR, although CT is more sensitive and specific in defining the anatomy of bony spinal fractures (see Fig. 19–4).

The strength of MR is imaging displaced bony fragments and their relationship to the thecal sac and cord. Sagittal T1WIs yield a clear anatomic picture of the relationship of the displaced or retropulsed fragments with the cord (see Fig. 19–3). The "myelogram" effect on sagittal T2WIs, especially with cardiac gating or flow compensation, demonstrates compression of the thecal sac because of superb contrast of low-signal cortical bone with high-signal CSF. Confirmation with axial views is helpful. T2-weighted axial images are helpful but time-consuming. However, low flip angle, gradient-refocused echo can be performed quickly and yield high-resolution, high-contrast T2WIs.

Associated complete or partial block from compression causes altered CSF flow dynamics. When compression of the subarachnoid space is great enough to dampen CSF pulsations (a "complete block"), the CSF within the spinal canal may have a higher signal as loss of normal CSF flow void results in T2 prolongation.[89–90] This is seen most prominently on nongated T2WIs below the level of the block. In contrast, turbulent CSF pulsations may occur with a partial block

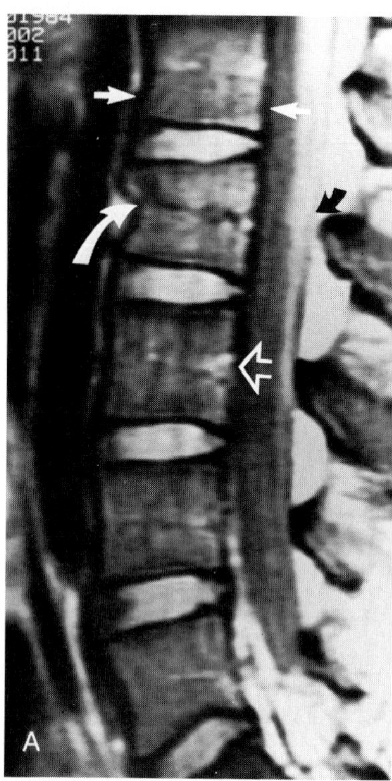


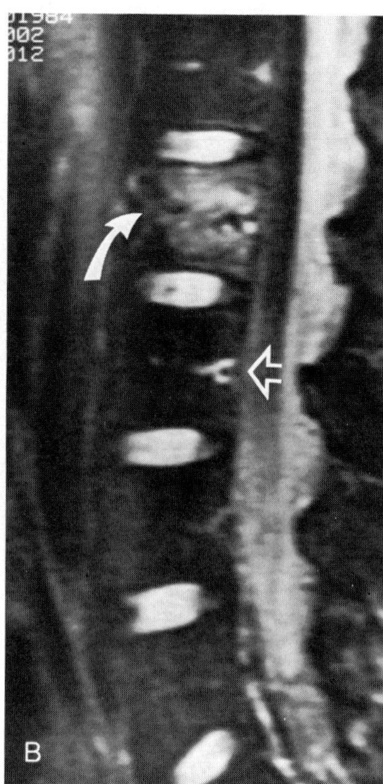


**Figure 19–9. Acute vertebral body fracture (1.5 T).** *A,* N(H)WI (TR 2000/TE 20). *B,* T2WI (TR 2000/TE 80). The transverse vertebral body fracture (curved white arrows) through the midportion of L2 at the conus level (black arrow) is an irregular, well-defined linear region of low signal on both images. It is most apparent on T1WI because of high lesion contrast with marrow fat. Cortical disruption anteriorly and loss of vertebral body height indicate a flexion compression mechanism. Osseous edema, manifested by long T2 is most apparent on the T2WI, but is inapparent on the N(H)WI which has negated the contrast effects of T1, T2, and proton density.

The anterior and posterior longitudinal ligaments, together with cortical bone, are identified as longitudinal stripes of hypointensity on N(H)WI (small white arrows). The basivertebral venous plexus (open arrows) enters the midportion of the vertebral body posteriorly. This normal structure should not be mistaken for a fracture. In this case, the fracture occurred through the venous plexus. (Courtesy of Neuroradiology Department, University of Cincinnati, Cincinnati, Ohio.)

that may result in a loss of signal at the level of the partial block.[90]

The stability of the spine depends upon both bony and ligamentous integrity.[91, 92, 95] The anterior and posterior longitudinal interspinous and supraspinous ligaments can be directly imaged as low-intensity structures on both T1 and T2WI (see Figs. 19–3 and 19–9). The ligamentum flavum has an intermediate signal on T1WI and a low signal on T2WI.[93] The extent of ligamentous disruption aids in classifying an injury as "stable" or "unstable" and aids in surgical management.[88] Reliability of MR in the establishment of preoperative ligamentous status has not been determined, although accurate diagnosis of ligamentous disruption has been reported.[88]

## Post-Traumatic Disk Herniation

Trauma may result in herniation of disk material. Most commonly, this results in posterior herniation similar to degenerative or idiopathic disk herniation. The MR findings associated with disk herniation are reviewed elsewhere; however, a few points deserve to be mentioned. Depending on its pretrauma status, an extruded disk may be normal or degenerated. When trauma causes herniation of a previously normal disk, MR will reveal a normal diskogenic signal on both T1WI and T2WI. More severe trauma may result in changes in disk morphology and signal.[88] The abnormal configuration of a traumatized disk can be identified on both T1WI and T2WI but because of image contrast, is more conspicuous on T2WI (see Figs. 19–1 and 19–3). Portions of disk material may extend into the fracture site through the disrupted annulus and vertebral body endplate (see Figs. 19–1 and 19–3). Sequestration by a disrupted posterior longitudinal ligament may cause disk edema, resulting in longer T1 and T2 relaxation times.[94] Intradiscal hematomas have been described.[88]

## Spinal Epidural Hematoma

Spinal epidural hematoma (SEH) is an uncommon event which may result from numerous causes including anticoagulation, bleeding diathesis, pregnancy, hypertension and atherosclerosis, SLE, AVMs, neoplasia, ankylosing spondylitis, rheumatoid arthritis, trauma (including birth trauma in neonates), lumbar puncture and spinal anesthesia, and "spontaneous."[102–111, 113, 114, 116, 118, 124–135, 141–153] Many patients with predisposing factors have varying degrees of minor trauma, including vigorous exercise, straining, coughing, or minor falls. Patients with seemingly minor trauma or "accentuated activities of daily living" have been referred to in the literature as having a "spontaneous" SEH.

The prevalence of SEH after major or minor trauma has been estimated to be between 1 per cent and 1.7 per cent.[111, 112] Associated vertebral injury is common. Children, because of the relative plasticity of their spinal columns, have a much lower prevalence of fracture-dislocation, even after major spinal trauma.[121, 122] The clinical presentation is usually one of acute neck or back pain often associated with a radiculopathy. There is typically a progression to severe neurologic deficit within hours to days, although rapid progression in minutes and more insidious, chronic progression have been described.[136–140] If the SEH occurs in the cervical spine, death from respiratory failure may occur.[113] When resulting from more severe trauma, SEH is usually associated with varying degrees of cord injury. Although cord damage may be irreparable, the development of an SEH represents a superimposed treatable insult. Spontaneous resolution is rare; the development of an SEH is a neurosurgical emergency requiring decompression.[107, 114–116] Early diagnosis and decompression is a critical factor in outcome determination.[117–120]

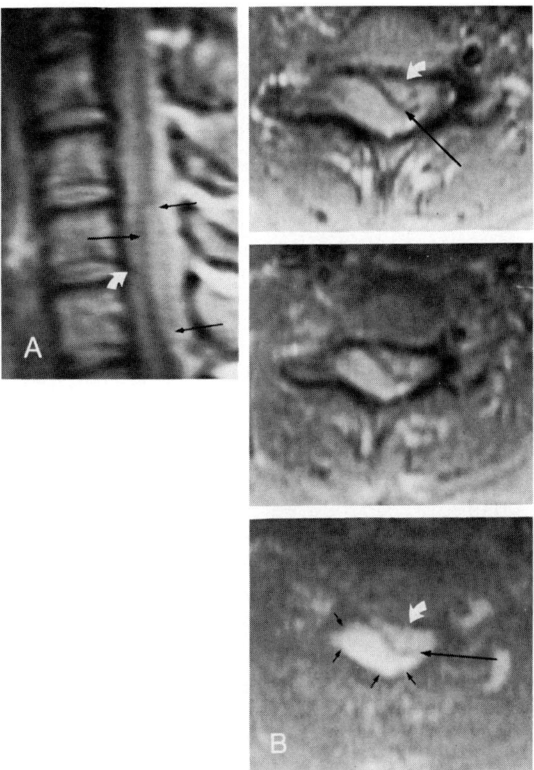


**Figure 19–10. Spinal epidural hematoma (SEH).** A 31-year-old woman in her second trimester developed sudden severe back pain and became acutely quadriparetic (1.5 T). *A*, Sagittal T1WI (SE TR 600/TE 20) shows a slightly hyperintense mass (between small black arrows) posterior to the cervical cord several segments long. The thin hypointense dura (long thin arrow) between the cord and the SEH supports an extradural location. In this sagittal view, the cord appears severely compressed (curved white arrow). *B*, Axial images T1WI (SE TR 600/TE 20) top, N(H)WI (SE TR 1800/TE 20) middle, T2WI (SE TR 1800/TE 80) bottom. The SEH (between small black arrows, bottom) is located posterolaterally on the right and causes mass effect with shift of the cord (curved white arrow) to the right. The SEH is intermediate to hyperintense on T1WI and hyperintense on T2WI. The hypointense dura (long black arrow) indicates the extradural nature of the hematoma.

Note that while there is mass effect and mild to moderate cord compression, the degree of cord compression on the sagittal view is misleading owing to displacement of the cord out of the imaging plane, illustrating the necessity of axial correlation. This case proved to be acute clot. The reason for the discordance between the acute clot and its atypical appearance by current "dogma" of high-field intracranial hematoma is unknown, but it is not uncommon in our experience with extra-axial spinal hematomata. The signal intensity changes of blood in this case are not incompatible with hyperacute hemorrhage.

### *MR Appearance*

Spinal epidural hematomas can be characterized by their morphology and abnormal signal. SEHs are mass lesions of variable length in the epidural space. Their epicenter is usually at the level of injury. They are most common in the thoracic and thoracolumbar spine. The spinal epidural space is composed of loose areolar tissue, which accounts for the tendency of SEHs to spread longitudinally over several cord segments (Fig. 19–10).[123] The overwhelming majority occur in a posterolateral or posterior position although unusually, they may occur anteriorly or circumferentially (Fig. 19–10). Axial images typically demonstrate a posterolateral, lenticular mass with obtuse angles causing mass effect, with cord compression and displacement to the opposite side. The low-signal dura can be identified separating the extradural mass from the cord. Identification of the dura is important, as it helps differentiate an extradural from a subdural hematoma. Sagittal images typically demonstrate a posteriorly located, "cigar-shaped" mass that extends over several segments. The cord is displaced anteriorly and to the opposite side. When the cord is laterally displaced, it may go out of a sagittally oriented imaging plane and thus appear falsely compressed on sagittal images; axial views are helpful to confirm the degree of compression (Fig. 19–10).

Signal abnormalities of aging blood in the epidural space, as with hematomas located elsewhere in the CNS, are age-dependent. However, unlike intracranial hematomas and hematomyelias, we have observed several acute SEHs that have demonstrated minimal hyperintensity on T1WI and hyperintensity or intermediate signal on T2WIs (Fig. 19–10; see also Fig. 19–1). The reason for this is unclear. Because SEHs are located adjacent to the subarachnoid space, their conspicuity varies. For instance, a high-signal SEH hematoma (short T1/long T2) may be difficult to differentiate from high-signal CSF on T2WI. T1WI will help separate the long T1 of CSF from the short T1 of the subacute SEH.

## Spinal Subdural Hematoma

Spinal subdural hematoma (SSH) is rare.[154–158, 177] Bleeding into the subdural space may result from anticoagulation[159] bleeding diathesis, trauma, iatrogenic (operations and LP's), tumor and AVM's, and "spontaneous."[155, 157, 159–174, 176, 177, 179–181] Trauma, accidental or iatrogenic, accounts for 46 per cent of SSHs.[167] They are commonly the result of minor trauma similar to that described with SEH. Clinical presentation is variable, dependent upon the involved level and time course. It may be acute, with sudden, severe pain followed by a radiculopathy and rapid paraplegia; subacute, with more gradual onset of pain and weakness over several weeks; or chronic, with minimal or no pain and gradual paraplegia over several months or years. SSH is more common in females (2:1) and is most common in the thoracic and thoracolumbar region.[158, 167] Calcification may occur.[177]

Unlike the epidural space, the subdural space does not contain large vessels; the source of bleeding is unknown.[158] The distinction between SEH and SSH may be difficult preoperatively. In fact, they commonly coexist.[175, 177, 181] Early diagnosis and decompression result in a better prognosis.[158, 176]

### *MR Appearance*

MR characteristics are the result of the abnormal mass and its abnormal signal. In the axial plane, SSHs typically have a convex outer margin and a concave inner margin, conforming to the shape of the spinal subdural space. An SSH usually extends over several cord segments. Because the hematoma is intradural, the low-signal dura does not separate the cord from the hematoma as it does with an SEH (Fig. 19–11). MR experience with the rare SSH has not been reported. However, the signal abnormalities associated with the hematoma are likely the same as those with SEH. Distinction between an SEH and SSH is difficult. The concave inner margin and the absence of the hypointense dura separating the hematoma from the cord help to differentiate between the two.

## Pseudotumor

"Pseudotumors" are fibrous granulation tissue and elastic fibers located in the anterior epidural space at the level of the craniovertebral junction that are thought to arise from chronic subluxation at C1–C2.[182, 183] Other causes of "pseudotumoral" extradural masses include SEH, pannus in rheumatoid arthritis, gout, fat deposition and pigmented villonodular synovitis.[184–188]

### *MR Appearance*

Fibrous tissue has a low water content[189] and contains tightly bound protons, resulting in a low to intermediate signal on T1WI and low signal on T2WI.[182] Compression and distortion of the subarachnoid space and brain stem by a low- or intermediate-signal, anterior epidural mass is identified (Fig. 19–12). Extradural fat (short T1/intermediate T2) can be distinguished from pseudotumor by its hyperintensity on T1WI. MR characterization of other pseudotumoral masses listed above has not yet been fully studied. Most neoplasms, in contrast with pseudotumors, have a high water content (long T1/T2) that makes them hyperintense on

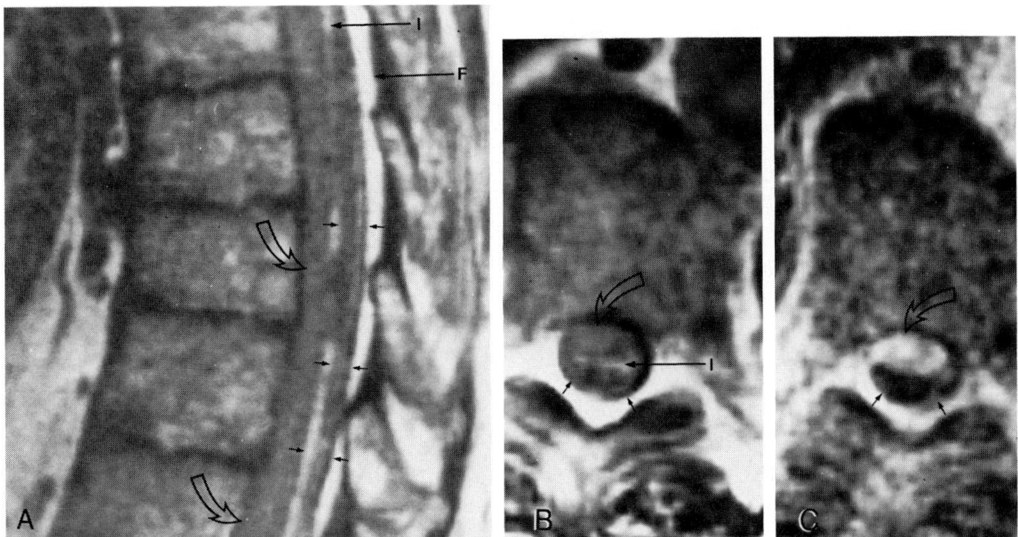


**Figure 19–11. Spinal subdural hematoma (SSH).** A 78-year-old man who after a fall from a chair developed acute LE paresis and an ascending thoracic sensory level (1.5 T). The MR was performed five days later.

*A,* Sagittal T1WI (SE TR 600/TE 25). *B* and *C,* Axial N(H)WI and T2WI (SE TR 2264/TE 30/60) with respiratory compensation show a long, crescentic hematoma (between small arrows) located anterior to epidural fat *(F)*, compressing and displacing the thecal sac anteriorly (open curved arrows). At surgery, a dry clot was found in the subdural space; the epidural space was normal. A subarachnoid clot was also present, which may account for the inhomogeneous signal within the dural tube. The high signal interface (I) between the cord and the SSH seen in *A* had no surgical counterpart. (Courtesy of N. Leeds, M.D. and R. Schepp, M.D., Dept. of Neuroradiology, Beth Israel Medical Center, New York, NY.)

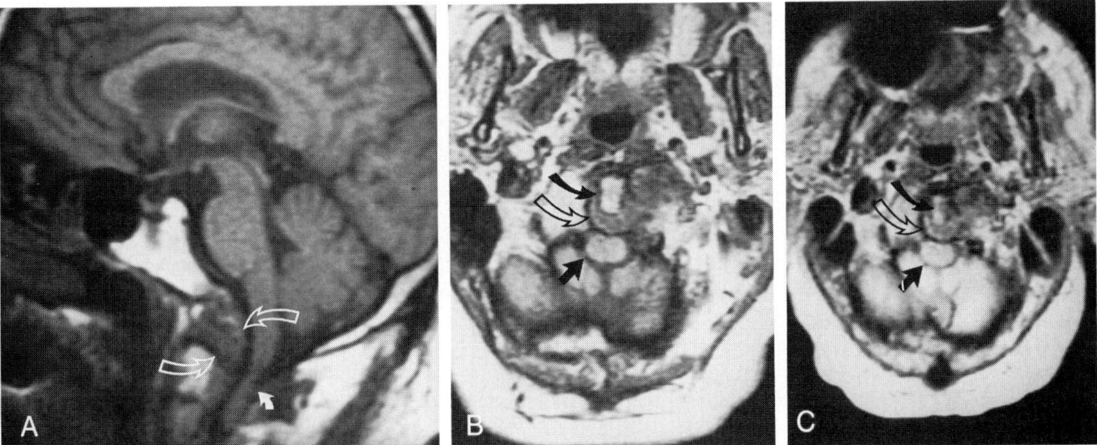


**Figure 19–12. Pseudotumor (1.5 T).** *A,* Sagittal T1WI (SE TR 600/TE 20) through the craniocervical junction shows a low signal mass (curved arrows) between the clival tip (basion) and dens, extending posteriorly to the body of C2. Extradural cord compression (small arrow), and displacement are present. *B,* Axial T1WI (SE TR 520/20) and *C,* N(H)WI (SE TR 2000/TE 20) at the level of the dens (curved black arrow) show the low signal mass on both images (open curved arrow), consistent with its fibrous histology. The pseudotumor extends around the dens in semilunar fashion, causing extradural cord (small arrow) compression. (Courtesy of Neuroradiology Department, University of Cincinnati, Cincinnati, Ohio.)

T2WI. Some neoplasms, however, may not have a long T2. Meningiomas with calcification and tumors with hemorrhagic foci may appear dark on T2 and may be difficult to differentiate from pseudotumors by signal intensity alone.

## TRAUMATIC NERVE ROOT AVULSION

Nerve root avulsion results from traction produced by violent motion of an extremity with forcible separation of the extremity from the spine.[190] This injury most commonly involves the brachial plexus but may occur with lumbosacral nerve roots as well.[204–207] Stretched beyond elastic limits, the nerve fails at its weakest point, the site of its attachment to the cord.[190, 193] Anatomically, nerve roots are contained within the endoneurium, a continuation of the pia. During their exit, the roots acquire a sleeve of arachnoid and dura, which only becomes attached at the dorsal root ganglia. The preganglionic nerve roots are separated from the dura and arachnoid by an extension of the subarachnoid space; thus the roots are only ensheathed by the thin endoneurium.[195] Beyond the ganglion, the dura becomes the tough, fibrous perineurium that helps protect the peripheral nerve from injury. With excessive traction, the nerve is pulled peripherally through the neural foramen, and the dura/arachnoid may tear. If traction continues, rupture of the unprotected nerve root results.

Dural rupture allows CSF to escape through the neural foramen into the surrounding soft tissues, causing a fibrotic response that usually closes the leak.[190–194, 208] This results in a CSF-containing outpouching, lined by meninges or scar, that communicates with the subarachnoid space—a "pseudomeningocele".[190–201] It is vital to assess the status of the plexus both anatomically and functionally because intradural nerve root disruption carries a poor prognosis, and traumatic plexopathies occur without disruption (for which the prognosis is good with proper rehabilitation).[192–201] Alternatively, the disruption may occur in an extradural location that may be amenable to surgery.[192, 196] Filling of the pseudomeningocele (PM) is the basis of myelographic diagnosis. However, correlation of pathology with myelography is imperfect, as dural tears and PMs may occur in the absence of nerve root avulsion, and nerve root avulsions may occur with normal myelograms.[193, 197, 202, 203] The failure of myelography to correlate with clinical and pathologic findings results primarily from its indirect visualization of the lesion. That is, identification of a PM (and thus a dural tear) is equated with an intradural avulsion injury. The avulsive lesion and status of the nerve root is not directly visualized.

### MR Appearance

MR appearances vary with the pathology. The dural tear is visualized as a CSF-containing structure extending a variable distance from the subarachnoid space. It may remain within the spinal canal or neural foramen, but it typically extends through the neural canal into the lateral paraspinal soft tissues (Fig. 19–13). Involvement of multiple contiguous nerve roots is more common than involvement of a single root.[191] Axial and coronal scans are the most helpful imaging planes. Axial images demonstrate the relationship of the subarachnoid space and the neural foramen to the PMs. Coronal images demonstrate their longitudinal relationship to the thecal sac and nerve roots in a manner similar to a myelogram.[210, 211] An uncomplicated traumatic meningocele has CSF signal characteristics (long T1/T2), and both T1WI and T2WI should be performed. Nongated T2WI may demonstrate higher signal of the CSF in the PM than in the thecal sac because of relatively decreased pulsation (and therefore less signal loss) within the PM.[211] Cardiac-gated T2WIs of the cervical spine are relatively free of flow artifacts and therefore allow higher resolution than nongated studies, although the flow artifact from dampened pulsations is lost. Axial fast-field images with a low flip angle yield quick T2WI with resolution comparable to that of T1WI. T2WIs offer high lesion contrast with surrounding soft tissues and cortical bone of the vertebral bodies and neural foramen. Oblique thin sections through the intervertebral foramen may be more sensitive to pathology in this region. The main differential diagnostic consideration is the neurofibroma. This mass within the neural foramen has a dumbbell, or tubular, appearance

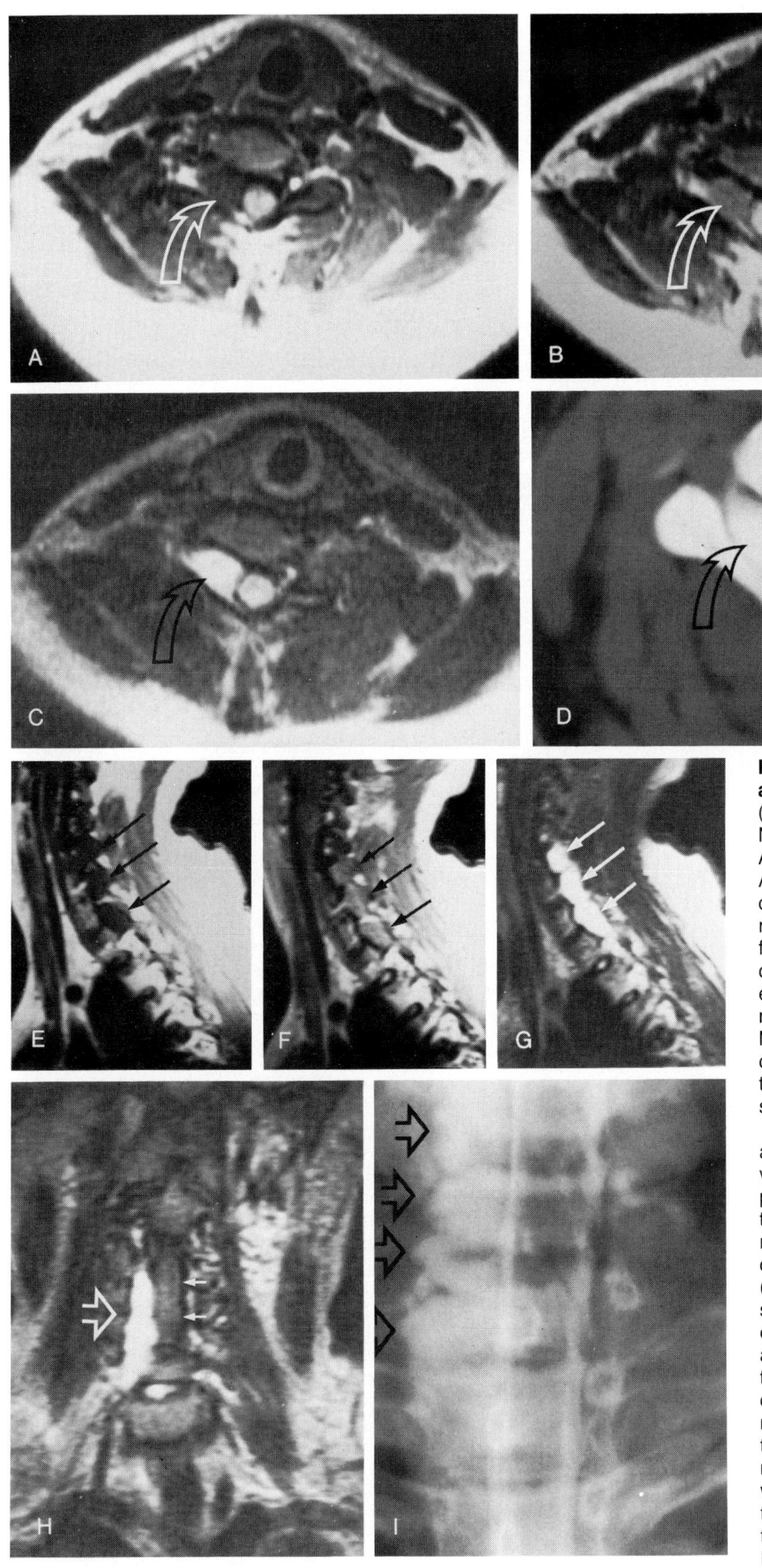


**Figure 19–13. Brachial plexus avulsion (1.5 T).** *A,* Axial T1WI (SE TR 400/TE 25); *B,* Axial N(H)WI (SE TR 1500/TE 25); *C,* Axial T2WI (SE TR 1500/TE 50). A fluid collection with CSF signal characteristics (open curved arrows) extends into the neural foramen, consistent with pseudomeningocele formation. The enlarged foramen from bone remodeling indicates chronicity. *D,* Metrizamide myelogram-CT demonstrates the communication of the pseudomeningocele with the subarachnoid space.

*E to G,* Sagittal T1WI, N(H)WI, and T2WI through the right intervertebral foramina show multiple pseudomeningoceles extending through the neural canals (arrows). Note the typical CSF signal on all images. *H,* Coronal T2WI (SE TR 1500/TE 50) from C4–C7 show the typical long T2 of CSF extending through the neural foramina (open arrow) to the right of the cord (small arrows), with cord displacement to the left. *I,* AP myelogram from C5–C7 shows the coronally oriented pseudomeningoceles (open arrows) filled with contrast originally placed in the subarachnoid space. (Courtesy of T. Seward, M.D., Bethesda North Hospital, and L. Eynon, M.D., Mercy Hospital, Cincinnati, Ohio.)

morphologically similar to a PM. However, signal characteristics are slightly different. Neurofibromas typically are hyperintense on T2WI, similar to the CSF-containing PM, but have an intermediate signal on T1WI when compared with the hypointensity of a PM.[212] Although the typical PM described above is the "hallmark" of avulsive injuries, other appearances may be manifest.

PMs may become quite large and cause bone remodeling or a large mass in the neck, supraclavicular region, or thorax.[208, 209] Extension of a "neck" of the large fluid collection into the neural foramen helps to distinguish a traumatic meningocele from other cystic collections. Avulsive injuries may result in scarring and irregularity of the margins of the subarachnoid space without the development of a PM. This scarring may take the form of a very small outpouching or even an irregular or convex mass effect upon the subarachnoid space.[191] Irregularity of the thecal sac is not specific for nerve root avulsion.

The goal of imaging in traumatic plexopathies is the direct identification of the avulsive lesion and its relationship to the dura and ganglion, instead of the indirect dural tear. MR commonly images both nerve roots and dorsal root ganglia using current surface coil technology and high-resolution scanning techniques.[213] Although the sensitivity of MR for the diagnosis of nerve root avulsion and accuracy in identifying the lesion site has not been established, the potential application of MR to this imaging task poses exciting possibilities.

## References

### *Post-Traumatic Myelopathy*

1. Anderson TE. Spinal cord contusion injury: experimental dissociation of hemorrhagic necrosis and subacute loss of axonal conduction. J Neurosurg 62:115, 1985.
2. Naseem M, Zachariah SB, Stone J, Russell E. Cervicomedullary hematoma: diagnosis with MR. AJNR 7:1096, 1986.
3. Obrador S, Dierssen G, Odoriz BJ. Surgical evacuation of a pontine-medullary hematoma: case report. J Neurosurg 33:82, 1970.
4. Kitahara T, Miyasaka Y, Ohwada T, et al. NSG. An operated case of cervical spontaneous hematomyelia. Abstract. No To Shinkei 10:675, 1982.
5. Kempe LG. Surgical removal of an intramedullary hematoma simulating Wallenberg's syndrome. J Neurol Neurosurg Psychiatr 27:78, 1964.
6. Post MJD. Computed tomography of spinal trauma. In Post MJD, ed. Computed Tomography of the Spine. Baltimore, Md. Williams & Wilkins, 1984:782.
7. Kao CC. Spinal cord cavitation after injury. In Windle WF, ed. The Spinal Cord and Its Reaction to Traumatic Injury. New York, M. Dekker, 1980:249.
8. Schneider RC, Cherry G, Pantek H. The syndrome of acute central cervical spinal cord injury. J Neurosurg 11:546, 1954.
9. Ducker TB, Lucas JT, Wallace CA. Recovery from spinal cord injury. In Weiss MH, ed. Clinical Neurosurgery. Vol. 30 1983:495.
10. Stillwell GK. The law of Laplace. Mayo Clinic Proc 48:863, 1973.
11. Dohrmann GJ, Wagner FC, Bucy PC. Transitory traumatic paraplegia: electron microscopy of early alterations in myelinated nerve fibers. J Neurosurg 36:407, 1972.
12. Kao CC, Chang LW. The mechanisms of spinal cord cavitation following spinal cord transection. Part 1. A correlated histochemical study. J Neurosurg 46:197, 1977.
13. Kao CC, Chang LW, Bloodworth JMB. The mechanism of spinal cord cavitation following spinal cord transection. Part II. Electron microscopic observations. J Neurosurg 46:745, 1977.
14. Allen AR. Surgery of experimental lesions of spinal cord equivalent to crush injury of fracture dislocation of spinal column. JAMA 57:878, 1911.
15. Brodkey JS, Miller CF, Harmody RM. The syndrome of acute central cervical spinal cord injury revisited. Surg Neurol 14:251, 1980.
16. Windle WF. Concussion, contusion, and severence of the spinal cord. In Windle WF, ed. The Spinal Cord and Its Reaction to Traumatic Injury. New York, M. Dekker, 1980:205.
17. Goodman JH, Bingham WG, Hunt WE. Ultra-structural blood-brain barrier alterations and edema formation in acute spinal cord trauma. J Neurosurg 44:418, 1976.
18. Bingham W, Goldman H, Friedman S, et al. Blood flow in normal and injured monkey spinal cord. J Neurosurg 43:162, 1975.
19. Dohrmann GJ, Wick KM, Bucy PC. Spinal cord blood flow patterns in experimental traumatic paraplegia. J Neurosurg 38:52, 1973.
20. Rivlin AS, Tator CH. Regional spinal cord blood flow in rats after severe cord trauma. J Neurosurg 49:844, 1978.
21. Sandler AN, Tator CH. Effect of acute spinal cord compression injury on regional spinal cord blood flow in primates. J Neurosurg 45:660, 1976.
22. Sandler AN, Tator CH. Review of the effect of spinal cord trauma on the vessels and blood flow in the spinal cord. J Neurosurg 45:638, 1976.
23. Chakeres DW, Flinckinger F, Bresnahan JC, et al. MR imaging of acute spinal cord trauma. AJNR 8:5, 1987.
24. Hackney DB, Asato R, Joseph PM, et al. Hemorrhage and edema in acute spinal cord compression: demonstration by MR imaging. Radiology 161:387, 1986.
25. Enzmann DR, Rubin JB, Wright A. Use of cerebrospinal fluid gating to improve T2-weighted images. Part I. The spinal cord. Radiology 162:763, 1987.
26. Enzmann DR, Rubin JB, DeLaPaz R, Wright A. Benefits and pitfalls in MRI scanning resulting from CSF pulsation. Radiology 161:773, 1986.
27. Citrin CM, Sherman JL, Gangarosa RE, et al. Phys-

iology of the CSF flow-void signal: modification by cardiac gating. AJR 148:205, 1987.
28. Bergstrand G, Bergström M, Nordell B, et al. Cardiac-gated MR imaging of cerebrospinal fluid flow. J Comput Assist Tomogr 9:1003, 1985.
29. Balériaux D, Deroover N, Hermanus N, et al. MRI of the spine. Diagn Imag Clin Med 55:66, 1986.
30. Weinstein M. Imaging of the spine: an overview. Spine Imaging Symposium. Chicago, Radiological Society of North America. 1986.
31. Nelson E, Gertz SD, Rennels ML, et al. Spinal cord injury. The role of vascular damage in the pathogenesis of central hemorrhagic necrosis. Arch Neurol 34:332, 1977.
32. Osterholm JL. The pathophysiological response to spinal cord injury: the current status of related research. J Neurosurg 40:5, 1974.
33. Yashon D, Bingham WG, Faddoul EM, et al. Edema of the spinal cord following experimental impact trauma. J Neurosurg 38:693, 1973.
34. Rossier AB, Foo D, Shillito J, et al. Posttraumatic cervical syringomyelia. Brain 108:439, 1985.
35. Williams B, Terry AF, Jones F, et al. Syringomyelia as a sequel to traumatic paraplegia. Paraplegia 19:67, 1981.
36. Barnett HJM, Jousse AT. Post-traumatic syringomyelia. In Vinken PJ, Bruyn EM, eds. Handbook of Clinical Neurology. New York, North-Holland Publishing Co., 1976.
37. Vernon JD, Chir B, Silver JR, et al. Post-traumatic syringomyelia. Paraplegia 20:339, 1982.
38. Barnett HJM, Botterell EH, Jousse AT, et al. Progressive myelopathy as a sequel to traumatic paraplegia. Brain 89:159, 1966.
39. Tator CH, Meguro K, Rowed DW. Favorable results with syringosubarachnoid shunts for treatment of syringomyelia. J Neurosurg 56:517, 1982.
40. Shannon N, Symon L, Logue V, et al. Clinical features, investigation and treatment of post-traumatic syringomyelia. J Neurol Neurosurg Psychiatr 44:35, 1981.
41. Griffiths ER, McCormick CC. Post-traumatic syringomyelia (cysticmyelopathy). Paraplegia 19:81, 1981.
42. Quencer RM, Green BA, Eismont FJ. Post-traumatic spinal cord cysts: clinical features and characterization with metrizamide computed tomography. Radiology 146:415, 1983.
43. Ducker TB, Kindt GW, Kempe LG. Pathological findings in acute experimental spinal cord trauma. Brain 98:159, 1966.
44. Cushing HW. Haematomyelia from gunshot wounds in the spine. Am J Med Sci 115:654, 1898.
45. Holmes G. Spinal injuries of warfare. Br Med J 2:769, 1915.
46. Greenfield JG. Syringomyelia and syringobulbia. In Greenfield's Neuropathology. Baltimore, Williams & Wilkins, 1976:668.
47. Escourolle R, Poirier J. Manual of Basic Neuropathology. Philadelphia, W. B. Saunders, 1973:19.
48. von Schulthess GK, Higgins CB. Blood-flow imaging with MR: spin phase phenomena. Radiology 157:687, 1985.
49. Bradley WG, Waluch VW. Blood flow: magnetic resonance imaging. Radiology 154:443, 1985.
50. Sherman JL, Barkovich AJ, Citrin CM. The MR appearance of syringomyelia: new observations. AJR 148:381, 1987.
51. Sherman JL, Citrin CM, Gangarosa RE, et al. The MR appearance of CSF pulsations in the spinal canal. AJNR 7:879, 1986.
52. Quencer RM, Morse BMM, Green BA, et al. Intraoperative spinal sonography: an adjunct to metrizamide CT in the assessment and surgical decompression of post-traumatic spinal cord cysts, AJNR 5:71, 1984.
53. Stevens JM, Olney JS, Kendall BE. Posttraumatic cystic and noncystic myelopathy. Neuroradiology 27:48, 1985.
54. Gebarski SS, Maynard FW, Gabrielson TO, et al. Posttraumatic progressive myelopathy. Radiology, 157:379, 1985.
55. Quencer RM, Sheldon JJ, Post MJD, et al. MRI of the chronically injured cervical spinal cord. AJR 147:125, 1986.
56. McArdle CB, Wright JW, Prevost WJ, et al. MR imaging of the acutely injured patient with cervical traction. Radiology 159:273, 1986.
57. Modic MT. Imaging of the spine. Spine Imaging Symposium, Radiological Society of North America, Chicago, 1986.
58. Axel L. Surface coil magnetic resonance imaging. J Comput Assist Tomogr 8:381, 1984.
59. Modic MT, Pavlicek W, Weinstein MA, et al. Magnetic resonance imaging of intervertebral disk disease. Radiology 152:103, 1984.
60. Han JS, Kaufman B, El Yousef SJ, et al. NMR imaging of the spine. AJNR 4:1151, 1983.
61. Kokmen E, Marsh WR, Baker HL. Magnetic resonance imaging in syringomyelia. Neurosurgery 17:267, 1985.
62. Lee BCP, Zimmerman RD, Manning JJ, et al. MR imaging of syringomyelia and hydromyelia. AJNR 6:221, 1985.
63. Pojunas K, Williams AL, Daniels D, et al. Syringomyelia and hydromyelia: magnetic resonance evaluation. Radiology 153:679, 1984.
64. Yeates A, Brant-Zawadzki M, Norman D, et al. Nuclear magnetic resonance imaging of syringomyelia. AJNR 4:234, 1983.
65. Barkovich AJ, Sherman JL, Citrin CM, et al. MR of postoperative syringomyelia. AJNR 8:319, 1987.
66. Brown JJ, van Sonnenberg E, Gerber KH, et al. Magnetic resonance relaxation times of percutaneously obtained normal and abnormal body fluids. Radiology 154:727, 1985.
67. Burton DR, Forsen A, Karlsrom G, et al. Proton relaxation enhancement in biochemistry. Prog Nucl Magn Reson Spectrosc 13:1, 1979.
68. Brant-Zawadzki M, Kelly W, Kjos B, et al. Magnetic resonance imaging and characterization of normal and abnormal intracranial CSF spaces. Neuroradiology 27:3, 1985.
69. Nakada T, Kwee IL, Palmaz JC. Computed tomography of spinal cord atrophy. Neuroradiology 24:97, 1982.
70. Donaldson I, Gibson R. Spinal cord atrophy associated with arachnoiditis as demonstrated by computed tomography. Neuroradiology 24:101, 1982.
71. Komaki S. Localized spinal cord atrophy: significance of its demonstration. Radiology 121:111, 1976.
72. Jirout J. Pneumographic examination of posttraumatic conditions and spinal cord atrophy of various causes. In Goree J, ed., Pneumomyelography. Springfield, Ill., Charles C Thomas, 1969: 237.
73. Shapiro R. Myelography, 4th ed. Chicago, Ill., Yearbook Medical Publishers, 1984:530.
74. Hoff J, Nishimura M, Pitts L, et al. The role of ischemia in the pathogenesis of cervical spondylotic myelopathy. Spine 2:100, 1977.

75. Dee GJ, Bello JA, Hilal SK. High field thin section nuclear magnetic resonance imaging of the cervical spine. Cardiovasc Intervent Radiol 8:283, 1986.
76. Brown-Sequard E. Lectures on the Diagnosis and Treatment of the Principal Forms of Paralysis of the Lower Extremities. Philadelphia, Collins, 1861.
77. Austin GM. The Spinal Cord 3rd ed. New York, Igaku Shoin, 1983:223.
78. Hyman RA, Edwards JH, Vacirca SJ, et al. 0.6 T MR imaging of the cervical spine: multislice and multiecho techniques. AJNR 6:229, 1985.
79. Masaryk TJ, Modic MT, Geisinger MA, et al. Cervical myelopathy: a comparison of magnetic resonance and myelography. J Comput Assist Tomogr 10:184, 1986.
80. Schenck JF, Foster TH, Henkes JL, et al. High-field surface coil MR imaging of localized anatomy. AJNR 6:181, 1985.
81. Meyer P, et al. Annual progress report VII (1978). In Calenoff L., ed. Radiology of Spinal Cord Injury. St. Louis, C. V. Mosby Co., 1981:181.
82. McArdle C, Wright JW, Prevost WJ, et al. MR imaging of the acutely injured patient with cervical traction. Radiology 159:273, 1986.
83. Rogers LF. In Calenoff L, ed. Radiology of Spinal Cord Injury. St. Louis, C. V. Mosby Co., 1981:85.
84. Riggins RS, Kraus JF. The risk of neurologic damage with fractures of the vertebrae. J Trauma 17:126, 1977.
85. Daffner RH, Deeb ZL, Rothfus WE. The posterior vertebral body line: importance in the detection of burst fractures. AJR 148:93, 1987.
86. Atlas SW, Regenbogen V, Rogers LF, et al. The radiographic characterization of burst fractures of the spine. AJR 147:575, 1986.
87. Calenoff L, Chessare JW, Rogers LF, et al. Multiple level spinal injuries: importance of early recognition. AJR 130:665, 1978.
88. McArdle CB, Crofford MJ, Mirkahraee M, et al. Surface coil MR of spinal trauma: preliminary experience. AJNR 7:885, 1986.
89. Enzmann DR, Rubin JB, DeLaPaz R, et al. Cerebrospinal fluid pulsation: benefits and pitfalls in MR imaging. Radiology 216:773, 1986.
90. Rubin JB, Enzman DR. Imaging of spinal CSF pulsation by 2DFT MR: significance during clinical imaging. AJNR 8:297, 1987.
91. McAfee PC, Yuan HA, Fredrickson BE, et al. The value of computed tomography in thoracolumbar fractures. J Bone Joint Surg (Am) 65:461, 1983.
92. Ferguson RL, Allen BL. A mechanistic classification of thoracolumbar spine fractures. Clin Orthop 189:77, 1984.
93. Reicher MA, Gold RH, Halbach VV, et al. MR imaging of the lumbar spine: anatomic correlations and the effects of technical variations. AJR 147:891, 1986.
94. Modic MT, Masaryk T, Boumphrey F, et al. Lumbar herniated disk disease and canal stenosis: prospective evaluation by surface coil MR, CT, and myelography. AJR 147:757, 1986.
95. Kilcoyne RF, Mack LA. Computed tomography of spinal fractures. Appl Radiol p. 40, March 1987.
96. McLean DR, Miller JDR, Allen, PBR, et al. Posttraumatic syringomyelia. J Neurosurg 39:485, 1973.
97. Post MJD, Quencer RM, Green BA, et al. Radiologic evaluation of spinal cord fissures. AJNR 7:329, 1986.
98. Cooper PR, Cohen W. Evaluation of cervical spinal cord injuries with metrizamide myelography-CT scanning. J Neurosurg 61:281, 1984.
99. Kulkarni MV, McArdle CB, Kopanicky D, et al. Acute spinal cord injury: MR imaging at 1.5 T. Radiology 164:837, 1987.
100. Mirvis SE, Borg U, Belzberg, H. MR imaging of ventilator-dependent patients: preliminary experience. AJR 149:845, 1987.
101. Kakulas, BA. Pathology of spinal injuries. Centr Nerv Syst Trauma 1:117, 1984.


***Spinal Epidural Hematoma***


102. Alderman DB. Extradural spinal cord hematoma. Report of a case due to dicumarol and review of the literature. N Engl J Med 255:839, 1956.
103. Cloward RB, Yuhl ET. Spontaneous intraspinal hemorrhage and paraplegia complicating dicumarol therapy. Neurology 5:600, 1955.
104. Jacobson I, MacCabe JJ, Harris P, et al. Spontaneous spinal epidural haemorrhage during anticoagulant therapy. Br Med J 1:522, 1966.
105. Locke GE, Giorgio AJ, Biggers SL, et al. Acute spinal epidural hematoma secondary to aspirin-induced prolonged bleeding. Surg Neurol 5:293, 1976.
106. Zuccarello M, Scanarini M, et al. Spontaneous spinal extradural hematoma during anticoagulant therapy. Surg Neurol 14:411, 1980.
107. Zilkha A, Irwin GA, Fagelman D. Computed tomography of spinal epidural hematoma. AJNR 4:1073, 1983.
108. Lanzieri CF, Sacher M, Solodnik P, et al. CT myelography of spontaneous spinal epidural hematoma. J Comput Assist Tomogr 9:393, 1985.
109. Costabile G, Husag L, Probst C. Spinal epidural hematoma. Surg Neurol 21:489, 1984.
110. Labadie EL. Spontaneous cervical epidural hematoma followed by disseminated intravascular coagulation. Ariz Med 31:417, 1974.
111. Foo D, Rossier AB. Post-traumatic spinal epidural hematoma. Neurosurgery 11:25, 1982.
112. Ducker T. Commentary. Neurosurgery 11:31, 1982.
113. Beatty RM, Winston KR. Spontaneous cervical epidural hematoma. J Neurosurgery 61:143, 1984.
114. Harik SI, Raichle ME, Reis DJ. Spontaneously remitting spinal epidural hematoma in a patient on anticoagulants. N Engl J Med 284:1355, 1971.
115. Pear BL. Spinal epidural hematoma. AJR 115:155, 1972.
116. Hernandez D, Vinuela F, Feasby TE. Recurrent paraplegia with total recovery from spontaneous spinal epidural hematoma. Ann Neurol 11:623, 1982.
117. Simmons EH, Grobler LJ. Acute spinal epidural hematoma. J Bone Joint Surg (Am) 60:395, 1978.
118. Haykal HA, Wang A, Zamani AA, et al. Computed tomography of spontaneous acute cervical epidural hematoma. J Comput Assist Tomogr 8:229, 1984.
119. Cooper DW. Spontaneous spinal epidural hematoma. J Neurosurg 26:343, 1967.
120. Grollmus J, Hoff J. Spontaneous spinal epidural hæmorrhage: good results after early treatment. J Neurol Neurosurg Psychiatr 38:89, 1975.
121. Burke DC. Spinal cord trauma in children. Paraplegia 9:1, 1971.
122. Burke DC. Traumatic spinal paralysis in children. Paraplegia 11:268, 1974.

123. Post MJ, Seminer DS, Quencer RM. CT diagnosis of spinal epidural hematoma. AJNR 3:190, 1982.
124. Priest WM. Epidural hæmorrhage due to hæmophilia causing compression of spinal cord. Lancet 2:1289, 1935.
125. Cromwell LD, Kerber C, Ferry PC. Spinal cord compression and hematoma: an unusual complication in a hemophiliac infant. AJR 128:847, 1977.
126. London GW, McKeever PE, Wiederholt WC. Spontaneous spinal epidural hæmatoma in alcoholism. Ann Intern Med 81:266, 1974.
127. Bidzinski J. Spontaneous spinal epidural hematoma during pregnancy. Case report. J Neurosurg 24:1017, 1966.
128. Yonekawa Y, Mehdorn HM, Nishikawa M. Spontaneous spinal epidural hematoma during pregnancy. Surg Neurol 3:327, 1975.
129. Cube HM. Spinal extradural hemorrhage. J Neurosurg 19:171, 1962.
130. Foo D, Chang YC, Rossier AB. Spontaneous cervical epidural hemorrhage, anterior cord syndrome, and familial vascular malformations. Neurology 30:308, 1980.
131. Müller H, Schramm J, Roggendorf W, et al. Vascular malformations as a cause of spontaneous spinal epidural hæmatoma. Acta Neurochir 62:297, 1982.
132. Solero CL, Fornari M, Savoiardo M. Spontaneous spinal epidural haematoma arising from ruptured vascular malformation. Acta Neurochir 53:169, 1980.
133. Dawson BH. Paraplegia due to spinal epidural haematoma. J Neurol Neurosurg Psychiatr 26:171, 1963.
134. Odom GL. Vascular lesions of the spinal cord. Malformations, spinal subarachnoid and extradural hemorrhage. Clin Neurosurg 8:196, 1962.
135. Harris DJ, Fornasier VL, Livingston KE. Hemangiopericytoma of the spinal canal. Report of three cases. J Neurosurg 49:914, 1978.
136. Scott BB, Quisling RG, Miller CA, et al. Spinal epidural hematoma. JAMA 235:513, 1976.
137. Tsai FY, Popp AJ, Waldman J. Spontaneous spinal epidural hematoma. Neuroradiology 10:15, 1975.
138. Hehman K, Norrell H. Massive chronic spinal epidural hematoma in a child. Am J Dis Child 116:308, 1968.
139. Maxwell GM, Puletti F. Chronic spinal extradural hematoma. Neurology 7:596, 1957.
140. Boyd HR, Pear BL. Chronic spontaneous spinal epidural hematoma: report of two cases. J Neurosurg 36:239, 1972.
141. Kosary IZ, Braham J, Shacked I, et al. Spinal epidural hematoma due to hemangioma of vetebra. Surg Neurol 7:61, 1977.
142. Ainsle JP. Paraplegia due to spontaneous extradural or subdural haemorrhage. Br J Surg 45:565, 1958.
143. Lougheed WM, Hoffman HJ. Spontaneous spinal extradural hematoma. Neurology 10:1059, 1960.
144. Sadka M. Epidural spinal haemorrhage, with a report of two cases. Med J Aust 2:669, 1953.
145. Agnetti V, Monaco F, Mutani R. Post-convulsive spinal epidural haematoma in ankylosing spondylitis. Eur Neurol 18:230, 1979.
146. Bohlman HH. Acute fractures and dislocations of the cervical spine: an analysis of three hundred hospitalized patients and review of the literature. J Bone Joint Surg (Am) 61A:1119, 1979.
147. Farhat SM, Schneider RC, Gray JM. Traumatic spinal extradural hematoma associated with cervical fractures in rheumatoid spondylitis. J Trauma 13:591, 1973.
148. Grisolia A, Bell RL, Peltier LF. Fractures and dislocations of the spine complicating ankylosing spondylitis. J Bone Joint Surg (Am) 49:339, 1967.
149. Lowrey JJ. Spinal epidural hematomas: experiences with three patients. J Neurosurg 16:508, 1959.
150. Towbin A. Latent spinal cord and brainstem injury in newborn infants. Develop Med Child Neurol 11:54, 1969.
151. Helperin SW, Cohen DD. Hematoma following epidural anesthesia. Anesthesiology 35:641, 1971.
152. Wittebol MC, van Veelen CWM. Spontaneous spinal epidural hæmatoma. etiological considerations. Clin Neurol Neurosurg 86:265, 1984.
153. Vallée B, Besson G, Gaudin J, et al. Spontaneous spinal epidural hematoma in a 22-month-old girl. J Neurosurg 56:135, 1982.


### *Spinal Subdural Hematoma*


154. Brandt RA. Chronic spinal subdural hematoma. Surg Neurol 13:121, 1980.
155. Gutterman P. Acute spinal subdural hematoma following lumbar puncture. Surg Neurol 7:355, 1977.
156. Paredes ESD, Kishore PRS, Ward JD. Cervical spinal subdural hematoma. Surg Neurol 15:477, 1981.
157. Stewart DH, Watkins ES. Spinal cord compression by chronic subdural hematoma. J Neurosurg 31:80, 1969.
158. Russell NA, Benoit BG. Spinal subdural hematoma. Surg Neurol 20:133, 1983.
159. Cloward RB, Yuhl ET. Spontaneous intraspinal hemorrhage and paraplegia complicating dicumerol therapy. Case report. Neurology 5:600, 1955.
160. Guthikonda M, Schmidek HH, Wallman LJ, et al. Spinal subdural hematoma: case report and review of the literature. Neurosurgery 5:614, 1979.
161. Kohli CM, Palmer AH, Gray GH. Spontaneous intraspinal hemorrhage causing paraplegia. A complication of heparin therapy. Ann Surg 179:197, 1974.
162. Russell NA, Maroun FB, Jacob JC. Spinal subdural hematoma occurring in association with anticoagulant therapy: report of a case and review of the literature. Can J Neurol Sci 8:87, 1981.
163. Tomarken JL. Spinal subdural hematoma. Ann Emerg Med 14:261, 1985.
164. Dunn D, Dhopesh V, Mobini J. Spinal subdural hematoma. A possible hazard of lumbar puncture in an alcoholic. JAMA 241:1712, 1979.
165. Edelson RN, Chernik NL, Posner JB. Spinal subdural hematomas complicating lumbar puncture. Occurence in thrombocytopenic patients. Arch Neurol 31:134, 1974.
166. Schiller F, Neligan G, Budtz-Olsen O. Surgery in hæmophilia. A case of spinal subdural hæmatoma producing paraplegia. Lancet 2:842, 1948.
167. Woolcot GJ, Grunnett ML, Lahey ME. Spinal subdural hematoma in a leukemic child. J Pediatr 77:1060, 1970.
168. Khosla VK, Kak VK, Mathuriya SN. Chronic spinal subdural hematomas. J Neurosurg 63:636, 1985.
169. Black PM, Zeruas NT, Caplan LR, et al. Subdural hygroma of the spinal meninges. Neurosurgery 2:52, 1978.
170. Russell NA, Mangan MA. Acute spinal cord compression by subarachnoid and subdural he-

matomas occurring in association with brachial plexus avulsion. J Neurosurg 2:410, 1980.
171. Jellinger K. Traumatic vascular disease of the spinal cord. In Vinken PJ, Bruyn GW, eds. Injuries of the Spine and Spinal cord. Part II. Handbook of Clinical Neurology. Vol. 12. New York, North-Holland Publishing Co., 1976:556.
172. Sokoloff J, Coel MN, Ignelzi RJ. Spinal subdural hematoma. Radiology 120:116, 1976.
173. Potts CS. Intradural cyst of the spinal meninges removed by operation. Remarks on the location of the spinal centers for testicular sensibilities. J Nerv Ment Dis 37:621, 1910.
174. Rader JP. Chronic subdural hematoma of spinal cord. N Engl J Med 253:374, 1955.
175. Edelson RN. Spinal subdural hematoma. In Vinken PJ, Bruyn GW, eds. Injuries of the Spine and Spinal cord, Part II. Handbook of Clinical Neurology. Vol. 26. New York, North-Holland Publishing Co., 1976:31.
176. Smith RA. Spinal subdural hematoma, neurilemmoma, and acute transverse myelopathy. Surg Neurol 23:367, 1985.
177. Rieth KG, Quindlen EA. Calcified chronic spinal subdural hematoma demonstrated by computed tomography. Spine 8:812, 1983.
178. Zilkha A, Nicoletti JM. Acute spinal subdural hematoma. J Neurosurg 41:627, 1974.
179. Sakata T, Kurihara A. Spontaneous spinal subdural hematoma. Spine 3:324, 1984.
180. Guy MJ, Zahra M, Sengupta RP. Spontaneous spinal subdural hematoma during general anesthesia. Surg Neurol 11:199, 1979.
181. Kirkpatrick D, Goodman SJ. Combined subarachnoid and subdural hematoma following spinal puncture. Surg Neurol 3:109, 1975.

### *Pseudotumor*

182. Sze G, Brant-Zawadzki MN, Wilson CR, et al. Pseudotumor of the craniovertebral junction associated with chronic subluxation: MR imaging studies. Radiology 161:391, 1986.
183. Prete PE, Henbest M, Michalski JP, et al. Intraspinal elastofibroma. Spine 8:800, 1983.
184. Kudo H, Iwano K, Yoshizawa H. Cervical cord compression due to extradural granulation tissue in rheumatoid arthritis. J Bone Joint Surg (Br) 66:426, 1984.
185. Leaney BJ, Calvert JM. Tophaceous gout producing spinal cord compression. J Neurosurg 58:580, 1983.
186. Badami JP, Hinck VC. Symptomatic deposition of fat in a morbidly obese woman. AJNR 4:684, 1982.
187. Guegan Y, Fardoun R, Launois B, et al. Spinal cord compression by extradural fat after prolonged corticosteroid therapy. J Neurosurg 56:267, 1982.
188. Kleinman GM, Dagi TF, Poletti CE. Villonodular synovitis in the spinal canal. J Neurosurg 52:846, 1980.
189. Cameron IL, Ord VA, Fullerton GD. Characterization of proton NMR relaxation times in normal and pathological tissues by correlation with other tissue parameters. Magn Reson Imag 2:97, 1984.

### *Traumatic Nerve Root Avulsion*

190. Taylor PE. Traumatic intradural avulsion of the nerve roots of the brachial plexus. Brain 85:579, 1962.
191. Yeoman PM. Cervical myelography in traction injuries of the brachial plexus. J Bone Joint Surg 50B:253, 1968.
192. Kewalramani LS, Taylor RG. Brachial plexus root avulsion: role of myelography. Review of diagnostic procedures. J Trauma 15:603, 1975.
193. Sunderland S. Mechanisms of cervical nerve root avulsion in injuries of the neck and shoulder. J Neurosurg 41:705, 1974.
194. Russell NA, Managan MA. Acute spinal cord compression by subarachnoid and subdural hematoma occurring in association with brachial plexus avulsion. J Neurosurg 52:410, 1980.
195. Sunderland S. Meningeal-neural relations in the intervertebral foramen. J Neurosurg 40:756, 1974.
196. Barnes R. Traction injuries of the brachial plexus in adults. J Bone Joint Surg 31B:10, 1949.
197. Davies ER, Sutton D, Bligh AS. Myelography in brachial plexus injuries. Br J Radiol 39:362, 1966.
198. Drake CG. Diagnosis and treatment of lesions of the brachial plexus and adjacent structures. Clin Neurosurg 11:110, 1963.
199. Mendelsohn RA, Weiner IH, Keegan JM. Myelographic demonstration of brachial plexus root avulsion. Arch Surg 75:102, 1957.
200. Murphey F, Hartung W, Kirklin JW. Myelographic demonstration of avulsing injury of the brachial plexus. AJR 58:102, 1947.
201. Murphey F, Kirklin JW. Myelographic demonstration of avulsing injuries of the nerve roots of the brachial plexus—a method of determining the point of injury and the possibility of repair. Clin Neurosurg 20:18, 1973.
202. Jaeger R, Whiteley WH. Avulsion of brachial plexus: report of six cases. JAMA 153:186, 1953.
203. Heon M. Myelogram: a questionable aid in the diagnosis and prognosis in avulsion of brachial plexus components by traction injuries. Conn Med 29:260, 1965.
204. Deans W, Leibrock LG, Bloch S, et al. Cerebrospinal fluid hypotension secondary to traumatic rupture of lumbosacral meninges. Surg Neurol 12:223, 1979.
205. Alker GJ, Glasauer FE, Zoll JG, et al. Myelographic demonstration of lumbosacral nerve root avulsion. Radiology 89:101, 1967.
206. Berberá J, Broseta J, Argüelles F, et al. Traumatic lumbosacral meningocele. J Neurosurg 46:536, 1977.
207. Barnett HG, Connolly ES. Lumbosacral nerve root avulsion: report of a case and review of the literature. J Trauma 15:532, 1975.
208. Gass H, Devadiga KV, Taptas JN. Supraclavicular cerebrospinal fluid effusion in brachial plexus avulsion injuries and iatrogenic omorrhea. J Bone Joint Surg 54A:1773, 1972.
209. Epstein BS, Epstein JA. Traumatic thoracic pseudomeningocele. Neuroradiology 3:46, 1971.
210. Armington WG, Harnsberger HR, Osborn AG, Seay AR. Radiographic evaluation of brachial plexopathy. AJNR 8:361, 1987.
211. Enzmann DR, Rubin JB, DeLaPaz R, et al. Cerebrospinal fluid pulsation: benefits and pitfalls in MR imaging. Radiology 161:773, 1986.
212. Burk DL Jr, Brunberg JA, Kanal E, et al. Spinal and paraspinal neurofibromatosis: surface coil imaging at 1.5 T. Radiology 162:797, 1987.
213. Flannigan BD, Lufkin RB, McGlade C, et al. MR imaging of the cervical spine: neurovascular anatomy. AJNR 8:27, 1987.

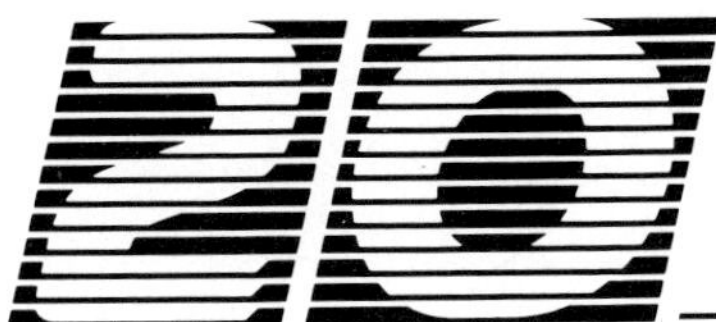

Steven E. Harms, M.D.

# ORBITAL MAGNETIC RESONANCE

Despite the relatively unrestricted access to the orbit by clinical examination, additional diagnostic imaging methods are often required to better define the anatomic location and to provide some additional insight into the etiology of the abnormality. When exact location of the mass is determined, the differential diagnosis can often be reduced to a few possibilities. The extent of the lesion can be outlined to stage the lesion and determine operability. Magnetic resonance (MR) is an excellent choice for displaying normal anatomy because of its inherently high soft tissue contrast and multiplanar capability.[1–11] A wide spectrum of pathologic entities involves the orbit. More recently, it has been discovered that in terms of orbital pathology, signal intensity characteristics provided on MR images (MRI) can also improve specificity.[12–32] The differential that is narrowed by the anatomic location can be further defined using these signal intensity patterns.

There are additional benefits of MRI over conventional imaging methods. MRI eliminates the use of ionizing radiation, which has well-known side effects, including cataractogenesis.[33] Radiation effects to the lens may be significant on CT, especially when multiple follow-up examinations for orbital tumors are considered.[34] No contrast agent is necessary for orbital MRI, and contrast-associated side effects can be eliminated. Artifacts secondary to high-density dental materials on coronal CT scans are not a problem on MRI. Artifacts near high-density bone that are frequently seen near the orbital apex on CT are not encountered on MRI.

The advantages of this method make MRI a principal imaging technique for evaluating most orbital masses. This chapter discusses normal orbital anatomy displayed by MRI, technical considerations for orbital MRI exams, and clinical applications.

## ANATOMY

The transverse (Fig. 20–1) and coronal (Fig. 20–2) anatomy of the normal orbit is reviewed as displayed by T1-weighted (T1WI) MRI. Multiple parameter dependent images are shown in Figure 20–3.[16, 17, 29, 30, 35–37] MRI signal characteristics of normal orbital constituents are summarized in Table 20–1.[16, 17, 29, 30]

The bony orbit is defined by seven bones: frontal, sphenoid, maxilla, zygoma, ethmoid, lacrimal, and palatine bones. Because of the low mobile proton density, cortical bone has almost no signal on MR images. Marrow fat can be seen as high signal on T1WI and moderate signal on T2-weighted images (T2WI). Multiple structures pass through the superior orbital fissure that connects the orbit with the middle cranial fossa, including the oculomotor (III), trochlear (IV), abducens (VI), and ophthalmic (first division of V) nerves and the superior and inferior ophthalmic veins. The inferior orbital fissure contains veins that connect the orbital venous system with the pterygoid plexus. The optic canal forms at the orbital apex. The optic nerve and ophthalmic artery pass through the optic canal.

The anterior soft tissues of the orbit are separated from the rest of the orbit by the septum that arises from the periosteum and attaches to the tarsal plates of the eyelids. The space anterior to the septum is thus

*Text continued on page 593*

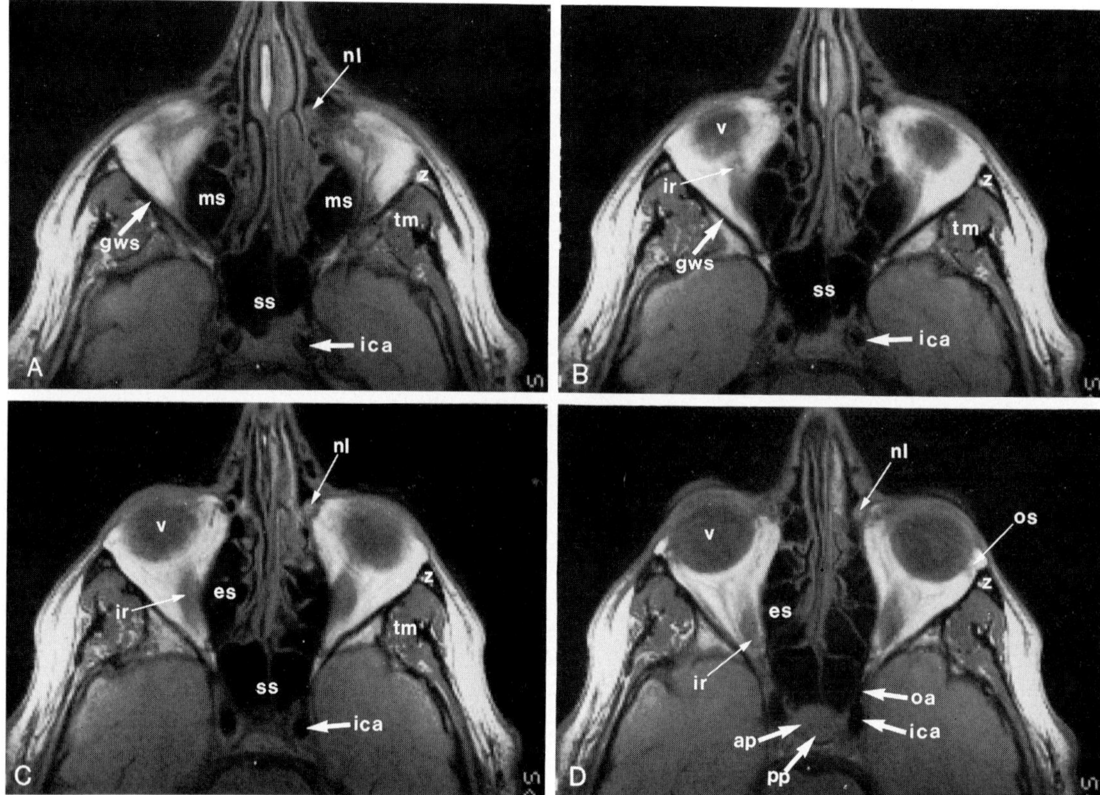


**Figure 20–1. Transverse anatomy.** *A* to *H*, Sequential transverse T1WI (TE 25/TR 300) of a normal orbit obtained with a 4-inch saddle coil and a selective 3DFT acquisition at 0.6 T. The slice thickness is 1.6 mm without interslice gaps. The following structures are labeled:

- a anterior chamber
- an nucleus of the lens (adult)
- ap anterior pituitary
- cb ciliary body
- cl central zones of the lens
- cr choroid and retina
- d dural sheath around the optic nerve
- es ethmoid sinuses
- gws greater wing of the sphenoid bone
- i infundibulum
- ica internal carotid artery
- iov interior ophthalmic vein
- ir inferior rectus muscle
- lc lamina cribrosa
- lpl lateral palpebral ligament
- lr lateral rectus muscle
- mpl medial palpebral ligament
- mr medial rectus muscle
- ms maxillary sinus
- nl nasolacrimal canal
- o optic nerve
- oa ophthalmic artery
- os orbital septum
- pp posterior pituitary
- s sclera
- ss sphenoid sinus
- tm temporalis muscle
- v vitreous
- z zygomatic bone

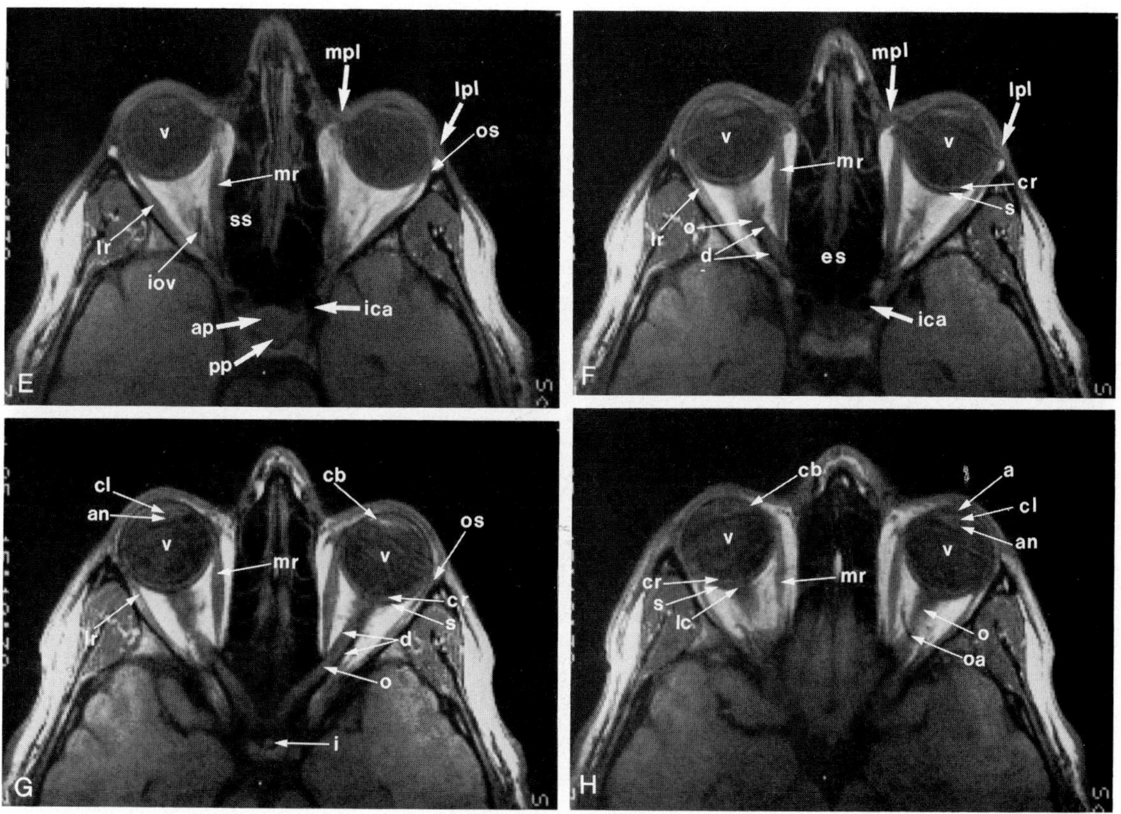


**Figure 20–1** *Continued*

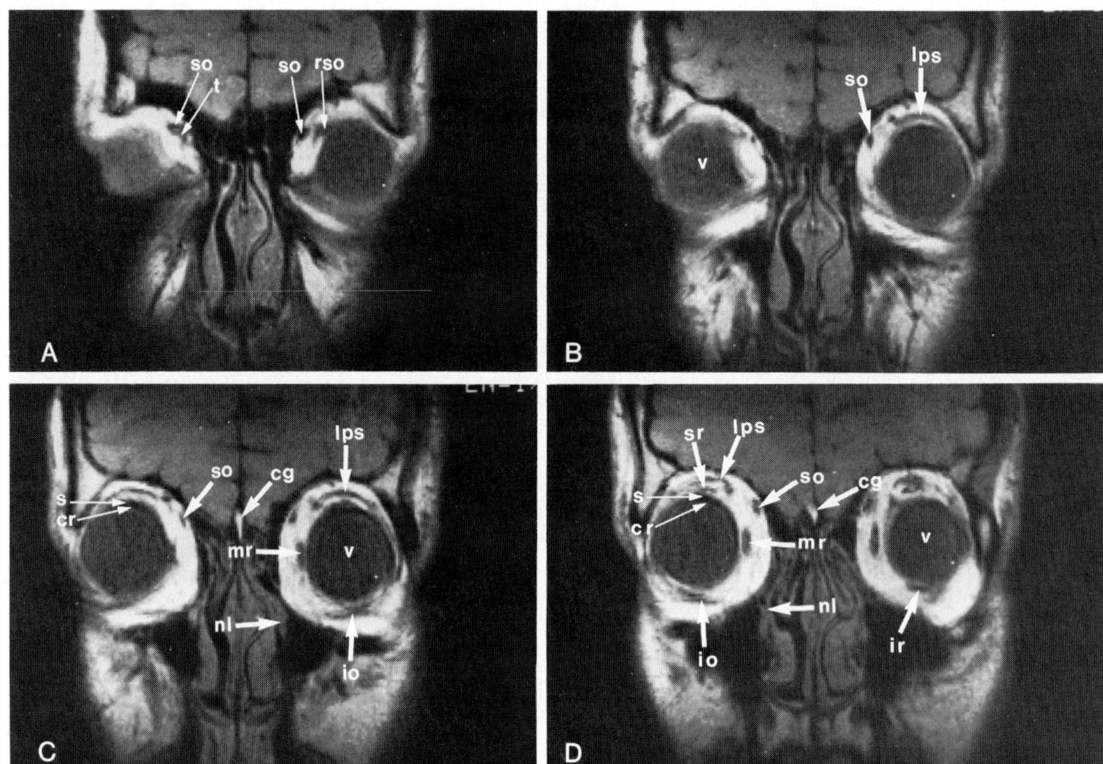


**Figure 20–2. Coronal anatomy.** *A* to I, Sequential coronal T1WI (TE 34/TR 600) of a normal orbit obtained with a 4-inch saddle coil and a 2DFT multislice acquisition using a slide thickness of 4 mm with a 10% interslice gap. The following structures are labeled:

| | |
|---|---|
| cg | crista galli |
| cr | choroid and retina |
| fn | frontal nerve |
| io | inferior oblique muscle |
| ir | inferior rectus muscle |
| lps | levator palpebrae superioris muscle |
| lr | lateral rectus muscle |
| mr | medial rectus muscle |
| nl | nasolacrimal duct |
| o | optic nerve |
| oa | ophthalmic artery |
| om | oculomotor nerve |
| rso | reflection of the superior oblique muscle |
| s | sclera |
| so | superior oblique muscle |
| sov | superior ophthalmic vein |
| sr | superior rectus muscle |
| t | trochlea |
| v | vitreous |

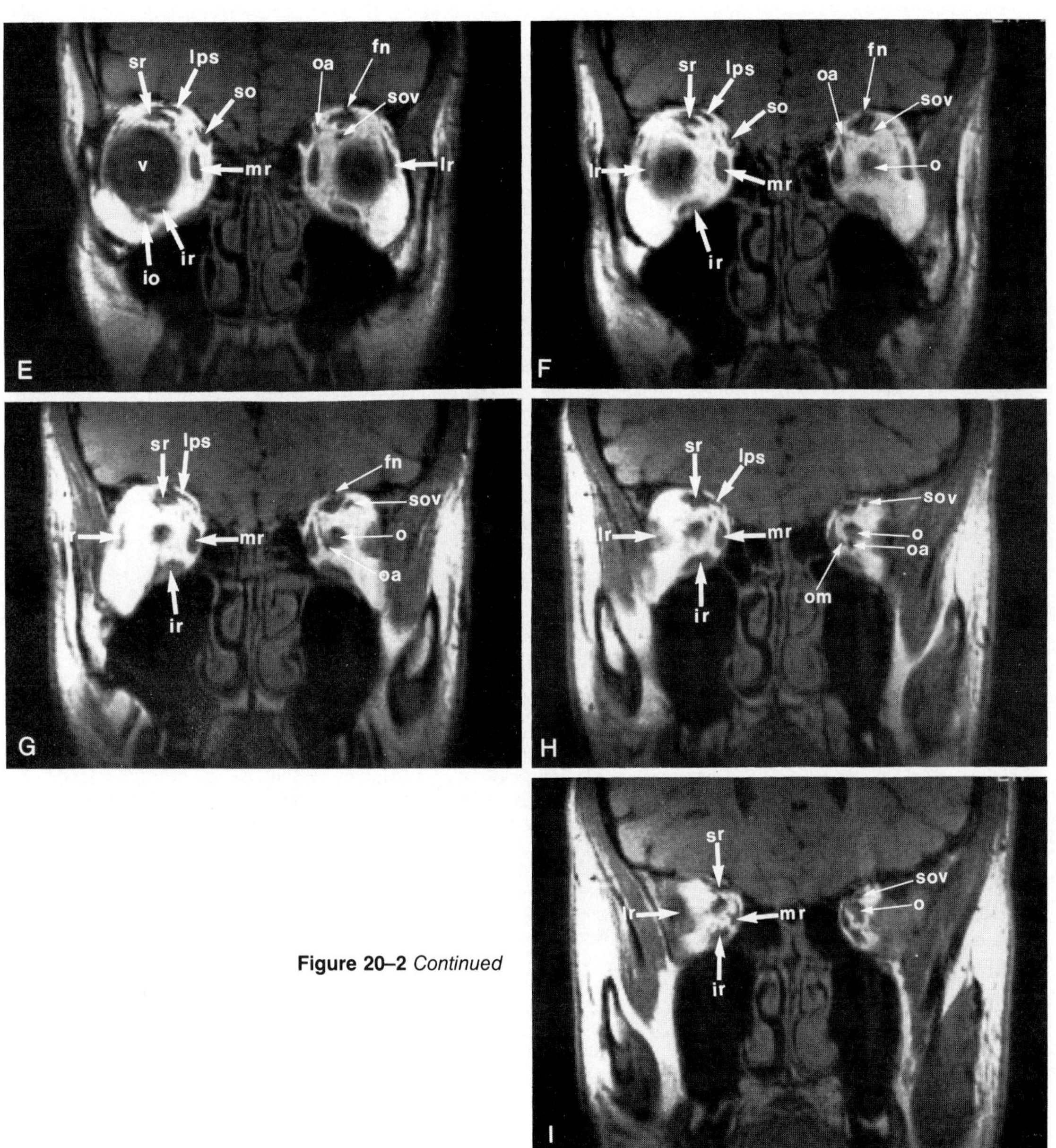


**Figure 20–2** *Continued*

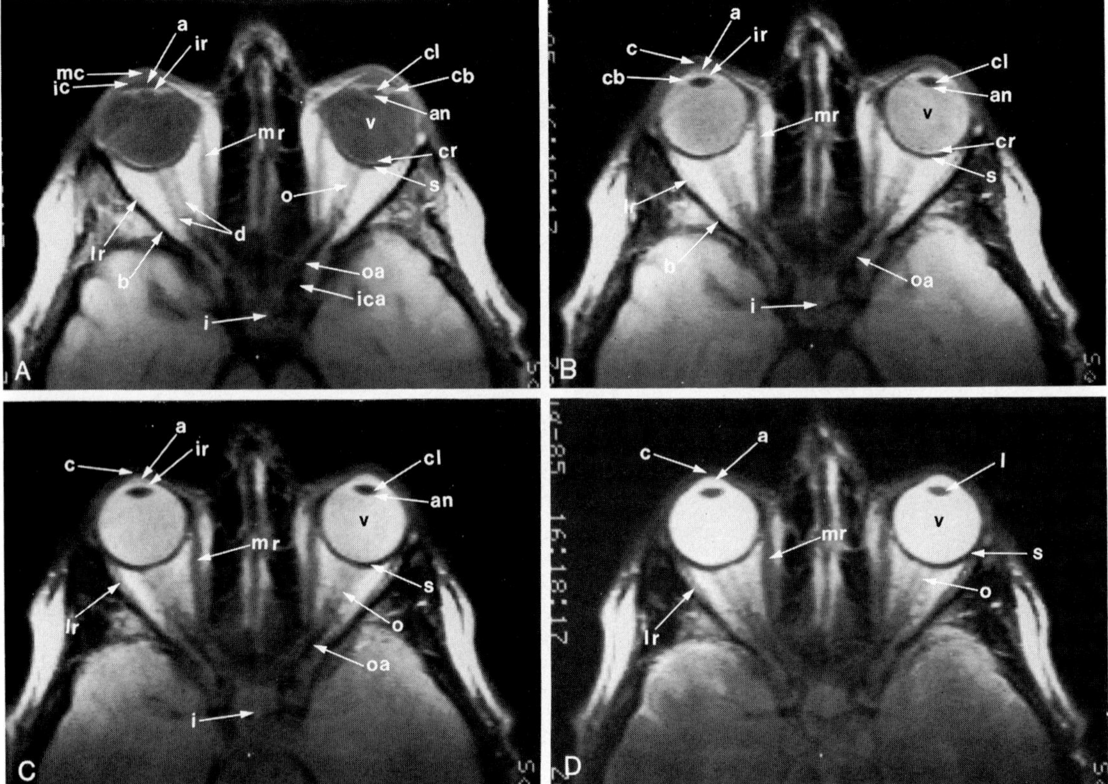


**Figure 20–3. Multiecho images.** A multiple spin-echo sequence using 4 echoes of TE 40, TE 80, TE 120, and TE 160 with a TR of 1000 produces varying parameter, weighted images in the same scan. Selective 3D acquisition was used. *A*, TE 40 image is more N(H) weighted with the vitreous having a low signal, but not as low as on T1WI (Fig. 20–1). *B*, TE 80, and *C*, TE 120, images have parameter weighting that results in the vitreous having a signal nearly equal to the brain. These images can be called "balanced" or "crossover" images. The TE 80 image is more N(H) weighted, and the TE 120 image is more T2 weighted. Most pathology will have a high signal on these images. Certain lesions, however, will be isointense and can thus be distinguished from other entities if these images are obtained. *D*, TE 160 image is heavily T2 weighted, with vitreous giving a very high signal compared with orbital fat. The following structures are labeled:

a anterior chamber
an nucleus of the lens (adult)
b cortical bone of the lateral orbital wall
c cornea
cb ciliary body
cl central nuclei of the lens
cr choroid and retina
d dural sheath around the optic nerve
i infundibulum
ica internal carotid artery
ic internal layer of the cornea
ir iris
l lens
lr lateral rectus muscle
mr medial rectus muscle
o optic nerve
oa ophthalmic artery
s sclera
v vitreous humor

**Table 20–1.** SIGNAL INTENSITIES OF NORMAL ORBITAL TISSUE

| Tissue | T1WI | T2WI | N(H)WI | Crossover |
|---|---|---|---|---|
| Vitreous | Low | High | Moderate to low | Isointense |
| Aqueous | Low | High | Moderate to low | Isointense |
| Ophthalmic artery | Low | Low | Low | Low |
| Ophthalmic veins | Low | Low | Low | Low |
| Cortical bone | Low | Low | Low | Low |
| Sclera | Low | Low | Low | Low |
| Bone marrow | High | Moderate | High | High |
| Orbital fat | High | Moderate | High | High |
| Muscles | Moderate | Low | Moderate | Moderate to low |
| Optic nerve | Moderate | Moderate | Moderate | Moderate |
| Cornea, external layer | Moderate | High | Moderate | — |
| Cornea, mid layer | Low | Low | Low | Low |
| Cornea, inner layer | High | — | High | — |
| Choroid, retina | High | — | High | — |
| Lens, external layer | High | High | High | High |
| Lens, inner zones | Low to moderate | Low | Low to moderate | — |
| Ciliary body | High | Low | High | — |
| Zonule | High | — | — | — |
| Iris | High | Low | High | — |

called the preseptal space. The space posterior to the septum, not including the globe, is called the retrobulbar space.

The lacrimal gland lies in the superior lateral quadrant of the orbit. The lacrimal sac lies in the lacrimal fossa, along the medial margin of the orbit. The nasolacrimal duct extends from the lacrimal sac and enters the nasal cavity beneath the inferior turbinate.

Six extrinsic muscles coordinate eye movements. The four rectus muscles (superior, inferior, medial, and lateral) arise at the orbital apex from the annulus of Zinn and insert into the sclera. The superior oblique muscle arises superomedial to the optic foramen, and extends between the superior and medial rectus muscles to the trochlea, in the anterior orbit. After passing through the trochlea, the superior oblique tendon courses posterolaterally to insert into the sclera. The inferior oblique muscle arises in the anterior medial aspect of the orbit, passing posteriorly and laterally beneath the inferior rectus muscle to insert on the posterolateral aspect of the globe. The inferior oblique muscle often cannot be distinguished from the inferior rectus muscle. The inferior oblique muscle and inferior rectus muscle together can be referred to as the inferior muscle group. Muscle has moderately high signal on T1WI and proton density-weighted image (N[H]WI) and is hypointense on T2WI owing to the relatively short T2 of muscle. Muscles are easily separated from the orbital fat, which has high signal on T1WI and moderate signal on T2WI. The extraocular muscles and their intermuscular membrane divide the retrobulbar space into the intraconal and extraconal compartments.

The optic nerve is divided into four segments: (1) an intracranial segment between the optic chiasm and optic canal, (2) an intracanalicular segment within the optic canal, (3) an intraorbital segment, and (4) an intraocular segment. The optic nerve is surrounded by meninges, and the subarachnoid space extends to the sclera. The optic nerve has moderately high signal on T1WI and N(H)WI and moderately low signal on T2WI.

The ophthalmic artery arises from the internal carotid artery as it emerges from the cavernous sinus. It passes through the optic canal within the dural sheath inferolateral to the optic nerve. Within the orbit, the ophthalmic artery crosses obliquely above the nerve to reach the medial aspect of the orbit between the superior oblique and medial rectus muscles. The superior ophthalmic vein arises in the medial part of the upper eyelid and courses in a posterolateral direction to penetrate the muscle cone in the mid orbit. It runs deep to the superior rectus muscle and passes through the superior orbital fissure to drain into the cavernous sinus. The inferior ophthalmic vein begins in a venous plexus near the floor and medial aspect of the orbit. It runs posteriorly above the inferior rectus muscle. It may join the superior ophthalmic vein or pass separately through the inferior orbital fissure to communicate with the pterygoid plexus. Because of the flow-void effect, most vessels have low signal on all MR images.

The globe comprises three tunics and the contents enclosed by them. From without inward, the three tunics are (1) the fibrous tunic, consisting of the sclera and cornea; (2) the vascular pigmented tunic comprising the choroid, ciliary body, and iris, forming together the uveal tract; and (3) the nervous layer, or retina.

The sclera is a firm fibrous layer that serves to maintain the form of the globe. The sclera has low signal on all MR images owing to the short T2 and low mobile proton density of fibrous tissue. The cornea has five layers, which are, from anterior to posterior (1) the corneal epithelium continuous with the conjunctiva, (2) the anterior limiting membrane (of Bowman), (3) the substantia propria, (4) the posterior limiting lamina (of Descemet), and (5) the endothelium of the anterior chamber. Multiple corneal layers can be seen on MRI. The external layer is isointense on the T1WI and N(H)WI and hyperintense on the T2WI. The middle layers are hypointense on all images. The inner layer is hyperintense on T1WI and N(H)WI.[29]

The choroid consists mainly of a dense capillary plexus that brings nutrients to the eye. On its external surface is a thin, nonvascular suprachoroid lamina consisting of connective tissue and pigmented cells. Pathologic processes may split the lamellae of the choroid to produce uveal effusions.

The ciliary body and iris are a direct anterior continuation of the choroid. These structures divide the eye into the anterior chamber filled with aqueous humor and the posterior chamber filled with vitreous humor. These fluid-filled chambers are hypointense on T1WI, mildly hypointense on N(H)WI, isointense on crossover images, and hyperintense on T2WI. The lens consists of concentric layers of elongated nonoverlapping cells that accrue peripherally throughout a person's life, much like tree rings. The lens has five concentric zones surrounded by an elastic capsule. From the center outward, these layers are (1) the embryonic nucleus, (2) the fetal nucleus, (3) the infantile nucleus, (4) the nucleus formed from the last weeks of fetal life to puberty, (5) the adult nucleus, and (6) the cortex that contains soft, young, superficial cells.[35–37] The lens contains 65% water and 35% protein, the latter in soluble and insoluble forms.[38, 39] The insoluble forms increase with age, zonal depth, and especially with cataracts.[40, 41] The external layer of the lens is hyperintense on all images owing to the increased mobile proton density attributed to a higher water content. The inner zones of the lenses have shorter T2 values than the cortex, resulting in lower signal on all images and especially on T2-weighted images.[29] Cortical cataracts result in increased water content and prolong cortical relaxation times. Nuclear cataracts have increased insoluble protein and do not affect the bound or free water to produce any change in relaxation times.[40, 41]

The ciliary body is concerned with the suspension of the lens and the mechanism of accommodation. It is also involved in the production of aqueous fluid for the anterior chamber and, probably, vitreous fluid for the posterior chamber. The ciliary body is highly innervated and well vascularized. Because of the high content of connective tissue and muscle resulting in an overall short T2, the ciliary body is hyperintense on T1WI and N(H)WI and is hypointense on T2WI. The zonule, the suspensory ligament from the ciliary body to the lens, can be seen as a high-signal strand on high-resolution T1WI.[29]

The iris is a delicate, pigmented diaphragm within the anterior chamber surrounding the pupil. This tissue has composition and signal intensity characteristics similar to the ciliary body.[29]

The retina is the very thin layer of the globe that comprises the sensory stratum of the eyeball. The retina and choroid cannot be separated on current MR images. These layers appear as a single layer having high signal on T1WI and N(H)WI compared with vitreous.[29]

## TECHNICAL CONSIDERATIONS

Several special considerations should be entertained when designing an imaging protocol for the orbit. The major categories are image plane selection, radio frequency (RF) coil selection, pulse sequence selection, acquisition selection, and miscellaneous factors.

### Image Plane Selection

MRI is not limited to the axial plane of CT; any desired imaging plane can be acquired by MRI. For orbital imaging, a good routine would probably consist of coronal and transverse images. Transverse images are effective at demonstrating anterior-posterior relationships such as the globe and the optic canal. Coronal images nicely demonstrate the extra-ocular muscles and relationships to the cone. Sagittal, and especially tilted sagittal, images along the optic nerve can be useful in showing pathology in the superior direction and along the optic nerve.

With the use of isotropic three-dimensional (3D) acquisitions and image processing, any desired view can be obtained from the same data set. Curved images and surface reconstructions are possible.[42] This process may be useful for careful surgical planning.

Thin sections are necessary for demonstrating many orbital lesions. A slice thickness of 5 mm or less is suggested.[17–19] The use of thin slices is especially critical when ocular pathology is considered. Using selective 3D techniques, we have obtained slice thicknesses of 0.6 mm.

### Radio Frequency Coil Selection

The major technologic advancement that allowed clinically useful MR imaging of the orbit was the development of surface coil imaging.[8, 9, 16, 17] A number of dedicated orbital surface coils have now been used and are commercially available. As the field progresses, these coils are expected to improve further in quality and sophistication. A number of orbital coils may be needed for optimal imaging.

Initially, only single-loop coils were used for a single orbit.[8, 9] In most cases, bilateral exams improve quality by having the opposite side for comparison.[16, 17, 31, 32] In some cases, such as inpatients with suspected retinoblastoma, evaluation of the opposite side is necessary to exclude disease.

A small coil may cover only the optic globe. This coil would be useful for evaluation of lens, corneal, or ciliary body pathology, but many tumor applications require thorough staging of the optic nerve. A larger coil diameter is necessary to penetrate as deep as the optic chiasm. Coils vary in size to fit children and adults.

### Pulse Sequence Selection

T1-weighted images are useful for demonstrating high-resolution orbital anatomy. These images can be accomplished with the use of a short TE and TR spin-echo sequence or inversion recovery.[43–47] Since only a relatively small number of slices is needed to cover the orbit and heavy T1 weighting is not necessary, a T1-weighted (T1W) spin-echo sequence serves this purpose well. Inversion recovery can be used if heavier T1 weighting or more slices with T1 weighting are required.[43] The use of short TI inversion recovery (STIR) sequences has been proposed as a method of achieving a nulling of fat signal for better T1WI of the retrobulbar region.[48, 49] For all T1W sequences, the TE should be kept as short as possible to reduce signal losses owing to T2 effects and to reduce motion artifacts.

Multiple spin-echo sequences are very useful in evaluating orbital pathology because of the multiple-parameter weighting that is possible (Fig. 20–3).[31, 32, 46] The variations in signal seen within the lesion at stages in the echo train can be used to help differentiate pathologic entities.[46] Long TR multiecho sequences produce images ranging from proton-density, or N(H) weighted (short TE), to T2 weighted (long TE). Short TR multiecho sequences produce images ranging from T1 weighted (short TE) to T2 weighted (long TE). Midrange echoes have diminished contrast between fluid and brain and are called "crossover" or "balanced" images. Crossover images are useful in evaluating T2 differences to further distinguish certain lesions that would not be possible on T2WI alone. In terms of timing parameter selection, short echo-refocusing times and more echoes will result in reduced motion artifacts compared with fewer echoes and longer echo refocusing times. For example, a TE 120 single echo will have far more motion artifacts than a TE 120 produced with four spin echoes. A T2W scan should have reduced fat signal compared with vitreous to allow separation of tumor extension within fat. This contrast can be achieved with a long TR (less T1 weighting), a long TE (more T2 weighting), or both. At 0.6 tesla (T), a TE 120/TR 2000 scan serves this purpose nicely. For certain 3D techniques, a shorter TR is desirable. In cases in which a short TR spin-echo sequence is used, a longer TE is required to achieve the same contrast effect. Adjustments will also have to be made for different field strengths. T2 contrast is more easily achieved at high field strengths owing to generally longer T2 values.

Gradient-echo sequences are now emerging as useful clinical methods.[50, 51] These can be a simple gradient-refocused echo (FLASH for fast low-angle shot) or a steady state (FISP for fast-imaging steady state precession and GRASS for gradient-echo acquisition in a steady state). The major advantages of these sequences relate to the reduced RF power imparted, allowing for reduced TRs and shorter scan times. In these sequences, T1 weighting is achieved with a wider tip angle and a shorter TR. T2 weighting is produced with a longer TE. N(H) weighting results in a narrow tip angle and a short TE. The chemical shift effects can be particularly bothersome with these sequences in the orbit owing to the mix of fat and fluid components. These chemical shift effects are more severe at high fields. Motion artifacts are also more severe than on standard spin-echo sequences. Magnetic susceptibility effects are not refocused on gradient echoes. Areas of high magnetic susceptibility differences may result in substantial signal loss when these gradient-echo sequences are employed. These magnetic susceptibility effects increase with the square of the magnetic field.

The chemical shift can be used to advantage when chemical shift–sensitive methods are used.[52, 53] The separation of tumor within high-intensity fat can be a problem on standard T1-weighted spin-echo sequences. When special chemical shift–sensitive methods are used, fat signal can be reduced to allow better visualization of tumors involving fat. These sequences perform better when a large chemical shift is present. This factor favors high field strength systems.[54]

Stimulated echoes (STEAM, for stimulated echo acquisition mode) can be used to obtain faster chemical shift images for faster 3D acquisitions.[55, 56] T1 and T2 weighting can be achieved in the same scan. Echo trains similar to a multiple-echo sequence can be obtained with longer echoes becoming more T1 dependent. Stimulated echoes refocus signals lost owing to magnetic susceptibility effects and may be superior to gradient-echo methods in these areas. The disadvantage of stimulated echoes is that the sequence has reduced signal-to-noise ratio (SNR) compared with standard spin echoes.

### Acquisition Method Selection

Fourier imaging method has become the standard acquisition technique on most commercial MR imagers.[43–47] This method can be used in two-dimensional (2D) or 3D modes.

In the 2D mode (see Fig. 20–2), Fourier imaging can be achieved in either the single slice or multislice mode. Slices are excited by a selective excitation utilizing a certain bandwidth RF pulse in the presence of a magnetic field gradient. The thinness of the slice is limited by the narrowness of the selection pulse and the strength of the slice selection gradient. Since very thin slices are ideal when imaging the orbit, these limitations may be severe on some instruments. Thinner slices can be produced by narrowing the bandwidth and increasing the TE. A longer TE results in more T2 weighting and a poorer SNR. Since the slice selection pulse is not perfectly square, optimal tip angles are not achieved uniformly through the slice and some tissue is excited outside the slice. In the multislice mode, these slice selection pulse imperfections necessitate gaps between slices. With thin slices, the bandwidth effect is more severe, requiring larger gaps between slices. This problem is reduced but not eliminated when more "square" pulse shapes are used. This problem is reduced when 2D examinations are obtained in the single-slice mode as is commonly performed when gradient-echo sequences are employed. Even gradient-echo sequences used in the multislice mode are improved since only 90° selection pulses are needed. Slice imperfections are more severe with 180° pulses.

In 2D multislice, the number of available slices per scan is limited by the TR. Very short TR sequences may not allow a sufficient number of slices. Very short TR gradient-echo sequences are often limited to the single-slice mode.

Selective 3D acquisitions solve some of the deficiencies encountered in 2D acquisitions (Figs. 20–1 and 20–3).[43, 46, 57, 58] In selective 3D, slices are not individually excited by a selective excitation at intervals throughout the TR, as in 2D methods. Instead, an entire slab is excited simultaneously with a selective excitation. Slices within the slab are encoded by phase-encoding gradients. In 3D acquisitions, there are inherently no gaps between slices. There is no practical limit to the ability to produce thin slices by this method. Slice thicknesses of 0.6 mm have been achieved with modest gradient strengths. Because the entire slice is excited simultaneously, the signal fall-off at the slice edge experienced in 2D methods is not a problem. More even tip angles across the slice result in better SNR. The use of 3D is an effective way of dealing with SNR problems, because the SNR for a 3D acquisition improves with the square root of the number of slices. The number of slices per scan is not limited by the TR as in 2D multislice. Short TR sequences used in fast scans are well suited to 3D techniques. Achieving a short TE is not a problem in 3D acquisitions, even with thin slices, because a narrow bandwidth excitation pulse is not required for thin slices.

There are some limitations to 3D acquisitions. The scan time lengthens with the number of slices. For long TR sequences, the scan time may become prohibitively long. Because T2W spin-echo sequences favor a long TR, selective 3D is practically limited to T1W spin-echo scans. T2 weighting can be achieved with very short TR fast scans. Combining 3D with a fast-scan sequence may compensate for the reduced SNR of the sequence and may achieve optimal efficiency for the scan. The greatest limitation of 3D is increased motion sensitivity. 3D is more motion sensitive than 2D methods because an extra phase-encoding axis is employed for slice encoding.

The 3D multislab acquisition method combines the attributes of 2D multislice and selective 3D.[59–61] Slabs are excited at different times during the TR interval similar to the 2D multislice method. Slices within those slabs are encoded with phase-encoding gradients similar to selective 3D acquisitions. The scan time for the 3D multislab examination is reduced by the number of slabs, compared with a selective 3D acquisition with the same number of slices. The SNR will improve with the square root of the number of slices per slab. There are no gaps between slices of the same slab, but there are gaps between slabs.

Emerging methods include the echo planar technique that utilizes rapidly changing gradients to achieve very fast images.[52] This method could effectively eliminate motion artifacts because of the very rapid scan time (as short as 30 msec per slice). This technique, however, has not yet been used for high-resolution imaging needed for orbital examinations. The hybrid echo-planar method combines some of the rapid imaging methods of echo planar with Fourier imaging methods.[63] The acquisition speed is improved at the expense of SNR. Because the very thin slice, high-resolution imaging required in orbital exams is currently SNR limited, this method is not expected to have a major impact in this area. Lower resolution scans may be acceptable, however, for biopsies or positioning in which speed is more important than resolution.

### Miscellaneous Technical Factors

Motion is a significant problem in orbital exams. Patients are asked to close their eyes, lie quietly, and avoid eye motion. We have found this method more effective than focusing on a point. As scan times get shorter, focusing on a still point may prove effective. With current scan times, most patients tire too easily, resulting in increased motion as they attempt to comply with our request. If motion remains a problem, increasing the number of signal averages in the pulse sequence will help. Lastly, some patients, especially children, will have to be sedated to undergo the exam.

Selection of the appropriate phase-encoding axis is important in reducing motion artifacts. For transverse scans, the phase encoding is achieved side to side. The motion artifacts from eyelid motion are then projected away from the critical orbital anatomy. If the anterior-posterior axis were phase encoded, motion artifacts from the lids and eye would propagate posteriorly through the rest of the orbit.

**Table 20–2.** SIGNAL INTENSITIES OF PRESEPTAL LESIONS

| Lesion | T1WI | T2WI |
|---|---|---|
| Cellulitis | Low | High |
| Basal cell carcinoma | Low | High |
| Granuloma | Low | Low |
| | or Low | High |
| | or High | High |

A high-resolution acquisition is achieved with gradient magnification. Photographic magnification of a low-resolution acquisition does not result in improved image resolution. If adequate SNR is not seen with higher resolution acquisition, the steps to improve the SNR previously outlined should be used rather than reducing resolution.[31, 32, 64] Many machines now offer the option of a rectangular matrix, or "strip scanning," in which resolution can be improved in the phase-encoding axis without increasing the number of phase-encoding steps. This method is effective in improving the resolution of transverse and coronal images without lengthening the scan time.

Some eye cosmetics contain iron oxide, especially those with brown or blue pigments. This small amount of material may have sufficient ferromagnetic content to severely distort MR images.[16, 65] Patients should remove all cosmetics prior to an orbital imaging examination. One patient with a history of metal working developed an ocular hemorrhage following an MRI examination as a result of movement of a metal fragment within the globe. All patients who have a history of metal working and therefore possibly have metal fragments in the eye should be screened before they enter the MR scan area.[66]

## PATHOLOGY

A wide spectrum of disease is encountered in orbital imaging. To narrow the differential diagnosis, the orbit is divided into compartments that help limit the number of diagnostic possibilities. These diagnostic groups are (1) preseptal lesions, (2) extraconal lesions, (3) extraocular muscle lesions, (4) intraconal lesions, (5) optic nerve and sheath lesions, and (6) ocular lesions. When the various clinical features and MRI characteristics are combined with the anatomic location, a highly specific diagnosis can often be made.

### Preseptal Lesions

The signal intensities of various lesions on MRI are summarized in Table 20–2.

Preseptal cellulitis produces swelling of the eyelids and periorbital soft tissues (Fig. 20–4). High signal can be seen from the soft tissues on T2W images. The orbital septum acts as a barrier to the spread of infection into the orbit. When the septum is breached by trauma, direct spread of infection, or thrombophlebitis, orbital cellulitis results (Fig. 20–5).[67–70] Clinically, proptosis, limited mobility of the globe, pain, and chemosis can occur with orbital cellulitis. Orbital cellulitis can be readily appreciated on T2WIs as areas of high signal extending deep to the orbital septum. Fluid collections, pus, or both are readily identified by MRI.

A variety of skin tumors involving the eyelids can require further imaging evaluation. Basal cell carcinoma is commonly encountered in this area (Fig. 20–6).[71] Cellulitis often accompanies these skin tumors, and distinction between tumor and edema can be difficult. Demonstration by MRI of invasion of the bone or retrobulbar area by the tumor usually poses no problem.

Granulomatous disease can produce mass lesions in the area. Possibilities include Wegener's granulomatosis, tuberculosis, and sarcoidosis.[72] Granulomas can have a variety of appearances on MRI. Well-defined lesions can have high signal on both T1WI and T2WI or low signal on T1WI and high signal on T2WI. Diffuse lesions typically have low signal intensity on both T1WI and T2WI, similar to other chronic inflammatory processes.

### Extraconal Lesions

Extraconal lesions can be further subcategorized into regions of origin: (1) bones, (2) sinuses, (3) lacrimal glands, and (4) other. The signal intensity characteristics of these lesions are summarized in Tables 20–3 to 20–5.

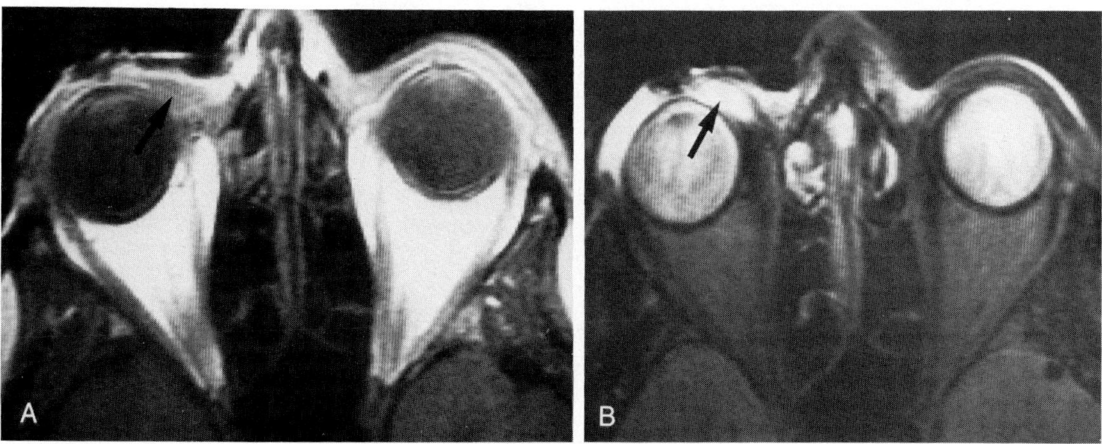


**Figure 20–4. Preseptal cellulitis.** Edema due to cellulitis is seen in the preseptal soft tissues (arrow). Homogeneous low signal is noted on *A*, T1WI (TE 30/TR 500), with homogeneous high signal on *B*, T2WI (TE 120/TR 2000). The orbital septum acts as a barrier to the spread of infection into the orbit.

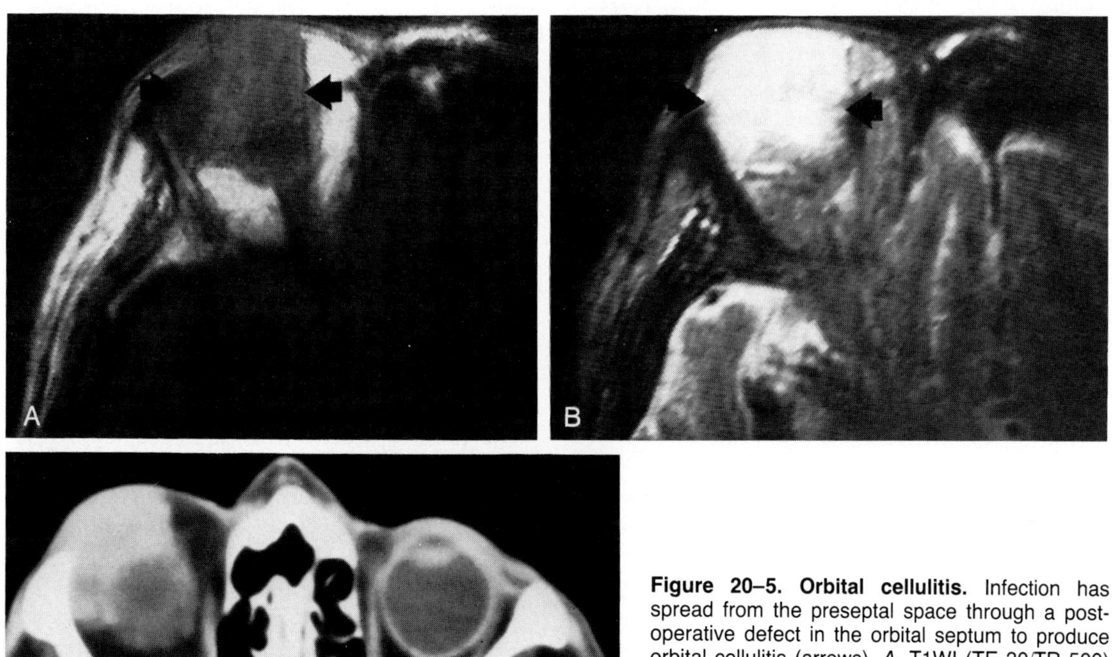


**Figure 20–5. Orbital cellulitis.** Infection has spread from the preseptal space through a postoperative defect in the orbital septum to produce orbital cellulitis (arrows). *A*, T1WI (TE 30/TR 500) shows a homogeneous low signal cellulitis that produces homogeneous high signal on *B*, T2WI (TE 120/TR 2000). *C*, A comparative CT scan is shown.

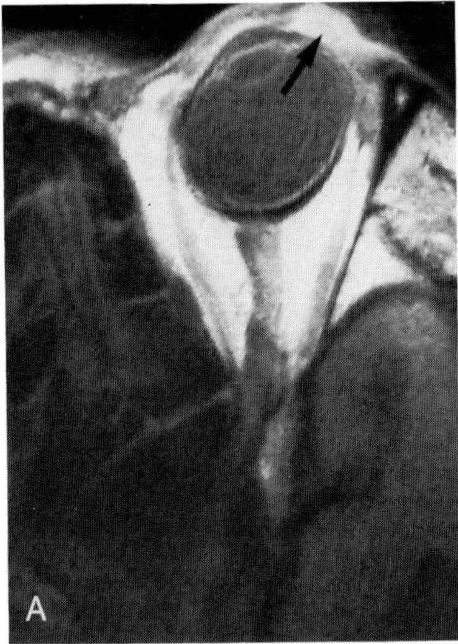

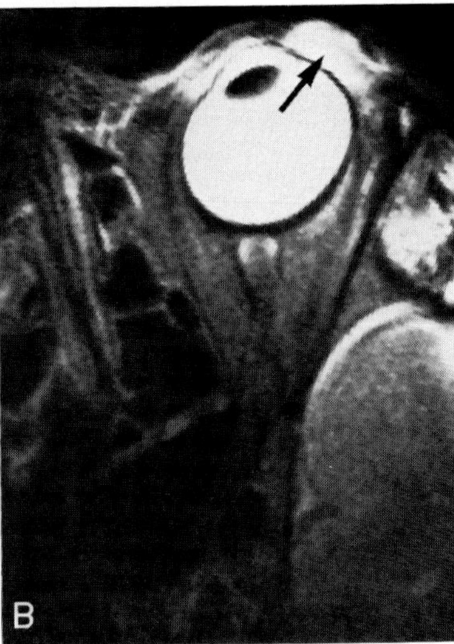


**Figure 20–6. Basal cell carcinoma.** A basal cell carcinoma is shown (arrow) involving the eyelid. This lesion is hypointense on *A*, T1WI (TE 30/ 500), and hyperintense on *B*, T2WI (TE 120/TR 2000). (From Sullivan JA, Harms SE. Characterization of orbital lesions by surface coil MR imaging. Radiographics 7:9–28, 1987, with permission.)

### *Bony Origin*

Fibrous dysplasia is probably a developmental mesodermal disorder; it is most frequently encountered in children and young adolescents. Clinically, fibrous dysplasia presents with headaches, facial asymmetry, and painless swelling. The superior lateral wall is most commonly involved of any of the bones comprising the bony margins of the orbit. Encroachment on the optic foramen can produce visual loss.[73–74] MRI shows bony enlargement by a lesion of low signal intensity on all images.[75] It may be difficult to separate fibrous dysplasia from hyperostosis secondary to an en plaque meningioma. These lesions are treated by plastic surgery. Radiation therapy is avoided since malignant degeneration can occur.

Osteomas most frequently arise in the paranasal sinus, usually the frontal sinuses, but can arise from the orbital wall. Gardner's syndrome should be suspected in any patient with an orbital osteoma. Visual symptoms can be produced from encroachment on the orbit.[76, 77] These lesions have low signal on all MR images (Fig. 20–7).[16, 17] Osteomas are not likely to be missed on MR images, but because of their dense calcifications, CT provides better visualization.

Ossifying fibromas are benign bone tumors that often arise in the paranasal sinuses adjacent to the orbit. These lesions are manifested as a painless facial swelling. The lesions may appear anatomically more aggressive than fibrous dysplasia.[78]

Chondrosarcomas arise from cartilaginous rests within the walls of the orbit and paranasal sinuses. Approximately 10% of chondrosarcomas occur in the bones of the face and cranium.[79] These lesions are usually slowly progressive and are not typically painful during their initial course. MRI of the chondrosarcoma usually shows mixed high and low signal on T2WI.[75] Evidence of invasion may be seen.

**Table 20–3.** SIGNAL INTENSITIES OF LESIONS OF BONY ORIGIN

| Lesion | T1WI | T2WI |
|---|---|---|
| Osteoma | Low | Homogeneous low |
| Fibrous dysplasia | Low | Homogeneous low |
| Hyperostosis 2° meningioma | Low | Homogeneous low |
| Osteoblastic osteosarcoma | Low | Inhomogeneous low |
| Giant cell tumors | Low | Low or high (cyst) |
| Metastatic | Low | Inhomogeneous, moderate to high |
| Chondrosarcoma | Low | Inhomogeneous, low to high |

**Table 20–4.** SIGNAL INTENSITIES OF LESIONS OF SINUS ORIGIN

| Lesion | T1WI | T2WI |
|---|---|---|
| Acute infection | Low | High |
| Lymphoma | Low | Homogeneous high |
| Squamous cell carcinoma | Low | Inhomogeneous low to moderate |
| Mucocele | High | High |

In contrast with chondrosarcomas, osteosarcomas rarely occur in this region. They can arise spontaneously or can be associated with Paget's disease or radiation therapy.[80] Clinically, these lesions are painful and have a rapid onset of symptoms. Osteoid matrix has low signal on all MR images.[75]

Giant cell tumors arising from the ethmoid bone can invade the orbit. These lesions could be low signal on both T1- and T2-weighted images or have a cystic component that enhances with T2 weighting.[75]

Hyperostosis may be seen with en plaque meningiomas. The meningiomas themselves may be very difficult to visualize by MRI, as they may appear isotense with adjacent neural tissue (Fig. 20–8). Contrast-enhanced CT may help sort out the hyperostosis resulting from a meningioma (Fig. 20–9) from fibrous dysplasia. As MRI contrast agents become available, contrast-enhanced MR may become the favored method of examination.[81]

Metastatic prostatic carcinoma and breast carcinoma can produce bony thickening of the orbital walls.[82] Most metastases produce higher signal on T2WI and can be distinguished from hyperostosis. An anatomically more aggressive-appearing lesion may also be noted.

### *Sinus Origin*

Orbital infections are most often due to spread from sinus infections, especially in children. In young children, orbital abscess is most often seen secondary to ethmoiditis. The orbital periosteum is loosely attached, and subperiosteal collections of pus accumulate near the site of sinus infection. In adolescents, frontal sinus infections can produce subperiosteal pus in the superior aspect of the orbit. Direct spread into the muscle cone is rare in the absence of trauma. Complications of orbital infection include septic thrombophlebitis, cavernous sinus

**Table 20–5.** SIGNAL INTENSITIES OF OTHER LESIONS OF EXTRACONAL ORIGIN

| Lesion | T1WI | T2WI | N(H)WI | Crossover |
|---|---|---|---|---|
| Carcinoma/ Sarcoma | Inhomogeneous low | Inhomogeneous high | Inhomogeneous high | Inhomogeneous high |
| Lymphoma | Homogeneous low | Homogeneous high | Homogeneous high | Homogeneous high |
| Hemangioma | Homogeneous low | Homogeneous high | Homogeneous high | Homogeneous high |
| Lymphangioma | Homogeneous low | Homogeneous high | Homogeneous high | Homogeneous high |
| Mixed/adenoma | Homogeneous low | Homogeneous high | Homogeneous high | Homogeneous high |
| Granuloma | Homogeneous low or high | Homogeneous low or high | Homogeneous low or high | Homogeneous low or high |
| Epidermoid | Low | High | Low | Isointense |
| Encephalocele | Low | High | Low | Isointense |
| Lipoma | High | Moderate | High | High |
| Dermoid* | High/moderate | Moderate/high | High/moderate | Isointense |
| Amyloid | Moderate | Low | — | — |
| Tolosa-Hunt | Low | Low | Low | Low |
| Pseudotumor | Low | Low | Low | Low |
| AVM | Low | Low | Low | Low |
| Hemorrhage (methemoglobin phase) | High | High | High | High |

*Nondependent/dependent fluid levels.

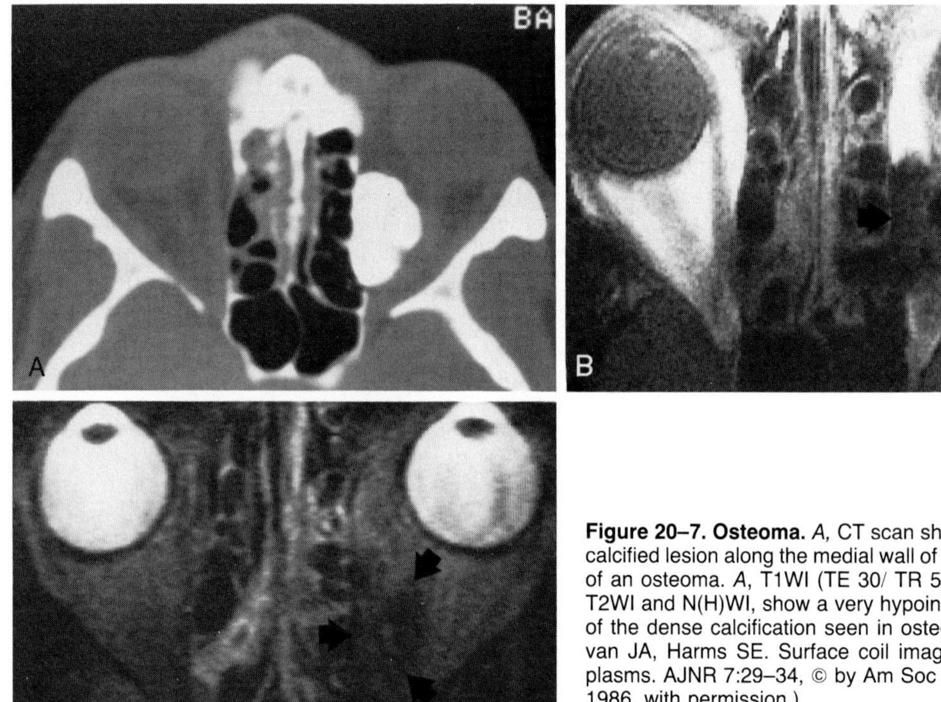

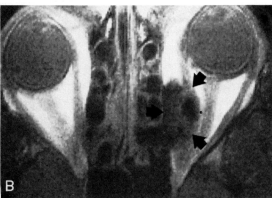

**Figure 20–7. Osteoma.** *A,* CT scan shows a well-defined calcified lesion along the medial wall of the left orbit typical of an osteoma. *A,* T1WI (TE 30/ TR 500), and *B* and *C,* T2WI and N(H)WI, show a very hypointense mass typical of the dense calcification seen in osteomas. (From Sullivan JA, Harms SE. Surface coil imaging of orbital neoplasms. AJNR 7:29–34, © by Am Soc of Neuroradiology, 1986, with permission.)

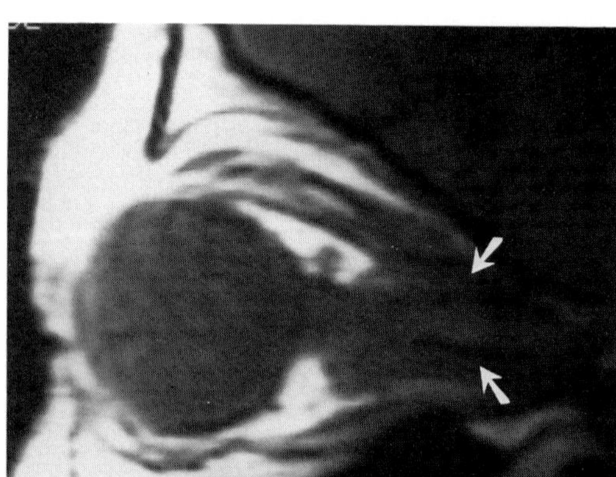

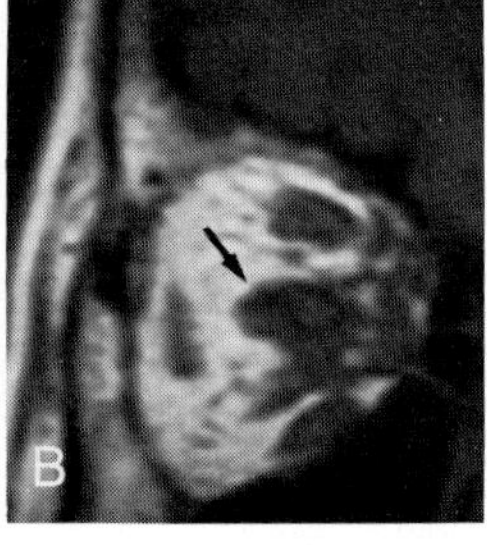

**Figure 20–8. Orbital meningioma.** *A,* Sagittal T1WI (TR 800/ TE 20). *B,* Coronal T1WI (TR 800/ TE 20). Surface coil T1WI with small field of view (FOV) (16 cm) allows one to delineate a mass (arrows) from the tubular-shaped optic nerve. The mass is virtually isointense with the optic nerve and appears to circumscribe the hypointense CSF or subarachnoid space around the nerve thus further confirming a diagnosis of meningioma rather than optic nerve glioma. (Courtesy of S.J. Pomeranz, M.D., Christ Hospital, Cincinnati, Ohio.)

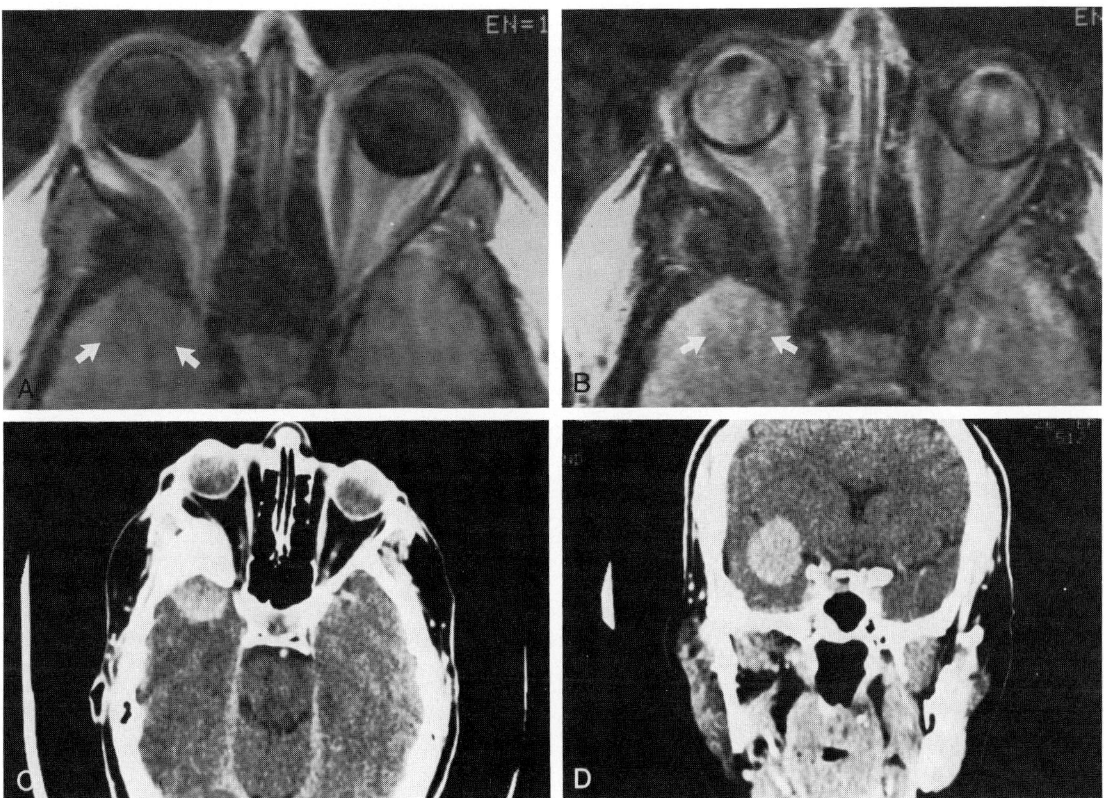

**Figure 20–9. Meningioma.** A thickened temporal wall of the orbit owing to hyperostosis from an adjacent meningioma is hypointense on *A*, N(H)-weighted image (TE 30/TR 1000), and *B*, T2WI (TE 100/TR 1000). The subtle, nearly isointense meningioma (arrows) is noted. The CT (*C,D*) scan easily shows the calcified meningioma.

thrombosis, intracranial epidural abscess, cerebritis, and intracerebral abscess.[67–70] Abscess (Fig. 20–10) is typically hypointense on T1WI and inhomogeneously hyperintense in T2WI.[17]

Neoplasms originating in the paranasal sinuses frequently invade the orbit. The most common of these lesions is squamous cell carcinoma. Anaplastic carcinoma and adenoid cystic carcinoma have also been known to involve the orbit. Less likely lesions that can invade the orbit are lymphoma, melanoma, plasmacytoma, inverting papilloma, fibrosarcoma, rhabdomyosarcoma, esthesioneuroblastoma, and leiomyosarcoma. Destruction of bone is a sign of tumor aggressiveness.[83] MR may provide more improved anatomic definition of these lesions compared with CT because of better soft tissue contrast and multiplanar imaging capability. The usual enhancement by a tumor on T2WI may not be seen with squamous cell carcinoma and other tumors with a high fibrous tissue content.

Mucoceles are produced by blockage of the ostium of the involved sinus. Smooth expansion of the sinus results, with thinning and remodeling of adjacent bone. The most frequent location is the frontal sinus, followed by the ethmoid sinus. A history of frequent sinus infections is common. Previous trauma is also often associated with the development of mucoceles. These lesions are filled with serous fluid that varies in protein content. Some mucoceles have fluid with a signal intensity approximating CSF.[84, 85] Many mucoceles, particularly longstanding lesions, have higher protein content, resulting in a shorter T1 and longer T2 that produce high signal on both T1WI and T2WI (Fig. 20–11). These lesions are then easily distinguished from other fluid-filled cysts.[17] Mucoceles can become infected, becoming mucopyoceles.

Granulomatous and mycotic infections involving the sinuses can secondarily involve the orbit. Granulomatous diseases include Wegener's granulomatosis, tuberculosis, and

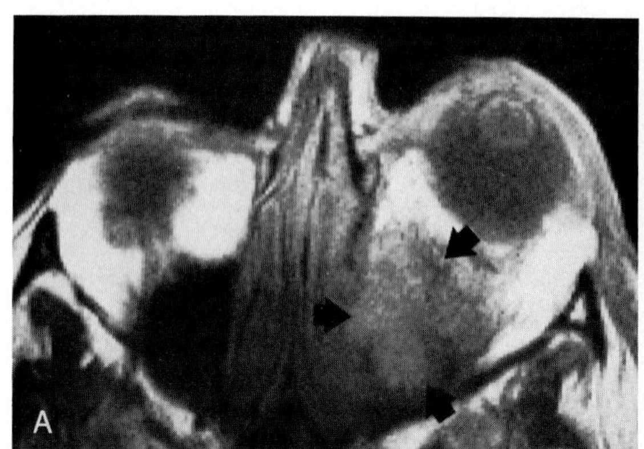


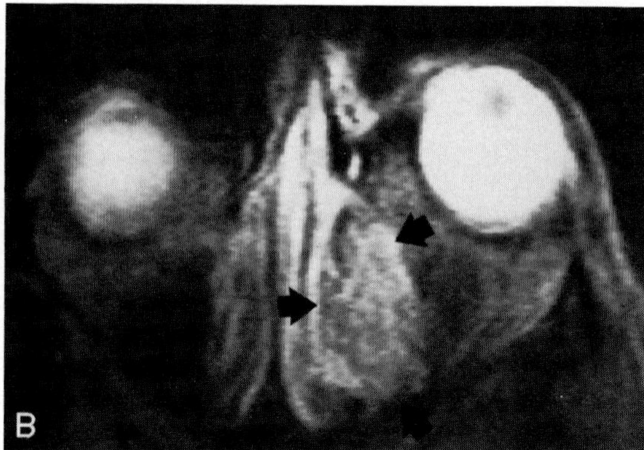


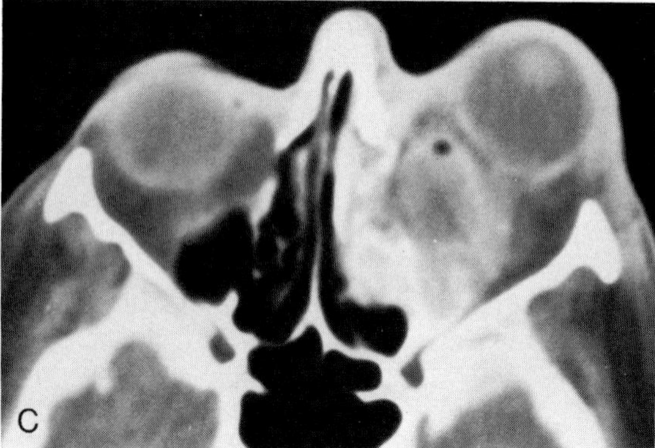


**Figure 20–10. Abscess.** An abscess (arrows) spreading from the adjacent maxillary sinus has a low signal on *A,* T1WI (TE 30/TR 500), and an inhomogeneous hyperintense signal on *B,* T2WI (TE 120/TR 2000). Gas is demonstrated within this fluid collection on *C*, CT scan. (From Sullivan JA, Harms SE. Surface coil imaging of orbital neoplasms. AJNR 7:29–34, © by Am Soc of Neuroradiology, 1986.)

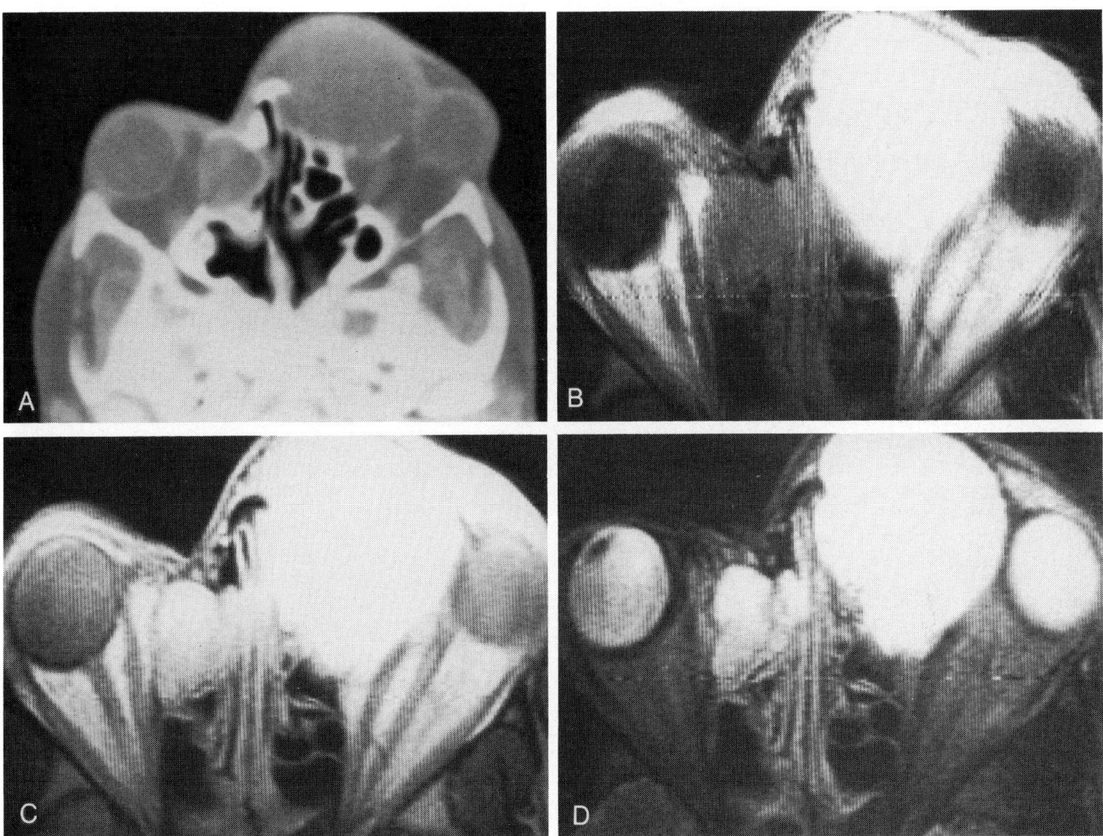


**Figure 20–11. Mucocele.** A 37-year-old man with progressive facial deformity following an automobile accident three years earlier presented with a large, homogeneous, expansile mass on *A*, CT scan. Differentiation between encephalocele and mucocele was difficult by CT. The lesion has a homogeneous high signal on *B,* T1WI (TE 30/TR 500); *C*, N(H)WI (TE 30/TR 1000); and *D,* T2WI (TE 120/TR 2000), which is typical of mucoceles. The CSF of an encephalocele would have a low signal on T1WI and N(H)WI. Additional N(H)WI (*E,F,G*) show the extent of this large mucocele. (From Sullivan JA, Harms SE. Surface coil imaging of orbital neoplasms. AJNR 7:29–34, © by Am Soc of Neuroradiology, 1986, with permission.)

*Illustration continued on following page*

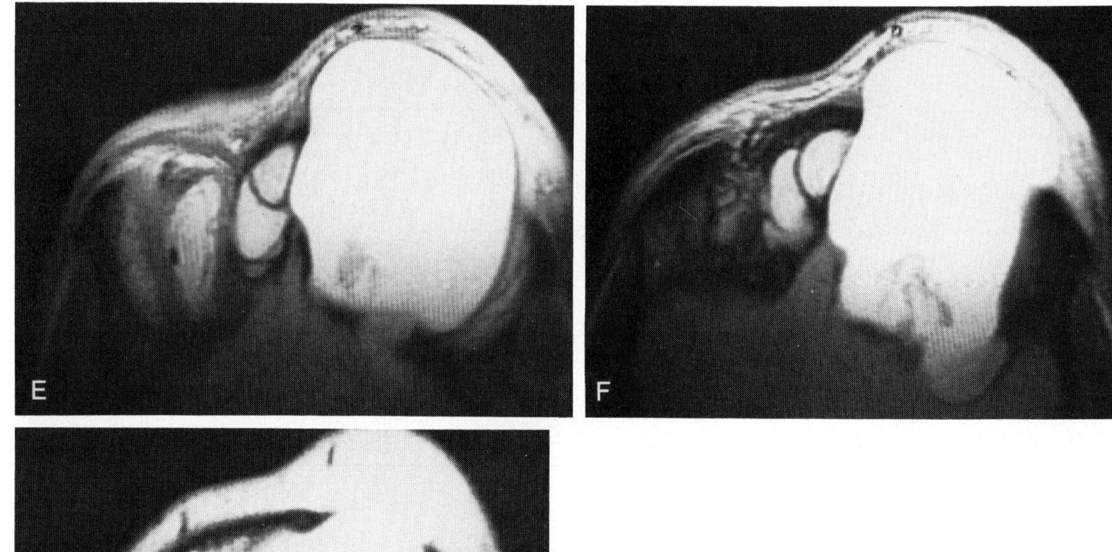


**Figure 20–11** *Continued*

sarcoidosis.[72, 73] Fungal infections include mucormycosis and aspergillosis.[86, 87]

### Lacrimal Gland Origin

About half of all tumors arising from the lacrimal gland are of epithelial origin. These are equally divided between mixed adenomas and various carcinomas. Adenoid cystic carcinoma is the most frequent carcinoma of lacrimal origin (Fig. 20–12). Masses of lymphatic origin range from benign lymphoid hyperplasia to malignant lymphoma. Inflammatory masses include dacryoadenitis and inflammatory pseudotumor.[88, 89] Benign mixed adenomas are well-defined masses that do not invade bone or the muscle cone. Typically, these lesions have homogeneous signal intensity with low signal on T1WI and high signal on T2WI. Malignant tumors tend to invade the orbital wall and muscle cone. These lesions have poorly defined margins and are inhomogeneous in signal intensity.[16, 17]

### Other Extraconal Origins

The lacrimal gland is the most frequent site of origin for lymphoma in the orbit, but lymphoma can occur in other areas as well. Lymphoma typically is an infiltrative mass having low signal on T1WI and high signal on T2WI. This lesion often can be distin-

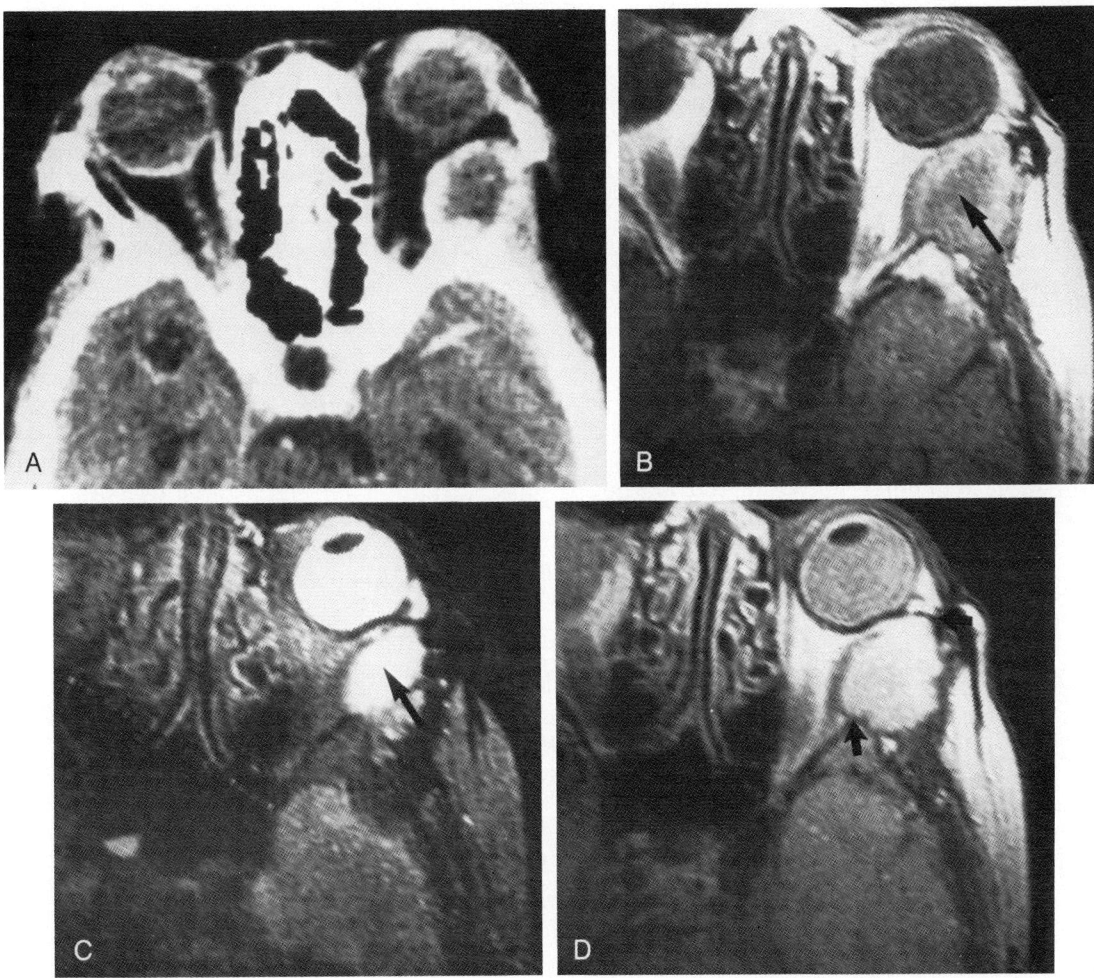


**Figure 20–12. Adenoid cystic carcinoma.** *A,* Enhanced CT shows an area of rim enhancement eroding the temporal wall of the orbit in this 73-year-old woman. *B,* T1WI (TE 30/TR 500) shows an inhomogeneous hypointense mass (arrow) with inhomogeneous hyperintensity on *C,* T2WI (TE 120/TR 2000). A central area of necrosis (arrow) is noted. *D,* Crossover (TE 90/TR 1500), shows homogeneous hyperintensity with good anatomical detail of the lateral soft tissue extension and medial rectus involvement (arrow). (From Sullivan JA, Harms SE. Surface coil imaging of orbital neoplasms. AJNR 7:29–34, © by Am Soc of Neuroradiology, 1986, with permission.)

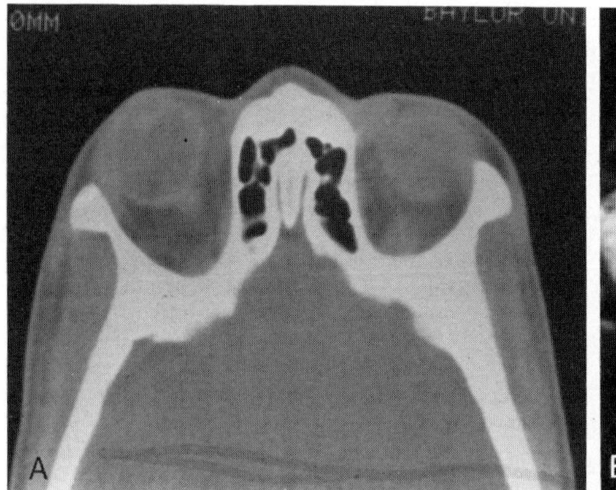

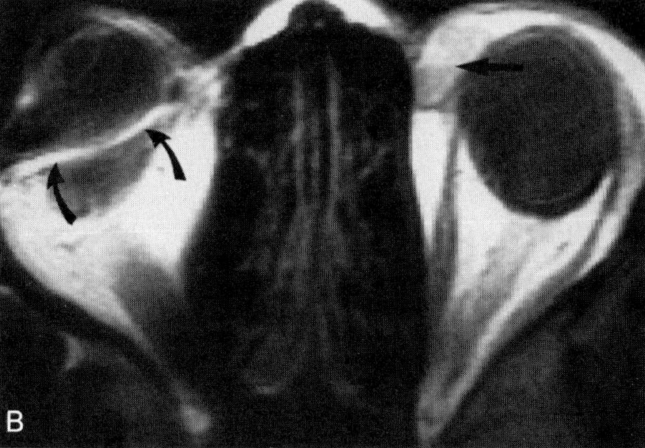

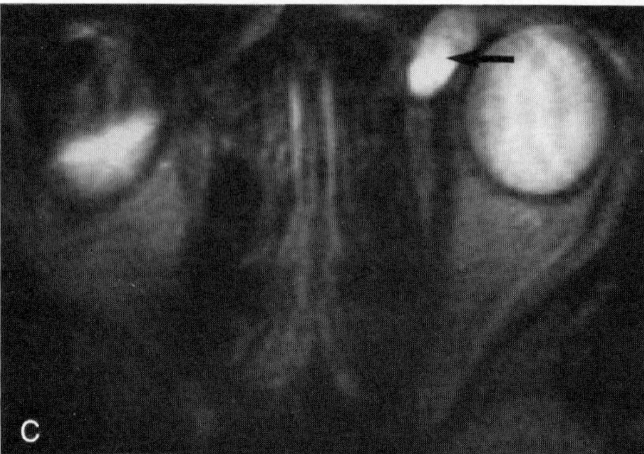

**Figure 20–13. Dermoid cyst.** *A,* CT scan shows a subtle soft tissue mass in the medial aspect of the left orbit. This lesion shows fluid level (arrow) on *B,* T1WI (TE 30/TR 500), and *C,* T2WI (TE 120/TR 2000). The nondependent fluid has fatlike signal characteristics with a high signal on T1WI and a moderate signal on T2WI. The dependent layer has fluid signal characteristics with a low signal on T1WI and a high signal on T2WI. The artifact in the right orbit (curved arrows) is due to eye cosmetics. (From Sullivan JA, Harms SE. Surface coil imaging of orbital neoplasms. AJNR 7:29–34, © by Am Soc Neuroradiology, 1986, with permission.)

guished from orbital pseudotumor, which has low signal on both T1WI and T2WI.[16, 25]

Dermoid cysts result from sequestration of epithelial tissue during embryogenesis. They are most frequently found in the lacrimal fossa but can occur anywhere in the extraconal orbit. These lesions are usually cystic and contain fluid and sebaceous components.[88, 90–94] On MRI fluid levels have often been demonstrated within these cystic masses that could not be seen by CT (Figs. 20–13 and 20–14). The nondependent fluid has fatlike signal characteristics with high signal on T1WI and moderate signal on T2WI. The dependent fluid was more waterlike with low signal on T1WI and high signal

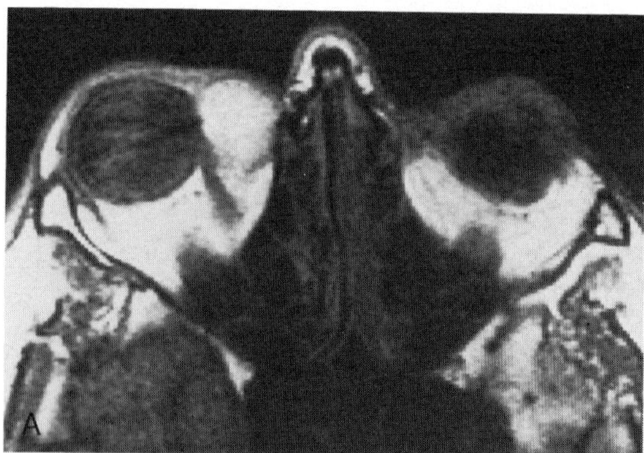

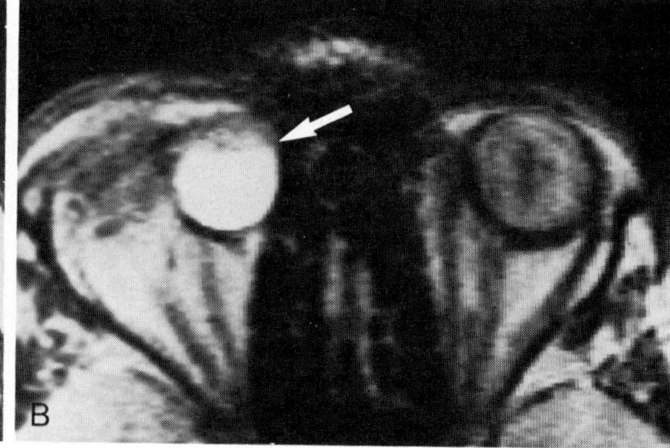

**Figure 20–14. Dermoid cyst.** A fat-fluid level (arrow) similar to Fig. 20–13 is noted on *A,* T1WI (TE 25/TR 250), and *B,* T2WI (TE 100/TR 1000).

on T2WI. If fluid levels are not demonstrated, the lesions in our series have high signal on both T1WI and T2WI (Fig. 20–15).[16, 17, 31]

Lipomas occur in the orbit.[91–95] These lesions are well-defined, soft, homogeneous masses having high signal on T1WI and moderate signal on T2WI. No fluid levels should be seen.

Epidermoid tumors are less common than dermoid cysts. These tumors are derived from epidermis. On multiecho MR images, the appearance of epidermoids is relatively characteristic. The signal intensity of epidermoid tumors tends to follow CSF on all images. These lesions can be separated from other high signal tumors on T2WI by looking at the shorter echo, N(H)WI, and crossover images in which the lesion is not enhanced relative to CSF (Fig. 20–16).[31, 45, 81] Most other tumors have high signal relative to CSF on N(H)WI and crossover images.

Encephaloceles can produce orbital mass effects.[96] The fluid within encephaloceles will follow CSF in signal intensity. Separation from epidermoid tumors should be based on anatomic characteristics and the homogeneous signal intensity of fluid.[31]

In Tolosa-Hunt syndrome, a lesion pathologically similar to orbital pseudotumor, involves the cavernous sinus and superior orbital fissure. Clinically, this lesion produces painful ophthalmoplegia.[97] This lesion usually responds to steroids, but similar responses have been seen in other conditions.[98] Low signal on both T1WI and T2WI, similar to orbital pseudotumor, is seen on MRI (Fig. 20–17).[31]

Obstruction of the nasolacrimal duct can lead to dilatation of the lacrimal sac (dacryocystitis). Obstructions can result from congenital stenosis, trauma, foreign bodies, and tumor. Filling defects within the lacrimal sac seen on dacryocystography have been associated with concretion of *Actinomyces israelii*.[99, 100] Homogeneous fluid can be seen in the distended nasolacrimal duct by MRI (Fig. 20–18).

Primary amyloidosis rarely can produce extraconal orbital masses.[101–104] Amyloid is characterized by the deposition of a homogeneous eosinophilic protein. On MRI these lesions may have moderate signal on T1WI and low signal on T2WI (Fig. 20–19).

A variety of vascular lesions can be found in the extraconal region. High-flow lesions have a low signal on all images owing to a flow-void effect. These lesions include carotid-cavernous fistulae and arteriovenous malformations.[90, 92] Enlargement of the orbital vessels and the rectus muscles is often associated. The presence of serpiginous tangles of vessels can be diagnostic. Slower flow in vascular malformation can result in higher signal. Very slow flow in hemangiomas has high signal on T2-weighted images. Lymphangiomas typically are less well defined and less homogeneous than hemangiomas. These lesions will be described in more detail in the intraconal section.[16, 17, 31]

A variety of other lesions can involve the extraconal orbit. Metastatic disease should be considered in patients with known primaries (Fig. 20–20). Primary sarcomas and neurofibromas can also occur in this region (Fig. 20–21).

## Extraocular Muscle Lesions

The signal intensity characteristics of lesions involving the extraocular muscles are summarized in Table 20–6.

Endocrine ophthalmopathy is the most common cause of enlarged extraocular muscles. The etiology of endocrine ophthalmopathy is poorly understood.[106, 107] This disease process is manifested by swelling and lymphocytic infiltration that produces proptosis and later fibrosis, restricting movement of the extraocular muscles.[108, 109] Endocrine ophthalmopathy occurs in individuals with controlled or uncontrolled hyperthyroidism and also in patients without hyperthyroidism.[110] The most common muscles of involvement in decreasing order of occurrence are inferior, medial, superior, and lateral rectus muscles.[111] The disease is bilateral in approximately 90% of cases by CT, but this involvement can be asymmetric.[111] Muscle enlargement typically is fusiform and characteristically tapers near the tendinous in-

**Table 20–6.** SIGNAL INTENSITIES OF EXTRAOCULAR MUSCLE LESIONS

| Lesion | T1 | T2 |
|---|---|---|
| Endocrine ophthalmopathy | Low | Low |
| Orbital myositis | Low | Low |
| Brown's syndrome | Low | Low |
| Rhabdomyosarcoma | Low | High |
| Lymphoma | Low | High |

*Text continued on page 614*

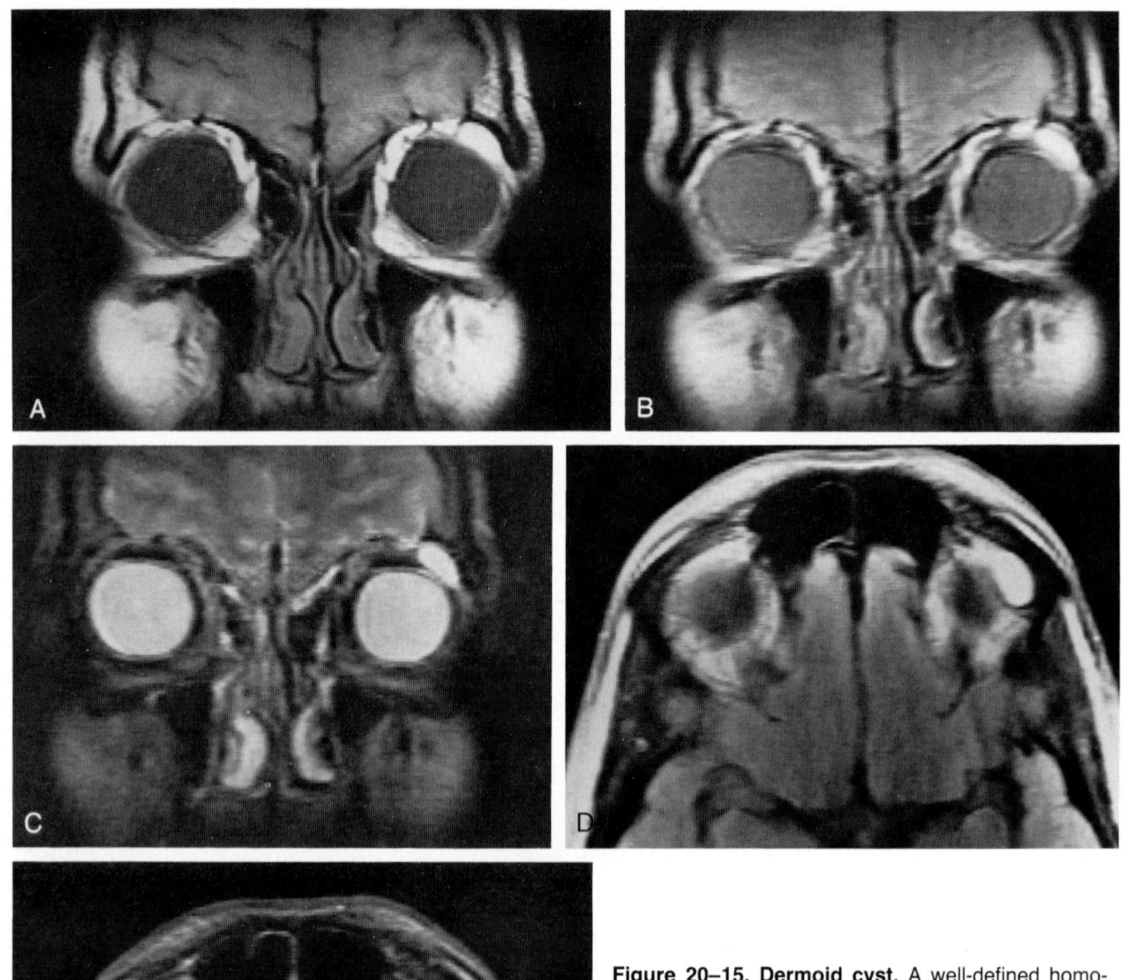


**Figure 20–15. Dermoid cyst.** A well-defined homogeneous, hyperintense mass is seen in the lateral left orbit on the coronal. *A,* T1WI (TE 30/TR 500), *B,* N(H)WI (TE 30/TR 2000), and *C,* T2WI (TE 120/TR 2000). No fluid levels can be demonstrated on the transverse, *D,* N(H)WI (TE 30/TR 2000), and *E,* T2WI (TE 120/TR 2000). This is an example of another appearance for a dermoid cyst.

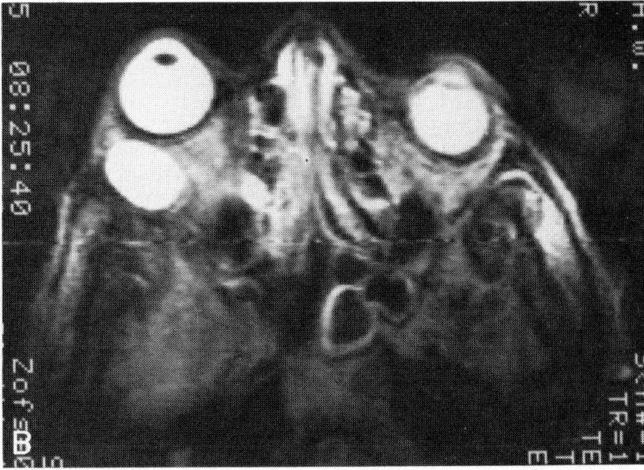


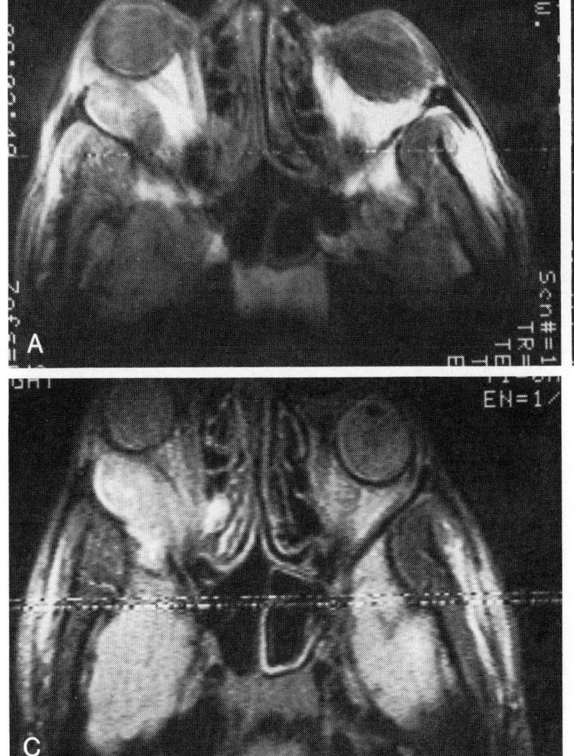


**Figure 20–16. Epidermoid.** A well-defined mass is seen along the lateral wall of the left orbit having a homogeneous low signal on *A,* T1WI (TE 26/TR 250), and a high signal on *B,* T2WI (TE 100/TR 1000). This appearance is not very different from many of the orbital lesions. To help differentiate this lesion, *C,* a crossover (TE 60/TR 1500) image was performed. On the crossover image, epidermoids are isointense, whereas most other lesions are hyperintense. (From Sullivan JA, Harms SE. Surface coil imaging of orbital neoplasms. AJNR 7:29–34, © by Am Soc Neuroradiology, 1986, with permission.)

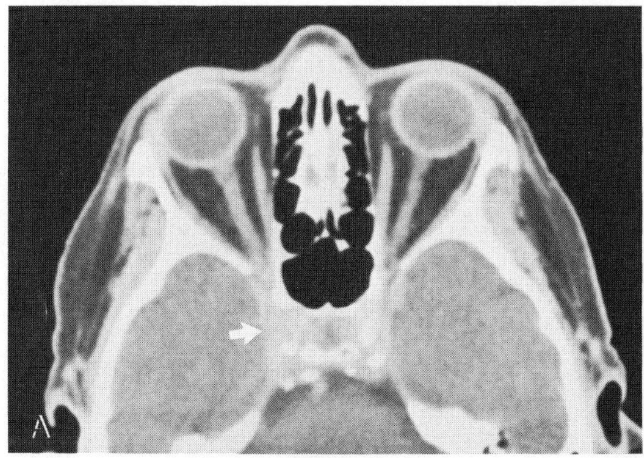


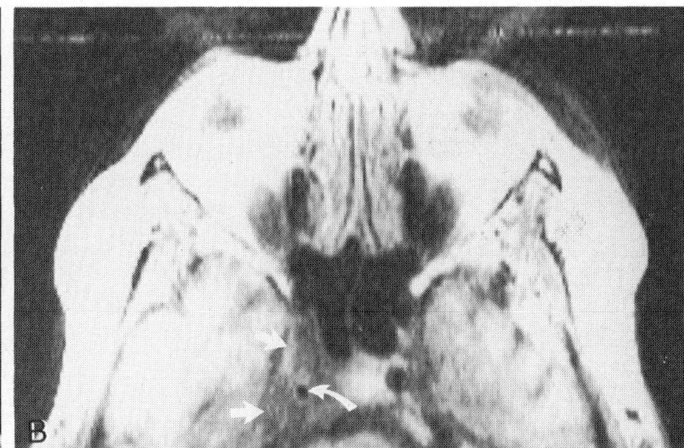


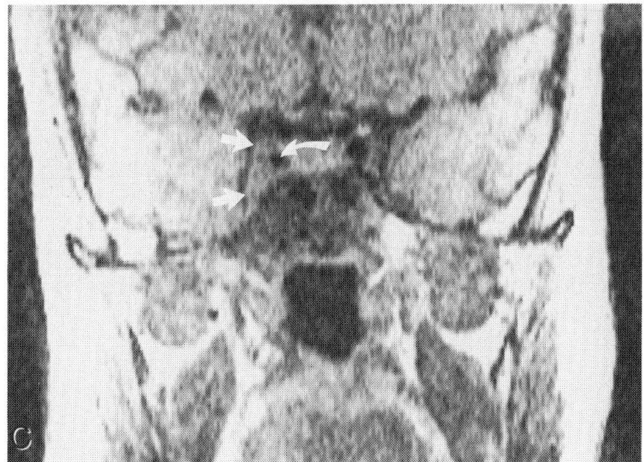


**Figure 20–17. Tolosa-Hunt syndrome.** *A,* CT scan shows a homogeneously enhancing mass involving the cavernous sinus (arrow). *B,* Transverse, and *C,* coronal T1WI (TE 25/TR 250), show an isointense mass (short arrows) surrounding the intracavernous carotid artery (curved arrow).

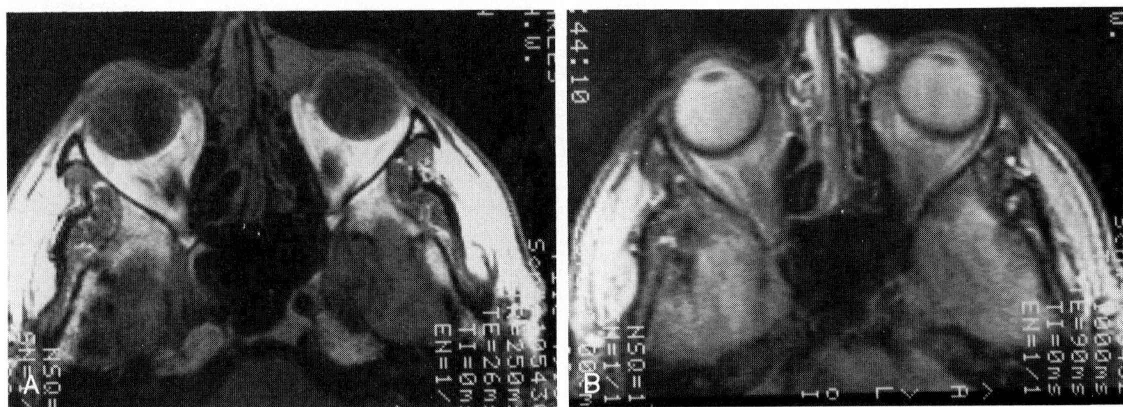

**Figure 20–18. Dacryocystitis.** Homogeneous hypointense fluid is seen in the distended lacrimal sac on *A*, T1WI (TE 25/TR 250), with homogeneous hyperintense fluid on *B*, T2WI (TE 90/TR 1000).

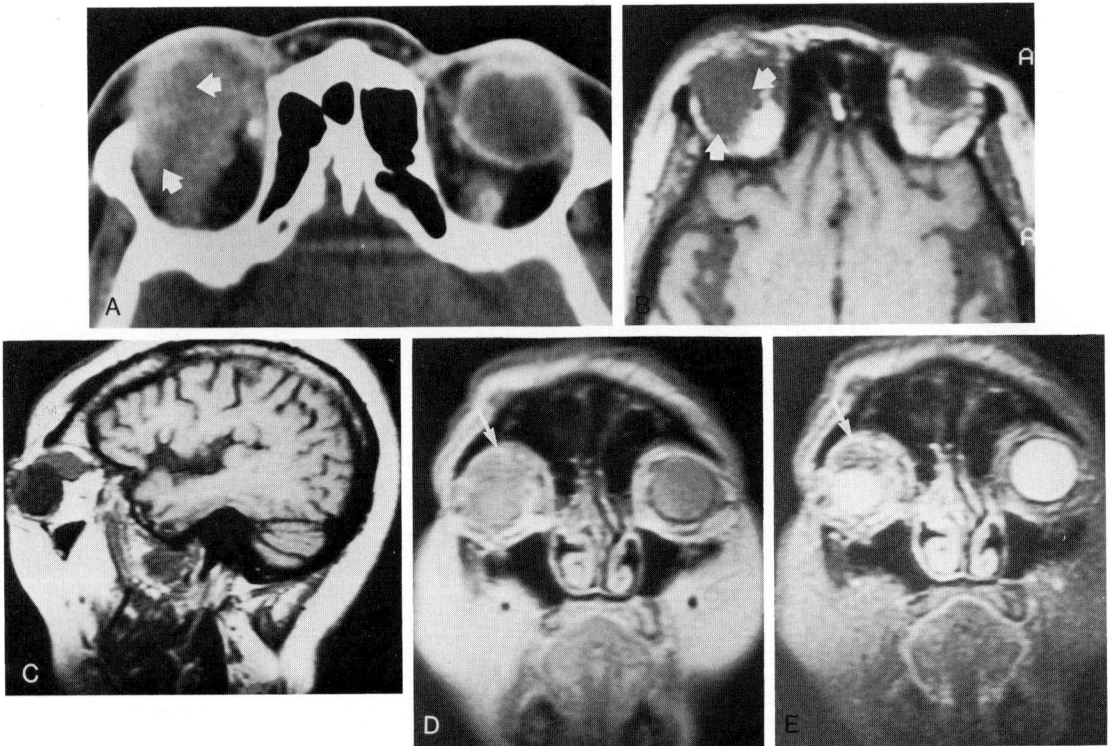

**Figure 20–19. Amyloidosis.** *A,* Contrast-enhanced CT scan shows an ill-defined extraconal mass (arrows). *B,* Axial T1WI (TE 25/TR 600), and *C,* sagittal T1WI (TE 25/TR 600), show a low-signal mass with much better anatomical definition (arrows) than CT. On coronal, *D,* N(H)WI, and *E,* T2WI, the mass (arrows) is hypointense. (Courtesy of S. J. Pomeranz, M.D., Christ Hospital, Cincinnati, Ohio.)

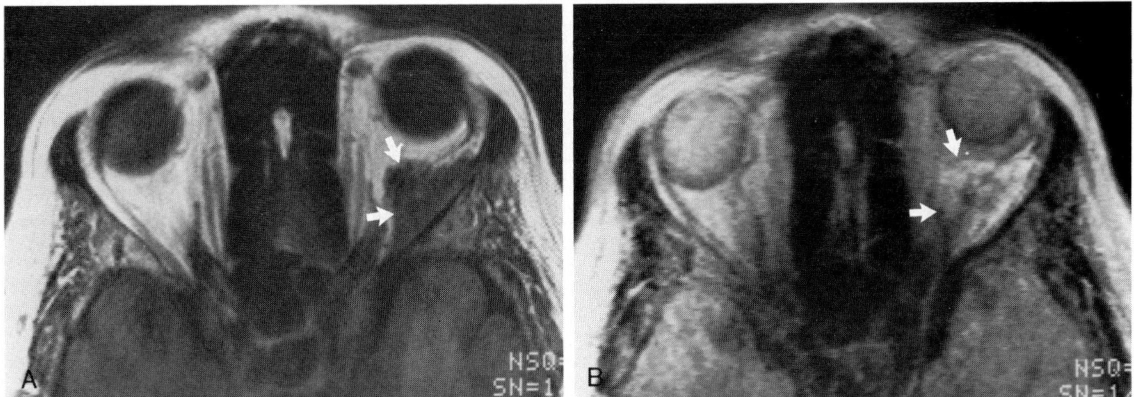


**Figure 20–20. Metastatic disease.** A mass (arrows) seen along the lateral aspect of the left orbit is homogeneous hypointense on *A,* T1WI (TE 25/TR 250), and is homogeneous and hyperintense on *B,* T2WI (TE 100/TR 1000).

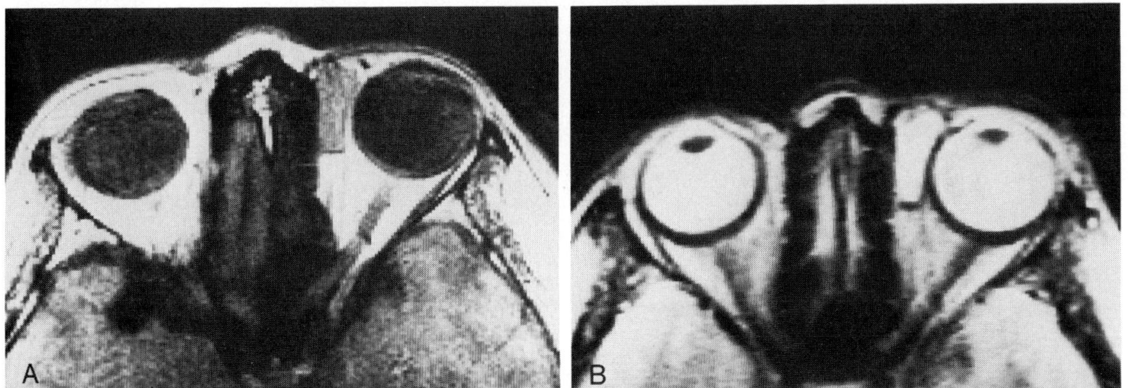


**Figure 20–21. Neurofibroma.** A well-defined neurofibroma is seen in the medial left orbit with a homogeneous low signal intensity on *A,* T1WI (TE 25/TR 250), and homogeneous high signal intensity on *B,* T2WI (TE 100/TR 2000). The sharply defined margins and homogeneous signal intensity on T2WI favor a benign lesion.

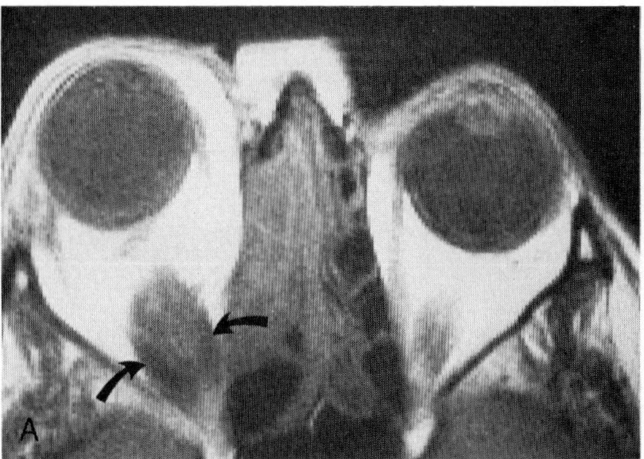

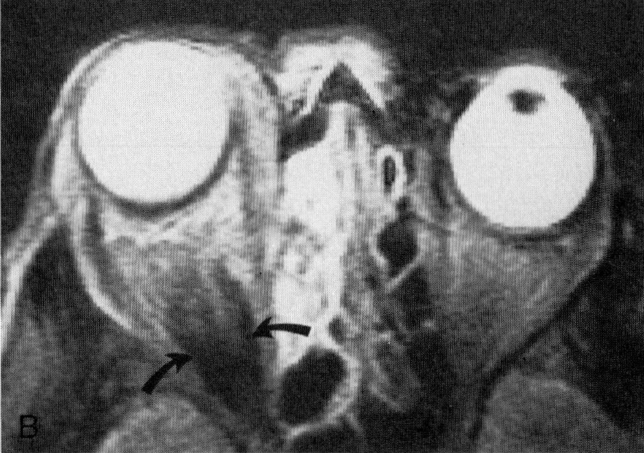

**Figure 20–22. Endocrine ophthalmopathy.** Fusiform enlargement of the inferior rectus muscle (arrows) is seen in this 53-year-old woman with unilateral proptosis and a history of Graves's disease. Hypointensity is seen on both *A,* T1WI (TE 30/TR 500), and *B,* T2WI (TE 120/TR 2000). (From Sullivan JA, Harms SE. Surface coil imaging of orbital neoplasms. AJNR 7:29–34, © by Am Soc Neuroradiology, 1986, with permission.)

sertion to the globe. On MRI the enlargement has moderate-to-low signal on both T1WI and T2WI (Figs. 20–22 and 20–23).[16, 17, 31] In addition to muscle enlargement, there is also increased orbital fat in patients with Graves's disease (Fig. 20–24).[111]

Orbital myositis is a subgroup of the nonspecific orbital inflammatory syndrome of orbital pseudotumor.[112–115] One or more extraocular muscles are affected by a diffuse infiltrate or inflammatory cells with well-differentiated lymphocytes predominating.[114, 116] The etiology is unknown, but the higher incidence in patients with systemic autoimmune disease suggests an immunologic mechanism.[113–115, 117] Initial CT reports indicated a typical unilateral process, but more recent findings indicate a high incidence of bilaterality.[112, 115, 118] Involvement of the tendon inserting on the globe may help

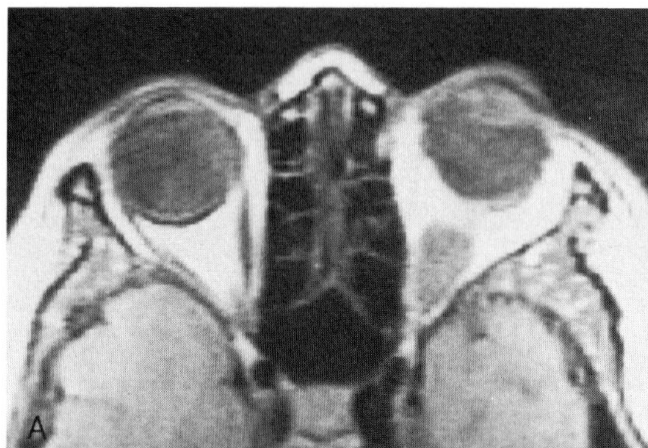

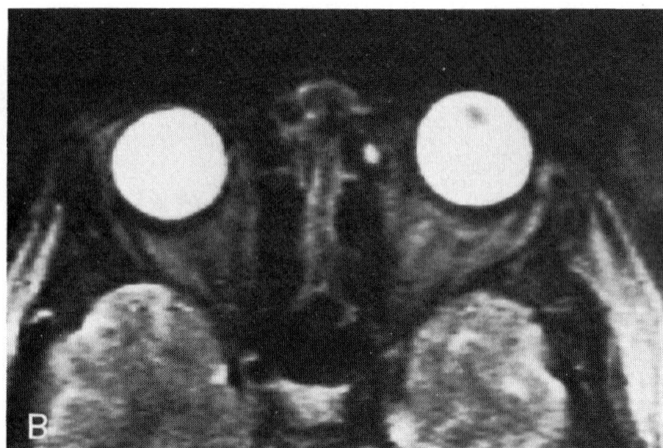

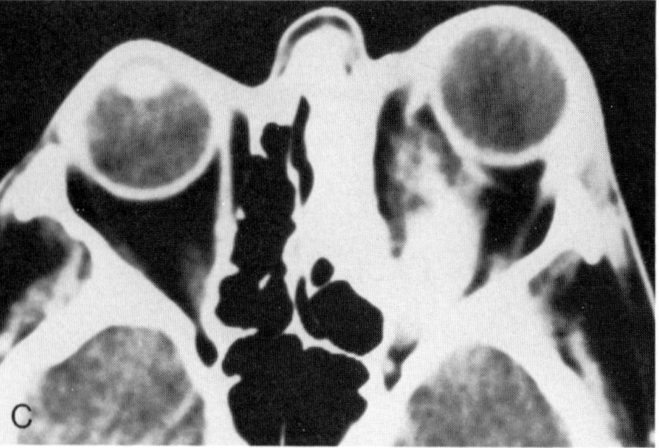

**Figure 20–23. Endocrine ophthalmopathy.** A low signal is seen from the enlarged inferior rectus muscle on *A,* T1WI (TE 25/TR 250), and *B,* T2WI (TE 100/TR 1000), typical of endocrine ophthalmopathy. Enlargement of the inferior rectus is also noted on *C,* CT scan.

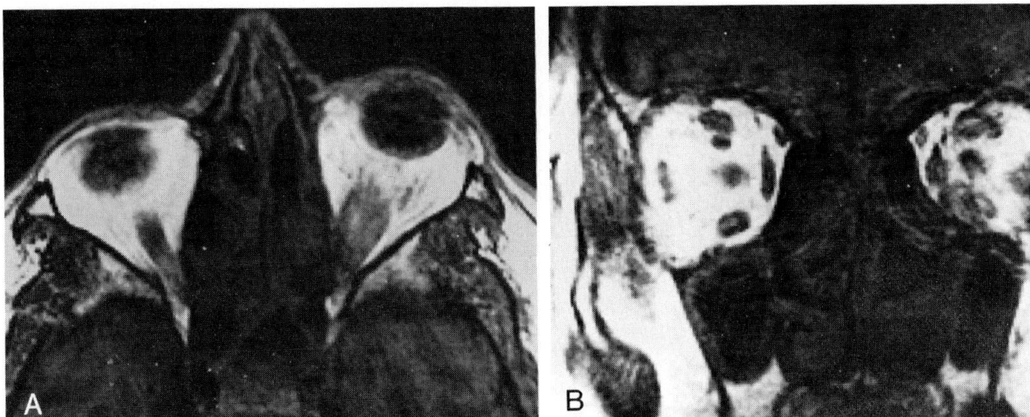


**Figure 20–24. Long-standing Graves's disease.** Increased high signal orbital and intramuscular fat is seen in the left orbit in this patient with long-standing, uncontrolled Graves's disease. High signal fat is seen within the inferior rectus muscle on *A*, transverse T1WI (TE 25/TR 250), and within all the rectus muscles on *B*, coronal T1WI (TE 25/TR 250).

distinguish myositis from endocrine ophthalmopathy that does not involve the tendons. Absence of tendon involvement does not however rule out myositis.[118, 119] Myositis tends to produce enlargement of muscles at the orbital apex, whereas endocrine ophthalmopathy tends to produce fusiform enlargement. Myositis involves the following muscles in decreasing frequency: medial, lateral, superior, and inferior rectus muscles.[118] MR shows enlargement of one or more extraocular muscles of low signal on both T1WI and T2WI similar to endocrine ophthalmopathy (Fig. 20–25).[16, 17, 31, 115]

Orbital lymphomas constitute less than 1% of all nodal and extranodal lymphomas. Differentiation from other lesions involving the extraocular muscles may be difficult by conventional imaging methods.[25] Most lymphomas enhance with heavy T2 weighting, distinguishing these lesions from endocrine ophthalmopathy and myositis, which have low signal on T2WI (Fig. 20–26).[25–31] Chloromas usually have high signal on T2WI, but in our series one case was not hyperintense on T2WI, probably secondary to responsive steroid therapy.

Brown's syndrome is characterized by the inability to raise the eye above horizontal level during adduction, but in the abducted position, full elevation is possible.[119] Congenital Brown's syndrome is due to a congenitally short or taut superior oblique tendon sheath complex.[120] Acquired Brown's

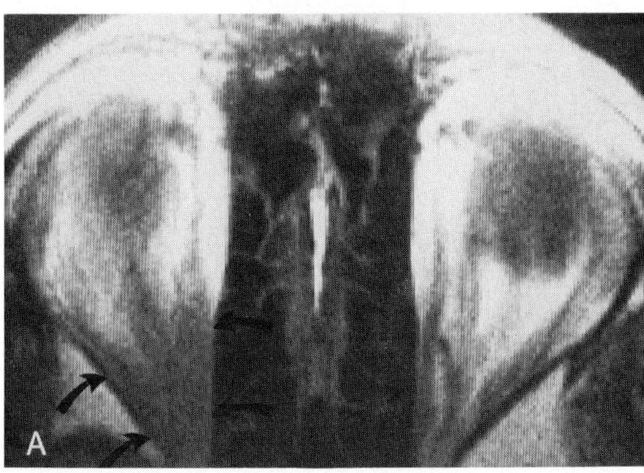


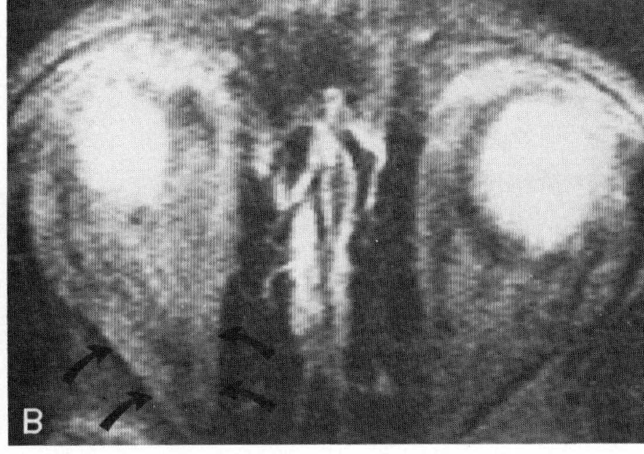


**Figure 20–25. Orbital myositis.** Orbital myositis (pseudotumor) is shown producing apical (arrows) enlargement of the extraocular muscles. Low signal intensity is seen on *A*, T1WI (TE 30/TR 500), and *B*, T2WI (TE 120/TR 2000). (From Sullivan JA, Harms SE. Surface coil imaging of orbital neoplasms. AJNR 7:29–34, © by Am Soc Neuroradiology, 1986, with permission.)

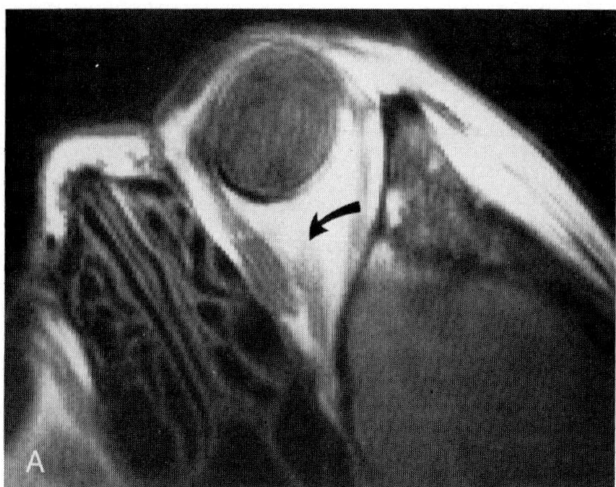


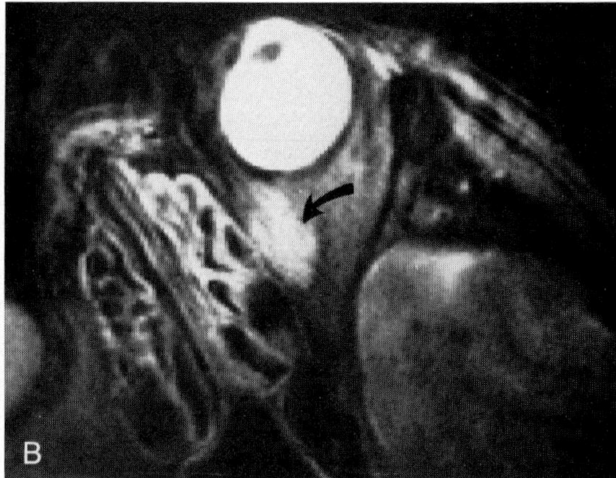


**Figure 20–26. Lymphoma.** An ill-defined mass (arrows) of homogeneous low signal intensity on *A,* T1WI (TE 30/TR 500), and high signal intensity on *B,* T2WI (TE 120/TR 2000), is typical of lymphoma. (From Sullivan JA, Harms SE. Surface coil imaging of orbital neoplasms. AJNR 7:29–34, © by Am Soc Neuroradiology, 1986, with permission.)

syndrome results from an impairment in the passage, usually by a mass within the superior oblique muscle tendon through the trochlea. Acquired Brown's syndrome can be either permanent or intermittent.[121, 122] MRI can directly image the tendon passing through the trochlea and evaluate anatomic defects (Fig. 20–27). The demonstration of an anatomic defect aids in the evaluation of potential corrective surgery, since a mass lesion in acquired Brown's syndrome is a correctable lesion and congenital Brown's syndrome is not surgically correctable.[31, 123]

Rhabdomyosarcoma is the most common primary orbital malignancy in children. Less than 10% of cases occur after the age of 16. The tumor is often large when discovered. Invasion of the adjacent intraconal space or extraorbital extension may be present.[92, 124] Most rhabdomyosarcomas have high signal on T2WI. Mixed patterns can occur in larger lesions.[75]

## Intraconal Lesions

The signal intensity characteristics of lesions involving the intraconal region are summarized in Table 20–7.

Cavernous hemangioma is the most common benign orbital neoplasm.[90, 92, 125–128] These lesions can occur anywhere within the orbit, but 83% are intraconal. The lesions appear twice as often in women as men, occurring in the second to fourth decades. These are well-demarcated, smoothly marginated, usually ovoid lesions that have homogeneous low signal on T1WI and high signal on T2WI (Figs. 20–28 and 20–29). Calcifications that are frequently seen on CT are usually not recognized on MRI.[16–18]

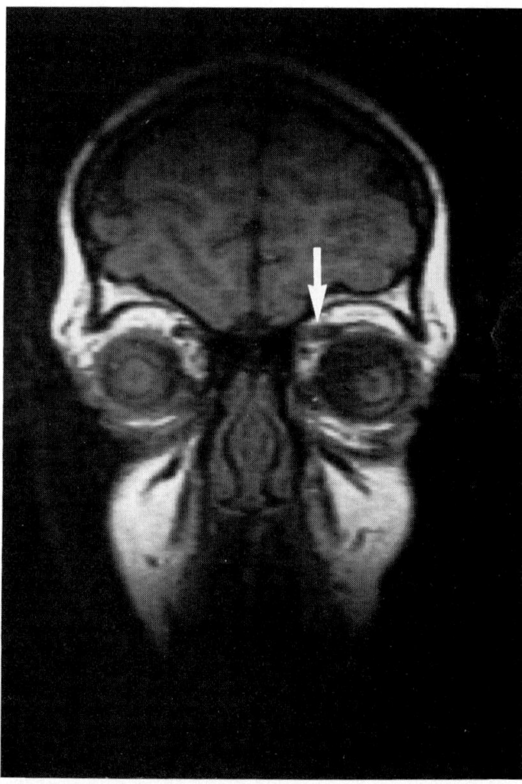

**Figure 20–27. Brown's syndrome.** Acquired post-traumatic Brown's syndrome is seen on MRI as an enlargement of the superior oblique muscle tendon (arrow) as it passes over the trochlea. Deviation of the lens, compared with the unaffected side, is also noted.

**Table 20–7.** SIGNAL INTENSITIES OF INTRACONAL LESIONS

| Lesion | T1 | T2 |
|---|---|---|
| Vascular malformations | Low | Low |
| Pseudotumor | Low | Low |
| Cavernous hemangioma | Homogeneous low | Homogeneous high |
| Lymphangioma | Homogeneous low | Homogeneous high |
| Lymphoma | Homogeneous low | Homogeneous high |
| Most sarcoma, carcinoma | Inhomogeneous low | Inhomogeneous high |
| Hemorrhage (methemoglobin phase) | High | High |
| Lipoma | High | Low |

Capillary hemangiomas occur primarily in infants. Most of these lesions are extraconal but can occur in the intraconal region. A feeding artery may be identified.[128]

Orbital lymphangiomas typically occur in a younger age group than cavernous hemangiomas.[128] Lymphangiomas can be well marginated like hemangiomas but are typically more diffuse. Heterogeneous low signal on T1WI with increased signal on T2WI can be seen by MRI (Fig. 20–30). Spontaneous hemorrhage is common.[128] Blood in the methemoglobin phase can be distinguished by the presence of high signal on both T1WI and T2WI.[129]

Hemangiopericytomas are slow-growing vascular neoplasms. About half of these lesions are malignant. The demonstration of infiltration into adjacent tissues would be helpful in distinguishing this lesion from hemangioma. Marked enhancement is seen on CT and may be difficult to separate from a meningioma. MRI should differentiate meningiomas from hemangiopericytoma on the basis of signal intensity differences.[23]

A variety of other lesions can involve the

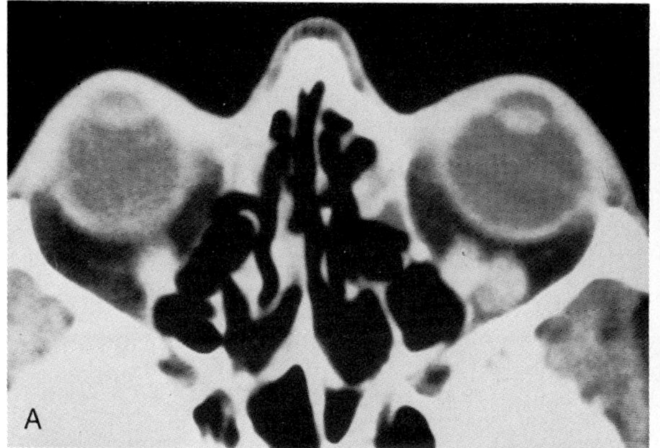


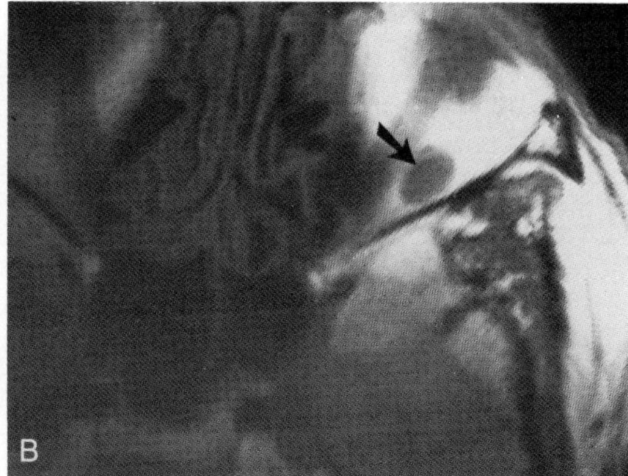


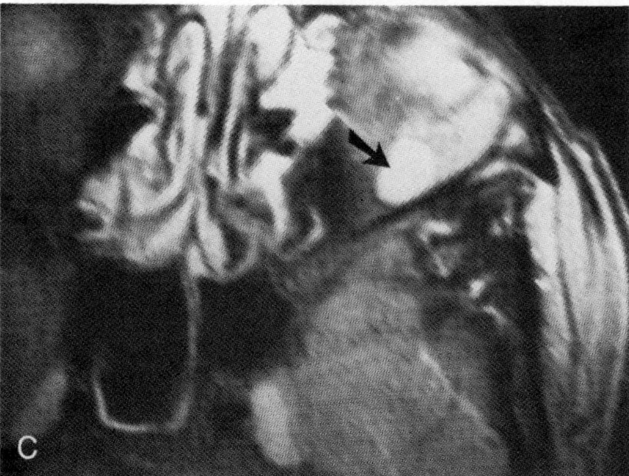


**Figure 20–28. Cavernous hemangioma.** A well-defined, homogeneously enhancing intraconal mass is seen on *A,* CT scan. The MRI shows a well-circumscribed homogeneous mass (arrow) that is hypointense on *B,* T1WI (TE 30/TR 500), and hyperintense on *C,* T2WI (TE 1220/TR 2000). (From Sullivan JA, Harms SE. Surface coil imaging of orbital neoplasms. AJNR 7:29–34, © by Am Soc Neuroradiology, 1986, with permission.)

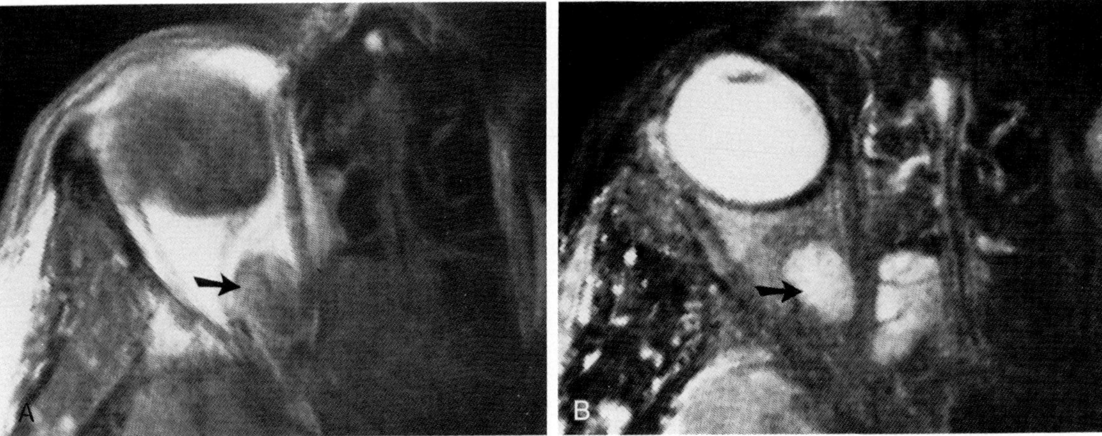

**Figure 20–29. Cavernous hemangioma.** A well-defined intraconal mass (arrow) with hypointense signal on *A,* T1WI (TE 30/TR 500), and hyperintense signal on *B,* T2WI (TE 120/TR 2000), is typical of cavernous hemangioma.

intraconal region. The signal intensity characteristics of lymphoma, leukemia, carcinomas, sarcomas, neurofibromas, lipomas, and vascular malformations are discussed elsewhere in this chapter (Fig. 20–31).

## Optic Nerve and Sheath Lesions

The signal intensity characteristics of lesions involving the optic nerve and sheath are summarized in Table 20–8.

Most optic nerve gliomas occur in childhood, with about half detected by the age of 5 years. These tumors are benign, slow-growing lesions that most commonly produce fusiform enlargement of the optic nerve. About 15% of patients with optic glioma show evidence of neurofibromatosis.[132] These tumors typically are homogeneously hypointense on T1WI and homogeneously hyperintense on T2WI. MRI is effective in demonstrating the degree of optic nerve involvement, particularly in the intracanalicular segment, where CT is impaired by bone artifacts.[29, 30]

Meningiomas most commonly occur in middle-aged women. These lesions may occasionally be encountered in children, in whom they are often associated with neurofibromatosis. Orbital meningiomas can be divided into three groups, depending on the

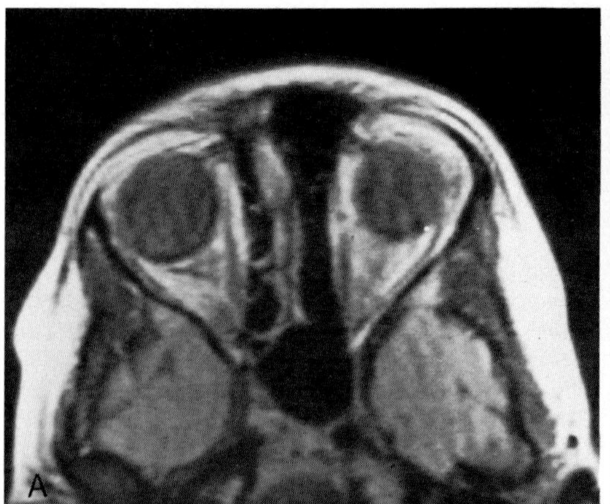

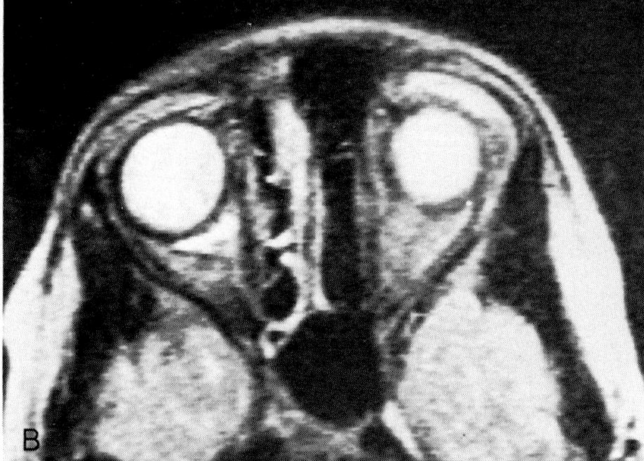

**Figure 20–30. Lymphangioma.** This intraconal mass is less well-circumscribed than the previously shown cases of hemangioma (Figs. 20–27 and 20–28). The mass has low signal intensity on *A,* T1WI, and high signal intensity on *B,* T2WI.

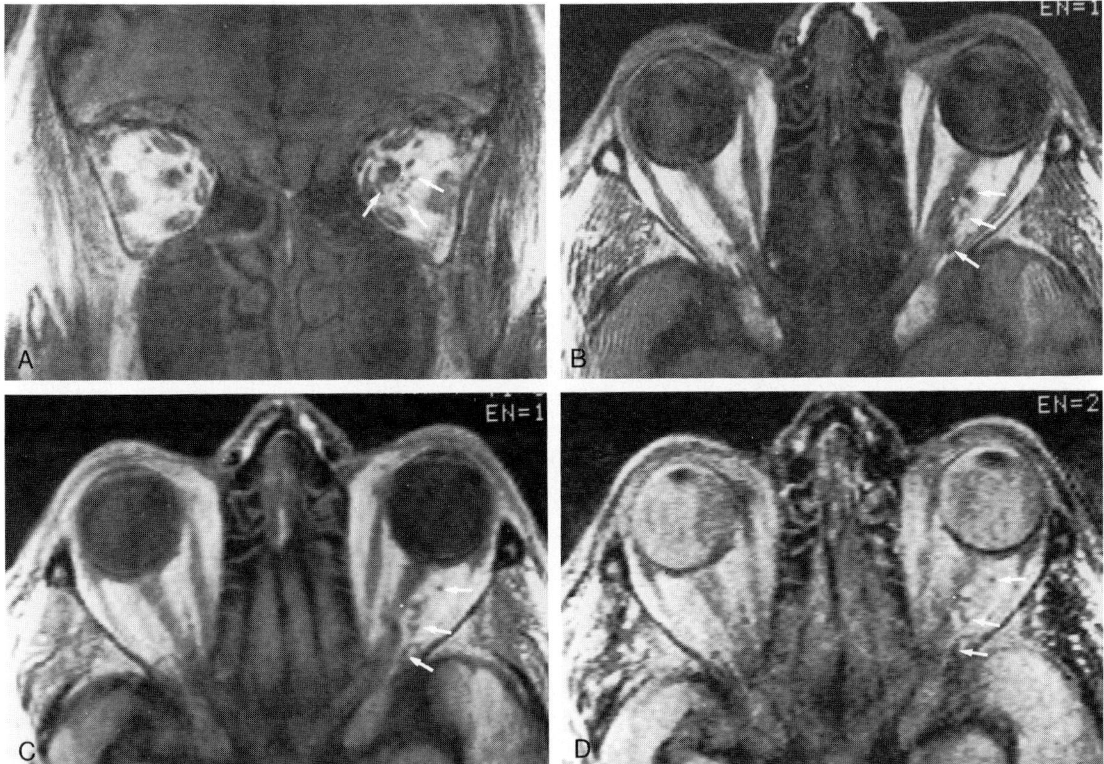


**Figure 20–31. Arteriovenous malformation.** Low signal serpiginous channels (arrows) are seen in the intraconal region on *A*, coronal; *B*, transverse T1WI (TE 25/TR 250); *C*, N(H)WI (TE 30/TR 1000); and *D*, T2WI (TE 100/TR 1000). The low intensity is due to rapid flows from the arteriovenous malformation.

site of origin: (1) dural sheath of the optic nerve, (2) intracranial origin extending into the orbit, and (3) arachnoid cells within the orbit.[133] On MRI meningiomas tend to be of low intensity to isointensity with optic nerve on all images (Figs. 20–9 and 20–32). Lower intensity can be seen in more densely calcified lesions. Occasionally, intracranial meningiomas have high signal on T2WI, but no orbital meningiomas with this pattern have been reported.[17, 24, 30]

Optic neuritis can be a manifestation of multiple sclerosis or an idiopathic acute inflammatory process. Focal lesions within the nerve can be seen in cases of MS in which associated periventricular plaques also are seen. In the idiopathic form, diffuse smooth enlargement results.[134] The presence of high signal on T2WI distinguishes this process from meningioma (Fig. 20–33).[24, 135, 136]

Optic nerve edema can be seen following radiation or central retinal vein occlusion, resulting in high signal on T2WI. Increased intracranial pressure can result in distentsion of the subarachnoid space surrounding the nerve. The normal signal from the nerve can be distinguished by MRI from the high signal CSF.[31]

Other lesions that can involve the optic

**Table 20–8.** SIGNAL INTENSITIES OF OPTIC NERVE AND SHEATH LESIONS

| Lesion | T1 | T2 | C | N(H) |
|---|---|---|---|---|
| Meningioma | Low to isointense | Low to isointense | Isointense | Isointense |
| Glioma | Low | High | High | High |
| Radiation change | Isointense | High | High | High |
| Optic neuritis | Isointense | High | High | High |

C = Crossover image; N(H) = proton density image.

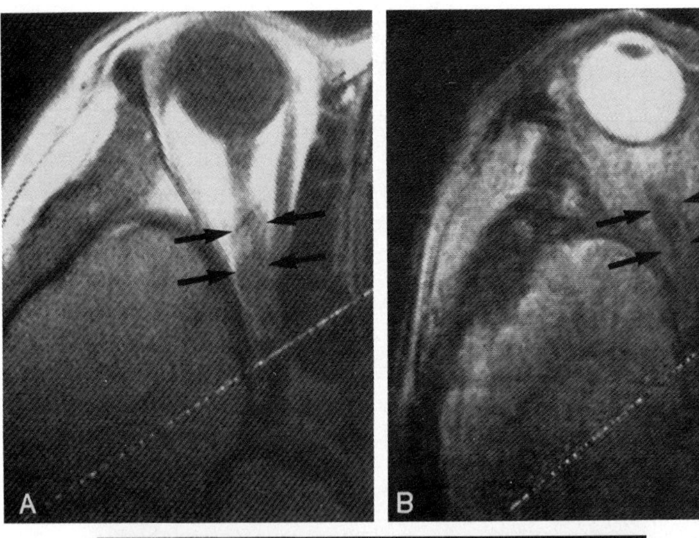

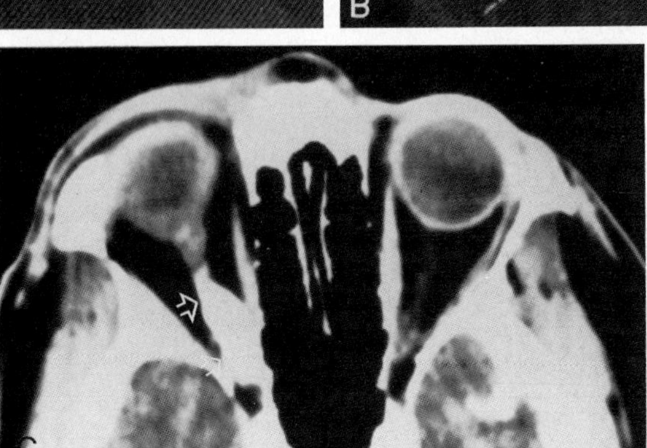

**Figure 20–32. Meningioma.** A mass can be seen surrounding the optic nerve (arrows) near the orbital apex. This mass has low signal on both *A,* T1WI (TE 30/TR 500), and *B,* T2WI (TE 120/TR 2000), typical of meningioma. The calcified mass (arrows) is much better seen on *C,* CT.

nerve include lymphoma, sarcoid, toxoplasmosis, tuberculosis, and syphilis.[24]

## Ocular Lesions

Ocular lesions can be further subcategorized clinically by the age of the patient. Certain ocular lesions tend to occur in childhood, and others are seen more frequently in adulthood. The signal characteristics of childhood ocular lesions are summarized in Table 20–9, and adulthood lesions are summarized in Table 20–10.

### *Ocular Lesions in Childhood*

Retinoblastoma is the most common intraocular tumor in children, occurring with a frequency of 1 in 17,000 to 34,000 live births. The tumor is congenital in origin, but few are recognized at birth. Two thirds of all cases are diagnosed by age 3 years. Bilateral disease is present in 30% of cases. In cases with bilateral disease, there is frequent familial history. Retinoblastoma is an autosomal dominant trait of variable penetrance. Other central nervous system tumors can occur with retinoblastoma, especially in cases of bilateral disease. The most common associated tumor is pineoblastoma (trilateral retinoblastoma). Retinoblastomas most com-

**Table 20–9.** SIGNAL INTENSITIES OF CHILDHOOD OCULAR LESIONS

| Lesion | T1 | T2 |
|---|---|---|
| Retinoblastoma | High | Low |
| Coats's disease | High | High |
| PHPV | High | High |
| Hemorrhage | High | High |
| Sclerosing endophthalmitis | High | High |
| Posterior scleritis | Low | Low |
| Osteoma | Low | Low |

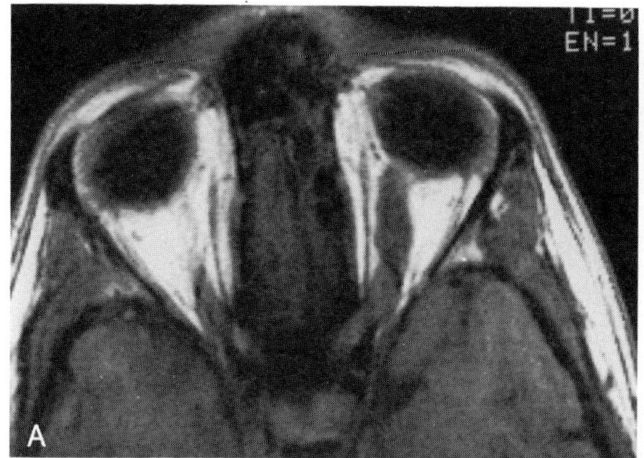


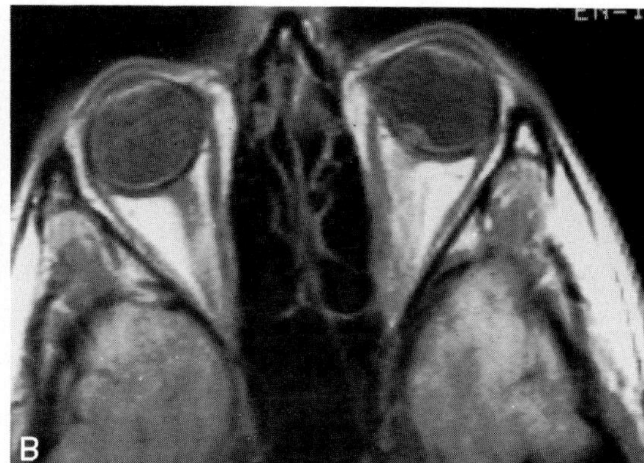


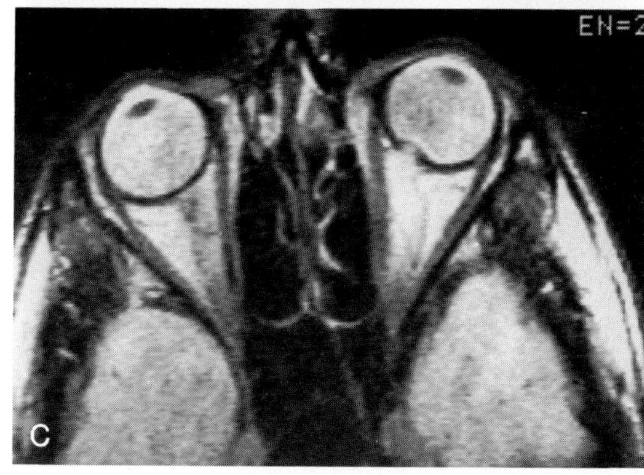


**Figure 20–33. Idiopathic optic neuritis.** Smooth diffuse enlargement of the optic nerve is shown to be isointense on *A,* T1WI (TE 25/TR 250), slightly hyperintense on *B,* N(H)WI (TE 30/TR 1000), and hyperintense on *C,* T2WI (TE 100/TR 1000).

monly present as leukokoria and diminished vision in the affected eye.[137–139]

Retinoblastoma may disseminate throughout the globe or extend along perineural and perivascular spaces, resulting in intraorbital and optic nerve spread. Extension of tumor into the subarachnoid space can facilitate spread throughout the central nervous system. Correct staging is important since tumors confined to the globe have a cure rate approaching 90%. For lesions that extend beyond the globe, the cure rate drops to 20%. These lesions are treated by enucleation, radiation therapy, or both. About 1% of lesions spontaneously regress.[140–142]

On computed tomography, calcification within retinoblastomas is common. These calcifications, however, are not specific and can occur in other tumors, inflammatory conditions, hypercalcemic states, and aging. The most important imaging consideration is accurate staging. The excellent soft tissue contrast provided by MRI allows more accurate staging of ocular disease (Fig. 20–34). The low signal sclera is easily separated from the intraocular mass. Invasion of the adjacent orbit is more easily determined. The optic nerve and sheath are well demonstrated by MRI. Retinoblastomas have high signal on T1WI and low signal on T2WI (Figs. 20–35 and 20–36). The unusual appearance on T2WI helps in differentiating this tumor from many other lesions that simulate retinoblastoma clinically.[4, 15–17]

**Table 20–10.** SIGNAL INTENSITIES OF ADULTHOOD OCULAR LESIONS

| Lesion | T1 | T2 |
|---|---|---|
| Melanoma | High | Low |
| Metastases | Moderate | Inhomogeneous high |
| Subretinal effusion | High | High |
| Hemorrhage (methemoglobin phase) | High | High |
| Phthisis bulbi | Low | Low |

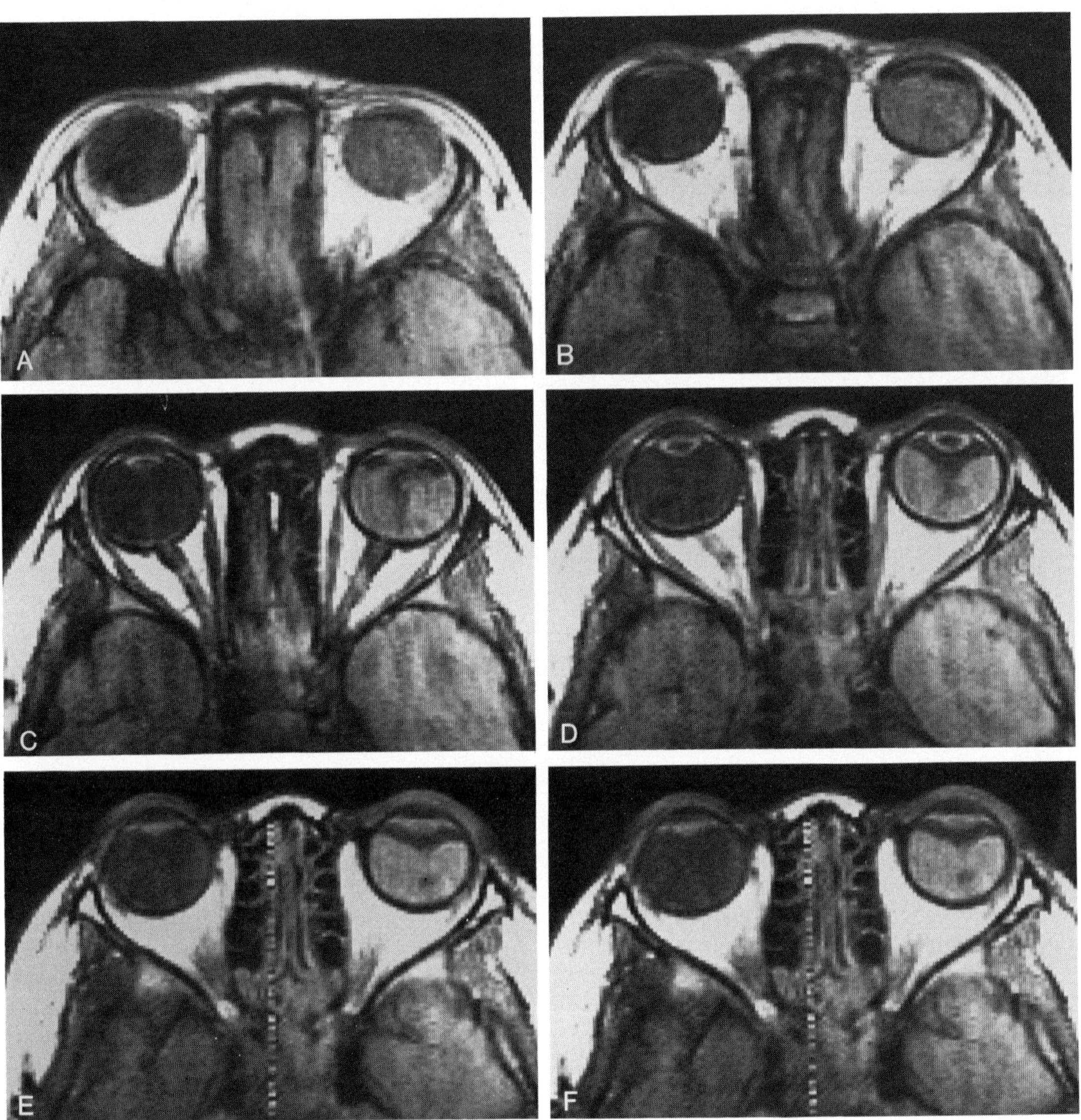


**Figure 20–34. Selective 3D imaging in retinoblastoma.** High-resolution, 1.6-mm sections without interslice gaps (*A–H*) allow accurate depiction of ocular anatomy in this patient with retinoblastoma. Low signal sclera is well separated from the ocular mass and effusion on this T1WI (TE 25/TR 250). *I–K*, NHWI (TE 30/TR 1000), and *L–N*, T2WI (TE 100/TR 1000), show the low signal intensity mass separate from the high signal effusion, but the anatomy is sacrificed on these thicker 5-mm 2DFT sections.

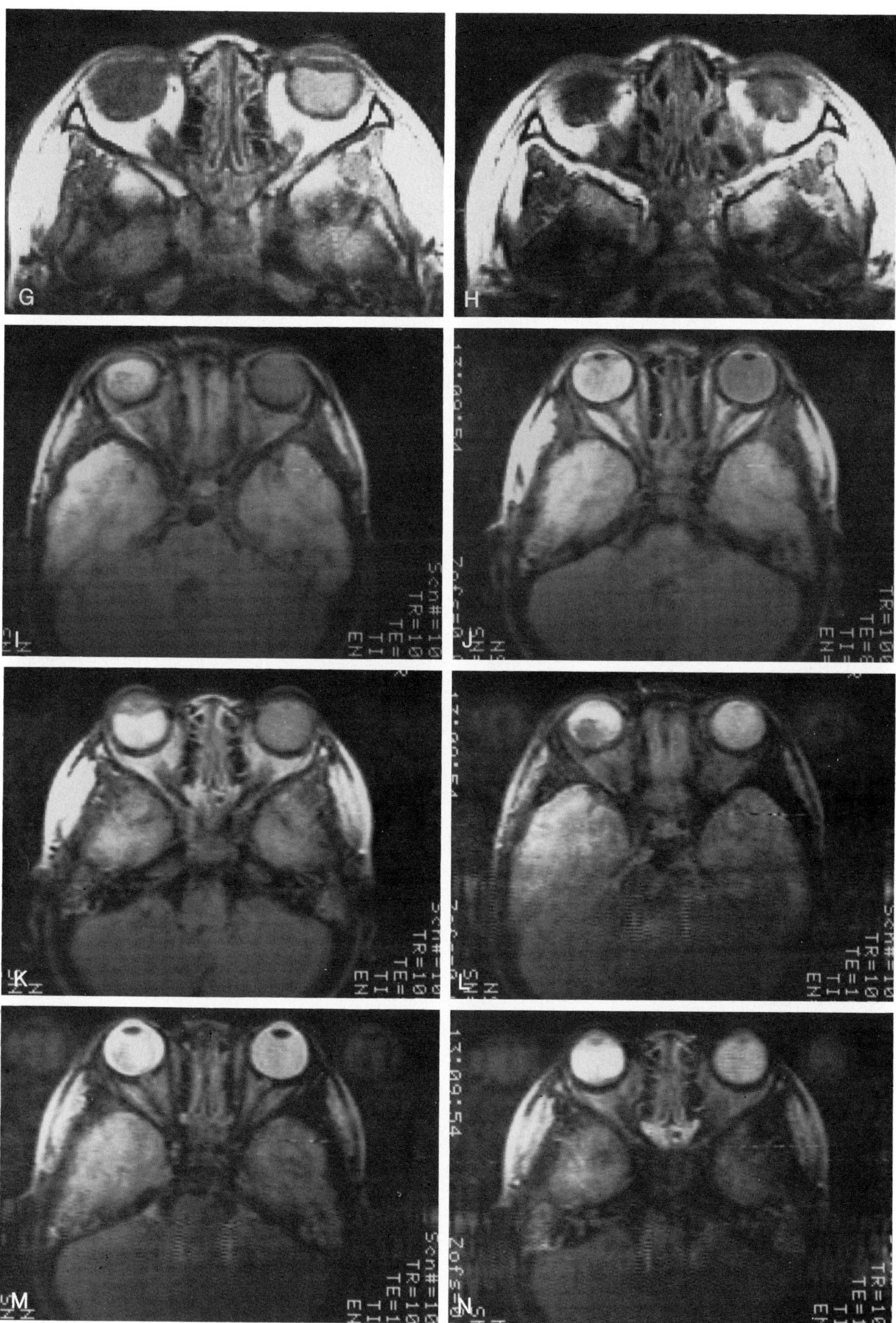


**Figure 20–34** *Continued*

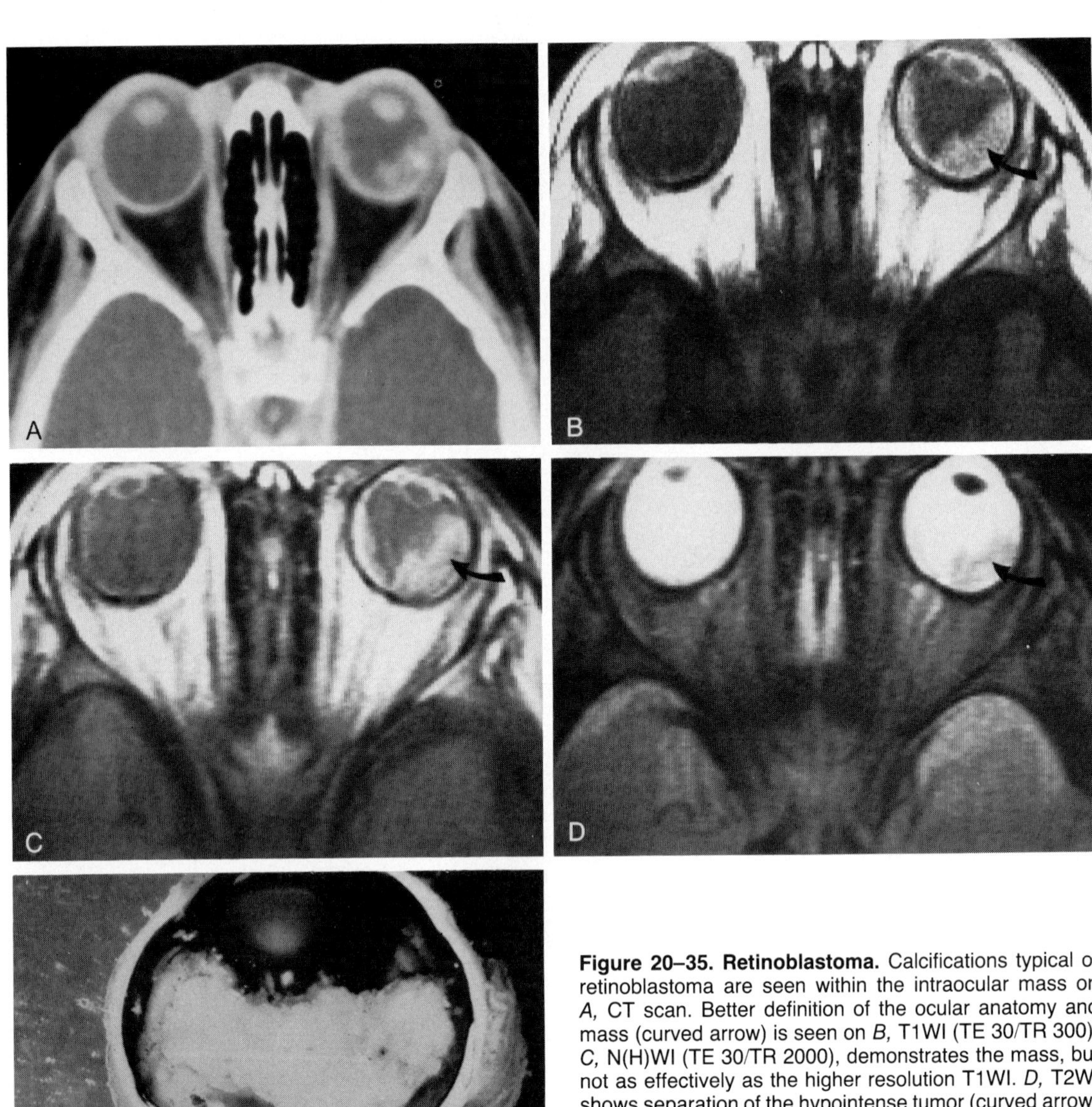

**Figure 20–35. Retinoblastoma.** Calcifications typical of retinoblastoma are seen within the intraocular mass on *A,* CT scan. Better definition of the ocular anatomy and mass (curved arrow) is seen on *B,* T1WI (TE 30/TR 300). *C,* N(H)WI (TE 30/TR 2000), demonstrates the mass, but not as effectively as the higher resolution T1WI. *D,* T2WI shows separation of the hypointense tumor (curved arrow) from the hyperintense subretinal effusion. *E,* The pathologic specimen reveals a large exophytic mass as demonstrated by MRI. (From Sullivan JA, Harms SE. Surface coil imaging of orbital neoplasms. AJNR 7:29–34, © by Am Soc Neuroradiology, 1986, with permission.)

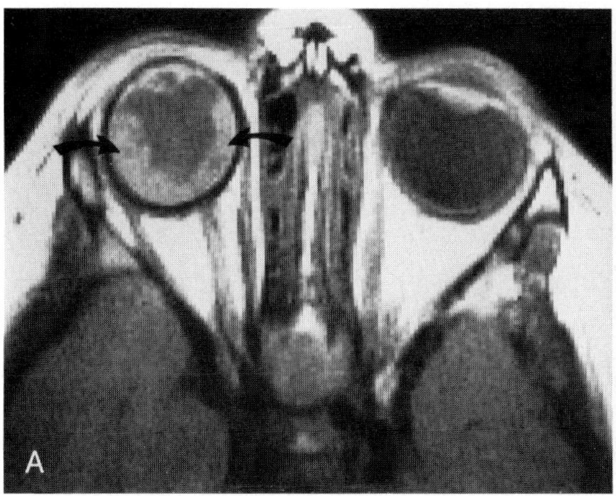


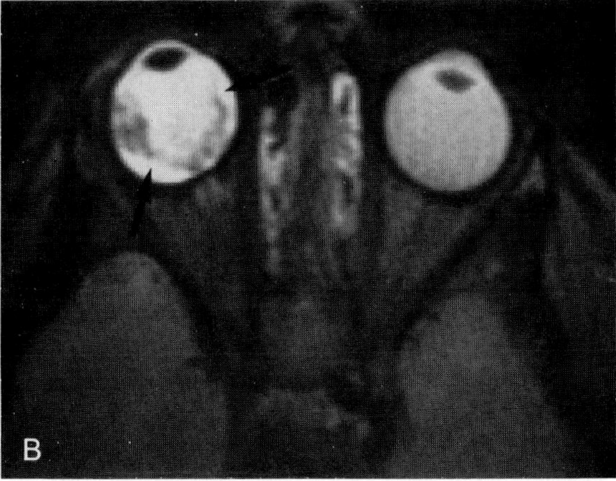


**Figure 20–36. Retinoblastoma.** The extent of the lesion is well staged (curved arrows) on *A*, high-resolution T1WI (TE 30/TR 500). The low signal tumor mass is separated from high signal subretinal effusion (arrows) on *B*, T2WI (TE 120/TR 2000). (From Sullivan JA, Harms SE. Surface coil imaging of orbital neoplasms. AJNR 7:29–34, © by Am Soc Neuroradiology, 1986, with permission.)

Uveal effusions are commonly seen with retinoblastoma. On CT it is difficult to distinguish these effusions from the mass. Most of these uveal effusions have high signal on both T1WI and T2WI.[16, 17] In designing MRI scan protocols, it is important to include the opposite orbit because of the high incidence of bilateral disease (Fig. 20–37).

Coats's disease is a primary retinal vascular anomaly characterized by telangiectasia and accumulation of lipoproteinaceous exudate in the retina and subretinal space. Clinically, Coats's disease presents as leukokoria in the same age group as retinoblastoma. Distinction from a neurotic retinoblastoma is difficult by clinical examination, sonography, and CT.[143] On MRI Coats's disease can be distinguished from retinoblastoma by the presence of homogeneous high signal on both T1WI and T2WI instead of the usual hypointense focus seen in cases of retinoblastoma on T2WI (Fig. 20–38).[15, 17]

Persistent hyperplastic primary vitreous (PHPV) is a congenital, frequently unilateral, persistence and hyperplasia of the embryonic hyaloid vascular system. The friability of the vessels leads to frequent intravitreal hemorrhage. This disorder appears at birth or in infancy.[144] Unilateral microphthalmos is noted with areas of high signal on both T1WI and T2WI (Fig. 20–39). Fluid levels may be seen. Norrie's disease is an X-linked recessive disorder frequently associated with seizures, hearing loss, mental retarda-

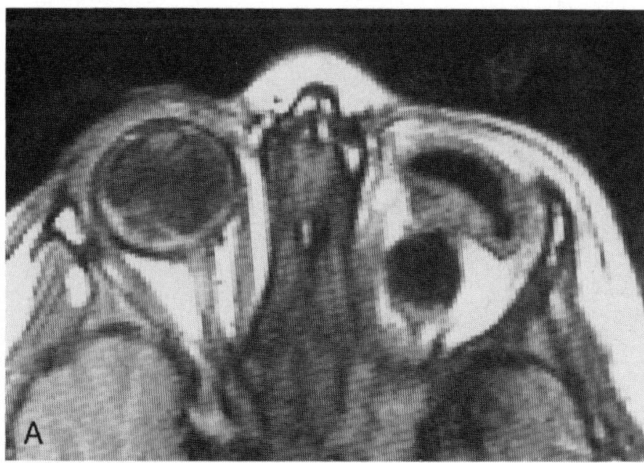


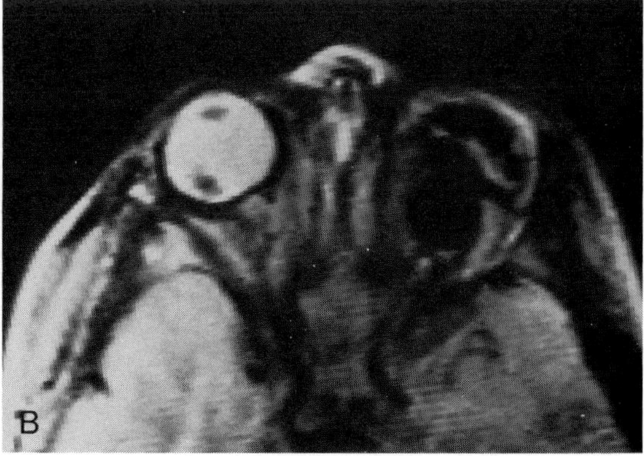


**Figure 20–37. Bilateral retinoblastomas.** A prosthesis is seen in the patient's left orbit following enucleation for retinoblastoma. Another retinoblastoma is seen on the right with typical findings on *A*, T1WI (TE 25/TR 250), and *B*, T2WI (TE 100/TR 1000).

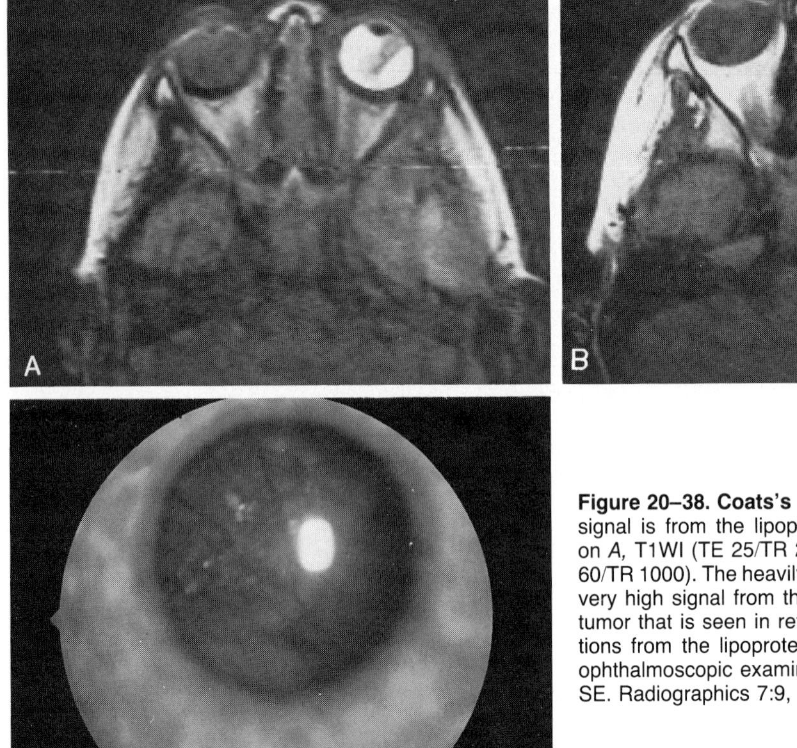

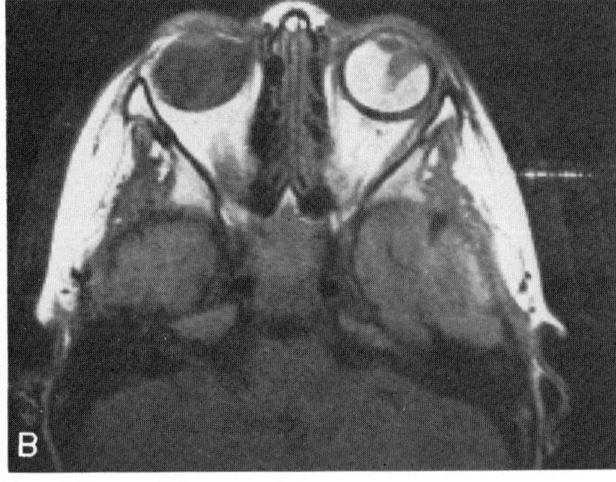

**Figure 20–38. Coats's disease.** The homogeneous high signal is from the lipoproteinaceous, subretinal exudate on *A,* T1WI (TE 25/TR 250), and the mildly *B,* T2WI (TE 60/TR 1000). The heavily T2WI (TE 120/TR 1000) showed very high signal from the lesion in contrast to low signal tumor that is seen in retinoblastoma. In this case, reflections from the lipoproteinaceous material is seen on *C,* ophthalmoscopic examination. (From Sullivan JA, Harms SE. Radiographics 7:9, 1987, with permission.)

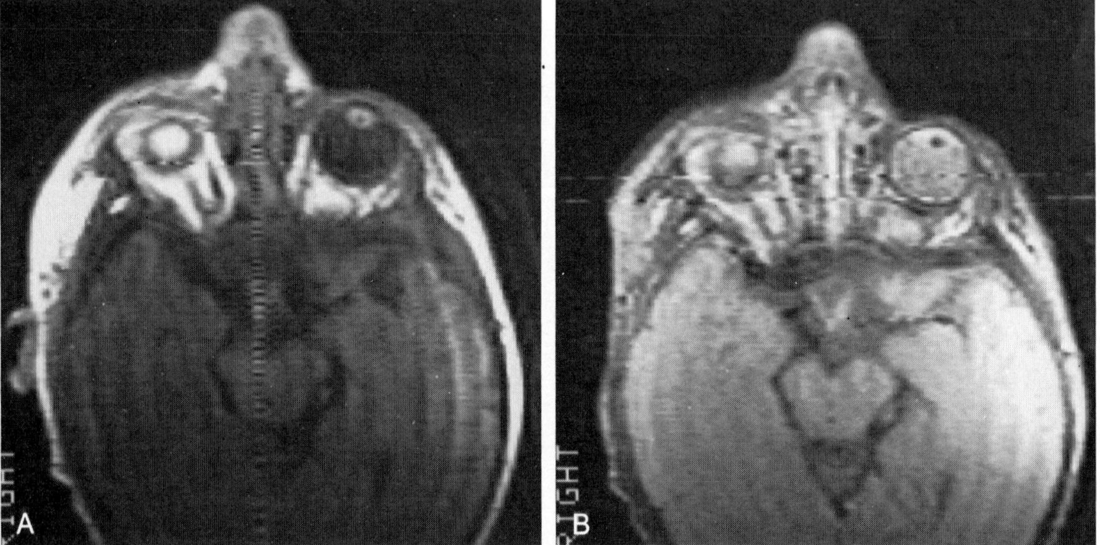

**Figure 20–39. Persistent hyperplastic primary vitreous.** A small right optic globe was noted at birth in this one-month-old child. Inhomogeneous high signal is seen from the affected globe on both *A,* T1WI (TE 25/TR 250), and *B,* T2WI (TE 120/TR 1000). (From Sullivan JA, Harms SE. Radiographics 7:9, 1987, with permission.)

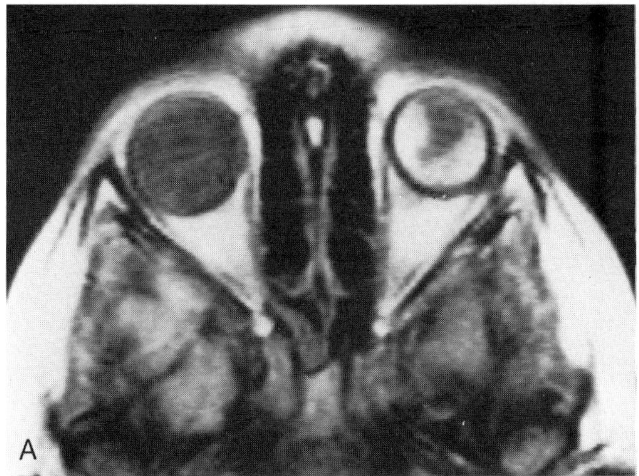


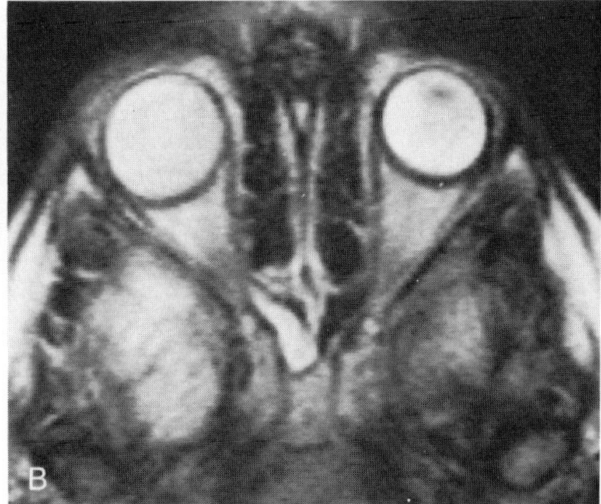


**Figure 20–40. Sclerosing endophthalmitis.** A high-signal ocular mass is seen on both *A,* T1WI (TE 25/TR 1250), and *B,* T2WI (TE 100/TR 1000), in this patient with visceral larva migrans.

tion, and cataracts. An appearance similar to PHPV is seen, and this disorder is considered by some to be an inherited form of PHPV.[17]

Sclerosing endophthalmitis is a well-defined sequela of the syndrome of visceral larva migrans. The granulomatous uveitis results following ingestion of puppy feces containing ova of the nematode, *Toxocara canis.*[145, 146] Three distinct lesions are seen: (1) posterior pale granuloma, (2) peripheral choroidal lesions with elevations of retinal folds, and (3) diffuse endophthalmitis with retinal detachment.[147] These lesions are hyperintense on both T1WI and T2WI (Fig. 20–40).[15] Enzyme-linked immunosorbent assay (ELISA) for *Toxocara* is diagnostic.[145, 146]

Several other ocular lesions rarely occur in childhood. Astrocytic hamartoma is usually a densely calcified benign tumor associated with tuberous sclerosis or neurofibromatosis. Optic drusen are asymptomatic masses composed of usually calcified hyaline-like material occurring near the surface of the optic disc.[141] Choroidal osteoma should also be in the differential diagnosis for a densely calcified, low signal intensity ocular mass.[148]

### *Ocular Lesions in Adulthood*

Uveal melanoma is the most common primary intraocular neoplasm. This tumor is seen most frequently in Caucasians between the ages of 50 and 70 years. The tumor is highly malignant and tends to metastasize either locally to the globe or optic nerve or systemically, especially to the liver, lung, and subcutaneous tissues. The overall mortality rate is about 40% at 5 years of age and 60% at 25 years of age.[149, 150] These lesions show high signal on T1WI and low signal on T2WI (Fig. 20–41). Low signal intensity on T2WI is presumably due to the T2 shortening effects of the stable free radicals found in melanin. This appearance is similar to retinoblastomas, but confusion between lesions should not occur because of the markedly different age groups affected. Melanomas often have associated uveal effusions that result in high signal on both T1WI and T2WI and are easily distinguished from the melanoma mass by MRI (Figs. 20–42 and 20–43). Melanoma usually is treated by enucleation, making accurate staging important.[16, 17, 19, 20, 22, 23, 28, 31]

The most important lesion to distinguish from melanoma is ocular metastasis. It is not uncommon for ocular metastasis to be manifested clinically before the discovery of the primary malignancy, especially in lung carcinoma. Metastases from renal, prostatic, testicular, pancreatic, and gastric primary tumors tend to appear clinically before the discovery of the primary tumors. Metastatic breast carcinoma to the eye is usually a late finding. It is important to differentiate ocular metastasis from melanoma to prevent unnecessary enucleation.[151–154] CT can only demonstrate a mass lesion.[155] On MRI ocular metastases have higher or equal signal compared with the vitreous on T1WI and mixed

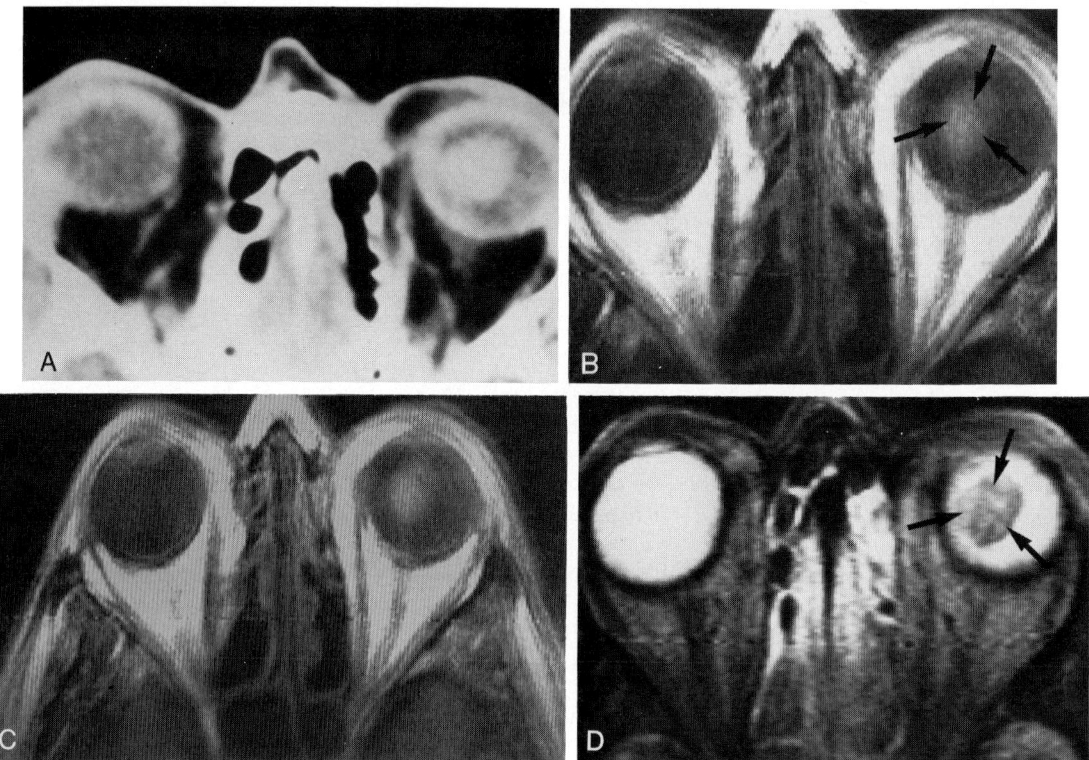


**Figure 20–41. Melanoma.** A hyperdense mass in the left globe is apparent on CT in *A*. A high signal intraocular mass (arrows) is seen on *B*, T1WI (TE 30/TR 500). The mass has lower signal than the vitreous on *D*, T2WI (TE 120/TR 2000). *C*, N(H)WI shows a high signal mass but provides no more information than the T1WI. (From Sullivan JA, Harms SE. Surface coil imaging of orbital neoplasms. AJNR 7:29–34, © by Am Soc Neuroradiology, 1986, with permission.)

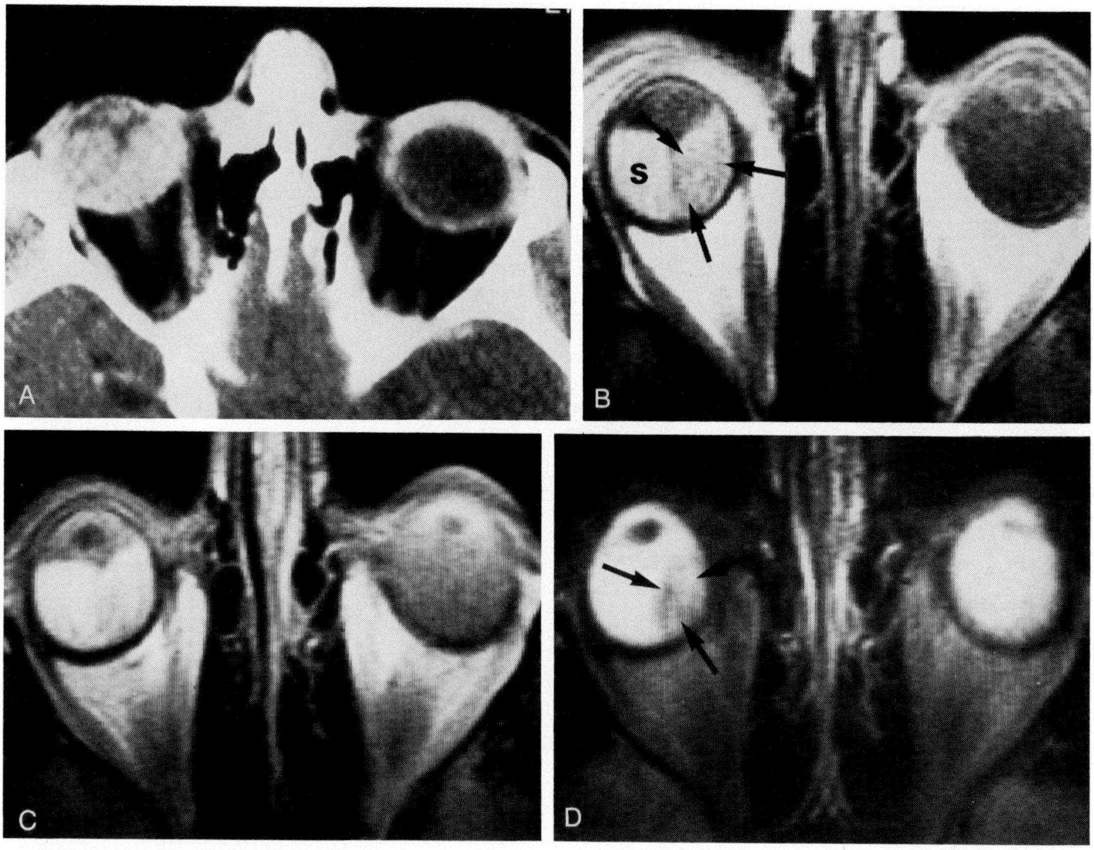

**Figure 20–42. Melanoma and effusion.** A mass fills almost the entire right optic globe on *A,* CT. The very high signal effusion (S) on *B,* T1WI (TE 30/TR 500); *C,* N(H)WI (TE 30/TR 1000); and *D,* T2WI (TE 120/TR 2000) is easily separated from the lower signal melanoma mass (arrows), especially on *D,* T2WI. (From Sullivan JA, Harms SE. Surface coil imaging of orbital neoplasms. AJNR 7:29–34, © by Am Soc Neuroradiology, 1986, with permission.)

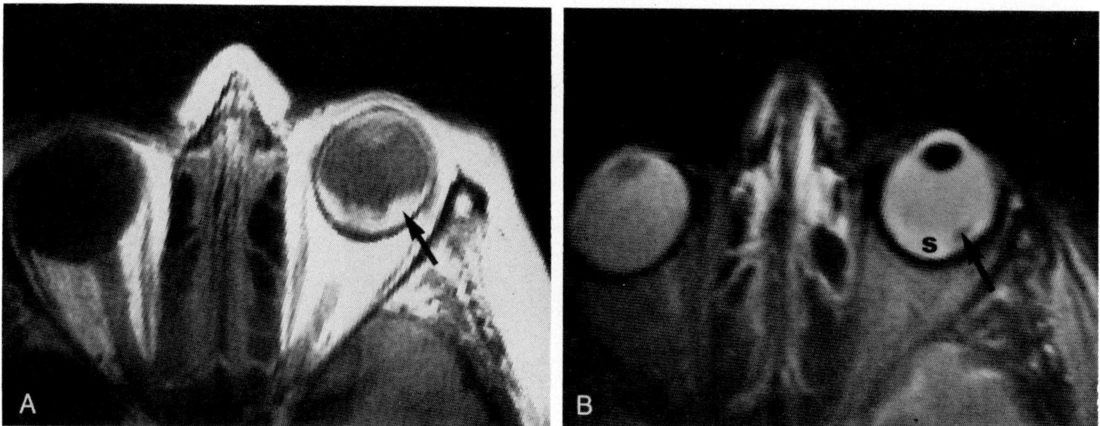


**Figure 20–43. Melanoma with retinal detachment.** The small melanoma mass (arrow) is difficult to separate from the subretinal effusion of *A,* T1WI (TE 30/TR 500), but is easily distinguished from the effusion (S) on *B,* T2WI (TE 120/TR 2000). (From Sullivan JA, Harms SE. Surface coil imaging of orbital neoplasms. AJNR 7:29–34, © by Am Soc Neuroradiology, 1986, with permission.)

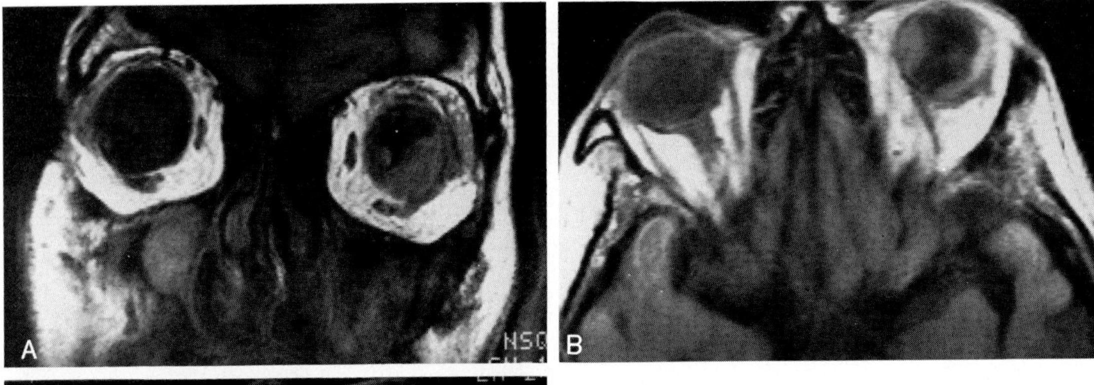


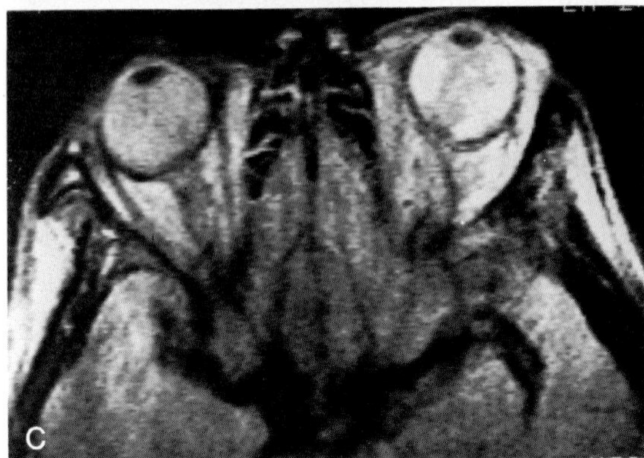


**Figure 20–44. Choroidal metastasis.** Metastatic carcinoma of the lung is shown on the coronal image, *A,* T1WI (TE 25/TR 250), as a hyperintense mass in patient's left globe. *B,* N(H)WI (TE 30/TR 2000), and *C,* T2WI (TE 100/TR 1000), also show a hyperintense mass that contrasts with the hypointense mass seen with melanoma (Figs. 20–40 to 20–42).

signal intensity on T2WI. Homogeneous, higher signal within the tumor is seen on T2WI in most metastases in contrast with the very low signal seen in melanoma (Fig. 20–44; see also Figs. 20–41 to 20–43). The tumor itself may be lower in signal on T2WI than the vitreous in some areas.[27] Retinal detachments often accompany ocular metastases. The subretinal fluid displays high signal on both T1WI and T2WI and is much higher in signal than tumor on both. MR therefore provides the ability to separate retinal detachment from tumor.[27, 155]

Other lesions to be considered are astro-

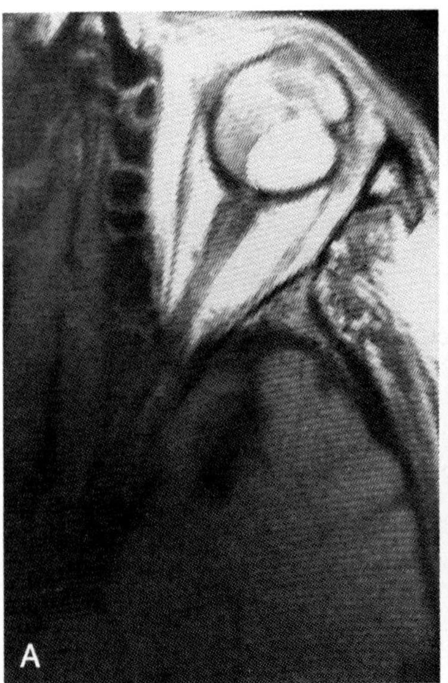


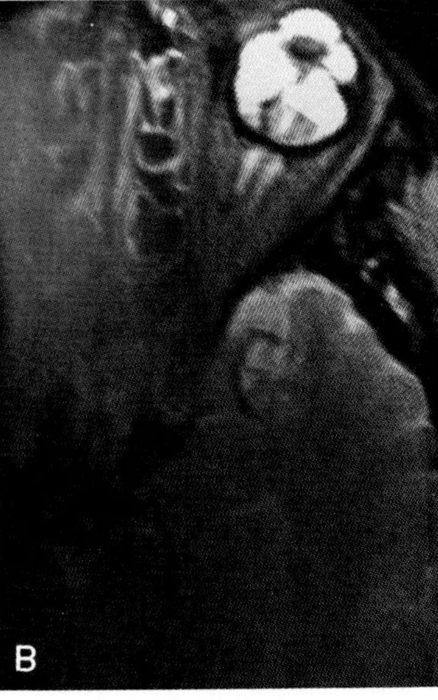


**Figure 20–45. Ocular hemorrhage.** In a patient with previous ocular trauma, hemorrhage in the methemoglobin phase is seen as areas of hyperintensity on *A,* T1WI (TE 30/TR 500), and *B,* T2WI (TE 120/TR 2000).

cytic hamartoma, choroidal osteoma, and drusen that may have very low signal due to dense calcifications.[141] Choroidal hemangioma, especially, should be considered in patients with Sturge-Weber syndrome.[141] Intraocular lymphoma can be seen in patients having acute leukemia, histiocytic lymphoma, Hodgkin's disease, or lymphocytic lymphoma.[27] Phthisis bulbi is a nonfunctioning globe that has contracted and calcified secondary to trauma or infection.[141, 156] Retinal detachments can be spontaneous or posttraumatic.[141] Subretinal effusions are easily detected by MRI. Hemorrhage in the methemoglobin phase (Fig. 20–45) is distinguished by the presence of high signal on both T1WI and T2WI.[16, 17]

## References


1. Li KC, Poon PY, Hinton P, et al. MR imaging of the orbital tumors with CT and ultrasound correlations. J Comput Assist Tomogr 8:1039, 1984.
2. Hawkes RC, Holland GN, Moore WS, et al. NMR imaging in the evaluation of orbital tumors. AJNR 4:254, 1983.
3. Han JS, Benson JE, Bonstelle CT, et al. Magnetic resonance imaging of the orbit: a preliminary experience. Radiology 150:755, 1984.
4. Sobel DF, Kelly W, Kjos BO, et al. MR imaging of orbital and ocular disease. AJNR 6:259, 1985.
5. Edward JH, Hyman RA, Vacirca SJ, et al. 0.6T magnetic resonance imaging of the orbit. AJNR 6:253, 1985.
6. Sobel DF, Mills C, Char D, et al. NMR of the normal and pathologic eye and orbit. AJNR 5:345, 1984.
7. Moseley I, Brant-Zawadzki M, Mills C. Nuclear magnetic resonance imaging of the orbit. Br J Ophthalmol 67:333, 1983.
8. Schenck JR, Hart HR, Foster TH, et al. Improved MR imaging of the orbit at 1.5 T with surface coils. AJNR 6:193, 1985.
9. Schenck JR, Foster TH, Henkes JL, et al. High-field surface-coil MR imaging of localized anatomy. AJNR 6:181, 1985.
10. Sassani JW, Osbakken MD. Anatomic features of the eye disclosed with nuclear magnetic resonance imaging. Arch Ophthalmol 102:541, 1984.
11. Gonzalez RG, Cheng H, Barnett P, et al. Nuclear magnetic resonance imaging of the vitreous body. Science 223:399, 1984.
12. Mosely J, Brant-Zawadzki M, Mills C. Nuclear magnetic resonance imaging of the orbit. Br J Ophthalmol 67:333, 1983.
13. Zimmerman RA, Bilaniuk LT, Yanoff M, et al. Orbital magnetic resonance imaging. Am J Ophthalmol 100:312, 1985.
14. Char DH, Sobel D, Kelly WM, et al. Magnetic resonance scanning in orbital tumor diagnosis. Ophthalmology 92:1305, 1985.
15. Haik BG, Louis LS, Smith ME, et al. Magnetic resonance imaging in the evaluation of leukocoria. Ophthalmology 92:1143, 1985.
16. Sullivan JA, Harms SE. Surface coil MR imaging of orbital neoplasms. AJNR 7:29, 1986.
17. Sullivan JA, Harms SE. Characterization of orbital lesions by surface coil MR imaging. Radiographics 7:9, 1987.
18. Bilaniuk LT, Schenck JR, Zimmerman RA, et al. Ocular and orbital lesions: surface coil MR imaging. Radiology 156:669, 1985.
19. Gomori JM, Grossman RI, Shields JA, et al. Choroidal melanomas: correlation of NMR spectroscopy and MR imaging. Radiology 158:443, 1986.
20. Peyman GA, Mafee MF. Uveal melanoma and similar lesions: the role of magnetic resonance imaging. Radiol Clin North Am 25:471, 1987.
21. Mafee MR, Peyman GA. Retinal and choroidal detachments: role of magnetic resonance imaging and computed tomography. Radiol Clin North Am 25:487, 1987.
22. Bilaniuk LT, Atlas SW, Zimmerman RA. Magnetic resonance imaging of the orbit. Radiol Clin North Am 25:509, 1987.
23. Mafee MF, Putterman A, Valvassori GE, et al. Orbital space-occupying lesions: role of magnetic resonance imaging and computed tomography—a review of 145 cases. Radiol Clin North Am 25:529, 1987.
24. Azar-Kia B, Nuheedy MH, Elias DA, et al. Optic nerve tumors: role of magnetic resonance imaging and computed tomography. Radiol Clin North Am 25:561, 1987.
25. Flanders AE, Espinosa GA, Mackiewicz DA, et al. Orbital lymphoma: role of CT and MRI. Radiol Clin North Am 25:601, 1987.
26. Wilbur AC, Dobben ED, Linder B. Paraorbital tumors and tumor-like conditions: role of CT and MRI. Radiol Clin North Am 25:631, 1987.
27. Peyster RG, Shapiro MD, Haik BG. Orbital metastasis: role of magnetic resonance imaging and computed tomography. Radiol Clin North Am 25:647, 1987.
28. Mafee MF, Peyman GA, Grissland JE, et al. Malignant uveal melanoma-simulating lesions: MR imaging evaluation. Radiology 160:773, 1986.
29. Gomori JM, Grossman RI, Shields JA, et al. Ocular MR imaging and spectroscopy: an ex vivo study. Radiology 160:201, 1986.
30. Daniels DL, Herfkins R, Gager WE, et al. Magnetic resonance imaging of the optic nerves and chiasm. Radiology 152:79, 1984.
31. Harms SE. Magnetic resonance imaging of the orbit. In Brady T, Edelman R, eds. Clinical Magnetic Resonance Imaging. Philadelphia, W. B. Saunders. In press.
32. Harms SE. Magnetic resonance imaging of the face, orbit and TMJ. In Partain CL, James AE, eds. Magnetic Resonance Imaging. Philadelphia, W. B. Saunders. In press.
33. Hall E. Radiobiology for the Radiologist. Hagerstown, Md., Harper & Row, 1978:351.
34. Rosenleranz G, Tellkamp H, Kohler K. Radiation exposure to the lens during CT of the orbital area. Digitale Bilddiagn 5:66, 1985.
35. Duke-Elder S. System of Ophthalmology. London, Kimpton, 1961.
36. Hogan MJ, Alvarado JA, Weddell JE. Histology of the Human Eye: An Atlas and Textbook. Philadelphia, W. B. Saunders, 1971.
37. Fine BS, Yanoff M. Ocular Histology: A Text and Atlas. Hagerstown, Md., Harper & Row, 1979.

38. Racz P, Tompa K, Pocsik I. The state of water in normal human, bird and fish eye lenses. Exp Eye Res 29:601, 1979.
39. Neville MC, Paterson CA, Rae JL, et al. Nuclear magnetic resonance studies and water "ordering" in the crystalline lens. Science 184:1072, 1974.
40. Racz P, Tompa K, Pocsik I. The state of water in normal and senile cataractous lenses studied by nuclear magnetic resonance. Exp Eye Res 28:129, 1979.
41. Pope JM, Chandra S, Balfe JD. Changes in the state of water in senile cataractous lenses as studied by nuclear magnetic resonance. Exp Eye Res 34:57, 1982.
42. Sherry CS, Harms SE. Spinal magnetic resonance imaging: multiplanar representations from a single high-resolution 3D acquisition. J Comput Assist Tomogr. In press.
43. Harms SE, Kramer DM. Fundamentals of magnetic resonance imaging. Crit Rev Diagn Imag 25:79, 1985.
44. Kramer DM. Basic principles of magnetic resonance imaging. Radiol Clin North Am 22:765, 1984.
45. Harms SE, Morgan TJ, Yamanashi WS, et al. Principles of nuclear magnetic resonance imaging. Radiographics 4:26, 1984.
46. Harms SE, Siemers PT, Hildenbrand P, et al. Multiple spin echo magnetic resonance imaging of the brain. Radiographics 6:117, 1980.
47. Rosen BR, Brady TJ. Principles of nuclear magnetic resonance for medical application. Semin Nucl Med 13:308, 1984.
48. Bydder GM, Young IR. MR imaging: clinical use of the inversion recovery sequence. J Comput Assist Tomogr 9:659, 1985.
49. Smith FW, Redpath TW, Parekh S, et al. Inversion recovery sequences for imaging the orbit. Program of Society of Magnetic Resonance in Medicine. Vol 4. 1986:1320.
50. Frahm J, Haase A, Matthari W. Rapid three-dimensional MR imaging using the FLASH technique. J Comput Assist Tomogr 10:363, 1986.
51. Haase A, Frahm J, Matthari W, et al. Rapid images and NMR movies. Program of Society of Magnetic Resonance in Medicine. London, August 19–23, 1985.
52. Dixon TU. Simple proton spectroscopic imaging. Radiology 153:189, 1984.
53. Frahm J, Haase A, Hanicke W, et al. Chemical shift selective MR imaging using a whole-body magnet. Radiology 156:441, 1985.
54. Roschmann P, Tischler R. Surface coil proton MR imaging at 2T. Radiology 161:251, 1986.
55. Frahm J, Merboldt KD, Hanicke W, et al. Stimulated echo imaging. J Magn Reson 64:81, 1985.
56. Haase A, Frahm J. NMR imaging of spin-lattice relaxation using stimulated echoes. J Magn Reson 65:481, 1985.
57. Harms SE, Muschler G. Three dimensional MR imaging of the knee using surface coils. J Comput Assist Tomogr 10:773, 1986.
58. Gallimore G, Harms SE. Three-dimensional magnetic resonance of the spine. J Comput Assist Tomogr 10:773, 1986.
59. Kramer DM, Comptom RA, Young HN. A volume (3D) analogue of 2D multislice or multislab MR imaging. Program Fourth Annual Meeting of the Society of Magnetic Resonance in Medicine. London, August 19–23, 1985.
60. Harms SE, Kramer DM. Clinical use of the 3D multislab acquisition method for imaging neurological disorders. Program of Society of Magnetic Resonance in Medicine. Montreal, August 18–22, 1986.
61. Wilk RM, Harms SE. Multislab 3DFT magnetic resonance imaging in temporomandibular joint imaging. Radiology. In press.
62. Mansfield P. Multi-planar image formation using NMR spin echoes. J Physol (Lond) 10:55, 1977.
63. Haacke EM, Bearden FH, Clayton JR, et al. Reduction of MR imaging time by the hybrid fast-scan technique. Radiology 158:521, 1986.
64. Wehrli FW, Hanal E. Orbital imaging factors determining magnetic resonance imaging appearance. Radiol Clin North Am 25:419, 1987.
65. Smith FW, Crosher GA. Mascara—an unsuspected cause of magnetic resonance imaging artifact. Magn Reson Imag 3:287, 1985.
66. Kelly WM, Paglen PG, Pearson JA, et al. Ferromagnetism of intraocular foreign body causes unilateral blindness after MR study. AJNR 7:243, 1986.
67. Weber AL, Mikulis DK. Inflammatory disorders of the paraorbital sinuses and their complications. Radiol Clin North Am 25:615, 1987.
68. Zimmerman RA, Bilaniuk LT. CT of orbital infection and its complications. AJR 134:45, 1980.
69. Leo JS, Halpern J, Sackler JP. Computed tomography in the evaluation of orbital infections. Comput Tomogr 4:133, 1980.
70. Fernbach SK, Naidich TP. CT diagnosis of orbital inflammation in children. Neuroradiology 22:71, 1981.
71. Firooznia H, Golimbu C. Computed tomography in evaluation of the orbits in patients with basal cell and squamous cell tumors of the face. In Gonzalez CA, Becker MH, Flanagan JC, eds. Diagnostic Imaging in Ophthalmology. New York, Springer-Verlag, 1986:303.
72. Fedukowiez HB, Stenson S. External infections of the eye. In Bacterial, Viral, Mycotic, and Noninfectious Immunologic Diseases, 3rd ed. East Norwalk, Conn., Appleton-Century-Crofts, 1985.
73. Fries JW. The roentgen features of fibrous dysplasia of the skull and facial bones. A critical analysis of thirty-nine pathologically proven cases. AJR 77:70, 1957.
74. Liakos GM, Walker CB, Carruth JAS. Ocular complications in craniofacial fibrous dysplasia. Br J Ophthalmol 63:611, 1979.
75. Harms SE, Greenway G. Musculoskeletal magnetic resonance. In Stark DD, Bradley WG, eds. Magnetic Resonance Imaging. St. Louis, C. V. Mosby. In press.
76. Whitson WE, Orcutt JC, Walkinshaw MD. Orbital osteoma in Gardner's syndrome. Am J Ophthalmol 101:236, 1986.
77. Newell FW. Osteoma involving the orbit. Am J Ophthalmol 31:1281, 1948.
78. Shields JA, Nelson LB, Brown JR, et al. Clinical computed tomography and histopathologic characteristics of juvenile ossifying fibroma with orbital involvement. Am J Ophthalmol 96:650, 1983.
79. Jones IS, Jakobiec FA. Diseases of the Orbit. Hagerstown, Md., Harper & Row, 1979.
80. Pagani JJ, Bassett LW, Winter J, et al. Osteogenic sarcoma after retinoblastoma radiotherapy. AJR 137:699, 1979.

81. Brant-Zawadzki M, Kelly W. Brain tumors. In Brant-Zawadzki M, Norman D. Magnetic Resonance Imaging of the Central Nervous System. New York, Raven Press, 1987:151.
82. Hesselink JR, Davis KR, Weber AL, et al. Radiological evaluation of orbital metastasis with emphasis on computed tomography. Radiology 137:363, 1980.
83. Weber AL, Stanton AC. Malignant tumors of the paranasal sinuses and radiologic clinical and histopathological evaluation of 200 cases. Head Neck Surg 6:761, 1984.
84. Natrig K, Larsen TE. Mucocoele of the paranasal sinuses: a retrospective clinical and histological study. J Laryngol Otol 92:1075, 1978.
85. Hesselink JR, Weber AL, New PF, et al. Evaluation of mucocoeles of the paranasal sinus with computed tomography. Radiology 133:377, 1979.
86. Marchevksy AM, Betton EJ, Gellar SA, et al. The changing spectrum of disease, etiology, an diagnosis of mucormycosis. Hum Pathol 11:456, 1980.
87. Green WR, Font RL, Zimmerman LE. Aspergillosis of the orbit. Arch Ophthalmol 83:302, 1969.
88. Hesselink JR, Davis KR, Dallow RL, et al. Computed tomography of masses in the lacrimal gland region. Radiology 137:363, 1980.
89. Stewart WB, Krobel GB, Wright JE. Lacrimal gland and fossa lesions: an approach to diagnosis and management. Ophthalmology 86:886, 1979.
90. Trokel SL, Hilal SK. Submillimeter resolution CT scanning of orbital diseases. Ophthalmology 87:412, 1980.
91. Wende S, Aulich A, Nover A, et al. Computed tomography of orbital lesions. A cooperative study of 210 cases. Neuroradiology 13:123, 1977.
92. Blei L, Chambers JT, Liotta LA, et al. Orbital dermoid diagnosed by computed tomographic scanning. Am J Ophthalmol 85:58, 1978.
93. Jacobs L, Weisbert LA, Kinkel WR: Computerized Tomography of the Orbit and Sella Turcica. New York, Raven Press, 1980.
94. Wachenheim A, van Damme W, Kosmann P, et al. Computed tomography in ophthalmology: density changes with orbital lesions. Neuroradiology 13:135, 1977.
95. Lloyd GAS. CT scanning in the diagnosis of orbital disease. Comput Tomogr 3:227, 1979.
96. Davidson RI, Kleinman PK. Anterior transorbital meningoencephaloceles: a defect in the pars orbitalis of the frontal bone. AJNR 1:579, 1980.
97. Glaser JS. Neuro-ophthalmology. Hagerstown, Md., Harper & Row, 1978.
98. Thomas JE, Yoss RF. The parasellar syndrome: problems in determining etiology. Mayo Clinic Proc 45:617, 1970.
99. Russell EJ, Czervionke L, Huekman M, et al. CT of the inferomedial orbit and the lacrimal drainage apparatus: normal and pathologic anatomy. AJNR 6:759, 1985.
100. Carbell W. The radiology of the lacrimal system. Br J Radiol 31:1, 1964.
101. Cohen MM, Lassell S. Amyloid tumors of the orbit. Neuroradiology 18:157, 1979.
102. Handousa A. Localized intraorbital amyloid disease. Br J Ophthalmol 38:510, 1959.
103. Howard GM. Amyloid tumors of the orbit. Br J Ophthalmol 50:421, 1966.
104. Raab E. Intraorbital amyloid. Br J Ophthalmol 54:445, 1970.
105. Gorman CA. Ophthalmopathy of Graves' disease. Editorial. N Engl J Med 308:453, 1983.
106. Gorman CA. Temporal relationship between onset of Graves' ophthalmopathy and diagnosis of thyrotoxicosis. Mayo Clin Proc 58:515, 1983.
107. Kodama K, Sikorska H, Bandy-Dafoe P, et al. Demonstration of a circulation autoantibody against a soluble eye-muscle antigen in Graves' ophthalmopathy. Lancet 2:1353, 1982.
108. Jensen SF. Endocrine ophthalmoplegia: is it due to myopathy or to mechanical immobilization? Acta Ophthalmol (Copenh) 49:679, 1971.
109. Volpe R. The thyroid. In Spittel JA Jr, ed. Clinical Medicine. Vol 8. Philadelphia, Harper & Row, 1984:1.
110. Enzmann DR, Donaldson SS, Kriss JP. Appearance of Graves' disease on orbital computed tomography. J Comput Assist Tomogr 3:815, 1979.
111. Forbes G, Gorman CA, Brennan MD, et al. Ophthalmopathy of Graves' disease: computerized volume measurements of the orbital fat and muscle. Radiology 7:651, 1985.
112. Slavin ML, Glaser JS. Idiopathic orbital myositis. A report of 6 cases. Arch Ophthalmol 100:1261, 1982.
113. Bullen CL, Young BR. Chronic orbital myositis. Arch Ophthalmol 100:1749, 1982.
114. Trokel SL, Hilal SK. Submillimeter resolution CT scanning of orbital diseases. Ophthalmology (Philadelphia) 87:412, 1980.
115. Atlas SW, Grossman RI, Savino PJ, et al. Surface-coil MR of orbital pseudotumor. AJNR 98:141, 1987.
116. Blodi FC, Gass JDM. Inflammatory pseudotumor of the orbit. Br J Ophthalmol 32:79, 1968.
117. Mottow LS, Jakobiec FA. Idiopathic inflammatory orbital pseudotumor in childhood. Arch Ophthalmol 96:1410, 1978.
118. Dresner SC, Rothfus WE, Slamovits TL, et al. Computed tomography of the orbital myositis. AJR 143:671, 1984.
119. Brown HW. Congenital structural muscle anomalies. In Allen JH, ed. Strabismus Ophthalmic Symposium. St. Louis, C. V. Mosby, 1950:205.
120. Brown HW. True and simulated superior oblique tendon sheath syndromes. Doc Ophthalmol 34:123, 1973.
121. Goldhammer Y, Smith LJ. Acquired intermittent Brown syndrome. Neurology 24:666, 1974.
122. Parks MM, Brown M. Superior oblique tendon sheath syndrome of Brown. Am J Ophthalmol 79:82, 1975.
123. Mafee MF, Folk ER, Langer BG, et al. Computed tomography in the evaluation of Brown syndrome of the superior oblique tendon sheath. Radiology 154:691, 1985.
124. Kennerdell JS, Ghoshhajra K. Computed tomography scanning of orbital tumors. Int Ophthalmol Clin 22:99, 1982.
125. Forbes GS, Sheedy PF II, Waller RR. Orbital tumors evaluated by computed tomography. Radiology 136:101, 1980.
126. Flanagan JC. Vascular problems of the orbit. Ophthalmology 86:896, 1979.
127. Lloyd GAS. CT scanning in the diagnosis of orbital disease. Computed Tomogr 3:227, 1979.
128. Davis KR, Hasselink JR, Dallow RL, et al. CT and ultrasound diagnosis of cavernous hemangioma and lymphangioma of the orbit. J Comput Assist Tomogr 4:98, 1980.

129. Gomori JM, Grossman RI, Golbert HI, et al. Intracranial hematomas: imaging by high-field MR. Radiology 157:87, 1985.
130. Jacobs L, Weisbert LA, Kinkel WR. Computed Tomography of the Orbit and Sella Turcica. New York, Raven Press, 1980.
131. Jones ES, Jakobiec FA. Diseases of the Orbit. Hagerstown, Md., Harper & Row, 1979.
132. Savojardo M, Harwood-Nash DCF, Tadmor R, et al. Gliomas of the intracranial anterior optic pathways in children: the role of CT, angiography, pneumoencephalography, and radionuclide brain scanning. Radiology 138:601, 1982.
133. Jakobiec FA, Depot MJ, Kennerdell JS, et al. Combined clinical and computed tomographic diagnosis of orbital glioma and meningioma. Ophthalmology 91:137, 1984.
134. Howard CW, Osher RH, Tomak RL. Computed tomographic features in optic neuritis. Am J Ophthalmol 89:699, 1980.
135. Rudick RA, Jacobs L, Kinkel PR, et al. Isolated idiopathic optic neuritis. Analysis of free kappa light chains in cerebrospinal fluid and correlation with nuclear magnetic resonance findings. Arch Neurol 43:456, 1986.
136. Jacobs L, Kinkel PR, Kinkel WR. Silent brain lesions in patients with isolated idiopathic optic neuritis: a clinical and nuclear magnetic resonance imaging study. Arch Neurol 43:452, 1986.
137. Danzier A, Price HI. CT findings in retinoblastoma. AJR 133:783, 1979.
138. Forbes GS, Earnest F IV, Waller RR. Computed tomography of orbital tumors, including late-generation scanning techniques. Radiology 142:387, 1982.
139. Zimmerman LE, Burns RP, Wankum G, et al. Trilateral retinoblastoma: ectopic intracranial retinoblastoma associated with bilateral retinoblastoma. J Pediatr Ophthalmol Strabismus 19:320, 1982.
140. Brown DH. The clinicopathology of retinoblastoma. Am J Ophthalmol 61:508, 1966.
141. Harris GJ, Williams AL, Reeser FH. Intra-ocular evaluation by computed tomography. Int Ophthalmol Clin 22:197, 1982.
142. Reese AB, Ellsworth RM. The evaluation and current concept of retinoblastoma therapy. Trans Am Acad Ophthalmol Otolaryngol 67:164, 1963.
143. Sherman JL, McLean IW, Brallier DR. Coat's disease, CT-pathologic correlation in two cases. Radiology 146:77, 1983.
144. Mafee MF, Goldbert MR, Valvassori GE, et al. Computed tomography in the evaluation of patients with persistent hyperplastic primary vitreous (PHPV). Radiology 145:713, 1982.
145. Armstrong EA, Smith TH, Harms SE. Brawny scleritis of the eye: correlation of CT and MRI anatomy. Presented at the European Society of Paediatric Radiology, 1985.
146. Brown DH. Ocular *Toxocara canis*. J Pediatr Ophthalmol 7:182, 1970.
147. Huntley CC. Visceral larva migrans. In Hoeprich PD, ed. Infectious Diseases. Philadelphia, Harper & Row, 1983:764.
148. Edwards MG, Pordell GR. Ocular toxocariasis studied by CT scanning. Radiology 157:685, 1985.
149. Danziger A, Price HI. CT findings in retinoblastoma. Am J Roentgenol 133:696, 1979.
150. Reese AB. Tumors of the Eye. New York, Harper & Row, 1976.
151. Zimmerman RA, Bilaniuk LT. Computed tomography in the evaluation of patients with bilateral retinoblastomas. J Comput Assist Tomogr 3:251, 1979.
152. Ferry AP, Font RL. Carcinoma metastatic to the eye and orbit: I. A clinicopathologic study of 227 cases. Arch Ophthalmol 92:276, 1974.
153. Font RL, Ferry R. Carcinoma metastatic to the eye and orbit. III. A clinicopathologic study of 28 cases metastatic to the orbit. Cancer 38:1326, 1976.
154. Hart W. Metastatic carcinoma to the eye and orbit. Int Ophthalmol Clin 2:465, 1962.
155. Bloch RS, Gartner S. The incidence of ocular metastatic carcinoma. Arch Ophthalmol 85:673, 1971.
156. Hesselink JR, Davis KR, Weber AL, et al. Radiological evaluation of orbital masses with emphasis on computed tomography. Radiology 137:363, 1980.
157. Kanz FG, Schwartz I. Intra-ocular calcium shadows: choroid ossification. Radiology 43:486, 1944.

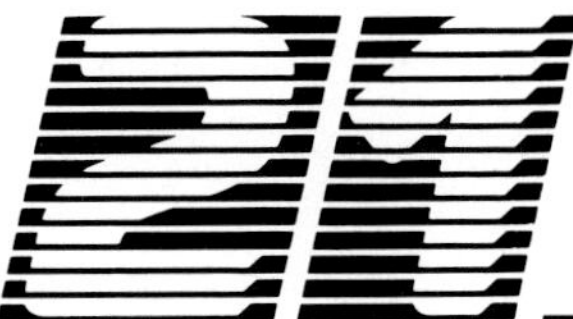

Stephen F. Quinn, M.D.

# MRI OF THE NASOPHARYNX

## ANATOMY

The nasopharynx is a tubular-shaped region marginated cephalad by the sphenoid sinus and clivus, caudad by a line drawn horizontally along the hard and soft palate, anteriorly by the nasal choanae, and posteriorly by the cervical spine and prevertebral muscles. The lateral extent of the nasopharynx includes the masticator, parapharyngeal, and carotid spaces.

There are three main compartments in the nasopharynx: medial, lateral, and posterior (Table 21–1; Fig. 21–1).

### Medial Compartment

The medial compartment is composed of all the nasopharyngeal structures on the airway side of the pharyngobasilar fascia (Fig. 21–2). The pharyngobasilar fascia extends from the cephalad boundary of the superior pharyngeal constrictor to the base of the skull and anterolaterally to the pterygoid plates.[1] On MRI the fascia can be identified as an area of signal void. Although the pharyngobasilar fascia is thin, it serves as a tough boundary in preventing the spread of disease. A process that penetrates the fascia usually is either malignant or an aggressive inflammatory lesion.[2]

**Table 21–1.** NASOPHARYNX COMPARTMENT AND SPACES

| |
|---|
| Medial compartment |
| Airway side of the pharyngobasilar fascia |
| Lateral compartment |
| Masticator space |
| Parapharyngeal space |
| Carotid space |
| Posterior compartment |
| Retropharyngeal space |
| Prevertebral space |

*Source:* Smoker WRK, Gentry LR. Semin US, CT, MR 7:107, 1986, with permission.

The medial compartment includes the nasopharyngeal mucosa, lymphoid tissue, and the levator veli palatini and salpingopharyngeus muscles.[1] The levator veli palatini muscle, which primarily originates from the temporal bone, passes through the pharyngobasilar fascia via the sinus of Morgagni and inserts into the middle segment of the soft palate. The salpingopharyngeus muscle originates from the torus tubarius and inserts on the posterolateral pharynx.[1] On MRI the levator and salpingopharyngeus muscles cannot be separated. Unlike CT, however, MRI can separate the tensor and levator palatini muscles.

The eustachian tube also passes through the foramen of Morgagni and opens into the nasopharynx anterior and inferior to the tip of the cartilaginous torus tubarius. The proximal portions of the eustachian tubes may be air filled, and the tori are often asymmetric. The lateral recesses or fossae of Rosemüller are posterior and superior to the tori and may also be asymmetric.[3, 4] The depth of the lateral recesses is in part dependent on the patient's age and the amount of lymphoid tissue present. The pharyngeal tonsils, which lie along the posterior wall, atrophy markedly by the end of adolescence but may persist to the second and third decades.[1–4]

At the level of the hard palate, the pharyngobasilar fascia is replaced by the superior constrictor and Passavant's muscle. These muscles marginate the posterolateral aspects of the airway. Passavant's ridge is a descriptive anatomic phrase describing the contracted superior pharyngeal constrictor and Passavant's muscles. The soft palate is raised against this ridge by the tensor and levator palatini muscles during swallowing.[1–4]

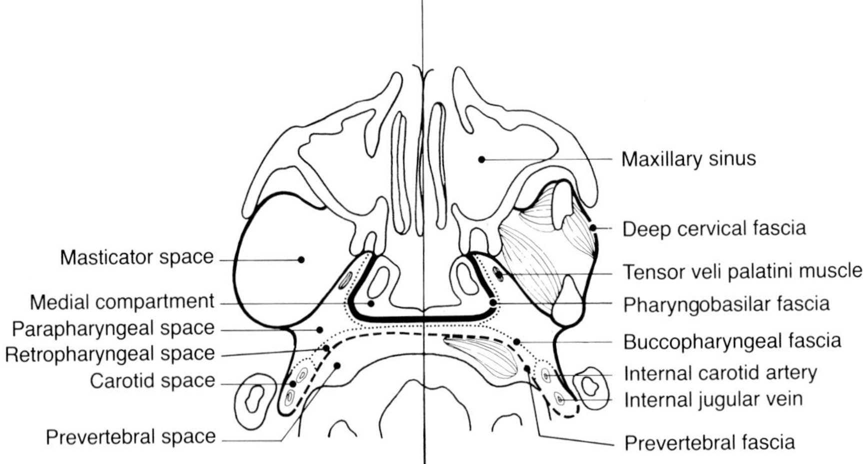


**Figure 21–1. The nasopharynx, separated into a series of compartments and spaces by fascial layers.** The compartments have respective differences in lesions and pathways of preferential spread. (Modified from Smoker WRK, Gentry LR. Semin US, CT, MR 7:107–130, 1986, with permission.)

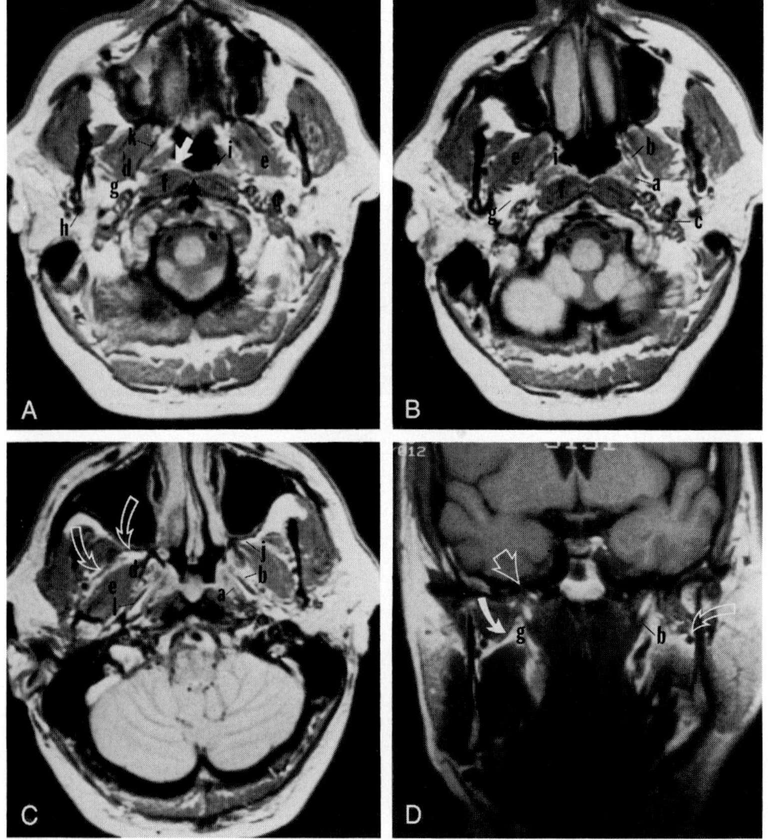


**Figure 21–2. Normal anatomy.** a: levator veli palatini muscle; b: tensor veli palatini muscle; c: carotid sheath; d: pterygoid plates; e: pterygoid muscles; f: prevertebral muscles; g: parapharyngeal space; h: retromandibular vein; i: torus tubarius; j: pterygoid palatine fossa; k: pharyngobasilar fascia; l: eustachian tube. *A,* (SE 2200/20). This axial section is at the junction of the oropharynx and the nasopharynx. The fascia is seen as a plane of signal void (black arrow). The mucosa of the airway (white arrow) is of higher signal intensity than the intermediate signal of muscle. *B* and *C,* Axial sections are increasingly more cephalad. The maxillary artery is seen traversing the masticator space and entering the PPF (open curved white arrows).

*D,* (TR 800 msec/TE 20 msec), same patient. Image in the coronal plane through the nasopharynx. The maxillary artery and vein are seen medial to the mandibular condyle (curved open arrow). The mandibular division (ICN) passes through the foramen ovale (open white arrow) and lateral to the medial pterygoid muscle (curved white arrow).

The foramen lacerum lies at the base of the medial pterygoid plate at the petrous apex. Meningeal branches of the ascending pharyngeal artery and the greater superficial petrosal nerve (eighth cranial nerve) pass through it. The foramen is filled with fibrocartilage and is in close proximity to the internal carotid artery as it leaves the carotid canal and enters the posterior cavernous sinus.[5, 6]

The pterygopalatine fossa (PPF) is a medial depression in the superior aspect of the pterygomaxillary fissure. It is delineated anteriorly by the posterior wall of the maxillary sinus, medially by the palatine bone, laterally by the masticator space, and posteriorly by the pterygoid plates.[3] The PPF serves as an interchange for multiple nerves via different foramina, canals, and fissures (Fig. 21–3).

The sphenopalatine ganglion, which is situated in the PPF posterior to the loop of the maxillary artery, is a parasympathetic ganglion containing nerve cell bodies that synapse with the fibers of the seventh cranial nerve and sensory and sympathetic fibers from other communicating nerves (e.g., maxillary nerve and sympathetic plexus via the vidian nerve).[7] The third part of the maxillary artery passes medially into the PPF via the pterygopalatine fissure and forms a characteristic loop. The maxillary artery gives off branches to the communicating foramina, canal, and fissures. The vascular branches share the name of the communicating channel they pass through (Fig. 21–4).[8, 9]

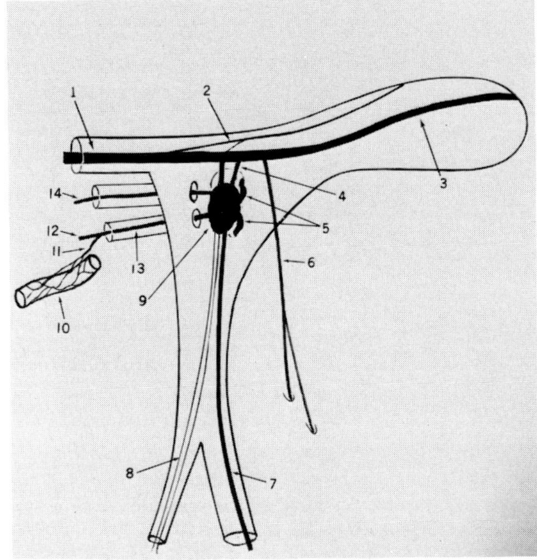


**Figure 21–3. The pterygopalatine fossa (PPF) which serves as an interchange for multiple nerves.**

1. Maxillary nerve (foramen rotundum)
2. Zygomatic nerve (infraorbital fissure)
3. Infraorbital nerve (infraorbital fissure)
4. Roots of ganglion
5. Posterior superior nasal nerve (sphenopalatine foramen)
6. Posterior superior alveolar nerve (sphenopalatine foramen)
7. Greater palatine nerve (greater palatine canal)
8. Lesser palatine nerve (lesser palatine canal)
9. Sphenopalatine ganglion
10. Sympathetic plexus on internal carotid
11. Deep petrosal nerve (sympathetic)
12. Greater superficial petrosal nerve (parasympathetic fibers from VII)
13. Nerve of pterygoid canal (vidian nerve) formed by 11 and 12 (pterygoid canal)
14. Pharyngeal nerve (pharyngeal canal).

(From Paff GH. Anatomy of the Head and Neck. Philadelphia, W. B. Saunders, 1973, pp. 141–146, with permission.)

## Lateral Compartment

The lateral compartment is composed of three spaces: the masticator, the parapharyngeal, and the carotid.

The masticator space is marginated by the superficial layer of deep cervical fascia.[1] (The term *infratemporal fossae,* which describes the cephalic extent of the masticator space, is not used in this discussion.) The four muscles of mastication are contained in this space: the lateral pterygoid muscle, which originates from the lateral pterygoid plate, infratemporal crest, and great wing of sphenoid and inserts on the mandibular condyle and articular disk of the temporomandibular joint; the medial pterygoid muscle, which originates from the medial side of the pterygoid plate pyramidal process of the palatine bone and inserts on the medial aspect of the mandibular ramus; the deep head of the temporalis muscle, which originates from the roof of the masticator space and infratemporal crest and inserts on the coronoid process and anterior mandibular ramus; and the masseter muscle, which originates from the zygomatic arch and inserts on the lateral mandibular ramus, angle, and condyle. These muscles are innervated by the mandibular division of the trigeminal (fifth) cranial nerve.[10] MRI is superior to CT in individually imaging muscles because it is more sensitive to the small amounts of intramuscular and intermuscular planes of fat.

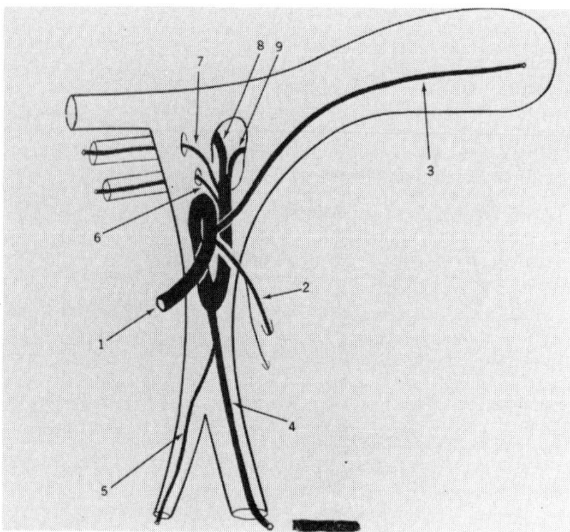


**Figure 21–4. The third part of the maxillary artery has a characteristic loop as it enters the PPF and lies anterior to the sphenopalatine ganglion.** The branches of the maxillary artery are named for the foramen through which they may pass.

1. Maxillary artery
2. Posterior superior alveolar artery
3. Infraorbital artery
4. Greater palatine artery
5. Lesser palatine artery
6. Artery of pterygoid canal, or vidian artery
7. Pharyngeal artery
8. Sphenopalatine artery (giving off in this specimen, a posterior nasal artery [9] while still in the fossa).

(From Paff GH. Anatomy of the Head and Neck. Philadelphia, W. B. Saunders, 1973, pp 141–146, with permission.)

The maxillary artery traverses the masticator space. The mandibular (first) segment travels first posteriorly then medially to the mandibular condyle, where it gives off the deep auricular and the tympanic branches posteriorly. More anteromedially, it gives off a middle meningeal branch of the foramen spinosum and the accessory meningeal to the foramen ovale, which passes superiorly. The inferior alveolar artery branches off inferolaterally into the mandibular foramen. The artery then passes into the pterygopalatine fossa.[8, 9]

The mandibular division of the fifth cranial nerve passes through the foramen ovale with the emissary vein, accessory meningeal artery (variable), middle meningeal veins (variable), and lesser superficial petrosal nerve (variable). The foramen ovale is situated in the posteromedial aspect of the masticator space, posterior to the lateral pterygoid plate. The foramen spinosum is posterolateral to the foramen ovale. The middle meningeal artery and recurrent (meningeal) branch of the mandibular nerve pass through this foramen.[5, 6]

The mandibular nerve gives off the medial pterygoid and the nervus spinosus nerves and divides into small anterior and larger posterior components. The smaller anterior division branches into two temporal nerves, a masseter nerve, a lateral pterygoid nerve, and a buccal nerve. The posterior division divides into the inferior alveolar nerve and lingual nerves. These travel between the lateral and medial pterygoid muscles.[7]

The lingual nerve, which is a branch of the mandibular division (V) of the fifth cranial nerve, combines with the chorda tympani, which is a branch of the eighth cranial nerve, to supply the anterior two thirds of the tongue with sensation (V) and taste (VII). Fibers from the chorda tympani also branch off to the submandibular and sublingual glands.[11]

The parapharyngeal space (PPS) is a triangular-shaped region in the lateral compartment. It extends from the skull base to the cornu of the hyoid bone. It abuts the pterygoid muscles anterolaterally; the pharyngobasilar fascia, tensor palatini muscles, and superior pharyngeal constrictor medially; the parotid posterolaterally; the carotid space posteriorly; and the retropharyngeal space posteromedially. The fascial margins of the PPS include the superficial layer of deep cervical fascia laterally, the middle layer of deep cervical fascia (buccopharyngeal) medially, and the three fascial layers of carotid sheath posteriorly.[1]

The PPS is a good anatomic landmark because it is usually symmetric and is primarily filled with fat. Some authors include the tensor veli palatini muscles in the anterior portion of the PPS. The PPS originates from the scaphoid fossa at the base of the medial pterygoid plate, the spine of the sphenoid bone, and the lateral margin of the eustachian tube. It hooks around the hamulus of the medial pterygoid plate and inserts on the membranous portion of the soft palate.[3]

The carotid space extends from the skull base to the aortic arch. It is enveloped by the deep, middle, and superficial layers of deep cervical fascia.[1] Depending on its location in the nasopharynx, the carotid space lies lateral to the cervical spine and prevertebral muscles. It is bordered anteriorly by the PPS, laterally by the styloid process and parotid, and—depending on its level—posteriorly by the cervical spine, skull base, or fat. The carotid sheath contains the ninth to twelfth cranial nerves, the internal jugular vein, the internal carotid artery, the sympathetic plexus, and the lymphatics.

### Posterior Compartment

The posterior compartment is composed of the retropharyngeal and prevertebral spaces. The retropharyngeal space is a potential space that lies between the middle (buccopharyngeal fascia) and deep (prevertebral fascia) layers of the deep cervical fascia. The high, medial, and the high lateral retropharyngeal lymph nodes are contained in the space.[1]

The prevertebral space is marginated posteriorly by the anterior longitudinal ligament and anteriorly by the deep layer of the deep cervical fascia. The longus colli, longus capitis, and rectus capitis muscles are contained in this space.[1]

## MRI OF THE NASOPHARYNX

Magnetic resonance imaging (MRI) of the nasopharynx has quickly gained recognition in head and neck imaging. Many authors have independently found MRI generally to be superior to CT in the nasopharynx.[12–19] The greatest singular advantage is the improved soft tissue contrast with MRI. With CT the superficial mucosa and lymphoid tissue cannot be separated from the nasopharyngeal musculature. With MRI T2-weighted images (T2WI) can separate these areas, because the superficial mucosa and lymphoid material have longer T2 relaxation times, making their signal more intense than muscle.

Like CT, fat is well seen with MRI. Fat has a short T1 relaxation time, making it bright on T1-weighted images (T1WI). The most important fat-containing region is the PPS. Fibrous tissue and fascial layers have low signal on both T1WI and T2WI.

Cortical bone has no signal, so that it appears black on MRI. Because of this, cortical abnormalities are better seen on CT. Spatial resolution of the bony foramina of the skull base seems to be somewhat better with CT than MRI. The intramedullary marrow has a bright signal on T1WI because of the marrow fat content. This is routinely seen in the pterygoid plates, which makes their identification easy.

Dental amalgam is usually not ferromagnetic and therefore does not present artifact. Certain dental appliances are ferromagnetic and cause a variety of distorting signal void artifacts.[13]

As with most pathological processes in the rest of the body, abnormal lesions in the nasopharynx tend to have longer T2 relaxation times than the surrounding soft tissues. Often abnormal nasopharyngeal lesions are isointense with the normal surrounding structures on T1WI, and T2WI is needed to accentuate tumor margins.

Lymph nodes are best differentiated from fat on T1WI because fat has a shorter T1 relaxation value (250 msec) than lymph nodes (400 to 500 msec).[13] Lymph nodes are best differentiated from muscles on T2WI because of the intermediate T2 relaxation values of muscle and the more prolonged T2 relaxation values of nodes. Pathologic nodes, either from reactive hyperplasia or neoplastic involvement, tend to have bright signal intensity from prolongation of T2 relaxation values.

Early data suggest that MRI will help sort through the difficult problems of post-treatment evaluations. Postsurgical and radiation changes make evaluation of nasopharynx difficult, but MRI can help differentiate fibrosis from scar and recurrent or residual tumor. Fibrosis tends to have diminished signal on all sequences, although hemorrhagic or edematous foci within the early phases of fibrous tissue can cause increased signal.[1]

### MRI Technique

The nasopharynx has been successfully imaged at low, intermediate, and high field strengths. The guidelines to successful imaging include use of surface and head coil, adequate matrix size, small slice thickness, pulse sequence optimization, sufficient number of averages or excitations, and adequate planes of imaging.

The type of coil used for imaging the nasopharynx depends on the equipment available. It seems that all the commercially available MRI units now have either a surface coil or head coil that allows adequate imaging of the nasopharynx.

A 256 × 256 matrix is currently used by most centers to obtain adequate anatomic detail. The matrix used will vary with field strength, surface coil, pulse sequence, and time constraints. The larger the matrix size in the y, or time-domain dimension, the longer the acquisition time.

The nasopharynx should be studied with sections in the 4 to 6 mm range. The signal-to-noise degradation with thinner sections can be offset by increasing the number of excitations or averages, which increases acquisition time.

Axial spin-echo T1WI (TR 400 to 800 msec/TE 20 msec) is usually obtained through the nasopharynx for good anatomic depiction. Axial spin-echo T2WI (TR > 2000/TE 20 to 40/40 to 80 msec) is obtained to help differentiate pathologic from normal and abnormal processes. Coronal and axial contrast-enhanced (CE) T1-weighted MR may be substituted for T2WI. If an abnormality is seen or there is a suspicion of a skull-base lesion, then T2-weighted coronal images are obtained. Sagittal sequences are often helpful, especially for midline lesions such as chordoma, encephalocele, or craniopharyngioma.

## Pathology

Because the differential diagnosis of nasopharyngeal processes changes according to the compartment involved, the discussion of pathology is organized by compartment.

### *Medial Compartment Abnormalities*

Ninety-eight percent of nasopharyngeal neoplasms are carcinomas, with squamous cell representing 80% of cases.[20] The use of subtypes *lymphoepithelioma* and *transitional cell carcinoma* to describe nonkeratinizing squamous cell carcinoma has fallen into disfavor. Although nonkeratinizing tumors tend to be more common and less well differentiated, the degree of keratinization does not necessarily correlate with tumor aggression.[20, 22] Eighteen percent of carcinomas are adenocarcinomas, adenocystic carcinomas, or other unclassified carcinomas.[20]

Nasopharyngeal carcinomas (NPC) usually arise in the posterosuperior aspect of the medial compartment.[21] NPC spread locally in five manners: (1) via the mucosa and submucosa, (2) along muscle bundles, (3) along fibro-fatty tissue planes, (4) along neurovascular bundles, and (5) along periosteal surfaces (Figs. 21–5 to 21–8).[2, 22, 23] Submucosal invasion of deglutitional muscles occurs and often goes understaged. This veritable anatomic conduit allows spread of tumor between the oropharynx and nasopharynx.[2] NPC may have a superficial exophytic component that can cause asymmetric soft tissue masses on MRI.

Posterior extension from the PPS into the carotid space can extend into the jugular fossa and cause deficits of cranial nerves IX to XII (jugular fossa syndrome).[1, 24, 25] Involvement of the cervical sympathetic plexus may cause Horner's syndrome.[2]

Lateral invasion from the PPS will extend into the masticator space. This may cause deficits of the lingual nerve, trismus, and pain. In late stages of disease, there is invasion of the masticator space muscles and mandible.[1]

NPC involvement of the skull base can occur through multiple pathways. Involvement of the carotid sheath and PPS permits cephalad extension into the skull via the carotid canal, the foramen lacerum, or both. Subsequent involvement of the cavernous sinus can produce deficits of cranial nerves III to VI.[1, 2, 4] Although adenocystic carcinomas are infamous for perineural spread, other carcinomas commonly spread in this manner as well. Erosions of the skull at points of muscular origins can occur as NPC travel along muscle groups (e.g., destruction of the pterygoid plate and basisphenoid secondary to involvement of the tensor and levator palatini muscles).[4, 26, 27]

Extension into bony foramina at the skull base can occur by following neurovascular bundles. For example, involvement of the trigeminal nerve may occur secondarily through the foramen ovale (mandibular nerve) or foramen rotundum (maxillary nerve). Neural involvement may cause ipsilateral atrophy of the masticator space musculature.[4] There is also an effect called postirradiation muscular atrophy that is often diffuse, corresponds to the treatment portal, and can involve the deglutitional as well as the masticator muscles.[3]

Nasopharyngeal carcinomas are typically not surgical lesions and are usually treated with radiation. MRI therefore is quite im-

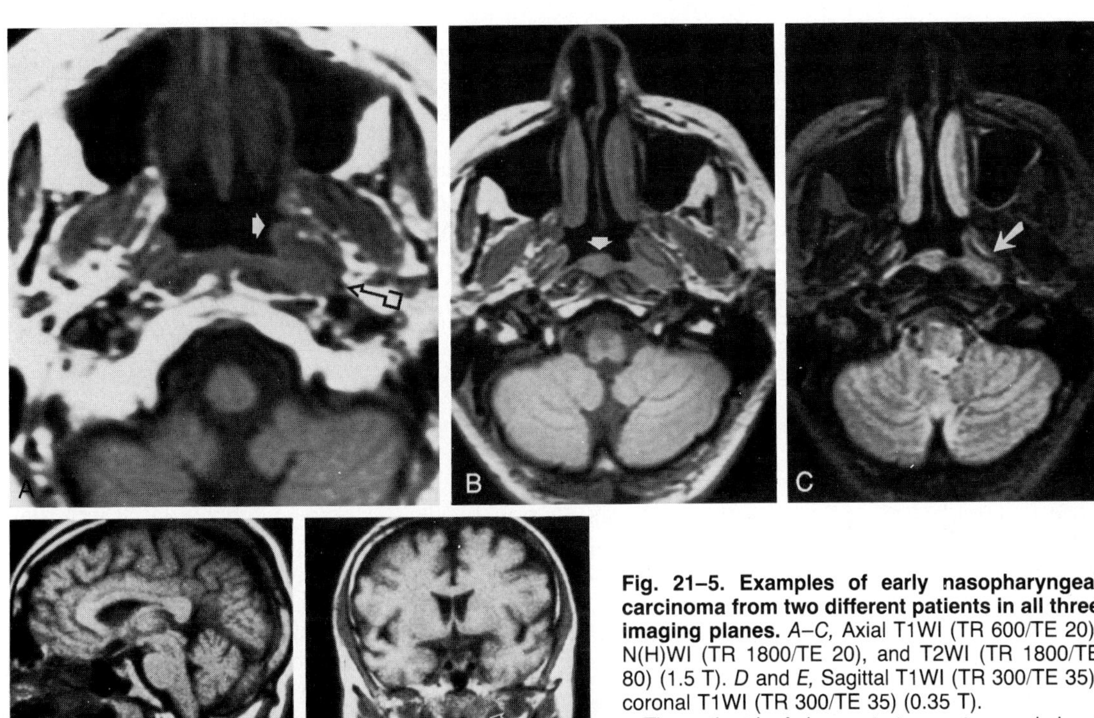

**Fig. 21–5. Examples of early nasopharyngeal carcinoma from two different patients in all three imaging planes.** *A–C,* Axial T1WI (TR 600/TE 20), N(H)WI (TR 1800/TE 20), and T2WI (TR 1800/TE 80) (1.5 T). *D* and *E,* Sagittal T1WI (TR 300/TE 35), coronal T1WI (TR 300/TE 35) (0.35 T).

The patient in *A* demonstrates contour and signal alteration of the left veli palatini musculature, the torus tubarius (arrow), the right fossa of Rosenmüller (open arrow), and the midline adenoidal pad region (arrow [*B*]). The patient in *D* and *E* demonstrates contour alteration in the adenoidal region on sagittal T1WI and in the left fossa of Rosenmüller on coronal T1WI (open arrow). Such contour alterations in the adenoidal region should not be present in an adult. (Courtesy of S. J. Pomeranz, M.D., Christ Hospital, Cincinnati, Ohio.)

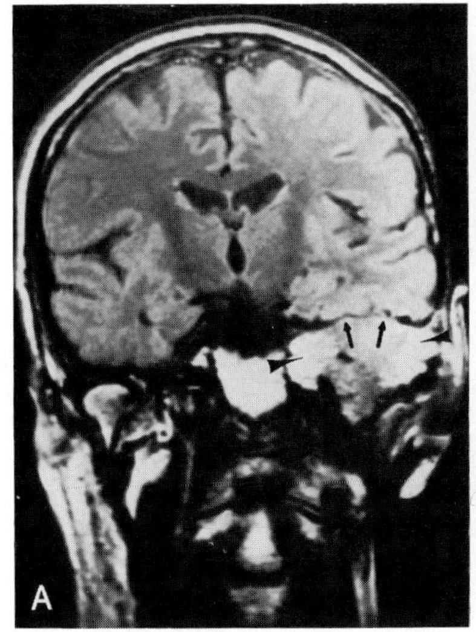

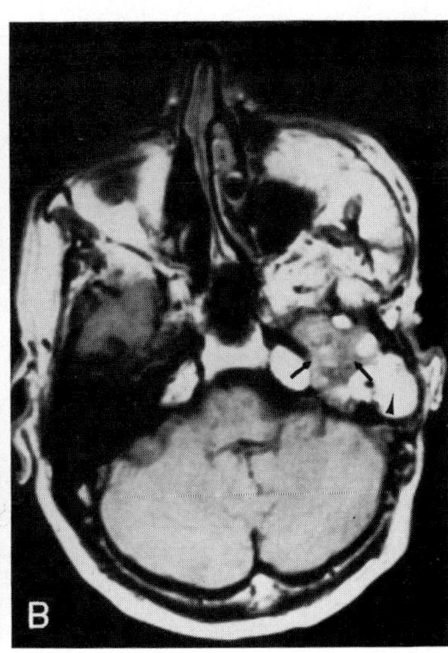

**Fig. 21–6. Nasopharyngeal carcinomas (NPC) growing along the course of the lateral pterygoid.** *A* (N[H]WI 2200/20), the NPC has grown along the fibers of the lateral pterygoid muscle and has invaded the floor of the temporal bone. *B* (N[H]WI 1500/20), the NPC has an extradural mass effect that is deforming the temporal lobe (arrows). The mastoid air cells are filled with fluid that is probably hemorrhagic (arrowheads).

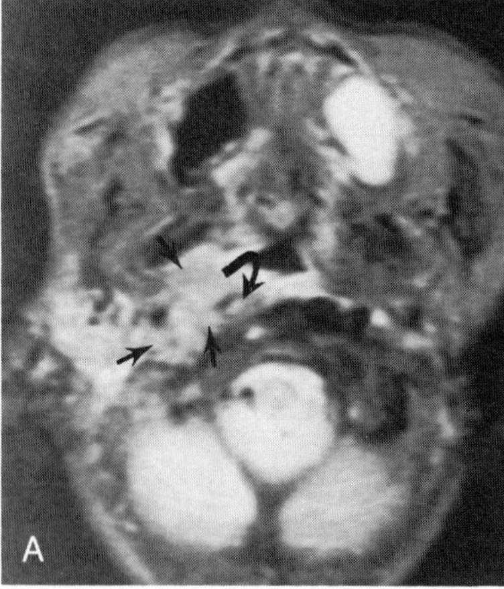


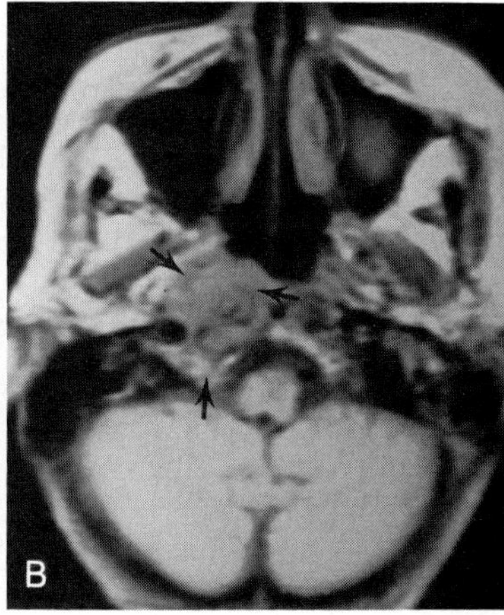


**Figure 21–7. Nasopharyngeal carcinoma (NPC) spread along fibrofatty planes.** *A* (N[H]WI 2200/20), the intermediate intensity NPC has broken out of the medial compartment into the lateral and posterior compartments, invading the carotid and parapharyngeal spaces (black arrows). *B* (T2WI 2200/100), at a slightly more caudal position, the high intensity nasopharyngeal carcinoma on this T2WI shows the lateral compartment spread (black arrows). There is a retropharyngeal node (curved black arrow). (Courtesy of S. J. Pomeranz, M.D., Christ Hospital, Cincinnati, Ohio.)

portant in identifying the site and extent of tumor. This information together with assessment of lymphadenopathy is important in staging, in designing radiation portals, and in the prognosis (Table 21–2).[2]

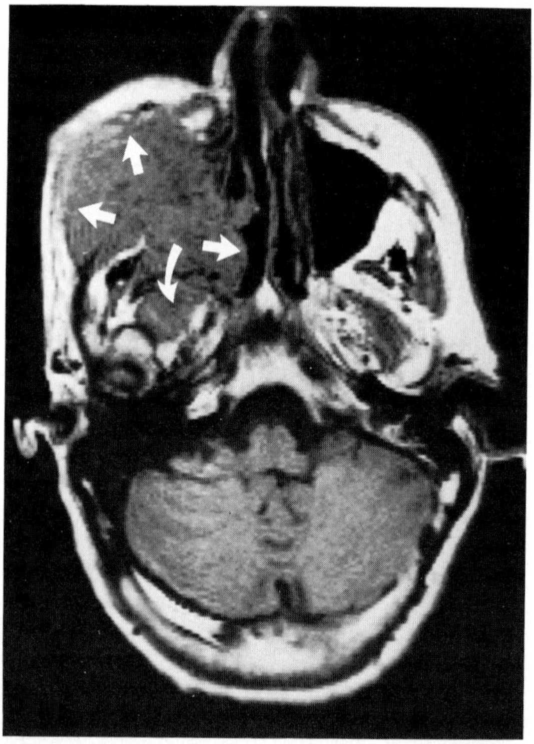

**Fig. 21–8. Nasopharyngeal carcinoma (NPC) spreading along posterolateral wall of maxillary antrum.** T1WI (TR 400 msec; TE 20 msec). The NPC spread through the maxillary antrum into the nasal cavity and soft tissues of the face (white arrows). There is invasion of the pterygoid muscles (curved white arrow). (Courtesy of Spencer Gay, M.D., University of Virginia Hospital, Charlottesville, Va.)

Rhabdomyosarcoma, the most common soft tissue sarcoma in the pediatric population, commonly occurs in the nasopharynx, a location second only to the orbit in frequency of involvement.[1, 29] Lymphomas, other sarcomas, melanomas, and plasmacytomas all can infrequently involve the medial compartment of the nasopharynx.[1]

**Table 21–2.** NASOPHARYNGEAL CARCINOMA STAGING

| | |
|---|---|
| **Primary Tumor and Adenopathy** | |
| Tis | Carcinoma in situ |
| T1 | Tumor confined to one site of nasopharynx or no tumor visible (positive biopsy only) |
| T2 | Tumor involving two sites (both posterosuperior and lateral walls) |
| T3 | Extension of tumor into nasal cavity or oropharynx |
| T4 | Tumor invasion of skull, cranial nerve involvement, or both |
| NX | Minimum requirements to assess the regional nodes cannot be met |
| N0 | No clinically positive node |
| N1 | Single clinically positive homolateral node 3 cm or less in diameter |
| N2 | Single clinically positive homolateral node more than 3 cm but not more than 6 cm in diameter, or multiple |
| | Clinically positive homolateral nodes, none more than 6 cm in diameter |
| **Distant Metastasis (M)** | |
| MX | Minimum requirements to assess the presence of distant metastasis cannot be met |
| M0 | No evidence of metastasis |
| M1 | Distant metastasis present<br>Specify |
| **Stage Grouping** | |
| Stage II | T2, N0, M0 |
| Stage III | T3, N0, M0 |
| | T1, or T2 or T3, N1, M0 |
| Stage IV | T4, N0 or N1, M0 |
| | Any T, N2 or N3, M0 |
| | Any T, any N, M1 |

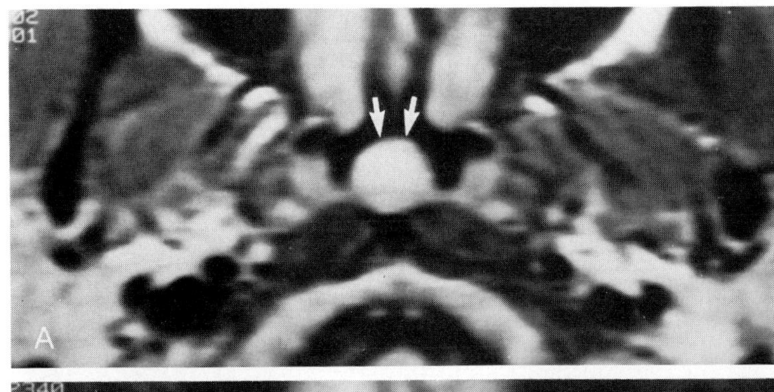


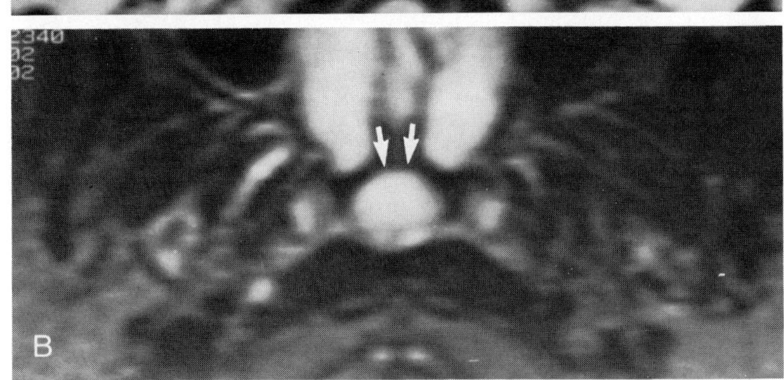


**Figure 21–9. Thornwaldt cyst.** *A* and *B,* Axial multiecho N(H)WI and T2WI (TR 2200/TE 20/100 msec). This cyst is situated high in the anterior nasopharynx, in the midline (arrows). Its signal intensity on the proton density and T2WI suggests that it may contain colloid material or mucin. (Courtesy of S. J. Pomeranz, M.D., Christ Hospital, Cincinnati Ohio.)

### *Benign Processes*

Abnormalities of the lymphoid tissue of the medial compartment are quite common. Lymphoid prominence is usually secondary to hyperplasia, either primary or secondary. Thornwaldt cysts, thought to originate in the pharyngeal bursa, are smooth walled, midline in location, and typically indent the posterosuperior aspect of the nasopharynx (Fig. 21–9).[2, 3]

Sphenoid sinus mucoceles, large nasal polyps, lipomas, transsphenoidal encephaloceles, chordomas, chondromas, craniopharyngiomas, and pituitary adenomas all can be manifested as nasopharyngeal masses.[1, 4]

Juvenile angiofibromas, although uncommon, are the most frequently encountered benign nasopharyngeal neoplasm. They probably arise near the sphenopalatine foramen and typically cause widening of the PPF and anterior bowing of the posterior wall of the maxillary antrum (Fig. 21–10). Juvenile angiofibromas tend to displace and thin the bone rather than cause irregular destruction. The neoplasm will travel through the ostia of the paranasal sinus and through the bony foramina, allowing intracranial spread (Table 21–3).[1, 4] On MRI the tumors have a signal that is isointense or slightly greater than muscle on T1WI. The signal increases somewhat on T2WI.

Juvenile angiofibromas can be confused

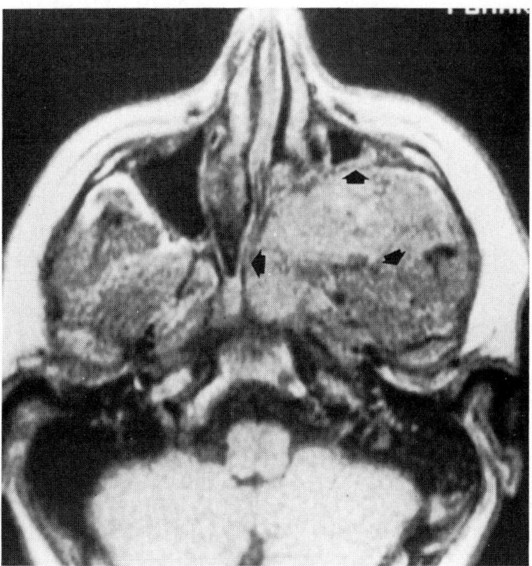

**Figure 21–10. Juvenile angiofibroma.** Axial T1WI (TR 800/TE 20 msec). The mass has extended from the pterygopalatine fossa to the nasal cavity medially, in the masticator space posterolaterally. The maxillary antrum is bowed and displaced anteriorly (arrows). (Courtesy of W. Hanafee, M.D., UCLA Medical Center, Los Angeles, Ca.)

**Table 21–3.** STAGES OF JUVENILE ANGIOFIBROMA

| Stage | Description of Spread |
|---|---|
| I | Localized |
| II | Nasal cavity and/or sphenoid sinuses |
| III | Superior masticator space, maxillary and ethmoid sinuses |
| IV | Intracranial (usually middle cranial fossa: cavernous sinus) |

with angiomatous polyps. The latter, unlike juvenile angiofibromas, tend to be hypovascular, originate in the nasal cavity, and at surgery tend to be less invasive.[1]

### Lateral Compartment Abnormalities

Abnormal processes in the masticator space often represent spread of infectious or neoplastic processes from the posterior and medial compartments. Infectious processes occurring here are usually odontogenic in origin.[1, 30] Unusual lesions such as chondrosarcomas and osteosarcomas may involve this space (Fig. 21–11).

Lesions that encroach on the PPS include those originating in the lateral compartment and those originating in the deep lobe of the parotid (Fig. 21–12). The latter are often dumbbell shaped. They pass through the stylomandibular gap and push the fat of the PPS medially.[4] The differentiation is important, as the surgical approach to the deep-lobe parotid and PPS lesions is different.[1, 31, 32]

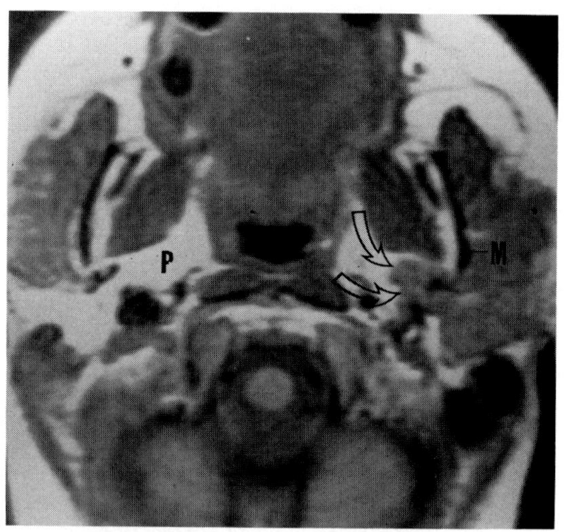


**Figure 21–12. Lymphoma of the parotid gland.** Axial T1WI (TR 600/TE 20 msec). The lymphomatous parotid gland extends through the stylomandibular gap and deforms the parapharyngeal space (arrows). M: mandible; P: parapharyngeal space.

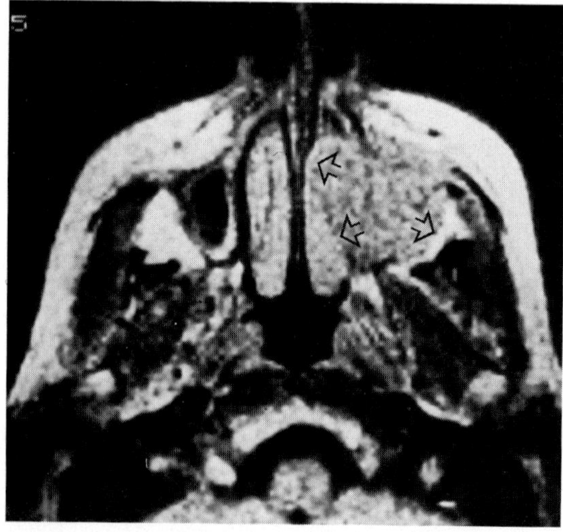

**Figure 21–11. Osteogenic sarcoma of maxillary antrum.** Axial (N[H]WI 1500/35 msec). The tumor has extended into the masticator space posterolaterally. There is effacement of the retrosinus fat and invasion of the nasal cavity (arrows). (Courtesy of S. J. Pomeranz, M.D., Christ Hospital, Cincinnati, Ohio.)

Deep-lobe parotid lesions require a transparotid approach, whereas the lateral compartment PPS lesion is approached transorally, submandibularly, or through a mandible-splitting procedure.[2, 33] The lesions originating in the PPS usually arise from accessory salivary tissue and are benign mixed tumors. Other lesions originating there include dermoids, chondromas, acinar cell carcinomas, and lymphoepitheloid tumors, brachial cleft cysts, lipomas, and parapharyngeal cysts.[1, 2, 20, 34, 35] These lesions tend to displace the carotid space posterolaterally.

Carotid space lesions are visually neurogenic in origin. These include schwannomas and neuromas originating from cranial nerves IX to XII and the sympathetic chain. They may displace the carotid artery medially, the internal jugular vein laterally, and the PPS fat anterolaterally.[1–4] On MRI the neoplasms may have bright signal on both T1- and T2-weighted images.

Paragangliomas or chemodectomas arise either from the jugular bulb (glomus jugulare) or vagus nerve (glomus vagale). Glomus jugulare tumors may cause destruction of the jugular fossa and extend either into the middle ear or intracranially through the jug-

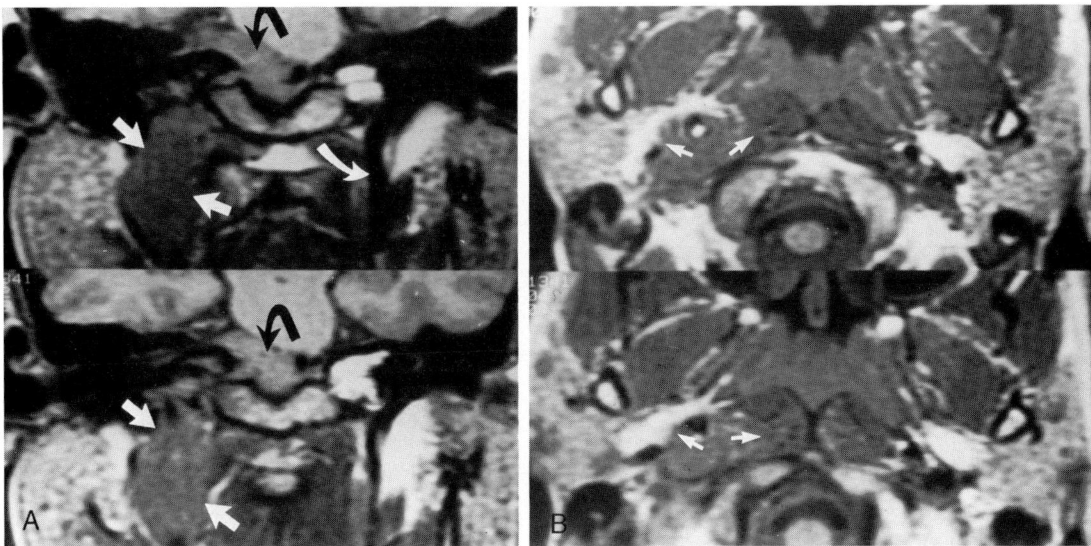

**Figure 21–13. Meningioma growing along the carotid sheath.** T1WI (TR 600/TE 20 msec). *A,* Coronal images show the intermediate-signal meningioma invading the jugular vein (white arrows) with intracranial, peripontine extension (black curved arrows). The left jugular vein (curved white arrow) is normal. *B,* Axial images show the meningioma displacing the parapharyngeal space and prevertebral muscles (white arrows) and invading the jugular vein. (Courtesy of S. J. Pomeranz, M.D., Christ Hospital, Cincinnati, Ohio.)

ular canal. Glomus vagale tumors arise caudal to the jugular foramen and push the carotid anteriorly.[4] Chemodectomas tend to have increased heterogeneous signal on T1WI and T2WI owing in part to areas of rapidly flowing blood with flow-void signal. Meningiomas may also grow to involve the carotid space (Fig. 21–13).

### Posterior Compartment Abnormalities

Fat and lymphatic components make up the vital structures of the retropharyngeal space and account for the type of lesions that occur there. Metastases from squamous cell carcinomas of the oropharynx and nasopharynx, lymphomas, suppurative lymphadenitis, hematomas, and abscesses may occur in this space.[1, 36]

Processes occurring in the prevertebral space usually arise in the vertebral bodies or skull base. Vertebral infections or neoplasms, primary or secondary, may involve the prevertebral space.[1]

### Lymphatic Spread

The lateral retropharyngeal, internal jugular, and spinal accessory nodes are first order drainage sites for the nasopharynx.[1, 2] In most cases, nodal masses over 3 cm are confluent nodes or tumor in soft tissues.[28] Squamous cell carcinomas tend to become necrotic when the nodal size exceeds 1.5 cm. Nonkeratinizing squamous cell carcinoma tends to produce larger nodes (> 2 cm) without significant necrosis. Lymphomas can produce marked nodal enlargement without necrosis.[2]

Lymphatic drainage in the nasopharynx is usually bilateral. Approximately 85% to 90% of patients have positive cervical nodes at presentation and 50% have bilateral disease. The drainage and portals for radiation treatment depend on histology, size, and distribution of the tumor.[2]

## References

1. Smoker WRK, Gentry LR. CT of the nasopharynx and related spaces. Seminars in US, CT and MR 7:107, 1986.
2. Mancuso AA, Hanafee WN. Nasopharynx and parapharyngeal space. In Mancuso AA, Hanafee WN, eds. Computed Tomography and Magnetic Resonance Imaging of the Head and Neck. Baltimore, Williams & Wilkins, 1985:428.
3. Silver AJ, Sane P, Hilal SK. CT of the nasopharyngeal region. Radiol Clin North Am 22:161, 1984.
4. Curtin HD. Nasopharynx, infratemporal fossa and skull base. In Carter BL, ed. Computed Tomography of the Head and Neck. New York, Churchill Livingstone, 1985:59.
5. Osborn AG, Harnsberger HR, Smoker WRK. Base of

the skull imaging. Seminars in US, CT and MR 7:91, 1986.
6. Whelan MA, Reede DL, Meisler W, et al. CT of the base of the skull. Radiol Clin North Am 22:161, 1984.
7. Paff GH. The pterygopalatine fossa. In Anatomy of the Head and Neck. Philadelphia, W. B. Saunders, 1973:141.
8. Paff GH. The maxillary artery and the contents of the infratemporal fossa. In Anatomy of the Head and Neck. Philadelphia, W. B. Saunders, 1973:64.
9. Allen WE, Kier EL, Rothman SLG. The maxillary artery: normal arteriographic anatomy. AJR 118:517, 1973.
10. Paff GH. The temporomandibular joint. In Anatomy of the Head and Neck. Philadelphia, W. B. Saunders, 1973:57.
11. Paff GH. Vessels and nerves to tongue, tonsils, glands and mucous membrane of oral region. In Anatomy of the Head and Neck. Philadelphia, W. B. Saunders, 1973:173.
12. Dillon WP, Mills CM, Kjos BO, et al. MRI of the nasopharynx. Radiology 152:731, 1984.
13. Dillon WP. MRI of head and neck tumors. Cardiovasc Intervent Radiol 8:275, 1986.
14. Glazer HS, Niemeyer JH, Balfe DM, et al. Neck neoplasms: MRI. Part I. Initial evaluation. Radiology 160:343, 1986.
15. Glazer HS, Niemeyer JH, Balfe DM, et al. Neck neoplasms: MRI. Part II. Post-treatment evaluation. Radiology 160:349, 1986.
16. Dillon WP. Applications of magnetic resonance imaging to the head and neck. Seminars in US, CT and MR 7:202, 1986.
17. Lloyd GAS, Phelps PD. Demonstration of tumours of the parapharyngeal space by magnetic resonance imaging. Br J Radiol 59:675, 1986.
18. Dietrich RB, Lufkin RB, Kangarloo H, et al. Head and neck MR imaging in the pediatric patient. Radiology 159:769, 1986.
19. Stark DD, Moss AA, Gamsu G, et al. Magnetic resonance imaging of the neck. Part I. Normal anatomy. Radiology 150:447, 1984.
20. Stark DD, Moss AA, Gamsu G, et al. Magnetic resonance imaging of the neck. Part II. Pathologic findings. Radiology 150:455, 1984.
21. Batsakis JH. Tumors of the Head and Neck: Clinical and Pathological Considerations, 2nd ed. Baltimore, Williams & Wilkins, 1979:188.
22. Lederman M. Cancer of the Nasopharynx: Its Natural History and Treatment. Springfield, Ill., Charles C Thomas, 1961:12.
23. Ballantyne AJ. Routes of spread. In Fletcher GH, MacComb WS, eds. Radiation Therapy in the Management of Cancers of the Oral Cavity and Oropharynx. Springfield, Ill., Charles C Thomas, 1962:91.
24. Gatenby RA, Mulhern CB, Strawitz J. CT-guided percutaneous biopsies of head and neck masses. Radiology 146:717, 1983.
25. Silver AJ, Mawad ME, Hilal SK, et al. Computed tomography of the nasopharynx and related spaces. II. Pathology. Radiology 147:733, 1983.
26. Mancuso AA, Som PM. The upper aerodigestive tract (nasopharynx, oropharynx, and floor of the mouth). In Bergeron RT, Osborn AG, Som PM, eds. Head and Neck Imaging Excluding the Brain. St. Louis, C. V. Mosby, 1984:374.
27. Dodd GD, Dolan PA, Ballantyne AJ, et al. The dissemination of tumors of the head and neck via the cranial nerves. Radiol Clin North Am 8:445, 1970.
28. Conley J, Dingman D. Adenoid cystic carcinoma in the head and neck (cylindroma). Arch Otolaryngol 100:81, 1974.
29. Beahrs OH, Myers MH. Pharynx. In Beahrs OH, Myers MH, eds. Manual for Staging of Cancer. Philadelphia, J. B. Lippincott, 1983:31.
30. Scott G, Harwood-Nash DC. Computed tomography of rhabdomyosarcomas of the skull base in children. J Comput Assist Tomogr 6:33, 1982.
31. Hardin CW, Harnsberger HR, Osborn AG, et al. CT evaluation of the normal and diseased masticator space. Radiology. In press.
32. Som PM, Biller HF, Lawson W, et al. Parapharyngeal space masses: an updated protocol based upon 104 cases. Radiology 153:149, 1984.
33. Stone DN, Mancuso AA, Rice D, et al. Parotid CT sialography. Radiology 138:393, 1981.
34. Som PM, Biller HF, Lawson W. Tumors of the parapharyngeal space: preoperative evaluation, diagnosis, and surgical approaches. Ann Otol Rhinol Laryngol (Suppl 80)90:3, 1981.
35. Bohman LG, Mancuso AA, Thomason J, et al. CT approach to benign nasopharyngeal masses. AJR 136:173, 1981.
36. Lawson VG, LeLiever WD, Makerwich LA, et al. Unusual parapharyngeal lesions. J Otolaryngol 8:241, 1979.

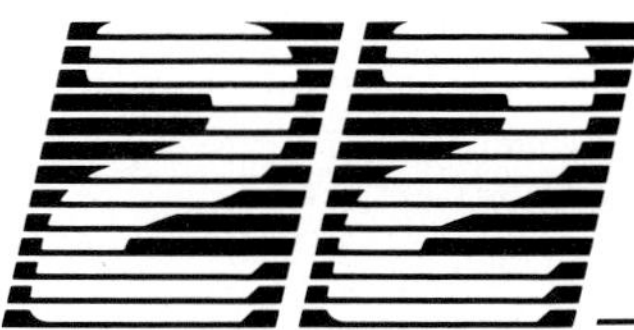

**Stephen F. Quinn, M.D.**

# MRI OF THE TEMPOROMANDIBULAR JOINT

Temporomandibular joint (TMJ) pain is quite common, affecting approximately 26% of patients in one survey of university students.[1] Symptoms usually begin in the second to fourth decades, and females are more commonly affected.[2]

Imaging techniques of the TMJ have traditionally used ionizing radiation. Fluoroscopic, plain,and tomographic radiographic techniques are also limited in evaluating soft tissue structures. Arthrography can delineate the contours of the meniscus and detect perforations but is technically difficult and painful.[3–5] CT is not invasive and can detect meniscal density but can be technically difficult and soft tissue detail is limited.[6, 7]

MRI has revolutionized TMJ imaging. It has unparalleled soft tissue resolution, allowing confident and consistent visualization of the meniscus.[8–14]

## MRI TECHNIQUE

The techniques discussed in this section are based on the author's experience using a 1.5 T superconducting magnetic resonance scanner (General Electric). A circular 3-inch diameter, receive only, planar surface coil is suspended horizontally above the TMJ with the head turned laterally. Also available are bilateral TMJ coils mounted on a head holder that function in parallel (simultaneously) or in series utilizing a remote switching device (Medical Advances, Inc). The patient's head should be rotated approximately 15° toward the surface coil so that the lateral pterygoid muscle is parallel to it.

We are currently using multiple partial flip angle images of the TMJ during different phases of opening to construct a "dynamic" sequence. The patient is positioned in the routine manner with a Burnet TMJ device in place (Fig. 22–1). One problem with the Burnett TMJ device is that there is no true closed mouth position. To have the device in place, there is at least a minor degree of opening. To circumvent this, we advise obtaining one sagittal sequence in the closed mouth position without the device in place.

A sagittal image using a gradient-recalled acquisition in the steady state pulse sequence (GRASS) is obtained each time the device is advanced two stops. The following parameters are used: Flip angle of 12°, 6 excitations, 256 × 256 matrix, TR 12 msec, TE 21 msec, 24-cm field of view, and 5-mm sections with no skip intervals. Approximately 12 to 20 images can be obtained, the number being decided by the patient's ability to open his or her mouth. Rapidly paging through the image sequence provides dynamic visualization of the TMJ and soft tissues. Fast-scan cine MR movies will soon be available (16 frames per second) for dynamic TMJ evaluation.

Occasionally, sagittal T1WI are obtained for better anatomic detail. The parameters used include TR 400 msec, TE 20 msec, 256 × 256 matrix, 12- or 14-cm field of view, 4 excitations, and 3-mm thick sections without gap.

If there is a suspicion of inflammatory disease such as postsurgical changes or an effusion, then relatively T2WI can be obtained. This will cause the areas of high water content to appear as regions of high signal intensity. A typical sequence for T2WI would be TR 2000 msec/TE 25–70 msec.

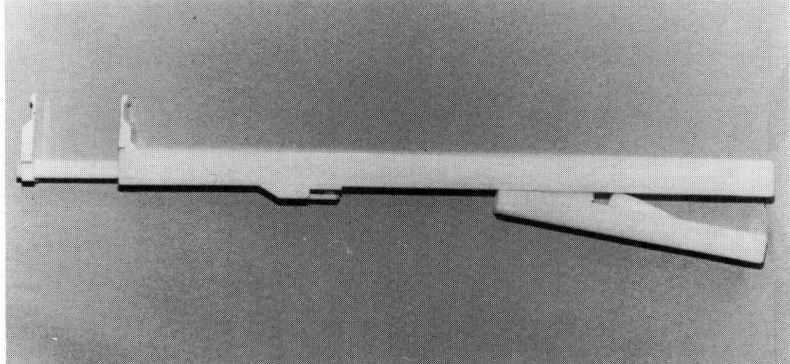

**Figure 22–1. Burnet TMJ device.** This device allows controlled opening, which is necessary to compile a series of static images, which are then used to construct a "dynamic" sequence. (Courtesy of Med Rad, Pittsburgh, Pa.)

## ANATOMY

The TMJ is a ginglymoarthroidal joint. That is, the bony surfaces of the joint both slide along their interfaces and have a hinge-joint function. The hinge movement is called rotation, and the anterior and posterior sliding movements are called translation. The normal anterior extent of translation varies from not reaching the articular eminence to moving completely into the infratemporal fossa.[15]

The TMJ is a synovial joint divided into superior and inferior compartments by a biconcave articular disc. The joint is enveloped by a capsule that is attached posteriorly to the inferior and posterior aspects of the glenoid fossa, inferiorly to the condylar neck, and anteriorly to the articular eminence.[16]

The superior belly of the lateral pterygoid muscle inserts on the anterior band of the articular disk by a fascial band, and the inferior belly of the lateral pterygoid muscle inserts on the condylar neck. The muscle bellies are separated by a fascial band.[16]

The mandibular condyle articulates with the articular eminence, not the glenoid fossa (Fig. 22–2). The fossa is filled with the bulbous portion of the posterior band and the bilaminar zone. The bilaminar zone has numerous blood vessels and nerves within it and serves as the posterior attachment to the anterior portion of the temporal bone.[5]

The areas of articulation, the posterior and inferior surfaces of the articular eminence and the anterosuperior surface of the mandibular condyle, are covered with fibrocartilage (Fig. 22–3). The bony trabeculations of the condyle and the articular eminence are aligned in a manner that designates them as weight-bearing joints. The biconcave articular disk, which is devoid of vessels and nerves, is situated between these articular surfaces.[17]

## NORMAL MRI FINDINGS

The superior and inferior bellies of the lateral pterygoid muscle can be recognized as separate structures divided by a low-signal fascial plane. The fascial band of the superior belly of the lateral pterygoid muscle can be recognized as a low-signal structure as it attaches to the anterior band of the meniscal complex. There is a fat pad anterior to the meniscal complex that can be used as an anatomic landmark.[13] The temporalis muscle can be seen coursing vertically anterior to the fossa (Fig. 22–4).

The posterior band, biconcave articular disk, and anterior band are low signal on MRI. The vascular bilaminar zone tends to be of intermediate signal and may be best seen on anterior translation.[13] The cortex of the mandibular condyle and articular eminence is low signal and its marrow is hyperintense on T1WI.

In the closed mouth position, the articular disk is situated between the posterior aspect of the glenoid fossa and the anterosuperior aspect of the mandibular condyle. The junction of the posterior band and disk should lie in a 12 o'clock position relative to the mandibular condyle. With anterior translation and rotation, the condyle and disk move forward, the disk articulating with the su-

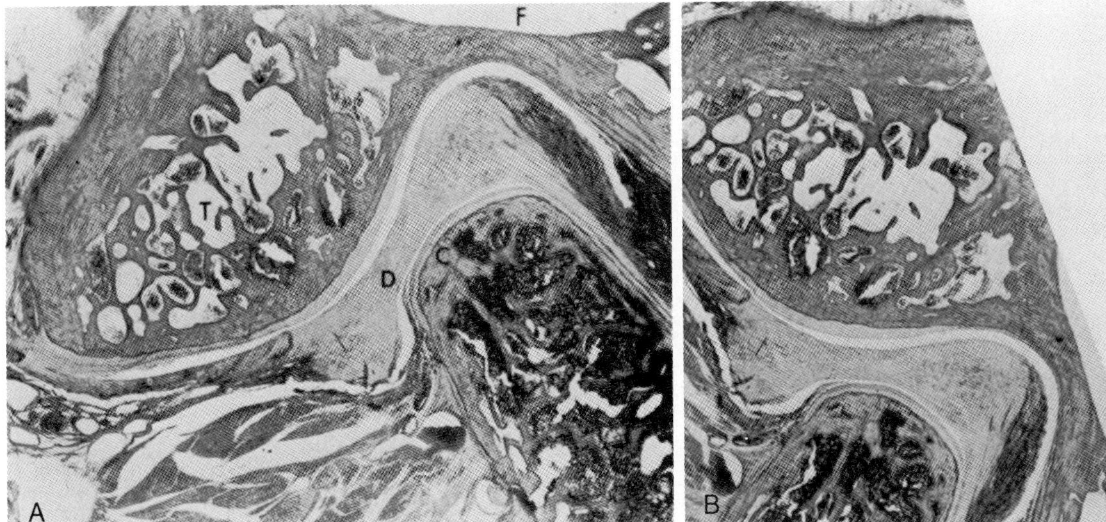


**Figure 22–2. Photomicrograph of the TMJ.** *A,* A photomicrograph of the TMJ taken by S. W. Chase shows the mandibular condyle–meniscus–articular eminence relationship. The articular disk (D), unlike many popular misconceptions, sits between the superoanterior fibrocartilage covering the condylar head (C) and posterior articular eminence. The condylar head therefore does not articulate with the glenoid fossa (F).

*B,* Only by rotating Chase's photomicrograph approximately 70° clockwise does the disk begin to assume a more superior relationship to the condyle. Note that the functional trabeculation is oriented along lines of stress, that is, beneath the fibrocartilage. (From Schemen P. In Gelb H, ed. Clinical Management of Head, Neck and TMJ Pain and Dysfunction. Philadelphia, W.B. Saunders, 1977, p. 196, with permission.)

perior aspect of the condyle and posterior aspect of the articular eminence (Fig. 22–5).

## Abnormal MRI Findings

The abnormal meniscus tends to lose its normal biconcave appearance and can vary in appearance from marked thinning to folding or having a globular configuration. Katzberg states that abnormal articular disks can lose signal intensity, which may be related in part to histologic calcification. The meniscus tends to lose its pliability and becomes stiffer.[13]

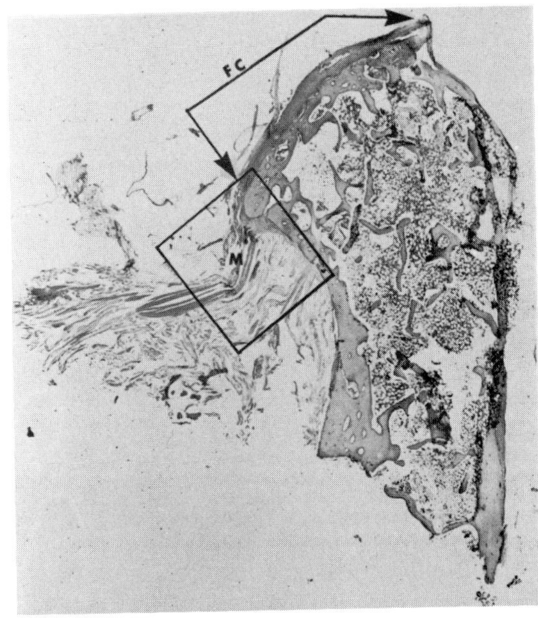


**Figure 22–3. Photomicrograph of TMJ fibrocartilage.** This sagittal histologic section of the mandible shows the cap of fibrocartilage (FC) covering the anterosuperior aspect of the condylar head. Fibers of the inferior belly of the lateral pterygoid (M) can be seen inserting into the mandible. (From Scheman P. In Gelb H, ed. Clinical Management of Head, Neck and TMJ Pain and Dysfunction. Philadelphia, W.B. Saunders, 1977, p. 194, with permission.)

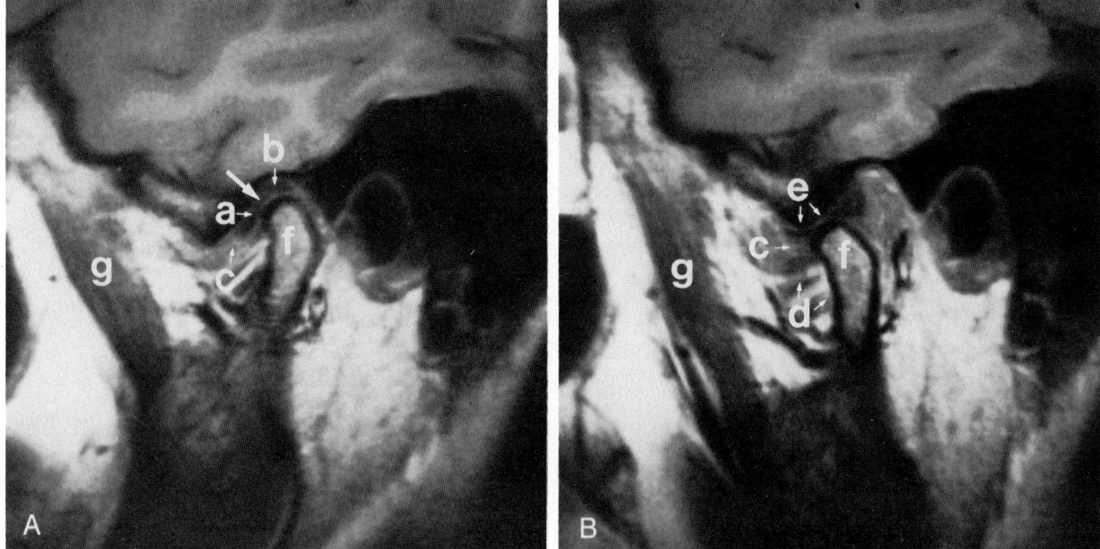


**Figure 22–4. Normal TMJ.** TR 400 msec/TE 20 msec. *A,* Closed mouth position. The low-intensity biconcave articular disk (large white arrow) is seen in its expected superoanterior relationship to the condylar head. *B,* Open mouth (partial) position. The articular disk (large white arrow in *A*) and condylar head have maintained their normal relationship. a: anterior band; b: posterior band; c: superior belly of lateral pterygoid; d: inferior belly of lateral pterygoid; e: articular eminence; f: condyle; g: temporalis muscle.

Katzberg also reports that in some abnormal joints there may be thickening of the fascial plane between the inferior and superior bellies of the lateral pterygoid muscle.[13] Associated inflammatory changes such as joint effusions can be seen as areas of increased signal on T2WI.

Bony changes such as ankylosis, osteochondromatosis, osteophytosis, erosions, and bony deformation can be detected on MRI.[8, 12, 18] Although cortical bone and articular disk are both of low signal intensity, there are sometimes ancillary findings to help sort out the anatomy. For example, marrow signal can outline an osteophyte, or joint fluid may separate disk from cortical overgrowth. A comparative study showed that MRI was capable of detecting bony abnormalities of the TMJ but was somewhat inferior to CT.[19]

MRI can reliably detect anterior dislocations of the meniscus. In the closed mouth position, the displaced meniscus is anterior and inferior to its expected position. The articular disk usually has an abnormal globular configuration (Fig. 22–6). The displaced meniscus can be in either a medial or a lateral position, and this can be determined by MRI.[13] The posterior band, which is normally seated in the 12 o'clock position relative to the condylar head, becomes displaced anteroinferiorly.

With adequate anterior translation, a reducing meniscus assumes a position superior to the condylar head. This reduction or capture of the disk occurs at the time of the audible click (Fig. 22–7).

A nonreducing anterior dislocation appears as a persistent globular area of decreased signal anteroinferior to the condylar head. The abnormal meniscus may become more prominent with anterior translation (Fig. 22–8). Restriction of movement either mechanically or because of pain may prevent anterior translation (closed lock), and the only movement may be rotational. To adequately assess condylar translation and rotation, at least 25mm of separation between central incisors should be present or produced with Burnet or another TMJ device.

Perforations of the meniscus have been described as areas of discontinuity in the disk, sometimes with osteophytes projecting through the tear.[8, 12] There is concern that small perforations will be missed on MRI (Fig. 22–9).

Harms described multiple cases of fibrous adhesions. These adhesions appear as foci of diminished signal that may not change in

*Text continued on page 655*

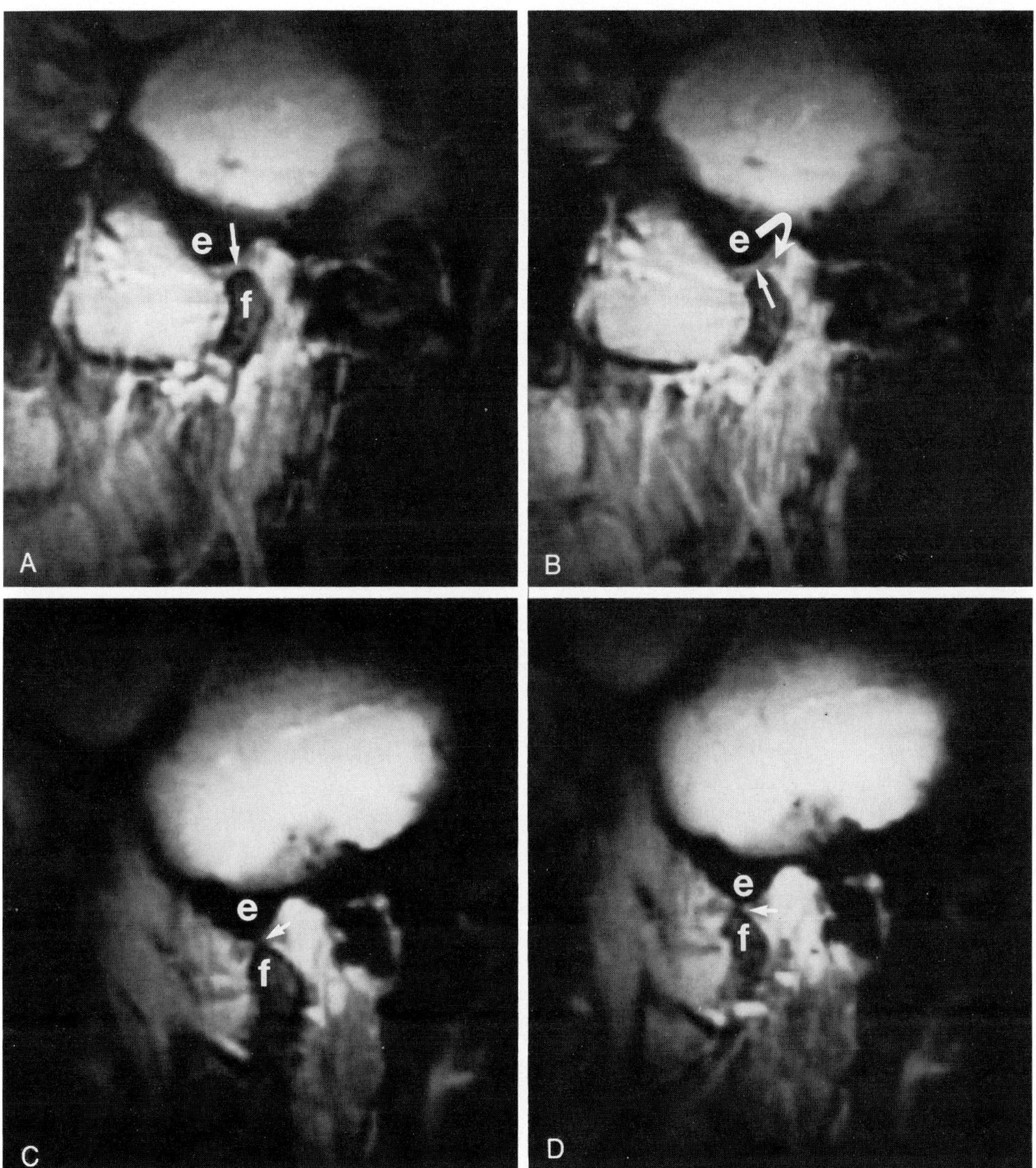


**Figure 22–5. Normal anterior translation.** "GRASS" sequence, using Burnet TMJ device (see text).

*A,* Partially opened. The condyle (f) has already translated anteriorly from its normal seat in the glenoid fossa. The biconcave articular disk (white arrow) has maintained its normal relationship with the condylar head.

*B,* With a slightly more anterior translation, the TMJ structures have maintained their normal relationships. The bilaminar zone (curved white arrow) is prominent.

*C,* The disk (arrow) is interposed between the articular eminence (e) and the 12 o'clock position of the condyle (f).

*D,* The condylar head (f) is anterior to the articular eminence (e), and the articular disk (white arrow) is beyond the 12 o'clock position.

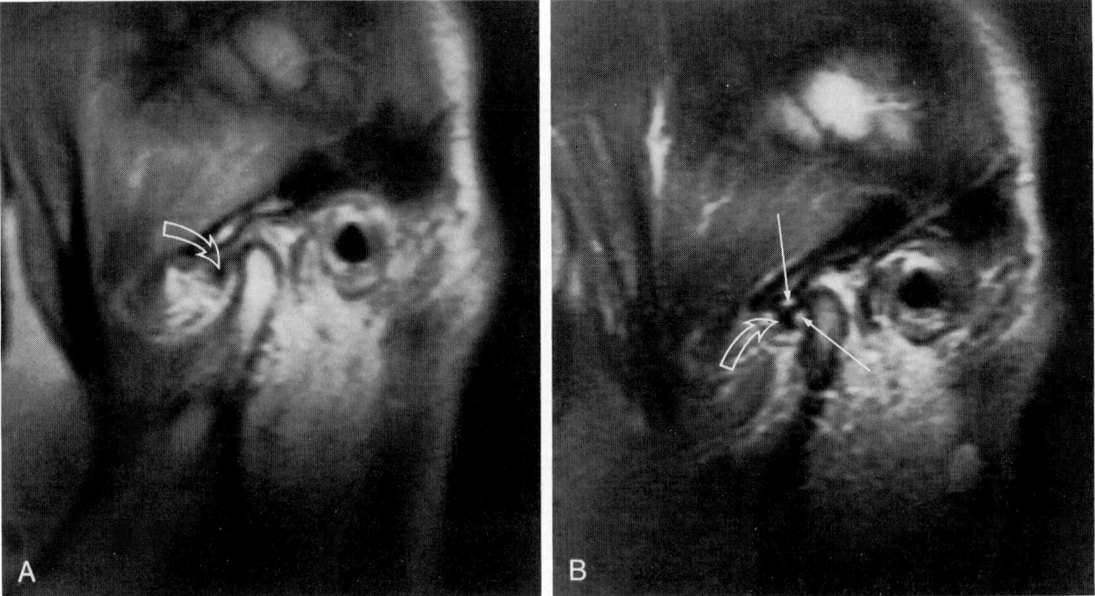

**Figure 22–6. Anterior subluxation.** *A* (SE N[H]WI 2000/20), in the closed mouth position, there is anterior displacement of the disk (open white arrow), which is lobulated in appearance. *B* (SE T2WI 2000/70), there is fluid in the anterior and inferior joint spaces (long white arrows). The high intensity of the joint fluid on this T2WI makes the articular disk more visible.

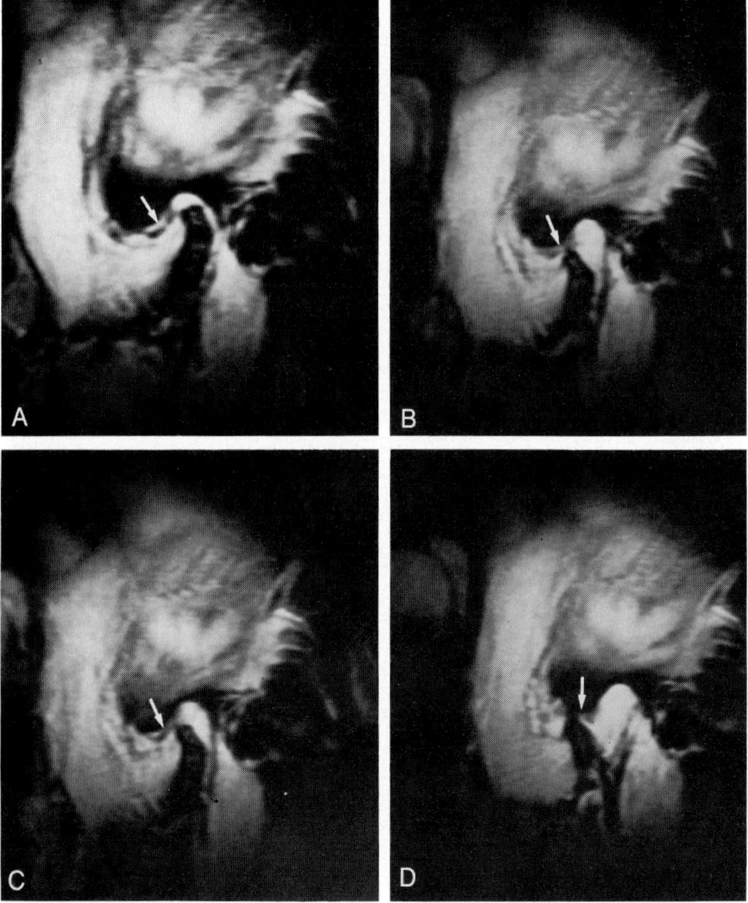

**Figure 22–7. Anterior dislocation with reduction.** Performed with "GRASS" sequence and Burnet TMJ device (see text). *A,* There is anterior displacement of the meniscus (arrow). *B* to *D,* With progressive anterior translation, there is late reduction when the meniscus is flush with the articular eminence (arrows).

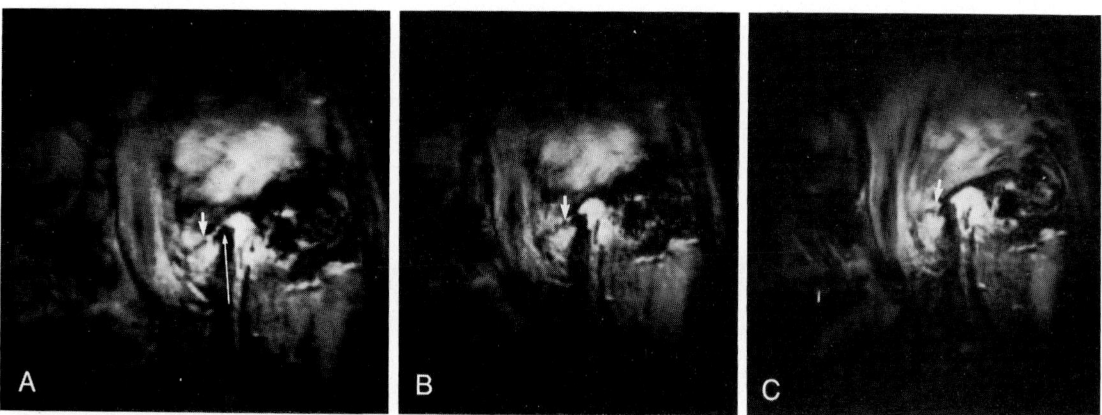


**Figure 22–8. Fixed anterior dislocation and probable meniscal perforation.** Performed with "GRASS" sequence and Burnet TMJ device (see text). *A,* There is anterior subluxation of the meniscus (short arrow). The mandibular condyle is deformed by degenerative changes (long arrow). *B,* With further anterior translation, the meniscus "accordions" still failing to reduce. *C,* At full anterior translation, the meniscus maintains an abnormal anterior position.

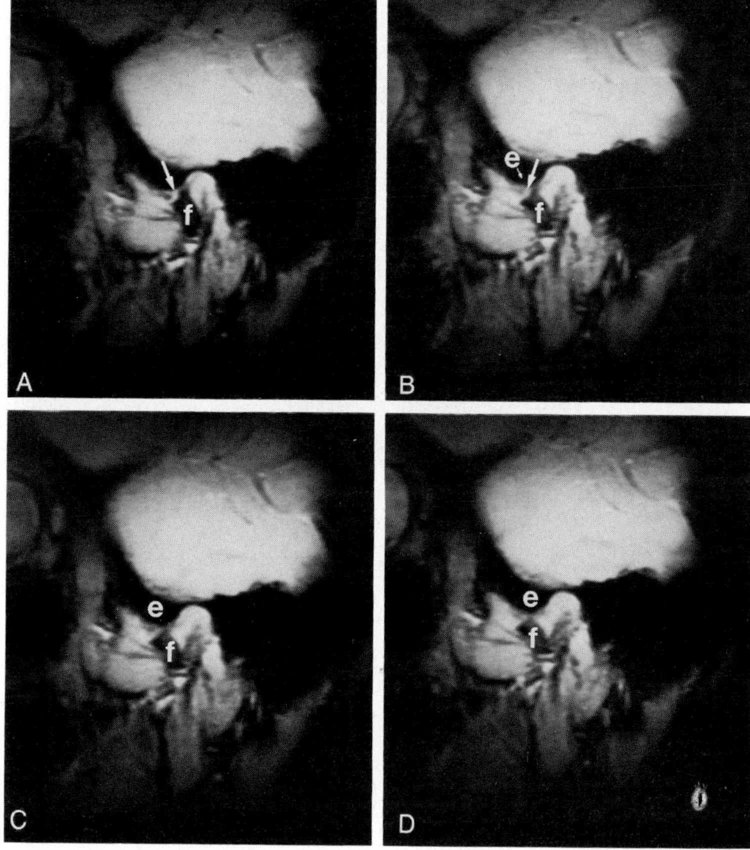


**Figure 22–9. Anterior displacement with late reduction and meniscal perforation.** Performed with "GRASS" sequence and Burnet TMJ device (see text). *A,* There is partial anterior translation of the mandibular condyle (f). The condylar head is deformed by degenerative changes. The meniscus is anteriorly displaced, and the discontinuity present is diagnostic of a perforation (arrow). *B,* With further anterior translation, the disk remains anteriorly displaced. *C,* With the condylar head at the articular eminence (e), there is continued anterior displacement. *D,* Only after the condyle (f) passes the articular eminence (e) is there capture of the meniscus.

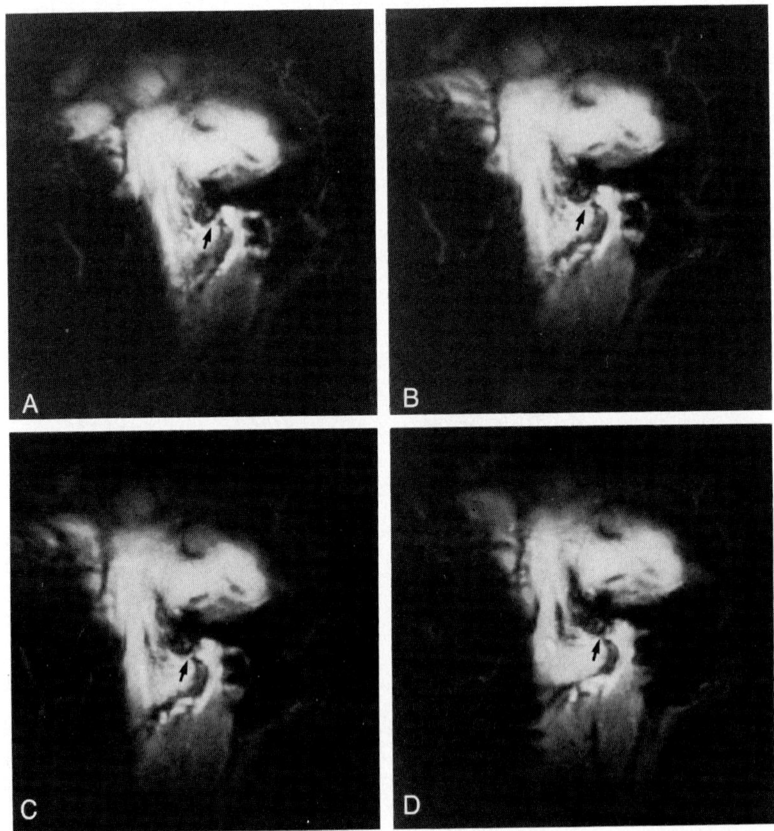


**Figure 22–10. Anterior subluxation of meniscus with fibrous adhesion to posterior articular eminence.** Performed with "GRASS" sequence and Burnet TMJ device (see text). *A,* There is mild anterior meniscal subluxation (arrow). *B* to *D,* With progressive anterior translation, the meniscus does not change in position, indicating the fibrous adhesion to the articular eminence. The shapes of the meniscus (flattened; poorly seen) and condylar head are abnormal, a sign of the chronicity of the condition. The range of the anterior translation is limited.

position with translation or rotation. The adhesions may cause fixation of the disk to adjacent bony structures (Fig. 22–10).[8, 12]

Katzberg has suggested that MRI may be able to detect postsurgical remodeling of the bilaminar zone from fibrovascular and fatty tissues into meniscal-like fibrous tissue.[13] These suggestions lend hope that MRI may be able to detect histologic derangement of the meniscus.

## References


1. Solberg WK, Woo MW, Houston JB. Prevalence of mandibular dysfunction in young adults. JADA 98:25, 1979.
2. Katzberg RW, Keith DA, Guralnick WC, et al. Internal derangements and arthritis of the temporomandibular joint. Radiology 146:107, 1983.
3. Katzberg RW, Dolwick MF, Helms CA, et al. Arthrotomography of the temporomandibular joint. AJR 134:995, 1980.
4. Dolwick MF, Katzberg RW, Helms CA, et al. Arthrotomographic evaluation of the temporomandibular joint. J Oral Surg 37:793, 1979.
5. Blaschke DD, Solberg WK, Sanders B. Arthrography of the temporomandibular joint: review of current status. JADA 100:388, 1980.
6. Thompson JR, Christiansen E, Hasso AN. Temporomandibular joints: high resolution CT evaluation. Radiology 150:105, 1984.
7. Sartoris DJ, Neumann CH, Riley RW. Temporomandibular joint. True sagittal CT with meniscus visualization. Radiology 150:250, 1984.
8. Harms SE, Wilk RM. Magnetic resonance imaging of the temporomandibular joint. Radiographics 7:521, 1987.
9. Katzberg RW, Schenck J, Roberts D, et al. Magnetic resonance imaging of the temporomandibular joint meniscus. Oral Surg 59:332, 1985.
10. Helms CA, Gillespy T, Sims RE, et al. Magnetic resonance imaging of internal derangement of the temporomandibular joint. Radiol Clin North Am 24:189, 1986.
11. Roberts D, Schenck J, Joseph P, et al. Temporomandibular joint: magnetic resonance imaging. Radiology 155:829, 1985.
12. Harms SE, Wick RM, Wolford LM, et al. The temporomandibular joint: magnetic resonance using surface coils. Radiology 157:133, 1985.
13. Katzberg RW, Besette RW, Tallents RH, et al. Normal and abnormal temporomandibular joint: MR imaging with surface coil. Radiology 158:183, 1986.
14. Westesson PL, Katzberg RW, Tallents RH, et al. Temporomandibular joint: comparison of MR images with cryosectional anatomy. Radiology 164:59, 1987.
15. Blaschke DP. The temporomandibular joint. In Osborn AG, Som PM, Bergeron RT, eds. Head and Neck Imaging. St. Louis, C.V. Mosby, 1984:251.
16. Paff GH. The temporomandibular joint. In Anatomy of the Head and Neck. Philadephia, W. B. Saunders, 1977:206.
17. Scheman P. Radiology and radiography of the temporomandibular articulation: Part I. In Gelb H, ed. Clinical Management of Head, Neck, and TMJ Pain and Dysfunction. Philadelphia, W. B. Saunders, 1977:206.
18. Nokes SR, King PS, Garcia R, et al. Temporomandibular joint chondromatosis with intracranial extension: MR and CT contributions. AJR 148:1173, 1987.
19. Westesson PL, Katzberg RW, Tallents RH, et al. CT and MR of the temporomandibular joint: comparison with autopsy specimens. AJR 148:1165, 1987.

# Appendix I
# SUMMARY OF EXAMINATION PREFERENCES

## CRANIAL EXAMINATION*

**Acute stupor or coma:** NCCT +/− CECT
**Base of skull and petrous bone:** NCCT +/− CECT; MR for soft tissue of neck, intracranial extension, or vascular/dural sinus invasion
**Congenital anomalies:** MR +/− CT (ultrasound for neonatal brain
**Demyelination/neurodegenerative disease:** MR
**Dural venous sinus disease/thrombosis:** MR
**Hydrocephalus/atrophy:** MR infratentorial; CT supratentorial; nuclear cisternography for normal-pressure hydrocephalus
**Inflammation/infection:** NCCT and CECT; MR for suspected herpes encephalitis only
**Internal auditory canal:** MR +/− CEMR only for equivocal cases
**Neoplasia, infratentorial:** MR +/− CEMR; NCCT for calcification (Ca) detection and bone destruction
**Neoplasia, supratentorial:** NCCT and CECT; MR for tumor versus hematoma, temporal lobe or high convexity lesions; CEMR for neoplasia versus radiation change
**New-onset seizures/temporal lobe epilepsy:** MR +/− CEMR
**Orbit:** CECT; MR only for retina, choroid, intracannalicular optic nerve, optic chiasm and optic tract, otherwise NCCT or CECT
**Phakomatoses:** MR +/− CEMR (except CT for tuberous sclerosis)
**Pineal region:** NCCT and CECT
**Sella/suprasellar/perisellar:** MR
**Stroke, infratentorial:** MR
**Stroke, supratentorial:** NCCT (MR only when hemorrhagic infarct is undiagnosable on NCCT [indeterminate CT numbers]) or negative CT
**Trauma, infratentorial:** MR +/− NCCT for bone assessment
**Trauma, supratentorial:** NCCT +/−MR; MR for suspected shear or extra-axial injury and negative CT; nuclear medicine or CT cisternography for CSF fistula
**Vascular (aneurysm/arteriovenous malformation:** MR +/− CEMR, infratentorial and temporal lobe; NCCT and CECT, supratentorial

*CECT: Contrast-enhanced computed tomography.
CEMR: Contrast-enhanced magnetic resonance.
MR: Magnetic resonance (noncontrast).
NCCT: Noncontrast computed tomography.
+/− indicates that examination may be adjunctive in diagnosis and occasionally positive or diagnostic when the primary examination is not.

## SPINAL EXAMINATION

**Craniocervical junction:** MR, conventional radiography +/− NCCT for skeletal anomalies +/− conventional tomography
**Disk disease:** MR in cervical, lumbar, and thoracic spine evaluation of young patients without spondylosis; in elderly patients with spondylosis, use high-resolution NCCT in lumbar and cervical regions but MR in thoracic spine; in elderly patients without spondylosis on conventional radiography, utilize MR; intrathecal water-soluable myelography followed by CT in selected cases of disk disease and extensive spinal stenosis/spondylosis
**Diskovertebral osteomyelitis:** MR and conventional radiography +/− CT
**Disk reprolapse:** MR + CEMR
**Metastasis:** MR for "complete block," myelopathy, pathologic versus nonpathologic vertebral collapse, "hot" vertebra on nuclear scintigraphy, and normal conventional radiography
**Myelopathy:** MR +/− CEMR
**Neoplasia, primary spinal cord:** MR +/− CEMR

**Neoplasia, primary spinal skeleton:** CT and conventional radiography; MR for chordoma staging and diagnosis
**Pediatric/anomalies/phakomatoses:** MR +/− CT
**Sacroiliitis:** NCCT and conventional radiography
**Spondylosis/radiculopathy/stenosis:** conventional radiography and NCCT +/− MR
**Trauma:** conventional x-ray and NCCT; water-soluble contrast myelography for root avulsion; MR for myelopathic hematomyelia, myelomalacia, cord cyst, and other post-traumatic intramedullary disease; intra-operative ultrasound for cyst localization and puncture

## ENT EXAMINATION

**Larynx:** CECT +/− MR
**Middle and external ear, skull base:** NCCT +/− CECT
**Parotid mass:** MR for staging of neoplasm and facial nerve localization; CT for inflammatory disease and sialolithiasis
**Pharynx and nasopharynx soft tissue:** MR +/− CEMR
**Temporomandibular joint:** MR

# Appendix II
# TECHNIQUES OF EXAMINATION

## DEFINITIONS*

**Cardiac gating (cardgate):** a method of synchronizing image acquisition during specific phases of the cardiac cycle; this is accomplished through synchronization with the R wave of QRS complex (ECG gating) or the mechanical action of blood pulsation (peripheral pulse gating)

**CEMR:** contrast-enhanced MR (gadopentatate dimeglumine [Berlex] in a dosage of 0.2 mL/kg or 0.1 mmol/kg, total dose not to exceed 20 mL); utilize T1WI single-echo imaging with CEMR and select the projection that optimally shows pathology on noncontrast MR; current scan intervals from completion of administration to completion of the scan series: 3 minutes (2 nex) to 6 minutes (4 nex); delayed scan, begun 8 minutes after contrast administration, optional in sella and postoperative spine; applications include brain, posterior fossa, and internal auditory canal

**Contiguous:** image acquisition of two distinct series acquired in direct sequence so that computer reprogramming for a second series is not required; imaging time is doubled; this is really a form of interleaving whereby sections do not overlap

**Flow compensation (FComp):** a gradient moment nulling technique that limits phase-related artifacts resulting from vascular or CSF motion (do not use flow comp with spin echo if aqueductal stenosis, dural venous sinus thrombosis, or arterial occlusive diseases are diagnostic considerations; flow comp may mask pertinent findings in such cases)

**Gap:** spacing between adjacent sections

**Gapless:** sections that are truly contiguous obtained in one series; imaging time is not doubled

**GRASS:** gradient-recalled acquisition steady state (TR 21–50/TE 12.5–40 msec/flip angle 5–50 degrees); this is a fast-scan, gradient-echo, reduced flip angle technique; parameters TR and TE may have to be varied, depending on number of slices, slice thickness, flip angle, and FOV chosen

**Interleaving:** the acquisition of two separate series in which slice locations are interlaced or overlapped with respect to one another, thus avoiding imaging gaps

**Nonorthogonal (oblique):** image planes that rotate around any of the three standard axial, sagittal, or coronal axes; brain examinations may be angulated along the canthomeatal line; spine para-axial sections may be obtained directly through the disk space, paracoronally through the cord or conus, and parasagittally, or perpendicular to the neural foramen; coronal sellar examination may be angled perpendicular to the gland, and in difficult cerebellopontine angle cases, oblique images parallel to the eighth nerve complex may be chosen

**No-phase wraparound:** allows scanning of small FOV without phase aliasing. This software selection reduces the number of excitations, averages, or repetitions by one-half, doubles the FOV chosen and doubles the imaging matrix

**Phase-frequency "swap":** an option utilized to project phase misregistration artifacts off an area of interest; since phase (y)-encoded information is prone to motion artifact and this artifact occurs in the phase direction, changing the axes of phase and frequency changes the orientation of this artifact; phase encoding is prone to aliasing or wraparound; therefore, when a swap is initiated, steps to minimize wraparound must be taken

**Respiratory compensation (RComp):** a form of ordered phase encoding that reduces periodic forms of motion-induced image noise

**Saturation (Sat):** the application of 90° presaturation pulses outside a region of interest; thus the signal artifacts from blood flowing into a region of interest are re-

*av: Averages.
FOV: Field of view.
nex: Excitations.
SC: Surface coil.
TE: Echo time.
TR: Repetition time.

duced; presaturation pulse can be applied in one plane (Sat 1) two planes (Sat 2) or three planes (Sat 3)

**Scout:** a scan series utilized for the purpose of localizing other anatomic projections (sagittal: multislice, single-echo T1WI [TR 300–1000/TE/20–35/msec]); 1 or ½ nex;† 10-mm, gap 2 mm; 24-cm FOV

**T1WI:** T1-weighted image (TR 300–600/TE 20–45 msec)

**T2WI:** T2-weighted image (TR 1500–3000/ TE 20–45 and 56–100 msec); this refers to a multiecho sequence that, although not technically correct, includes a first-echo spin or proton-density image and a more heavily T2-weighted second-echo image

## EXAMINATION PROTOCOLS‡

### Screening Brain

(scout)

**Axial:** multislice; multiecho T2WI (TR 1500–3000/TE 20–40 and 56–100 msec; 2 nex; 5-mm, gap 2 mm; 20-cm FOV; oblique angle parallel to orbitomeatal line, optional at operator's discretion for all heads; FComp (omit FComp in cases in which dural sinus thrombosis is suspected)

### Higher Resolution Brain

For first-time seizures, refractory partial epilepsy/arteriovenous malformation, multiple sclerosis plaque, patients with prior normal CT (scout)

**Coronal:** multislice multiecho T2WI; 2 nex; 5-mm, gap 2 mm; 20-cm FOV; FComp

**Axial:** multislice; multiecho T2WI; 2 nex; 5-mm, gap 2-mm; 20-cm FOV; FComp

**Axial or Coronal CEMR:** multislice, single-echo T1WI (TR 300–1000/TE 20–35 msec); 2 to 4 nex; 5-mm, gap 1 or 2 mm; 20 to 24-cm FOV (optional for first-time seizures; neoplasm, primary or metastatic; prior normal NCCT, CECT, NCMR and strong clinical suspicion of pathology)

### Posterior Fossa (Cerebellum)

(scout)

**Axial:** Multislice; multiecho T2WI; 2 nex; 5-mm, gap 1–2 mm; 20-cm FOV; FComp

**Coronal:** multislice; multiecho T2WI; 2 nex; 5-mm, gap 1–2 mm; 20-cm FOV; FComp

†One average (av) equals two excitations (nex).

‡**Note:** All protocols are acquired with 128 × 256 matrix unless otherwise specified.

**Axial or Coronal CEMR:**protocol same as high resolution brain

### Posterior Fossa (Brain Stem)

(scout)

**Axial:** same as posterior fossa (cerebellum)

**Sagittal:** multislice; multiecho T2WI; 2 or 4 nex; 3-mm (or 5-mm), gap 1 mm; 20-cm FOV; FComp (omit FComp to assess aqueductal patency)

### Skull Base and Foramen Magnum

(scout)

**Coronal** (for middle and anterior cranial fossa skull base): multislice, multiecho T2WI; 2 nex; 5-mm, gap 1–2 mm; 20-cm FOV; FComp

**Coronal** (optional for middle and anterior fossa skull base): multislice, single-echo T1WI 4 nex; 3-mm, gap 1 mm; 20-cm FOV through specified small region-of-interest

**Sagittal** (optional for foramen magnum) or **axial** (optional for perisellar region):same as T1WI coronal skull base protocol

**Axial** (for high resolution of small brain stem/foramen magnum lesions) multislice, multiecho T2WI 4 nex; 5-mm, gap 1 mm; 20-cm FOV; FComp; CEMR is optional

### Cerebellopontine Angle [CPA]

(scout)

**Coronal:** central section placed over the posterior one-third of the C2 dens; multislice, single-echo T1WI; 4 nex; 3-mm, gapless; 20-cm FOV; 128 × 256; 256 × 256–matrix optional alternative with 24-cm FOV (3-mm, gap 1 mm, 16-cm FOV; 6 nex; 128 × 256 is also an alternative optional high resolution protocol)

**Axial:** Same as Coronal, preceding; central section location chosen from previous coronal with parameters identical to coronal section

**Axial and/or Coronal CEMR:** one may repeat above axial and coronal T1WI immediately after contrast administration

**Axial or coronal** (optional for problem case only): multislice, multiecho T2WI; 4 nex; 3-mm, gap 1.5 mm; 20 FOV; FComp

**Axial and coronal surface coil (SC)** (optional for problem cases only): multislice, single-echo T1WI; 4 nex; 3-mm, gapless; 16-cm FOV; use oblique images tangent to neural complex when one nerve is studied

**Sella** (alternative protocol at lower field, see Sella section):

(scout): a sellar scout is *not* performed since the initial diagnostic sagittal view may be performed by centering on the nasion; begin with the sagittal view

**Sagittal:** multislice, single-echo T1WI; 4 or 6 nex; 3-mm, gapless; 16-cm FOV
**Coronal:** multislice, single-echo T1WI; 4 or 6 nex; 3-mm, gapless; 16-cm FOV
**Coronal** (optional): multislice; multiecho T2WI; 2 nex or 4 nex; 3-mm or 5-mm, gap 1 mm; 20-cm FOV; F Comp

**Cervicolumbar Spine Disk/Radiculopathy**

**Coronal SC (scout):** multislice, single-echo T1WI; 1 or 2 nex; 5-mm, gap 2-mm; 24-cm FOV; center over midline to substitute a sagittal scout
**Sagittal SC** (may be substituted as scout instead of coronal SC): multislice, single-echo T1WI; 4 nex; 5-mm or 3-mm, gapless; 20 to 24-cm FOV, depending on number of vertebral levels to be viewed; with 5-mm, 24-cm FOV and 4 nex; 256 × 256 matrix may be used
**Sagittal SC fast scan (cervical only):** multislice, single-echo GRASS (TR 20–70/TE 12.5 msec/flip 5°–30°; 4 nex; 5-mm, gapless; 24-cm FOV; FComp; 256 × 256 matrix
**Axial SC oblique (lumbar only):** multislice; single-echo T1WI; 4 nex; 5-mm, gapless; 24-cm FOV; 128 × 256 matrix; 256 × 256 matrix optional
**Axial SC oblique fast scan (cervical spine only):** multislice; single-echo GRASS (TR 20–70/TE 12.5 msec/flip 5°–30°) 4 nex; 5-mm, gapless; 24-cm FOV; FComp (TR will vary with number of slices required)
**Sagittal SC oblique (optional):** parameters the same as sag SC T1WI; angle perpendicular to neural foramen to evaluate foraminal encroachment; Sat 2

**Cervicolumbar Postoperative Spine; Lumbar Spondylosis and Stenosis Cervicolumbar Neoplasia or Myelopathy***

**SC sagittal:** multislice, single-echo T1WI; 2 nex; 5-mm, gap 2 mm; 24-cm FOV (center slice positioned over midline)
**Sagittal SC:** multislice, multiecho T2WI; 4 nex; 5-mm, gap 1–2 mm (3-mm sections optional in cervical spine); 24-cm FOV; FComp
**Axial SC:** multislice; multiecho T2WI; 4 nex 5-mm, gap 1–2 mm; 24-cm FOV; Sat 2
**Sagittal SC finger-pulse or ECG gated** (optional for cervical cord infarct, trauma, myelitis, and intramedullary cord neoplasm; may be substituted for above sagittal SC): multi-slice, multiecho T2WI; 1 or 2 nex; 5-mm, gap 1 mm; 24-cm FOV; TR gated to every second or third beat, depending on heart rate; Fcomp optional
**Sagittal SC oblique** (optional for foraminal evaluation): multislice, single-echo T1WI; 4 nex; 5-mm, gap 1 mm; 24-cm FOV; Sat 2
**Sagittal SC CEMR** (optional for postoperative spine and myelopathy): scan 1–5 minutes post-infusion; multislice, single-echo T1WI; 2 nex; 5-gap 2 mm; 24-cm FOV

**Thoracic Spine**

(screen; no clinical level given)
(scout)
**Whole-volume body coil:** multislice, single-echo T1WI; 5-mm or 3-mm, gapless; 2 nex; 40–48 cm FOV; RComp optional
**Sagittal:** multislice, multiecho T2WI; 2 nex; 5-mm, gap 1 mm; 32–40 cm FOV; FComp; if negative, STOP; if positive, defer to axial SC on thoracic high-resolution protocol at the level in question

**Thoracic Spine**

(high resolution; approximate clinical level given)
(scout)
**Sagittal SC:** multislice; single-echo T1WI; 5-mm, gap 1–2 mm; 1 nex; 40–48 cm FOV for level localization; RComp optional
**Sagittal SC:** multislice, multiecho T2WI; 5-mm (or 3-mm), gap 1 mm; 2 or 4 nex; 24-cm FOV; FComp
**Axial SC:** multislice, single-echo T1WI; 5-mm, gap 1 mm; 4 nex; 24 (or 20)-cm FOV; RComp and Sat 2
**Axial SC** (optional or may be substituted for axial SC T1WI): multislice, multiecho T2WI; 4 nex; 5-mm (or 3-mm), gap 1 mm; 24-cm FOV; RComp and FComp (optional)
**Sagittal SC finger-pulse, ECG gated:** (Optional for cord infarct, trauma, myelitis, or intramedullary neoplasm; may be substituted for sagittal SC T2WI) multislice, multiecho T2WI; 5-mm, gap 1 mm; 1 or 2 nex; 24-cm FOV; TR gated to every second or third beat, depending on heart rate; either RComp or FComp optional

**Complete Spine**

(for spinal block)

**BODY COIL PROTOCOL**

**Sagittal:** multislice, single-echo T1WI; 3-mm (or 5-mm), gapless; 2 nex; 40- to 48-cm FOV; Sat 2; RComp
**Axial** (through selected abnormal level on sagittal view): multislice, multiecho T2WI;

*Open FOV (24–32 cm) on sagittal SC series of lumbar spine examination if extensive lumbar stenosis involving higher levels or conus disease is suspected.

4 nex; 5-mm, gap 2 mm; 28- to 32-cm FOV; RComp and FComp (optional)

**Rectangular Surface Coil Protocol**

**Sagittal SC:** cervicothoracic multislice; single-echo T1WI; 5- or 3-mm, gapless; 4 nex; 32-cm FOV; Sat 2

**Sagittal SC:** thoracolumbar multislice, single-echo T1WI; 5- or 3-mm, gapless; 4 nex; 32-cm FOV; Sat 2

**Axial SC:** (through selected abnormal level on sag) multislice, multiecho T2WI; 4 nex, 5-mm, gap 1–2 mm; 24-cm FOV; RComp and Sat 2

**TMJ**

**Coronal SC†:** multislice, single-echo T1WI; 5-mm, gap 1 mm; 2 nex; 18-cm FOV for disk localization and diagnosis of medial/lateral dislocation

**Sagittal Condylar Oblique SC Open and Closed Mouth Views, Bilateral:** multislice, single-echo T1WI (TR 800/TE 20 msec); 3-mm, gapless; 12-cm FOV; 4 nex; 128 × 256 matrix

**Sagittal Oblique SC Fast-Scan Gradual:** (flip angle 13°, TR 34/TE 17 msec); 5-mm, gapless; 4 nex; 256 × 256 matrix; best slice is selected from T1WI, and 6 to 8 gradual mouth opening positions (one slice per position) are scanned with rubber bite plate or Burnet Med Rad TMJ device (Med Rad, Inc)

†Examination is performed with bilateral, parallel, automatically switched, dedicated TMJ coil on all sequences except gradual opening series (one side scanned at a time).

**Optic Pathway (Globe, Nerves, Chiasm, Tracts)‡**

**Sagittal:** multislice, single-echo T1WI; 10-mm, gap 2 mm; 1 nex; 24-cm FOV

**Coronal:** (perpendicular to optic nerve; scan globe to chiasm) multislice, single-echo; 3-mm, gap 1 mm; 4 nex; 16-cm FOV; 256 × 256 optional

**Axial oblique:** (tangential to optic nerves) multislice, multiecho T2WI; 3-mm, gap 1 mm; 4 nex; 20-cm FOV; FComp; 128 × 256 matrix

**Globe/Anterior Orbital Cone**

**Sagittal SC:** multislice; single-echo T1WI; 10-mm, gap, 2 mm; 1 nex; 24-cm FOV

**Coronal SC:** multislice, single-echo T1WI; 5-mm, gap 1 mm; 4 nex; 16-cm FOV; 256 × 256 optional

**Axial SC oblique** (parallel to optic nerves): multislice, single-echo T1WI; 3-mm, gap 1 mm or gapless; 4 nex; 14-cm to 16-cm FOV; 256 × 256 optional

**Axial or coronal SC:** (select orientation that best shows pathology) multislice; multiecho T2WI; 3-mm (or 5-mm), gap 1 mm; 4 nex; 20-cm FOV; FComp

**Sagittal SC oblique optional** (parallel to optic nerves): multislice, single-echo T1WI; 3-mm, gap 0.5 mm; 4 nex; 16-cm FOV; 256 × 256 matrix optional

‡Performed in standard head coil.

# INDEX

*Note:* Page numbers in *italics* refer to illustrations; page numbers followed by t refer to tables.